Mayo Clinic Medical Neurosciences

Organized by Neurologic Systems and Levels

FIFTH EDITION

Mayo Clinic Medical Neurosciences

Organized by Neurologic Systems and Levels

FIFTH EDITION

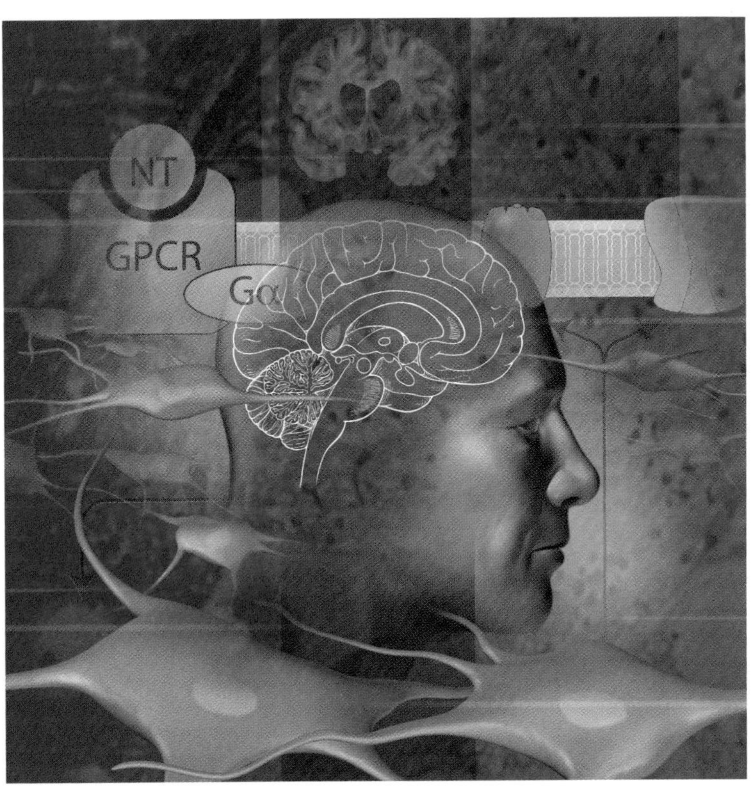

Eduardo E. Benarroch, MD
Jasper R. Daube, MD
Kelly D. Flemming, MD
Barbara F. Westmoreland, MD

MAYO CLINIC SCIENTIFIC PRESS
AND INFORMA HEALTHCARE USA, INC.

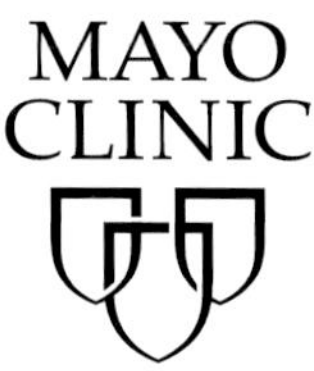

ISBN-13 9781420045161

For order inquiries, contact Informa Healthcare, Kentucky Distribution Center, 7625 Empire Drive, Florence, KY 41042 USA.

E-mail: orders@taylorandfrancis.com.

www.informahealthcare.com

Library of Congress Cataloging-in-Publication Data

Mayo Clinic medical neurosciences: organized by neurologic systems and levels. -- 5th ed. / edited by Eduardo E. Benarroch ... [et al].

p. ; cm.

Rev. ed. of: Medical neurosciences. 4th ed. / Eduardo E. Benarroch ... [et al.]. c1999.

Includes bibliographical references and index.

ISBN-13: 978-1-4200-4516-1 (pb : alk. paper)

ISBN-10: 1-4200-4516-4 (pb : alk. paper) 1. Nervous system--Diseases--Diagnosis. 2. Neurosciences. I. Benarroch, Eduardo E. II. Mayo Clinic. III. Medical neurosciences. IV. Title: Medical neurosciences.

[DNLM: 1. Nervous System Diseases. 2. Nervous System. WL 140 M473 2007]

RC348.M43 2007

616.8--dc22

2007036058

Care has been taken to confirm the accuracy of the information presented and to describe generally accepted practices. However, the authors, editors, and publisher are not responsible for errors or omissions or for any consequences from application of the information in this book and make no warranty, express or implied, with respect to the contents of the publication. This book should not be relied on apart from the advice of a qualified health care provider.

The authors, editors, and publisher have exerted efforts to ensure that drug selection and dosage set forth in this text are in accordance with current recommendations and practice at the time of publication. However, in view of ongoing research, changes in government regulations, and the constant flow of information relating to drug therapy and drug reactions, the reader is urged to check the package insert for each drug for any change in indications and dosage and for added warnings and precautions. This is particularly important when the recommended agent is a new or infrequently employed drug.

Some drugs and medical devices presented in this publication have Food and Drug Administration (FDA) clearance for limited use in restricted research settings. It is the responsibility of the health care providers to ascertain the FDA status of each drug or device planned for use in their clinical practice.

Printed in Canada

Dedicated To

The medical students and residents of the College of Medicine, Mayo Clinic, who provided the stimulus for this venture by teaching us as we have taught them, who have helped us refine our objectives and methods of presentation, and who through their enthusiasm have encouraged us to prepare another edition of this book.

Preface

The first edition of Medical Neurosciences, published in 1978, presented an organization of knowledge of the nervous system based on the neurologist's approach to clinical problems. For medical students and residents alike, this framework served as an effective foundation on which to build knowledge in the classroom and at the bedside. Continued advances in knowledge of the nervous system required updating the text through the previous four editions.

Increasingly rapid expansion in understanding the normal brain and its response to disease over the past eight years demanded an even greater revision for this, the Fifth Edition. The increasing complexity of our knowledge of the nervous system also required changes in the format and presentation of the information.

Chapters have been reordered to improve the integration of neurochemistry and neuropharmacology and reorganized to facilitate student grasp of the large sections of knowledge, for example, the posterior fossa and supratentorial chapters have each been subdivided. Major sections have been added on gross anatomy. The format of each chapter consists of Objectives, Introduction, Overview, and text. Clinical problems have been integrated into the text. Detailed supplemental information has been identified in each chapter.

The need to present the vast array of current knowledge of the nervous system required new diagrams of anatomy and histology, including new magnetic resonance and computed tomographic images to correlate with basic anatomy. Many concepts are clarified further by new figures and the abundant use of color throughout. Sections have been added to introduce newly identified immunologic and genetic neurologic disorders. Examples of details of new knowledge are particularly evident in the pathology of vascular disorders and clarifications of the physiology of the motor system.

This edition, like its predecessors, is the product of the authors. However, it could not have been accomplished without the contributions of many others, especially medical students and faculty here and elsewhere. We need to particularly acknowledge the residents who have assisted in teaching our introduction to the neurosciences to first- and second-year medical students, and the faculty who have contributed to this edition: Joseph Parisi, MD, Division of Neuropathology; Clifford Jack, MD, Division of Neuroradiology; Michael Silber, MD, Division of Sleep Medicine; Peter Dyck, MD, Division of Peripheral Nerve; and Andrew Engel, MD, Division of Neuromuscular Diseases. The superb teams in the Section of Scientific Publications and Media Support Services have added immeasurably to the quality of the book: O. Eugene Millhouse, PhD, Roberta Schwartz, Traci Post, Alissa Baumgartner, Karen Barrie, Jim Tidwell, Jim Rownd, and Jim Postier. Special thanks need to go to the original authors whose concepts are carried on in the soul of the book: Burton A. Sandok, MD, and Thomas J. Reagan, MD.

This is an exciting time in the study of the nervous system and its disorders; we hope the readers will be stimulated to explore further.

Eduardo E. Benarroch, MD
Jasper R. Daube, MD
Kelly D. Flemming, MD
Barbara F. Westmoreland, MD

Author Affiliations

Eduardo E. Benarroch, MD
Consultant, Department of Neurology, Mayo Clinic, Rochester, Minnesota; Professor of Neurology, College of Medicine, Mayo Clinic

Jasper R. Daube, MD
Consultant, Department of Neurology, Mayo Clinic, Rochester, Minnesota; Professor of Neurology, College of Medicine, Mayo Clinic

Kelly D. Flemming, MD
Consultant, Department of Neurology, Mayo Clinic, Rochester, Minnesota; Assistant Professor of Neurology, College of Medicine, Mayo Clinic

Barbara F. Westmoreland, MD
Consultant, Department of Neurology, Mayo Clinic, Rochester, Minnesota; Professor of Neurology, College of Medicine, Mayo Clinic

Table of Contents

PART I

Survey of the Neurosciences

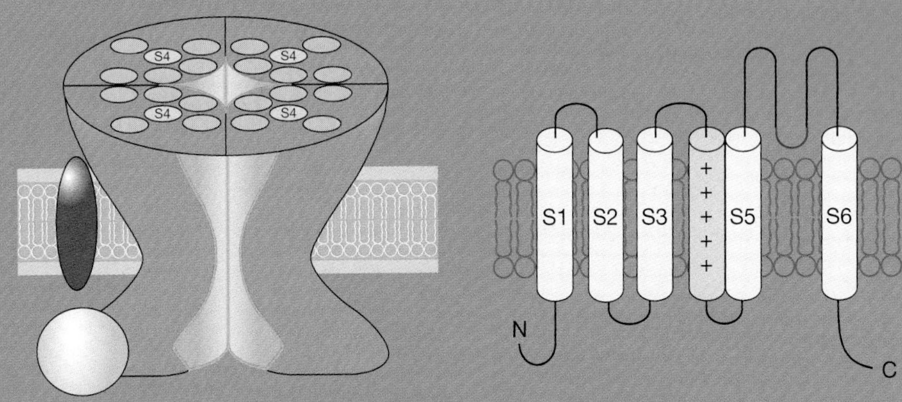

Chapter 1

Integrated Neuroscience for the Clinician

Objectives

1. Define the following: problem solving, pattern recognition, inductive reasoning, and hypothesis.
2. Given any clinical problem, develop a series of hypotheses that allows you to understand the cause of the problem.
3. Identify and describe the type of reasoning used to generate and test these hypotheses.
4. Name the four major levels and the seven major systems of the nervous system.

Introduction

Neurologic disorders are common, and all clinicians must be capable of recognizing and managing them. Many steps are required in solving a neurologic problem. Patients seldom present to their physician with a well-defined diagnosis for which appropriate therapy can be readily dispensed. Instead, they present with an array of symptoms and signs that constitute a clinical problem the physician must attempt to resolve.

Overview

Generally, a problem can be solved by using one of two methods:

1. *Pattern recognition*: If the problem is similar to or identical to one encountered previously and the solution is recalled, one moves quickly to an answer.
2. *Inductive reasoning*: Logical analysis is applied by tracing the problem to its source through a series of steps based on knowledge of the underlying structure and function.

Both methods have a critical step in common that is used throughout one's medical career, namely, *hypothesis testing*.

- When a problem looks like one encountered before, one can hypothesize that the solution is likely to be the same and develop a scheme to test the hypothesis.
- When a problem is not clearly understood but some of the underlying components are understood, one can propose a hypothesis about the mechanism of the problem based on an analysis of that knowledge and then test the hypothesis.

The solution of a clinical neurologic problem, as in any area of medicine, requires knowledge of anatomy, physiology, and pathophysiology. In this book, the body of information contained in the basic neurologic sciences is organized in the format used by clinicians to deal with diseases of the nervous system, that is, the levels and systems of the nervous system (Table 1.1).

Organization of the Nervous System

A clinician who examines a patient who has a neurologic disorder (i.e., one involving the brain, spinal cord, nerves,

Table 1.1. The Levels and Systems of the Nervous System

Levels
Supratentorial
Posterior fossa
Spinal
Peripheral
Systems
Sensory
Motor
Internal regulation
Consciousness
Cerebrospinal fluid
Vascular

or muscles or some combination of these) may use pattern recognition or inductive reasoning. Inductive reasoning uses distinct pieces of information to reach a conclusion.

The medical history of a 55-year-old woman includes the following:

- Distribution of the symptoms—numbness and weakness of the left side of her face, left arm, and left leg and headache. *Hypothesis*—the lesion is on the right side at the supratentorial level.
- Chronologic account of the evolution of the symptoms with time (the temporal profile)—the symptoms were of abrupt onset. *Hypothesis*—the lesion is focal and vascular.
- The neurologic examination confirmed the distribution of the impairment and shows that the patient is confused. *Confirmation*—the lesion is localized on the right side of the brain and accompanied by brain swelling and hypertension.

Patients with neurologic disease often have symptoms of changes in sensation, strength, movement, thinking, or consciousness. The physical examination usually documents precisely the function that is impaired, and this can be related to specific areas of the nervous system, as follows:

- Numbness or loss of the ability to perceive sensations—evidence of disease of the sensory system that extends from the limbs to the brain
- Weakness or inability to move normally—evidence of disease of the motor system that extends from the brain to the limbs
- Hypertension—evidence of a disorder involving the internal regulation system
- Confusion—evidence of involvement of the consciousness system
- Signs of brain swelling—evidence of involvement of the cerebrospinal fluid system
- Acute onset—evidence of a disorder of the vascular system

In the example here, the process is most likely an intracranial hemorrhage on the right side of the brain.

Throughout the neurologic interview and the examination, the clinician is constantly organizing and reorganizing the collected data to arrive at hypotheses about the identity and mechanism of the disorder. In the preceding example, the hypothesis of a right cerebral hemorrhage was reached because the temporal profile of abrupt onset is common with vascular disorders, and weakness and numbness on the left side of the body often are due to disease of structures that are controlled by the opposite side of the brain (the supratentorial level).

The physician must answer three questions:

- Is there disease involving the nervous system?
- If so, where is the disease located?
- What kind of disease is it (that is, what is the pathology of the disease)?

Clinical Problem 1.1.

You walk into your room and find your friend lying limp and motionless on the floor. As you approach and attempt to assess the situation and offer aid, you have several thoughts about what might have happened.

a. Describe the thoughts and the reasoning that contributed to each of them.

Clinical Problem 1.2.
You are sitting quietly in a chair with your legs crossed and notice a numb-tingling feeling in your right lower leg. On attempting to rise from the chair, you are unable to move the right leg normally.

a. What hypotheses have you developed about the possible causes?
b. Describe the reasoning that contributed to each of them.

The first question is often one of the most difficult to answer because the answer depends not only on the knowledge to be presented in this book but also on experience with disease involving all other body systems. This book focuses primarily on answering the two simpler questions:

- Where is the lesion located?
- What is its pathology?

Neurologic diseases include all the major pathologic categories that affect other organ systems and can involve one or several areas of the human nervous system. However, adequate management of neurologic problems can be based on answering two questions: Where is the problem? What is the problem? The elaboration and analysis of these specific questions form the major objectives in the study of medical neuroscience. The answers to these questions are based on knowledge of the anatomy of the nervous system (Fig. 1.1), physiology of the nervous system, the usual patterns of disease, and the forms of treatment available. This simplified approach to neurologic disease is the one customarily used by many neurologists, and it includes two questions that address where the problem is (disease), and two questions that address what the problem is (pathology):

1. Is the responsible disease located at
    - The supratentorial level?
    - The posterior fossa level?
    - The spinal level?
    - The peripheral level?
    - More than one level?

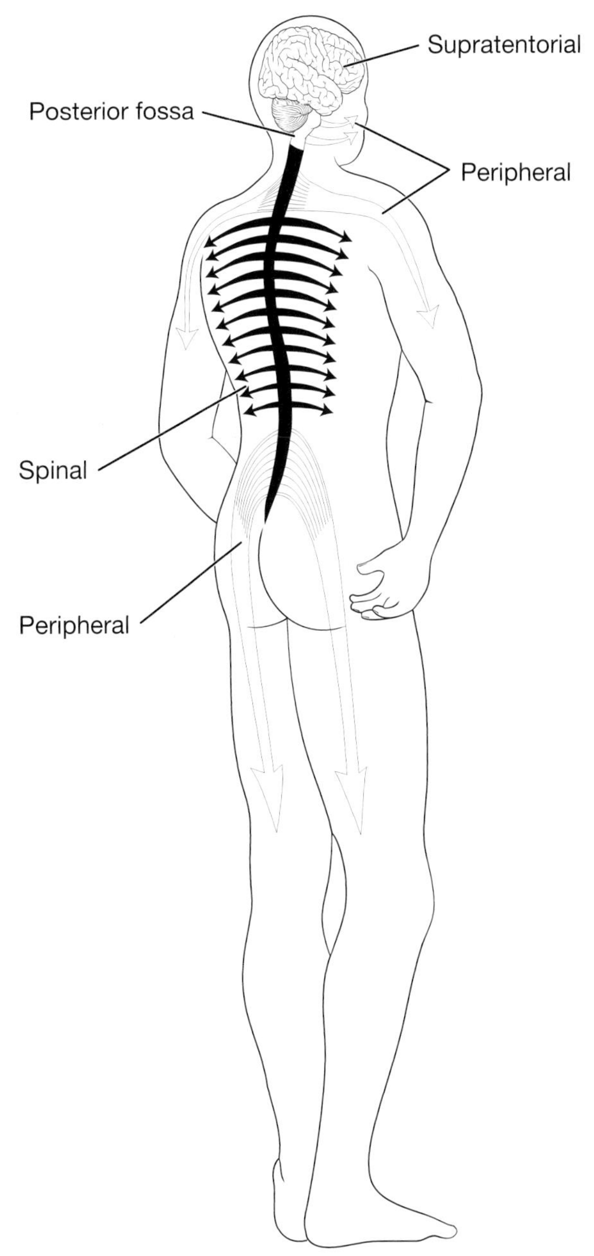

Fig. 1.1. Levels of the neuraxis. The supratentorial level includes the cerebral hemispheres and portions of cranial nerves I and II within the skull. The posterior fossa level includes the brainstem, cerebellum, and portions of cranial nerves III through XII within the skull. The spinal level includes the spinal cord and portions of nerve roots contained within the vertebral column. The peripheral level includes portions of both cranial and peripheral nerves that lie outside the skull and spinal column and the structures innervated by these nerves.

2. Is the responsible disease
   - Focal and located on the right side of the nervous system?
   - Focal and located on the left side of the nervous system?
   - Focal but involving midline and contiguous structures on both sides of the nervous system?
   - Diffuse and involving homologous, symmetric, noncontiguous areas on both sides of the nervous system?
3. Is the responsible disease
   - Some form of mass lesion?
   - Some form of nonmass lesion?
4. Is the lesion most likely
   - Vascular?
   - Degenerative (genetic)?
   - Inflammatory-immunologic?
   - Neoplastic?
   - Toxic-metabolic?
   - Traumatic?
   - Congenital-developmental-genetic?

The primary objective of this book is to provide the information necessary to answer these questions for any clinical problem that involves the nervous system and to provide a description of the mechanism by which the patient's symptoms and findings are produced by the underlying disorder.

Organization of the Book

The solution of a neurologic problem requires three levels of knowledge.

Section I provides general information necessary to understand the anatomy and physiology of the nervous system, how neurologic disorders are diagnosed, and how the disease process is identified.

The rest of the text is organized to enable precise topographic localization by relating the patient's functional impairment to a system and a level.

Section II defines, describes, and provides information for localization to one of the seven longitudinal systems.

Section III defines, describes, and provides information for localization to one of the four levels of the nervous system.

Each chapter begins with a chapter outline, list of objectives, introduction, and overview, and each ends with clinical problems for self-assessment. A list of additional readings is provided.

The clinician must first understand the methods used to diagnose a neurologic disorder. How is a lesion localized, and to what do the anatomical terms used to describe localization refer? How is a pathologic or etiologic diagnosis determined, and what do the terms used to describe them mean? These questions require general knowledge of the diagnostic principles of neurologic disorders as the principles relate to the anatomy, physiology, and pathology of the nervous system. Anatomy is better understood through a study of the development of the nervous system. Chapters 2 through 5 provide the basic vocabulary and background knowledge necessary to begin solving clinical problems. These chapters cover the following subjects:

Chapter 2—Developmental Organization of the Nervous System: Neuroembryology

Chapter 3—Diagnosis of Neurologic Disorders: Anatomical Localization

Chapter 4—Diagnosis of Neurologic Disorders: Neurocytology and the Pathologic Reactions of the Nervous System

Chapter 5—Diagnosis of Neurologic Disorders: Transient Disorders and Neurophysiology

Chapter 6 discusses the functional organization of the systems in terms of the chemical agents used for transmission and modulation of neural activity and provides an additional method of classifying neurologic function.

Chapter 6—Synaptic Transmission and Neurochemical Systems

Longitudinal Systems

Detailed knowledge of the anatomy and physiology of the nervous system is required for precise diagnosis of a neurologic disorder. The clinician usually relies first on the patient's symptoms and signs to identify which of the longitudinal subdivisions of the nervous system is involved. These longitudinally organized groups of structures are called systems within the nervous system, with each one subserving a specific function. Section II describes the anatomy, physiology, and clinical expression of disease as it affects the following major longitudinal systems:

Chapter 7—The Sensory System
Chapter 8—The Motor System
Chapter 9—The Internal Regulation System
Chapter 10—The Consciousness System
Chapter 11—The Cerebrospinal Fluid System
Chapter 12—The Vascular System

Correlation of the symptoms and signs with the appropriate system permits localization of the disease process in one dimension.

Levels of the Neuraxis

The final step in localizing a lesion requires defining where along its length a longitudinal system is involved. Although a more precise localization can be made in many cases, most clinicians classify the disorder according to one of four major regions defined by the bony structures surrounding much of the nervous system. Section III explores the ways in which functions in each major system are integrated and modified at each of the following levels:

Chapter 13—The Peripheral Level
Chapter 14—The Spinal Level
Chapter 15—The Posterior Fossa Level
Chapter 16—The Supratentorial Level

In all three sections, there is repetition of material, with each subsequent section building on the basic information presented earlier to provide amplification and emphasis. This approach to clinical neurologic problems can be used for any neurologic problem and is particularly useful for problems that are new, unfamiliar, or unusual to the clinician. Although the identification of diseases by recognition of a particular syndrome sometimes can be very efficient, the method of hypothesis testing and inductive reasoning presented herein is consistently more accurate and more reliable.

Additional Reading

Albanese MA, Mitchell S. Problem-based learning: a review of literature on its outcomes and implementation issues. Acad Med. 1993;68:52-81. Erratum in: Acad Med. 1993;68:615.

Cholowski KM, Chan LK. Cognitive factors in student nurses' clinical problem solving. J Eval Clin Pract. 2004;10:85-95.

Custers EJ, Stuyt PM, De Vries Robbe PF. Clinical problem analysis (CPA): a systematic approach to teaching complex medical problem solving. Acad Med. 2000;75:291-7.

Elstein AS, Schwartz A. Clinical problem solving and diagnostic decision making: selective review of the cognitive literature. BMJ. 2002;324:729-32. Erratum in: BMJ. 2006;333:944.

Engel GL. Clinical observation: the neglected basic method of medicine. JAMA. 1965;192:849-52.

Kassirer JP, Gorry GA. Clinical problem solving: a behavioral analysis. Ann Intern Med. 1978;89:245-55.

Kempainen RR, Migeon MB, Wolf FM. Understanding our mistakes: a primer on errors in clinical reasoning. Med Teach. 2003;25:177-81.

Mandin H, Harasym P, Woloschuk W. Clinical problem solving and the clinical presentation curriculum. Acad Med. 2000;75:1043-5.

Maudsley G, Strivens J. Promoting professional knowledge, experiential learning and critical thinking for medical students. Med Educ. 2000;34:535-44.

Stuyt PM, de Vries Robbe PF, van der Meer JW. Why don't medical textbooks teach? The lack of logic in the differential diagnosis. Neth J Med. 2003;61:383-7.

Whitfield CF, Mauger EA, Zwicker J, Lehman EB. Differences between students in problem-based and lecture-based curricula measured by clerkship performance ratings at the beginning of the third year. Teach Learn Med. 2002;14:211-7.

Chapter 2

Development of the Nervous System (Neuroembryology)

Objectives

1. Describe the formation of the neural tube and neural crest.
2. On a transverse section of the neural tube, identify the ventricular, subventricular, and marginal zones and the alar and basal plates.
3. List the five major subdivisions of the cephalic portion of the neural tube, their associated central cavities, and the major adult structures derived from them.
4. Name the major proliferative zones of the embryonic, fetal, and adult nervous systems.
5. Describe the major processes involved in the differentiation of neuronal and glial cells.
6. Describe the mechanism of radial migration.
7. Describe the main elements that determine axonal growth, target recognition, dendritic differentiation, and synaptogenesis.
8. Describe the formation of the peripheral nervous system and how its connections with the central nervous system are formed.
9. List examples of disorders of neural tube closure, ventral induction, neuronal migration, and neuronal maturation.

Introduction

The study of neuroscience begins with a survey of the development of the nervous system because it provides a framework and background for understanding the anatomy and function of the nervous system in the adult. The eventual location and connectivity of the structures in the brain, spinal cord, and peripheral nervous system reflect the orderly development of the nervous system. The molecular mechanisms involved in each developmental process of the nervous system have been elucidated by studying simple organisms. The results of these studies can be extended to the nervous system of mammals, including humans. Developmental neurobiology helps in understanding the pathogenesis of developmental neurologic abnormalities that are encountered not only in the newborn and pediatric periods but also later in life.

Overview

The development of the nervous system involves several consecutive and partially overlapping processes. These include neural induction and formation of the neural tube, patterning of the neural tube in the longitudinal and transverse axes, cell proliferation and differentiation, programmed cell death, neuronal migration, axonal growth and pathfinding, target recognition and synaptogenesis, and myelination (Fig. 2.1). Neural development is controlled by soluble signals from the mesoderm, target-derived growth factors, and adhesion molecules. These substances control the expression of transcription factors that regulate genes involved in determining neuronal or glial fates. These substances also control the dynamics of cytoskeletal proteins required for axonal and dendritic growth (Fig. 2.2).

The formation of the neural tube begins on the 18th

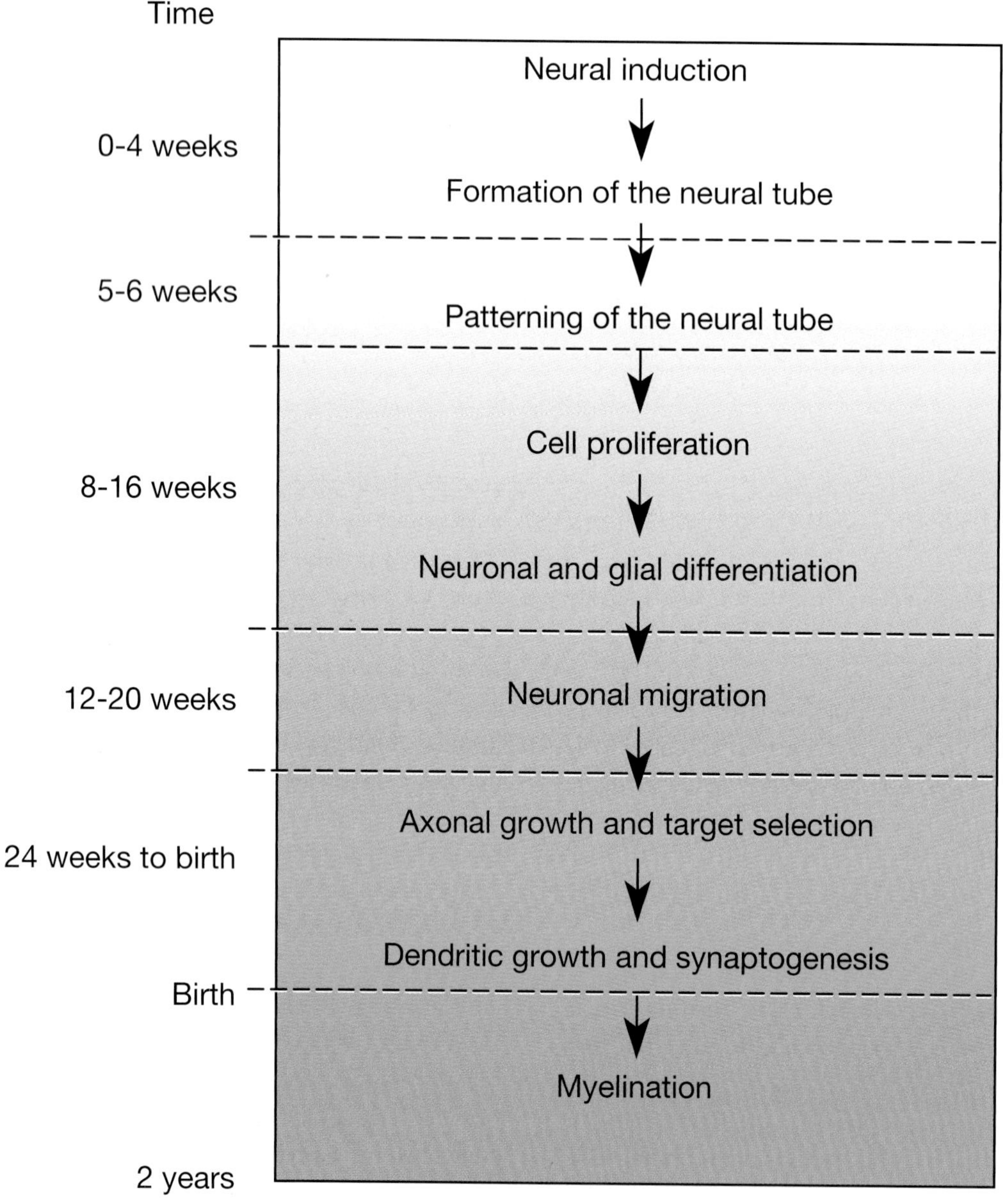

Fig. 2.1. Stages and timing of development of the nervous system. Note that there is partial temporal overlap of the different processes.

day of gestation. The two-layered embryo that consists of ectoderm and endoderm is transformed into a three-layered embryo by the outgrowth of mesoderm. The *notochord*, a specialized column of mesodermal cells, grows forward from the anterior end of the primitive streak (Hensen node). The ectoderm overlying the notochord is induced to form the *neural plate*, which thickens and folds into the *neural tube*. The entire central nervous system develops from the neural tube by the mechanism of regional differentiation along the longitudinal (rostrocaudal or anteroposterior) and transverse (dorsoventral) axes. Through longitudinal differentiation, the neural tube gives rise to three primary divisions: prosencephalon, mesencephalon, and rhombencephalon. These then

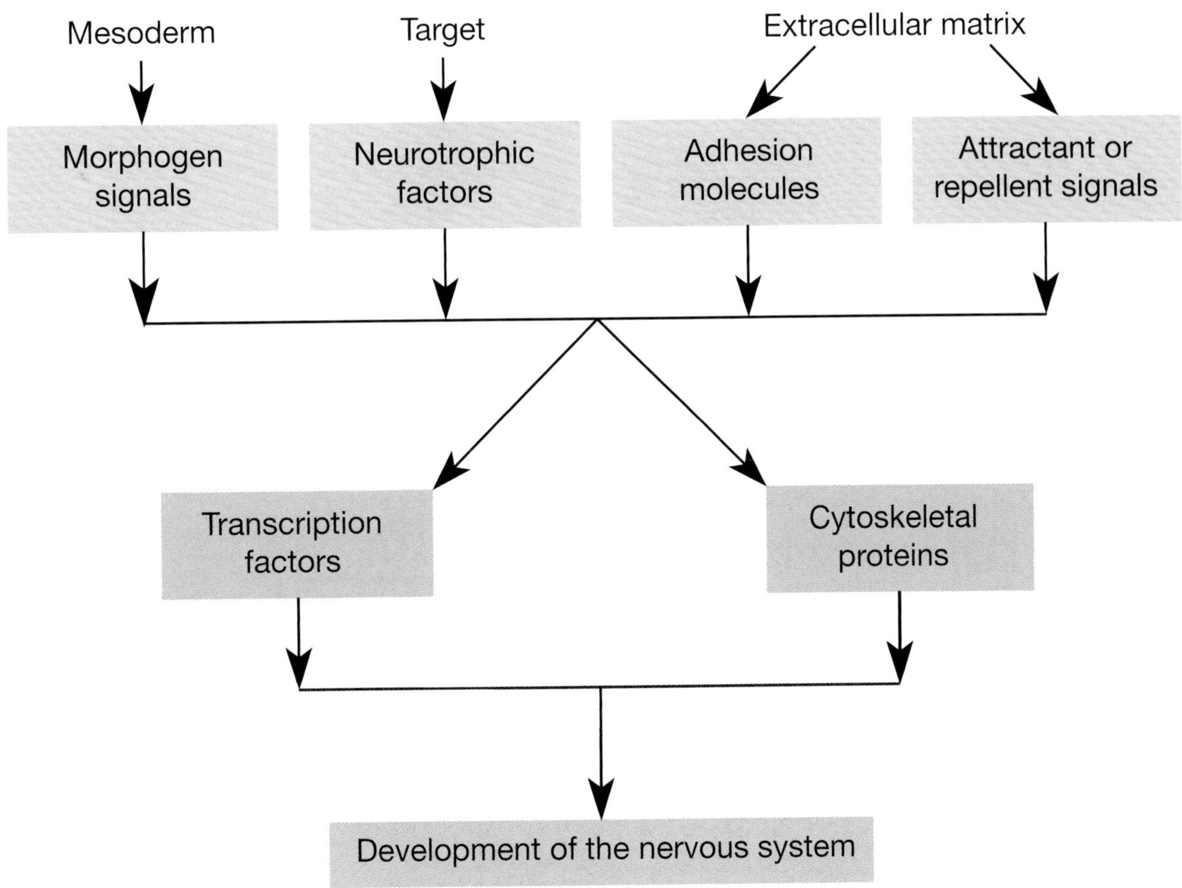

Fig. 2.2. Signals involved in the development of the nervous system.

differentiate into five divisions: *telencephalon* (cerebral hemispheres), *diencephalon* (thalamus and hypothalamus), *mesencephalon* (midbrain), *metencephalon* (pons), and *myelencephalon* (medulla) (Fig. 2.3). The junction between the mesencephalon and the metencephalon, called the *isthmus*, together with the *rhombic lip* of the metencephalon, gives rise to the cerebellum. As a consequence of transverse differentiation, the neural tube has a dorsal region, the *alar plate*, and a ventral region, the *basal plate*. The alar plate gives rise to all sensory neurons, cerebellum, and cerebral hemispheres, and the basal plate gives rise to motor neurons and the hypothalamus. The cavity of the neural tube forms the central canal at the spinal cord level and more complex fluid-filled spaces, the *ventricular system*, at cephalic levels.

Cell columns called the *neural crest* separate from the neural tube and form a major portion of the peripheral nervous system. The cells of the neural crest differentiate into dorsal root ganglia, autonomic ganglia, and Schwann cells (peripheral glia). The cranial nerves are derived from both the neural crest and specialized regions of ectoderm called *placodes*.

Throughout the length of the neural tube, primitive neuroectodermal cells proliferate and differentiate into neurons, astrocytes, oligodendrocytes, and ependymal cells. Neuronal precursors (neuroblasts) migrate to their genetically coded location, guided by adhesion molecules and glial cells. The axons grow toward their targets and establish specific synaptic connections with the appropriate neurons. These connections are stabilized by the activity of the synapse and the presence of target-derived factors. The strength of these connections continues to

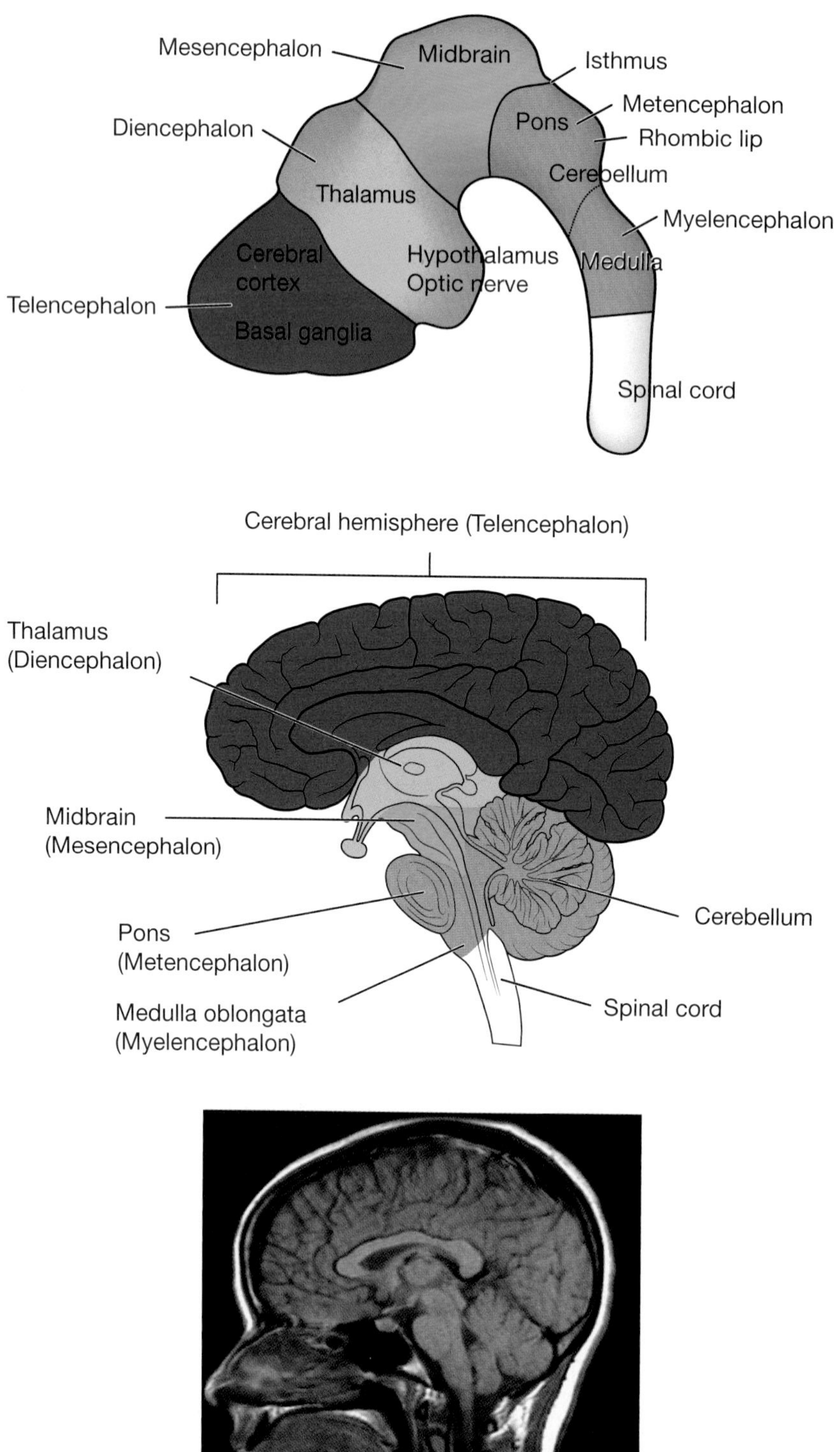

Fig. 2.3. Subdivisions of the primitive nervous system and their derivatives in the adult brain, as shown in a midsagittal magnetic resonance image of the brain. (Modified from Benarroch EE. Basic neurosciences with clinical applications. Philadelphia: Elsevier; 2006. Used with permission of Mayo Foundation for Medical Education and Research.)

change in an activity-dependent manner throughout life. Many axons become myelinated by oligodendrocytes in the central nervous system and by Schwann cells in the peripheral nervous system. Myelination is completed during the first several years of postnatal life.

The subdivisions of the neural tube are the precursors of three of the four major anatomical levels in the adult: supratentorial (telencephalon and diencephalon), posterior fossa (mesencephalon, metencephalon, and myelencephalon), and spinal (spinal cord). The fourth, or peripheral, level consists of a combination of efferent fibers that grow out from the posterior fossa and spinal levels and neural crest derivatives that include somatic and visceral afferent neurons and postganglionic autonomic neurons (Table 2.1). The neuroectodermal derivatives of the neural tube and neural crest give rise to the sensory, motor, internal regulation, and consciousness systems. Mesodermal tissues surround the neural tube and form the meninges, which in conjunction with the ventricular system form the cerebrospinal fluid system. Mesoderm that surrounds and grows into the neural tube forms the vascular system.

Many environmental factors, such as maternal infections and toxins, may affect each step in the development of the nervous system. The manifestations vary according to the stage of development when the insult occurs. For example, impairment of the developmental process during the first 4 weeks affects closure of the neural tube, whereas impairment later during fetal life postnatally affects synaptic organization or myelinogenesis.

Notable points are the following:

1. Development of the nervous system involves induction and formation of the neural tube and neural crest, regionalization, proliferation, differentiation, migration, axonal growth, synaptogenesis, and myelination.
2. The different stages of development are controlled by signals from the mesoderm, growth factors, and adhesion molecules, which regulate gene transcription and cytoskeletal function.
3. The neural tube gives rise to neurons and glial cells of the central nervous system and the neural crest gives rise to neurons and Schwann cells of the peripheral nervous system.

Table 2.1. Derivatives of the Neural Tube and Neural Crest

Level	Primary division	Precursor	Derivative	Cavity
Supratentorial	Prosencephalon (forebrain)	Telencephalon	Cerebral cortex Basal ganglia	Lateral ventricle
		Diencephalon	Thalamus Hypothalamus Pineal gland Neurohypophysis Retina	Third ventricle
Posterior fossa	Mesencephalon (midbrain)	Mesencephalon	Midbrain	Aqueduct of Sylvius
	Rhombencephalon (hindbrain)	Metencephalon	Pons Cerebellum	Fourth ventricle
		Myelencephalon	Medulla	Fourth ventricle
Spinal	Caudal neural tube	Spinal cord	Spinal cord	Central canal
Peripheral	Neural crest	Neural crest	Dorsal root ganglia Autonomic ganglia Adrenal medulla Enteric nervous system Schwann cells	

4. Genetic or environmental mechanisms may affect each stage of development, producing distinct clinical disorders that depend on the time the injury occurs.

Formation and Regional Differentiation of the Neural Tube

Formation of the Neural Tube

The central nervous system of vertebrates arises from the dorsal midline ectoderm of the vertebrate gastrula. The transformation of these ectodermal cells into neural cells is *neural induction*. It results in the formation of the neural plate. The neural tube is formed in 7 to 10 days, beginning on the 18th day of gestation.

Primary and Secondary Neurulation

The initial step in the formation of the neural tube is a thickening of the ectoderm in the dorsal midline overlying the notochord. This thickening forms the neural plate. The lateral edges of the neural plate thicken more rapidly than the center and begin to roll toward the midline, creating the neural groove, which has lateral margins, the *neural folds* (Fig. 2.4). The midline of the neural plate becomes anchored to the underlying axial mesoderm, forming a hinge around which the neural folds elevate. By days 22 to 24, the process of elevation is followed by fusion of the neural folds. This fusion forms the neural tube. The classic view of fusion is that it starts at the level of the future cervical region and extends zipper-like toward the head (cephalad) and toward the tail (caudad), until the entire tube is closed. The unfused areas at the two ends of the tube (before complete closure) are called *neuropores*. The anterior neuropore closes on days 24 to 26, and the posterior neuropore, on days 25 to 28. An alternative view is that fusion is initiated at five different sites along the embryo. In humans, fusion concludes at the end of the fourth week of gestation. Epidemiologic, clinical, and experimental evidence indicates that *folic acid* has a critical role in neural tube closure. This vitamin is routinely prescribed to pregnant women to prevent neural tube defects.

The formation of the neural tube as far caudally as the future S2 level is called *primary neurulation*. The caudal portion of the neural tube develops from a cell mass called the *caudal eminence*, which is located at approximately the future S2 level. The cavity of the neural tube extends into the caudal eminence. This process is called *secondary neurulation*, and it gives rise to the lower sacral cord, including the conus medullaris, and the filum terminale.

As the neural tube is being formed by fusion of the neural folds, the skin ectoderm also fuses, thus covering the dorsal surface of the neural tube. Ultimately, the two ectodermal derivatives, neural tube and skin, are separated by the growth of intervening mesodermal derivatives, bone and muscle. Cell columns derived from the original junction of the skin and neuroectoderm form the neural crest, which later differentiates into important components of the peripheral nervous system. Parallel with the neural tube, the mesodermal cells on each side become segmented into aggregates, the somites, from which the dermis, bone, and muscle arise.

- Neural induction is the transformation of ectodermal cells into the neural plate.
- Closure of the neural tube is complete at the end of the fourth week of gestation in humans.
- Cell columns derived from somatic and neural ectoderm form the neural crest.
- The somites give rise to the dermis, bone, and muscle.

Longitudinal Subdivisions of the Neural Tube

Even before the neural tube is entirely closed, longitudinal differentiation begins. At the same time, the cephalic, or head, end of the neural tube becomes larger than the caudal end, producing an irregularly shaped tubal structure. Continued differential growth along the length of the neural tube results in the formation of three cavities at the cephalic end of the tube. These are the primary brain vesicles: the prosencephalon (forebrain), mesencephalon (midbrain), and rhombencephalon (hindbrain). These three vesicles further differentiate into five subdivisions, which persist in the brain of the mature nervous system and evolve, through the processes of cellular proliferation, migration, and differentiation, into the major

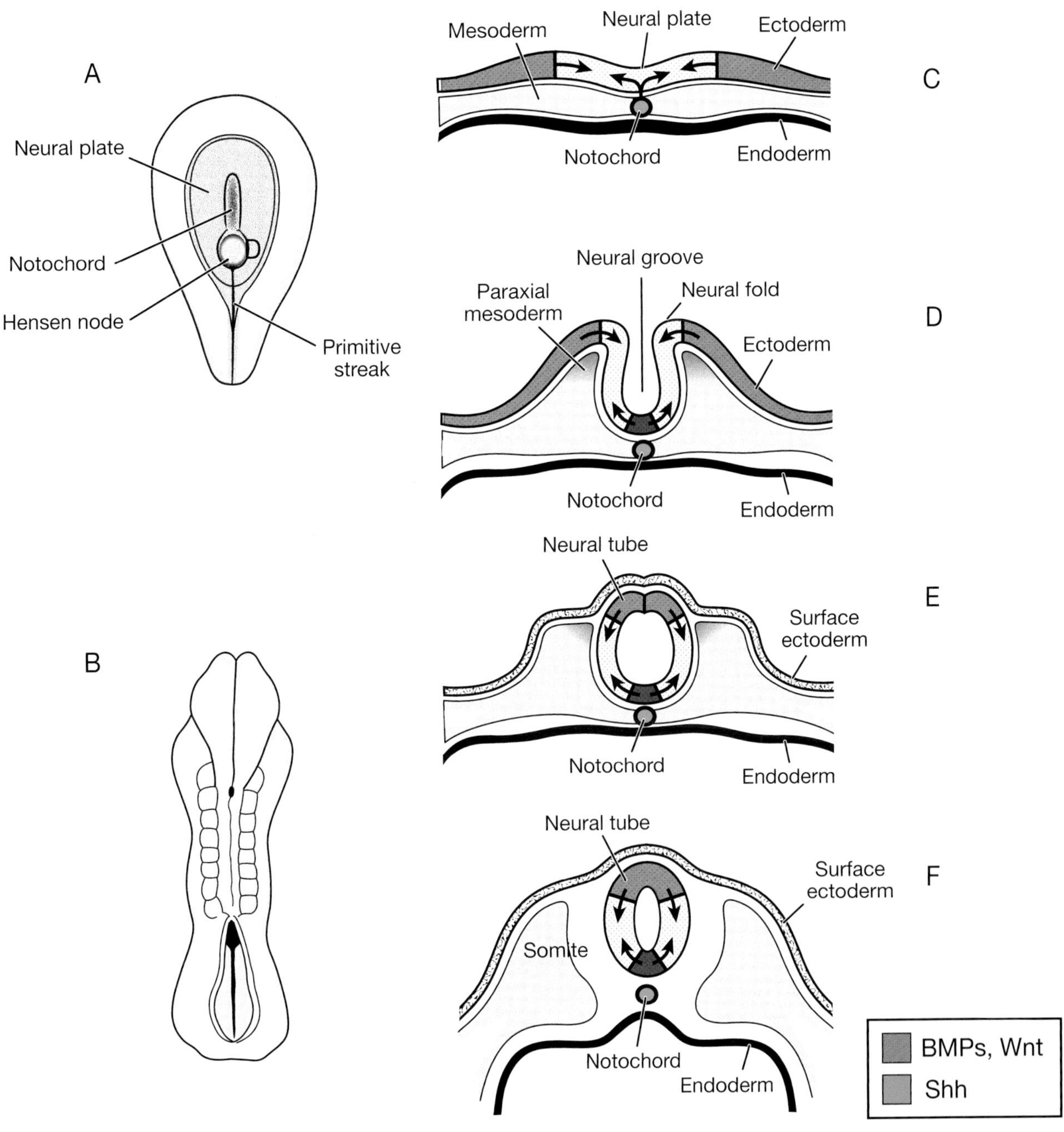

Fig. 2.4. Formation of the neural plate and neural tube. Dorsal view of the neural plate (*A*) and neural tube (*B*). Cross sections showing the formation of the neural plate (*C*), neural folds (*D*), and closure of the neural tube (*E* and *F*). BMP, bone morphogenic protein; Shh, Sonic hedgehog.

elements in the adult nervous system listed in Table 2.1. The caudal end of the neural tube undergoes much less modification as it forms the spinal cord. A central remnant of the internal cavity of the neural tube remains in each of these derivatives and forms the different components of the ventricular system (Fig. 2.5).

Between the third and fifth weeks of gestation, development differs remarkably along the length of the neural tube. The most complex changes occur at the cephalic end of the embryo. They are the result of three processes: the formation of flexures, the development of special structures in the head, and differential growth rates (Fig. 2.6).

> Three bends, or flexures, occur in the neural tube. The cervical flexure occurs between the spinal cord and myelencephalon in a ventral direction, the pontine flexure occurs in the metencephalon in a dorsal direction, and the midbrain flexure occurs in the mesencephalon in a ventral direction. These flexures produce a widening of the transverse axis of the neural tube in the rhombencephalon. The sum of the three flexures leaves only a slight bend in the mature brain at the diencephalon-mesencephalon junction and at the medulla-spinal cord junction.

- Longitudinal differentiation of the neural tube gives rise first to three primary vesicles: prosencephalon (forebrain), mesencephalon (midbrain), and rhombencephalon (hindbrain).
- The prosencephalon gives rise to the telencephalon and diencephalon, the mesencephalon to the midbrain, and the rhombencephalon to the metencephalon and myelencephalon.
- The central cavity of the neural tube remains as the ventricular system.

Mechanisms of Induction and Patterning of the Neural Tube

Neural induction and the initial patterning of the neural tube into forebrain, midbrain, hindbrain, and spinal cord are intimately intertwined. The cells in the early neural plate and neural tube acquire their regional identity from exposure to regionally restricted signals secreted by surrounding cells of the mesoderm and ectoderm. These signals, called morphogens, are secreted by several *patterning centers*, including the dorsal ectoderm, paraxial mesoderm, anterior visceral endoderm, prechordal mesoderm, and notochord, and operate along the longitudinal (rostrocaudal) and transverse (dorsoventral) axes of the embryo (Fig. 2.7).

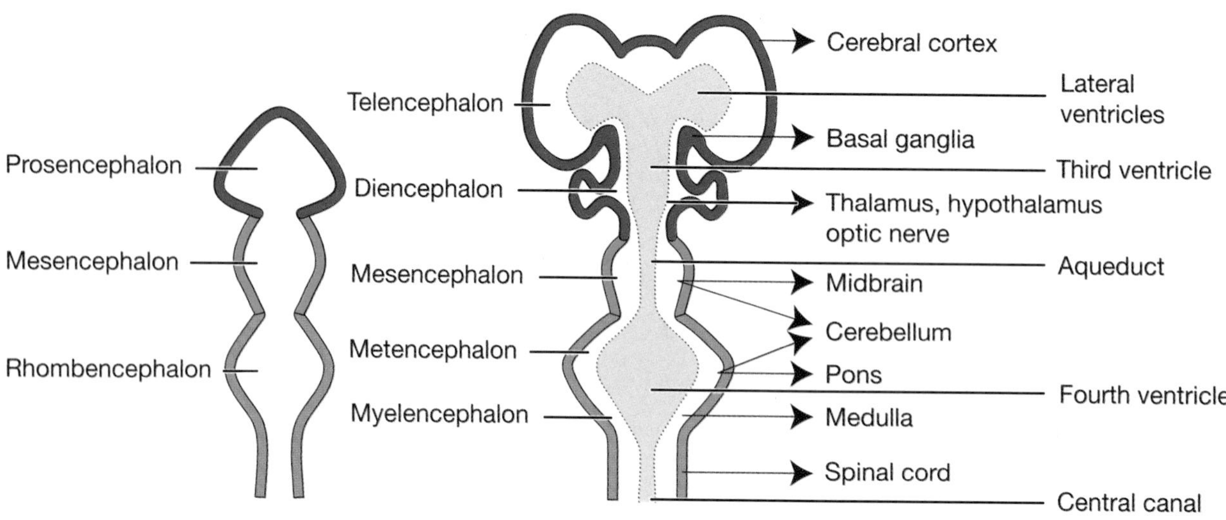

Fig. 2.5. Formation of the major brain vesicles of the neural tube. *Left*, Stage of three primary vesicles. *Right*, Stage of five major vesicles.

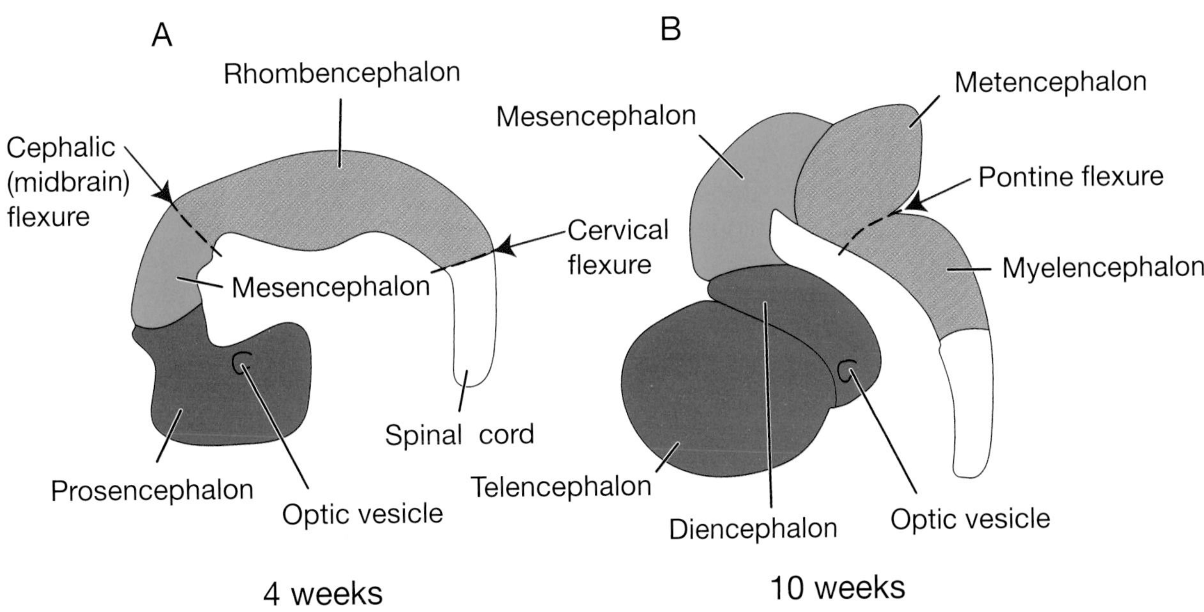

Fig. 2.6. Flexures (*arrows*) of the neural tube as primary (*A*) and secondary (*B*) brain vesicles are formed.

Neural induction involves the activity of an *organizer*, which in mammals corresponds to *Hensen node*. In addition, the *anterior visceral endoderm*, which underlies the future neural plate, is required for induction of the formation of the forebrain. Induction and patterning of the nervous system occur in several steps. During a first step, the anterior visceral endoderm and precursors of the node elicit early neural induction and specify the forebrain. During a final step called *caudalization*, or *posteriorization*, signals from the node specify the midbrain, hindbrain, or spinal cord.

The morphogen signals involved in induction and regionalization of the neural tube include fibroblast growth factors, bone morphogenetic proteins, Wnt proteins (the name is derived from *Drosophila* wingless and mouse Int-1), Sonic hedgehog, and retinoic acid. These molecules act as gradient signals in several combinations to direct cell fates by inducing the expression of transcription factors. The transcription factors that regulate cell fate and regionalization belong to several families, including the homeobox and basic helix-loop-helix families. All these transcription factors regulate expression of surface receptors and signal transduction pathways that control, at several successive steps, neural induction, regional patterning, cell fate determination, migration, axon guidance, targeting, and synaptogenesis.

Fibroblast growth factor has a critical role in neural induction by inactivating a constitutive "antineurogenic" signal mediated by bone morphogenetic proteins that repress neural differentiation in ectodermal cells. After the initial steps of induction and specification of the forebrain, caudalizing signals from the node, including retinoic acid, allow specification of the midbrain, hindbrain, or spinal cord. Sonic hedgehog is critical for ventral differentiation of the neural tube, and bone morphogenetic proteins and Wnt proteins are critical for dorsal differentiation and formation of the neural crest. The Eph family of receptors and their ephrin ligands mediate cell contact-dependent signaling and are involved primarily in the generation and maintenance of patterns of cell organization in the developing nervous system.

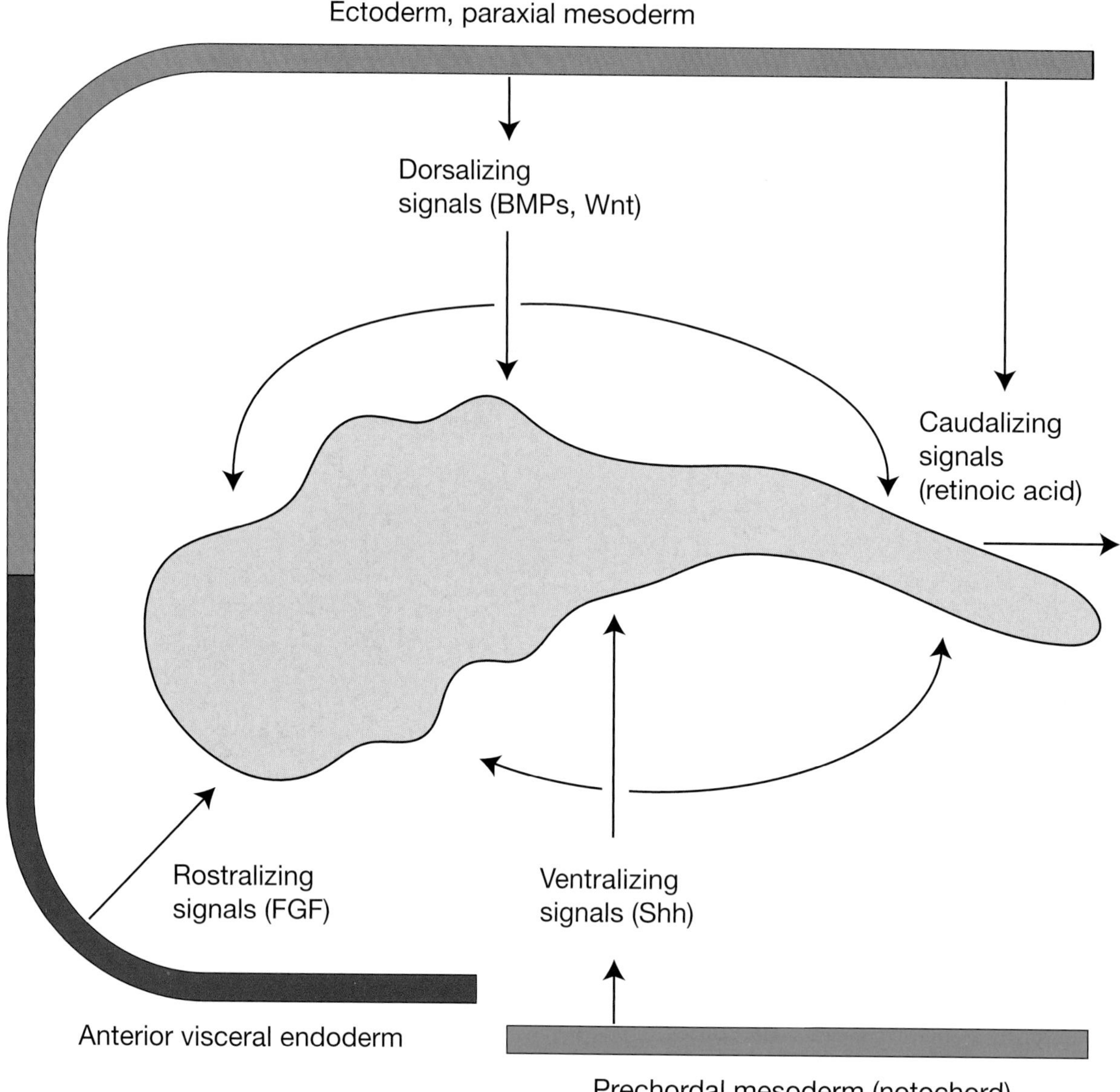

Fig. 2.7. Morphogen signals and transverse differentiation of the neural tube. Dorsalizing signals from the paraxial mesoderm include bone morphogenetic proteins (BMPs) and Wnt proteins. The critical ventralizing signal is Sonic hedgehog (Shh). Rostral differentiation requires fibroblast growth factor (FGF) signals, and caudal differentiation involves retinoic acid. (Modified from Benarroch EE. Basic neurosciences with clinical applications. Philadelphia: Elsevier; 2006. Used with permission of Mayo Foundation for Medical Education and Research.)

- Neural induction and patterning of the neural tube depend on morphogen signals secreted by patterning centers derived from the mesoderm and anterior endoderm.

Branchial Arches and Placodes

Two types of specialization occur in the cephalic region of the embryo. The first of these is the development of *branchial arches*. These arches contribute to the formation of structures in the head and neck, such as the facial muscles. The motor and sensory neurons that innervate structures derived from the branchial arches are located in the rhombencephalon. The second specialization is the appearance of complex sensory structures. The neural tube induces the overlying epithelium to form placodes. The *olfactory placode* is induced at the level of the prosencephalon and gives rise to the olfactory receptors. At the level of the rhombencephalon, the *otic placode* generates the receptors for hearing and balance and the *epibranchial placodes* generate the receptors for taste. The receptors for vision arise directly from the diencephalon.

Longitudinal and Transverse Differentiation of the Neural Tube

Longitudinal Differentiation

The initial step of regionalization is the establishment of an anteroposterior axis and the subdivisions of the brain vesicles. This involves selective expression of several transcription factors in response to signals secreted by specific patterning centers. One of these centers is the *anterior neural ridge*, which is located at the junction between the prosencephalon and the nonneural ectoderm. This center secretes signals necessary for the subdivision of the forebrain into the telencephalon and diencephalon. Another patterning center is the *isthmic organizer*, or isthmus, which is at the junction between the midbrain and hindbrain. It is necessary for the development of the mesencephalon and metencephalic structures (pons and cerebellum). The anteroposterior patterning of the hindbrain that gives rise to the pons and medulla proceeds through the generation of eight transient, lineage-restricted compartments called *rhombomeres*.

> The appearance of rhombomeres requires the segment-restricted expression of genes encoding transcription factors of the homeobox family, such as those encoded by the *Hox* genes. The segmental expression of *Hox* genes that determines the correct patterning of the caudal hindbrain is regulated by concentration gradients of retinoic acid.

Transverse Differentiation

As the neural tube enlarges and rostrocaudal patterning occurs, the neural tube undergoes anatomic and functional differentiation in the transverse plane. In a transverse section, the region of the neural tube nearest the thoracic and abdominal cavities is described as *ventral* and the region farthest from them, as *dorsal*. Within each longitudinal subdivision of the neural tube, cell fate is differentially determined in the dorsal and ventral zones. The differential proliferation of cells in the dorsal and ventral regions on each side results in the formation of a longitudinal groove, the *sulcus limitans*, in the lateral wall on each side of the neural canal. The sulcus limitans divides the neural tube into a dorsal region, or alar plate, and a ventral region, or basal plate (Fig. 2.8). As cell precursors proliferate, most of them accumulate laterally in the wall of the neural tube so that the middorsal and midventral areas are relatively thin and constitute the *roof plate* and *floor plate*, respectively.

> The dorsalizing signals that determine the alar plate arise from the dorsal ectoderm and paraxial mesoderm and are then propagated by the roof plate after neural tube closure. These signals include bone morphogenetic proteins and Wnt proteins. The ventralizing signal that determines the basal plate is secreted by the notochord and the prechordal mesoendoderm and is later propagated by the floor plate. This signal is mediated by Sonic hedgehog.

The alar plate gives rise to all sensory neurons in the spinal cord and brainstem. These neurons receive peripheral sensory information from derivatives of the somites (i.e., skin, muscle, joints, and bone) or the endoderm (i.e., internal organs) and relay this information to higher levels of the central nervous system. The term *afferent* is used to describe nerve fibers that conduct information from the periphery toward the central nervous system. These neurons and pathways constitute the sensory system. The growth of the alar plate of the prosencephalon results in large cerebral hemispheres, which almost completely surround the derivatives of the diencephalon. The cerebral cortex, basal ganglia, and thalamus are all derived from the alar plate. The cerebellum arises from the proliferation of cells of the alar plate, called the *rhombic lip*, in the metencephalon and eventually covers the dorsal surface of the entire rhombencephalon.

The basal plate gives rise to the motor neurons of the brainstem and spinal cord. These neurons are *efferent*, that is, they conduct impulses away from the central nervous system. Motor neurons and pathways concerned with the control of striated skeletal muscle constitute the somatic motor system. Those concerned with the control of internal organs form the visceral motor system. The basal plate of the diencephalon gives rise to the hypothalamus, posterior pituitary, and optic nerve.

- The alar plate gives rise to all sensory neurons in the spinal cord and brainstem and to the cerebellum, thalamus, basal ganglia, and cerebral cortex.
- The basal plate gives rise to all the motor neurons in the brainstem and spinal cord and to the hypothalamus and retina.

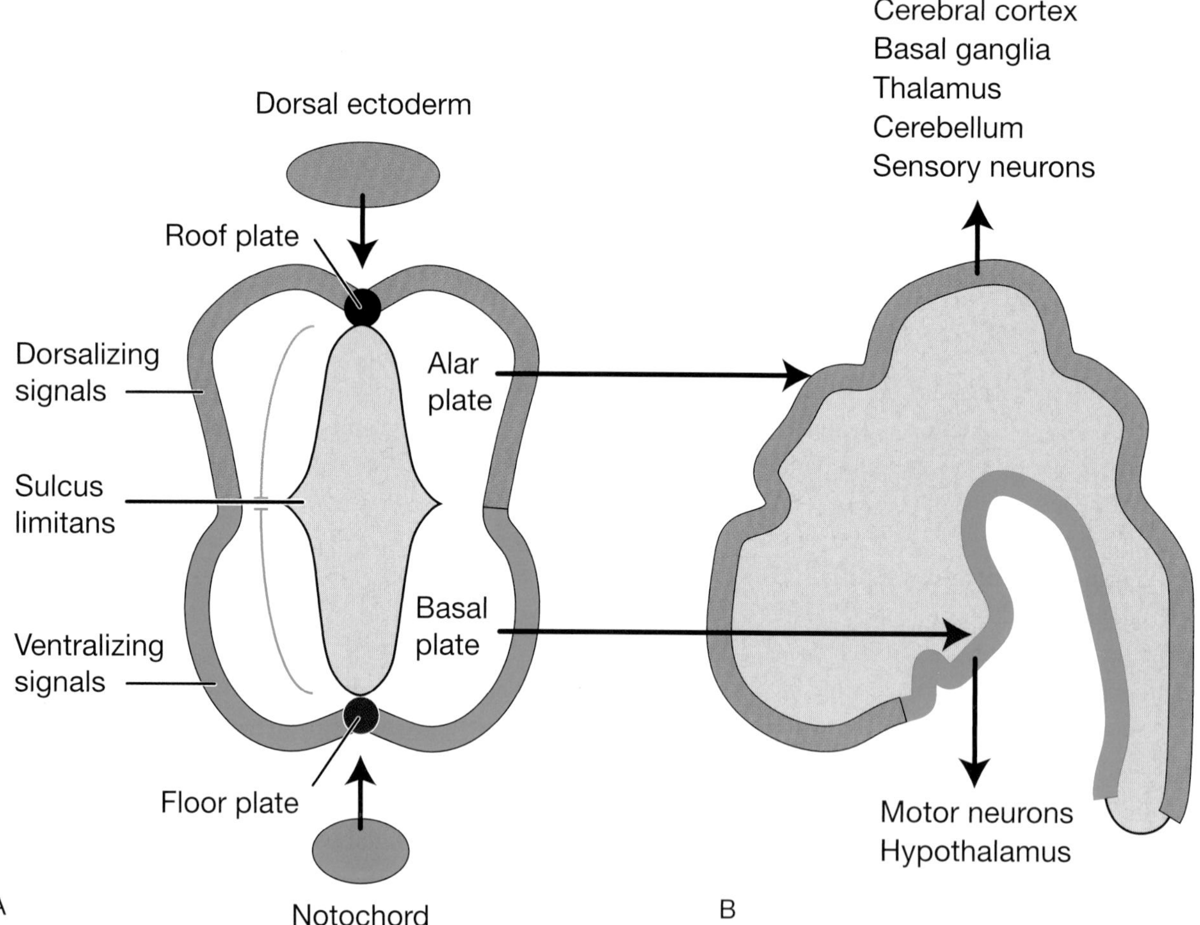

Fig. 2.8. Transverse differentiation of the neural tube. *A*, Dorsalizing signs from the dorsal ectoderm are propagated by the roof plate and elicit differentiation of the alar plate. Ventralizing influences from the notochord are propagated by the floor plate and elicit differentiation of the basal plate. There is antagonistic interaction between the dorsalizing and ventralizing signals. The boundary between the alar and basal plates is marked by the sulcus limitans. *B*, Derivatives of the alar and basal plates. (Modified from Benarroch EE. Basic neurosciences with clinical applications. Philadelphia: Elsevier; 2006. Used with permission of Mayo Foundation for Medical Education and Research.)

Cell Proliferation, Differentiation, and Migration

Through four processes that occur in concert, the cells that make up the mature nervous system accumulate in sufficient number, develop into the appropriate type of cells, move to specific sites, and make specific connections with other cells. These four processes are called proliferation, migration, differentiation, and maturation.

Cell Proliferation

Fine Structure of the Neural Tube

The wall of the primitive neural tube initially consists of a single layer of *neuroepithelial cells* that are derived from the ectoderm and form a pseudostratified epithelium. These cells have an apical-basal polarity, with the apical portion in contact with the central cavity and the basal portion in contact with the outer surface of the tube. This pseudostratified epithelium constitutes the primary germinative, or proliferative, layer that is called the *ventricular zone* (Fig. 2.9). About midway through embryogenesis, the ventricular zone is much reduced in size and mitotically active cells accumulate in the *subventricular zone*, which provides large populations of neurons and glial cell precursors. The cytoplasmic processes of these precursor cells extend radially to the outer limits of the tube, forming the *marginal zone*. Cells that migrate from the subventricular to the marginal zone make up the fourth, or *intermediate*, zone of the tube. The prominence of the zones varies at different levels of the neural tube and during different stages of development.

Primary and Secondary Germinal Matrices

The ventricular zone is the primary germinative, or proliferative, zone early during development. During early neurogenesis, the neuroepithelial cells of this zone divide symmetrically along a vertical cleavage plane and form two identical daughter cells, thus exponentially expanding the neuroepithelial cell population. In sequential phases of neurogenesis, the cell cycle progressively lengthens and the neuroepithelial cells gradually stop proliferating and start differentiating into other cell types. At this stage, the neuroepithelial cells divide asymmetrically along a horizontal cleavage plane, which results in an asymmetric distribution of molecules in the two daughter cells. The apical daughter cell remains in the ventricular zone and the basal daughter cell migrates from this zone toward the marginal zone. Mitotically active cells accumulate in the subventricular zone, which becomes the secondary germinative center. In the adult brain, the subventricular zone is called the *subependymal zone*, and the ventricular zone becomes reduced to a single layer of ependymal cells. The subventricular zone of the telencephalon is conspicuous until late in gestation and may be the site of neurogenesis in the adult brain.

Both the ventricular and subventricular zones contain two types of proliferative cells: stem cells and progenitor cells. The *stem cells* have unlimited capacity for self-renewal and multipotential ability to differentiate into neurons, astrocytes, or oligodendrocytes in vitro. The *progenitor cells* are proliferative cells with limited capacity of self-renewal and are often unipotent. There is evidence that the *radial glia* is able to generate neurons during development. Radial glial cells are generated in the ventricular zone in the early embryo and have several properties similar to those of neuroepithelial cells. In the mammalian brain, most radial glia persists until the late perinatal period and then disappears within weeks or days after birth, when the cells transform into mature astrocytes.

- The primitive neural tube consists of ventricular, subventricular, and marginal zones.
- The ventricular zone is the primary germinative zone and contains pluripotent neuroepithelial stem cells.
- The neuroepithelial cells of the ventricular zone are stem cells that give rise to progenitors of neurons and glial cells that accumulate in the subventricular zone.
- The marginal zone consists of the radially extended cytoplasmic processes of cells of the ventricular and subventricular zones.
- The radial glia, derived from neuroepithelial cells, may generate neurons during embryogenesis and then differentiate into mature astrocytes.
- The subventricular zone adjacent to the lateral ventricles may support neurogenesis in the adult brain.

Developmental Cell Death

Many neuronal and glial precursors created during the proliferative phase are removed through programmed cell

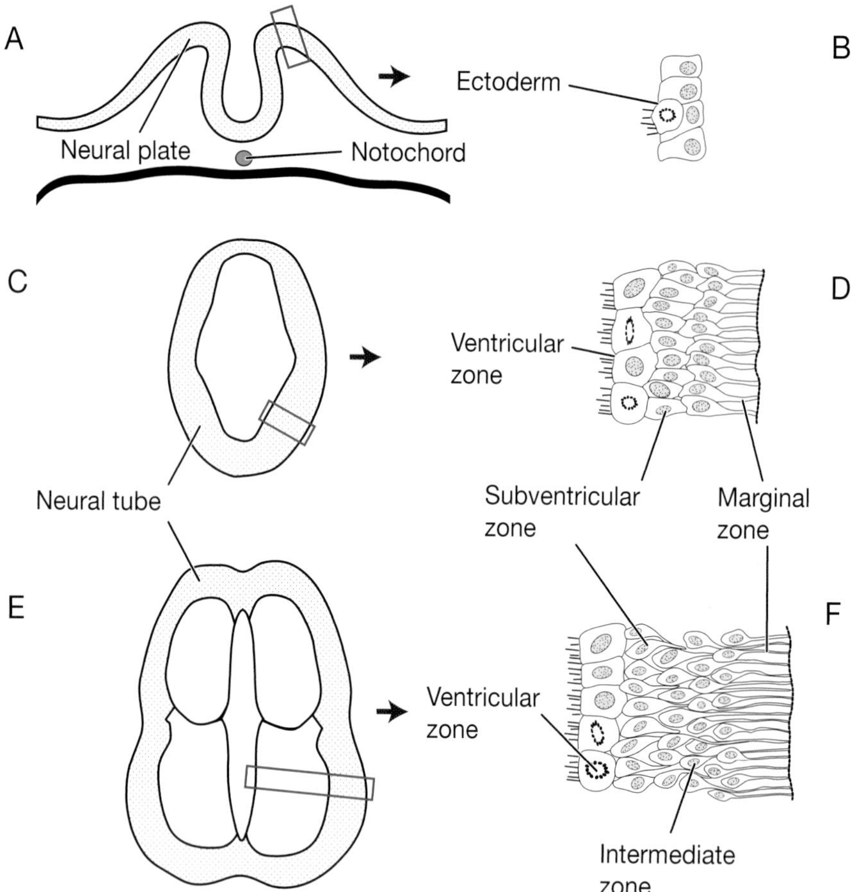

Fig. 2.9. Differentiation of the cell layers in the primitive neural tube, with a high power view on the *right* and a cross section of the tube shown on the *left*. *A* and *B*, The early neural plate is a single layer of ciliated neuroepithelial cells. *C* and *D*, Formation of layers of cells by proliferation and outward migration. The neuroepithelial cells form the ventricular zone, the proliferating and migrating immature neurons and glial cells form the subventricular zone, and the processes of these cells form the marginal zone. *E* and *F*, Further differentiation of the cell layers, showing an expanded subventricular zone and an intermediate zone consisting of migrating immature neurons.

death, or apoptosis. The main stimulus for programmed cell death during development is deprivation of *growth factors*. These factors are soluble proteins produced by target and glial cells; they promote the expression of genes required for neuronal survival, growth, and differentiation. Many of these genes encode proteins that inhibit apoptosis.

Growth factors have several roles during development; they not only promote cell survival but also participate in differentiation and contribute to the control of axonal growth and synaptogenesis. For example, nerve growth factor is critical for the survival and differentiation of sympathetic ganglion neurons, small dorsal root ganglion neurons, and cholinergic neurons in the forebrain; brain-derived neurotrophic factor, for neurons in the cranial nerve ganglia and several regions in the brain; and glial-derived neurotrophic factor, for dopaminergic neurons in the midbrain. Platelet-derived growth factor and fibroblast growth factor promote the proliferation of glial-restricted precursors. Later, ciliary neurotrophic factor induces cells to form astrocytes, and thyroid hormone induces cells to form oligodendrocytes.

- Many proliferating neuronal and glial precursors undergo programmed cell death.
- The main stimulus for programmed cell death during development is deprivation of growth factors.
- Growth factors are soluble proteins produced by target and glial cells; they promote the expression of genes required for cell survival, growth, and differentiation.

Cell Determination: Specification of Cell Types and Subtypes

Specification of Neuronal Fate

The progenitor cells that are initially multipotent gradually become restricted in potential to develop into either a neuron or a particular type of glial cell. Neurons and glial cells are generated from common precursors in a temporally coordinated matter. Generally, neurons are generated first, followed by glial cells (Fig. 2.10). Specification of cell types involves the actions of growth factors and transcription factors that regulate the expression of *proneural genes*. Vertebrate proneural genes are often expressed in restricted progenitor domains and are implicated in the specification of neuronal subtypes. An essential role of proneural proteins is to restrict their own activity to single progenitor cells and to inhibit their own expression in adjacent cells, thus preventing these cells from differentiating into neurons. This is achieved in part through a process called lateral inhibition, which involves the evolutionarily conserved *Notch* signaling pathway.

Notch is a transmembrane protein that after binding to ligands encoded by proneural genes undergoes cleavage of its intracellular domain, which is then translocated to the nucleus, where it inhibits expression of proneural genes. Through this mechanism, proneural gene expression is restricted to single cells that enter a neuronal differentiation pathway, whereas the target cells become committed to a glial fate.

Specification of Glial Fate

Several extracellular factors instruct progenitor cells toward a glial fate decision. Glial cell precursors give rise to astrocytes and oligodendrocytes. Downstream effectors of these molecules have dual functions in that they activate gliogenic differentiation and simultaneously inhibit neurogenic differentiation. The radial glia gives rise to astrocytes in the adult brain. Oligodendrocytes arise primarily from precursors located in two narrow ventral columns of neuroepithelium that are on either side of the floor plate and extend all along the spinal cord, hindbrain, midbrain, and caudal forebrain.

- Specification of a neuronal or glial fate involves the actions of growth factors and transcription factors.
- Proneural genes promote development of neurons at the expense of glial cells.

Neuronal Migration

In the developing nervous system, neurons migrate from their site of origin in the germinal centers to their final destination, where they mature and develop functional connections. Neuronal migration requires dynamic changes in the neuronal cytoskeleton. It is guided by interactions between neurons and the microenvironment, including glial cells and the extracellular matrix. These interactions are mediated by several adhesion and guidance molecules.

Radial Migration

Radial migration is critical for the formation of laminated structures such as the cerebral cortex (Fig. 2.11). Radial migration follows the radial organization of the germinative zones in the neural tube and involves the radial glia, which provides a scaffold for the directed migration of postmitotic neurons in the brain.

Radial migration involves several stages and signals. Mobilization of neuronal progenitors and their ongoing migration along the radial glial pathway involves several proteins associated with the cytoskeleton, including filamin-1, doublecortin, and LIS-1 (so-named because its deficit produces lissencephaly). Formation of the different laminae in the cerebral cortex and the cerebellum depends on reelin, which provides a stop signal to migrating neurons.

Tangential Migration

Tangential migration of neural precursors from the subventricular zone of the rostral forebrain is important for development of the olfactory bulb. Tangential migration is also involved in the formation of the *external granular cell layer* of the cerebellum. This is a secondary germinal matrix that originates at the end of gestation and is the source of granule cells in the cerebellum.

- The radial glia provides a scaffold for radial migration of immature neurons to the cerebral cortex.
- Radial migration involves several stages and signals and depends on proteins associated with the cytoskeleton.
- Tangential migration is involved in the formation of the external granular cell layer of the cerebellum and the olfactory bulb.

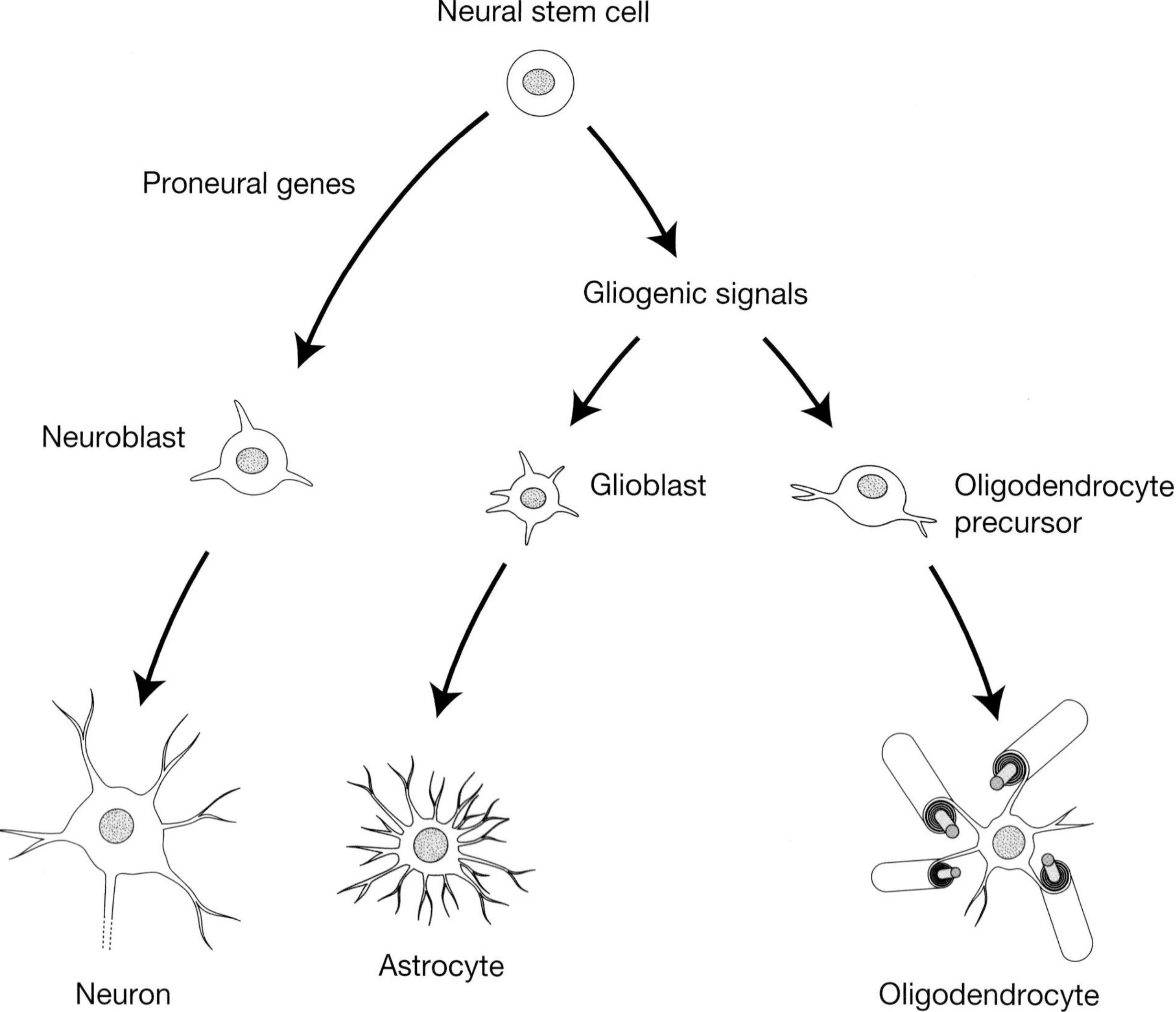

Fig. 2.10. Progressive determination of cell fate in the nervous system. Expression of proneural genes determine differentiation into neurons and prevents the glial cell fate. Gliogenic signals determine the precursors of oligodendrocytes and astrocytes.

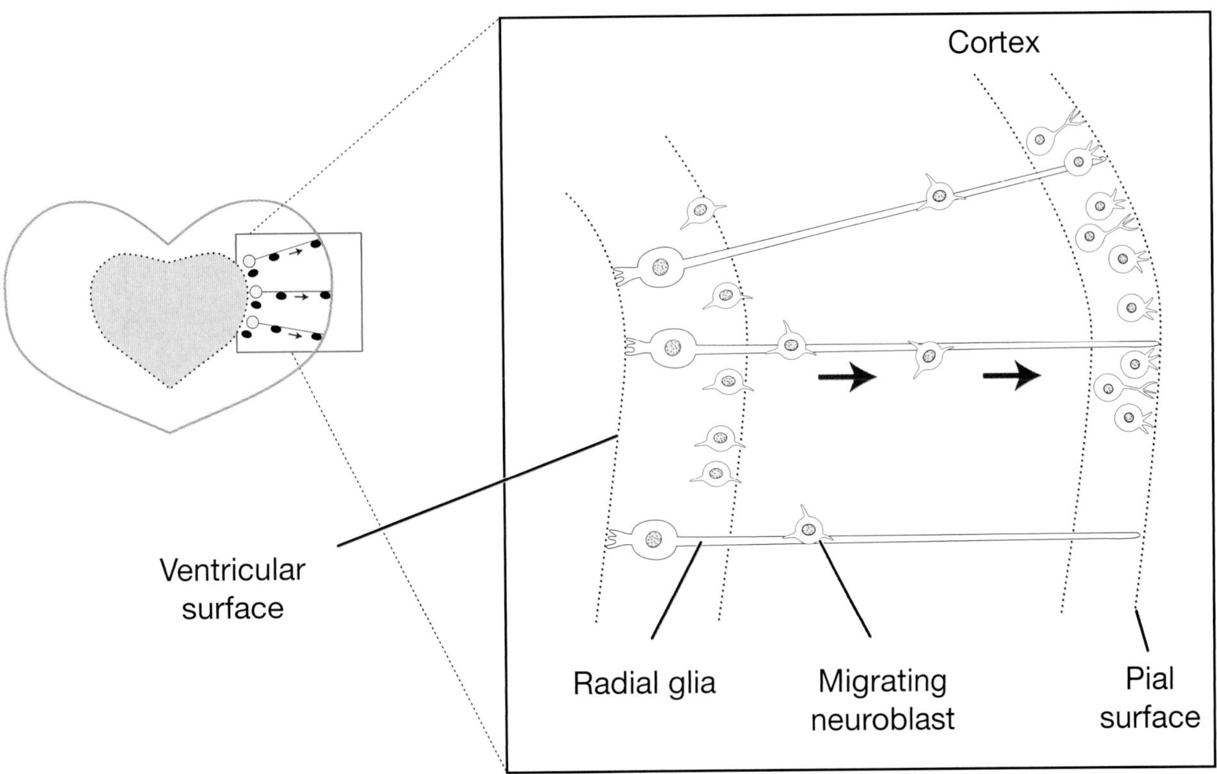

Fig. 2.11. Radial migration is critical for the formation of the cerebral and cerebellar cortices. Formation of the cerebral cortex involves migration of precursors of pyramidal cells from the ventricular zone to the periphery, toward the pial surface. This depends on the radial glia, whose processes span the entire width of the neural tube.

Neuronal Maturation

After a neuron has reached its final location in the central nervous system, it establishes appropriate contacts with other neurons, both locally and at a distance. It does this by extending processes called neurites. Most neurites become *dendrites*, which receive information coming from other nerve cells. One neurite, the *axon*, ultimately reaches a specific target. The contact between the axon of a neuron and the dendrites of the neuronal target is called a *synapse*. Synapses are the basis for transmission of information in the nervous system (Fig. 2.12). Maturation of the nervous system involves mechanisms of axonal growth, dendritic development, and synaptogenesis. These are dynamic processes that persist throughout life and are critical for mechanisms of learning and repair in the nervous system.

Axonal Growth and Pathfinding

The Growth Cone

Neurons grow by extending axons and dendrites guided by an expanded terminal structure called the *growth cone* (Fig. 2.13). Neuronal growth cones recognize extracellular guidance signals and translate them into neurite growth. The growth cone of the axon continuously changes shape and direction. Growth cone motility depends on extensive rearrangements of the cytoskeleton.

> The axonal growth cone explores the environment by extending and retracting weblike sheets of membrane, called lamellipodia, and fingerlike processes, called filopodia. The formation of lamellipodia and filopodia depends on dynamic

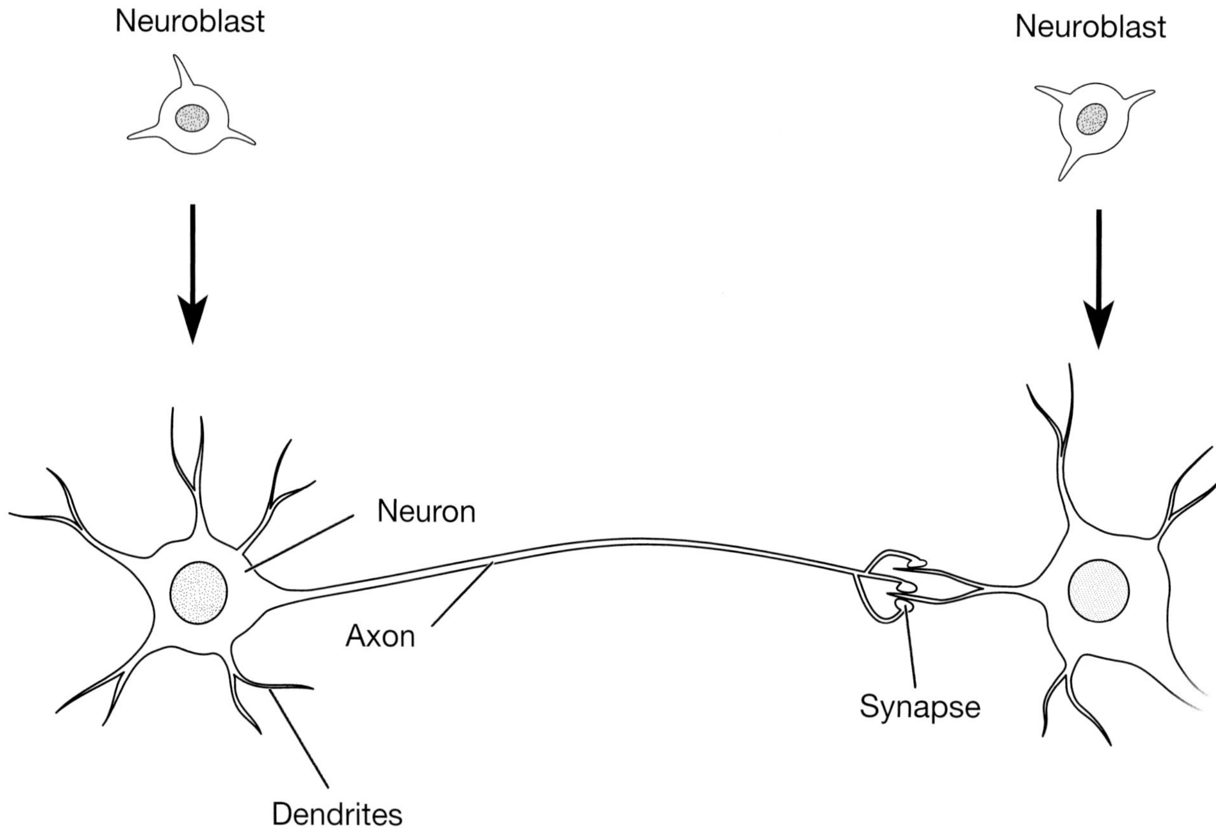

Fig. 2.12. Progressive neuronal differentiation involves extension of dendrites and axons and formation of synaptic contacts.

rearrangements of the actin cytoskeleton and microtubules regulated by small guanosine triphosphate-binding proteins of the Rho family.

Guidance Signals for the Axon

Growth cones are guided to their targets by the interaction of various chemoattractant or chemorepellent signals that may act as short- or long-range environmental cues. These signals include secreted substances, adhesion molecules, and components of the extracellular matrix.

There are four conserved families of guidance molecules that regulate, through specific receptors, the cytoskeletal dynamics of the growth cone and thus determine its behavior. They are netrins, semaphorins, ephrins, and Slits. Netrins, Slits, and some semaphorins are secreted molecules; other semaphorins and ephrins are expressed at the cell surface. Netrins can act as chemoattractants or chemorepellents, but semaphorins, ephrins, and Slits are primarily repellents. The integration of these signals determines growth cone behavior, such as advancing, turning, withdrawing, and target recognition. Target-derived growth factors also provide chemoattractant signals to the axons.

- Neurons grow by extending axons and dendrites guided by growth cones.
- Growth cones change shape and direction through rearrangements of the cytoskeleton.
- Axonal growth cones are guided to their targets by the interaction of various chemoattractant or chemorepellent environmental cues.

Dendritic Growth and Synaptogenesis

Once the axon reaches its target, it forms a synapse. In the central nervous system, axons make synaptic contacts with the dendrites or cell bodies of the target neuron. Each neuron receives multiple synapses, and the richness of synaptic contacts determines the ability of the neuron to receive and process information critical for function of the nervous system.

Development of Dendritic Arborizations

Dendrites grow through a steady process of extension and branching. Dendritic growth generally occurs after outgrowth of the axon. Dendritic branching, like axonal branching, is regulated by local cues that affect the dynamics of the cytoskeleton. In many areas of the central nervous system, excitatory synapses are made on small protrusions of the dendrites called *dendritic spines*. The final

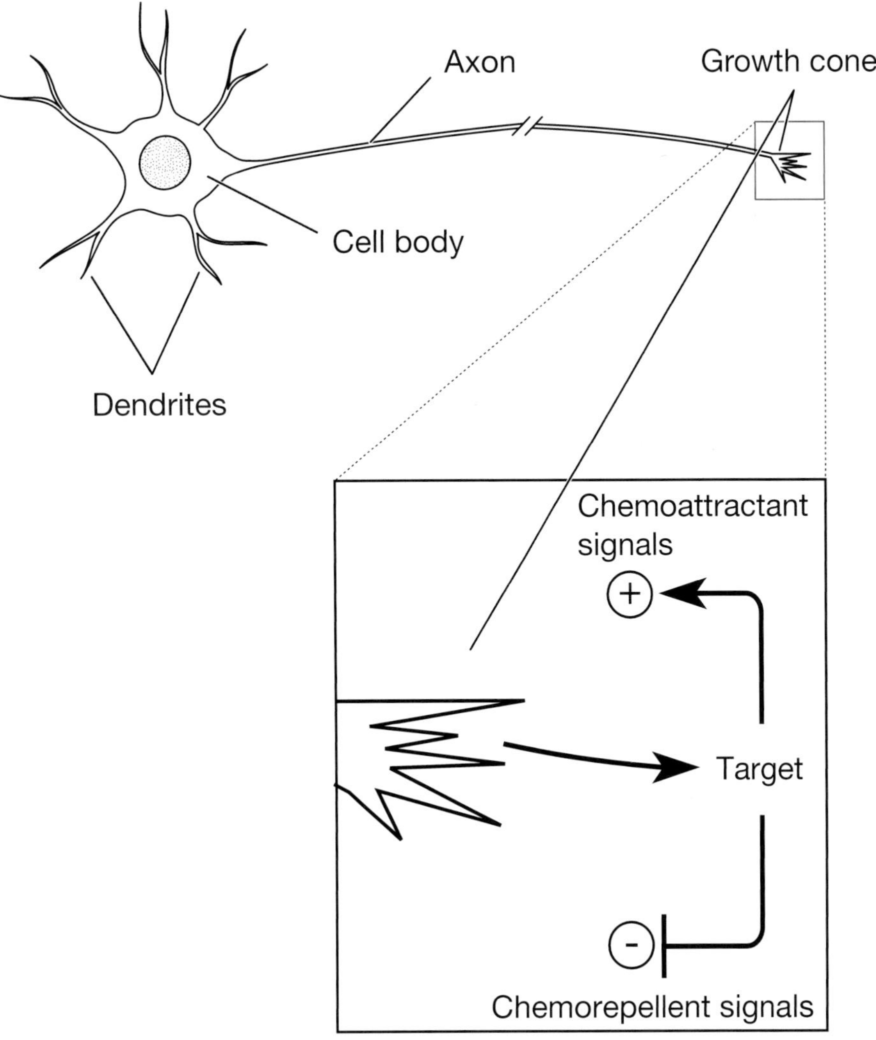

Fig. 2.13. Neurons extend processes, called growth cones, that respond to environmental signals for growth. Axonal growth and pathfinding depend on dynamic changes in the cytoskeleton of the axonal growth cone in response to chemoattractant or chemorepellent signals from the environment, including target cells, glia, and nonneural structures.

form and extent of the dendritic arborizations result from interactions between genetic factors and environmental cues. Dendritic spines undergo rapid structural modifications in response to synaptic activity, which fine-tunes dendritic growth and branching (Fig. 2.14). The selective growth or pruning of dendritic arbors is guided by the specific patterns of activity of their inputs.

Establishment and Stabilization of Synaptic Connections
The earliest pattern of synapses formed between functionally related neuronal groups may be imprecise and inadequate for normal function. As maturation proceeds, the synaptic pattern is modified and refined by the elaboration and strengthening of some connections and the atrophy and elimination of others. There is evidence that the onset of electrical activity in the nervous system and the pattern of synaptic excitation of the target neuron are critical for the formation and stabilization of mature synaptic connections. This *activity-dependent plasticity* refines axonal projections and synaptic connections by eliminating exuberant projections and strengthening functionally relevant connections. Immature neurons that do not establish appropriate functional contact are eliminated through programmed cell death. Synapse elimination also involves pruning and retraction of many axons that initially impinge on a neuron.

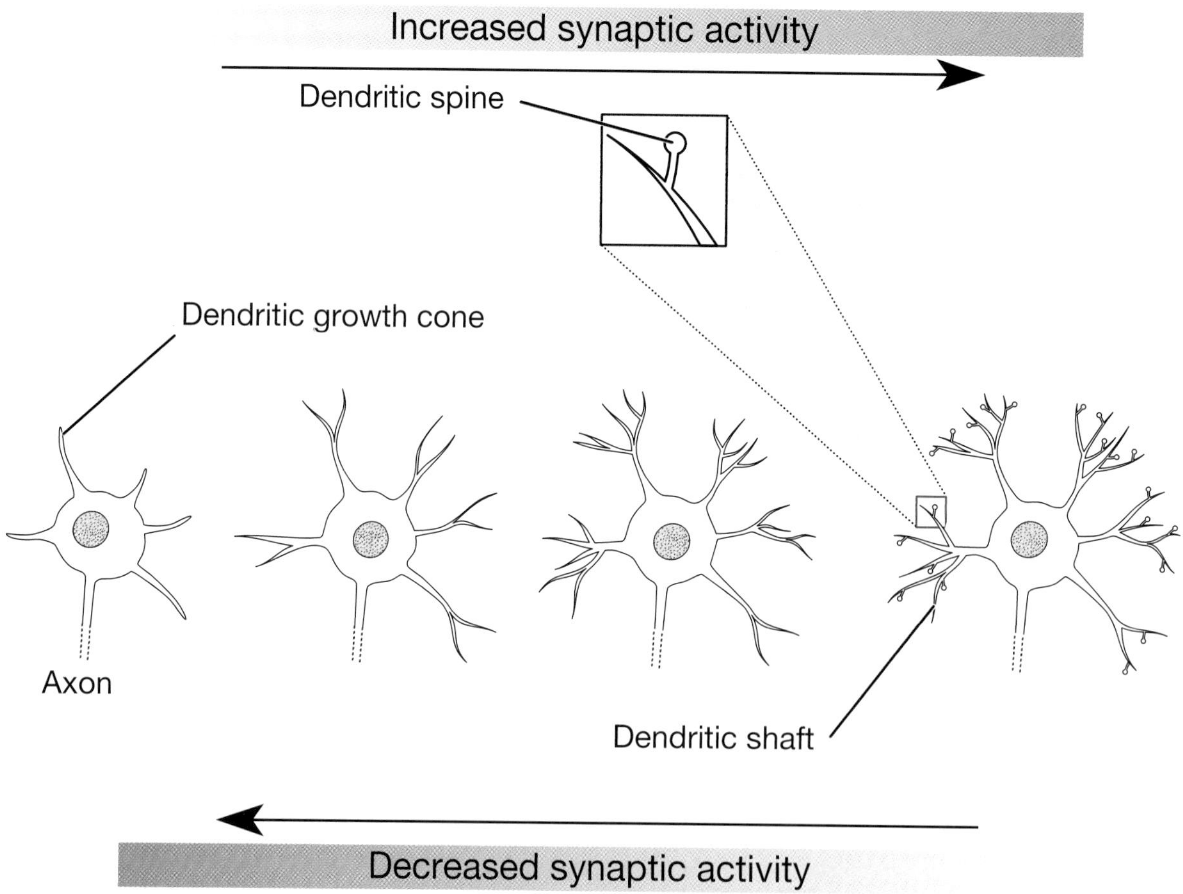

Fig. 2.14. Growth and differentiation of the dendrites are determined by environmental signals, particularly synaptic activity. Use-dependent growth of dendritic arborizations, including dendritic spines, is critical for synaptogenesis in the nervous system. This dynamic process remains throughout life. Loss of activity reverses this process, leading to loss of synaptic connectivity and function.

In many areas of the brain, the effects of sensory experience on development and organization of specific circuits is significant during a brief postnatal interval called the *critical period*. For example, deprivation of visual input during this critical period prevents the normal development of visual cortex.

This process of use-dependent synaptic remodeling is not only critical during development but persists throughout life. It has far-reaching implications, not only in normal processes such as learning and refinement of motor and sensory skills, but also in many pathologic situations, such as epilepsy, pain, and recovery after injury to the nervous system.

- Dendritic branching and the formation of dendritic spines result from interactions between genetic factors and environmental cues.
- The selective growth or pruning of dendritic arbors is guided by the specific patterns of activity of their inputs.
- Activity-dependent plasticity refines axonal projections and synaptic connections by eliminating exuberant projections and strengthening functionally relevant connections.
- Use-dependent synaptic remodeling persists throughout life and is critical for learning and recovery from injury.

Establishment of the Structure of the Mature Central Nervous System

At all levels, the central nervous system consists of a ventricular cavity surrounded by ependymal cells (derived from the primitive ventricular zone), *gray matter* (derived mostly from the subventricular zone and containing the cell bodies and dendrites of neurons), and *white matter* (consisting of axons). Both gray matter and white matter contain glial cells. As the result of differential proliferation, differentiation, and migration within the neural tube, the structure of the ventricular system and the gray and white matter varies at each level of the mature central nervous system. These unique changes occur during the fourth to sixth weeks of development.

The neurons in the central nervous system form four longitudinal systems: the motor system, sensory system, internal regulation system, and consciousness system. Neurons of the future midbrain, pons, medulla, and spinal cord are arranged into longitudinal somatomotor, visceromotor, viscerosensory, and somatosensory columns that exhibit a segmental organization.

In addition to the four longitudinal systems, two essential support systems derived from the mesoderm are formed during embryogenesis: the cerebrospinal fluid system and the vascular system. The primitive neural tube is surrounded by layers of connective tissue, called *meninges*, that encase the central nervous system. The innermost layer, the *pia mater*, is intimately adherent to the outer wall of the tube during development and to the external surface of the mature brain and spinal cord. Angiogenic mesodermal elements penetrate the substance of the neural tube through this layer and form an extensive vascular network. In certain areas of the thin roof plate of the rhombencephalon, diencephalon, and telencephalon, the pia mater and its accompanying blood vessels grow into the ventricular cavity and carry a layer of ependyma with them to form the *choroid plexuses*. Choroidal epithelial cells are specialized ependymal cells that produce *cerebrospinal fluid*, which fills the central canal and ventricular system. Surrounding the pia mater is a layer of loose connective tissue called the *arachnoid*, which, in turn, is surrounded by a thick layer called the *dura mater*.

- The gray matter contains the cell bodies and dendrites of the neurons, the white matter contains the axons, and both contain astrocytes and oligodendrocytes.
- The meninges and cerebral blood vessels are derived from the mesoderm.

Spinal Level

Organization of the Spinal Cord

As the caudal end of the neural tube develops into the spinal cord, it remains basically the same as that of the primitive nervous system. The central canal becomes obliterated, and the shape of the gray matter is modified. The spinal gray matter becomes subdivided into a *dorsal horn*, which is from the alar plate, and the *ventral horn*, which is from the basal plate (Fig. 2.15). The dorsal horn contains sensory neurons that receive input from dorsal root ganglion neurons (neural crest derivatives) that innervate the somites (skin, muscle, and skeleton) and visceral organs (derived from the endoderm). The dorsal root ganglion neurons that innervate somites are *general somatic afferents* and those that innervate viscera are *general visceral afferents*. The ventral horn contains motor neurons that innervate the skeletal muscle derived from the somites. The axons of these neurons constitute *somatic efferents* (also referred to as "general" somatic efferents). The dorsal and ventral horns are connected by the *intermediate gray matter*, which contains different classes of interneurons, including at thoracic, lumbar, and sacral levels the preganglionic neurons that control the function of the viscera; these are *general visceral efferents*. This regionally restricted generation of different neuronal subtypes involves a process of patterning in the dorsoventral axis, followed by further elaboration of neuronal identity.

The marginal layer of the primitive neural tube becomes the white matter of the spinal cord, a dense layer of nerve fibers consisting of the axons of spinal neurons and ascending or descending axons that connect the spinal cord with more rostral areas.

- The dorsal horn of the spinal cord is derived from the alar plate and contains sensory neurons that send ascending axons to other areas of the central nervous system.
- The dorsal horn neurons receive somatic and visceral afferent inputs from neurons in the dorsal root ganglia (derived from the neural crest).
- The ventral horn contains motor neurons whose axons innervate the skeletal muscles derived from somites (somatic efferents).
- The intermediate gray matter of the spinal cord contains interneurons and preganglionic neurons whose axons (general visceral efferents) innervate the autonomic ganglia (derived from the neural crest).

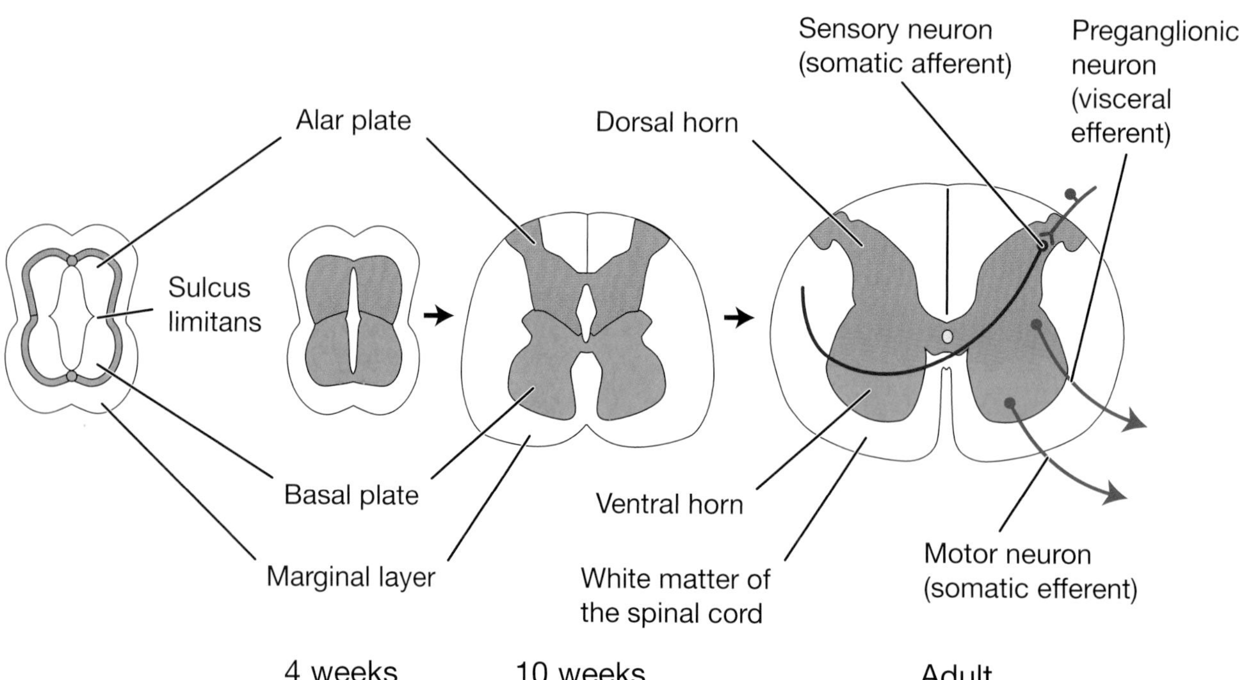

Fig. 2.15. Transverse section of the neural tube showing early regional differentiation. Transverse section of the spinal cord at 4 weeks, 10 weeks, and adult.

- The white matter of the spinal cord contains ascending and descending axons that interconnect spinal cord neurons with other areas of the central nervous system.

Relation Between the Spinal Cord and Vertebral Column
The meninges surround the spinal cord and form a subarachnoid space. Bone surrounding spinal cord forms the *vertebral column*. The longitudinal growth of the vertebral column is much faster than that of the spinal cord (Fig. 2.16). In the third fetal month, the spinal cord extends the entire length of the vertebral canal; at birth, it terminates at the lower border of the third lumbar vertebra; and in adults, it terminates near the upper border of the second lumbar vertebra. Therefore, to perform a lumbar puncture in a newborn infant, the needle must be inserted at a very low level to avoid puncturing the spinal cord. The differential rate of growth between the spinal cord and vertebral column places the spinal cord segments above the vertebral segments of the corresponding number. Because the spinal nerves

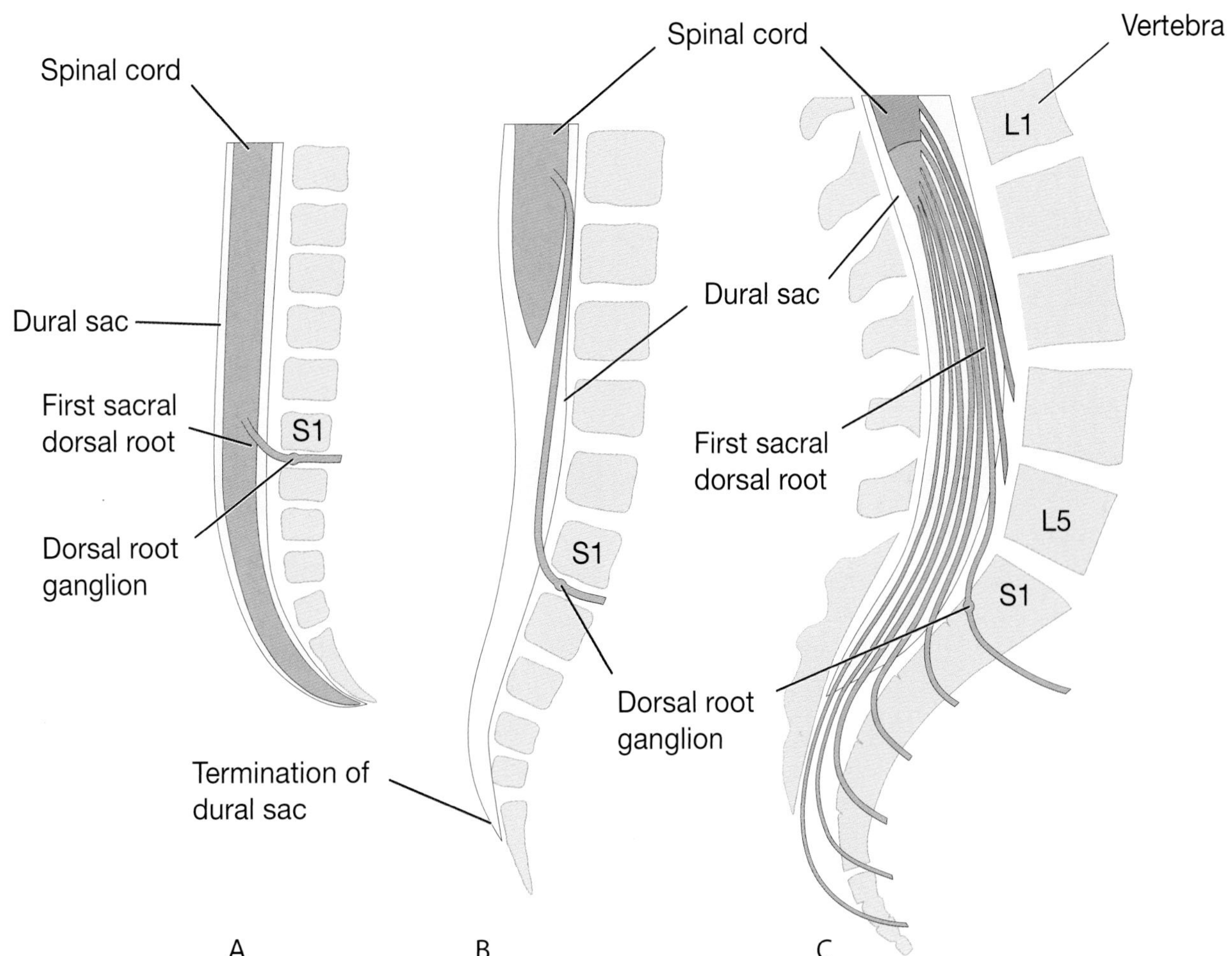

Fig. 2.16. The location of the caudal end of the spinal cord in the vertebral column at, *A*, 12 weeks, *B*, birth, and *C*, childhood. The first sacral dorsal root in *B* and *C* is representative of the spinal roots that form the cauda equina. (Modified from Moore KL, Persaud TVN. The developing human: clinically oriented embryology. 8th ed. Philadelphia: Saunders; 2008. Used with permission.)

emerge between the embryologically established vertebral bodies, the lower nerve roots progressively elongate, forming the *cauda equina* of adults.

- The spinal cord terminates at the lower border of the third lumbar vertebra at birth and near the upper border of the second lumbar vertebra in adults.

Posterior Fossa Level

The mesoderm that surrounds the cephalic end of the embryonic nervous system forms the skull and meninges that enclose and protect the brain within the cranial cavity. In concert with the formation of the primary brain vesicles and flexures, folds of meninges that ultimately become tough dural septa are formed. A major horizontal fold of dura mater forms at the level of the mesencephalon. This fold eventually covers the dorsal surface of the cerebellum and is called the *tentorium cerebelli*. The region of the cranial cavity below the plane of this tentorium is the posterior cranial fossa, which contains structures derived from the mesencephalon and rhombencephalon (metencephalon and myelencephalon) that give rise to the brainstem and cerebellum.

Brainstem

The lower portion of the brainstem is derived from the rhombencephalon. As the flexures develop in the rhombencephalon, the alar plates of the myelencephalon and metencephalon rotate laterally, the roof plate becomes greatly thinned, and the central cavity opens out into a rhomboid-shaped space, the *fourth ventricle* (Fig. 2.17). This rotation produces a change in the relation of the alar and basal plates, so that the alar plate lies lateral to the basal plate. The sulcus limitans, a groove in the floor of the fourth ventricle in the *medulla* (Fig. 2.18) and the *pons*, marks the junction between the alar and basal plates

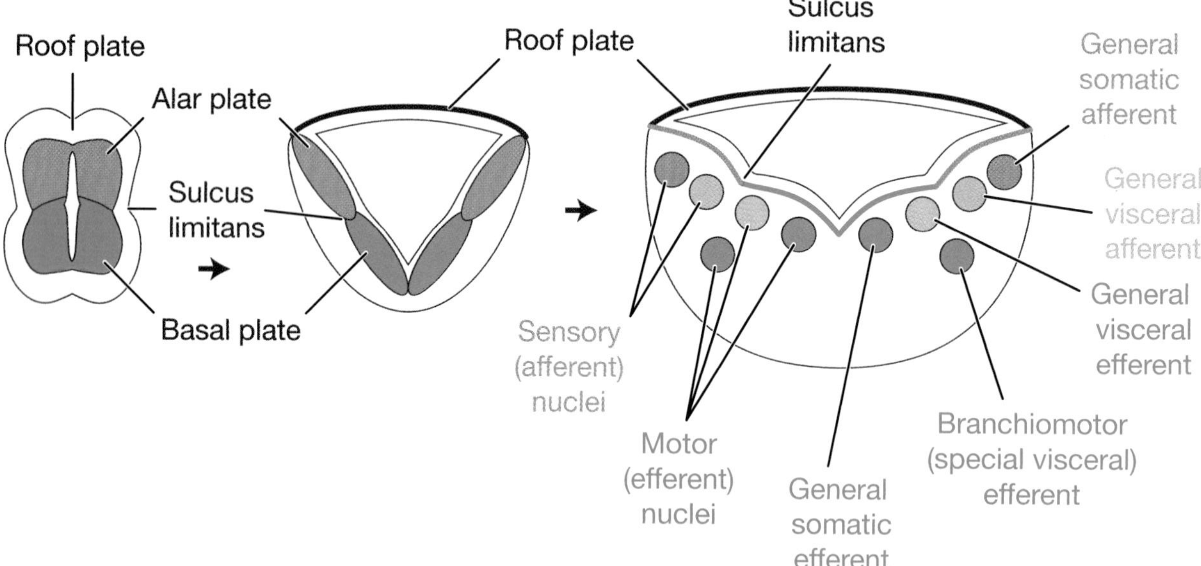

Fig. 2.17. As the flexure develops in the rhombencephalon, the alar plates of the myelencephalon and the metencephalon rotate laterally, the roof plate becomes greatly thinned, and the central cavity opens out into a rhombic-shaped space, the fourth ventricle. This rotation changes the relation of the alar and basal plates, so that the alar plate lies lateral to the basal plate, with the sulcus limitans marking their junction in the floor of the fourth ventricle in the adult medulla and pons. Therefore, in both the medulla and pons, motor neurons are located medially and sensory neurons laterally in relation to the sulcus limitans, with the visceral motor and visceral sensory neurons located in between.

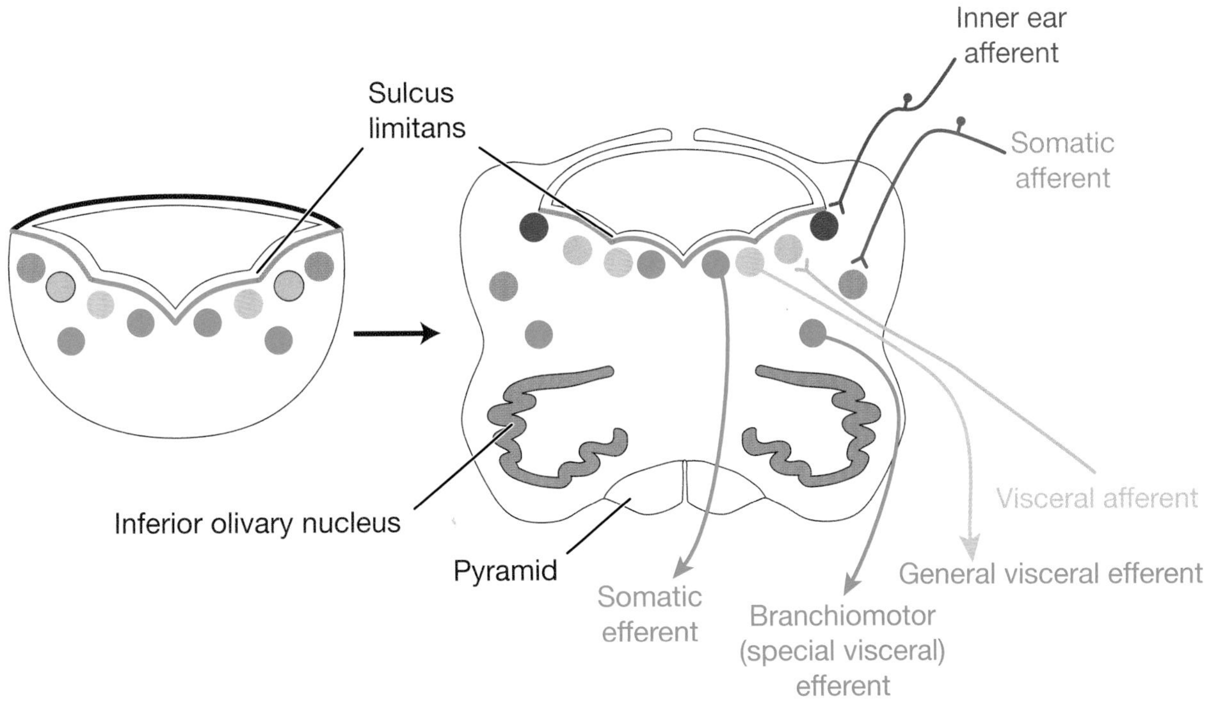

Fig. 2.18. Derivatives of the alar plate and basal plate in the medulla.

(Fig. 2.19). Therefore, both in the medulla and pons, motor neurons are located medially and sensory neurons laterally in respect to the sulcus limitans. The visceral motor and visceral sensory neurons are located in between the somatic motor and somatic sensory neurons. Motor and sensory neurons in the brainstem form functionally specific longitudinal columns that correspond to the different neuronal groups found in the spinal cord. Thus, like the spinal cord, the basal plate of the brainstem gives rise to motor neurons that innervate derivatives of the somites (extraocular and tongue muscles) and form the general somatic efferent column and preganglionic neurons that innervate the autonomic ganglia and form the general visceral efferent column. In the medulla and pons, there is an additional group of neurons that innervate facial, laryngeal, and pharyngeal muscles derived from the branchial arches. These *branchiomotor neurons* constitute the so-called *special visceral efferent* column (a misnomer). In the medulla and pons, the alar plate gives rise to different types of sensory neurons. In addition to sensory neurons that receive input from somatic derivatives of the face (general somatic afferent column) or from visceral organs (general visceral afferent column), there are neurons that receive input from taste receptors (so-called *special visceral afferents*) and from inner ear organs related to hearing and balance (so-called *special somatic afferents*). All these functional columns occupy a predictable position at each level of the brainstem.

The junction between the thinned roof plate and the alar plate is the *rhombic lip* (Fig. 2.19). Proliferation and migration of cells from the rhombic lip result in the formation of important derivatives of the alar plate, including the *inferior olivary nucleus* in the medulla (Fig. 2.18), the *pontine nuclei* in the pons (Fig. 2.19), and the granule cells in the cerebellum. The cerebellum comes to overlie the entire fourth ventricle and rhombencephalon. In the mesencephalon, which becomes the midbrain, the basic relationships seen in the spinal cord persist (Fig. 2.20). The central cavity is a small canal, the *aqueduct of Sylvius*. As the alar and basal plates differentiate into specialized sensory and motor structures, they become known as the *tectum* and *tegmentum*, respectively. The tegmentum

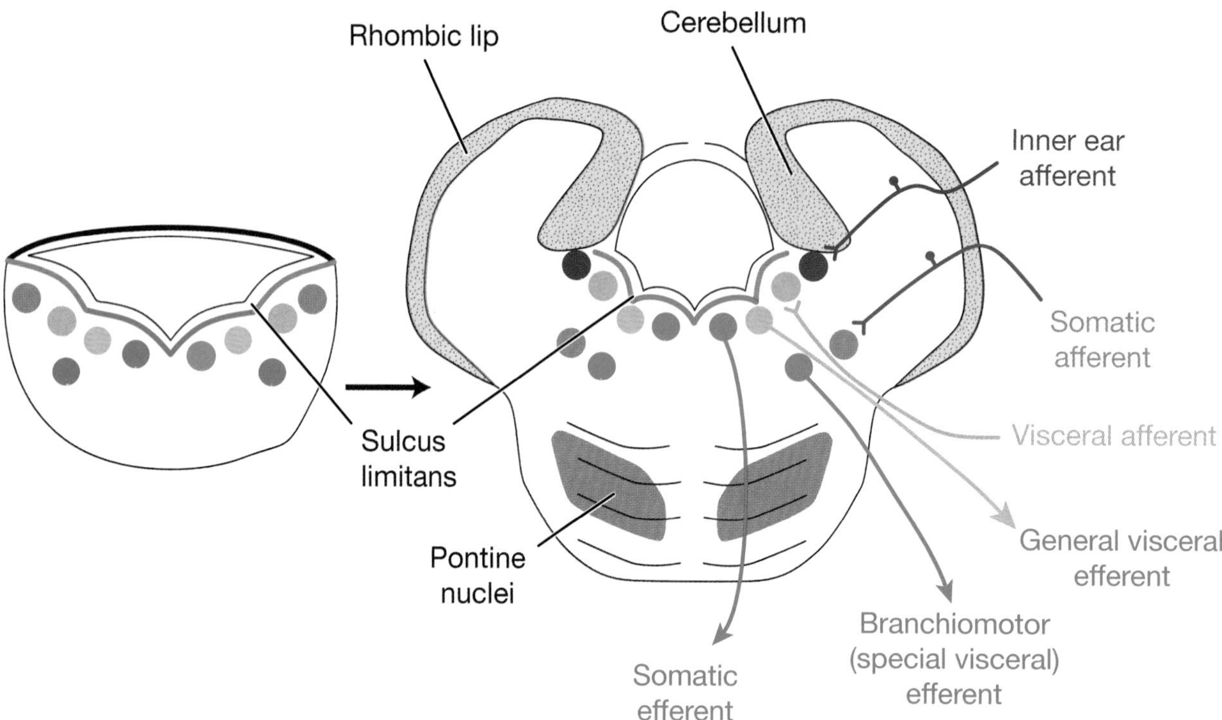

Fig. 2.19. Derivatives of the alar plate and basal plate in the pons. The junction between the thinned roof plate and the alar plate is the rhombic lip. Proliferation and migration of cells from the rhombic lip result in the formation of important derivatives of the alar plate, including the inferior olivary nucleus in the medulla, the pontine nuclei in the pons, and the granule cells in the cerebellum.

of the midbrain and rostral pons contain neurons that are part of the consciousness system. Dense bundles of longitudinal axons descend from the cerebral cortex and form part of the motor system. These cortical motor axons are in the most ventral portion of the brainstem, forming the *cerebral peduncles* at the level of the midbrain (Fig. 2.20), the *basis pontis* at the level of the pons (Fig. 2.19), and the *pyramids* at the level of the medulla (Fig. 2.18).

Cerebellum

The development of the cerebellum depends critically on inductive signals secreted by cells in the isthmus at the junction of the midbrain and hindbrain. These signals mark the site of induction of the cerebellar rhombic lip. This specialized germinative epithelium arises relatively late during development at the interface between the neural tube and the roof plate of the fourth ventricle. The cerebellum consists of the cerebellar cortex and deep cerebellar nuclei. Neurons in the cerebellum originate from the ventricular neuroepithelium at the level of the isthmus and rhombic lip (Fig. 2.21). The isthmus gives rise to the Purkinje cells of the cerebellar cortex and the cells of the cerebellar nuclei. The rhombic lip gives rise to the granule cells.

The granule cell precursors form a thin layer of proliferating cells, the external granular layer, which migrate tangentially over the cerebellar surface. After birth, the granule cell precursors rapidly proliferate in the external granular layer. These immature neurons then migrate radially past the Purkinje cell layer to form the granular layer of the adult cerebellar cortex.

- **The posterior fossa level includes the brainstem and cerebellum.**

- The brainstem includes the midbrain (derivative of the mesencephalon), pons (derivative of the metencephalon), and medulla (derivative of the myelencephalon).
- The brainstem motor nuclei are located medially, and the sensory nuclei are lateral.
- The descending cortical motor axons form the cerebral peduncles (midbrain), basis pontis (pons), and pyramids (medulla).
- The central cavity of the neural tube becomes the aqueduct of Sylvius (midbrain) and the fourth ventricle (pons and medulla).
- The cerebellum originates from the isthmus at the junction of the midbrain and hindbrain and the rhombic lip (metencephalon).

Supratentorial Level

The portion of the cranial cavity located above the tentorium cerebelli contains the two derivatives of the prosencephalon, the telencephalon and diencephalon (Fig. 2.22).

General Organization of the Telencephalon

The telencephalon is from the alar plate and gives rises to the *cerebral hemispheres*. The telencephalon consists of two main components called the dorsal telencephalon, or *pallium*, and the ventral telencephalon, or *ganglionic eminence*. The pallium gives rise to all the pyramidal neurons of the cerebral cortex. The ganglionic eminence gives rise to the *striatum* and *globus pallidus* and to the interneurons of the cerebral cortex. One component of the striatum, the caudate nucleus, forms the lateral walls of the *lateral ventricles*, which are the ventricular cavities of the telencephalon (Fig. 2.22). The roof of the lateral ventricles is formed by a large system of axons that connect the two cerebral hemispheres, the *corpus callosum*.

An important step in forebrain development is the formation of the dorsal midline roof plate, which depends on dorsalizing signals. In a normal 7- to 8-week human fetus, the telencephalic vesicles, precursors of the cerebral hemispheres, expand more rapidly than the midline roof plate. Because of the rapid rate of proliferation of the cells

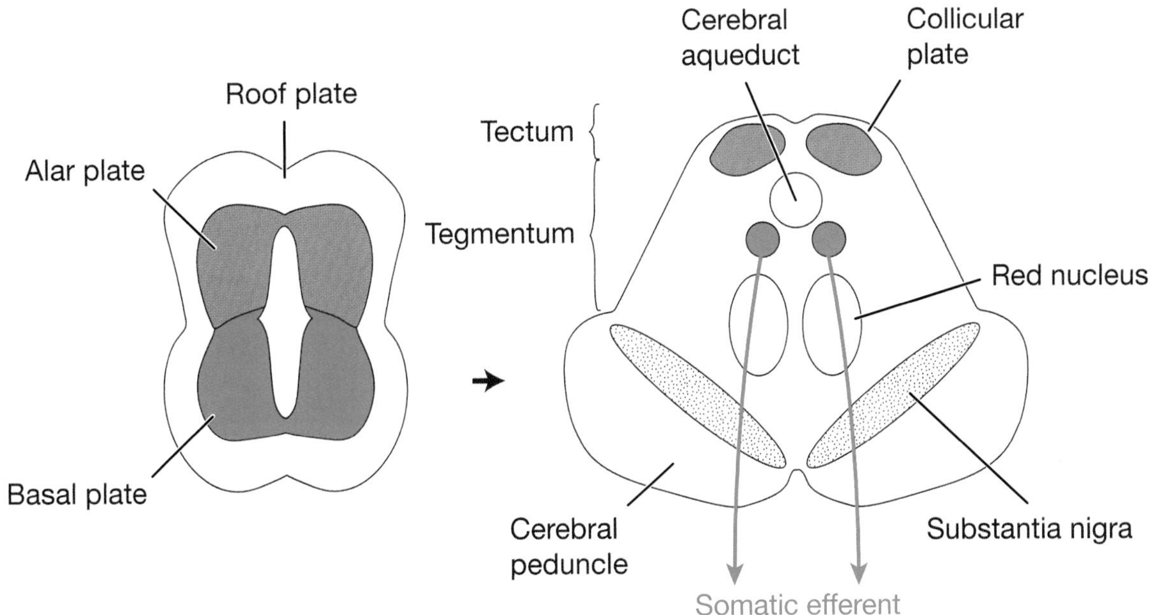

Fig. 2.20. In the mesencephalon, which becomes the midbrain, the basic relations seen in the spinal cord persist. The central cavity here is a small canal, the aqueduct of Sylvius. As the alar and basal plates differentiate into specialized sensory and motor structures, they become known as the *tectum* and *tegmentum*, respectively.

in the dorsal part of the vesicle, each telencephalic vesicle grows posteriorly, laterally, and ventrally to form a C-shaped structure. This shape is obvious in several structures of the cerebral hemispheres, especially the lateral ventricles and caudate nucleus (Fig. 2.23).

Cerebral Cortex

The cerebral cortex consists of pyramidal cells that arise from the ventricular zone and reach the cortex by radial migration and interneurons that arise primarily from the ganglionic eminence and reach the cortex by tangential migration. Two important features of the cerebral cortex are its laminar structure and its organization into functional columns. Both of these features depend on radial migration of the undifferentiated pyramidal cells from the ventricular zone. The organization and connectivity pattern of the adult cerebral cortex are the result of a progressive developmental differentiation from the most primitive areas, which constitute the *limbic cortex* (including the *hippocampus*) on the medial aspect of each hemisphere, through intermediate areas (referred to as *paralimbic cortex*) to the most differentiated areas, or *neocortex*, located on the convexity of each hemisphere (Fig. 2.24).

The most developed cortex contains a typical laminar pattern consisting of six laminae or layers. There are three waves of migration during the development of the cerebral cortex. The first

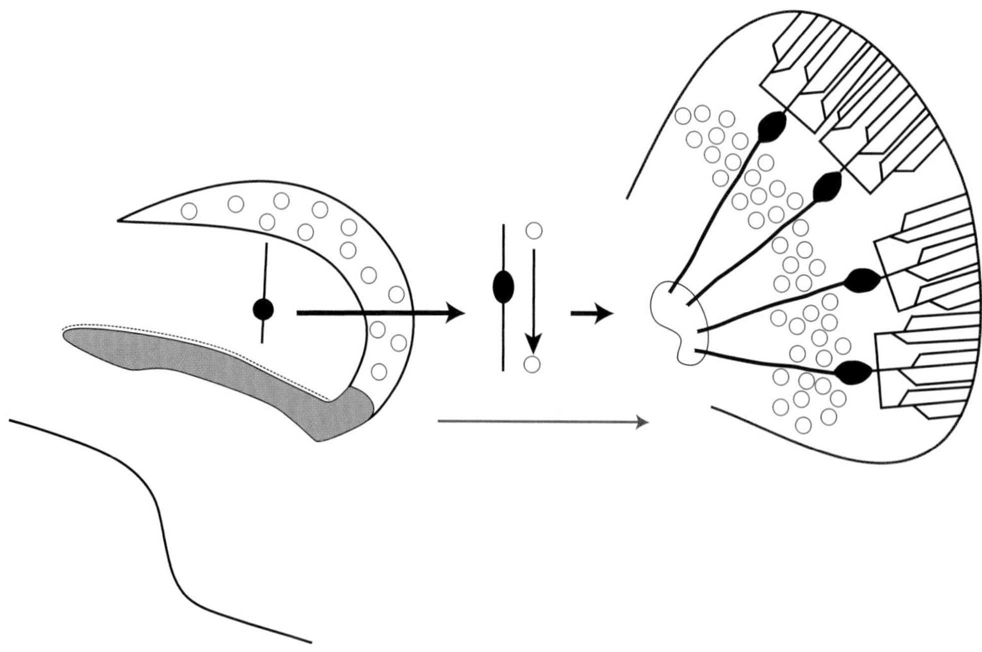

Fig. 2.21. Neurons in the cerebellum originate from two sources: from the ventricular neuroepithelium at the level of the isthmus and from the rhombic lip. The isthmus gives rise to the Purkinje cells of the cerebellar cortex and the cells of the cerebellar nuclei. The rhombic lip gives rise to the granule cells of the cerebellum. The immature granule cells form a thin layer of proliferating cells, the external granular layer, that migrate tangenitally over the cerebellar surface. After birth, there is rapid proliferation of immature granule cells in the external granular layer. These cells then initiate their radial migration past the Purkinje cell layer to form the granular layer of the adult cerebellar cortex.

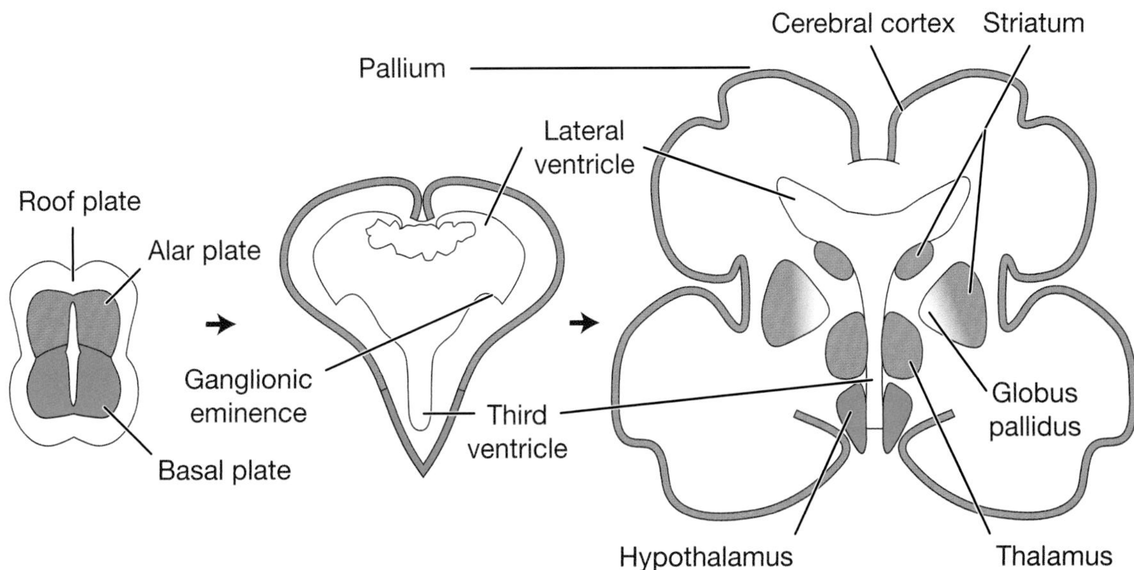

Fig. 2.22. The telencephalon is derived from the alar plate and gives rises to the cerebral hemispheres. The dorsal telencephalon, or pallium, gives rise to all the pyramidal neurons of the cerebral cortex, and the ventral telencephalon, or ganglionic eminence, gives rise to the striatum and globus pallidus. The diencephalon consists of the thalamus (dorsal diencephalon) and the pineal gland, which are derived from the alar plate, and the hypothalamus and subthalamus (ventral diencephalon), which are derived from the basal plate. The diencephalon also gives rise to the optic nerve and neurohypophysis.

migratory wave forms the most superficial layer, which contains the earliest cortical neurons. The second wave forms a transient subplate. The third wave forms the cortical plate between the marginal zone and the subplate. It is the precursor of all the other layers of the cerebral cortex. Within the cortical plate, the different laminae develop in a sequence such that the earlier generated cells are located in deeper laminae and the later generated cells, in more superficial laminae. This process is the inside-out pattern of migration (Fig. 2.25).

The increase in the mass of the brain as a whole is accompanied by a marked increase in the total surface area of the cerebral cortex, to about 2,300 cm^2 at maturity. If the surface remained smooth, the capacity of the cranial cavity would have to be increased several times to accommodate the brain. This is compensated for by the complex folding of the surface of the brain, which begins with the formation of the lateral sulcus (sylvian fissure) at about 50 days of gestation. The development of the normal pattern of fissures and secondary and tertiary gyri is nearly complete at 40 weeks of gestation.

The specialized sensory structures concerned with olfaction are also derived from the telencephalon. The olfactory placode gives rise to the olfactory epithelium. Immature neurons of the subventricular zone in the most anterior portion of the lateral ventricles migrate tangentially to form the olfactory bulb.

- The supratentorial level includes derivatives of the telencephalon and diencephalon.
- The telencephalon gives rise to the cerebral cortex, basal ganglia, and olfactory bulb.
- The more primitive areas of the cerebral cortex are located on the medial aspect of each hemisphere and are part of the limbic system.
- The neocortex develops later and forms the large lateral surface of each cerebral hemisphere.
- The earlier generated pyramidal cells are located in deeper laminae in the mature cortex and later

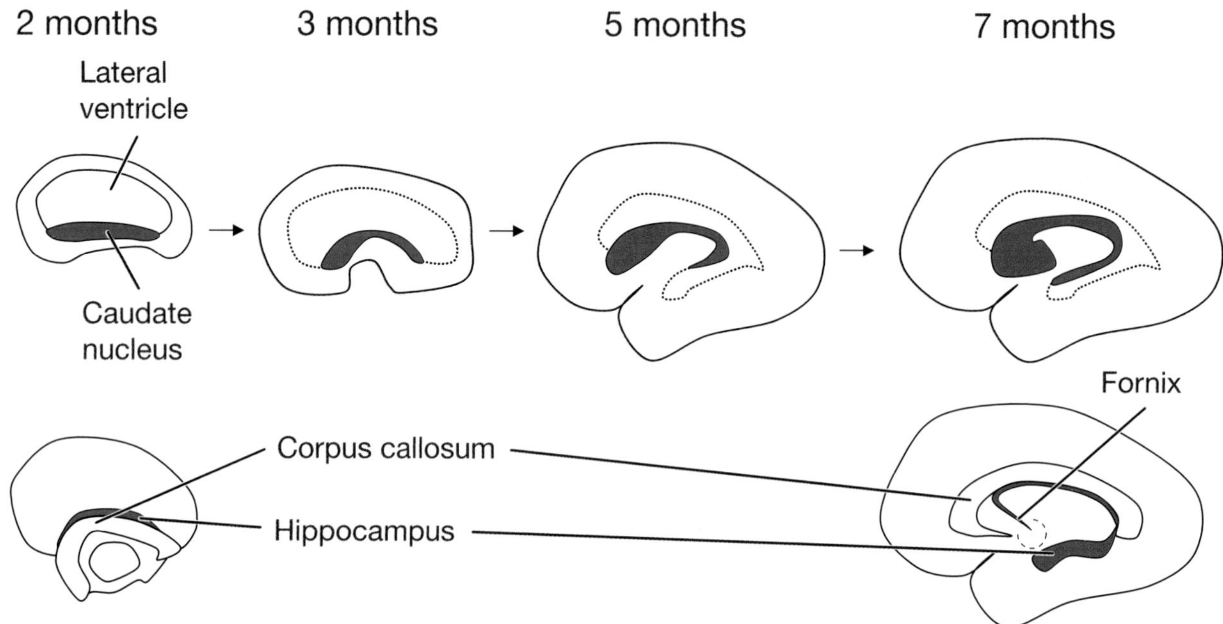

Fig. 2.23. The rapid rate of proliferation of the cells in the dorsal part of each telencephalic vesicle results in the tissue sweeping posteriorly, laterally, and ventrally. This broad sweep and cellular migration give the cerebral hemispheres and lateral ventricles a C-shaped configuration, which is obvious in several structures such as the corpus callosum, striatum, and fornix (axons from neurons in the hippocampus).

generated cells, in more superficial laminae.

- The basal ganglia (striatum and globus pallidus) are derived from the ganglionic eminence.
- The lateral ventricles form the ventricular system of the telencephalon.
- Many structures of the telencephalon, including the lateral ventricles, corpus callosum, and caudate nucleus have a C-shaped configuration that reflects the rapid expansion of the telencephalon during development.

Diencephalon

The diencephalon consists of the *thalamus* (dorsal diencephalon) and *epithalamus* (pineal gland), which are derived from the alar plate, and the *hypothalamus* and *subthalamus* (ventral diencephalon), which are from the basal plate. The neural canal in the diencephalon becomes a slitlike midline cavity, the *third ventricle*, which is in communication with the lateral ventricle of each cerebral hemisphere through the *foramen of Monro* and with the aqueduct of Sylvius in the midbrain (Fig. 2.22).

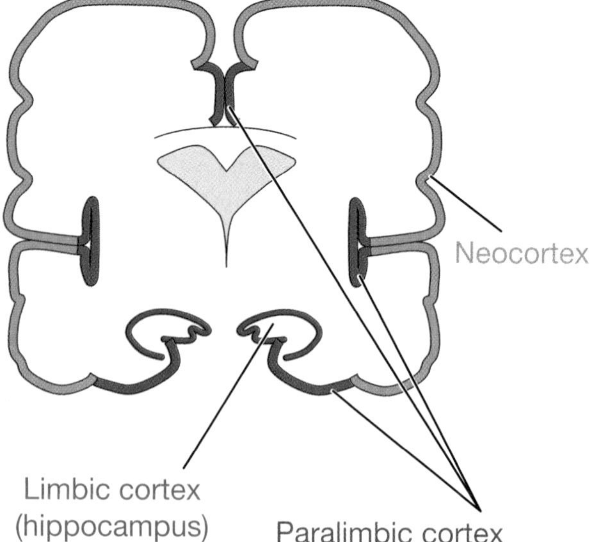

Fig. 2.24. There is a progressive differentiation of the cerebral cortex from the most primitive areas, or limbic cortex (including the hippocampus), through intermediate areas (paralimbic cortex) to the most differentiated cortex, or neocortex.

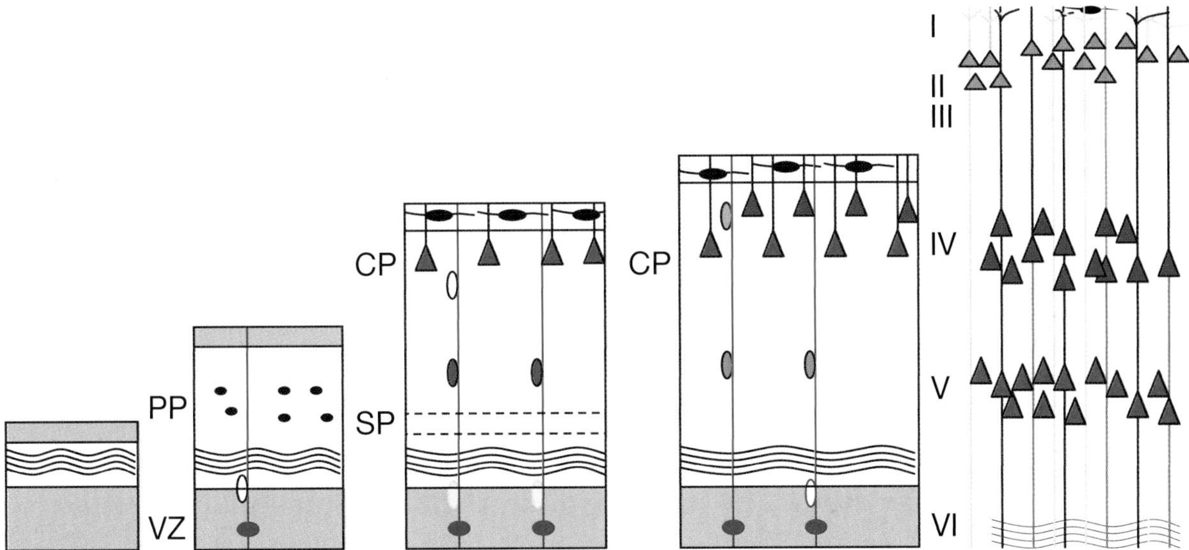

Fig. 2.25. The neocortex has a typical laminar pattern consisting of six laminae or layers. Three waves of migration occur during cortical development. Two early waves form a preplate (PP). The first migratory wave forms the most superficial layer, which contains the earliest cortical neurons. The second wave forms a transient subplate (SP). The third wave forms the cortical plate (CP), which is the precursor of all the other layers of the cortex. Within the cortical plate, the different laminae develop in a sequence such that the earlier generated cells occupy deeper laminae and later generated cells occupy more superficial laminae. This process is known as the inside-out pattern of migration. SP, subplate; VZ, ventricular zone. I-VI, cortical layers. (From Benarroch EE. Basic neurosciences with clinical applications. Philadelphia: Elsevier; 2006. Used with permission of Mayo Foundation for Medical Education and Research.)

Two specialized cranial structures are derived from the diencephalon, and each depends on the interaction of neural tissue with other tissue. The eye develops from tissue derived from paired lateral outgrowths of the diencephalon and from the overlying ectoderm in contact with these outgrowths. The diencephalon gives rise to the *retina* and optic nerves, and the ectoderm gives rise to other components of the eye. The *pituitary gland*, an endocrine gland, has a dual origin. A midline ventral outgrowth of the diencephalon, called the infundibulum, produces the neurohypophysis (posterior pituitary gland), whereas the oral ectoderm, or *Rathke pouch*, gives rise to the adenohypophysis (anterior pituitary gland).

- The diencephalon gives rise to the thalamus, hypothalamus, retina and optic nerve, neurohypophysis, and pineal gland.
- The third ventricle forms the ventricular system of the diencephalon.

Late Stages of Development of the Central Nervous System

Birth is an artificial landmark in the process of growth and development of the central nervous system. The process is a continuum that begins with the formation of the neural plate and proceeds late into the second decade, when the brain reaches its maximal weight.

Brain Growth

Cell Growth

After the second trimester, cellular proliferation contributes little to brain growth. The increase in brain weight, from about 380 g at 40 weeks of gestation to about 1,400 g at 18 years of age, is accounted for by two major factors: cell growth and myelination.

There is a progressive increase in the volume of individual cells, especially neurons. With an increase in diameter from 5 μm for a neuronal precursor to 50 μm for a mature neuron, the volume of the cell body increases as much as 1,000-fold. The overall effect of the increase in length, diameter, and complexity of cell processes on the volume of the central nervous system is enormous. A parallel process that contributes to the growth of the brain and especially to its functional maturation is the elaboration and refinement of connections between neuronal groups. Similar considerations apply to glial and other supporting cells.

Neurogenesis and Gliogenesis in the Adult Brain

Although it is traditionally accepted that the number of neurons in the adult nervous system are determined by about 36 weeks of gestation, there are two well-characterized germinal centers in the adult forebrain where neurogenesis continues throughout life: the subependymal cell layer in the most rostral part of the lateral ventricle, which gives rise to cells of the olfactory bulb, and the subgranular cell layer of the dentate gyrus of the hippocampus, which provides granule cells to the hippocampus. In the transition from birth to adulthood, there is an attenuation of glial progenitor cell proliferation and migration, and most glial cells produced in adulthood are oligodendrocytes. There is evidence for the presence of multipotential common glial progenitor cells in the white matter of the adult brains. Subcortical white matter progenitor cells produce primarily oligodendrocytes, whereas spinal cord progenitor cells produce an equal number of oligodendrocytes and astrocytes.

- The increase in brain weight from about 380 g at birth to about 1,400 g in the adult depends primarily on a progressive increase in the volume of individual cells and myelination.
- Neurogenesis may still occur in two areas of the adult brain: in the subependymal cell layer at the rostral end of the lateral ventricles and in the subgranular cell layer in the dentate gyrus of the hippocampus.

Myelination

The other important influence on both the anatomical growth and physiologic maturation of the central nervous system is the progressive myelination of the axons by the oligodendrocytes (Fig. 2.26). The formation of myelin sheaths around axons in the central nervous system begins early in the second trimester and continues into early adult life. Oligodendrocyte proliferation, maturation, and survival occur at distinct stages and are regulated by local environmental signals, including thyroid hormones.

The period of most rapid myelination occurs between the third trimester and about 2 years of age. This corresponds to the period of most rapid brain growth and most rapid physiologic maturation. The myelination of the various tracts and regions of the central nervous system follows a well-defined, orderly sequence. Myelination generally progresses from caudal to rostral, dorsal to ventral, and central to peripheral. The progression of this sequence correlates well with the progression of physiologic maturation and the development of specific functions and skills.

For example, in the corticospinal tract (the major direct projection from the cerebral cortex to the motor neurons of the spinal cord), the proximal portions of the axons begin to myelinate at about 36 weeks of gestation. However, the cerebral cortex has almost no control over motor function at birth. Myelination of the corticospinal tract progresses during the first 2 years of life, and this correlates with the progressive acquisition of motor skills, first of the upper extremities (grasping, manipulating objects) and then of the lower extremities (standing, walking, running). Myelination of the cerebral hemispheres starts in the caudal or posterior region (occipital lobe) and progresses toward the rostral or anterior region (the frontal lobe). In general, the areas of the brain involved in highly differentiated functions (association areas) are the last to myelinate.

- The formation of myelin in the central nervous system depends on oligodendrocytes.
- Myelination in the central nervous system begins early in the second trimester and peaks between the third trimester of development and about 2 years of age.
- Myelination in the central nervous system follows an orderly sequence that correlates with the development of specific functions and skills.
- In general, the areas of the brain involved in highly differentiated functions (association areas) are the last to myelinate.

Differentiation of the Peripheral Nervous System

The derivatives of the neural tube outlined above become the central nervous system contained within the bony skull and spinal column. The peripheral nervous system is largely a derivative of the neural crest, and the peripheral neuromuscular structures are from three sources: neural crest cells, somites, and axonal outgrowths of neurons in the central nervous system. All these structures outside the spinal column and skull are at the peripheral level.

Neural Crest

As the neural tube closes, cells split from the neural tube and ectoderm and form two columns of cells along the junction between the surface ectoderm and the neural tube. These cell columns form the neural crest. As the neural tube separates from the overlying ectoderm, the neural crest cells proliferate and migrate along specific pathways to their peripheral destinations. At the target sites, they differentiate into diverse groups of cells (Fig. 2.27).

The neural crest gives rise to three of the four components of the peripheral nervous system: dorsal root ganglia, autonomic ganglia, and Schwann cells. *Dorsal root ganglia* are collections of cell bodies of sensory neurons. These neurons send axons peripherally to all areas of the body to gather sensory information and centrally into the alar plate to transmit the sensory information into the central nervous system. Therefore, these neurons are the initial neurons of all somatosensory pathways.

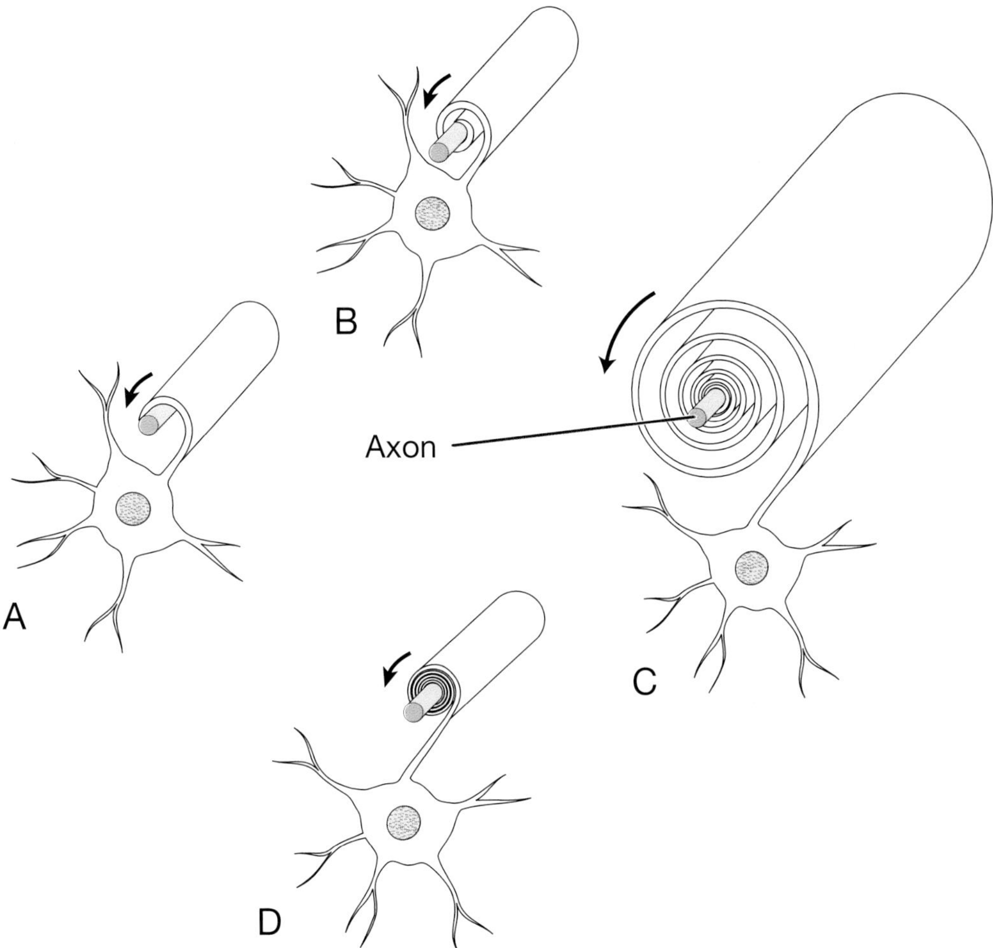

Fig. 2.26. Process of myelination of nerve fibers in the central and peripheral nervous systems. A layer of cytoplasm wraps around the axon (*A*) and then encircles it repeatedly (*B* and *C*). Condensation of layers of cytoplasm forms myelin (*D*).

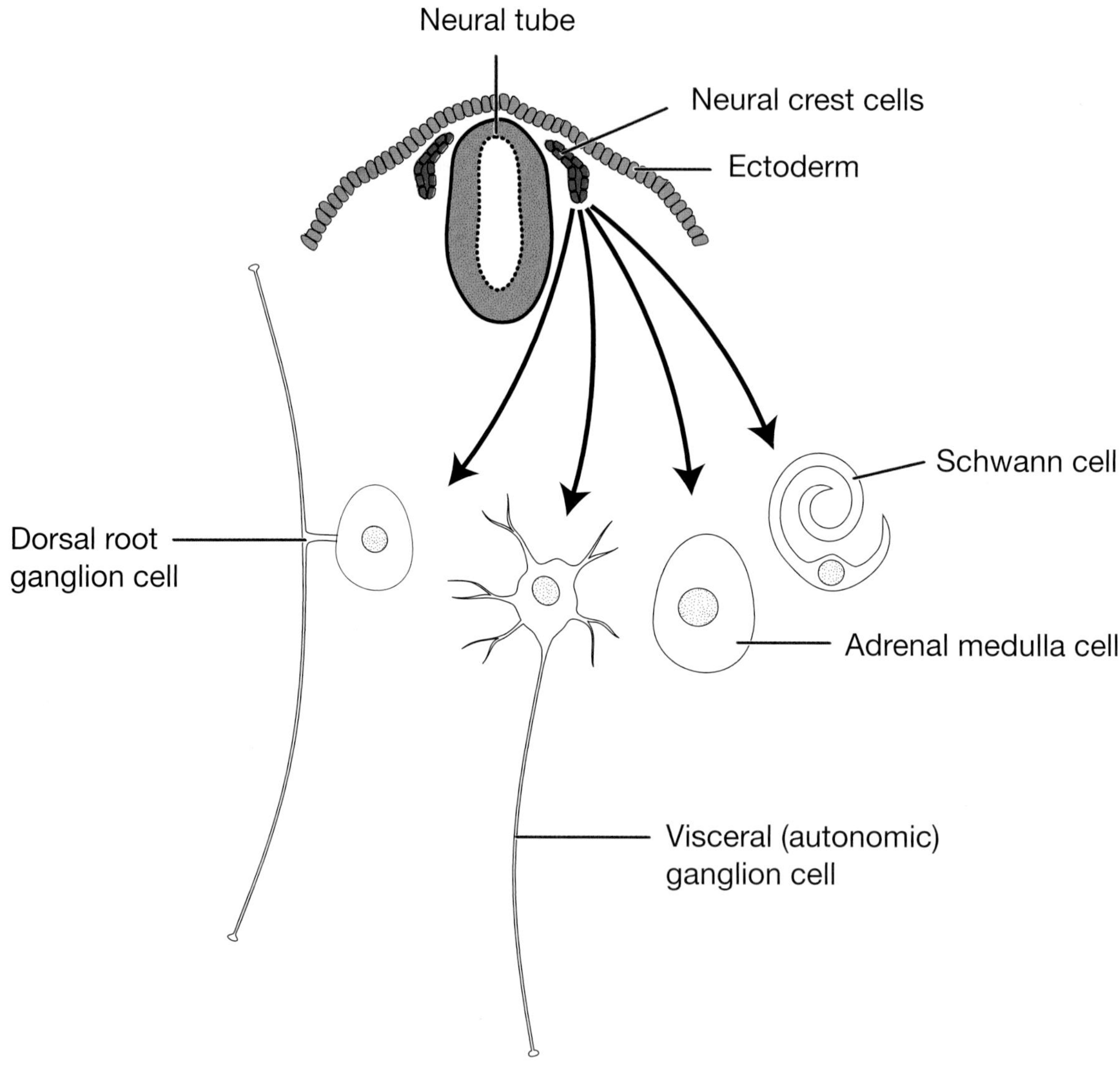

Fig. 2.27. Derivatives of neural crest cells, which are formed at the junction of the neural tube and covering ectoderm.

The *autonomic ganglia* are collections of cell bodies of neurons in the trunk and head that send out axons to innervate all the internal organs. The autonomic ganglia receive connections from preganglionic neurons derived from the basal plate of the brainstem and spinal cord.

Sympathetic ganglia are distributed on both sides and in front of the vertebral column, whereas parasympathetic ganglia are located close to the effector organ. The same precursor that gives rise to the sympathetic ganglia produces the chromaffin cells of the adrenal medulla. The neural crest also gives rise to neurons that populate the walls of the gut and form the enteric nervous system.

After the migration of neural crest cells and a series of cell divisions, a subpopulation of cells becomes *Schwann cell* progenitors and continues to proliferate and populate peripheral nerves.

The survival of Schwann cell precursors depends on signals from the axon. Later during development, immature Schwann cells diverge into two types: myelinating Schwann cells that wrap large-diameter axons and nonmyelinating Schwann cells that ensheathe and accommodate many small-diameter axons. This process of phenotypic differentiation is determined by the axon.

The neural crest also gives rise to the *melanocytes* of the skin and to cells that form the connective tissue of the face and neck.

Somites

As the neural tube closes, the embryonic mesoderm lateral to the tube becomes segmented into cell masses known as *somites* (Fig. 2.28). The somites differentiate into three components. The ventromedial portion of the somite forms the *sclerotome*. Sclerotomes differentiate into the cartilage and bone that form the vertebrae of the vertebral column and base of the skull surrounding the central nervous system. The notochord becomes incorporated into the ventromedial extensions of the sclerotomes and thus remains ventral to the neural tube. The notochordal remnant within the vertebral column is the *nucleus pulposus* of the intervertebral disk. The dorsomedial portion of the somite forms the *myotome*. Myotomes form the striated skeletal muscle of the body, except for the striated muscle that comes from the branchial arches in the head and neck. The primordial muscle cells of the myotomes migrate peripherally to form the muscles of the trunk and limbs. The lateral portion of the somite forms the *dermatome*. Cells from each dermatome migrate peripherally to form the dermis, the connective tissue layer of the skin.

Components of the Peripheral Nerves

The peripheral nerves consist of axons that connect the central nervous system with the peripheral structures. The nerves that form at the spinal level and innervate the trunk and limbs are called *spinal nerves* and those that form at the posterior fossa level and innervate cranial and facial structures are called *cranial nerves*. Both types are composed of mixtures of sensory and motor axons.

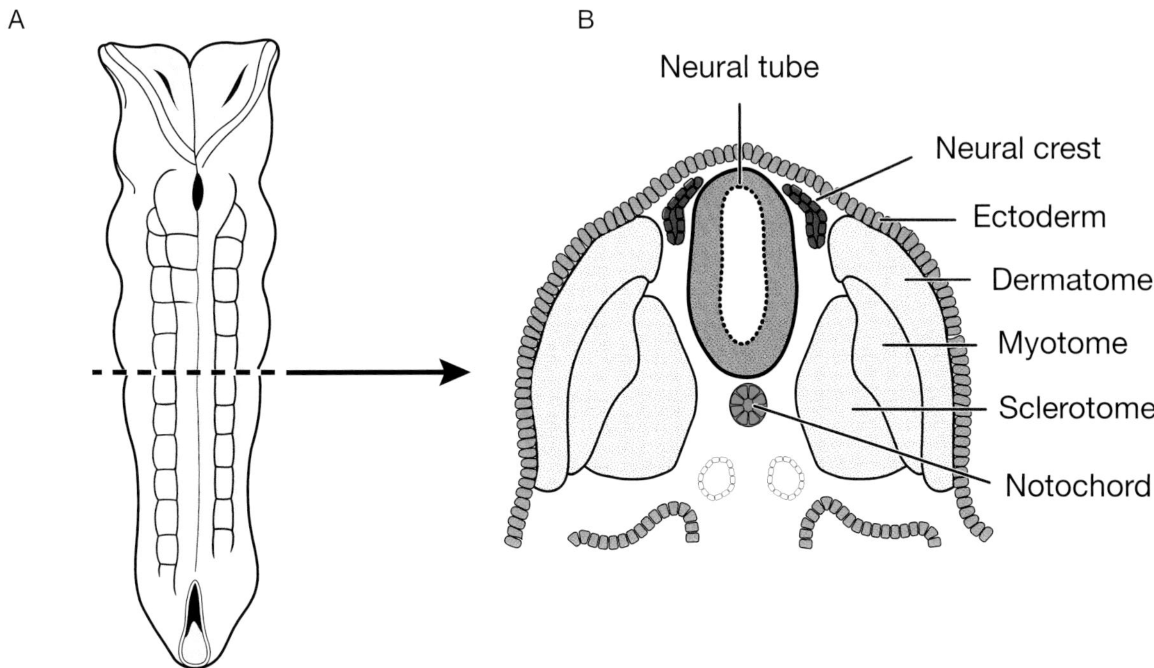

Fig. 2.28. Formation of myotomes, sclerotomes, and dermatomes from somites in a 4-week embryo. *A*, Whole embryo. *B*, Transverse section (level indicated by horizontal line in *A*).

Connections between the peripheral structures and the central nervous system generally are established by the growth of axons from sensory neurons derived from the neural crest into the alar plate of the neural tube and by the outgrowth of axons from motor neurons derived from the basal plate to peripheral effector structures.

The alar plate and basal plate neurons are arranged in functionally distinct afferent and efferent columns that extend longitudinally through the spinal cord and brainstem. The peripheral sensory input from structures derived from the somites terminate in the *general somatic afferent* column. Afferents from visceral structures (derived from the mesoderm or endoderm) terminate in the *general visceral afferent* column. The motor axons that innervate muscles derived from somites are somatic efferents that arise from basal plate neurons, which form the *general somatic efferent* column. The output to the autonomic ganglia controlling the visceral organs arises from the *general visceral efferent* column. Thus, a typical spinal nerve consists of four types of axons (Fig. 2.29). Sensory axons from dorsal root ganglion neurons (neural crest) that innervate the somites (somatic afferents) or visceral organs (general visceral afferents) terminate in the dorsal horn of the spinal cord (alar plate). Axons from motor neurons of the ventral horn (basal plate) join the peripheral nerve to innervate the skeletal muscles of the limbs and trunk (somatic efferents). Axons from preganglionic neurons innervate the sympathetic ganglia (neural crest), which send axons to the blood vessels and visceral organs (general visceral efferents).

The same general principle applies to cranial nerves. However, unlike spinal nerves, the composition of each cranial nerve varies according to its function. Some cranial nerves contain only general somatic efferents that arise from the general somatic efferent column of the brainstem and innervate extraocular or tongue muscles. However, many cranial nerves have multiple functional components. For example, some cranial nerves contain general somatic afferent axons from somites of the face, general visceral afferent axons from visceral organs, special visceral afferent axons that convey input from taste buds derived from placodes, branchiomotor (*special visceral efferent*) axons that innervate facial muscles arising from the branchial

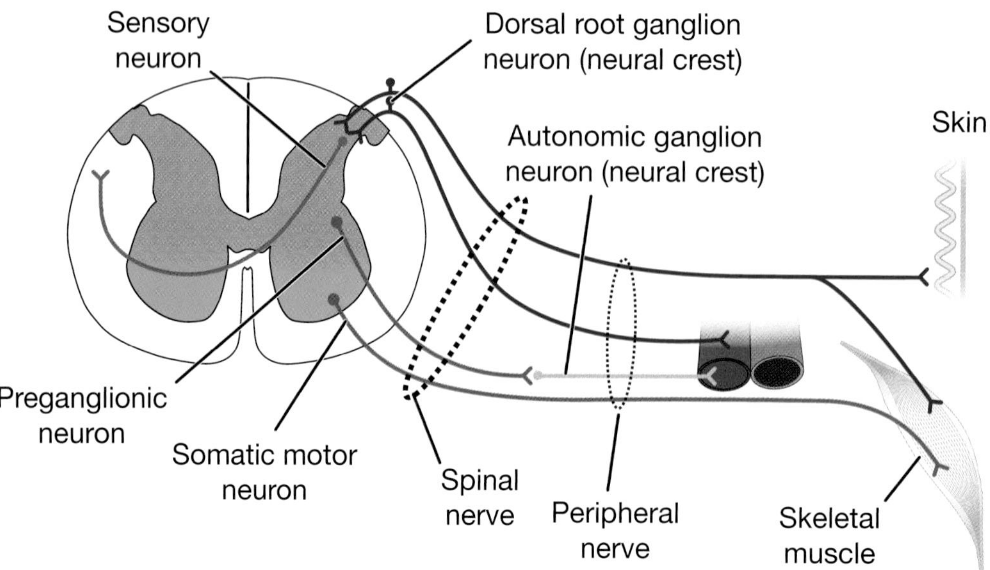

Fig. 2.29. Formation of spinal nerves by the combination of axons derived from basal plate neurons and axons from dorsal root ganglia derived from the neural crest.

arches, and general visceral efferent axons that innervate the exocrine glands or other visceral effectors. One cranial nerve contains special afferents arising from the inner ear (a derivative of the otic placode) that terminate in a separate column of cells derived from the alar plate in the lower pons and medulla. The arrangement of the different functional columns in the spinal cord and brainstem is shown in Figures 2.17–2.20. Table 2.2 summarizes the classification of the functional components of nerves on the basis of embryologic origin and destination.

- The neural crest gives rise to the dorsal root ganglia, autonomic ganglia, enteric nervous system, adrenal chromaffin cells, Schwann cells, melanocytes, and cells that form the connective tissue of the face and neck.
- The somites give rise to cartilage and bone of the vertebral column and base of the skull (sclerotome); the muscles of the tongue, trunk, and limbs (myotome); and the dermis of the skin (dermatome).
- Connections between the periphery and the central nervous system are established by neurons derived from the neural crest whose axons extend into the alar plate and by neurons derived from the basal plate whose axons innervate muscles (derived from the mesoderm) or autonomic ganglia (derived from the neural crest).
- The alar plate and basal plate neurons are arranged into afferent and efferent cell columns that extend longitudinally through the brainstem and spinal cord.
- The peripheral nerves consist of somatic afferents, visceral afferents, somatic efferents, and visceral efferents.
- Essentially all components of a peripheral nerve, including the Schwann cells, are derived from the neural crest.
- The motor axons that innervate the skeletal muscles are derived from the basal plate.

Clinical Correlations

Although some developmental processes occur more or less simultaneously, they can be subdivided into six stages, according to the dominant process at that stage (Table 2.3). Many genetic factors, such as chromosomal abnormalities or defects in DNA replication or transcription,

Table 2.2. Classification of the Functional Components of Spinal and Cranial Nerves on the Basis of Embryologic Origin and Destination

Type	Subtype	Tissue innervated	Tissue origin
Afferent (sensory)	Somatic	Skin, muscle, bone, joints	Somites
	Visceral	Visceral organs	Endoderm
		Taste receptors	Placode
	Special	Olfactory epithelium	Placode
		Hair cells	Placode
Efferent (motor)	Somatic	Striated muscle of limbs, trunk, tongue, and eyes	Somites
	Visceral	Smooth muscle	Nonsomite mesoderm and endoderm
		Heart	
		Exocrine glands	
	Branchiomotor	Striated muscle of mandible, face, pharynx, and larynx	Branchial arches

Table 2.3. Major Stages of Development and the Corresponding Developmental Disorders

Stage	Weeks of gestation	Major morphologic events	Examples of disorders
Dorsal induction (primary neurulation)	3-4	Neural tube closure Neural crest formation	Anencephaly Encephalocele Craniorachischisis Meningocele Spina bifida
Ventral induction	5-6	Cranial neural crest formation Forebrain and face formation Optic placodes, olfactory placodes Diencephalon formation	Holoprosencephaly Craniofascial anomalies
Neuronal and glial proliferation and early differentiation	8-16	Cellular proliferation in ventricular and subventricular zones Early differentiation of neuroblasts and glial cell precursors	Microcephaly
Migration	12-20	Radial migration	Heterotopia Lissencephaly Pachygyria Microgyria Schizencephaly Agenesis of corpus callosum
Differentiation	24 to birth	Alignment and orientation of cortical neurons Axonal growth Synaptogenesis Glial differentiation	Cortical dysplasia Dendritic hypoplasia Down syndrome Rett syndrome
Myelination	24 to 2 years postnatal	Oligodendrocyte membrane synthesis	Dysmyelination (leukodystrophy)

or environmental factors, such as maternal infections (including those due to human immunodeficiency virus 1 or rubella), medications (e.g., many antiepileptic drugs), toxins (e.g., alcohol or cocaine), cigarette smoking, and diabetes mellitus, may affect each step of development of the nervous system. The clinical manifestations reflect the stage of development that is affected.

Disorders of Closure of the Neural Tube

The first stage of development is the formation of the neural tube (also called dorsal induction). This occurs during the third and fourth weeks of embryogenesis. Genetic or acquired injury of the embryo during this period results in failure of closure of the neural tube, referred to as *neural tube defects*. They are manifested by defects in the dorsal midline, often obvious on the surface, and may occur at all levels of the neuraxis with several degrees of severity (Fig. 2.30). At the lumbosacral level, the mildest form is *spina bifida occulta*, a defect that affects only the vertebral arch and occurs

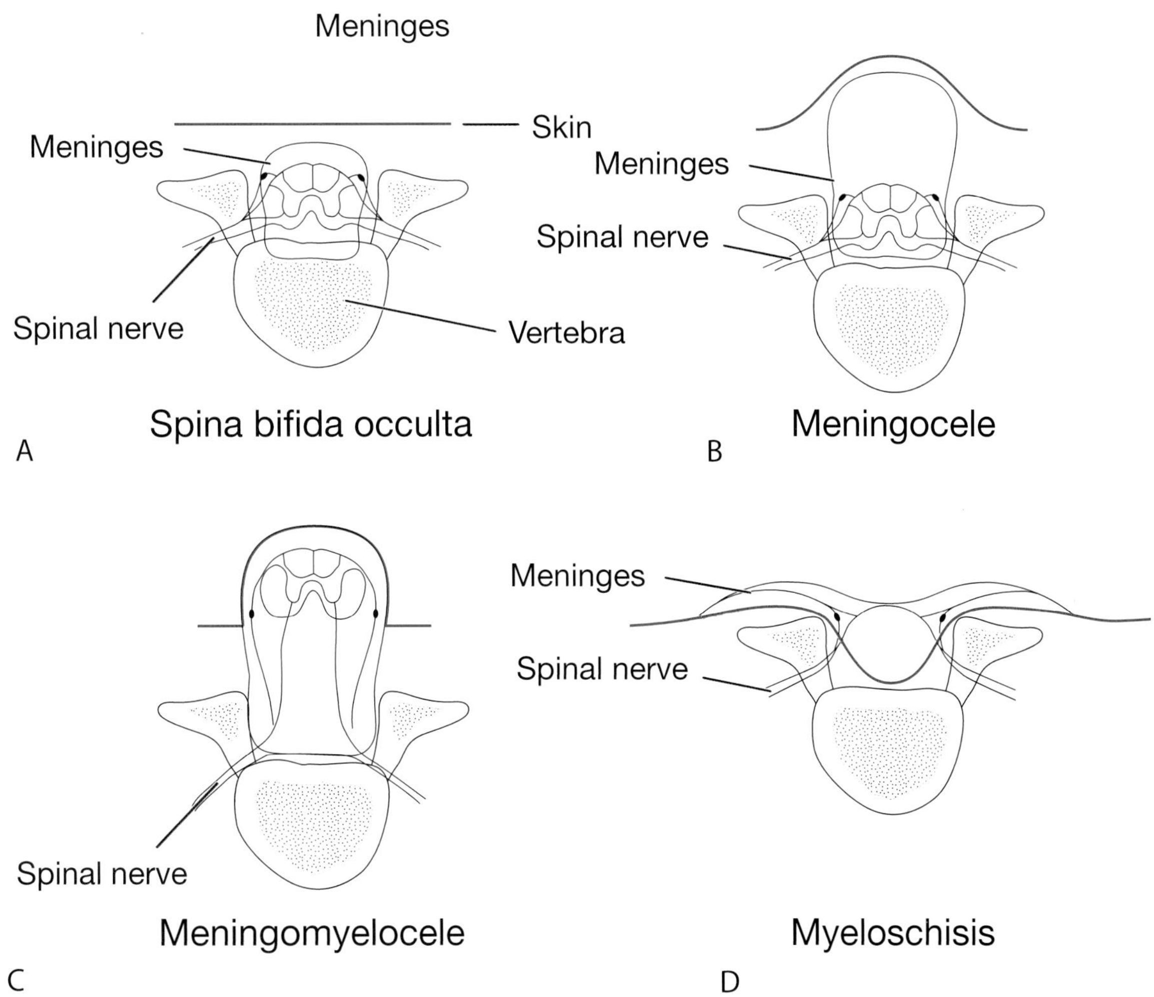

Fig. 2.30. Examples of failure of fusion at the spinal level. *A*, Spina bifida occulta with incomplete vertebral arch. *B*, Meningocele with outpouching of a fluid-filled sac of meninges and skin. *C*, Meningomyelocele with sac containing abnormal neural tissue. *D*, Myeloschisis with no closure and a deformed neural plate open to the surface.

in up to 10% of otherwise normal subjects. Progressively more severe disorders are *meningocele* (protrusion of a meningeal sac through the bone defect), *meningomyelocele* (protrusion of a meningeal or skin-covered spinal cord), and *myeloschisis* (the spinal cord is completely exposed because of a defect of the overlying skin and bone). Similar disorders occur at the rostral end of the neural tube and cause *cranium bifidum*, *cranial meningocele*, *meningoencephalocele*, and *anencephaly* (exposed or absent brain). The most severe defect is a completely open neural tube and dorsal midline, termed craniorachischisis.

Neural tube defects are multifactorial disorders that may be due to genetic or environmental factors or some combination of both. There is risk for recurrence within families. Environmental influences include maternal obesity, diabetes mellitus, and use of anticonvulsant drugs. Deficiency of folic acid may be important in the pathogenesis of these disorders. These disorders can be diagnosed early during pregnancy with ultrasonography and measurement of the level of alpha-fetoprotein in maternal serum. Folic acid supplementation is now recommended for all pregnant women.

Clinical Problem 2.1.

A newborn girl has a large bulging mass over the lower portion of the spinal column. No skin covers this mass, and ill-defined neural structures can be seen through the glistening membranes of the fluid-filled mass. The infant does not move her legs.

a. What stage of the embryologic process was not completed in this child?
b. What embryonic structures are involved and at what stage in development?
c. Which types of functions are probably absent in this child?
d. What is the name of this child's disorder?
e. Name four examples of failure of fusion at the spinal level. How do they differ?
f. What is prescribed to pregnant women to prevent this condition?

Disorders of Ventral Induction

The second stage of central nervous system development occurs during the fifth and sixth weeks. This stage, sometimes called *ventral induction*, is characterized by the formation of the telencephalon in conjunction with cranial, facial, and neck structures derived from the branchial arches. Defects that occur during this stage can cause severe abnormalities in the formation of the telencephalon and craniofacial structures. *Holoprosencephaly* is a developmental disorder characterized by failure of the normal midline separation of the two hemispheres, resulting in a single forebrain with a single ventricle and continuity of the gray matter across the midline. The cerebral hemispheres and basal ganglia are incompletely separated to varying degrees. There is also loss of midline structures of the head and face, ranging in severity from a single central incisor or nostril, to midfusion of the lateral ventricles, to complete *cyclopia*.

Holoprosencephaly has been associated with several factors, including poorly controlled maternal diabetes mellitus, toxins such as retinoic acid and ethanol, chromosomal abnormalities, and genetic disorders involving the Sonic hedgehog signaling pathway or the formation of the dorsal roof plate.

Clinical Problem 2.2.

A baby is born with a single midline eye and dies a few days after birth. Examination of the brain showed that the two cerebral hemispheres failed to separate.

a. What is the name of this disorder?
b. Impairment of what developmental process may produce this condition?
c. What signal is critical for ventral induction of the neural tube?

Disorders of Proliferation

The third stage of development is dominated by proliferative activity of the ventricular and subventricular zones and reaches a peak during the 8th to 16th week of gestation. Genetic or acquired disorders that decrease the proliferation of neurons and glia or increase apoptosis (or both) manifest with *microcephaly* (small head).

Clinical Problem 2.3.

A child is born with an unusually small head and low-set ears but normally developed facies. At the end of 1 year, the child's head has grown but is still well below normal. Also, the child has failed to acquire the usual motor and social milestones for age.

a. What is this child's condition called?
b. What stage of development was probably affected in this child?
c. What are the proliferative zones of the neural tube?

In less severe cases, genetic or environmental causes may lead to failure to elaborate the proper number and types of synapses, which may account for some cases of mental retardation in persons with grossly normal brains.

In contrast, disorders of excessive proliferation or decreased apoptosis (or both) are manifested by *megalencephaly* (large brain) or with abnormal proliferation of abnormal cell types. This proliferation may be non-neoplastic, giving rise to *hamartomas*, or neoplastic, giving rise to tumors.

Cell proliferation is regulated by the balance between proliferative signals that facilitate the cell cycle and signals that either prevent the cells from entering the cell cycle or facilitate apoptosis. Genes encoding for these proliferative signals, including growth factors, their receptors, and transduction molecules, are referred to as oncogenes. In contrast, genes that encode for antiproliferative signals are referred to as tumor suppressor genes. One important example is neurofibromin 1, which is mutated in patients with neurofibromatosis type 1.

Because the skin, nervous system, and retina are derived from the ectoderm, it is not unexpected that genetically determined disorders may affect them together. At least some of these disorders, known as *neurocutaneous disorders*, are due to mutation of tumor suppressor genes (Table 2.4). Many of these disorders are inherited in an autosomal dominant fashion and produce, in addition to hamartomas or neoplasms in the nervous system, similar lesions in other organs, including the liver, kidney, and heart.

Clinical Problem 2.4.

A 4-year-old boy is evaluated for seizures and mild mental retardation. He has red lesions on his face and white spots (phakomas) in the retina, as seen with an ophthalmoscope. Magnetic resonance imaging of the head shows an area of abnormal thickening of the cerebral cortex and multiple nodular regions in the area adjacent to the ependyma of the lateral ventricles.

a. What is the name of this disorder?
b. What is the basis for involvement of the skin, eyes, and brain in this and related disorders?
c. What is the basis for susceptibility to brain neoplasms in this and similar disorders?

Table 2.4. Examples of Neuroectodermal Dysplasias Associated With Mutations of Tumor Suppressor Genes

Disease	Nervous system tumors	Skin manifestations	Eye manifestations
Neurofibromatosis type 1	Cutaneous neurofibromas Optic glioma Meningiomas Schwannoma Ependymoma	Café au lait spots	Pigmented hamartomas in the iris (Lisch nodules)
Tuberous sclerosis	Cortical hamartomas Subependymal giant cell astrocytoma	Adendoma sebaceum Depigmented patches Subungual fibromas	Retinal nodular hamartomas (phakomas)
von Hippel-Lindau disease	Hemangioblastoma of the cerebellum or spinal cord (or both)		Retinal hemangioblastoma

Disorders of Neuronal Migration

The fourth stage of central nervous system development is the radial migration of neurons, which is most active from the 12th to 20th week of gestation. Pathologic processes affecting the fetus during this period of development may cause malformations attributable to disorders of arrested migration. The disorders of radial migration that affect the development of the cerebral cortex can be classified according to the stage of development when they occur.

Heterotopia consists of agglomerates of morphologically normal neurons in an abnormal site and constitute the most common neuronal migration disorder in humans. Most patients come to medical attention because of seizures. *Lissencephaly* (smooth brain) comprises a heterogeneous group of conditions that is manifested pathologically and radiographically as a simplification or complete loss of gyri and sulci.

Heterotopia can be readily diagnosed with magnetic resonance imaging. For example, periventricular (or subependymal) heterotopia reflects complete failure of migration and results in persistent accumulation of nodules of mature-appearing neurons in the periventricular region in the adult brain. Double cortex, or subcortical band heterotopia, results from the accumulation of mature-appearing neurons in the subcortical white matter. Many of these disorders are due to mutations of genes that encode proteins that interact with the neuronal cytoskeleton and are critical for radial migration, including filamin 1, doublecortin, and LIS-1.

Clinical Problem 2.5.

A 10-year-old boy presents with a history of seizures and moderate mental retardation. Magnetic resonance imaging suggests that there is an abnormal pattern of gray matter around the ventricles of the brain.

a. What is the name of this disorder?
b. What stage of development is likely affected in this child?
c. At what time of gestational development did this likely occur?
d. What is lissencephaly?

Clinical Problem 2.6.

A 2-year-old girl is brought to the physician because of delayed development. Examination showed persistent median epicanthic folds and spots in the iris, short extremities with incurved fifth digits of the hand, and hypoplastic middle phalanges. There is evidnece of delayed neurologic milestones. Magnetic resonance imaging of the brain shows a small brain for age, but no other abnormalities.

a. What is this syndrome called?
b. What late neurologic stage of development might be affected?
c. What are other examples of this group of disorders?

Related to the disorders of migration are the disorders of cortical organization. *Polymicrogyria* refers to cerebral cortex that contains multiple small gyri. *Schizencephaly* refers to the presence of a unilateral or bilateral cleft that extends from the pial surface of the cortex to the ventricular surface. Polymicrogyria and schizencephaly can be caused by acquired disorders, such as prenatal viral infection or vascular insufficiency in utero, and genetic disorders.

Disorders of Dendritic Growth and Synaptogenesis

The fifth stage of development of the nervous system is dominated by the differentiation of neurons and glia. This process includes physical growth, elaboration of dendrites and dendritic spines, and development of synapses and extends from the sixth gestational month to maturity. Synaptic remodeling persists throughout life. Widespread disturbances of these processes during development do not usually lead to obvious gross malformations but rather to functional disturbances that range from learning disabilities to mental retardation.

Clinical Problem 2.7.

A 3-year-old boy is evaluated for progressive impairment of his gait and speech and loss of intellectual milestones over the past year. Magnetic resonance imaging of the head suggests a lack of myelin formation in the parieto-occipital regions of the cerebral hemispheres.

a. What major stage of brain development was likely affected to produce this disorder?
b. What is the name given to this group of disorders?
c. What is the source of myelin in the central nervous system and in the peripheral nervous system?

Mental retardation is highly heterogeneous both in its severity and etiology, which includes both genetic and environmental factors. Genetic causes range from chromosomal abnormalities to single-gene mutations. Genetic and environmental conditions associated with mental retardation commonly produce abnormalities in the dendrites of cortical neurons. A frequent finding in patients with mental retardation is a decrease in the number and length of dendritic branches and aberrant morphology of the dendritic spines. Important examples are Down syndrome, Rett syndrome, fragile X syndrome, and other X-linked forms of mental retardation. Several progressive metabolic disorders that affect primarily the cerebral cortex produce abnormalities of the dendrites. For example, phenylketonuria is associated with a decrease in dendritic arborizations and abnormal spine morphology.

Disorders of Myelination

The sixth stage of development is associated with myelination of the central nervous system. This process extends from the last half of gestation up to age 18 years and is most evident from birth to age 2 years. Genetic or acquired diseases that affect this process result in myelin either not forming or, once formed, degenerating because of faulty structure. Genetic disorders in this category are called *leukodystrophies*. Although they usually occur in the first 2 years of life, they may also be manifested later, even in early adulthood.

Disorders Affecting the Neural Crest

Disorders that affect the development of neural crest derivatives, including dorsal root ganglia, autonomic ganglia, and Schwann cells, may produce several forms of *hereditary peripheral neuropathies*.

Impairment of Schwann cell differentiation leads to demyelinating hereditary sensory and motor neuropathies. Impairment of development of dorsal root ganglion and sympathetic ganglion cells may lead to hereditary sensory and autonomic neuropathies. This can be manifested by congenital insensitivity to pain and inability to sweat (anhidrosis).

Clinical Problem 2.8.

A 4-year-old boy is evaluated because he has sustained injuries in his feet without being aware of them. He cannot exercise in a hot environment because he is unable to sweat. Examination shows a lack of sensation in the lower limbs and dry skin.

a. What neurons are likely affected in this child?
b. What is their origin?
c. What are other derivatives of this embryonic structure?

- Impairment of dorsal induction during the first 4 weeks of development produces neural tube defects, such as myelomeningocele.
- Impaired development of the prosencephalon and cranial structures produces holoprosencephaly.
- Impaired proliferation of neuronal and glial precursors during development produces microcephaly.

- Mutations in genes encoding for tumor suppressor genes may result in exaggerated proliferation of neurons and glia, resulting in hamartomas or neoplasms.
- In many of these disorders, brain abnormalities are associated with abnormalities of the eyes and skin.
- Disorders of radial migration result in heterotopy and lissencephaly.
- Disorders affecting dendritic development or synaptogenesis produce mental retardation.
- Disorders of myelination produce leukodystrophies.
- Disorders affecting development of Schwann cells produce hereditary demyelinating sensory and motor neuropathies.
- Disorders affecting development of the dorsal root ganglia and autonomic ganglia produce hereditary sensory and autonomic neuropathies.

Additional Reading

Barkovich AJ, Kuzniecky RI, Jackson GD, Guerrini R, Dobyns WB. Classification system for malformations of cortical development: update 2001. Neurology. 2001;57:2168-78.

Brody BA, Kinney HC, Kloman AS, Gilles FH. Sequence of central nervous system myelination in human infancy. I: an autopsy study of myelination. J Neuropathol Exp Neurol. 1987;46:283-301.

Gleeson JG, Walsh CA. Neuronal migration disorders: from genetic diseases to developmental mechanisms. Trends Neurosci. 2000;23:352-9.

Jessell TM, Sanes JR. Development: the decade of the developing brain. Curr Opin Neurobiol. 2000;10:599-611.

Rubenstein JL, Anderson S, Shi L, Miyashita-Lin E, Bulfone A, Hevner R. Genetic control of cortical regionalization and connectivity. Cereb Cortex. 1999;9:524-32.

Shatz CJ. The developing brain. Sci Am. 1992;267:60-7.

Chapter 3

Diagnosis of Neurologic Disorders: Anatomical Localization

Objectives

1. Know the types and functions of the cells of the nervous system and be familiar with the terms nuclei, ganglia, fasciculus, and tract.
2. Define the boundaries of the major anatomical levels (supratentorial, posterior fossa, spinal, and peripheral), and identify the major anatomical structures contained in each level.
3. Given a cross-section specimen, identify the approximate area of the neuraxis to which the specimen belongs (i.e., cerebral hemisphere, midbrain, pons, medulla, cerebellum, or spinal cord [cervical, thoracic, lumbar, or sacral]).
4. Given a clinical problem, answer the following two questions:
   a. The signs and symptoms contained in the protocol are most likely the manifestation of disease at which of the following levels of the nervous system?
      - Supratentorial level
      - Posterior fossa level
      - Spinal level
      - Peripheral level
      - More than one level
   b. Within the level you have selected, the responsible lesion is most likely
      - Focal, on the right side of the nervous system
      - Focal, on the left side of the nervous system
      - Focal, but involving the midline and contiguous structures on both sides of the nervous system
      - Nonfocal and diffusely located

Introduction

The diagnosis of neurologic disorders is a skill that requires the application of basic scientific information to a clinical problem. As knowledge about the nervous system increases, more complicated neurologic problems can be solved in more sophisticated ways; however, the basic approach to the solution of all neurologic problems remains unchanged. In arriving at a solution, three questions must be answered: 1) Is there a lesion involving the nervous system? 2) Where is the lesion located? 3) What is the histopathologic nature of the lesion?

Answering the first question is the most difficult because it requires familiarity not only with clinical neurology but also with other disciplines of medicine. In time, as the manifestations of neurologic disorders become better known, the neurologic origin of certain symptoms will be identified with increasing confidence.

To answer the question "Where is the location of the lesion that has caused the signs and symptoms?" requires an understanding of the organization of the nervous system and an ability to relate the patient's description and the physician's observations of dysfunction to a particular area or areas in the nervous system.

In addition to localizing a lesion in an area in the nervous system, the physician must determine the nature of the lesion. An infarction (stroke), tumor, or abscess may lead to similar signs and symptoms. The manner in which these symptoms evolve, that is, the temporal profile, provides the clues to distinguish these disorders and to predict the histopathologic changes responsible for the observed abnormality.

A physician highly skilled in neurologic-anatomical diagnosis is capable of localizing a lesion in the nervous system to within millimeters of its actual site. Although this type of skill is laudable, it is often more than is required of even the practicing neurologist. For proper patient management in most clinical situations, it is sufficient to decide whether the responsible lesion is producing dysfunction in one or more longitudinal systems, to relate the abnormalities to one (or more) of several gross anatomical levels, and to determine whether the presumed lesion is on the right side, on the left side, or in the midline or is diffuse and involves homologous areas bilaterally. Neurologic disorders may affect one or more of the following systems: cerebrospinal fluid system, sensory system, motor system, internal regulation system, consciousness system, and vascular system. Neurologic disorders occur at one or more of the following levels: supratentorial, posterior fossa, spinal, and peripheral.

Familiarity with these major systems and levels will aid in the diagnosis of neurologic disorders. Each system and level are discussed in further detail in subsequent chapters; this chapter discusses the anatomy of the levels.

- When solving clinical problems, first ask yourself, is it neurologic?
- Second, where does it localize to?
    - Anatomical level (supratentorial, posterior fossa, spinal, peripheral)
    - Focal or diffuse
    - Left, right, or midline
- Third, what type of pathology?
    - Onset (acute, subacute, chronic)
    - Course (improving, static, progressive)
    - What system(s) is involved (cerebrospinal fluid, sensory, motor, internal regulation, consciousness, vascular)

Overview

Neurons and Glial Cells

Neurons are the fundamental cells of the nervous system. They function to receive and transmit information to parts of the nervous system. They are specialized in function. Some neurons transmit sensory information from the periphery to the central nervous system and are designated *afferent* neurons. Other neurons innervate skeletal muscle, organs, smooth muscle, or glands and are designated *efferent* neurons. An actual nerve is a bundle of neuronal axons and may contain both afferent and efferent fibers. The cranial nerves and spinal nerves are examples.

Glial cells are supporting cells of the nervous system. *Astrocytes* function to repair the central nervous system. *Microglia* also serve a role in response to disease. *Oligodendroglia* in the central nervous system and *Schwann cells* in the peripheral nervous system function to myelinate axons. Myelin allows increased speeds of conduction.

The Human Nervous System

The *central nervous system* refers to the brain and spinal cord. The *peripheral nervous system* consists of the cranial nerves and spinal nerves once they have exited the skull and vertebral column, respectively.

Protective Coverings of the Central Nervous System

The major structures of the central nervous system, the brain and spinal cord, are surrounded by three fibrous connective tissue linings called *meninges* and are encased in a protective bony skeleton. The brain, consisting of derivatives of the primitive telencephalon, diencephalon, mesencephalon, metencephalon, and myelencephalon, is enclosed in the skull, and the spinal cord is situated in the spinal column (Fig. 3.1). Cranial and peripheral nerves must pass through these surrounding investments to reach more peripheral structures.

The major anatomical levels discussed below are defined by the meninges and bony structures to which they are related. The divisions between the anatomical levels used in this book are not exact, and there is some divergence from strict anatomical definitions given in other textbooks. However, as defined, the levels have boundaries that are clinically useful in understanding neurologic disorders.

The floor of the human skull is divided into three distinct compartments (fossae) on each side: anterior,

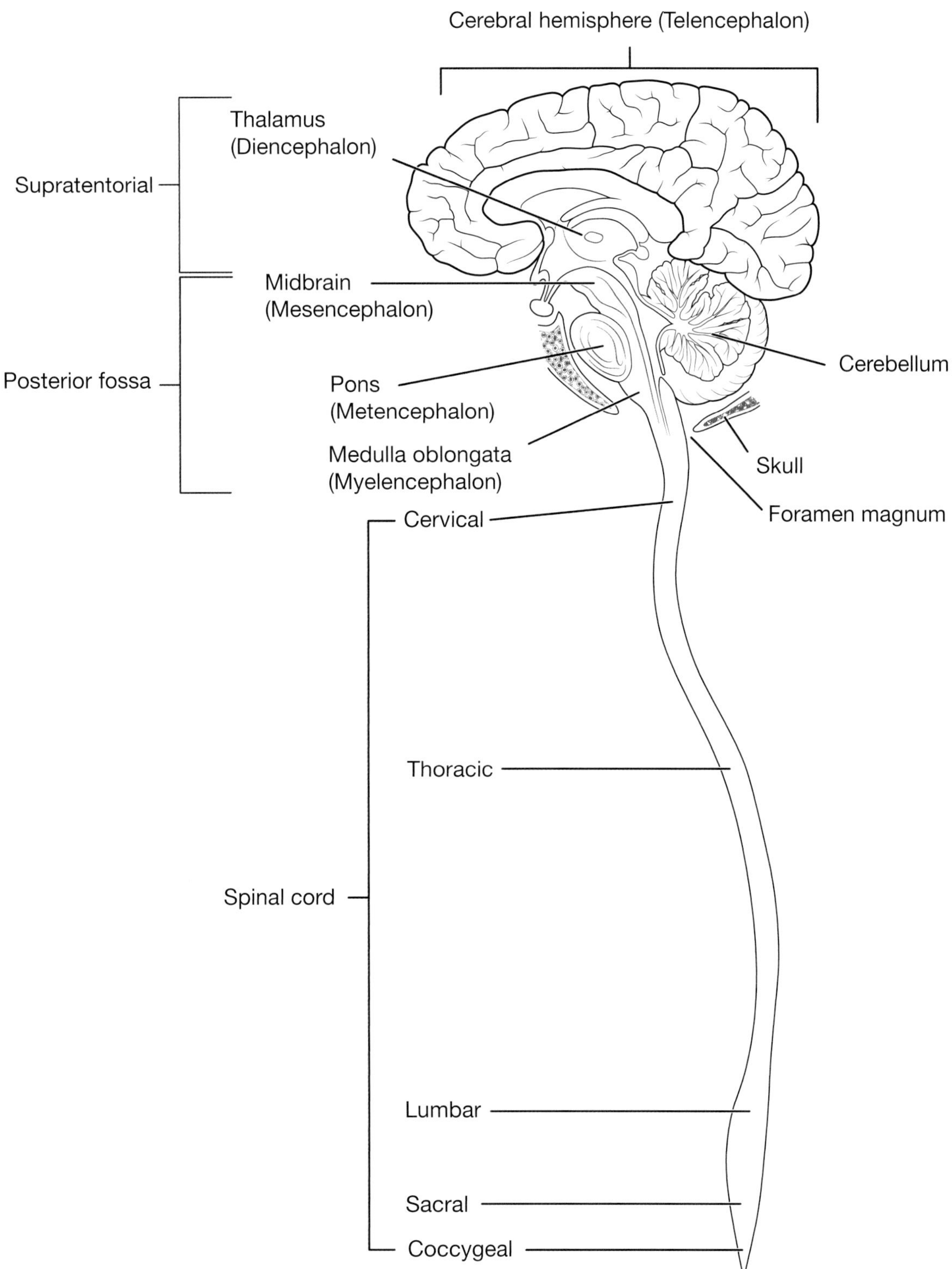

Fig. 3.1. Medial view of the brain and spinal cord illustrating the major levels: supratentorial, posterior fossa (with brainstem and cerebellum), and spinal level. The peripheral level is not shown.

middle, and posterior (Fig. 3.2). A rigid membrane, the tentorium cerebelli, separates the anterior and middle fossae from the posterior fossa (Fig. 3.3). The tentorium lies in a nearly horizontal plane and is attached laterally to the petrous ridges and posteriorly to the occipital bone. The portion of the nervous system located above the tentorium cerebelli constitutes the supratentorial level. The portion of the nervous system below the tentorium cerebelli is infratentorial and designated as the posterior fossa.

Supratentorial Level

Structures within the skull above the tentorium cerebelli can be designated as supratentorial. The major anatomical structures of this level are derivatives of the telencephalon and diencephalon and consist primarily of the cerebral hemispheres, basal ganglia, thalamus, hypothalamus, and cranial nerves I (olfactory) and II (optic).

Posterior Fossa Level

Structures located within the skull below the tentorium cerebelli but above the *foramen magnum* (the opening of the skull to the spinal canal) constitute the posterior fossa level. These structures, the midbrain, pons, medulla, and cerebellum, are derivatives of the mesencephalon, metencephalon, and myelencephalon. Cranial nerves III through XII are located in the posterior fossa. Anatomically and physiologically, these nerves are analogous to other peripheral nerves; however, functionally they are intimately related to the mesencephalon, metencephalon, and myelencephalon and, thus, are studied

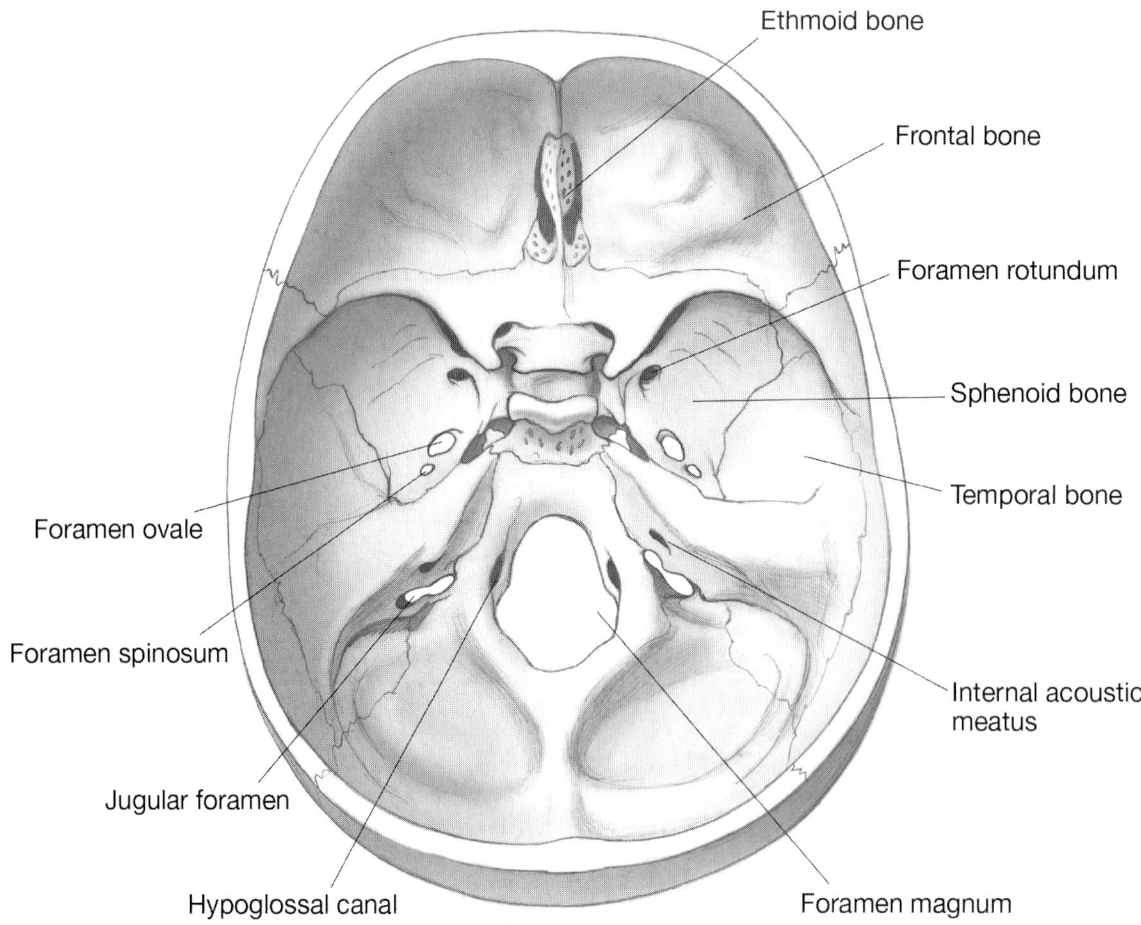

Fig. 3.2. Base of the cranial cavity viewed from above, illustrating the major cranial fossae, bones of the base of the skull, and the foramina.

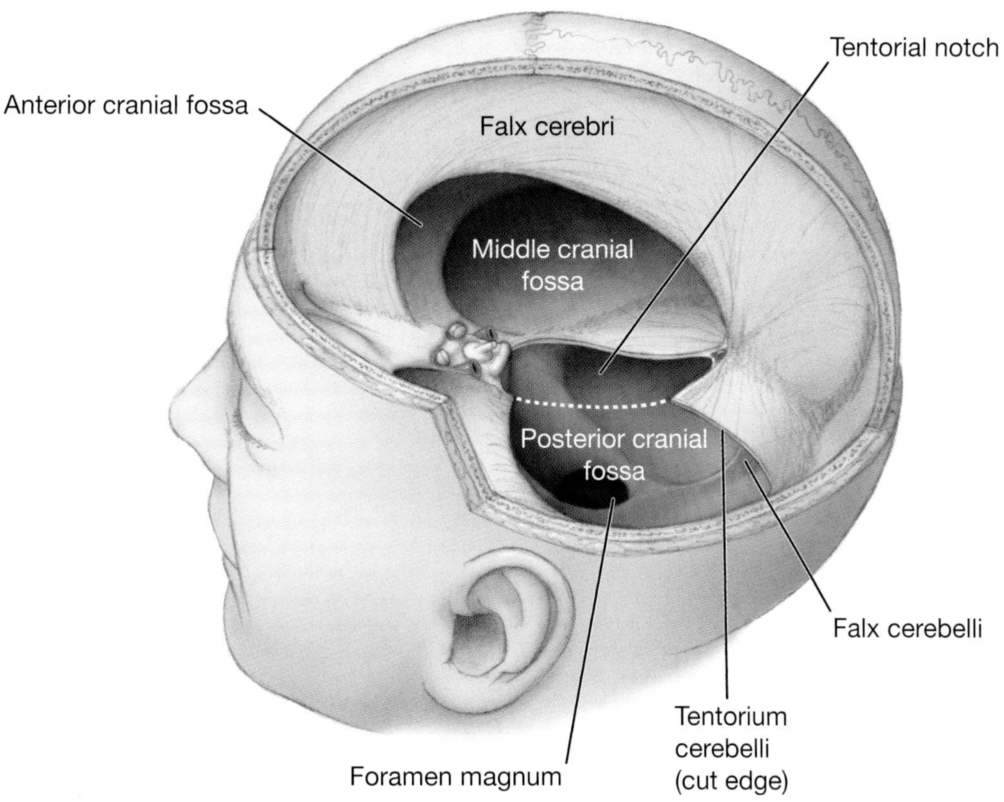

Fig. 3.3. Reflections of the dura mater forming the falx cerebri and tentorium cerebelli. Structures located above the tentorium cerebelli are part of the supratentorial level, and those located below the tentorium cerebelli but above the foramen magnum are part of the posterior fossa level.

together with the structures of the posterior fossa. The segments of cranial nerves contained in the bony skull are considered part of the posterior fossa level. After these nerves emerge from the skull, they are part of the peripheral level.

Spinal Level

The portion of the central nervous system located below the foramen magnum of the skull but contained in the vertebral column constitutes the spinal level (Fig. 3.4). This level has a considerable longitudinal extent, reaching from the skull to the sacrum. However, the spinal cord itself (the major structure at the spinal level) does not extend that entire length. A series of spinal nerves arise in the spinal canal and exit through the intervertebral foramina. Nerves contained in the bony vertebral column and in the intervertebral foramina are part of the spinal level. After these nerves leave the vertebral column, they become part of the peripheral level. The vertebral column itself is part of the spinal level.

Peripheral Level

The peripheral level includes all neuromuscular structures located outside the skull and vertebral column, including the cranial and spinal nerves, their peripheral branches, and the structures (including muscle) that are innervated by these nerves. The autonomic ganglia and nerves are also part of the peripheral level.

Longitudinal Systems

Many functional systems traverse several levels of the anatomical horizontal levels. Each system has well-defined anatomical structures that function together for a specific purpose. These include the cerebrospinal

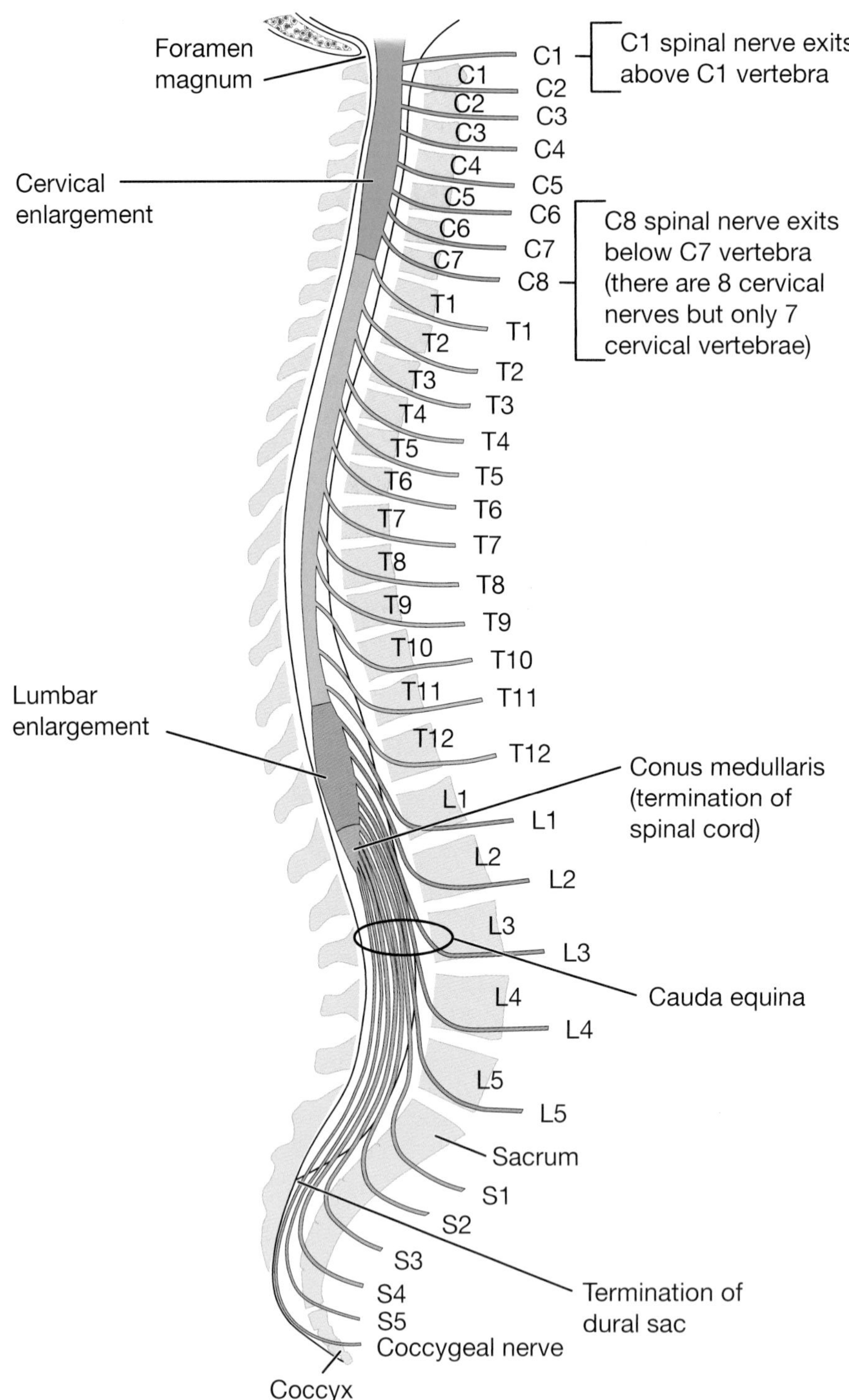

Fig. 3.4. Lateral view of structures at the spinal level. This level includes the spinal cord, the nerve roots contained in the vertebral column, and the vertebral column itself.

fluid system, motor system, sensory system, consciousness system, internal regulation system, and vascular system.

Cells of the Nervous System: Neurons and Glial Cells

The central and peripheral nervous systems are composed of neurons and supporting cells, known as glial cells. These concepts are introduced here but expanded upon in more detail in Chapter 4.

The fundamental cells of the nervous system designed to receive and transmit information to and from areas of the nervous system are *neurons*. A neuron is composed of dendrites, a cell body, and an axon (Fig. 3.5). *Dendrites* may have extensive branches and receive information from other cells. Information is processed or integrated in the cell body, which contains the nucleus, mitochondria, Golgi bodies, and Nissl substance. Groups of cell bodies arranged in functional units are known as *nuclei* when they lie within the central nervous system. For example, neurons innervating facial muscles have cell bodies located within the *facial nucleus*. Neurons are also arranged in sheets of gray matter that cover the cerebral hemispheres (*cortical gray matter*, or *cerebral cortex*) and cerebellum (*cerebellar cortex*). When the cell bodies lie outside the central nervous system, they are called *ganglia*. For instance, groups of cell bodies of axons that transmit sensory information from the limbs reside in the *dorsal root ganglia*. The axon, which is usually singular, transmits the modified information from the cell body to other neurons. This information is transmitted to another neuron at the *synapse*, a contact point between two neurons (Fig. 3.5). The presynaptic axon releases neurotransmitters that contact the postsynaptic dendrites of another cell or cells. In the case of an axon that transmits information to a muscle cell, the axon terminates on a *motor end plate*.

Certain aspects of neuronal shape differ from one another and, thus, neurons can be classified on the basis of their morphology. Neurons may be multipolar, bipolar, or unipolar. Multipolar refers to the multiplicity of dendritic processes. These cells typically have a single axon. Bipolar neurons have two processes, a dendrite and an axon. Unipolar neurons have a single conducting process and a cell body.

Although all neurons have the basic function of conveying information, they are specialized for various functions. For example, some neurons receive input from sensory receptors and transmit input from the periphery (limbs and organs) to the central nervous system. Other neurons innervate skeletal muscle. Still other neurons innervate organs and glands.

Sensory information transmitted by a neuron from the periphery to the central nervous system is designated as an *afferent* projection. Information projected to the periphery from the central nervous system is designated as *efferent*. Afferent information enters the central nervous system dorsally in the spinal cord. The cell bodies of these neurons lie outside the central nervous system and are called the *dorsal root ganglia*. Efferent information exits the central nervous system ventrally in the motor roots of the spinal cord. Where the dorsal sensory root and ventral motor root come together is known as a *spinal nerve*. There are 31 pairs of spinal nerves. Because of the development of the neural tube at the level of the brainstem and the presence of the fourth ventricle, afferents enter the brainstem laterally and efferent fibers leave it more medially. Nerves exiting or entering the brain or brainstem are known as *cranial nerves*. There are 12 pairs of cranial nerves.

Cranial and spinal nerves can be divided into categories depending on their embryologic origin or common structural and functional characteristics. These include three motor and four sensory types (Table 3.1).

Visceromotor fibers are efferent fibers that innervate smooth muscle, cardiac muscle, or glands. These nerves collectively form the autonomic nervous system, so designated because it regulates unconscious motor control. The autonomic nervous system includes *sympathetic* and *parasympathetic* components (Fig. 3.6). These systems are discussed in detail in other chapters. However, the basic circuitry is briefly outlined here. Parasympathetic nuclei are located in either the brainstem (cranial nerves III, VII, IX, and X) or at the sacral level of the spinal cord. Nuclei in the hypothalamus are involved in the control of sympathetic nuclei (preganglionic neurons) in the thoracic and lumbar levels of the spinal cord. Both preganglionic parasympathetic and sympathetic nerves synapse in a ganglion. From here, a second order (postganglionic)

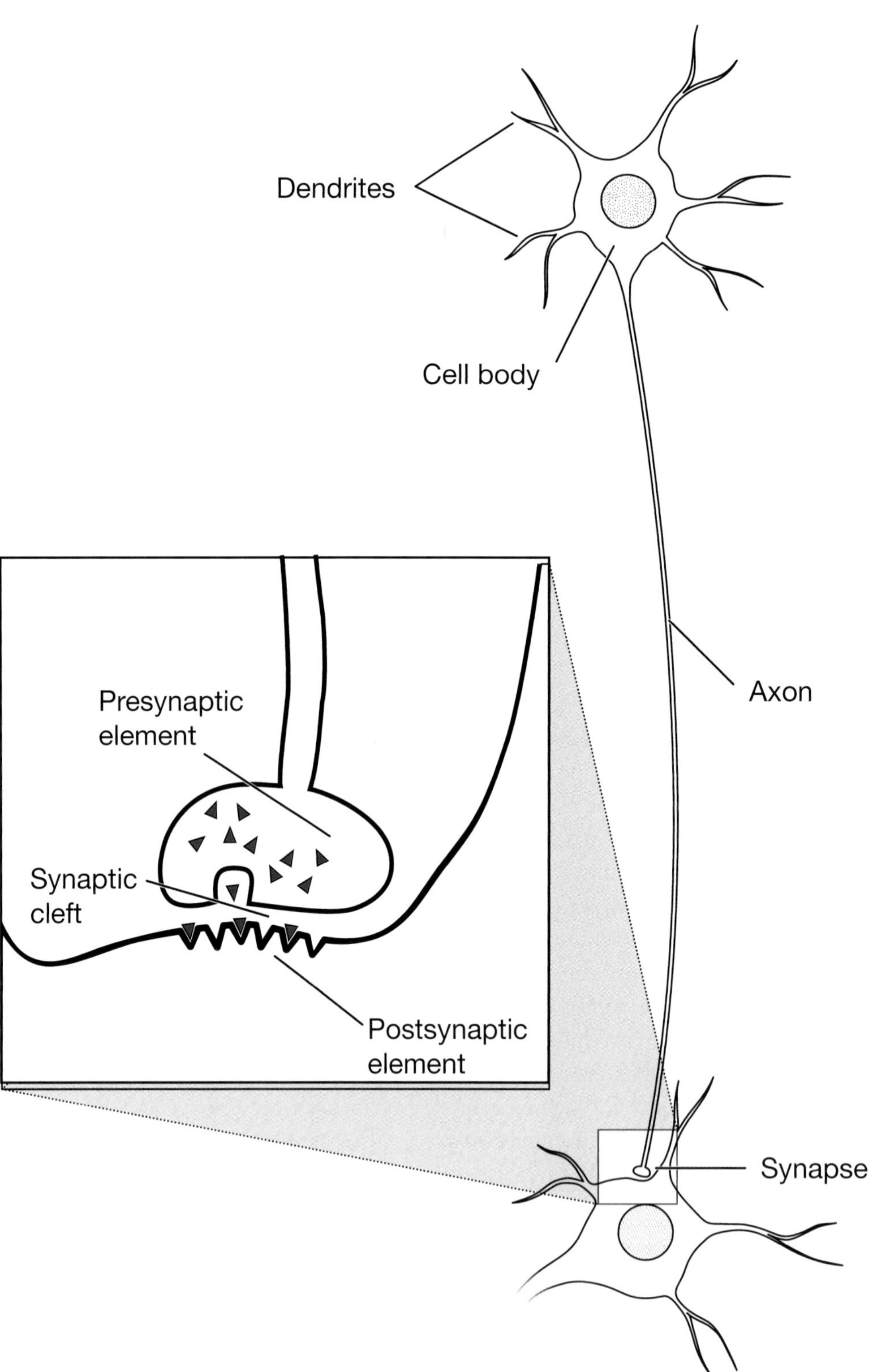

Fig. 3.5. Neuron with synapse.

Table 3.1. Functional Components of Cranial and Spinal Nerves

Type	Description	Example
General somatic efferent	Innervate muscle derived from somites	Spinal nerves Cranial nerves III, IV, VI, XII
Special visceral efferent	Innervate muscle derived from brachial arches	Cranial nerves V, VII, IX, X, XI
General visceral efferent	Innervate mesoderm- or endoderm-derived structures, including smooth muscle, organs, and glands	Spinal nerves (sacral segment) Cranial nerves III, VII, IX, X
General somatic afferent	Subserve sensory information from somite-derived structures, including skin, joints, mucosal membranes, dura mater	Spinal nerves Cranial nerves V, IX, X
Special visceral afferent	Subserve sensation from ectoderm-derived structures (taste and smell)	Cranial nerves I, VII, IX, X
Special somatic afferent	Subserve sensation from special senses derived from ectoderm (vision, balance, hearing)	Cranial nerves II, VIII
General visceral afferent	Subserve sensory function from endoderm-derived organs	Spinal nerves Cranial nerves IX, X

neuron sends its axon to innervate the designated structure. In the case of sympathetic nerves, the preganglionic axons are relatively short and synapse in sympathetic chain ganglia. Postganglionic sympathetic fibers are longer. Conversely, preganglionic parasympathetic axons are long relative to the postganglionic axons and synapse in ganglia that lie near the target organ.

A typical nerve is composed of the axons of many neurons (Fig. 3.7). Some nerves may be composed solely of motor neuron axons. Other nerves, such as the vagus nerve, may have mixed components, including special visceral efferents, general visceral efferents, general somatic afferents, special visceral afferents, and general visceral afferents.

Glial cells are the supporting cells of the nervous system. In the central nervous system, the glial cells include astroglia, oligodendroglia, and microglia. Astrocytes function in repair of the central nervous system. Microglia also serve a role in response to disease. They migrate to a site of damage and are involved in phagocytosis of pathogens and diseased neurons. Oligodendroglia form myelin sheaths around axons in the central nervous system.

Myelin is a spiral of membrane that surrounds axons, insulating them and increasing conduction rate. In the brain and spinal cord, *white matter*, which consists of axons, is so-named because of the appearance of the myelin sheaths. Tracts are formed by axons of neurons with a common destination. For example, the corticospinal tract is formed by axons with cell bodies in a specific area of the cerebral cortex. These axons descend through the cerebral hemisphere and brainstem to synapse on ventral horn cells in the spinal cord. The terms *fasciculus*, *peduncle*, and *lemniscus* also refer to axons traveling in a specific region of the central nervous system, but these structures may consist of a single tract (e.g., the medial lemniscus) or multiple tracts (e.g., the cerebral peduncle). For example, the *cerebral peduncle* contains the corticospinal and the corticopontocerebellar tracts.

In the peripheral nervous system, *Schwann cells* myelinate axons, although not every axon is myelinated. For instance, postganglionic autonomic fibers and fibers carrying pain and temperature sensation are either unmyelinated or lightly myelinated.

- Neurons are the fundamental cells of the nervous system designed to receive and transmit information.

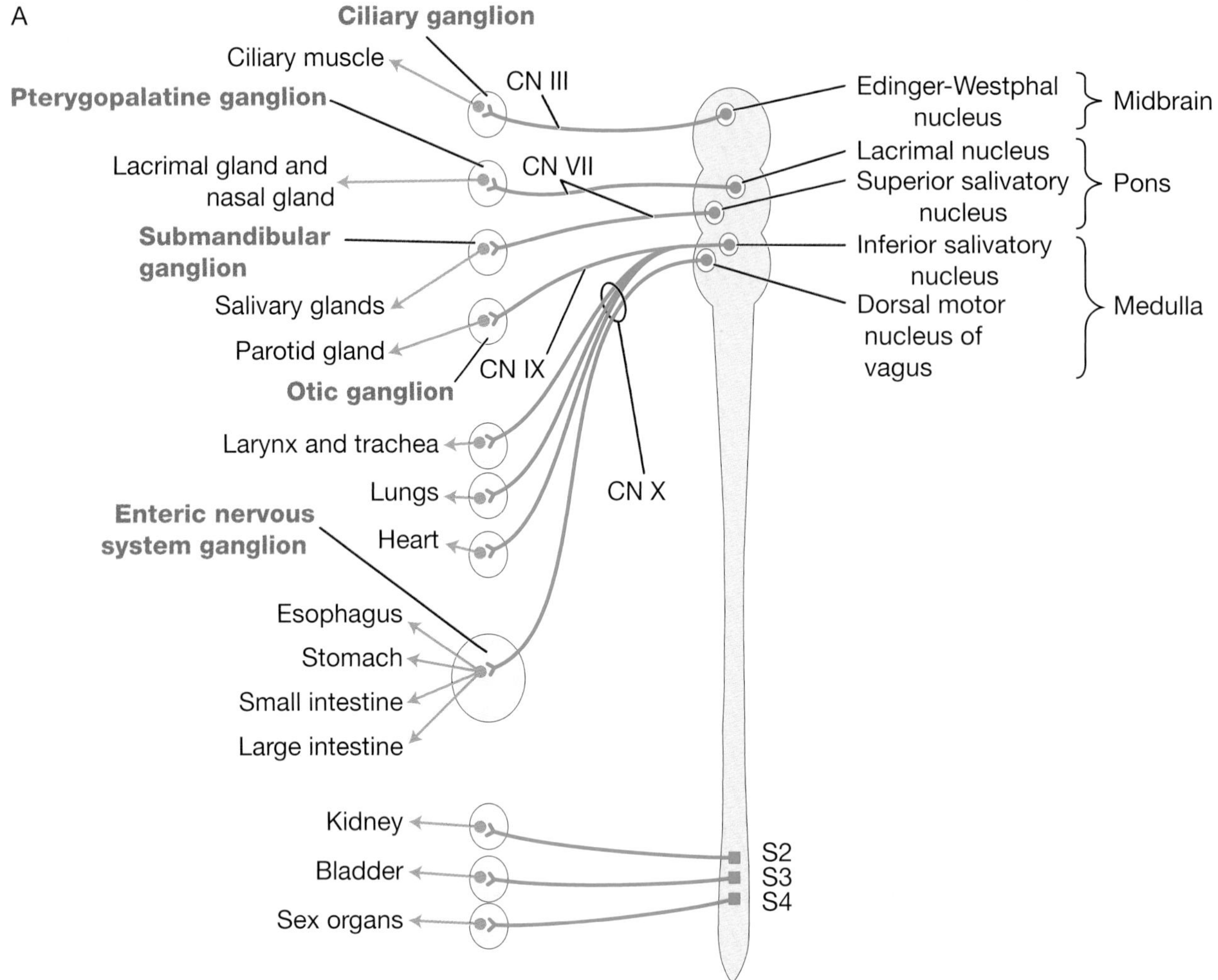

Fig. 3.6. Schematic representation of the autonomic nervous system. *A*, The parasympathetic division and, *B*, the sympathetic division. Note that preganglionic parasympathetic fibers begin in the cranial and sacral regions (*A*), and preganglionic sympathetic fibers begin in the thoracic and lumbar regions (*B*).

- Neurons are specialized to receive sensory information (afferent) or to provide motor output (efferent) to skeletal muscle, smooth muscle, glands, or organs.
- A nucleus is a group of cell bodies with similar function lying within the central nervous system.
- A ganglion is a group of cell bodies with similar function lying outside the central nervous system.
- Oligodendroglia myelinate axons in the central nervous system, and Schwann cells myelinate axons in the peripheral nervous system.
- A tract is a group of axons with a common destination.

The Human Nervous System

The nervous system is generally divided into the central and peripheral nervous systems. The central nervous system consists of the brain and spinal cord encased within the skull and vertebral column, respectively. The peripheral nervous system consists of the nerves that connect peripheral structures such as muscle, glands, and sensory receptors to the central nervous system.

The central nervous system may be further divided into horizontal levels: supratentorial (telencephalon and diencephalon), infratentorial or posterior fossa (mesencephalon, metencephalon, and myelencephalon), and

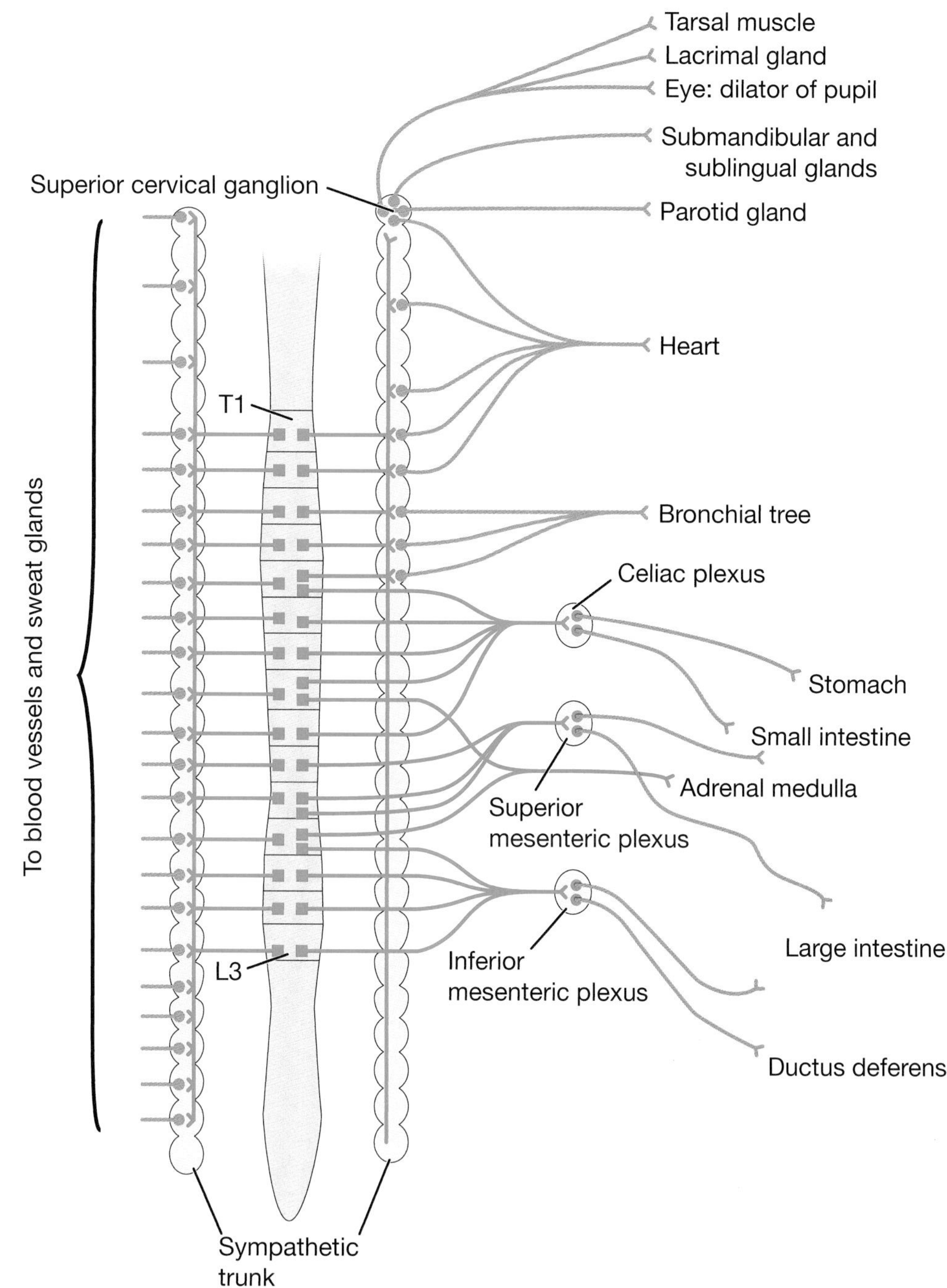

spinal (Fig. 3.1). The designation of supratentorial and infratentorial is based on the anatomy of the skull and the protective coverings or meninges surrounding the brain. The floor of the human skull (Fig. 3.2) is divided into three distinct compartments (*fossae*) on each side: anterior, middle, and posterior. A rigid membrane, the *tentorium cerebelli*, separates the anterior and middle fossae from the posterior fossa (Fig. 3.3). The tentorium lies in a nearly horizontal plane and is attached laterally to the petrous ridges and posteriorly to the occipital bone. The portion of the nervous system located above the tentorium cerebelli constitutes the *supratentorial* level. The portion

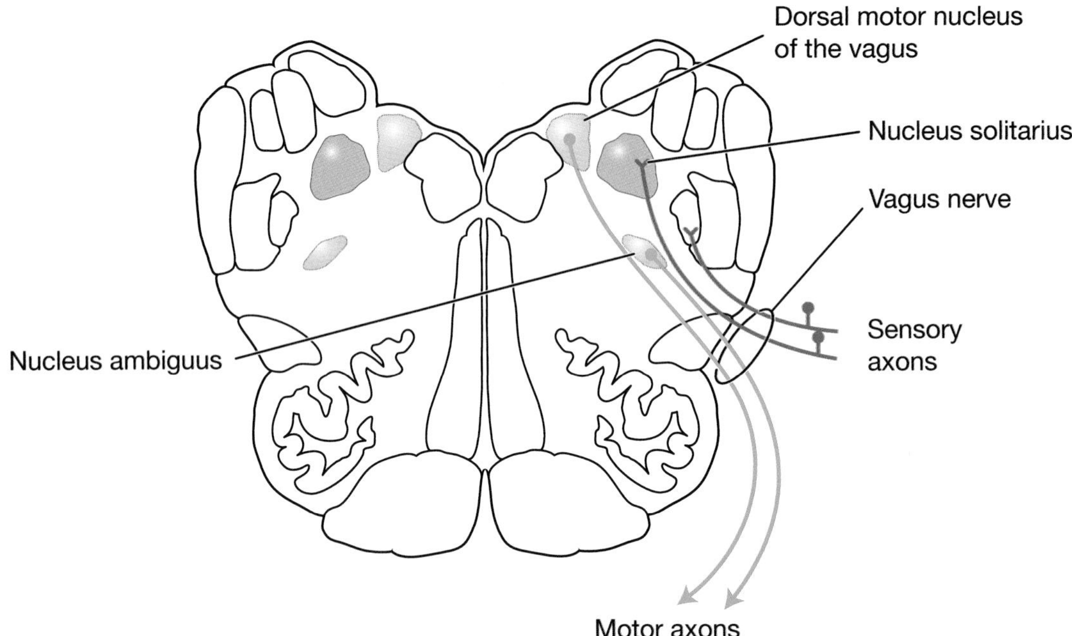

Fig. 3.7. The vagus nerve is an example of a mixed nerve containing both sensory and motor axons.

of the nervous system below the tentorium cerebelli is *infratentorial*, also designated as the posterior fossa.

The peripheral nervous system consists of cranial nerves and spinal nerves that connect the central nervous system with the periphery. There are 12 pairs of cranial nerves and 31 pairs of spinal nerves.

- Central nervous system = brain, spinal cord, and their protective coverings.
- Peripheral nervous system = cranial and spinal nerves after they have exited the skull and vertebral column, respectively.

Protective Coverings of the Central Nervous System

Skull

The skull is formed by the union of several bones and can be grossly subdivided into 1) the facial bones and orbits, 2) the sinus cavities within the bones that form the anterior aspect of the skull, and 3) the cranial bones (Fig. 3.8). The cranial bones surround the brain in the cranial cavity and provide a nonyielding protective covering for the brain. In contrast to other protective structures in the body, the cranial bones severely limit the expansion of the brain, even when expansion occurs in response to specific pathologic processes.

The cranial cavity is formed by the *frontal*, *parietal*, *sphenoid*, *temporal*, and *occipital* bones. The bones forming the base of the cavity are shown in Figure 3.2. When the base of the cranial cavity is viewed from above, three distinct areas are noted: the anterior, middle, and posterior fossae. In addition, there are symmetrically placed holes (foramina) in the base of the skull through which the cranial nerves emerge to innervate peripheral structures (Table 3.2).

Vertebral Column

The vertebral column consists of individual vertebral bodies separated by disks and connected by ligaments. Similar to the spinal cord, the vertebral column is divided into five separate levels. There are 7 *cervical*, 12 *thoracic*, and 5 *lumbar* vertebral bodies. There are five *sacral* vertebrae, which are fused, and one *coccygeal* vertebra. The vertebral body of each segment is unique (Fig. 3.9). Several ligaments connect the vertebral bodies, ensuring

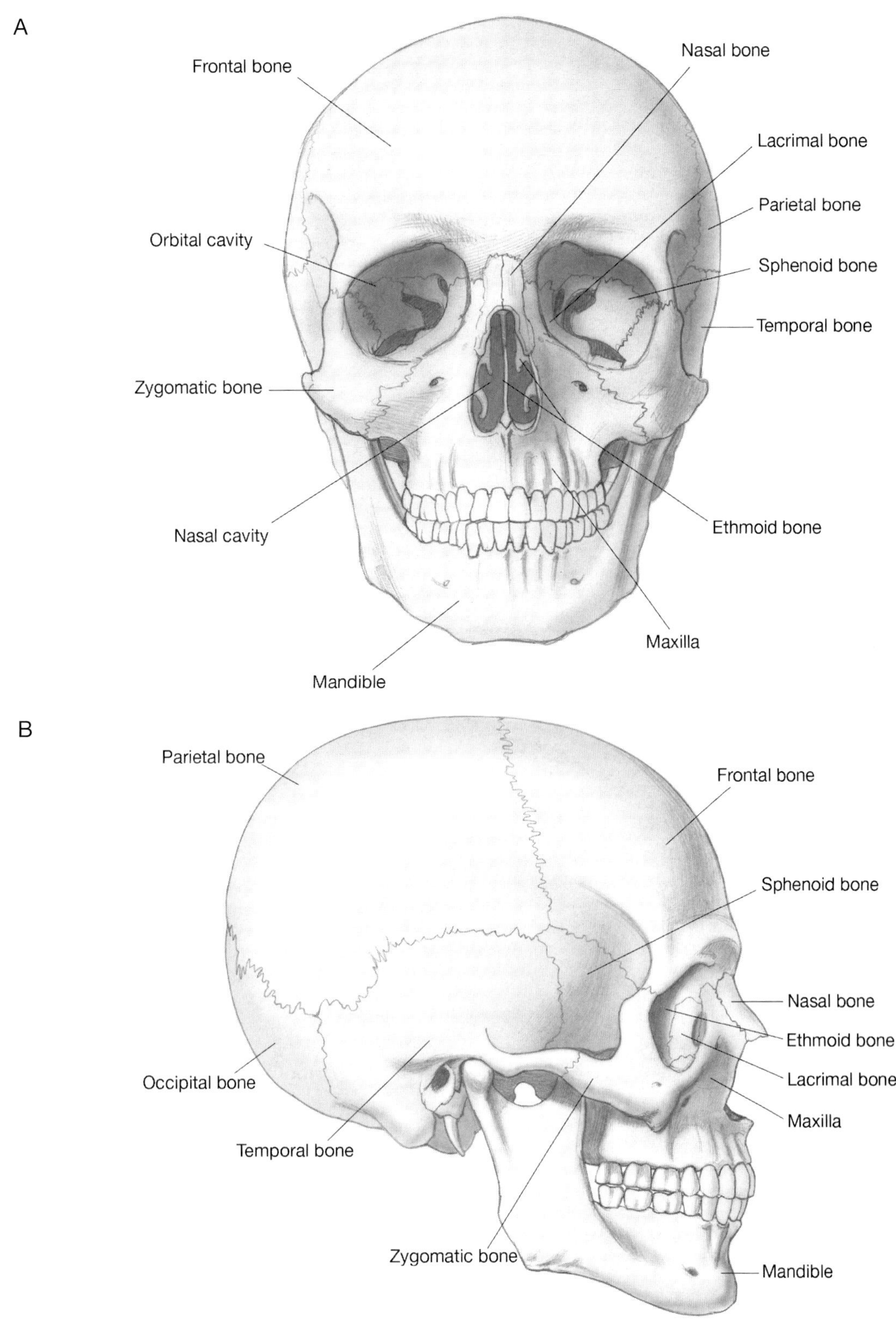

Fig. 3.8. Anterior (*A*) and lateral (*B*) views illustrating major bones of the skull. Hollow sinus cavities are located within frontal, ethmoid, sphenoid, and maxillary bones.

Table 3.2. Cranial Foramina and Associated Structures

Foramen	Associated structures
Cribriform plate of ethmoid bone	Olfactory nerves (CN I)
Optic foramen	Optic nerve (CN II)
	Ophthalmic artery
Superior orbital fissure	Oculomotor (CN III), trochlear (CN IV), abducens (CN VI) nerves and ophthalmic division of trigeminal nerve (CN V)
Foramen rotundum	Maxillary division of trigeminal nerve (CN V)
Foramen ovale	Mandibular division of trigeminal nerve (CN V)
Carotid canal	Sympathetic nerves
	Internal carotid artery
Foramen spinosum	Middle meningeal artery and vein
Internal acoustic meatus	Facial (CN VII) and vestibular and auditory nerves (CN VIII)
	Internal auditory artery
Jugular foramen	Glossopharyngeal (CN IX), vagus (CN X), and spinal accessory (CN XI) nerves
	Jugular vein
Hypoglossal canal	Hypoglossal nerve (CN XII)
Foramen magnum	Medulla, spinal accessory nerve (CN XI)
	Vertebral artery, anterior and posterior spinal arteries

CN, cranial nerve.

stability and flexibility of the spinal column (Fig. 3.10). These include the supraspinous, interspinous, and anterior and posterior longitudinal ligaments and ligamentum flavus.

Meninges

The meninges are an important supporting element of the central nervous system and include the dura mater, arachnoid, and pia mater (Fig. 3.11). The outermost fibrous membrane, the *dura mater*, consists of two layers of connective tissue that are fused, except in certain regions where they separate to form the intracranial *venous sinuses* and *septae*. Septae are folds of the dura mater that separate the cranial cavity into distinct fibrous barriers. Examples include the *falx cerebri*, which is located between the two cerebral hemispheres, and the *tentorium cerebelli*, which demarcates the superior limit of the posterior fossa. The delicate, filamentous *arachnoid* lies beneath the dura mater and appears to be loosely applied to the surface of the brain. *Pacchionian granulations* (arachnoid villi) are small tufts of arachnoid invaginated into dural venous sinuses, especially along the dorsal convexity of the cerebral hemispheres, superior to the longitudinal (interhemispheric) fissure. Many of the major arterial channels can be seen on the surface of the brain beneath the arachnoid. The innermost layer, the *pia mater*, is composed of a very thin layer of mesoderm that is so closely attached to the brain surface it cannot be seen in gross specimens.

Several important potential and actual spaces are found in association with these meningeal coverings. Between the bone and the dura mater is the epidural space, and beneath the dura mater is the subdural space. Normally, the bone, dura mater, and arachnoid are closely applied to one another so that the epidural and subdural spaces are potential spaces; however, in certain disease states, blood or pus may accumulate in these potential spaces. Beneath the arachnoid is the *subarachnoid space*, which surrounds the entire brain and spinal cord and is filled with cerebrospinal fluid. The ventricular system of the brain communicates with the subarachnoid space

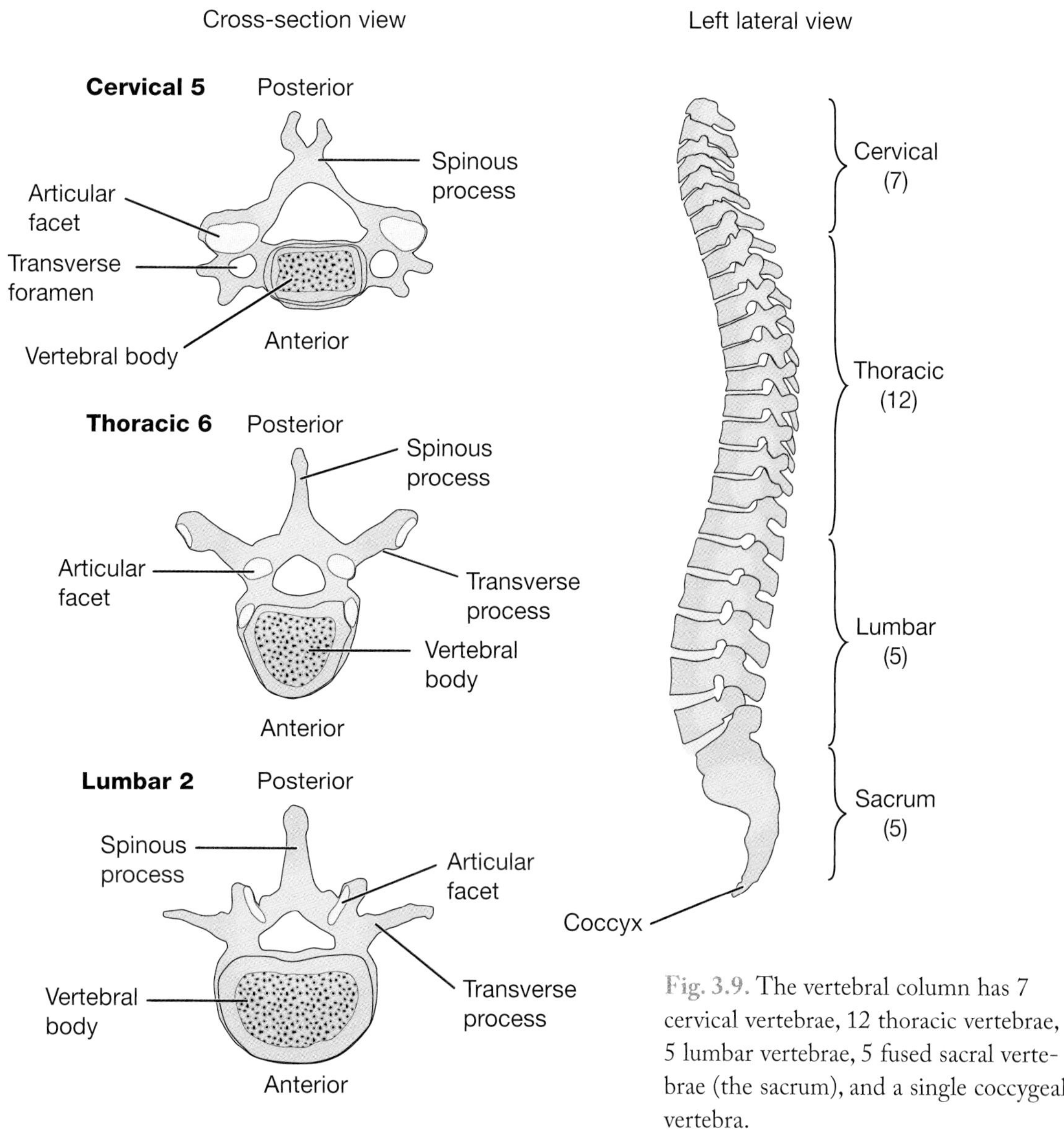

Fig. 3.9. The vertebral column has 7 cervical vertebrae, 12 thoracic vertebrae, 5 lumbar vertebrae, 5 fused sacral vertebrae (the sacrum), and a single coccygeal vertebra.

through foramina in the roof of the fourth ventricle (Fig. 3.12).

The spinal cord is surrounded by meninges similar to those that surround the brain. Exterior to the dura mater is the epidural space, an actual space that contains fat and venous plexuses. Between the arachnoid, adjacent to the inner surface of the dura mater, and the pia mater is the subarachnoid space, which contains the cerebrospinal fluid. The spinal pia mater is applied closely to the surface of the spinal cord but is visible as the *denticulate ligaments* that extend on either side between the origins of the spinal nerve roots. These ligaments join the arachnoid at intervals and are inserted into the dura mater. The dural sac and subarachnoid space end at the level of the second sacral vertebra (Fig. 3.13). The pia mater continues caudally as a filamentous membrane (the *filum terminale interna*) from the end of the spinal cord (the *conus medullaris*). It fuses with the dural sac at the level of the second sacral vertebra and attaches to the dorsal surface of the coccyx as the sacrococcygeal ligament.

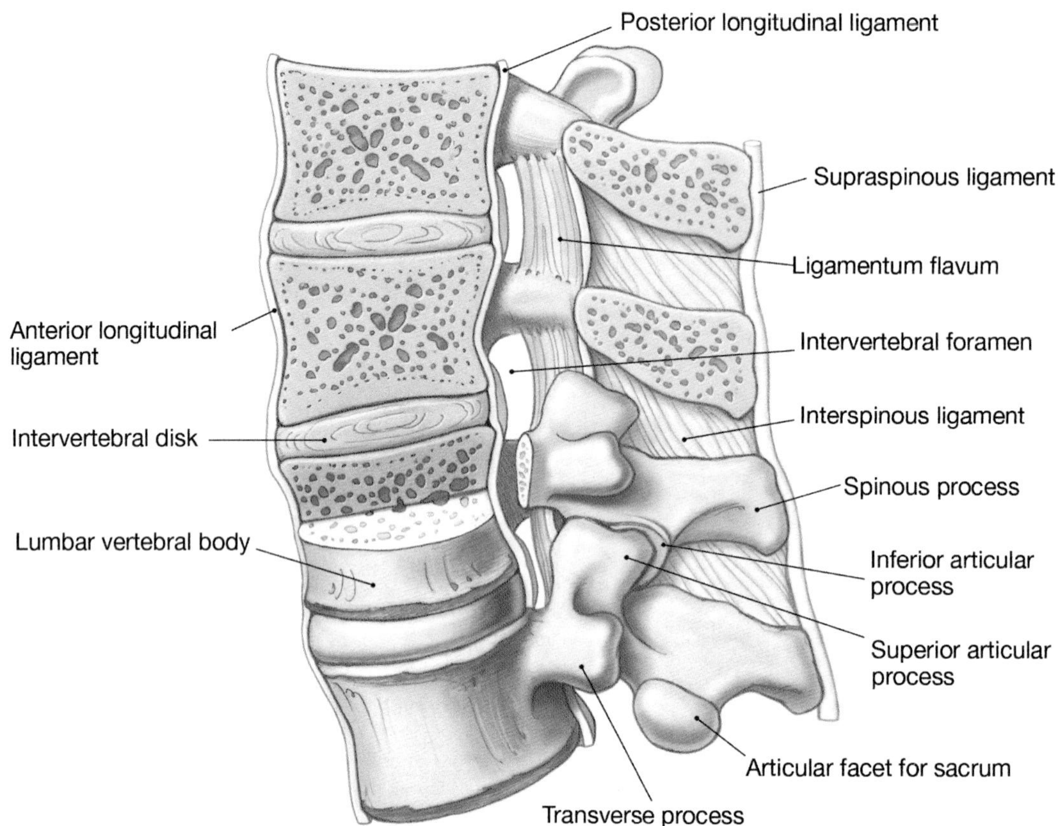

Fig. 3.10. The stability of the spine depends on several ligaments, including the anterior and posterior spinal ligaments, ligamentum flavum, the interspinous ligaments, and the supraspinous ligament.

Gross Neuroanatomy—Horizontal Levels

The Supratentorial Level

The major structures at the supratentorial level are the cerebral hemispheres, basal ganglia, diencephalon (thalamus and hypothalamus), and cranial nerves I (olfactory) and II (optic).

Cerebral Hemispheres

Through a process of growth and proliferation, the telencephalic structures differentiate into the cerebral hemispheres. The *longitudinal* (interhemispheric) *fissure* separates the cerebrum into two cerebral hemispheres. The surface of each hemisphere is convoluted: the folds are known as *gyri* and the grooves that separate them are called *sulci*. Certain grooves are more prominent, deeper, and more constant and are known as *fissures*. The sulci and fissures help identify the lobes of the brain and demarcate certain functional areas.

The four anatomical lobes of the brain, the *frontal*, *parietal*, *temporal*, and *occipital* lobes, are defined by specific fissures and sulci. The boundaries of these lobes are listed in Table 3.3 and illustrated in Figure 3.14. The *limbic lobe* is sometimes designated as a lobe because its parts are interconnected functionally. It lies on the medial surface of the brain. The *insula* is an involuted portion of cerebral cortex deep within the lateral sulcus.

The frontal lobe, the largest lobe, extends from the frontal pole posteriorly to the central sulcus. The *lateral sulcus* (*sylvian fissure*) separates the frontal lobe from the temporal lobe inferiorly. The frontal lobe contains the *precentral gyrus*, which extends vertically, and the *superior*, *middle*, and *inferior frontal gyri*, which extend horizontally. Continuing on the medial surface of the hemisphere, the

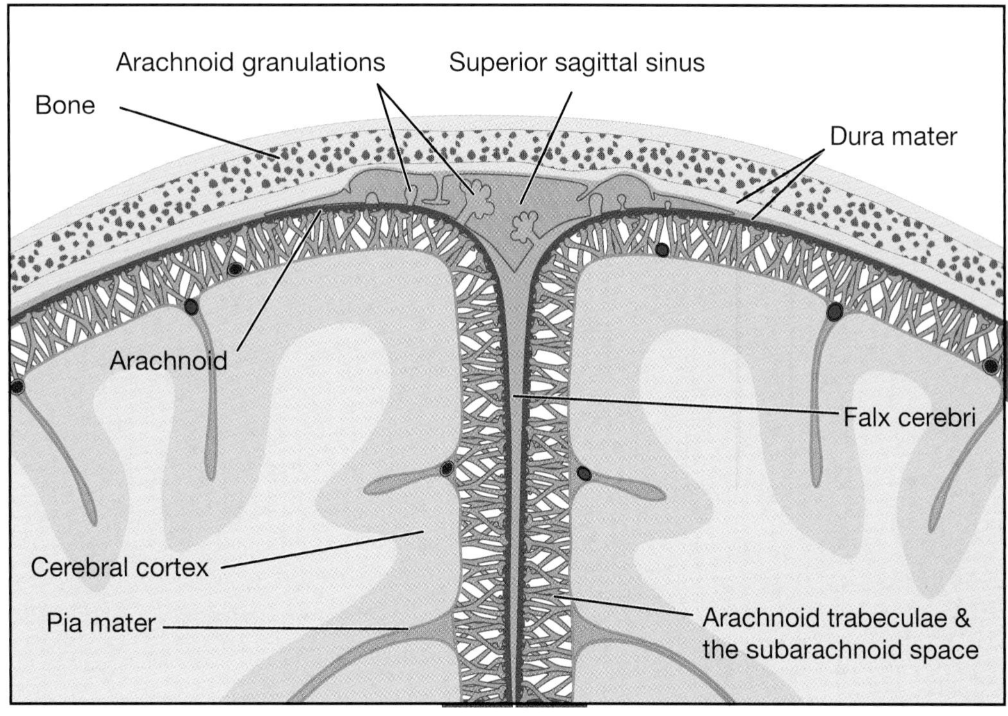

Fig. 3.11. Meninges and meningeal spaces. Coronal section through the paramedian region of the cerebral hemispheres.

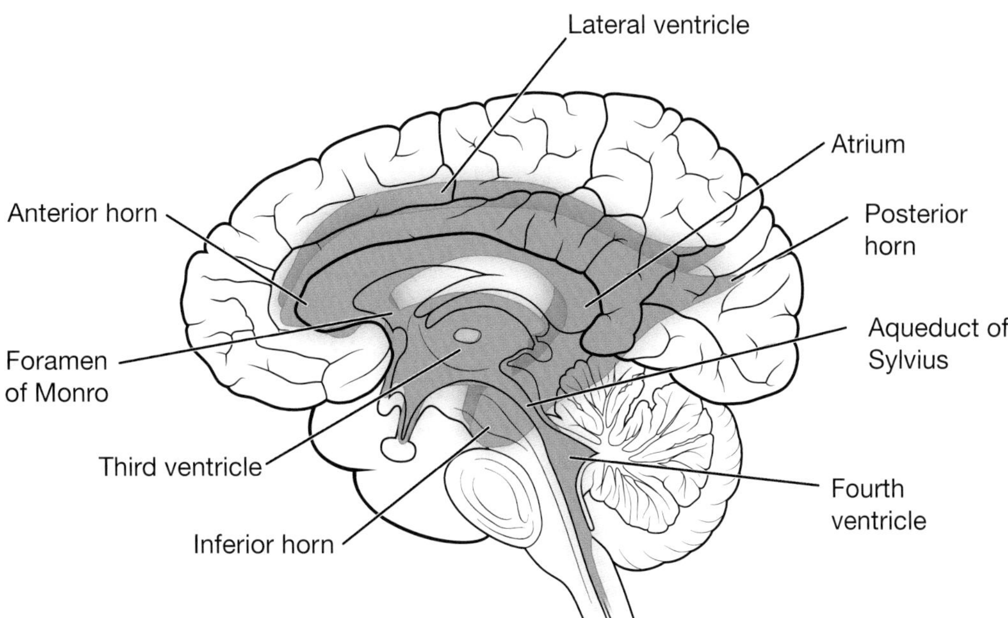

Fig. 3.12. Ventricular system. Cerebrospinal fluid is formed by choroid plexuses in the ventricles. This fluid circulates from the lateral to the fourth ventricle and enters the subarachnoid space through the foramina of Luschka and Magendie.

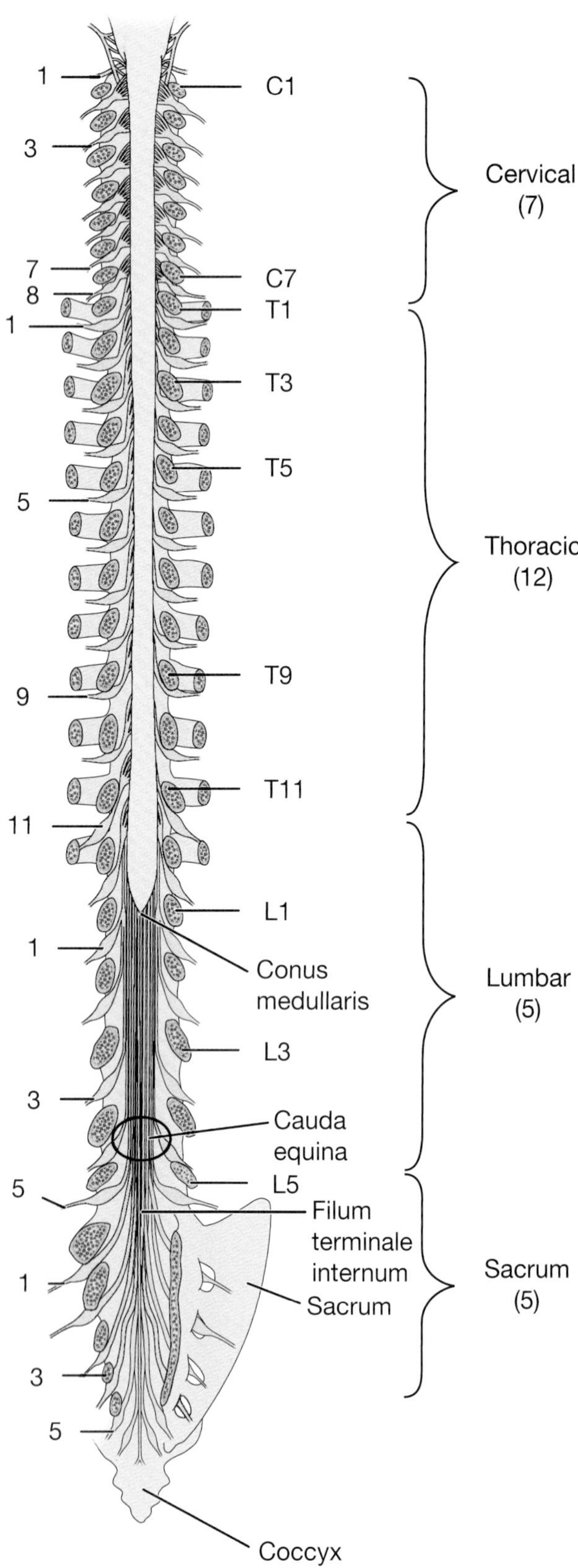

Fig. 3.13. Dorsal view of the spinal level. The spinal cord terminates between vertebrae L1 and L2 and is enlarged at the cervical and lumbrosacral levels. These enlargements correspond to the segments that innervate the upper (cervical enlargement) and lower (lumbosacral enlargement) limbs. The roots form the spinal nerves, which exit through the intervertebral foramina. The cervical roots exit above the corresponding vertebra, and the eighth cervical root exits between vertebrae C7 and T1. The rest of the roots exit below the corresponding vertebra. Because of the difference in length between the spinal cord and the spinal canal, the lumbar and sacral roots of the conus medullaris travel a relatively long distance in the subarachnoid space before exiting through their corresponding foramina. These roots form the cauda equina.

superior frontal gyrus extends to the *cingulate gyrus*. Functionally, the frontal lobe can be divided into several major components: primary motor cortex (precentral gyrus), the premotor and supplementary motor areas, frontal eye fields, the area of Broca (language), and prefrontal cortex (the large area anterior to the precentral gyrus and premotor and supplementary motor areas) (Table 3.3).

The *central sulcus* separates the frontal and parietal lobes. The *parieto-occipital sulcus* forms the boundary between the parietal and occipital lobes. The parietal lobe can be divided anatomically into the postcentral gyrus, which extends vertically along the lateral hemispheric surface, and the inferior and superior parietal lobules, also located laterally. The *paracentral lobule* and *precuneus* are on the medial surface of the parietal lobe. Functionally, the postcentral gyrus, also known as primary sensory cortex, receives incoming sensory information from the contralateral face and limbs. In the dominant hemisphere, a portion of the inferior parietal and the superior temporal gyrus subserve language function. The majority of the parietal lobe contains somatosensory association areas and integrates sensory information from all modalities.

The temporal lobe is separated from the frontal lobe by the sylvian fissure. The temporal lobe is further divided into the *superior*, *middle*, and *inferior temporal gyri*. The superior temporal gyrus continues laterally toward the insula as the temporal operculum. Functionally, the temporal lobe contains the primary auditory cortex,

Wernicke area, and, medially, the hippocampus and amygdala. The latter structures are related functionally to the limbic lobe (Table 3.3).

The parieto-occipital sulcus divides the occipital lobe from the parietal lobe. The medial occipital lobe can be divided into the *cuneus* and *lingual* gyri. The occipital lobe contains the primary visual cortex and visual association cortices.

The *limbic lobe* is the ring of cortex on the medial aspect of each cerebral hemisphere that includes the

Table 3.3. Lobes of the Brain

Lobe	Anatomical boundaries	Functional components
Frontal	Central sulcus separates frontal and parietal lobes Lateral sulcus (sylvian fissure) separates frontal and temporal lobes Important gyri include precentral gyrus and superior, middle, and inferior frontal gyri	Prefrontal cortex Integrate motivational cues with complex objects, events, and sequences Motivation, judgment, planning, personality Supplementary motor and premotor areas Motor programming of complex movement Primary motor cortex (precentral gyrus) Contralateral voluntary movement Frontal eye fields Voluntary conjugate movement of eyes Broca area Language
Parietal	Central sulcus separates frontal and parietal lobes Parietal lobe is bounded inferiorly by lateral sulcus, which separates parietal and temporal lobes Parieto-occipital sulcus separates parietal and occipital lobes Important gyri include postcentral, supramarginal, and angular gyri	Primary somatosensory cortex (postcentral gyrus) Contralateral sensation of face and limbs Somatosensory association cortex Complex somatosensory information Sensorimotor integration (angular and supramarginal gyri and inferior parietal lobule)
Temporal	Separated from frontal and parietal lobes by lateral sulcus Important gyri are superior, middle, and inferior temporal gyri	Primary auditory cortex Hearing Auditory association cortex Auditory processing Hippocampus Memory Wernicke area Language
Occipital	Parieto-occipital sulcus separates parietal and occipital lobes	Primary visual cortex Visualize contralateral visual field Visual association cortex Integrate visual information, including interpretation of shape, color, size, motion, and orientation

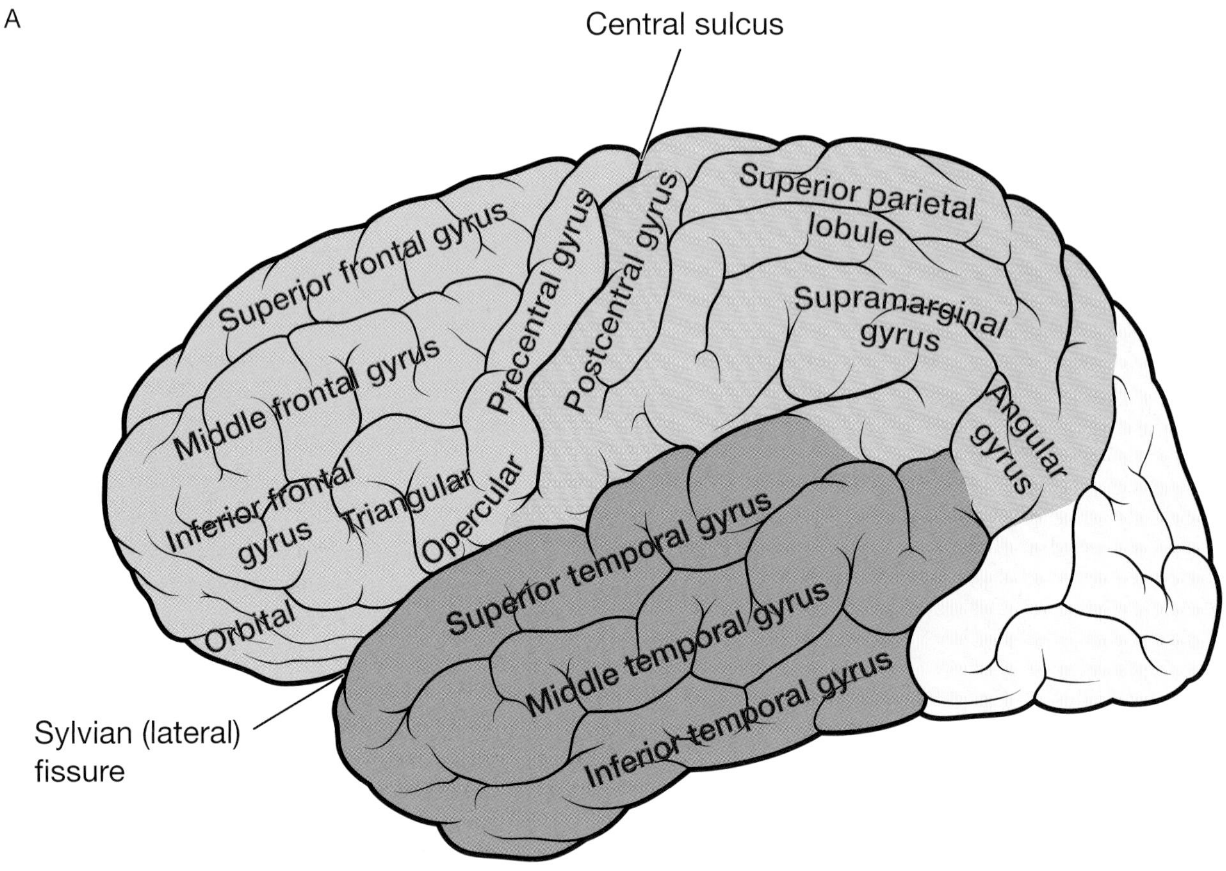

Fig. 3.14. Lateral (*A*) and medial (*B*) surfaces of the cerebral hemisphere illustrating the major gyri and sulci and division of the hemisphere into five major lobes: frontal, parietal, temporal, occipital, and limbic.

cingulate gyrus, parahippocampal gyrus, uncus, and hippocampus. Functionally, these structures and the hypothalamus, thalamus, basal forebrain, and prefrontal cortex belong to the *limbic system*. This system participates in the control of autonomic function, arousal, motivated behavior, emotion, learning, and homeostasis.

Many large tracts in the white matter interconnect areas of the cortex. *Association fibers* connect one area of cerebral cortex with another area in the same hemisphere. *Commissural fibers*, such as the *corpus callosum*, connect areas of the cerebral cortex in opposite hemispheres (Fig. 3.15). *Projection fibers* project to deep structures, for example, the thalamus.

Basal Ganglia

The basal ganglia, composed of the *caudate nucleus*, *putamen*, and *globus pallidus*, are part of the motor system. A large and important area of white matter, the *internal capsule*, passes between these central nuclear masses and connects the cerebral cortex and lower structures (Fig. 3.16). The basal ganglia function in motor programming and initiation of motor programs.

Diencephalon

The diencephalon represents a zone of transition between the cerebral hemisphere at the supratentorial level and the structures in the posterior fossa. The diencephalon

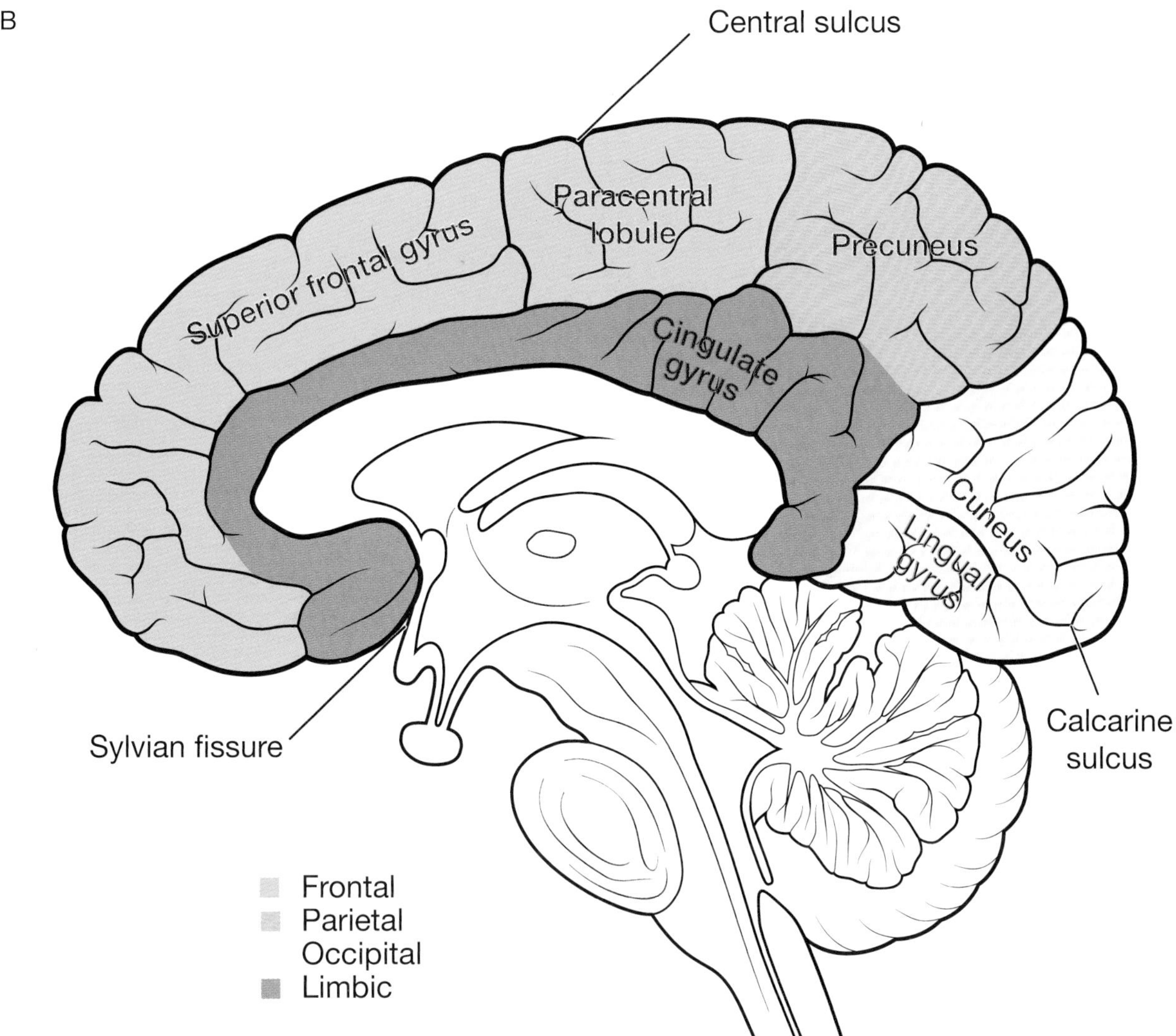

consists of the thalamus, hypothalamus, optic pathways, and pineal body. It is divided into left and right halves by the third ventricle. At the base of the hypothalamus is an important neuroendocrine structure, the hypophysis, or *pituitary gland*, which is located in the middle of the skull in the bony sella turcica. All these structures are at the supratentorial level.

The *thalamus* is a relay center in the central nervous system. That is, it receives and sends integrated information to motor and sensory areas of cerebral cortex. It also has a role in memory, consciousness, and limbic functions. The thalamus consists of two masses on either side of the third ventricle and, in many brains, connected by the mass intermedia. Laterally, the thalamus extends to the posterior limb of the internal capsule (Fig. 3.16).

The *hypothalamus* is ventral to the hypothalamic sulcus, which is in the wall of the third ventricle, and extends from the optic chiasm anteriorly to the mammillary bodies posteriorly (Fig. 3.17). The hypothalamus is connected with many regions of the cerebral cortex, especially with the limbic system, and the pituitary gland. It is part of the internal regulatory system, integrating sensory input with an autonomic, visceral, or hormonal response. Its functions include temperature regulation, sexual behavior and reproduction, metabolic homeostasis, emotional response, sleep, and diurnal variations.

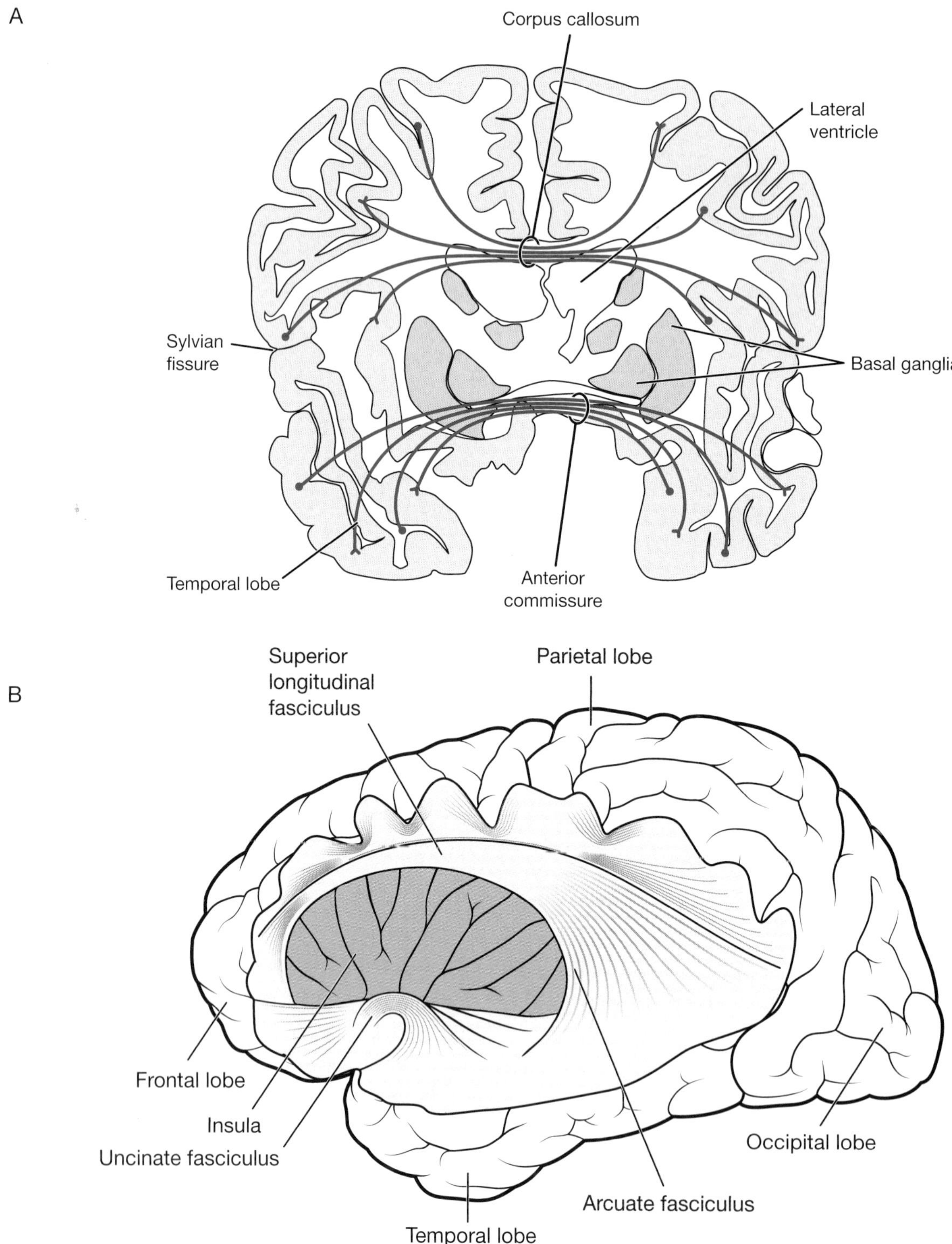

Fig. 3.15. *A*, White matter tracts that connect the cerebral cortex of one hemisphere with that of the other hemisphere are known as commissural fibers. Examples include the anterior commissure and corpus collosum. *B*, White matter tracts that connect one area of cerebral cortex with another area within a hemisphere are called association fibers. Examples include the superior longitudinal fasciculus, uncinate fasciculus, and arcuate fasciculus.

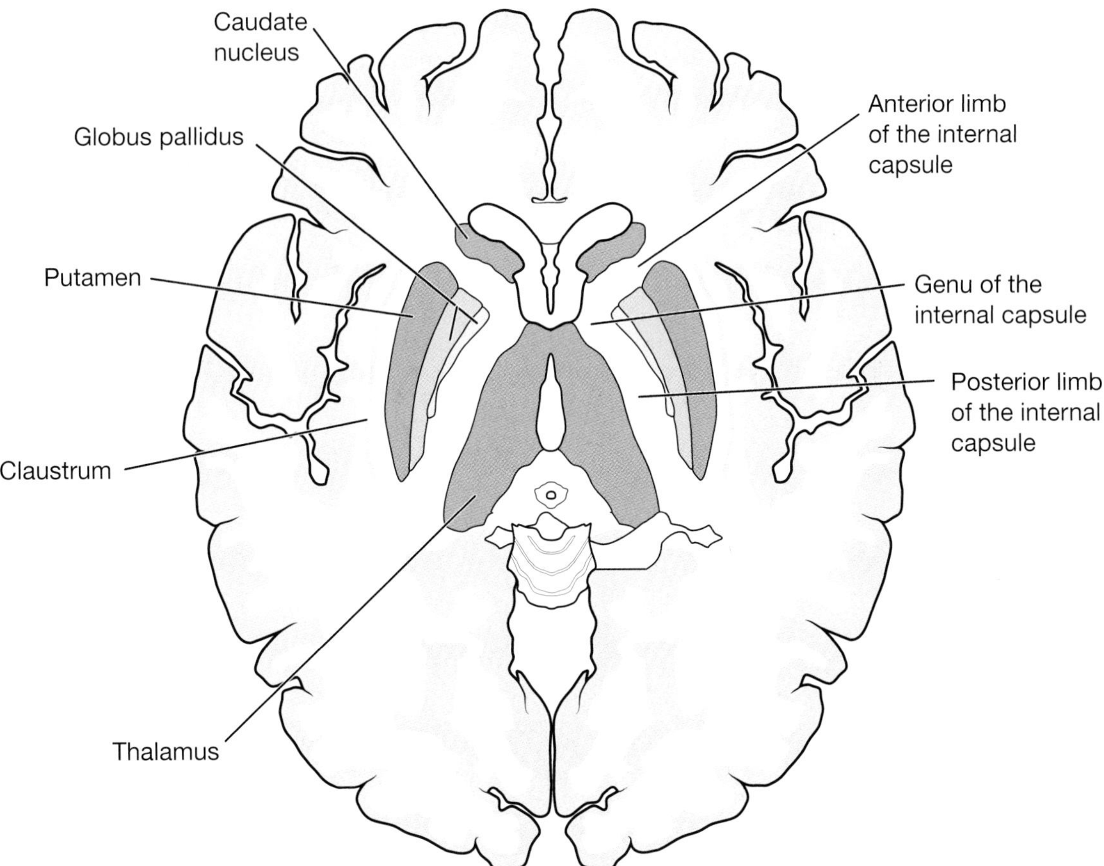

Fig. 3.16. Axial view through the cerebral hemispheres showing the deep structures. The thalamus is medial to the posterior limb of the internal capsule. The putamen and globus pallidus are lateral to the internal capsule. The caudate nucleus is medial to the anterior limb of the internal capsule.

The pineal body secretes melatonin. The production of melatonin is influenced by the hypothalamic detection of cycles of light and dark.

Cranial Nerves I and II

The olfactory bulb and tract (cranial nerve I) are located at the base of each frontal lobe and subserve the sense of smell. The olfactory nerves pass from the nasal cavity through the cribriform plate and synapse in the olfactory bulb.

The optic nerves (cranial nerve II) develop as an outgrowth of the primitive diencephalon. The optic pathway from the orbit consists of the optic nerve, optic chiasm, and optic tract. The intracranial portions of cranial nerves I and II are at the supratentorial level.

Figure 3.18 introduces the anatomy of the supratentorial region as seen in coronal sections.

The Posterior Fossa Level

The major structures contained in this level are the brainstem, cerebellum, and origins of cranial nerves III through XII.

Brainstem

The term *brainstem* is not a precise anatomical term and has been defined in different ways. However, the term is used so often in neurologic discussions that one must be familiar with it. As defined here, the brainstem is the portion of the brain that remains after removal of the cerebral hemispheres and cerebellum (Fig. 3.19).

Cephalad from the spinal cord, the brainstem includes

the medulla oblongata (myelencephalon), pons (metencephalon), and midbrain (mesencephalon). Only the pontine portion of the metencephalon is part of the brainstem; the cerebellum is excluded.

The transition between the spinal cord and the medulla is at the level of the foramen magnum. At this level, the decussation of the pyramidal tracts is apparent on the ventral surface of the medulla. The medulla extends rostrally to the pons.

The pons extends from the pontomedullary junction to an imaginary line just below the exit of cranial nerve IV. It is divided into the *tegmentum* and *basilar* areas.

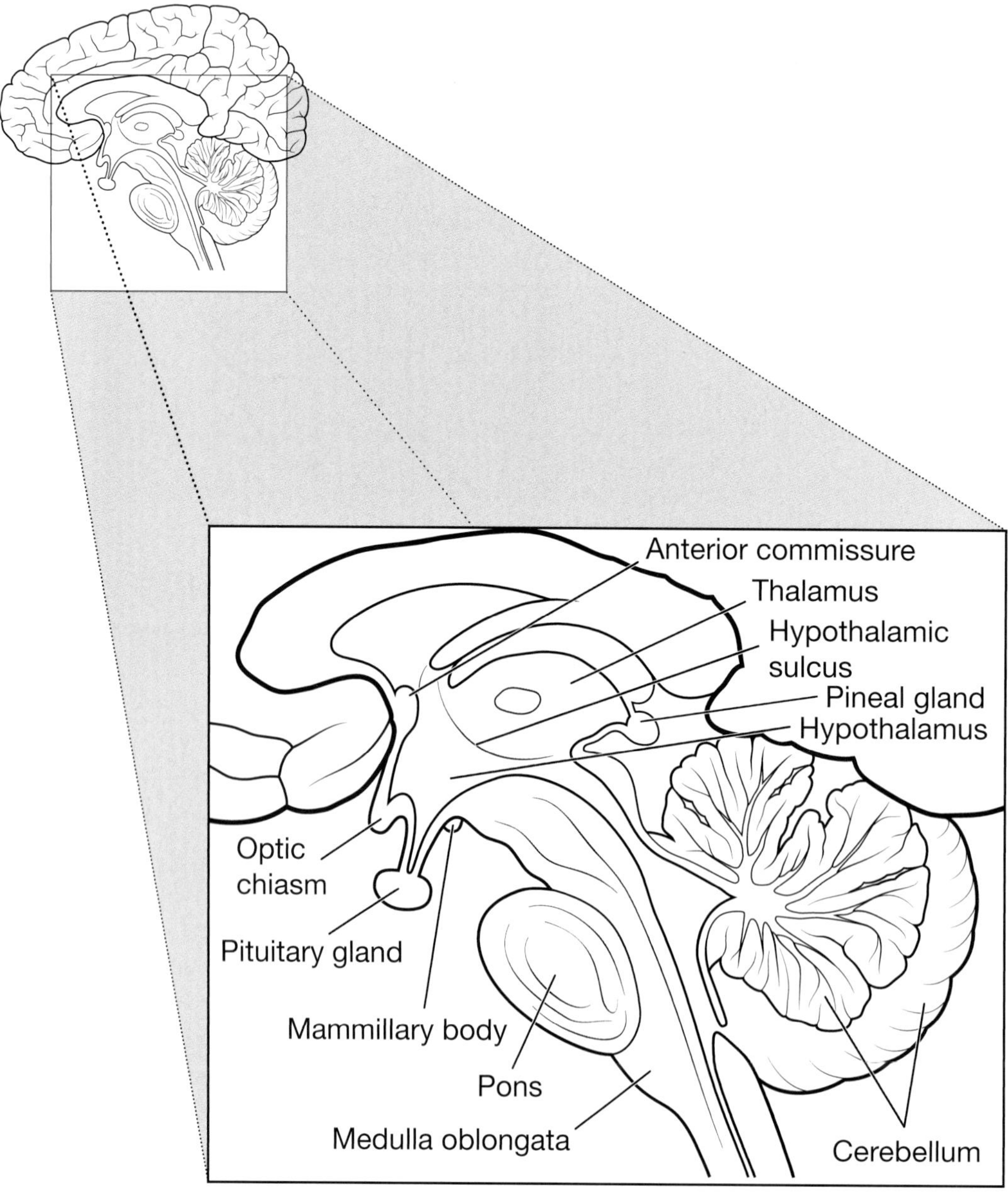

Fig. 3.17. Midsagittal section of the brain showing the region of the hypothalamus (enlarged diagram). The hypothalamus lies on either side of the third ventricle between the optic chiasm and mammillary bodies. It is ventral to the thalamus and separated from it by the hypothalamic sulcus.

The area of numerous nuclei and intermingled pathways ventral to the aqueduct and fourth ventricle is the tegmentum. The large distinct cerebral and cerebellar white matter pathways in the ventral region below the tegmentum make up the base, or basilar region, of the pons.

The midbrain extends from the pons-midbrain junction to the diencephalon. In this text, the diencephalon is not considered part of the brainstem. The *superior colliculus* is used to demarcate the upper border of the brainstem. The red nucleus and substantia nigra are located in the upper mesencephalon and extend into the posterior diencephalon, thus overlapping the supratentorial and posterior fossa levels. The midbrain is divided dorsoventrally into three regions. The area dorsal to the aqueduct of Sylvius is the *tectum*; its major structures are the superior and inferior colliculi (collectively known as the corpora quadrigemina). The *tegmentum* is the region ventral to the aqueduct and extends to the cerebral peduncles. The *basal region* of the midbrain consists mainly of the large crus cerebri, or cerebral peduncles.

Cerebellum

The cerebellum consists of two *hemispheres*, a midline *vermis*, and a small *flocculonodular lobe* (Fig. 3.20). The cerebellar surface is more highly convoluted than the surface of the cerebral hemisphere, with the folds called *folia*. The cerebellum is derived from the metencephalon and, thus, is associated structurally with the pons. The cerebellum lies dorsal to the fourth ventricle, the pons, and the medulla. It is important in the coordination of motor output.

Cranial Nerves III Through XII

Emerging from the brainstem are 10 pairs of cranial nerves (Fig. 3.19). (Cranial nerves I and II are not contained in the posterior fossa.) The names, location, and general function of all the cranial nerves are summarized in Table 3.4.

Cross sections of the brainstem and cranial nerves are shown in Figure 3.21.

The Spinal Level

The major structures contained in the spinal level are the spinal cord, the origins of the spinal nerves within the vertebral column, and the vertebral column.

The adult spinal cord begins rostrally from the caudal margin of the medulla at the level of the foramen magnum and terminates opposite the caudal margin of the first lumbar vertebra. Thus, the spinal cord does not extend the entire length of the spinal canal. Throughout much of the length of the spinal cord, a spinal segment is not adjacent to its corresponding vertebral segment.

The spinal cord exhibits cervical and lumbosacral enlargements. Cross sections show a relative increase in gray matter in these two regions, accounting for the relative enlargement in these areas. Thirty-one pairs of spinal nerves are attached to the spinal cord by dorsal (posterior) and ventral (anterior) nerve roots. Segmentally, there are 8 cervical, 12 thoracic, 5 lumbar, 5 sacral, and 1 coccygeal spinal nerves on each side. At their origins, the nerve roots consist of multiple filaments, which on the posterior (dorsal) surface of the cord are attached along a relatively constant groove, the *posterior lateral sulcus*. The dorsal and ventral roots of each spinal nerve join as they enter the intervertebral foramen of the spine. After leaving the spinal cord, the roots of the lumbar and sacral spinal nerves go caudally several vertebral segments toward their exit. A collection of spinal nerve roots contained in the lumbosacral spinal canal is known as the cauda equina (Fig. 3.4). Although most spinal nerves have both a ventral (motor) root and dorsal (sensory) root, the first cervical nerve often has only a motor root, and the first coccygeal nerve and the fifth sacral nerve have only a sensory root. Surrounding the spinal cord is the *vertebral column*, consisting of 7 cervical, 12 thoracic, and 5 lumbar vertebrae, the fused sacrum, and the coccyx (Fig. 3.9).

The spinal cord levels are illustrated in Figure 3.22.

The Peripheral Level

The major structures of the peripheral level are the somatic nerves, the autonomic nerves and ganglia, the neuromuscular junctions, the muscles of the skeleton, and the peripheral sensory receptors. The *spinal nerves*, as they emerge from the vertebral column, enter the peripheral level. Spinal nerves are formed by the joining of dorsal and ventral roots and thus contain somatic and autonomic motor and sensory nerve fibers. Spinal nerves branch into posterior and anterior divisions as they enter the peripheral level. Fibers

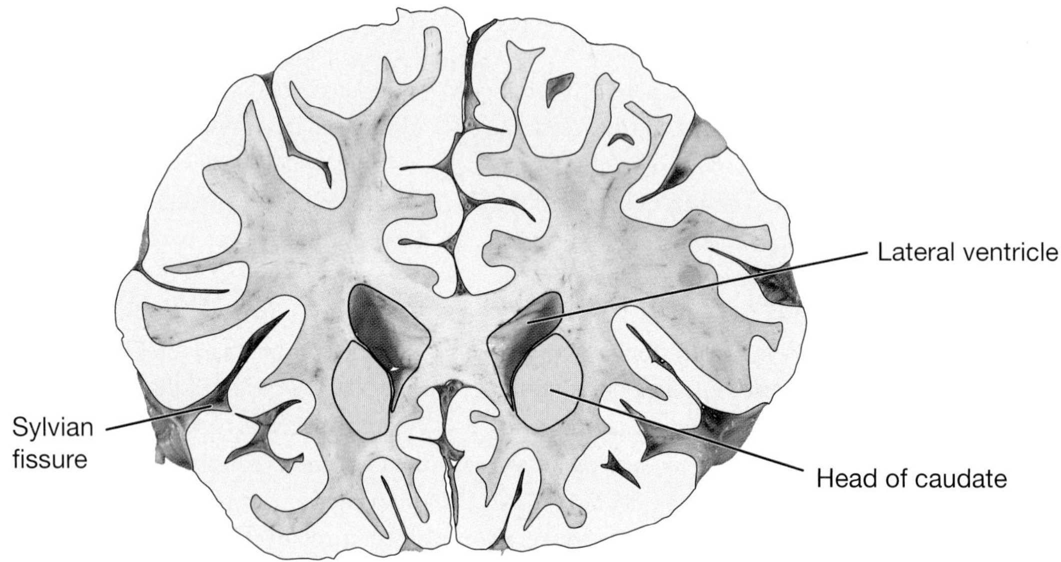

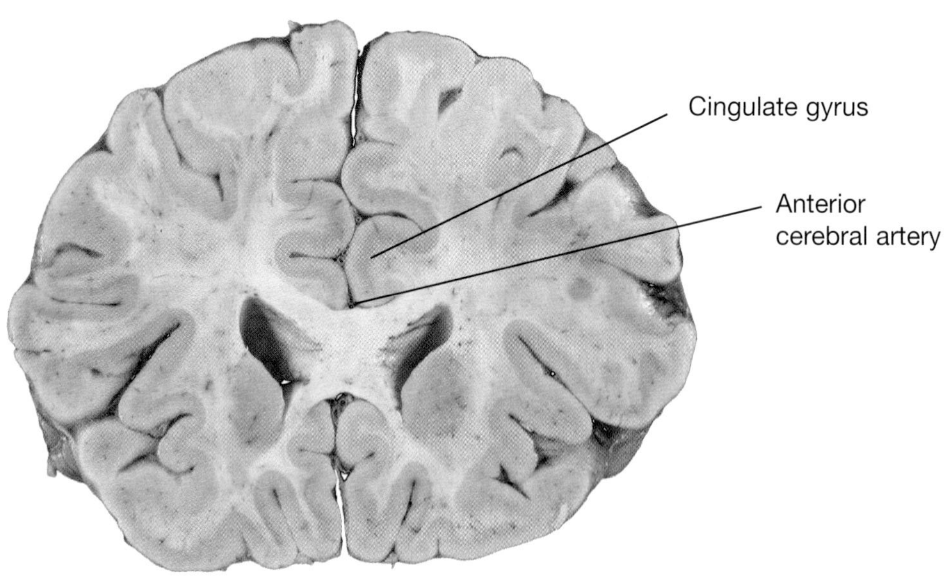

Fig. 3.18. Atlas of coronal sections through the cerebral hemispheres.

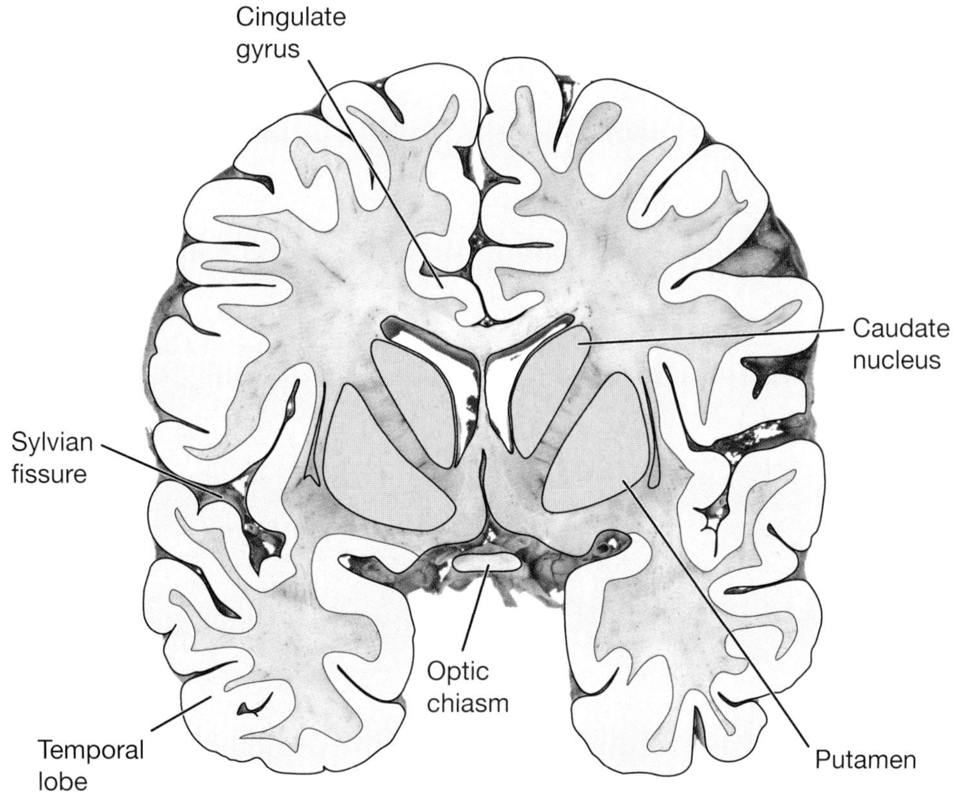
Cingulate gyrus
Caudate nucleus
Sylvian fissure
Optic chiasm
Temporal lobe
Putamen

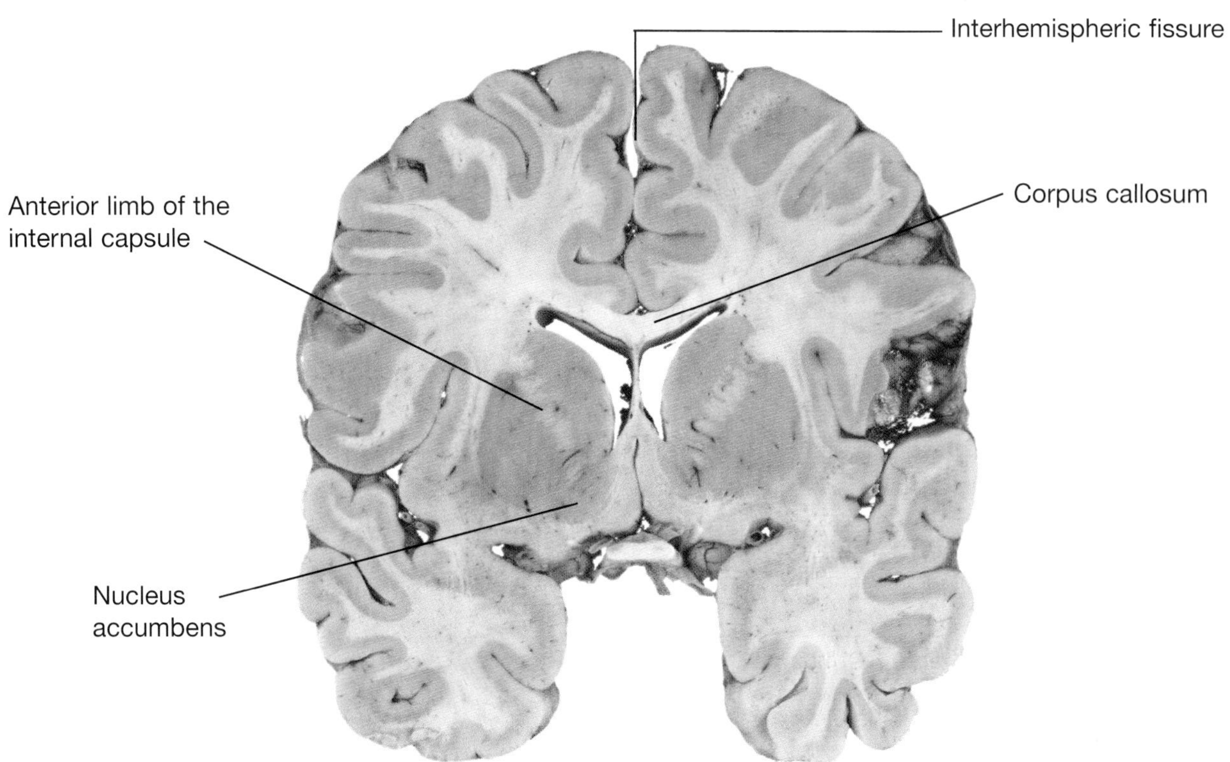
Interhemispheric fissure
Anterior limb of the internal capsule
Corpus callosum
Nucleus accumbens

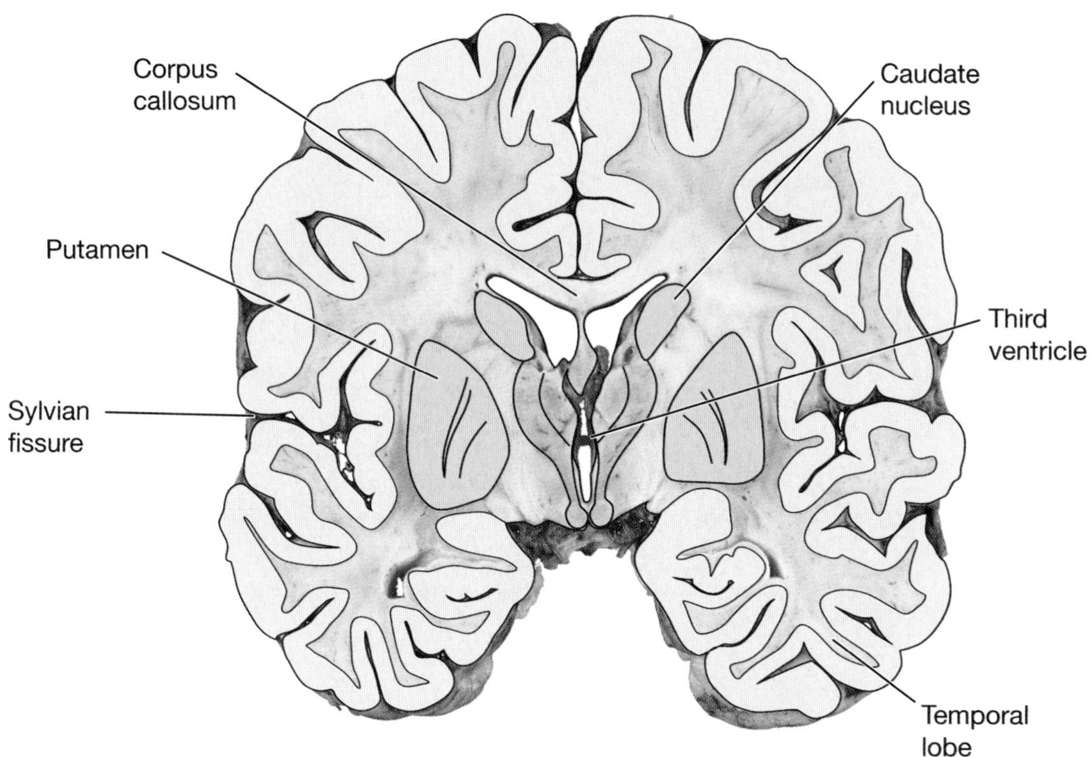
Corpus
callosum
Caudate
nucleus
Putamen
Third
ventricle
Sylvian
fissure
Temporal
lobe

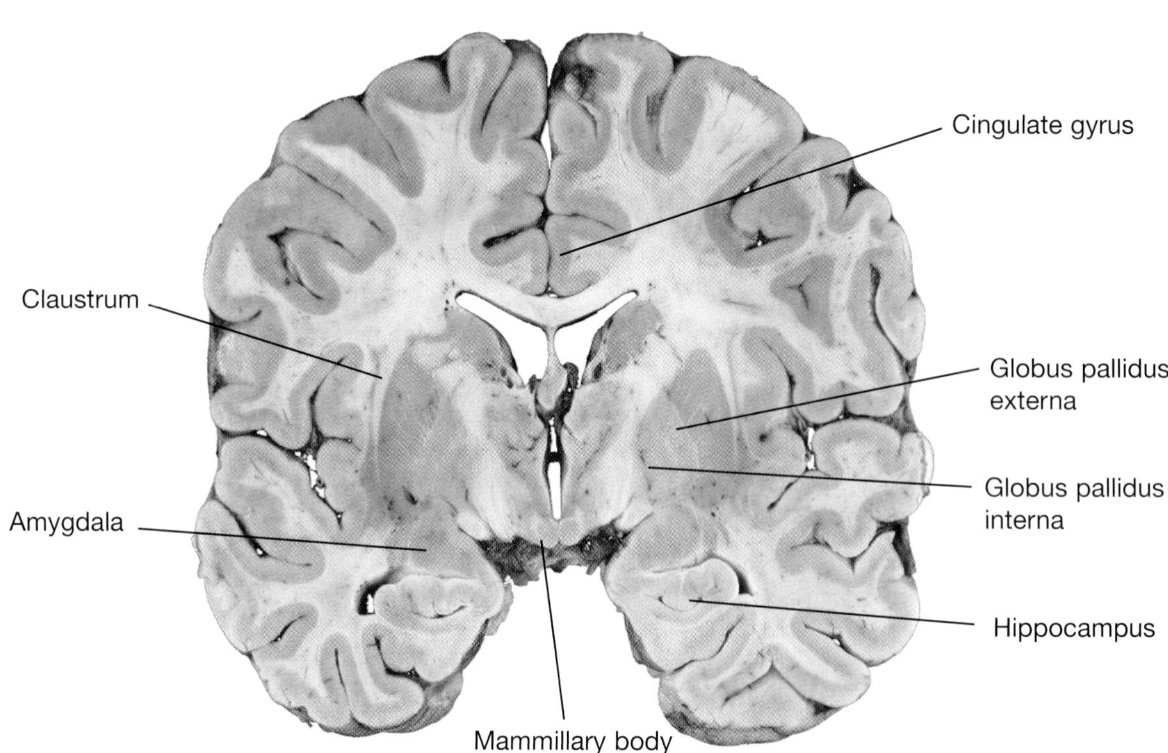
Cingulate gyrus
Claustrum
Globus pallidus
externa
Globus pallidus
interna
Amygdala
Hippocampus
Mammillary body

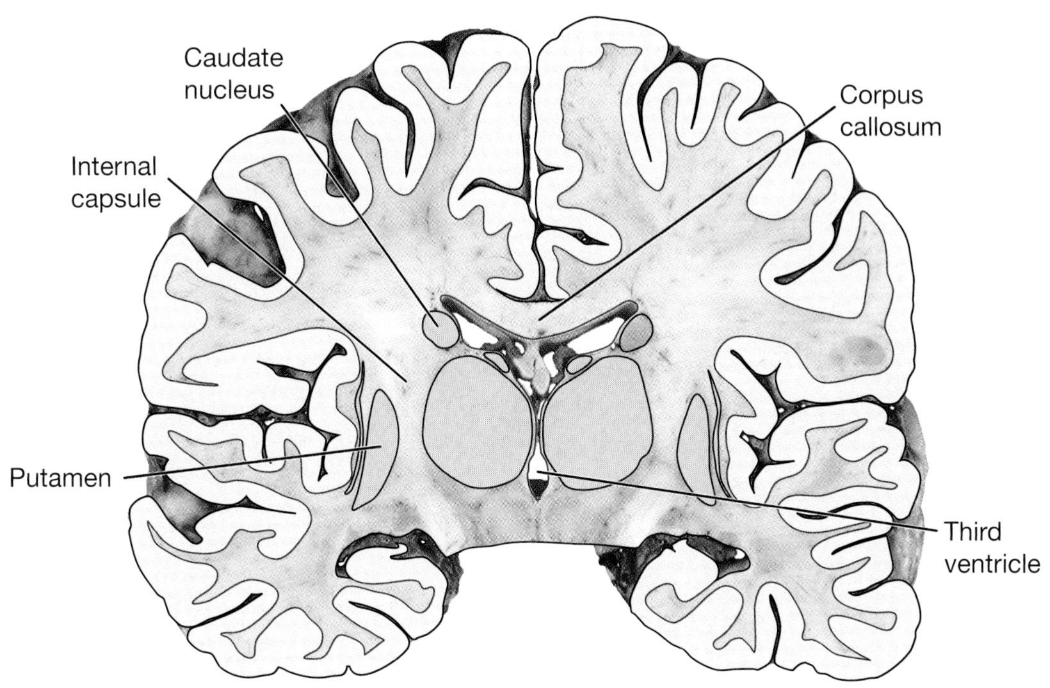
Caudate nucleus
Corpus callosum
Internal capsule
Putamen
Third ventricle

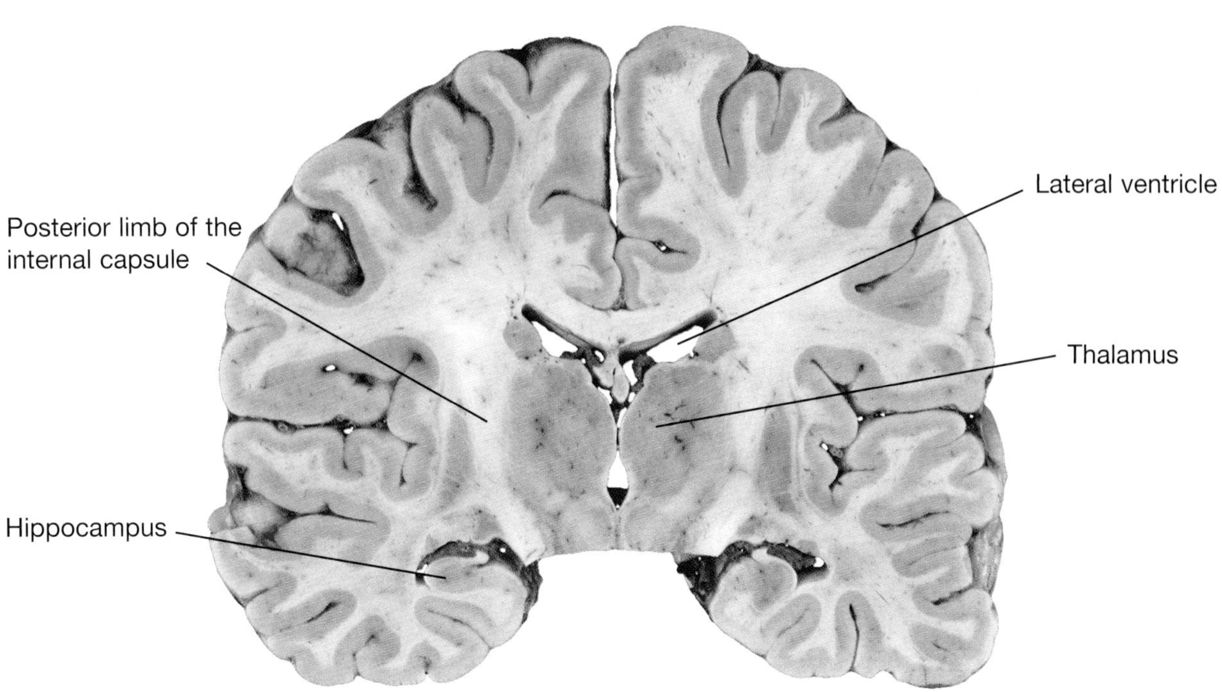
Lateral ventricle
Posterior limb of the internal capsule
Thalamus
Hippocampus

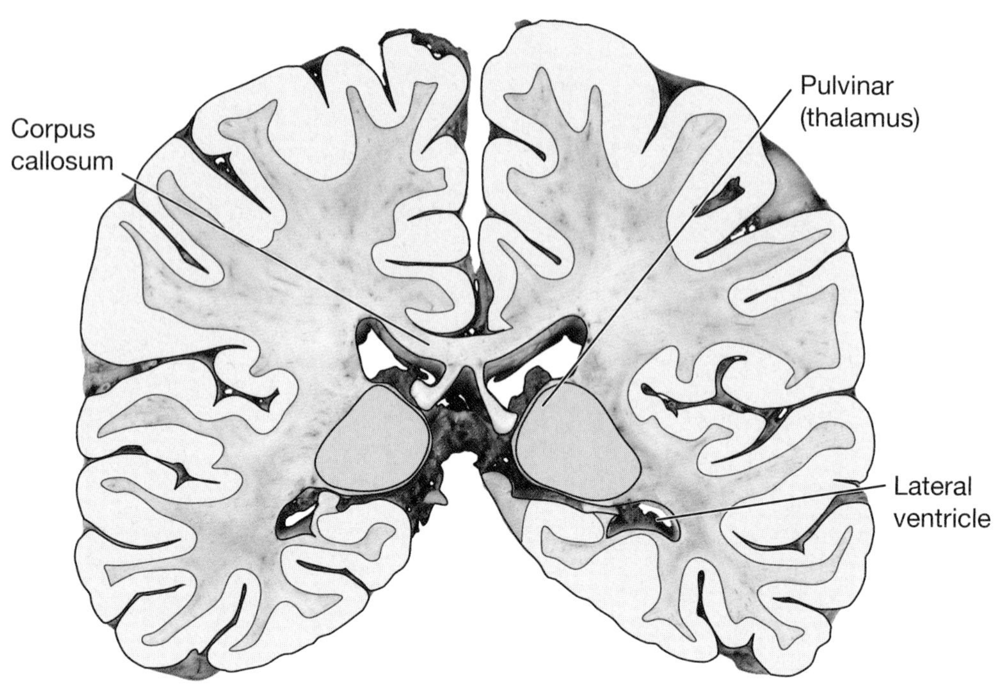
Corpus
callosum
Pulvinar
(thalamus)
Lateral
ventricle

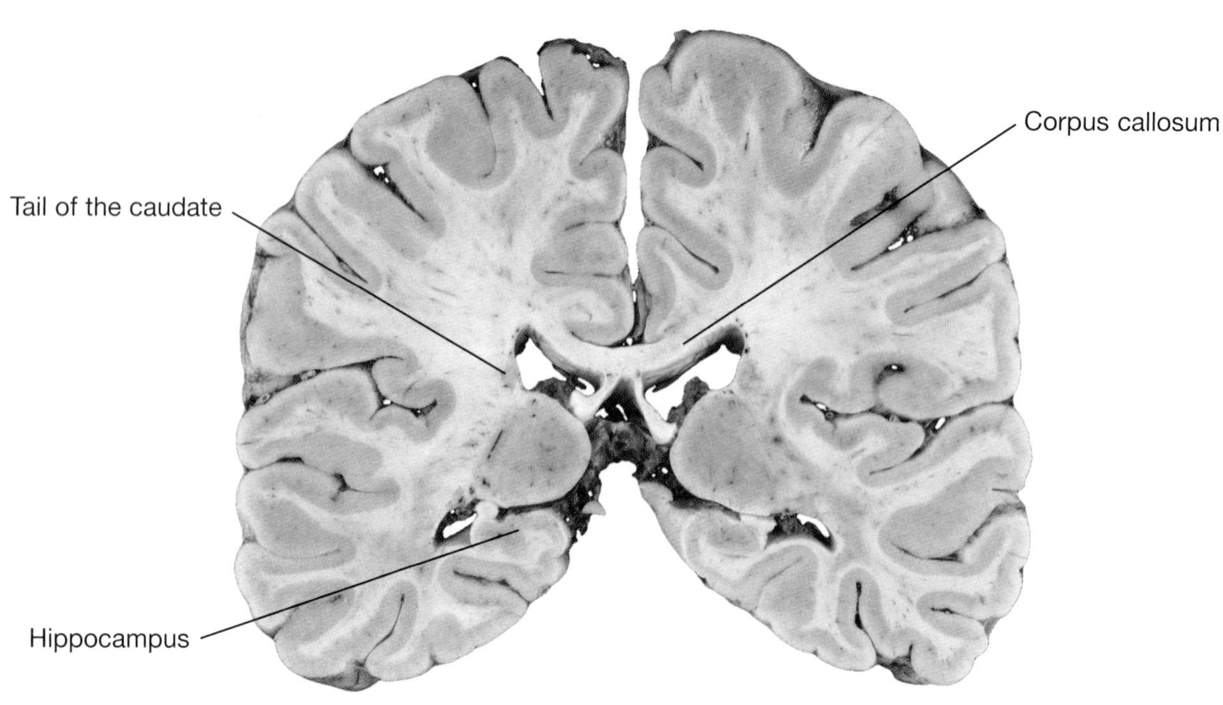
Corpus callosum
Tail of the caudate
Hippocampus

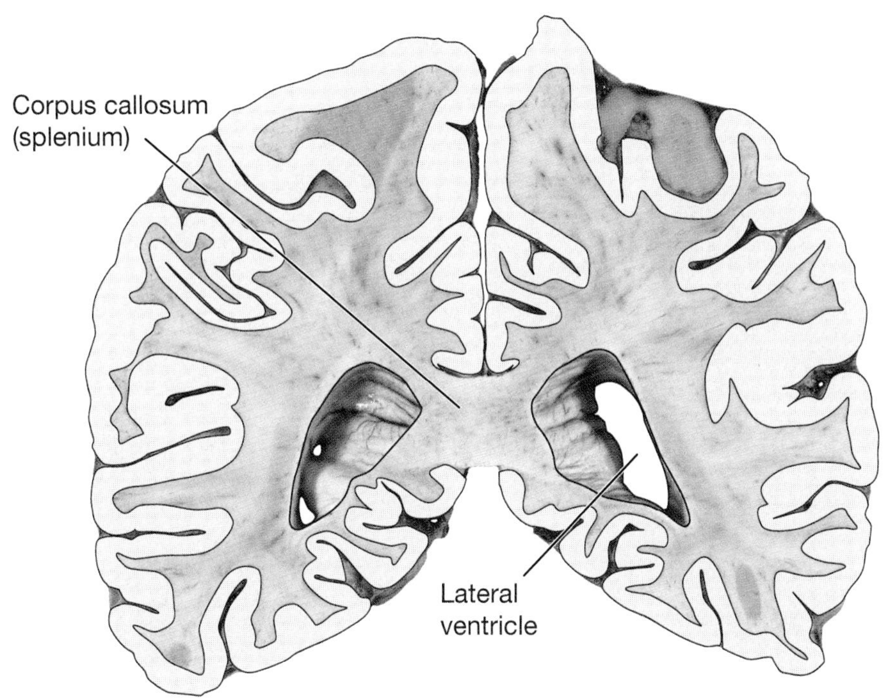
Corpus callosum
(splenium)
Lateral
ventricle

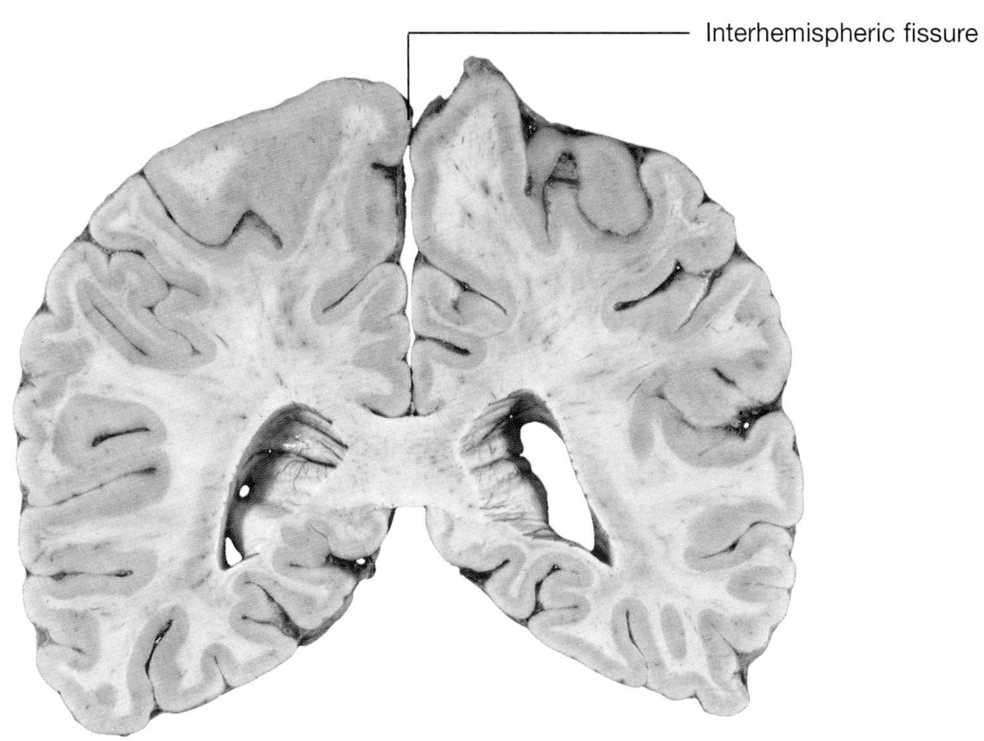
Interhemispheric fissure

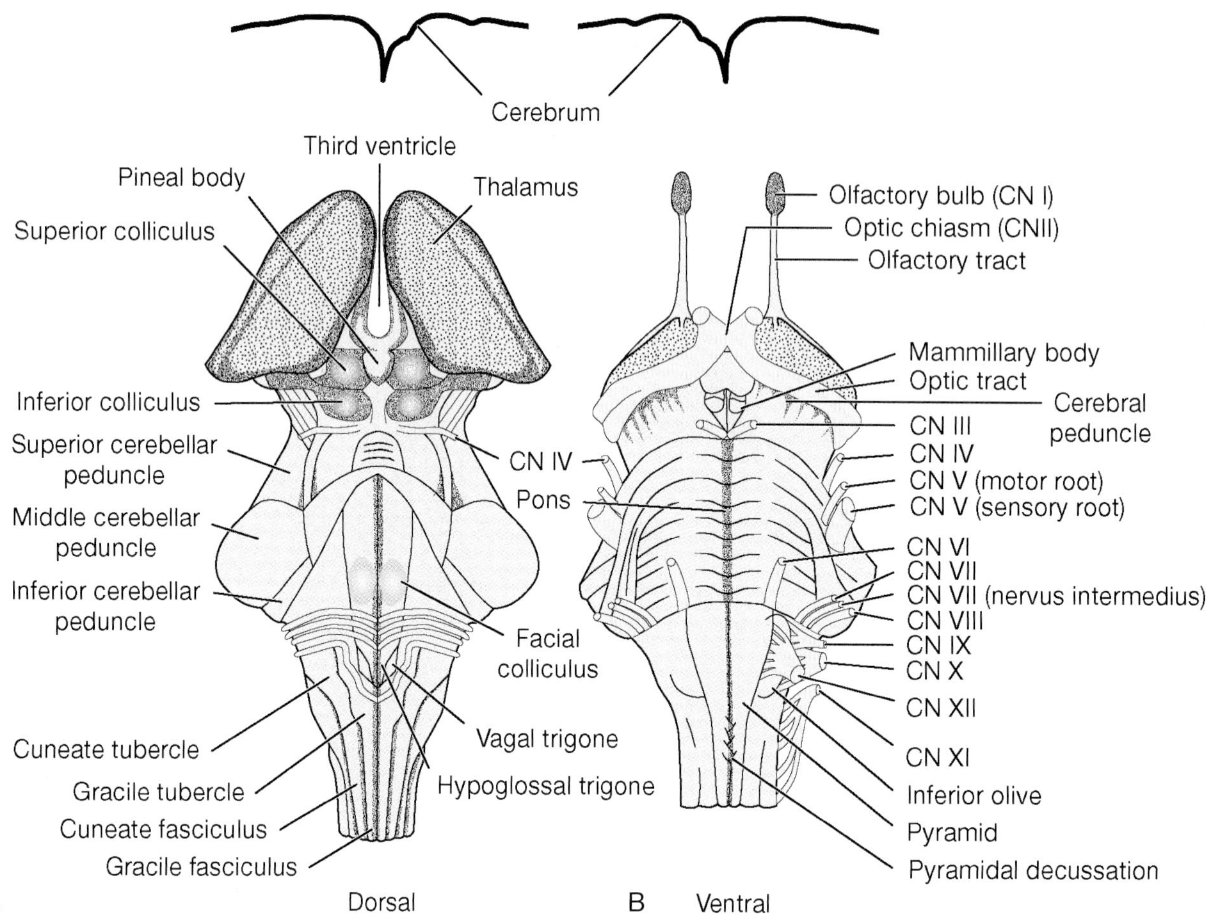

Fig. 3.19. Dorsal (*A*) and ventral (*B*) views of the brainstem and cranial nerves. CN, cranial nerve.

of the anterior divisions en route to the limbs come together and are rearranged into plexuses. The brachial plexus, located in the axillary region, redistributes the fibers to the major nerves of the upper extremities: the median, ulnar, radial, axillary, and musculocutaneous nerves. The lumbosacral plexus, located in the lower abdominal cavity and pelvis, redistributes the fibers to the major nerves in the lower extremities: the femoral, obturator, and sciatic nerves. The sciatic nerve divides into the tibial and peroneal nerves.

- The supratentorial level consists of the cerebral hemispheres, basal ganglia, thalamus, hypothalamus, and cranial nerves I and II.
  - Each cerebral hemisphere is composed of four anatomical lobes (frontal, parietal, temporal, and occipital) and one functional lobe, the limbic lobe.
  - The basal ganglia are paired nuclei deep in the hemisphere; they have a role in motor programming.
  - The thalami are located medially to the posterior limb of the internal capsule; they function as a relay station of information going to and coming from the cerebral cortex.
  - The hypothalamus is an important structure that integrates an autonomic, hormonal, or behavioral response with sensory input.
- The posterior fossa consists of the brainstem, cerebellum, and cranial nerves III–XII.
  - The brainstem consists of the medulla, pons, and midbrain.

Table 3.4. Location and General Function of the Cranial Nerves

	Cranial nerve	Anatomical relationship	Function
I	Olfactory	Cerebral hemisphere	Smell
II	Optic	Diencephalon	Vision
III	Oculomotor	Midbrain	Eye movement Pupil constriction
IV	Trochlear	Midbrain	Eye movement
V	Trigeminal	Pons	Facial sensation Mastication
VI	Abducens	Pons	Eye movement
VII	Facial	Pons	Facial movement Taste Lacrimation, salivation
VIII	Cochlear-vestibular	Pons, medulla	Hearing, equilibrium
IX	Glossopharyngeal	Medulla	Pharyngeal movement Taste Visceral sensory
X	Vagus	Medulla	Pharyngeal and laryngeal movement Visceral motor to organs Visceral sensory
XI	Spinal accessory	Spinal cord, medulla	Shoulder and neck movement
XII	Hypoglossal	Medulla	Tongue movement

  - The cerebellum has two hemispheres, a midline vermis, and a flocculonodular lobe; it has a role in coordination of motor acts.
- The spinal level consists of the spinal cord and its protective coverings.
- The peripheral level consists of cranial and spinal nerves.

Gross Neuroanatomy—Longitudinal Systems

The gross anatomical features of each major level have been reviewed. Here, some of these same structures are discussed in relation to the major longitudinal systems, which are described in detail in subsequent chapters.

The Cerebrospinal Fluid System

Structures included in the cerebrospinal fluid system are the meninges (the dura mater, arachnoid, and pia mater), the meningeal spaces (epidural, subdural, and subarachnoid), the ventricular system, and the cerebrospinal fluid. This system occurs at the supratentorial, posterior fossa, and spinal levels. It provides both a cushion and buffer for the central nervous system and helps maintain a stable environment for neural function.

Located within the depth of the brain is the *ventricular system*, which is derived from the primitive embryonic neural canal. Cerebrospinal fluid is formed in the lateral, third, and fourth ventricles by the choroid plexus and circulates throughout the ventricles and subarachnoid space.

The cavity contained within each cerebral hemisphere is the lateral ventricle, which communicates with the cavity of the diencephalon, the third ventricle, through the *foramen of Monro*. The caudal end of the third ventricle narrows into the cavity of the mesencephalon, the *aqueduct of Sylvius*, which leads into the fourth ventricle. The ventricular system communicates with the subarachnoid space through the two lateral *foramina of Luschka* and the *central foramen of Magendie* (all located in the walls of the fourth ventricle). The portion of the primitive central canal of the spinal cord becomes obliterated in the mature human nervous system and is usually identified only as a cluster of ependymal and glial cells in the central region of the spinal cord.

The Sensory System

The sensory system receives somatosensory information from the external environment and transmits it to the central nervous system (afferent), where it can be processed and used for adaptive behavior. Elements of the somatosensory system are found at all major levels and include the peripheral receptor organs; afferent fibers traveling in cranial, peripheral, and spinal nerves; dorsal root ganglia; ascending pathways in the spinal cord and brainstem; portions of the thalamus; and the thalamocortical radiations that terminate primarily in the sensory cortex of the parietal lobe. In addition, structures related to the special sensory systems (vision, taste, smell, hearing, and balance) are located at the supratentorial, posterior fossa, and peripheral levels.

The Motor System

The motor system initiates and controls activity in the somatic muscles. Components of this system include the motor cortex and other areas of the frontal lobes; descend-

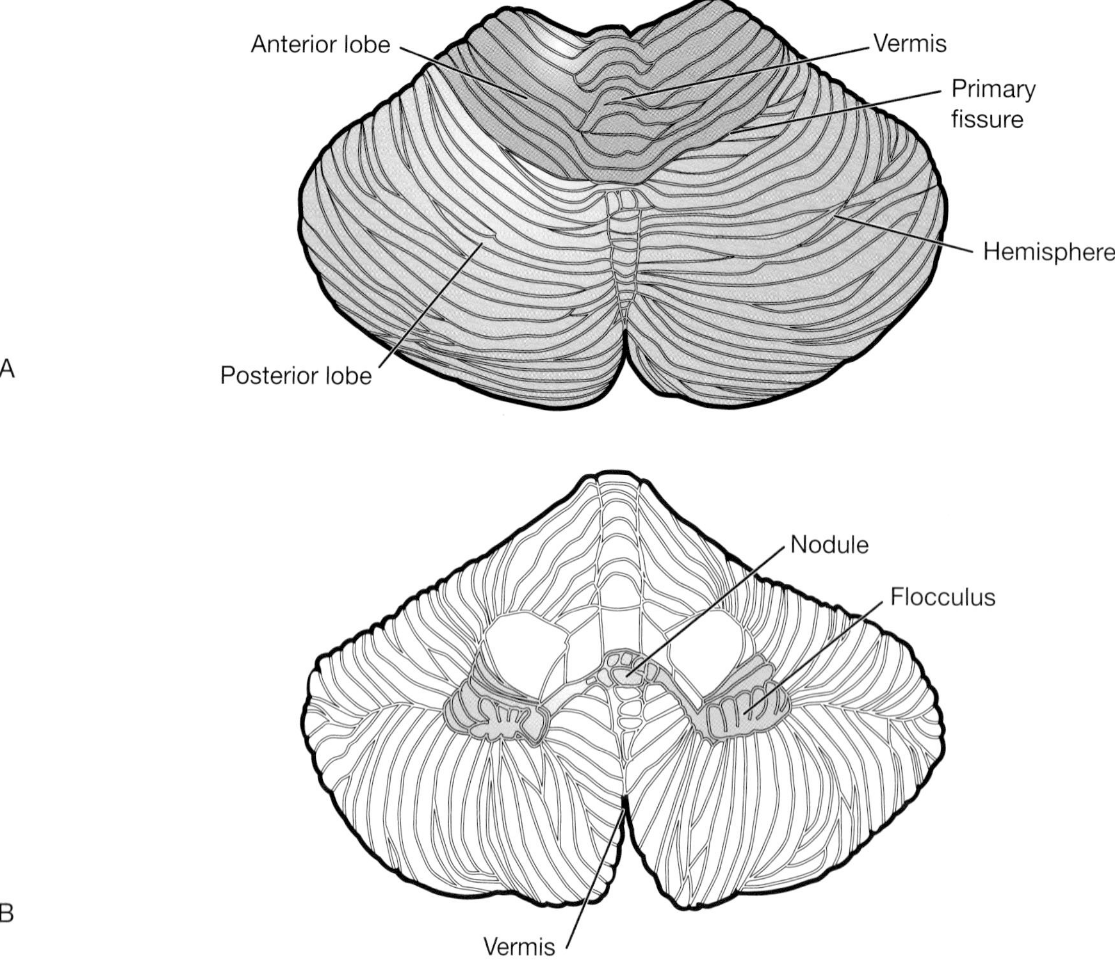

Fig. 3.20. Dorsal (*A*) and ventral (*B*) views of the cerebellum. Note that the ventral surface of the cerebellum cannot be seen unless the brainstem is removed.

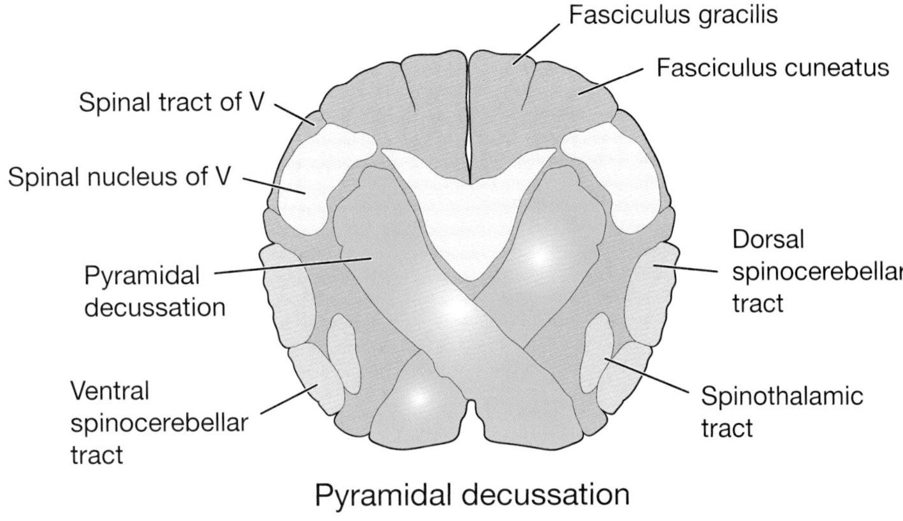

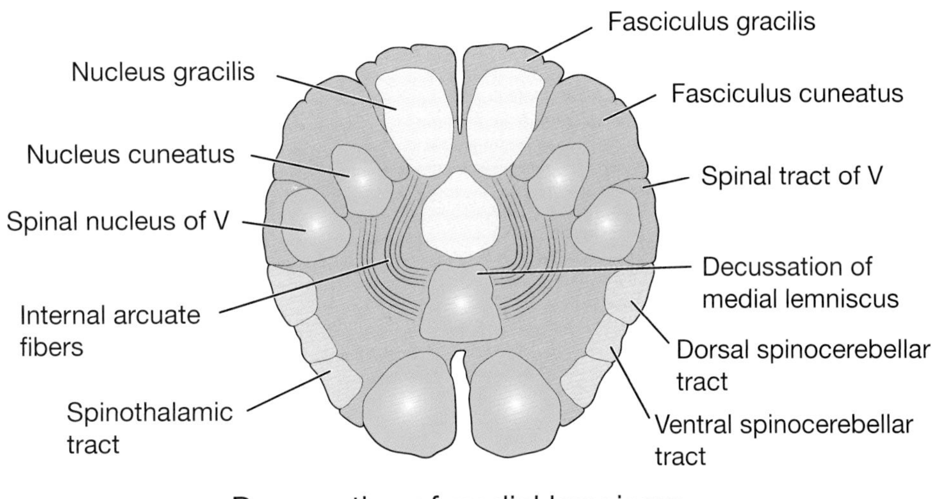

Fig. 3.21. Atlas of horizontal sections through the brainstem.

ing pathways that traverse the internal capsule, cerebral peduncles, medullary pyramids, and other areas of the brainstem; portions of the spinal cord, including the ventral horns; ventral roots; efferent fibers traveling in both peripheral and cranial nerves; and muscle, the major effector organ of the motor system. Also included in this system are the cerebellum and basal ganglia and related pathways. Thus, the motor system is present at all major levels and is directly involved in the performance of all motor activity mediated by striated musculature.

The Internal Regulation System

The internal regulation system consists of the structures in the nervous system that monitor and control the function of visceral glands and organs. It contains both afferent and efferent components, which interact to maintain the internal environment (homeostasis). The system has major representation at all levels of the nervous system. Important structures include areas of the limbic lobe and hypothalamus (supratentorial level); the *reticular formation* and fibers traveling in cranial nerves (posterior fossa

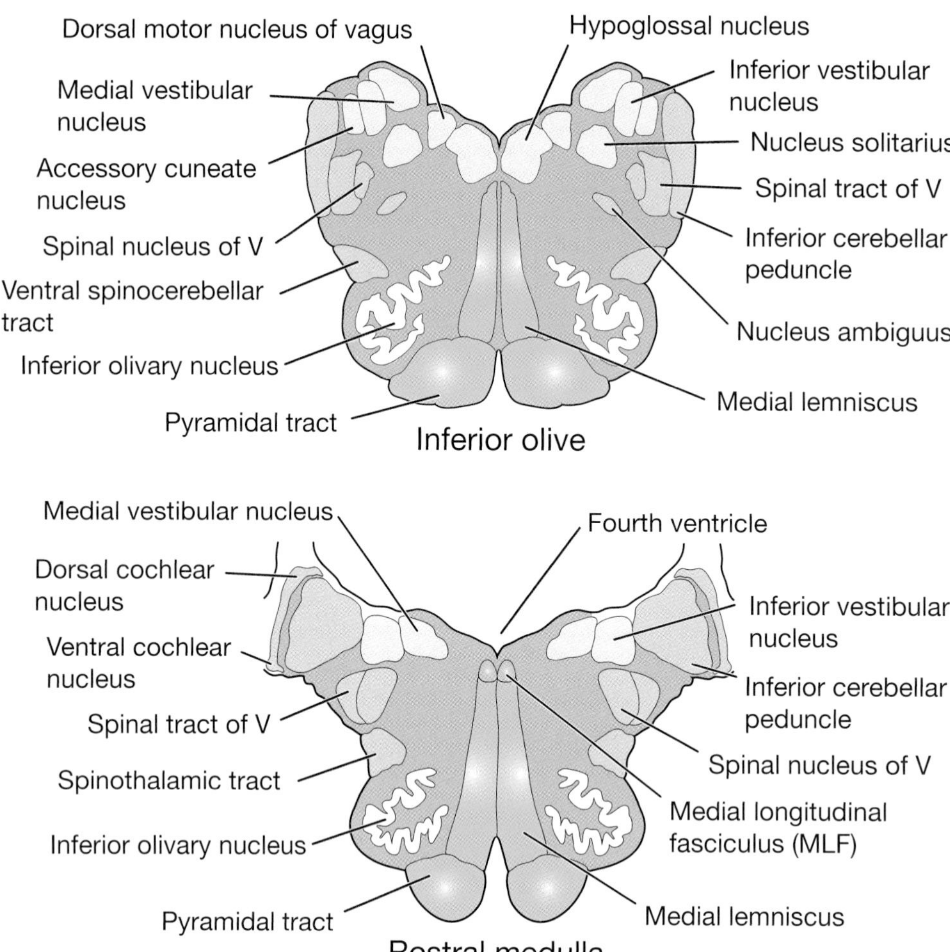

level); longitudinal pathways in the spinal cord and brainstem; and numerous ganglia, receptors, and effectors in the peripheral level.

The Consciousness System

Functioning as an additional afferent system, the consciousness system allows a person to attend selectively to and perceive isolated stimuli. This system maintains various levels of wakefulness, awareness, and consciousness. Structures contained within this system are found only at the posterior fossa and supratentorial levels and include portions of the central core of the brainstem and diencephalon (reticular formation and ascending projectional pathways), portions of the thalamus, basal forebrain, and pathways that project diffusely to the cerebral cortex. All lobes of the cerebral hemispheres are part of this system.

The Vascular System

Each organ in the body must have blood vessels to provide a relatively constant supply of oxygen and other nutrients and to remove metabolic waste. The vascular system is found at all major levels of the nervous system and includes the arteries, arterioles, capillaries, veins, and dural sinuses. These supply supratentorial, posterior fossa, spinal, and peripheral nervous system structures.

Blood enters the skull through two arterial systems. The brain is supplied by the posteriorly located *vertebrobasilar* system and the anteriorly located *carotid* system. A series of anastomotic channels at the base of the brain, known as the *circle of Willis*, provides communication between these two systems.

The *internal carotid artery* and its major branches, the *anterior cerebral* and *middle cerebral arteries*, are at the base of

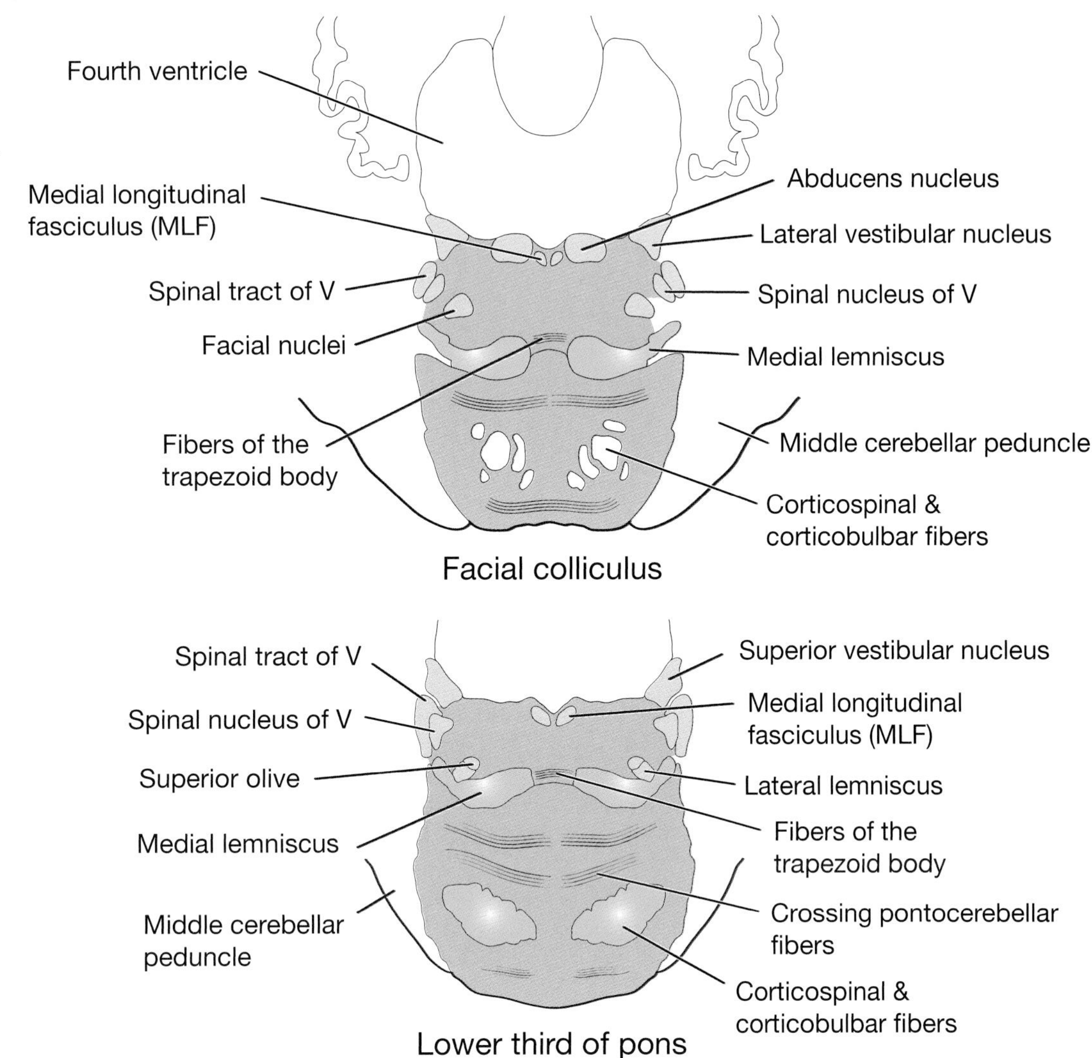

the brain (Fig. 3.23). The anterior cerebral arteries are connected to one another by the small anterior communicating artery and continue in the midline between the two hemispheres to supply blood to the medial surface of each hemisphere. The middle cerebral artery courses laterally between the temporal and frontal lobes and emerges from the insula in the sylvian fissure. Its branches spread over and supply blood to the lateral surface of the hemisphere.

Blood is also carried to the brain by the two *vertebral arteries*, which enter the skull through the foramen magnum and join at the caudal border of the pons to form the *basilar artery* (Fig. 3.23). Branches from these arteries are normally the sole arterial supply to the occipital lobe, the inferior surface of the temporal lobe, thalamus, midbrain, pons, cerebellum, medulla, and portions of the cervical spinal cord. The *posterior inferior cerebellar arteries* are branches of the vertebral arteries, and the *anterior inferior cerebellar* and *superior cerebellar arteries* are branches of the basilar artery.

The basilar artery continues cephalad and divides into the posterior cerebral arteries. The posterior communicating arteries usually arise as branches of the posterior cerebral arteries and join these vessels with the internal carotid arteries to complete the circle of Willis.

Blood leaves the head by way of veins (Fig. 3.24) that course over the cerebral hemispheres to converge into large channels, the venous sinuses, contained within the layers of the dura mater. The most prominent of these sinuses are the *superior sagittal sinus* and *inferior sagittal sinus*, which extend longitudinally from front to back in the falx cerebri between the cerebral hemispheres. The major venous

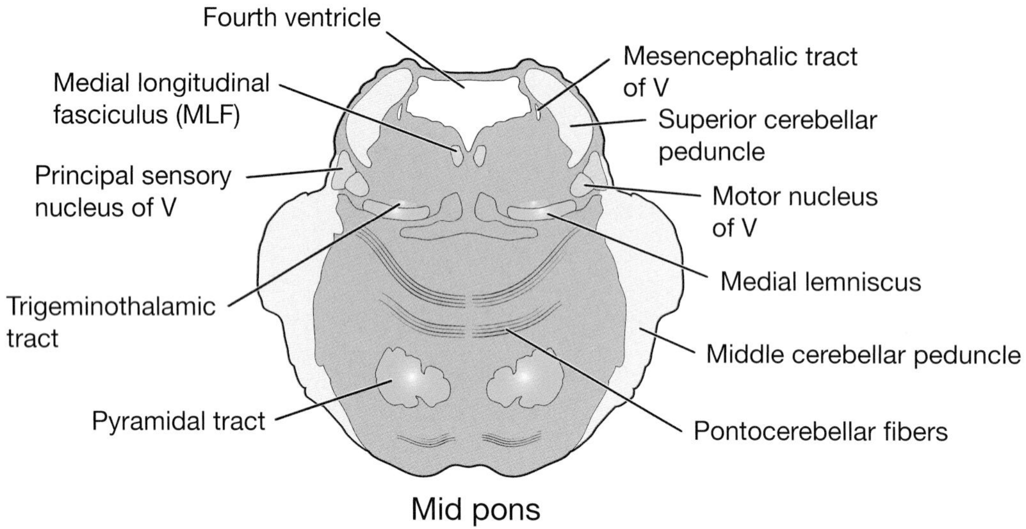

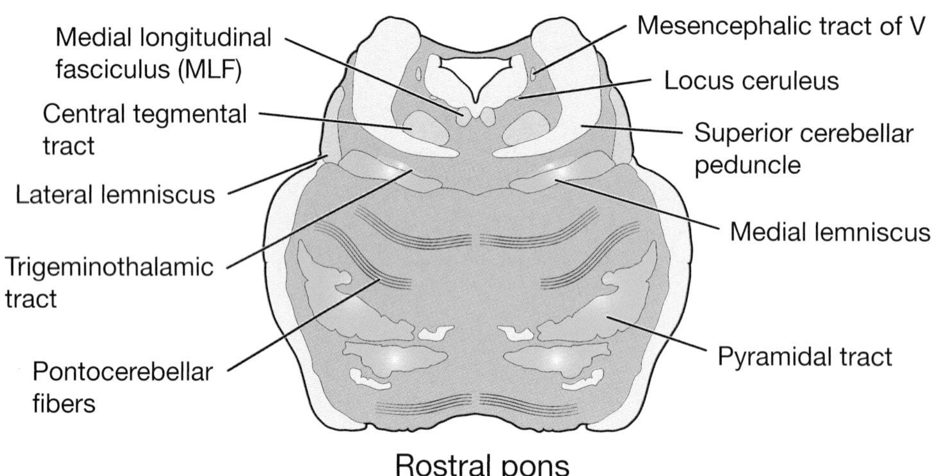

channels merge in the occipital region and form the *transverse* and *sigmoid sinuses*, which exit the skull through the jugular foramen as the internal jugular veins.

- Cerebrospinal fluid is produced in the ventricular system and flows into the subarachnoid space around the brain and spinal cord, thereby cushioning these structures. It is reabsorbed into the venous system.
- The sensory system is composed of four types of afferent information, each with a specific receptor type and pathway from the periphery into the central nervous system. The general somatic afferent pathway synapses in the thalamus before terminating in the primary sensory cortex.
- The motor system comprises the motor unit and cortical and associated subcortical structures (basal ganglia, cerebellum, red nucleus, and vestibular system).
- The internal regulation system is composed of structures that monitor and control the function of the visceral glands and organs.
- The consciousness system is related to important structures in the supratentorial (cerebral hemispheres, thalamus) and posterior fossa regions (reticular formation).
- The internal carotid artery and its major branches, including the anterior and middle cerebral arteries, supply blood to the major regions of the cerebral hemispheres. The vertebrobasilar system and branches

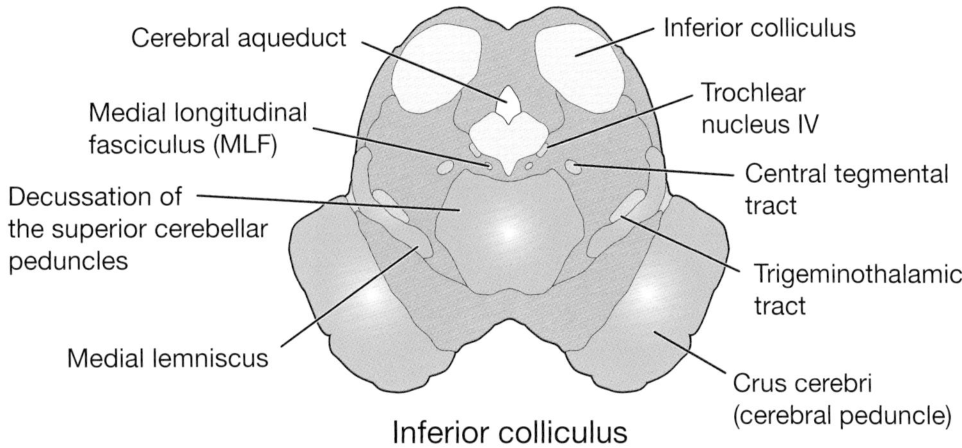

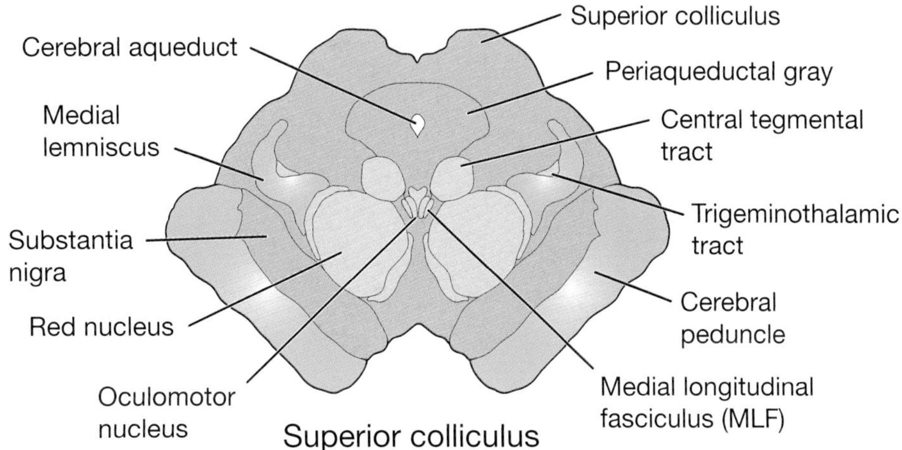

supply the posterior fossa and the inferior temporal and occipital lobes of the brain.

Introduction to Neuroimaging

Many imaging modalities are available for noninvasively visualizing anatomical structures of the brain and spinal cord. Images may be presented in various planes, as shown in Figure 3.25.

Computed tomography shows the anatomical structure of the brain, skull, spinal cord, and vertebral column. It provides excellent detail of the bones but less detail about the soft tissue and parenchyma of the brain, especially in areas where thick bone causes distortion or artifact of the soft tissue. *Magnetic resonance imaging* is superior to computed tomography for visualizing details of the soft tissue and brain parenchyma. Nerve roots may also be visible with magnetic resonance imaging. Computed tomography and magnetic resonance imaging of the brain are compared in Figure 3.26.

Arteries can be visualized anatomically with *angiography* and *ultrasonography*. Noninvasive angiographic techniques include magnetic resonance angiography (Fig. 3.27) and computed tomographic angiography. These techniques can also visualize the venous system (*venography*). Arteriography, or "conventional angiography," is a technique in which contrast dye is injected through a catheter into arteries of the brain and radiographs made at specified time intervals. Both the arterial and venous phases can be visualized. Ultrasonography can also be used to evaluate the vasculature, although it is limited in that only certain blood vessels can be imaged with this method.

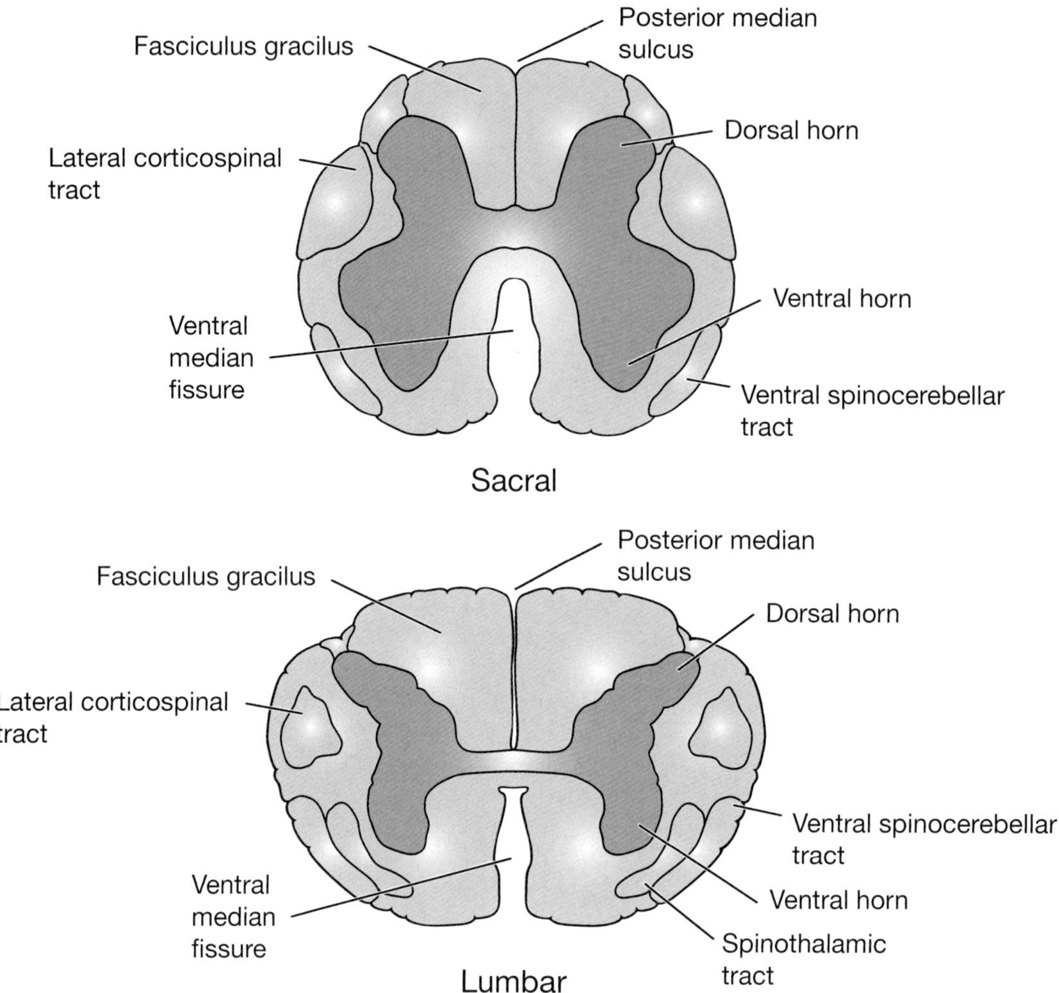

Fig. 3.22. Atlas of cross sections through levels of the spinal cord.

General Principles of Connectivity: Approach to Clinical Problem Solving

Neurologic diagnosis includes identification of the anatomical location and pathology of the disorder. Through the use of problem-solving skills that are already familiar and the assignment of some functional significance to the anatomical structures discussed in this chapter, one can begin to solve clinical neurologic problems by identifying the anatomical location.

In certain respects, an analogy may be drawn between the nervous system and an electrical circuit. The nervous system can be considered a series of electrical cables laid out according to a specific plan (Fig. 3.28). Leading to and from the cerebral hemispheres are two parallel intersegmental cables (representing a longitudinal system) that conduct impulses from one segment to another. Scattered along these intersegmental cables are several smaller branching segmental wires. As in an electrical circuit, damage (a lesion) anywhere along the course of the main intersegmental cables causes malfunction in all areas beyond that point, but damage to a segmental wire causes malfunction only within that segment. This analogy can be applied to the human nervous system: the higher centers exert control or receive information from the body segments through long intersegmental pathways and one cerebral hemisphere is associated with function on the opposite side of the body.

Anatomical diagnosis first requires the ability to relate the patient's signs and symptoms to specific longitudinal

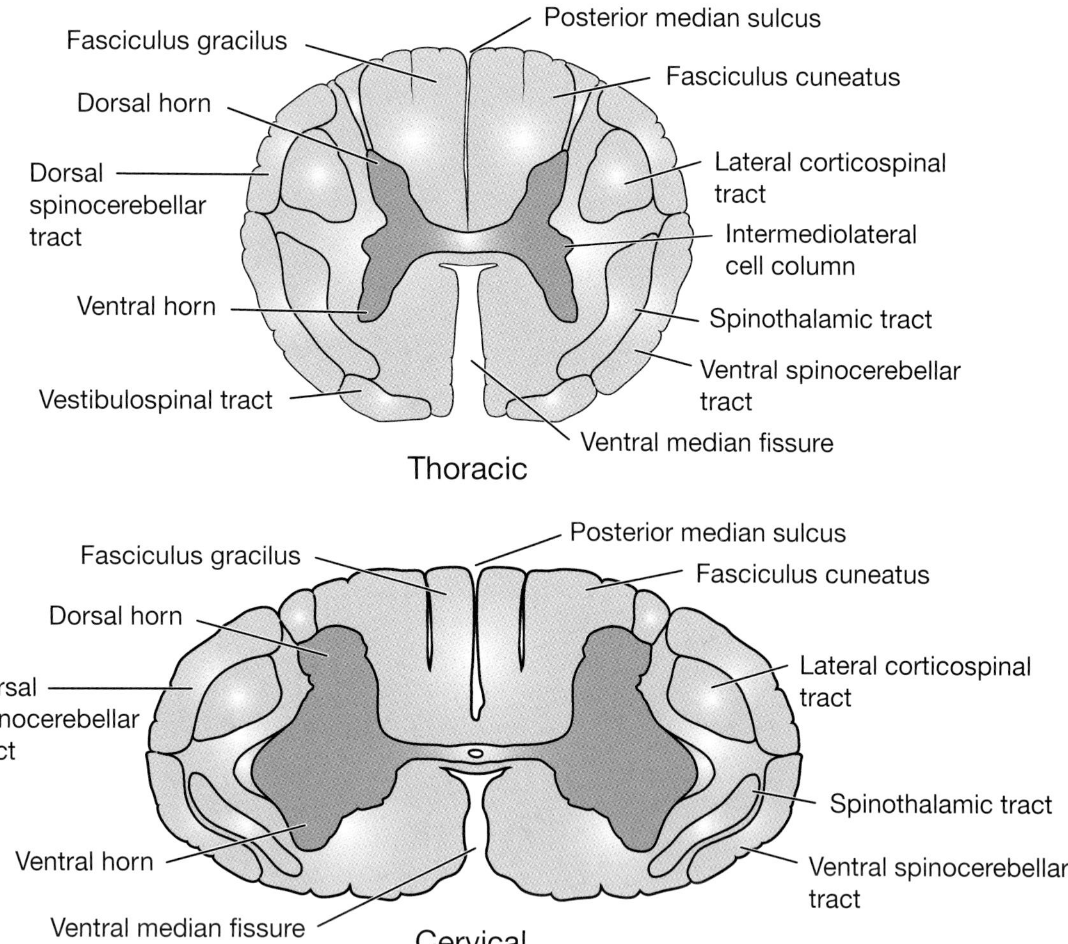

systems within the nervous system. Neurologic diagnosis relies mainly on the symptoms of dysfunction in the sensory, motor, and consciousness systems. Symptoms of dysfunction in the sensory system consist of altered sensation, described by the patient as pain, numbness, tingling, or loss of sensation. Symptoms of dysfunction in the motor system consist primarily of weakness, paralysis, incoordination, shaking, or jerking. Lesions of the consciousness system, which is located only at the supratentorial and posterior fossa levels, are expressed as altered states of consciousness and coma. The presence of any of these or related symptoms identifies the longitudinal system involved in a disease.

Localization is determined by the level of the nervous system in which the pathway function is interrupted. To aid in localization, the functions of each of the major anatomical levels are described in the following sections and are schematically represented in Figure 3.29 and summarized in Table 3.5.

Peripheral Level

The spinal and cranial nerves (after emerging from the vertebral column and skull) and the structures they innervate constitute the major components of the peripheral level. Each emerging nerve defines a specific segment. A lesion in one of these nerves alters all function within that segment but has no effect on functions carried to and from other segments. Thus, with a peripheral lesion, the loss of sensation and muscle weakness in a focal area are common. Often, peripheral nerve damage is not complete and the sensation of pain is produced. Therefore, in addition to sensory loss and muscle weakness, pain in a segmental distribution is an important clue to a lesion at the peripheral level.

- Peripheral lesions cause an ipsilateral segmental deficit (usually sensory or motor or both).

Spinal Level

The spinal cord has two functions. It is the structure from which nerves to individual segments of the limbs and trunk originate, and it transmits information to and from higher centers. Therefore, lesions at the spinal level may alter segmental function in the region of the abnormality and alter intersegmental function below the level of the lesion. Except in complete transections of the spinal cord, all functions are not altered equally; however, even under those circumstances, the characteristic combination of segmental loss of function at the site of the lesion and intersegmental loss below the lesion usually can be identified.

The spinal cord is a narrow structure that contains the major intersegmental pathways for both sides of the neuraxis (nervous system). Therefore, with spinal lesions, bilateral involvement from a single focal lesion is not uncommon. Because of the length of the spinal column, specific segmental functions can be assigned to certain

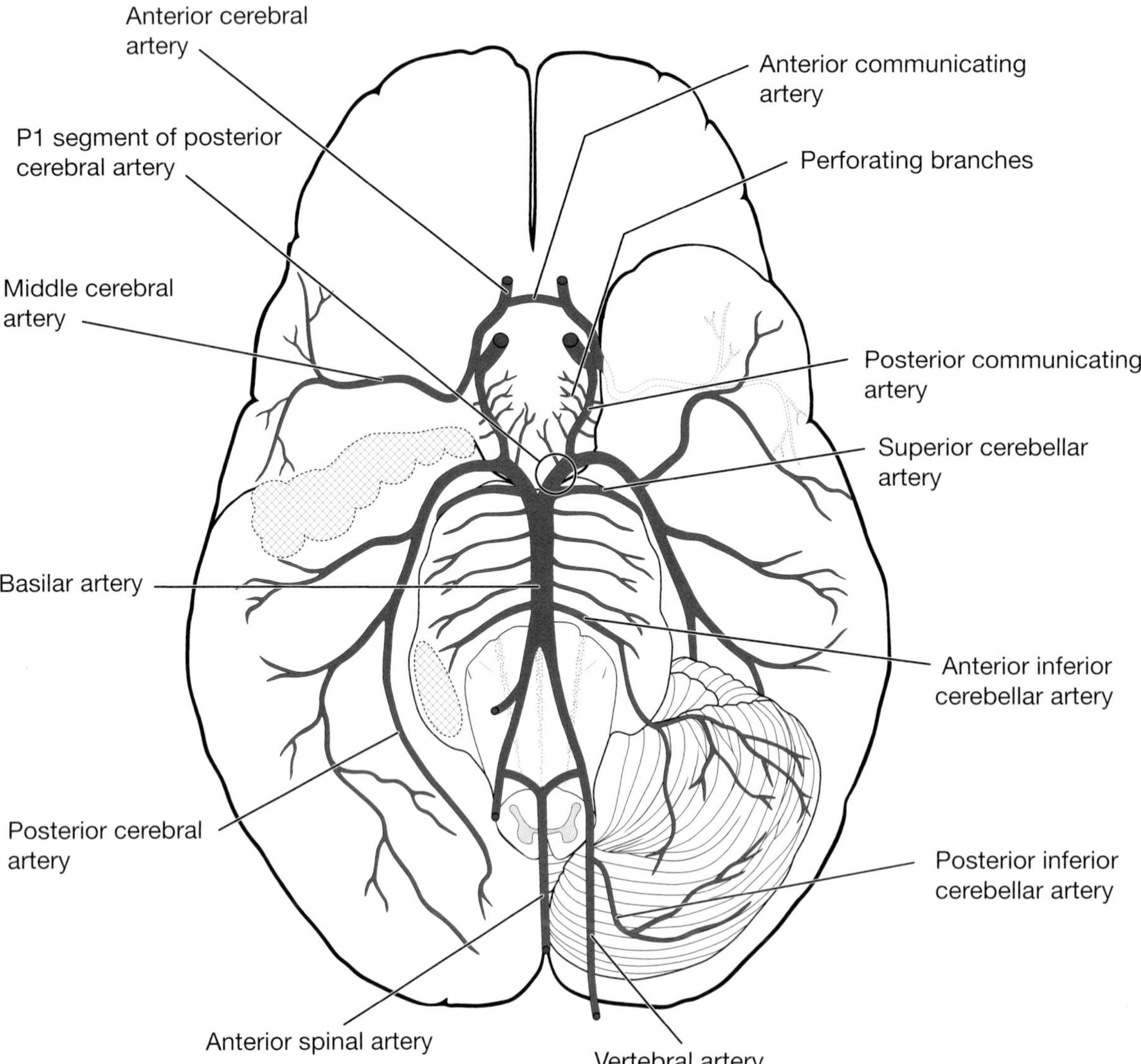

Fig. 3.23. The major cerebral arteries as visualized on the base of the brain.

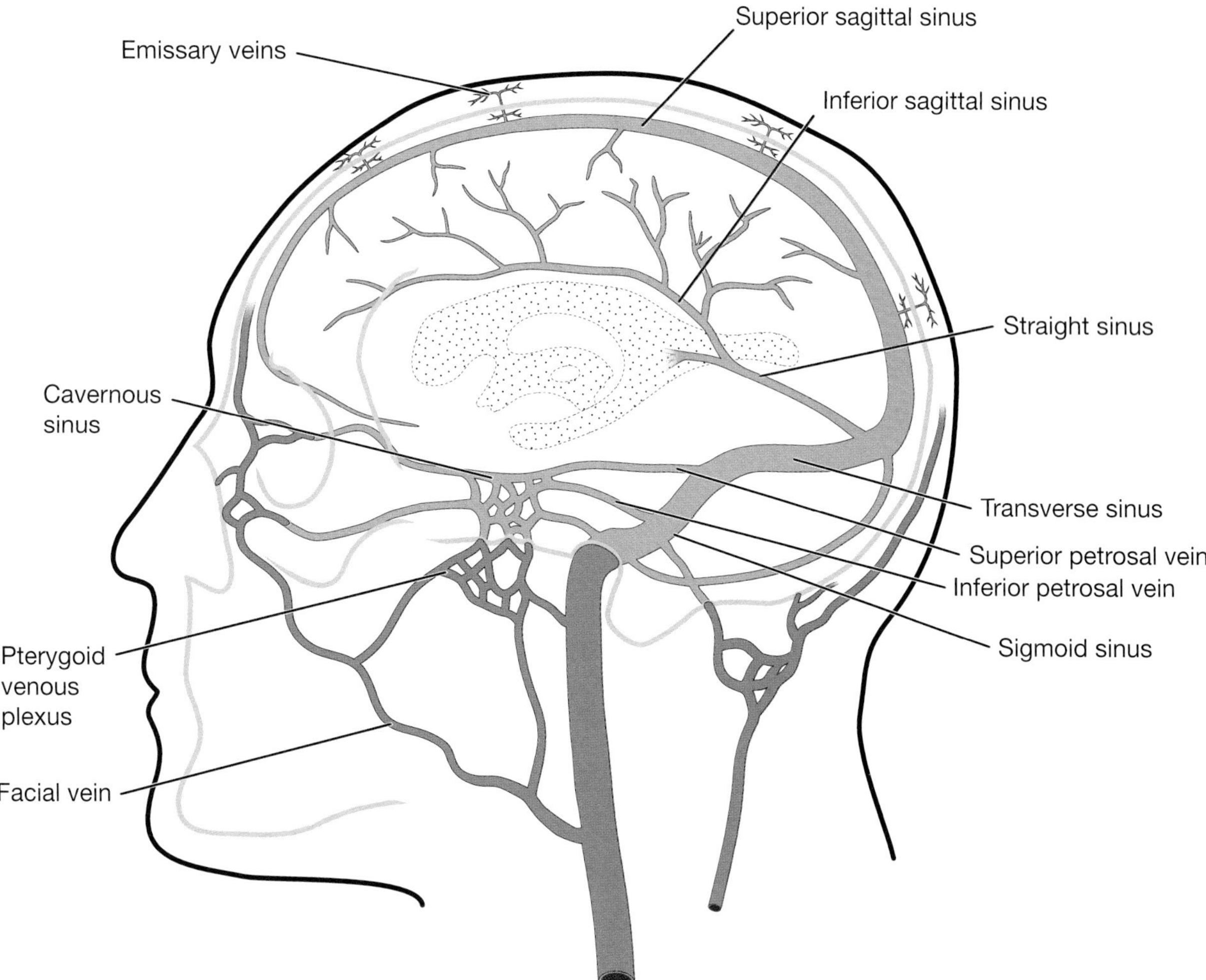

Fig. 3.24. Cerebral veins. Blood circulating over the cerebral cortex collects in the superior sagittal sinus; blood from deeper structures enters other venous sinuses. The direction of flow is toward the confluence of sinuses in the occipital region and then toward the internal jugular veins by way of the transverse and sigmoid sinuses.

levels. The upper portion of the spinal cord (cervical segments) is related primarily to arm function, the midportion is related to trunk function, and the lower portion (lumbar segments) is related to leg function.

- Cervical segments affect arm function; lumbar segments affect leg function; and sacral segments affect bladder, bowel, and sexual functions.
- A lesion of the spinal cord may result in segmental dysfunction at a particular level, but it may also interfere with intersegmental function (i.e., descending motor or ascending sensory tracts) below the level of the lesion.

Posterior Fossa Level

The cranial nerves mediate segmental function for the head and arise in the posterior fossa. Therefore, lesions at the posterior fossa level produce segmental and intersegmental disturbances, just as at the spinal level. The segmental nerves of the brainstem are the cranial nerves, which control movement and sensation in the head (Table 3.5). Brainstem lesions often alter these segmental functions. Also, because the brainstem is an area where intersegmental pathways cross or have crossed the midline, a characteristic pattern is often seen with focal lesions. Lesions of the posterior fossa cause loss of segmental head function

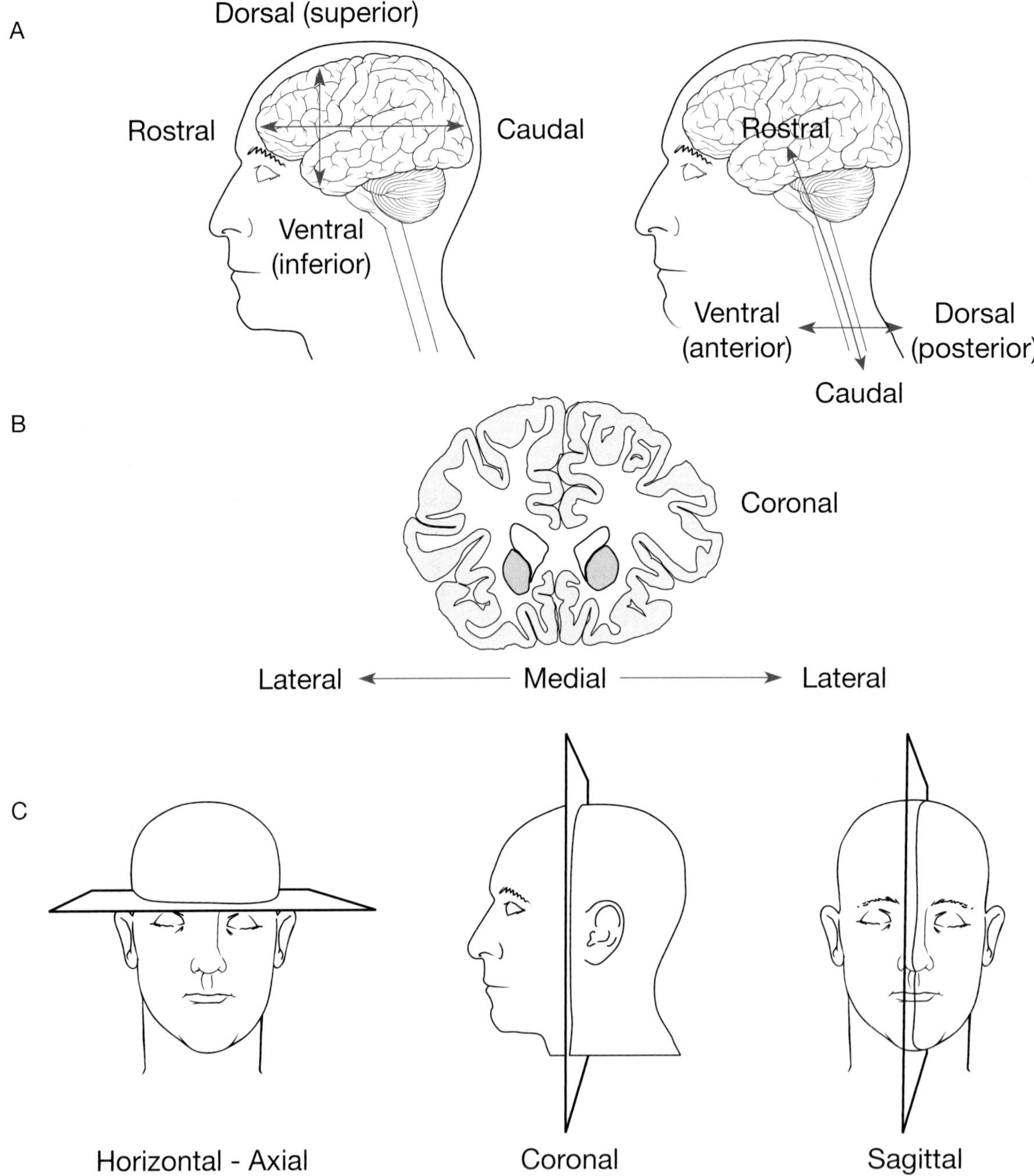

Fig. 3.25. *A* and *B*, The nomenclature used to describe the location of anatomical structures. *C*, The planes in which structures may be visualized radiographically and pathologically.

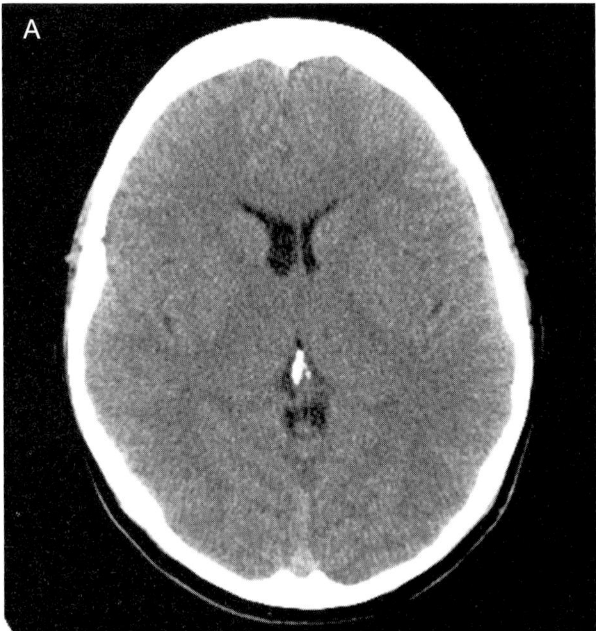

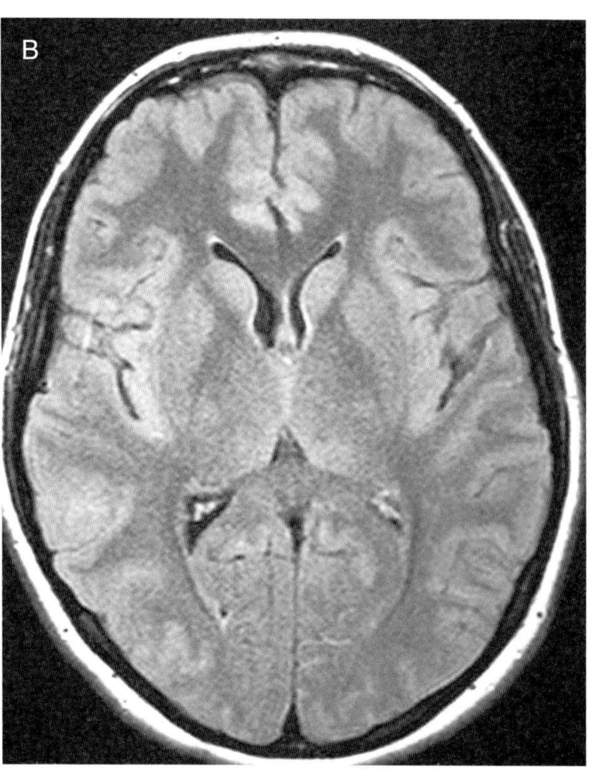

Fig. 3.26. Axial sections through the level of the internal capsule. *A*, Computed tomographic scan. *B*, Magnetic resonance image, T2/FLAIR sequence.

ipsilateral (same side) to the lesion; if the lesion also involves intersegmental pathways, it causes loss of intersegmental function on the side of the body contralateral (opposite) to the lesion (Fig. 3.29). Extensive lesions in the brainstem may affect the consciousness system and produce coma.

The cerebellum influences motor coordination. The left cerebellar hemisphere influences the left limbs and the right cerebellar hemisphere, the right limbs. The midline, or vermis, of the cerebellum influences posture (axial musculature).

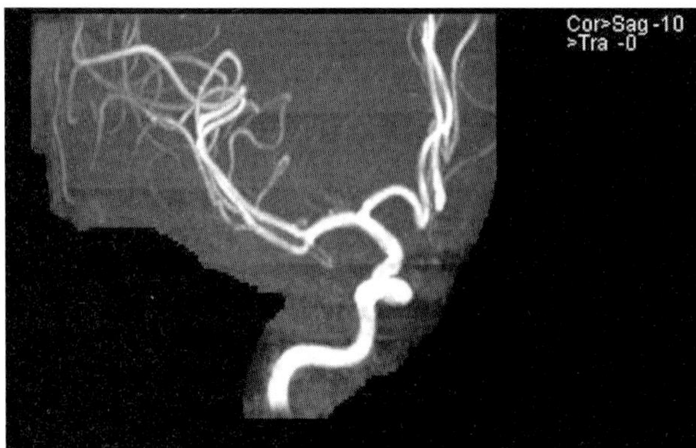

Fig. 3.27. Magnetic resonance angiographic image (sagittal view) showing the vasculature of the anterior circulation.

- Cranial nerve lesions (of the nuclei or ganglia) result in *ipsilateral* segmental dysfunction.
- A lesion of the brainstem may result in segmental dysfunction at a particular level (e.g., a cranial nerve lesion), but it may also interfere with intersegmental function (ascending sensory and descending motor tracts) below the level of the lesion.
- The cerebellum influences motor coordination on the *ipsilateral* side.

Supratentorial Level

Each cerebral hemisphere exerts control over the opposite side of the body. Therefore, supratentorial lesions are associated with loss of intersegmental sensory or motor function on the opposite side of the body. In addition, some functions are associated almost exclusively with

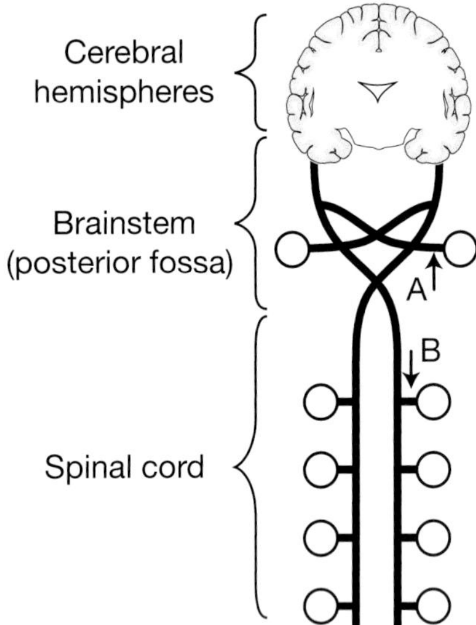

Fig. 3.28. Major nervous system connections. *A*, Cranial nerves; *B*, peripheral nerves. Note long intersegmental pathways leading to and from higher centers and multiple, short segmental pathways (cranial and peripheral nerves) to the peripheral level.

the supratentorial level and may be considered segmental functions of this level. These functions are language (almost always localized to the left side of the brain), memory, intelligence, cognition, olfaction, and vision. When abnormal, these functions help to further localize the disorder to the supratentorial level (Fig. 3.29). Extensive lesions involving the structures of the supratentorial level may alter consciousness and produce coma.

The basal ganglia influence the initiation and sequencing of motor programs in addition to exerting influence over certain behavior. The right basal ganglia influence the left side of the body and vice versa.

- A cerebral hemisphere lesion results in *contralateral* body (motor or sensory or both) dysfunction because of the interruption of intersegmental pathways (descending motor pathways and ascending sensory pathways).
- The cerebral cortex has very specific segmental functions, including language, cognition, memory, vision, visual-spatial perception, and personality.
- A basal ganglia lesion may result in *contralateral* body dysfunction.

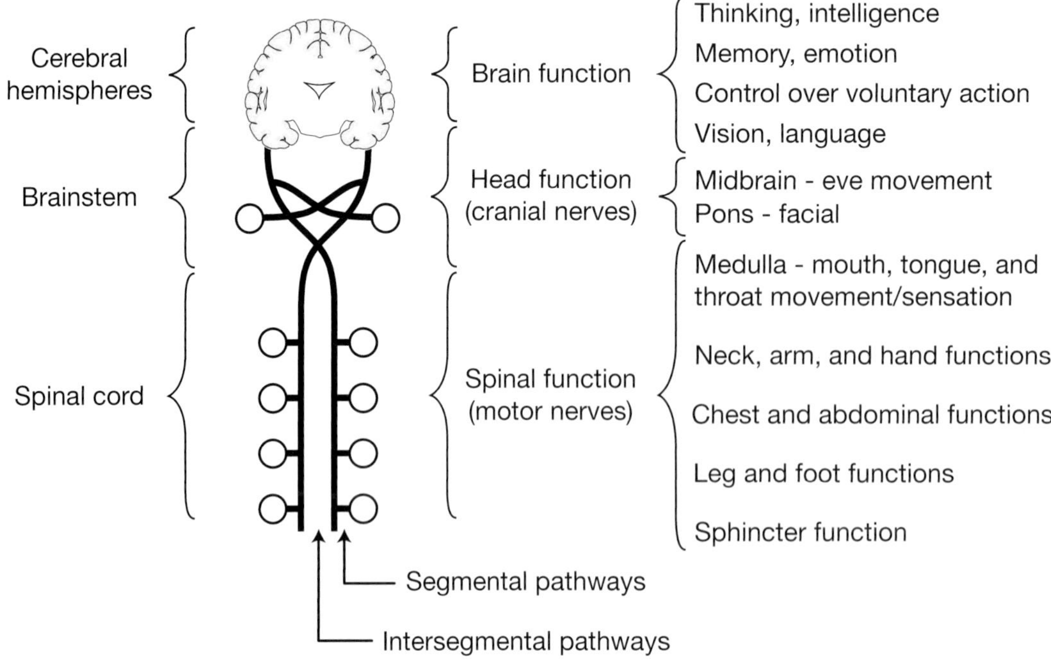

Fig. 3.29. Summary of the functions associated with the major anatomical levels.

Precise localization is possible when an area can be identified in which both segmental and intersegmental functions are altered in one or more systems. The major features to be determined in the anatomical diagnosis of neurologic disorders are the following:

1. Anatomical level: Are the segmental features or intersegmental features characteristic of lesions in the supratentorial, posterior fossa, spinal, or peripheral level?
2. Focal or diffuse: Is the lesion confined strictly to a well-circumscribed area? If so, it would be considered a focal lesion. Certain pathologic conditions such as stroke or multiple sclerosis often form discrete focal lesions. A diffuse lesion may involve only a single level or multiple levels. In general, a lesion is considered to be diffuse if it involves bilateral regions in the nervous system without extending across the midline as a single, circumscribed lesion. Certain pathologic conditions affect the nervous system in a more diffuse manner. An example is meningitis, which is an infection of the meninges that surround the brain and spinal cord. Therefore, the symptoms may also be diffuse. Thus, knowing if a nervous system process is focal or diffuse can aid in determining a potential cause.

Table 3.5. Summary of Clinical Findings by Level

Level	**Clinical finding**		**Segmental signs at level**
Supratentorial	Loss of sensation and/or weakness of face and body *contralateral* to the lesion	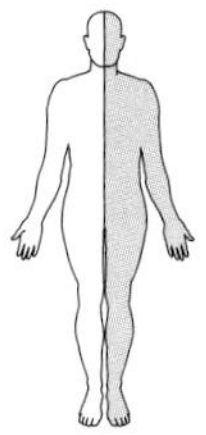	Vision Olfaction Cognition Memory Intelligence Behavior Seizures
Posterior fossa	Loss of sensation and/or weakness of face *ipsilateral* to the lesion and of the body *contralateral* to the lesion *Ipsilateral* cranial nerve deficit Cerebellar incoordination *ipsilateral* to the lesion	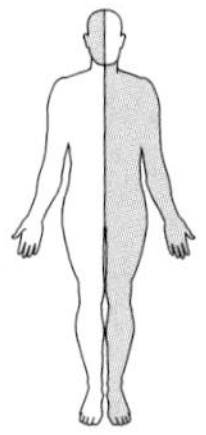	Hearing Vertigo Diplopia (double vision) Dysarthria (slurred speech) Dysphagia (swallowing difficulty)
Spinal	Sensory level Loss of pain and temperature *contralateral* to the lesion Weakness *ipsilateral* to the lesion Loss of position sense and vibration *ipsilateral* to the lesion	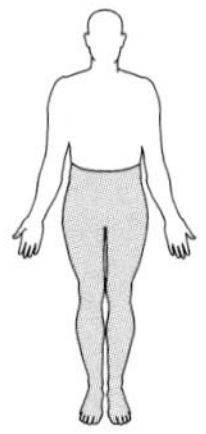	Neck or back pain Meningeal signs (stiff neck)
Peripheral	Loss of sensation to all modalities in the distribution of a single root or nerve or stocking/glove pattern Muscle weakness confined to a single root or nerve	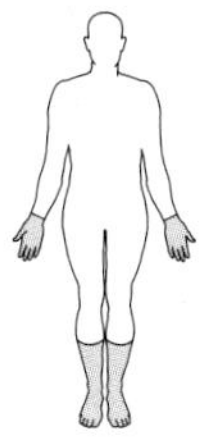	Limb pain Sensory or motor deficit confined to single nerve distribution

Clinical Problems

The following is a series of case histories of neurologic disorders. The problems were selected to illustrate examples of involvement of different regions of the nervous system. Read each history carefully. Although you do not yet know each specific pathway in the nervous system, the segmental and intersegmental signs and symptoms you have learned can help you localize the problem. On the basis of the information presented, try to answer the question "Where is the location of the lesion?"

1. Anatomical level (supratentorial, posterior fossa, spinal, or peripheral)?
2. Focal or diffuse?
3. Left, right, or midline?

Clinical Problem 3.1.

A 19-year-old man was in an automobile accident. Two weeks later, he gradually developed progressive headaches and personality changes, with reduced motivation. His family also noted that his right face seemed to droop and he had mild weakness of his right arm and leg.

Where is the location of the lesion?

Clinical Problem 3.2.

A 24-year-old woman was in an automobile accident. When examined, she had complete loss of sensation from the level of the arms downward. She could not move her hands or legs and had no sensation below the armpits. She was incontinent.

Where is the location of the lesion?

Clinical Problem 3.3.

Over several years, a 42-year-old man noted the onset of ringing in his right ear and then loss of hearing in that ear. He also experienced right facial weakness and decreased sensation. In the weeks before his examination, he noted stiffness and weakness of his left arm and leg.

Where is the location of the lesion?

Clinical Problem 3.4.

A 46-year-old laborer noted numbness and pain in the first 3 digits of his right hand with use. He also had weakness of his right thumb (opponens pollicis) but not of other muscles of the hand.

Where is the location of the lesion?

Clinical Problem 3.5.

A 26-year-old man awoke and noted that all the muscles on the left side of his face seemed to be paralyzed. Sensation was normal, although he was aware of an inability to taste on the left side of his tongue. He had no other difficulties. Six weeks later, he noted gradual and continued improvement.

Where is the location of the lesion?

Clinical Problem 3.6.

A 21-year-old college woman developed a diffuse body rash, fever, and headache. One day later, she began to complain of neck and back pain, especially with neck flexion. After 2 days, she developed reduced level of consciousness as well as continuing to have fever.

Where is the location of the lesion?

Additional Reading

Haines DE, editor. Fundamental neuroscience. 2nd ed. New York: Churchill Livingstone; 2002.

Rhoton AL Jr. The supratentorial cranial space: microsurgical anatomy and surgical approaches. Neurosurgery. 2002;51(4 Suppl 1):S1-iii.

Chapter 4

Diagnosis of Neurologic Disorders: Neurocytology and the Pathologic Reactions of the Nervous System

Objectives

1. Describe the origin of neurons, astrocytes, oligodendrocytes, ependymal cells, microglia, and Schwann cells.
2. Describe the components and functions of the neuronal secretory system, cytoskeleton, and axonal transport.
3. Describe the basic components of synapses and the functions of dendritic spines.
4. Name the cells that give rise to myelin sheaths in the central and peripheral nervous systems, and describe the general organization and function of myelin sheaths.
5. Describe the general functions of astrocytes, ependymal cells, and the blood-brain barrier.
6. Describe the main differences and mechanisms of necrosis and apoptosis.
7. Describe the morphology and mechanisms of ischemic cell change and central chromatolysis.
8. Name the inclusion bodies found in Alzheimer disease and Parkinson disease.
9. Describe wallerian degeneration.
10. Describe the differences in axonal regeneration in the peripheral and central nervous systems.
11. Describe the pathologic reactions affecting myelin sheaths.
12. Describe the pathologic reactions of astrocytes and ependymal cells.
13. Describe the general mechanisms of inflammation.
14. Describe the general mechanisms of neoplastic transformation in the nervous system.
15. Describe the different types of cerebral edema.
16. Describe the clinical and pathologic features of vascular disease, inflammatory disease, neoplastic disease, metabolic or toxic disease, and traumatic disease.
17. On a photograph, be able to recognize neurons, astrocytes, oligodendrocytes, microglia, ependymal cells, ischemia and infarction, neoplasia, diffuse inflammation, abscess formation, amyloid plaques, neurofibrillary tangles, and Lewy bodies.
18. In a clinical situation, be able to answer the following four questions:
    a. The signs and symptoms contained in the medical record are most likely the manifestation of disease at which of the following levels of the nervous system?
        i. Supratentorial level
        ii. Posterior fossa level
        iii. Spinal level
        iv. Peripheral level
        v. More than one level
    b. Within the level you have selected, the responsible lesion is most likely:
        i. Focal, on the right side of the nervous system
        ii. Focal, on the left side of the nervous system
        iii. Focal, but involving midline and contiguous structures on both sides of the nervous system
        iv. Nonfocal and diffusely located
    c. The principal pathologic lesion responsible for the symptoms is most likely:
        i. Some form of mass lesion

ii. Some form of nonmass lesion

d. The cause of the responsible lesion is most likely:

i. Vascular

ii. Inflammatory

iii. Neoplastic

iv. Degenerative

v. Toxic-metabolic

vi. Traumatic

Introduction

The principles of anatomical localization are introduced in Chapter 3. Anatomical localization, however, is but one part of the diagnosis of neurologic disorders; it is also necessary to determine the pathologic features of the lesion involved. Identification of the pathologic condition requires knowledge of the cellular elements of the nervous system (neurocytology), the molecular and biochemical bases of their function, and the ways in which these cells react to noxious stimuli (pathologic reactions).

Two major factors must be considered in describing lesions of the nervous system:

1. The *topography* of the lesion: the anatomical location of the pathologic process and a judgment about whether the abnormality is
   a. *Focal:* strictly confined to a single circumscribed anatomical area
   b. *Diffuse:* distributed over wide areas of the nervous system. A diffuse lesion may involve only a single level (e.g., supratentorial or spinal), or it may be distributed over multiple levels. A diffuse lesion involves bilaterally symmetrical areas in the nervous system, without extending across the midline as a single, circumscribed lesion.
2. The *morphology* of the lesion: the gross and histologic appearance of the abnormal area and a judgment about whether the pathologic process is a
   a. *Nonmass:* one that alters cellular function in the area of the lesion but does not interfere significantly with the performance of neighboring cells by virtue of its size or volume
   b. *Mass:* one that not only alters cellular function in the area of the lesion but also is of sufficient size and volume to interfere with the functioning of neighboring cells by compressing, damaging, or destroying the cells.

Integration of the *topographic* and *morphologic* descriptions provides a precise pathologic diagnosis. When patients are examined clinically, tissue is not available for study; yet, on the basis of the signs and symptoms and the *temporal profile* of their evolution, the nature of the responsible pathologic lesion can be deduced. This chapter provides the information necessary to accomplish this task.

Overview

The nervous system is composed of neurons and glial cells derived from the neuroectoderm and supporting cells derived from the mesoderm. The functional units of the nervous system are *neurons*. They have two important and interrelated functions: signaling and trophism. The survival of neurons depends on several factors, including adequate supply of glucose and oxygen, mitochondrial metabolism, processing of intracellular proteins, and transport of proteins along the axon and dendrites, both from the cell body toward the periphery and vice versa. Impairment of any of these processes may result in neuronal injury or death. Mature neurons do not proliferate, but they can undergo adaptive changes in response to injury. Most disease processes that affect neurons produce neuronal degeneration or neuronal loss.

Proper neuronal function also requires that neurons interact with their environment, which consists of glial cells and extracellular fluid. The neuroglia consists of true glial cells (macroglia), ependymal cells, and microglia. The macroglia is derived from the neuroectoderm and includes the *astrocytes* and *oligodendrocytes* in the central nervous system (derived from the neural tube) and the *Schwann cells* in the peripheral nervous system (derived from the neural crest). The astrocytes provide metabolic support to neurons, regulate the neuronal microenvironment, and participate in signaling, development, and repair mechanisms. Oligodendrocytes in the central nervous system and Schwann cells in the peripheral nervous system are responsible for the formation of the myelin sheaths around axons.

The central nervous system is surrounded by cerebrospinal fluid, which is produced by the epithelium of the *choroid plexus* (a derivative of the ependyma). Ependymal cells line the entire ventricular system and provide a selective barrier between the ventricular fluid and the brain substance. Noxious stimuli may produce a loss of ependymal cells. The central nervous system receives its nutrition through capillaries that are joined by tight junctions and form the *blood-brain barrier*, which is critical for maintaining the normal composition of brain extracellular fluid. The *microglia* is derived from the bone marrow and migrates into the central nervous system. These cells normally are few in number, but they can proliferate rapidly in response to injury to become scavenger cells, or *macrophages*. The nervous system is surrounded by the meninges, which are of mesodermal origin.

- Neurons are the functional units of the nervous system for signaling and trophic function.
- Astrocytes regulate the neuronal microenvironment, and oligodendrocytes and Schwann cells produce myelin sheaths in the central and peripheral nervous systems, respectively.
- The survival of neurons and neuroectodermal supporting cells depends on the supply of glucose and oxygen, energy metabolism, and the ability to process and transport intracellular proteins.

Disease processes may affect the functions and morphology of these cells in a very specific way. For example, acute energy failure results in the swelling of astrocytes, whereas other diseases are often associated with astrocytic proliferation, which results in *gliosis* (the scar tissue of the central nervous system). Disease processes that affect oligodendrocytes or Schwann cells are associated with myelin breakdown and loss (*demyelination*). Disorders that affect the endothelial cells increase the permeability of the blood-brain barrier. Differences in the histologic features of these disorders form the morphologic basis for the various clinical features of neurologic diseases.

The signs and symptoms produced by these disorders reflect the anatomical location and histologic evolution of the underlying pathologic lesion. The presumptive pathologic basis of a particular constellation of neurologic signs or symptoms is based on two main features: 1) the anatomical location of the abnormality (focal, multifocal, or diffuse) and 2) the temporal profile of its onset (i.e., acute, subacute, or chronic) and evolution (i.e., stable, improving, relapsing-remitting, or progressive).

According to the underlying cause, lesions that affect the nervous system can be classified as vascular, inflammatory, neoplastic, degenerative, toxic, metabolic, or traumatic. All these pathologic processes produce a loss of neurons and other cells of the nervous system by two morphologically distinguishable mechanisms: *necrosis* and *apoptosis*. The predominant mechanism of cell death depends on several factors, including the temporal profile of the insult, and both mechanisms may coexist in some conditions. An important concept is that the development of focal and progressive neurologic manifestations indicates the presence of a *mass lesion*, regardless of the underlying etiology (vascular, inflammatory, or neoplastic).

Vascular disease may be of several pathologic types, but they are all associated with sudden alteration in structure and function. Therefore, vascular disease is always acute in onset (i.e., within 24 hours) and may be focal and either nonprogressive (infarct) or progressive (intracerebral hemorrhage or a mass lesion) or it may be diffuse (subarachnoid hemorrhage or anoxic encephalopathy). *Inflammatory* disorders reflect the development of a rapid but not immediate cellular response to foreign pathogens invading the nervous system (*infections*) or to exogenous or endogenous antigens (*immune disorders*). Therefore, these disorders are generally *subacute* in onset (usually from 24 hours up to 4 weeks). Infections commonly present with a subacute, progressive deficit that may be focal (abscess, or a mass lesion) or diffuse (meningitis or encephalitis). Immune disorders are generally multifocal or diffuse, with a subacute or chronic temporal profile.

Neoplastic transformation and proliferation of cells result in a gradually enlarging, localized mass that affects surrounding tissue. Thus, neoplasia is manifested clinically as a focal progressive (mass) deficit with a chronic (longer than 1 month) evolution. *Degenerative* disorders are characterized by the gradual loss of neurons in widespread areas of the nervous system and, thus, are diffuse, chronic progressive diseases. *Metabolic* and *toxic* disorders alter neural function over widespread areas and, therefore, produce diffuse signs and symptoms. Depending on the responsible cause, these symptoms may have an acute, subacute, or chronic temporal profile. *Traumatic* lesions are usually of acute onset, reflecting the immediate damage of tissue, and may produce focal or diffuse deficits. At times, the delayed effects of traumatic lesions may produce clinical symptoms with the pattern of a chronic, progressive lesion.

- The presumptive diagnosis of a neurologic disorder depends on its anatomical localization and temporal profile.
- Focal and progressive neurologic deficits suggest the presence of a mass lesion.
- Vascular disorders produce acute deficits, which may be focal or diffuse and nonprogressive (ischemia) or progressive (hemorrhage).
- Inflammatory disorders produce subacute progressive deficits, which may be focal or diffuse.
- Neoplasia produces focal, chronic, and progressive deficits.
- Neurodegenerative disorders produce diffuse, chronic, and progressive deficits.
- Metabolic or toxic disorders produce diffuse deficits, which may be acute, subacute, or chronic.
- Traumatic lesions produce acute (immediate) focal or diffuse deficits that are stable or improve, but they may also manifest as chronic, progressive disorders.

Structural Elements of the Nervous System

The nervous system is composed of three basic categories of cells: 1) neurons, which are derived from the neuroectoderm (neural tube and neural crest) and are the major functional units of the nervous system; 2) supporting cells of neuroectodermal origin (astrocytes, oligodendrocytes, and ependymal cells from the neural tube, and Schwann cells from the neural crest); and 3) supporting cells of mesodermal origin (microglia, vascular endothelium, and meninges). The structure of all these cell types and their interrelationships have been studied extensively at the light microscopic and electron microscopic levels.

Neural tissue is routinely studied with light microscopy by using thin sections stained to emphasize certain features of cells. For example, nucleic acids react with basic dyes such as cresyl violet (Nissl method), whereas the lipids of the myelin sheath are stained by Luxol fast blue. Silver impregnation techniques, developed by the neuranatomists Golgi and Ramon y Cajal, provide details about the structure of neurons and glia. Histochemical and immunocytochemical techniques allow the localization of specific chemical substances in neurons and other elements of the nervous system. In situ hybridization allows the detection of a messenger ribonucleic acid (mRNA) encoding the protein of interest in these cells.

Neurons

Neurons are the most important structural elements and functional units of the nervous system. They generate and conduct electrical activity, transmit information required for the moment-to-moment function of the nervous system, and exert long-term effects required for storage of this information. Normal mature neurons do not undergo cell division, but throughout life they can undergo adaptive changes in morphology and function in response to activity or injury.

Neuronal Cell Body

Neurons have certain common features that are demonstrated most readily by the largest neurons such as the motor neurons of the ventral horn of the spinal cord (Fig. 4.1). Neurons consist of three main elements: the cell body (or soma), axon, and dendrites. The cell body is the metabolic and trophic center of the neuron. It varies in size and shape and, in motor neurons of the ventral horn, can be as large as 100 μm in diameter. Neurons typically have an irregular shape and contain a large spherical nucleus with a prominent nucleolus (Fig. 4.2). The nucleus appears to be relatively clear, or vesicular, because of the dispersion of the chromatin. The lack of dense chromatin, or heterochromatin, in neurons is typical of cells that are highly biosynthetic.

The cytoplasm surrounding the nucleus constitutes the cell body, or *perikaryon*, which contains the same

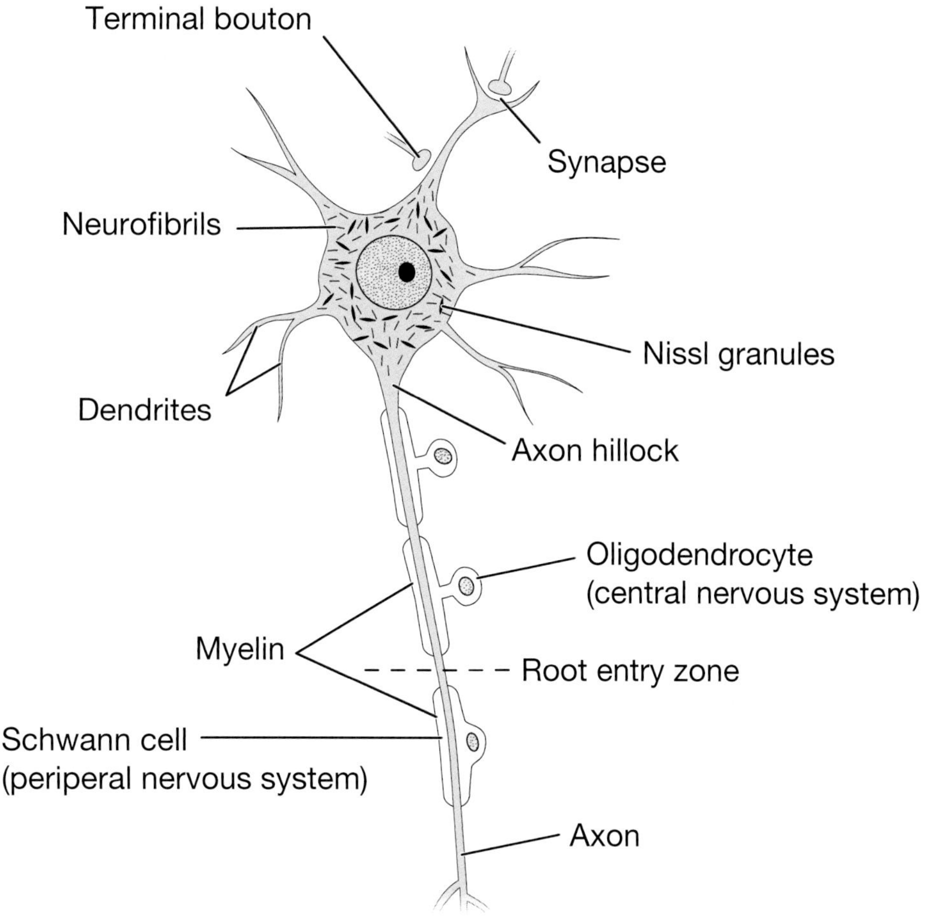

Fig. 4.1. General features of a prototypical neuron (spinal motor neuron).

types of organelles for metabolism as does the cytoplasm of other cell types. These include an elaborated system of membrane cisterns, including the rough endoplasmic reticulum and its associated ribosomes, the smooth endoplasmic reticulum, and the Golgi apparatus. The rough endoplasmic reticulum and ribosomes produce the appearance, at the light microscopic level, of dense basophilic bodies called *Nissl granules* (Fig. 4.2). The proteins synthesized in the rough endoplasmic reticulum follow a secretory pathway through the smooth endoplasmic reticulum and Golgi complex, where they undergo several modifications before becoming incorporated into various vesicles that finally are targeted for insertion in different cell membranes. The mitochondria are the center of oxidative energy metabolism. Lysosomes are

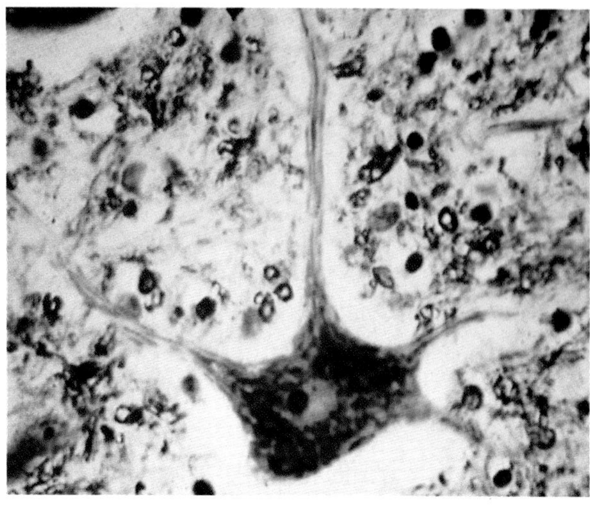

Fig. 4.2. Spinal motor neuron. (Nissl stain; ×400.)

involved in the degradation of macromolecules, including large carbohydrates and complex lipids.

The smooth endoplasmic reticulum has several functions in the neurons, including intracellular calcium homeostasis. It is able to take up calcium from the cytosol and release it in response to different signals. Mitochondria are critical for energy metabolism in neurons, producing the adenosine triphosphate (ATP) required for essentially all functions of the cell. Mitochondria contain their own DNA (mitochondrial DNA) that, unlike nuclear DNA, is transmitted exclusively by the mother.

- Neurons consist of a cell body, dendrites, and axon.
- The neuronal cell body contains a large clear nucleus, prominent nucleolus, and rough endoplasmic reticulum that forms Nissl granules.
- Proteins synthesized in the rough endoplasmic reticulum follow a pathway through the smooth endoplasmic reticulum and Golgi complex and are incorporated into vesicles for targeting and insertion in different cell membranes.
- Mitochondria contain their own DNA and are critical for energy metabolism.

The neuronal *cytoskeleton* is a semirigid matrix composed of filamentous proteins that determine cell morphology, biochemical topography of the membrane, and intracellular transport. The cytoskeleton includes the *microfilaments*, *neurofilaments*, and *microtubules* (Fig. 4.3). Microfilaments determine and maintain the cell shape. Microtubules are necessary for transport of vesicles containing proteins from one part of the cell to another. Neurofilaments form the *neurofibrils* that are characteristic of neurons (Fig. 4.4).

The components of the cytoskeleton are formed by the polymerization of subunits and are distributed throughout the cell body and all the processes of the neuron. The microfilaments are 5 nm in diameter and consist of polymers of actin. Through their interactions with a large variety of actin-binding proteins, microfilaments determine the cell shape and distribution of proteins in the cell membrane. The microtubules are 20 to 30 nm in diameter and consist of polymers of tubulin; they are important for intracellular transport mechanisms. Polymerization of microtubules, required for normal transport, is regulated by microtubule-associated proteins, particularly tau proteins. The neurofilaments are 10 nm in diameter and constitute the intermediate cytoskeletal filaments that are unique to nerve cells. They form a conspicuous fibrillar component of the cytoplasm of the cell body and the axon called neurofibrils, which can be demonstrated with silver stains. The functions of the cytoskeletal proteins are regulated by the state of phosphorylation of their associated proteins.

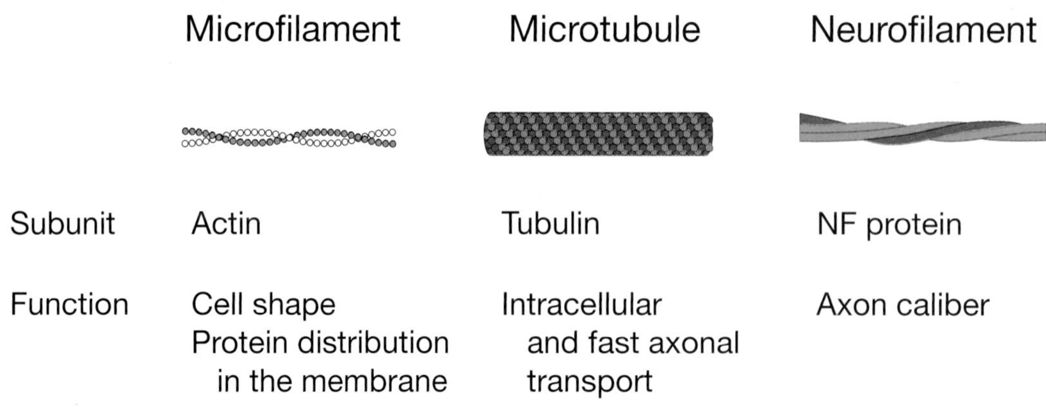

Fig. 4.3. Components of the neuronal cytoskeleton. NF, neurofilament.

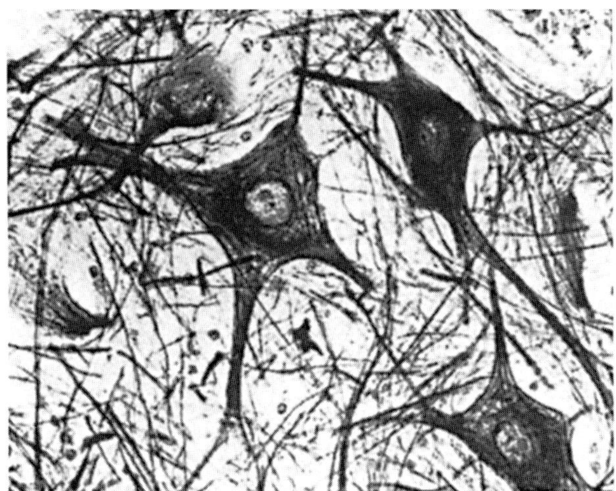

Fig. 4.4. Spinal motor neuron showing numerous neurofibrils streaming through the cytoplasm of the cell body and processes. The background contains processes of other neurons. (Bodian stain; ×400.)

- The cytoskeleton consists of microfilaments, microtubules, and neurofilaments.
- Actin microfilaments are critical for maintenance of cell shape.
- Microtubules are necessary for intracellular transport.
- The presence of Nissl granules and neurofibrils distinguish neurons from other cells in the nervous system.

Axon and Dendrites

The *axon* and *dendrites* are processes that extend outward from the neuronal cell body. Neurons contain a variable number of dendrites and only one axon. The number, length, and branching of these processes vary markedly from one type of neuron to another. The dendrites and axons differ in several important properties (Fig. 4.5).

Neurons of the central nervous system have one or, usually, many dendrites. The dendrites extend a relatively short distance from the cell body and generally branch repeatedly. Dendrites are in a sense the antennae of the nerve cell, and they transmit incoming signals toward the cell body. Many dendrites of neurons in the central nervous system have small projections called *dendritic spines*.

The *axon* conducts electrical activity and trophic influences away from the cell body and toward another neuron in the central nervous system or toward an effector organ (muscle or gland) in the periphery. Axons consist of three elements: the initial segment, the conducting segment (axon proper), and the axon terminal. The region of the cell body from which the axon arises, called the *axon hillock*, lacks Nissl granules and appears relatively pale in routine stains (Fig. 4.2). This narrows into the initial segment, which is the site of initiation of the electrical impulse that is propagated (conducted) along the axon. From the axon hillock, the axon extends outward for distances that vary from a few millimeters to several feet. Axons also vary in diameter, and this depends primarily on the number and separation of neurofilaments in the axon. The terminal arborizations of the axon contain the synaptic terminals that contact the target cell.

All neuronal mRNA and protein synthesis occur in the cell body and, to a lesser extent, in the dendrites. In contrast, the integrity of the axons absolutely requires proteins synthesized in the cell body and transported down the axon. *Axonal transport* is a complex process, with distinct sets of proteins moving as coherent waves down the axon at different rates (Fig. 4.6). Fast axonal transport moves membrane- and vesicle-contained proteins between the cell body and the synaptic terminal. *Fast anterograde transport* moves synaptic and other membrane proteins to the axon terminals, and *fast retrograde transport* moves proteins incorporated by the synaptic terminal from the environment to the neuronal cell body. Fast axonal transport depends on the microtubules, which form the tracks for the fast transport of organelles over long distances, and molecular *motor proteins*, which provide an energy-dependent movement of the vesicles along the microtubules. *Slow axonal transport* moves cytoskeletal components and other cytoplasmic proteins to the axon and axon terminals. There is also a different transport mechanism for mitochondria.

With fast anterograde transport, membrane organelles travel to the axon terminal at a rate of 200 to 400 mm/day. Important examples of specific constituents of fast anterograde transport are synaptic vesicles, neurotransmitter receptors, and ion channels. The motor proteins for fast anterograde transport are members of the kinesin family. Fast

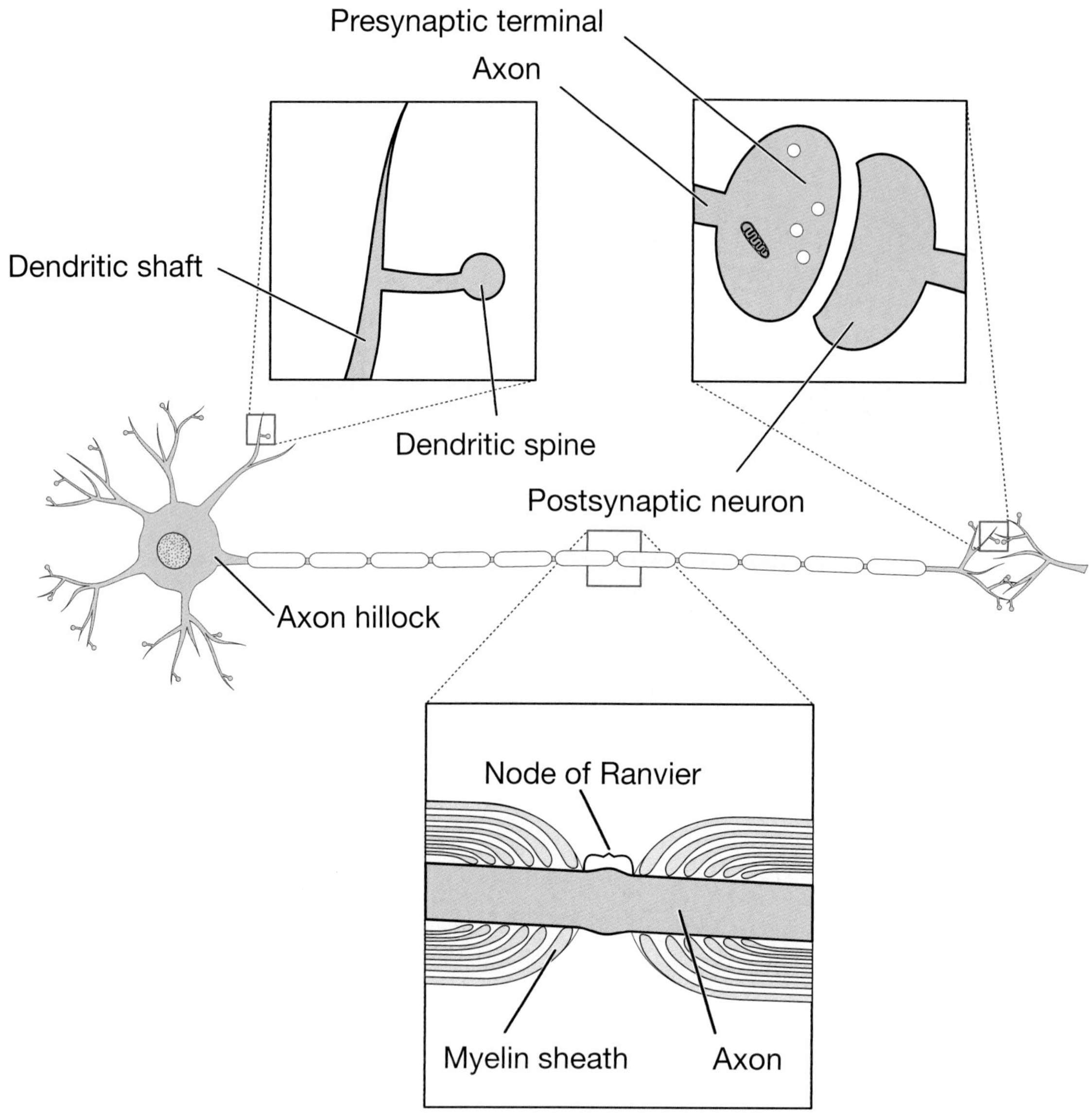

Fig. 4.5. Structural and functional components of a typical neuron. (Modified from Benarroch EE. Basic neurosciences with clinical applications. Philadelphia: Elsevier; 2006. Used with permission of Mayo Foundation for Medical Education and Research.)

retrograde transport (200-300 mm/day) facilitates membrane recycling and provides a pathway for the transmission of signals from the neuronal environment to the neuronal cell body. A typical example is the retrograde transport of nerve growth factor and its receptor. Viruses and toxins (tetanus, botulism) access the nervous system through retrograde transport. The motor molecules for fast retrograde transport are cytoplasmic dyneins. Slow axonal transport includes two subcomponents. One component consists primarily of polypeptides associated with microtubules and moves at a rate of 0.2 to 1 mm/day. The second component is composed of proteins of the actin microfilament network and soluble cytoplasmic proteins and moves at a rate of 2 to 8 mm/day.

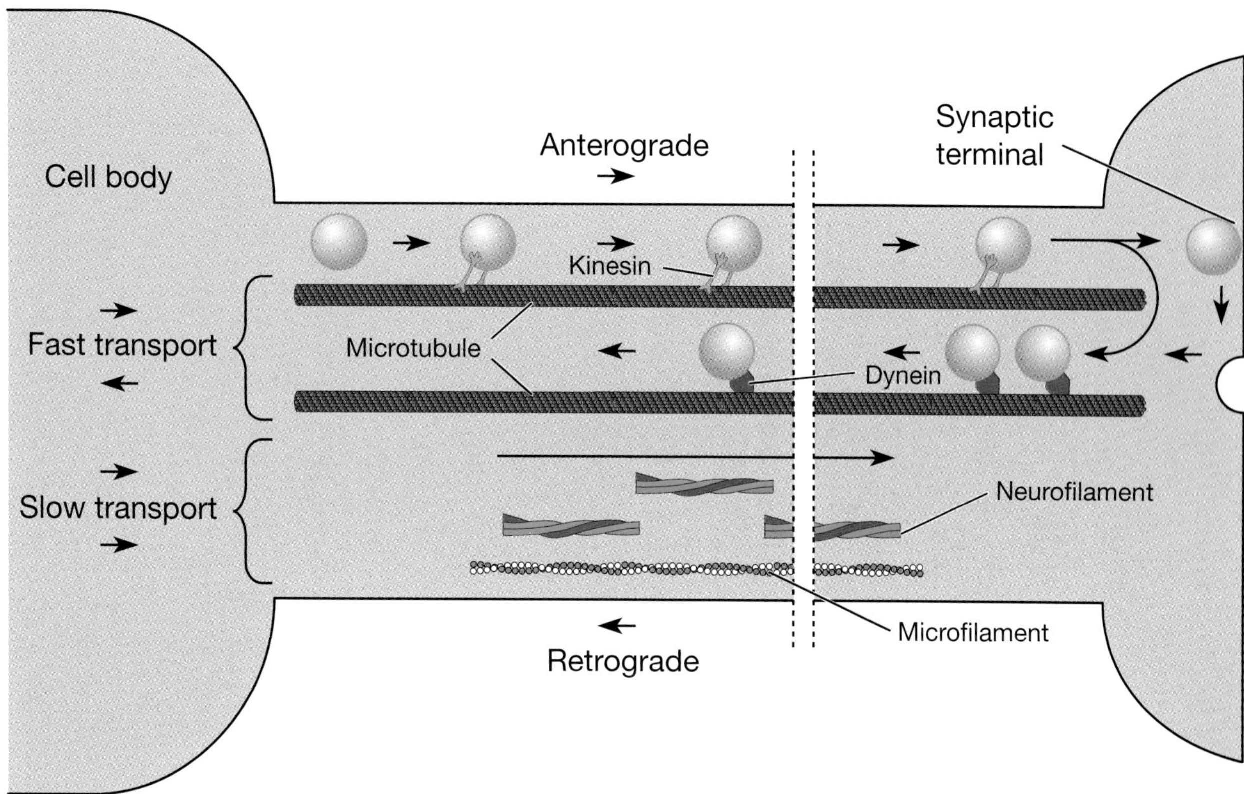

Fig. 4.6. Mechanisms of fast and slow axonal transport. (Modified from Benarroch EE. Basic neurosciences with clinical applications. Philadelphia: Elsevier; 2006. Used with permission of Mayo Foundation for Medical Education and Research.)

Many axons of the central and peripheral nervous systems are surrounded by a myelin sheath and are called *myelinated axons*. In general, these axons have a large diameter and are specialized for rapid conduction of electrical signals. The formation and structure of the myelin sheath is described in the next section. Other axons lack a myelin sheath and are called *unmyelinated axons*.

- Dendrites are the main receptive surface of the neuron.
- The axon is specialized to conduct electrical activity and trophic influences away from the neuronal cell body.
- Axonal transport is critical for survival of the axon and for bidirectional interactions of the neuron with its environment.
- Fast axonal transport depends on microtubules and energy-dependent motor proteins.

Synapses

Communication between neurons occurs at specialized regions called *synapses* (Fig. 4.7). The most common types of synapses in the nervous system are *chemical synapses*. They consist of a *presynaptic* element and a *postsynaptic* element that are separated by a space, called the *synaptic cleft*, 200 to 300 Å wide. In most synapses, the presynaptic element is the axon terminal, which may be enlarged to form a terminal *bouton* or *varicosity*. Synaptic terminals harbor *synaptic vesicles*, which contain the chemical neurotransmitter responsible for transfer of the signal from the presynaptic to the postsynaptic cell.

The axon terminal of a neuron usually forms a synapse with the dendrites or cell body of another neuron. In the central nervous system, many axons synapse with dendritic spines (Fig. 4.7). Synapses do not always occur at the terminal end of an axon but may form in places where an axon passes by a dendrite or cell body. These are called *en passant* synapses. Some synapses may occur between dendrites or between two axon terminals. Some synapses in the brain are made by direct bridges, or *gap junctions*, that allow direct transfer of electrical information between cells. These are called *electrical synapses*. The dendritic tree and cell body of the neuron may be covered by hundreds of synapses from numerous sources. An axon may branch repeatedly and form synapses on many other neurons. This convergence and divergence of information provides the basis for the complexity and flexibility of the function of the nervous system. In the periphery, chemical transmission occurs between the axons and effector structures, including skeletal muscles (*neuromuscular junction*) and visceral targets (autonomic *neuroeffector junctions*).

Synapses are not only sites of transmission of information but also the sites of bidirectional trophic communication between neurons and their target cells.

> There are several examples of trophic interactions between neurons and their targets in both the central and peripheral nervous systems. For example, target-derived signals, such as nerve growth factor, bind to receptors on the axon terminal and are retrogradely transported to the neuronal cell body, where they are critically important for cell survival and differentiation. Other trophic factors, such as brain-derived neurotrophic factor, are released from presynaptic terminals, bind to receptors on dendrites, and stimulate dendritic branching and synaptogenesis.

- Communication between neurons occurs primarily at the level of chemical synapses.
- Axon terminals harbor synaptic vesicles containing the chemical transmitter.
- Synapses are sites of bidirectional trophic communication.

The Plasma Membrane

The properties of the plasma membrane allow neurons to selectively detect and integrate synaptic and other environmental signals and to transmit these signals to other cells. The plasma membrane is a lipid bilayer that has a characteristic structure and composition. Phospholipids

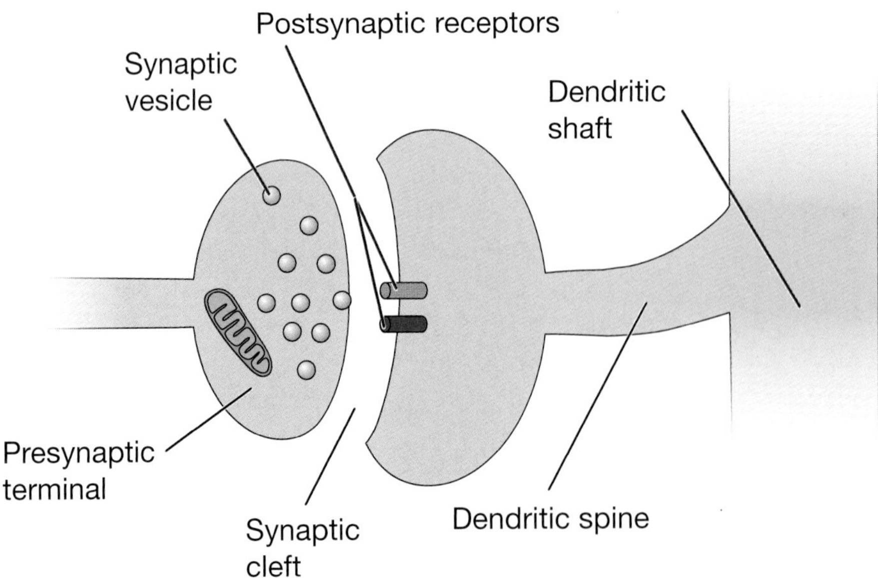

Fig. 4.7. Representation of a typical excitatory synapse in the central nervous system. (Modified from Benarroch EE. Basic neurosciences with clinical applications. Philadelphia: Elsevier; 2006. Used with permission of Mayo Foundation for Medical Education and Research.)

constitute the majority of the lipids and are involved in several functions. Several transmembrane proteins, including ion channels, ion pumps, transporters, receptors, gap junction proteins, and adhesion molecules, are critical for neuronal integrity and function and for interactions between a neuron and its environment. All these proteins are distributed heterogeneously in the plasma membrane, and this topographically selective distribution depends on their interaction with the actin cytoskeleton.

Ion channels allow the passive flux of ions across the membrane, driven by their electrochemical gradient, and are critical for electrical signaling within the nervous system. Ion pumps are critical for maintenance of intracellular ionic composition, and their function critically depends on ATP. Transporters allow the incorporation of nutrients, such as glucose and amino acids, or chemical transmitters into the cell. Receptors are proteins that bind to a chemical transmitter and initiate a synaptic response. Gap junction proteins (connexins) allow rapid intercellular communication between neurons and astrocytes. Adhesion molecules allow structural interactions among neurons, glia, and extracellular matrix proteins. These adhesive interactions are critical during development and have a major role in structural plasticity and repair mechanisms following injury.

Morphologic and Functional Diversity of Neurons

Neurons vary greatly in size and shape from one region of the nervous system to another (Fig. 4.8). From a functional standpoint, they can be grouped into three major categories: afferent, motor, and interneurons. Afferent neurons convey information from the periphery to the nervous system, and motor neurons send commands to muscles and glands. The most abundant neurons in the central nervous system are interneurons, which either process information locally or convey information from one region to another. The first type is called *local interneurons* and the second type is called relay, principal, or *projection neurons*. Neurons in each of these categories vary greatly in shape, size, and chemical transmitter. However, neurons that have a similar function or are located in a given region often resemble each other structurally and biochemically. The morphology of neurons is best defined using Golgi techniques.

Bipolar neurons in sensory receptor organs and T-shaped pseudonipolar neurons in the dorsal root ganglia are sensory neurons. Multipolar neurons are characteristic of the brain, spinal cord, and peripheral autonomic nervous system. According to the pattern of the axonal projection, neurons in the central nervous system are subdivided into Golgi type II, or local circuit neurons, with axons that arborize within a nucleus or region of the brain, and Golgi type I, or projection neurons, which send axons over long distances. Important examples of projection neurons are the pyramidal cells of the cerebral cortex and Purkinje cells of the cerebellum. Both types of cells have large dendritic trees with multiple dendritic spines. In contrast, the large motor neurons of the ventral horn of the spinal cord have large dendritic arborizations but lack dendritic spines.

Supporting Cells of Neuroectodermal Origin

Oligodendrocytes, Schwann Cells, and Myelin Sheaths

Oligodendrocytes and Schwann cells are discussed together because they share an important function: they form the insulating sheaths called *myelin*. Myelin consists of multiple tightly wrapped spirals of membrane that ensheath large-diameter axons. Oligodendrocytes form myelin in the central nervous system, and Schwann cells form it in the peripheral nervous system. The myelin sheath is composed of fundamental, radially arranged subunits, each corresponding to a single layer of plasma membrane derived from the myelin-forming cell. This spiral layering is the result of the apposition and fusion between the intracellular or extracellular surfaces of the membrane (Fig. 4.9). A key feature is the *compaction* of the sheath between the membrane surfaces. The juxtaposed inner leaflets of the plasma membrane form the *major dense line*. The juxtaposed outer leaflets form the minor dense line, or *intraperiod line*. In noncompacted regions of myelin, the intracellular leaflets of membrane are not fused.

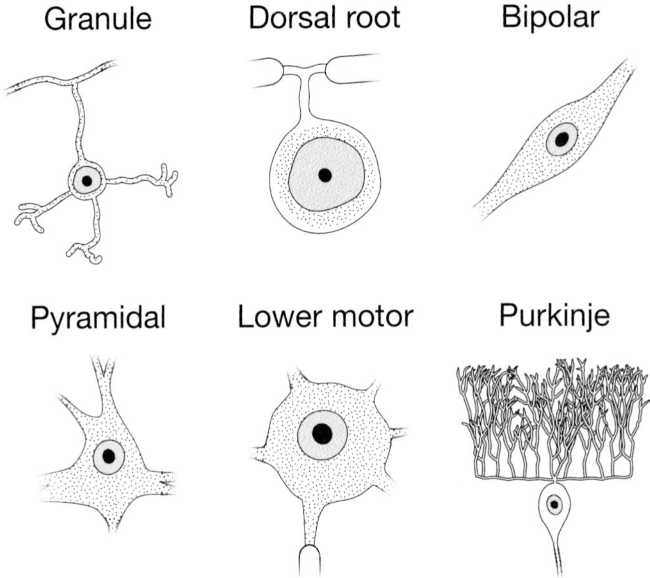

Fig. 4.8. Different sizes and configurations of neurons. Purkinje cell as visualized with the Golgi method.

Myelin structure and compaction depend on the presence of several myelin proteins produced by Schwann cells and oligodendrocytes. Important examples are myelin-associated glycoprotein, which serves as an adhesion molecule between myelin and the axon, myelin protein zero, which is critical for myelin compaction in the peripheral nervous system, and myelin basic protein and proteolipid protein, which participate in myelin compaction in the central nervous system. Mutations of the genes encoding for these proteins result in structural abnormalities of myelin.

The myelin sheath is interrupted at the *nodes of Ranvier* (Fig. 4.10). These regions contain clusters of sodium channels that are responsible for the rapid propagation of nerve impulses along the axon. Between the node of Ranvier and the compact myelin, called the *internode*, is a region of noncompacted myelin called the *paranode*. The distance between the nodes of Ranvier varies directly with the thickness of the myelin sheath of the axon.

■ The myelin sheath consists of multiple tightly wrapped spirals of membrane surrounding an axon.

■ Myelin is formed by oligodendrocytes in the central nervous system and by Schwann cells in the peripheral nervous system.

There are important differences between myelin sheaths in the peripheral and central nervous systems (Fig. 4.10). In peripheral axons, each segment of myelin, including the internode and paranodal regions, is formed by a single Schwann cell. In transverse sections of a peripheral nerve, most axons are surrounded by a myelin sheath (Fig. 4.11). The plasma membrane of an individual Schwann cell invests a single axon and wraps around it, forming a single internode (Fig. 4.12). The number of spirals that the Schwann cell process makes around the axon determines the thickness of the myelin sheath. In very small axons, the Schwann cell membrane may simply invest them once and make no turns at all. These axons are considered unmyelinated fibers. A single Schwann cell may invest a segment of several unmyelinated fibers in this way (Fig. 4.13). The Schwann cells are surrounded by a basal lamina, which provides a structural support that guides axonal regeneration after injury of the peripheral nerve.

There are important interactions between the Schwann cell and axon. The phenotype of Schwann

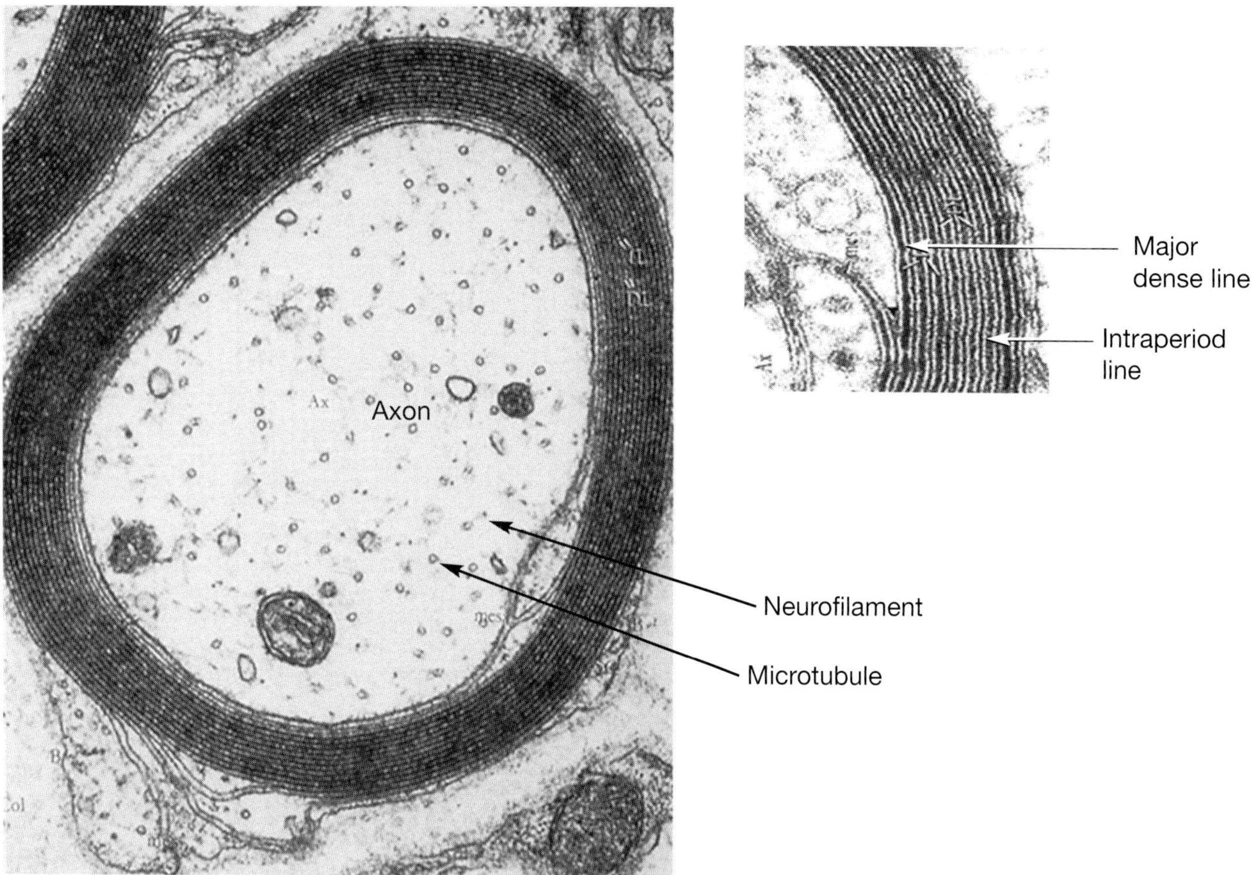

Fig. 4.9. Electron micrograph showing a typical myelinated axon and the structure of compact myelin.

cell (i.e., myelinating or nonmyelinating) after it migrates from the neural crest depends on trophic influences from the axon. In turn, Schwann cells contribute to the survival and differentiation of axons and guide them and regulate their architecture and the distribution of ion channels.

Oligodendrocytes are derived from the neural tube and are present in both gray and white matter. In routine histologic preparations of central nervous system tissue, oligodendrocytes are recognized as small, round nuclei with a dense chromatin network and unstained cytoplasm (producing the appearance of a clear halo around the nucleus) (Fig. 4.14). Their morphology is better delineated in silver-stained preparations (Fig. 4.15). Oligodendrocytes have cytoplasmic extensions that wrap around an axon and fuse, forming the major dense line and intraperiod lines of central myelin. There are two major differences between central and peripheral myelin: 1) a single oligodendrocyte contributes to the myelin sheath around several axons in its vicinity, whereas a Schwann cell myelinates a single segment of only one axon and 2) no basement membrane surrounds oligodendrocytes or central axons. These two differences are among the more significant factors in the different abilities that central and peripheral axons have to regenerate after axonal injury.

- Important trophic interactions occur between the Schwann cell and axon.
- Each Schwann cell interacts with one axon and contributes to the formation of a single internode.
- Processes from a single oligodendrocyte contribute to the myelin sheath of several axons near the cell.

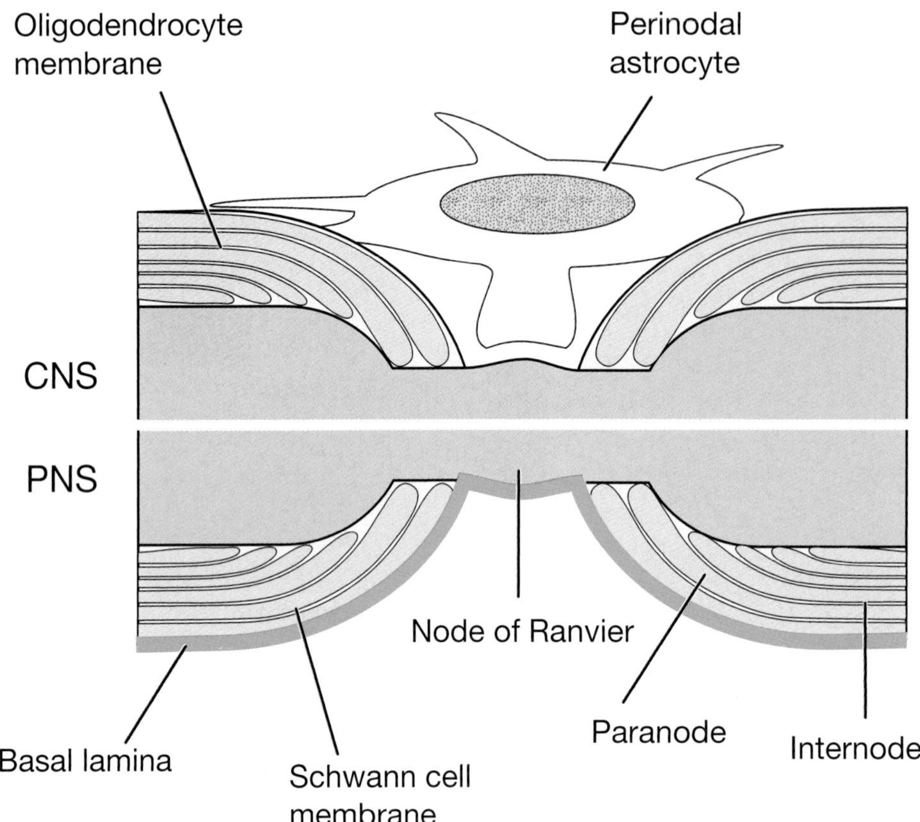

Fig. 4.10. Functional compartments of the myelinated axons in the central (CNS) and peripheral (PNS) nervous systems. In the central nervous system, the myelin sheath is formed by oligodendrocytes, each contributing to one internode of several axons. In the peripheral nervous system, each Schwann cell forms a single node of one axon. Peripheral, but not central, axons are surrounded by a basal lamina. Processes from the perinodal astrocyte interact with the axonal membrane of the node of Ranvier. (Modified from Benarroch EE. Basic neurosciences with clinical applications. Philadelphia: Elsevier; 2006. Used with permission of Mayo Foundation for Medical Education and Research.)

Astrocytes

Astrocytes are critical to the function of the central nervous system. They have multiple interactions with neurons: they support neuronal migration during development, provide substrates for neuronal energy metabolism, maintain the chemical microenvironment, contribute to the regulation of synaptic transmission and the coupling of local blood flow to neuronal activity, and participate in the response to injury and repair of the nervous system. Astrocytes are easily recognized in histologic sections of central nervous system tissue stained with hematoxylin and eosin by their oval nuclei, which are slightly larger and less densely stained than those of oligodendroglia (Fig. 4.14). Astrocytes typically extend five to eight major processes that branch in appendages, giving astrocytes a starlike appearance. This becomes apparent when they are stained with metallic impregnation methods or immunostained for *glial fibrillary acidic protein*, the intermediate filaments of astrocytes (Fig. 4.16).

Astrocytes are arranged linearly along the cerebral microvessels and send one or more expanded processes, called *foot processes*, to abut on the wall of a capillary (Fig. 4.16). A nearly continuous sheath of astrocytic foot processes surrounds the capillary network. This organization emphasizes the important role of astrocytes in providing substrates for neuronal metabolism and allows astrocytes to function as conduits for the transport of water, ions, and other molecules between the extracellular

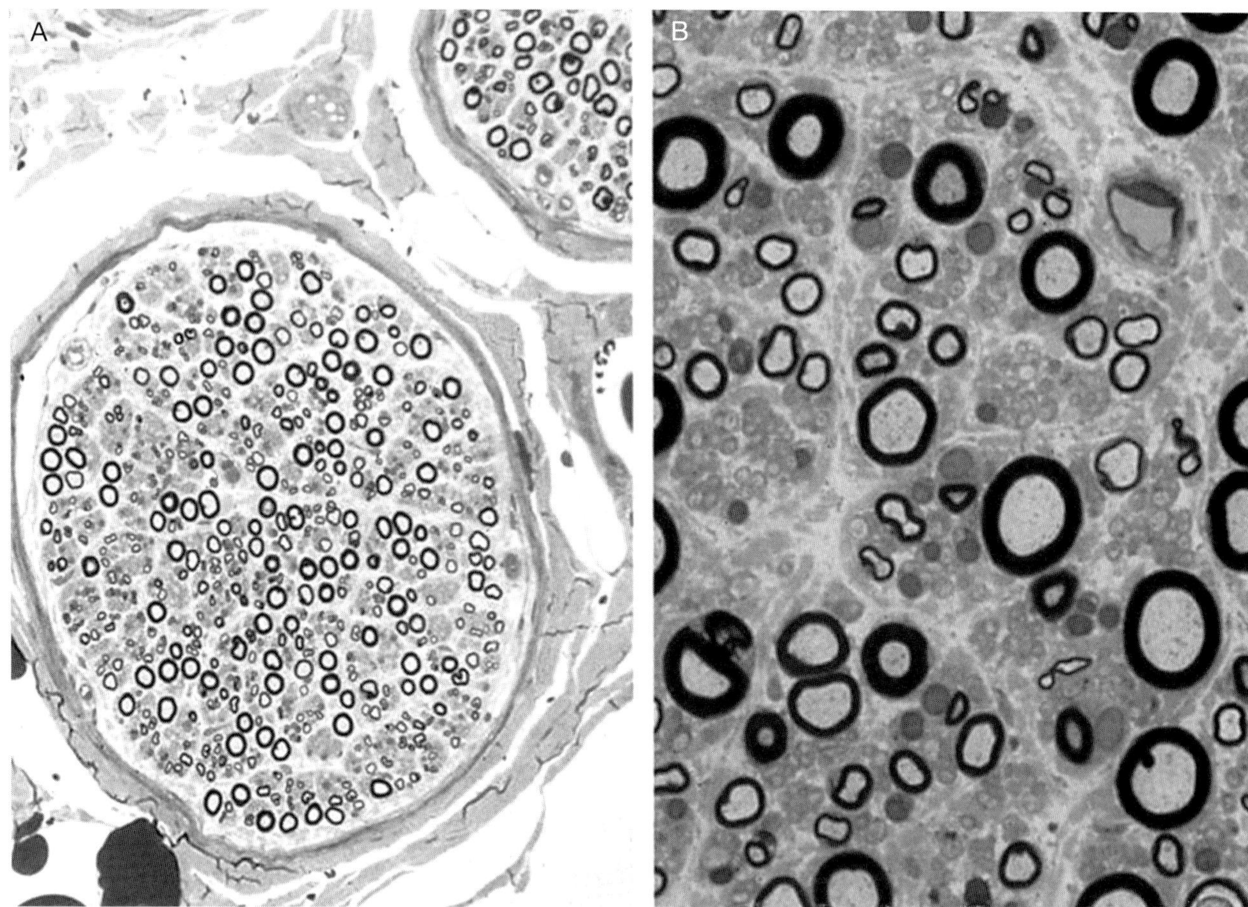

Fig. 4.11. Light micrographs of a transverse 1-μm–thick section of a normal human sensory (sural) nerve. *A*, Cross section of a fascicle and, *B*, a higher-power view showing the spectrum of myelinated fibers and less distinct profiles of Schwann cells containing unmyelinated fibers.

environment and the capillaries. Astrocytes also have a critical role in the coupling of cerebral blood flow to neuronal activity and metabolism. Astrocytes are connected extensively by gap junctions, forming a syncytium-like organization. Communication within this multicellular syncytium is rapid and coordinated and allows reciprocal interactions of signals across neuronal and astrocytic networks.

Neurons release neurochemical signals, including glutamate and potassium ions (K^+), that reach the astrocytes through the extracellular fluid. Neuronal activity triggers several changes in the astrocytes including influx of K^+ ions, increase in cell volume, activation of glucose metabolism, and increase in intracellular concentrations of calcium ions (Ca^{2+}). The astrocytes, in turn, provide glucose and lactate to support energy metabolism in neurons. They also regulate the neuronal microenvironment by removing glutamate and other neurochemical transmitters from the synapse and buffering extracellular K^+ to maintain neuronal excitability, prevent the accumulation of ammonia by synthesizing glutamine from glutamate, and release vasodilator substances, such as nitric oxide, that increase local blood flow in response to neuronal activity. Astrocytes communicate with each other through gap junctions and the release of ATP. Thus, astrocytes have a critical role in

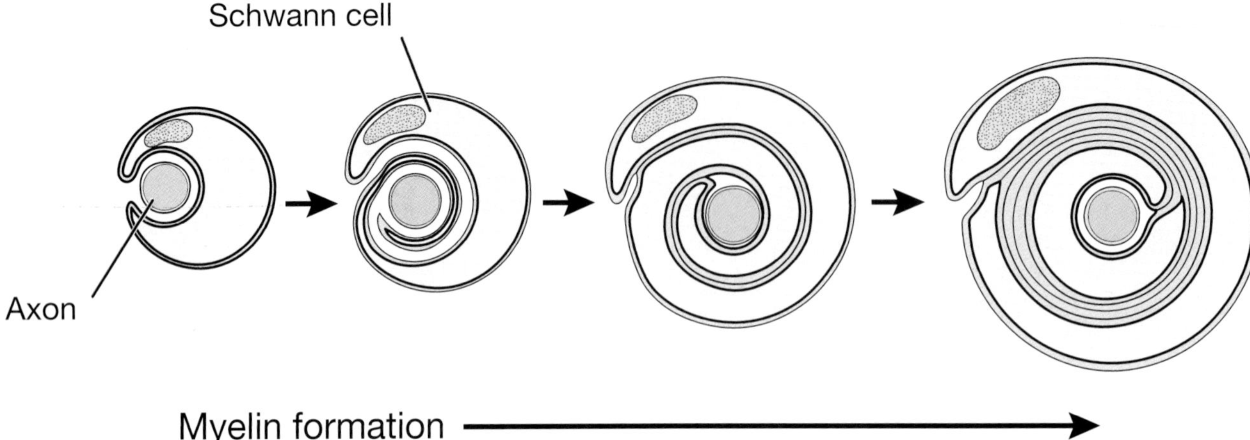

Fig. 4.12. Progressive steps in myelination of an axon by a Schwann cell.

maintaining the tight coupling among neuronal activity, energy metabolism, and cerebral blood flow required for function of the nervous system.

- Astrocytes form a network interconnected by gap junctions and have foot processes that ensheath brain capillaries.
- Reciprocal astrocyte-neuronal interactions are critical for the normal functioning of the nervous system.
- Astrocytes support neuronal metabolism, regulate the composition of the extracellular fluid, and participate in the coupling of cerebral blood flow with neuronal activity.

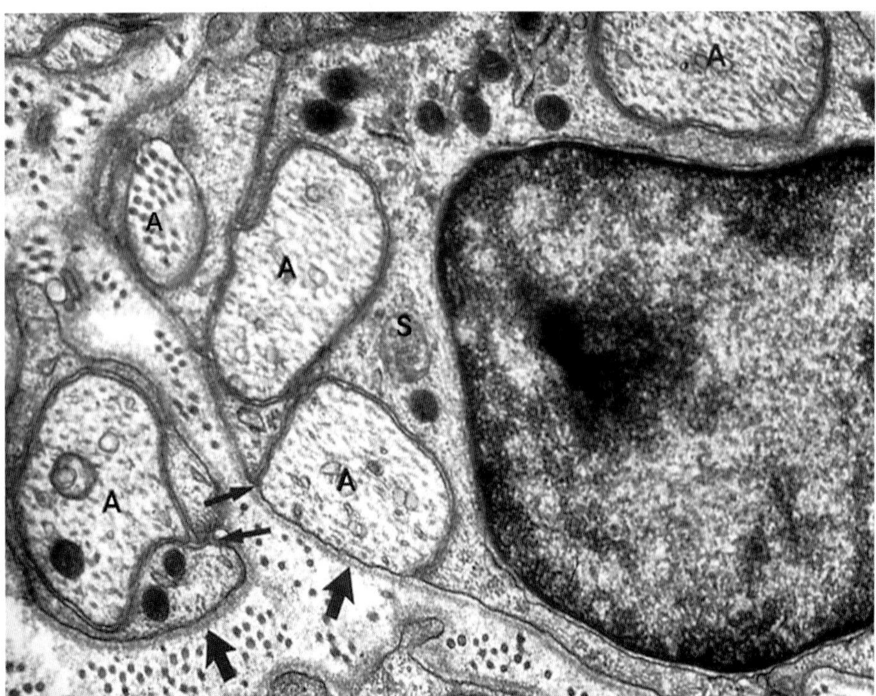

Fig. 4.13. High-power view of unmyelinated axons (A) invested by a single Schwann cell (S). Thick arrows, basement membrane; thin arrows, Schwann cell tongue around axon.

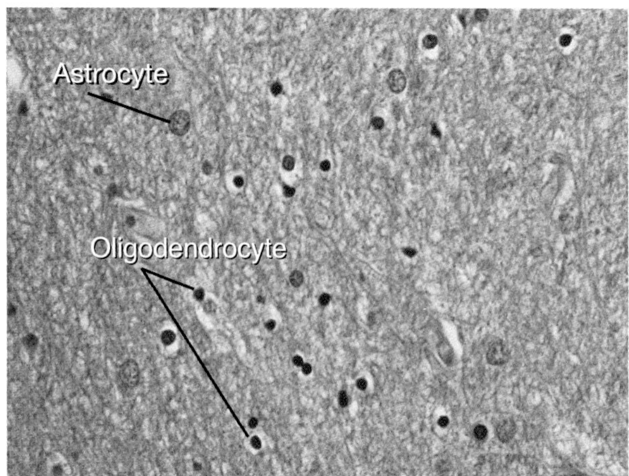

Fig. 4.14. Section of brain white matter showing nuclei of astrocytes and oligodendrocytes.

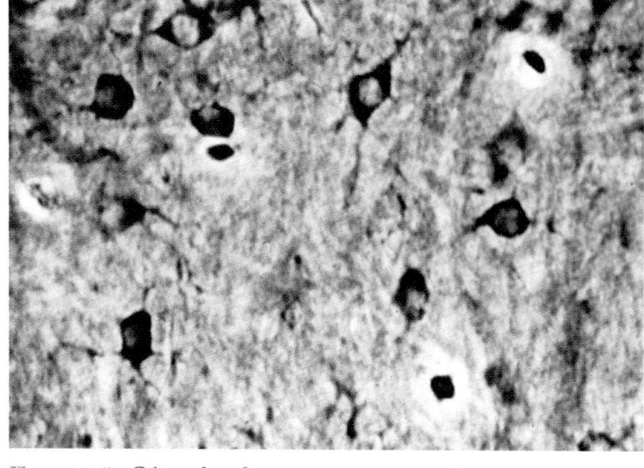

Fig. 4.15. Oligodendrocytes as seen with a silver stain technique.

Ependymal Cells

Ependymal cells are derived from the neuroepithelial cells of the ventricular zone of the neural tube. They form a single layer of ciliated columnar epithelial cells that lines the entire ventricular system of the cerebral hemispheres and brainstem of the mature brain (Fig. 4.17). The central canal of the adult spinal cord is usually obliterated and represented by a disorganized nest of ependymal cells. Tight junctions between adjacent ependymal cells form a selective barrier that prevents the free passage of substances between the ventricular fluid and the brain parenchyma. The ependyma gives rise to the *choroid plexus*, which produces the cerebrospinal fluid (Fig. 4.18).

The choroid plexus is formed when the thinned roof plate, consisting of a layer of ependymal cells, invaginates into the ventricular cavity together with vascular and connective tissue derived from the pia mater. These invaginations eventually form many small tufts that consist of the ventricular surface lined by cuboidal choroid epithelium derived from the ependyma and a core of richly vascular connective tissue (Fig. 4.18). The free surface of the choroidal cells has numerous microvilli, and its membrane ion pumps allow the passage of ions, accompanied by water, from the blood to this cell, leading to formation of cerebrospinal fluid, which is then secreted into the ventricular system.

- The ependyma forms the lining of the wall of the ventricles and gives rise to the choroid plexus, which secretes cerebrospinal fluid.

Supporting Cells of Mesodermal Origin

Cerebral arteries, arterioles, venules, and veins do not differ structurally from vessels of similar size and function in other organs. Capillaries are composed of a single layer of endothelial cells surrounded by a basement membrane. Capillaries of the nervous system are unique in their ultrastructure and physiology (Fig. 4.19). Unlike capillaries in all other organs, capillaries in the nervous system lack pores, and their adjacent endothelial cells are joined by tight junctions. This creates a barrier to the diffusion of solutes between the endothelial cells and provides the anatomical substrate of the *blood-brain barrier*. In the central nervous system, the capillaries are invested by a nearly continuous layer of astrocytic foot processes. Only the capillary basement membrane separates the plasma membrane of the astrocyte from that of the endothelial cell. Interactions between astrocytes and endothelial cells are critical for development and maintenance of the blood-brain barrier.

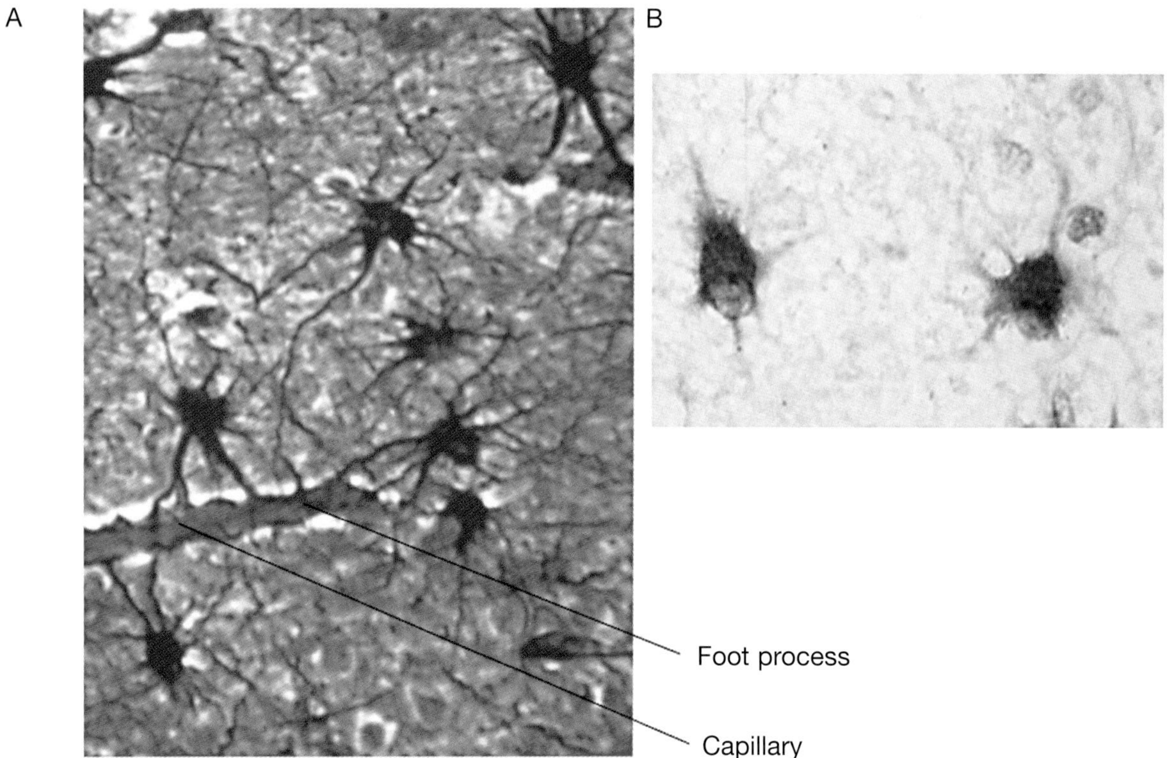

Fig. 4.16. *A*, Astocytes as seen with a gold sublimate stain. Note the many astrocytic foot processes ending on capillary walls. (Cajal stain; ×400.) *B*, Astrocytes identified with immunocytochemical staining for glial fibrillary acidic protein. (×600.)

The blood-brain barrier maintains the chemical composition of the brain extracellular fluid relatively independent of changes in the chemical composition of the blood. The ability of different blood-borne substances to cross this barrier varies widely with different classes of molecules. The maintenance of the tight junctions between capillary endothelial cells and the active transport mechanisms critical to the function of the blood-brain barrier are energy dependent and require a constant supply of ATP. Therefore, breakdown of this barrier is a common and early pathologic response to almost any form of injury to the central nervous system, including trauma, ischemia, inflammation, and pressure from mass lesions.

The capillaries of peripheral nerves (endoneural capillaries) are also nonfenestrated and joined by tight junctions, providing a blood-nerve barrier, which is similar in function to the blood-brain barrier. Ganglia, in contrast, have fenestrated capillaries, making them more susceptible to blood-borne toxins.

- Tight junctions between endothelial cells in brain capillaries form the blood-brain barrier.
- Astrocytic foot processes surround the capillaries and maintain blood-brain barrier function.

Microglia

Microglial cells are mesodermal cells of monocyte lineage that migrate into the central nervous system along with blood vessels from the mesoderm surrounding the neural tube. In normal brains, these cells are inconspicuous and are seen in hematoxylin and eosin–stained sections as scattered, small, elongated, darkly staining nuclei (Fig. 4.20). Resident microglia undergoes little turnover with hematogenous monocytes and are scattered throughout the parenchyma. Perivascular microglia occurs within the perivascular basal lamina and undergoes turnover with hematogenous monocytes.

Connective Tissue

Other than vascular structures, the parenchyma of the central nervous system is almost devoid of fibrous connective tissue elements. Therefore, fibroblasts rarely participate in reactive or reparative processes (scar formation) in diseases of the central nervous system. The central nervous system is surrounded by three connective tissue membranes called *meninges*. The two inner membranes, the pia mater and arachnoid, are the leptomeninges and are very thin and delicate. The space that separates the pia mater (which covers the surface of the brain and spinal cord) from the arachnoid is called the *subarachnoid space*, which communicates with the ventricular system, contains cerebrospinal fluid, and harbors the arteries that supply the central nervous system. The outer membrane, the dura mater (or pachymeninx), is thick and tough.

The peripheral nerves are rich in fibrous connective tissue. Each myelinated nerve fiber in a peripheral nerve is invested by a thin layer of collagen, the *endoneurium*; groups of nerve fibers are bound together in fascicles by the *perineurium*. The fascicles that comprise a nerve trunk are surrounded by a thick sheath called the *epineurium*. The three connective tissues are analogous to the three layers of the meninges (pia mater, arachnoid, and dura mater) and are continuous with them at the spinal nerve level.

- Microglial cells are mesodermal cells of monocyte lineage.

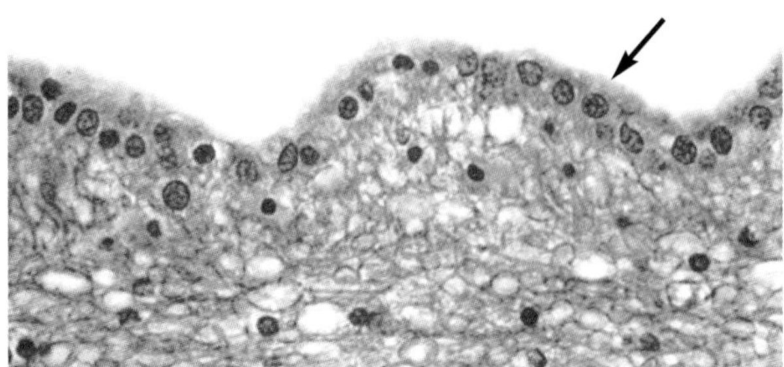

Fig. 4.17. Ependymal lining of the ventricle. Note the continuous layer of columnar cells with cilia (*arrow*) on the free (ventricular) border. (H&E; ×100.)

- The pia mater, arachnoid, and dura mater in the central nervous system and the endoneurium, perineurium, and epineurium in the peripheral nervous system are derived from the mesoderm.

Mechanisms of Injury of the Nervous System

Each of the cellular elements of the nervous system may undergo pathologic changes in response to disease states. In some conditions, the pathologic alteration may affect primarily neuronal function, without changes in the physical appearance of the cell. This produces transient neurologic disorders. In many diseases, however, the physical appearance of the cell is altered, and cells undergo changes that reflect either the damage caused by the pathologic process or their reaction to it. Some of these morphologic changes are nonspecific and may be seen in many entirely different types of diseases. Other changes may be specific and indicate a particular type of disease or even a specific disease entity. In most pathologic conditions, the various cell types react in concert, and the pathologic diagnosis is derived from analysis of the total tissue reaction.

Cell Survival Mechanisms Potentially Affected By Disease

The pathologic appearance of cells shown by light or electron microscopy ultimately reflects changes in the structure

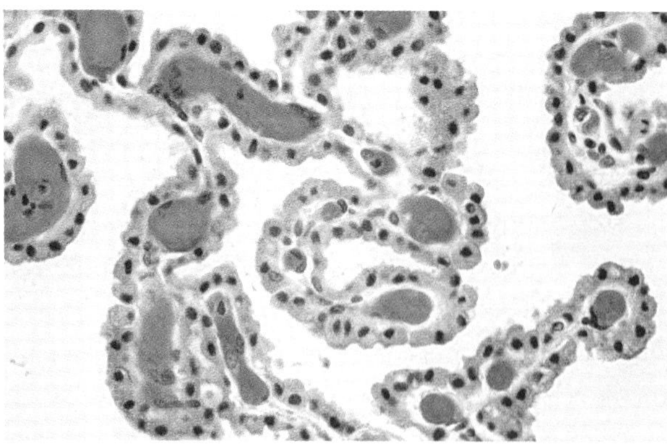

Fig. 4.18. Choroid plexus. Each tuft consists of a core containing a dilated capillary surrounded by a small amount of connective tissue and covered by choroidal epithelial cells. (H&E; ×100.)

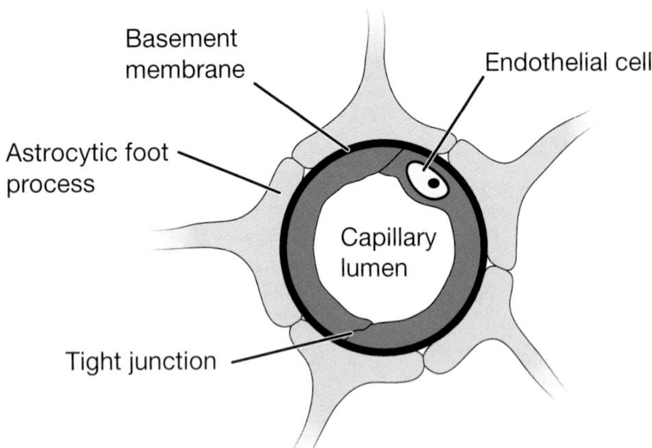

Fig. 4.19. Nonfenestrated capillary of the central nervous system. Endothelial cells are joined by tight junctions that form the blood-brain barrier and are surrounded by a basement membrane and a sheath of astrocytic foot processes.

and arrangement of molecules in the cell. In some diseases, the mechanism of cell injury or death is genetically programmed. However, in most disease processes, damage to cells results from extrinsic factors, such as the loss of availability of essential nutrients, the entry of toxic substances into the cell, or the attachment of antibodies to the cell membrane. Many disorders reflect a genetic susceptibility to injury by environmental factors. Any of these mechanisms can initiate a cascade of events that finally produces cell damage and death.

Genetic Determinants of Neuronal Phenotype and Survival in the Nervous System

Regulation of DNA duplication, DNA transcription into messenger RNA (mRNA), processing of mRNA, translation of the mRNA into proteins, and post-translational processing of these proteins into functional molecules are critical for brain growth and development, function, survival, and response to injury in the nervous system. Appropriate transmission of genetic information depends on the accurate duplication of DNA during the cell cycle and the segregation of the resultant sister chromatids during mitosis.

> Progression through the cell cycle is tightly regulated at specific checkpoints, which ensures that damaged DNA does not propagate. Failure of checkpoint control may result in cell death, abnormal proliferation, and passage mutations. Cell cycle progression is driven by sequential activation of cyclin-dependent kinases that phosphorylate proteins critical for DNA synthesis and cell division, and it is negatively regulated by inhibitors that arrest the cycle at a particular stage. The responses to DNA damage include cell cycle arrest and blockade of DNA replication, facilitation of DNA repair, and activation of programmed cell death.

The coordinated pattern of activation and inactivation of gene expression determines neuronal phenotype, plasticity, and information storage. This is controlled by special proteins called *transcription factors* that bind to specific sequences of DNA. Another important process is post-transcriptional processing of mRNA, including splicing of sequences encoding for proteins (exons) from noncoding sequences (introns). A defective DNA template (mutation) results in impaired transcription or processing of mRNA. This leads to lack of expression or abnormal structure or function of a specific gene product, such as an enzyme or a structural or regulatory protein. Genetic defects may be compatible with normal cell function for long periods, but ultimately they cause damage to the metabolic machinery or structural integrity of the cell, with eventual loss of function.

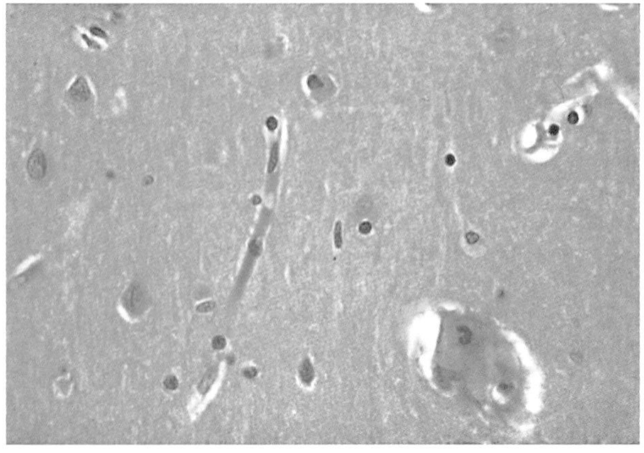

Fig. 4.20. Section of the brain white matter showing the nuclei of scant microglial cells.

- Brain development, function, survival, and response to injury require normal control of DNA duplication, transcription into mRNA, mRNA processing, and its translation into proteins.
- Control of the cell cycle at specific checkpoints prevents the propagation of damaged DNA.
- Transcription factors and mRNA processing are critical for normal gene expression.
- Mutations that affect cell cycle control, mRNA transcription, or mRNA processing impair the production or function of critical cell proteins.

Protein Processing, Transport, and Destruction

Post-translational processing, intracellular transport, and regulated destruction of proteins are essential for function and survival of neurons and other cells of the nervous system. These functions may be impaired by numerous genetic or acquired disorders. These disorders may affect the secondary structure of proteins, elicit oxidative damage of the proteins, impair normal protein processing and destruction, or compromise transport of proteins within the cell. This may lead to the accumulation of abnormal proteins in the form of *cell inclusions*.

Under normal conditions and because of environmental stresses, nascent or mature proteins are subject to misfolding, unfolding, and aggregation. A group of proteins known as heat shock proteins bind to nascent proteins to prevent their premature folding and destruction. Many aspects of cellular function require regulatory turnover of proteins involving protein degradation by the ubiquitin-proteasome system. Ubiquitin is a small protein that tags the target protein for degradation by a cytosolic enzymatic complex, the proteasome. Failure to eliminate ubiquinated proteins results in aggregates that form cell inclusions and disrupt cellular homeostasis. The lysosomes are also essential in the destruction of proteins and other complex molecules such as glycogen and sphingolipids.

- Genetic or acquired disorders that affect the structure, processing, destruction, or transport of proteins may lead to the accumulation of cell inclusions.

Energy Metabolism and Ionic Homeostasis

The brain comprises approximately 2% of body weight; yet, in the wake resting state, it accounts for 20% of a person's total energy consumption. This reflects the critical dependence of the nervous system on the blood supply of glucose and oxygen for ATP production to maintain its function and survival. ATP is important for maintaining ionic homeostasis, cell volume, electrical excitability, and synaptic function. Other energy-dependent processes include regulation of cytosolic calcium, axonal transport, and processing of denatured proteins.

Neuronal activity, local blood flow, and glucose metabolism are tightly coupled, and this coupling depends on interactions among neurons, surrounding astrocytes, and local blood vessels. Most communication in the brain involves rapid transmission at excitatory synapses mediated by the amino acid L-glutamate. Approximately 80% of the ATP consumed by the sodium ion (Na^+), K^+-ATPase, a membrane pump that restores the ionic gradients and membrane potentials altered by excitatory transmission. This ATP-dependent pump also prevents excessive accumulation of glutamate in the synaptic space and excessive activation of postsynaptic receptors, which may result in excessive accumulation of Ca^{2+} in the cytosol. Intracellular Ca^{2+} is tightly regulated by several ATP-dependent mechanisms, including the extrusion of Ca^{2+} from the cell and intracellular buffering by the smooth endoplasmic reticulum and mitochondria.

- Oxidative metabolism of glucose in the mitochondria is vital for cell survival in the nervous system.
- Most ATP consumption in the nervous system is for fueling the Na^+, K^+-ATPase to restore the ion gradients altered by excitatory neurotransmission and neuronal activity.
- ATP is also critical for preventing excessive accumulation of glutamate in the synaptic space and excessive accumulation of Ca^{2+} in the cytosol.

Mechanisms of Cell Death in the Nervous System

Neurons, glial cells, and endothelial cells may follow at least two separate pathways for cell death, *necrosis* and *apoptosis*, which differ morphologically and biochemically (Table 4.1). Despite differences, the absolute distinction between these two processes is an oversimplification, because a pathologic condition may elicit either or both of these processes according to its intensity and temporal profile (Fig. 4.21). In general, when the insult is severe and abrupt and ATP is rapidly depleted, the cell dies of necrosis. Slower processes, in which ATP is still available, can activate the intrinsic apoptotic program in the cell. The mitochondria are critically involved in both processes; failure of oxidative phosphorylation causes ATP depletion in necrosis, and the release of some intramitochondrial constituents triggers the cascade of apoptosis.

Necrosis

Necrosis reflects an underlying pathologic process that produces an abrupt and severe loss of supply of oxygen or glucose for ATP production (e.g., hypoxia, hypoglycemia, or ischemia), excessive mechanical strain (e.g., traumatic injury), or excessive increase in neuronal energy demands (e.g., prolonged seizures). The acute depletion of ATP leads to neuronal damage from excessive accumulation of L-glutamate. This process, called *excitotoxicity*, involves activation of glutamate receptors, accumulation of cytosolic Ca^{2+}, activation of Ca^{2+}-triggered cascades, generation of oxygen free radicals, and mitochondrial failure. Cells undergoing necrotic cell death show mitochondrial swelling, dilatation of the endoplasmic reticulum, and extensive vacuolization of the cytoplasm. The chromatin becomes coarse and clumpy, which is followed by loss of nuclear staining. The cells swell and eventually lyse, releasing their contents into the surrounding tissue and triggering an inflammatory response.

> Without oxygen or glucose, mitochondrial production of ATP stops, ATP stores are quickly depleted, and several functions become impaired. Without the energy necessary to fuel the Na^+, K^+ pump, the ionic gradients cannot be maintained and the neurons become depolarized. This results in the loss of neuronal excitability and the massive release of glutamate. Energy shortage also impairs glutamate uptake by astrocytes. Excessive build-up of glutamate at synapses eventually leads to necrotic death of synaptic target neurons. The consequences of energy failure are initially functional and potentially reversible. If the cause is not corrected, these changes are followed by the accumulation of Ca^{2+} in the cytosol and mitochondria, which triggers irreversible changes such as the destruction of cellular, mitochondrial, and other membranes; disorganization of the cytoskeleton, and degradation of DNA. Accumulation of Ca^{2+} in the mitochondria impairs the respiratory chain and ATP production and leads to the formation of oxygen free radicals. Calcium activates several phospholipases, which together with oxidative stress, destroy membrane phospholipids. Calcium activates the production of nitric oxide, which reacts with oxygen free radicals and results in further oxidation and nitration of several essential proteins. Calcium also activates calpains, which are proteases that destroy the submembrane cytoskeleton, microtubules, and neurofilaments, and endonucleases that cause DNA damage. The accumulation of lactate from anaerobic glucolysis leads to a decrease in intracellular pH, which depresses neuronal activity, elicits cell swelling, and enhances the production of free radicals.

Apoptosis

Apoptosis is a form of programmed cell death that is essential for normal development and tissue homeostasis. However, when implemented erroneously under certain abnormal conditions, it results in pathologic cell loss. Important triggers of apoptosis include DNA mutations, inflammatory mediators, abnormal accumulation of intracellular proteins, and oxidative stress. The apoptotic machinery consists of two main steps: 1) activation of "death receptors," or the release of mitochondrial triggers of apoptosis, particularly *cytochrome c*, and 2) activation of autocatalytic proteolytic cascades involving proteolytic enzymes called *caspases*, which result in DNA damage and nuclear fragmentation (Fig. 4.21). Cells undergoing apoptosis shrink but the condensed cytoplasm contains normal-appearing organelles; the nucleus shrinks and the chromatin condenses (*pyknosis*) and collapses into patches against the nuclear membrane. The cell finally breaks into dense spheres called *apoptotic bodies*. The DNA fragmentation, margination of chromatin along the inner aspect of the nuclear envelope, membrane blebbing, and phagocytosis of the apoptotic bodies by neighboring cells, in the absence of inflammation, distinguish apoptosis from necrosis.

Caspases are cysteine proteases that trigger DNA fragmentation and disassemble the nuclear laminae and the submembrane cytoskeleton. The caspase-mediated apoptotic cascade may be triggered by cytokines released during inflammation, DNA damage, oxidative stress, or accumulation of Ca^{2+} in the mitochondria. Accumulation of intramitochondrial Ca^{2+} leads to the opening of a large permeability transition pore that allows the release of cytochrome *c* from the inner mitochondrial membrane into the cytosol. In the cytosol, cytochrome *c* interacts with a caspase activator and triggers apoptosis. The Bcl-2 proteins are important in regulating the mitochondrial pathway for apoptosis. The balance of activity between proapoptotic and antiapoptotic members of the Bcl-2 family determines whether the mitochondrial permeability transition pore will open, cytochrome *c* will be released, and caspase will be activated.

- Cell death in the nervous system occurs by the mechanisms of necrosis and apoptosis.
- The mechanism of cell death depends on the temporal profile and what triggers the injury.
- Necrosis involves mechanisms of glutamate-induced excitotoxicity.
- Apoptosis results from the activation of caspases.

Table 4.1. Features of Necrosis and Apoptosis

Feature	Necrosis	Apoptosis
Cause	Acute, severe injury (energy failure, trauma)	DNA damage, inflammation, neurodegeneration
Pattern	Foci of numerous cell types affected	Individual cell affected
Cell volume	Increased early (cell swelling), then shrinkage (dead red cell)	Decreased
Membrane integrity	Compromised early	Persists after late in the process
DNA damage	Degradation	Internucleosomal cleavage
Nucleus	Chromatin margination	Pyknosis
Inflammatory changes	Yes	No
Apoptotic bodies	No	Yes
Mitochondrial involvement	Swelling Impairment of respiratory chain	Opening of permeability transition pore Release of cytochrome *c*
Mechanism	Glutamate-induced excitotoxicity, accumulation of intracellular Ca^{2+}, oxidative stress	Activation of death receptors, oxidative stress, DNA damage or mitochondrial release of cytochrome *c* and other mediators resulting in activation of caspases
Effector molecules	Calcium-activated phospholipases, proteases, and endonucleases	Caspases

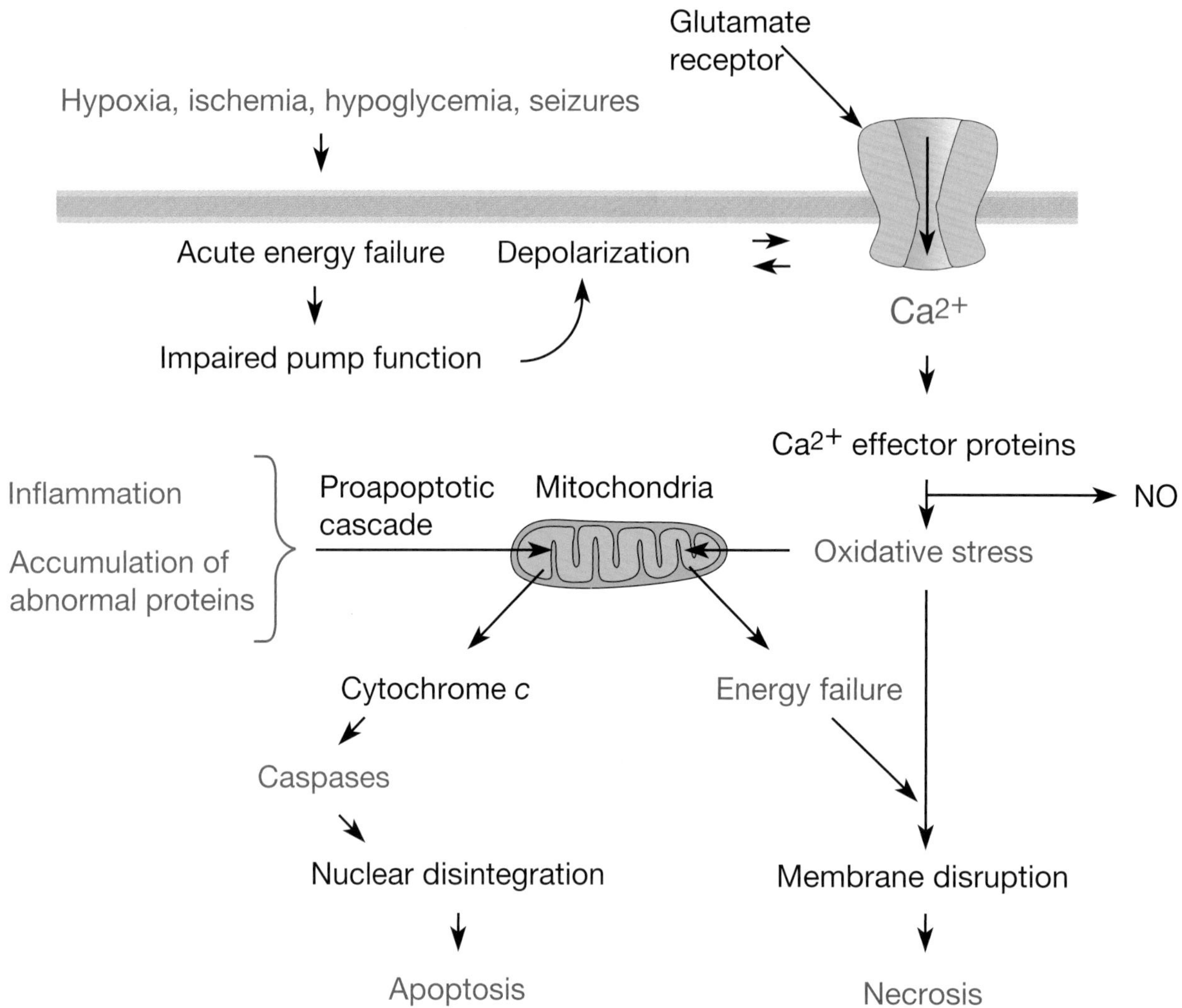

Fig. 4.21. Main mechanisms involved in necrosis and apoptosis. Ca^{2+}, calcium ions; NO, nitric oxide. (Modified from Benarroch EE. Basic neurosciences with clinical applications. Philadelphia: Elsevier; 2006. Used with permission of Mayo Foundation for Medical Education and Research.)

Reactions of the Structural Elements

Pathologic Reactions of Neurons

Nonspecific Reactions

The physiologic or metabolic abnormalities associated with conditions that lead to death, the catabolic processes that proceed after death (*autolysis*), and the procedures involved in obtaining and processing brain tissue post mortem can all distort the appearance of neurons. Therefore, almost any histologic section of brain tissue contains some neurons that deviate from the normal in size, shape, and affinity for stains. Both shrunken, dark-staining neurons and swollen, pale-staining neurons are often encountered. Neuronal loss is a nonspecific change that may occur from any form of severe damage to a neuron. Under pathologic circumstances, neuronal loss is usually accompanied by a reaction of other tissue elements (astrocytes and microglia), which marks the site of damage. Neuronal changes of a more specific type can accompany certain pathologic processes and, when present, can help define the pathophysiologic basis for the disorder.

Ischemic Cell Change

Ischemic cell change (Fig. 4.22) is a readily recognized morphologic change in neurons that occurs in response to oxygen deprivation and cessation of oxidative metabolism. From 8 to 12 hours after the insult, the neuron becomes smaller, its outline becomes more sharply angular, the cytoplasm becomes distinctly eosinophilic, and the nucleus shrinks and is homogeneously dark when stained. This is an irreversible change (i.e., a "red, dead neuron") and the end result is complete dissolution of the cell.

> The typical morphologic features of ischemic cell change may be preceded briefly by acute swelling of the neuron. This is associated with microvacuolation of the cytoplasm from swelling of the endoplasmic reticulum and mitochondria, as shown with electron microscopy.

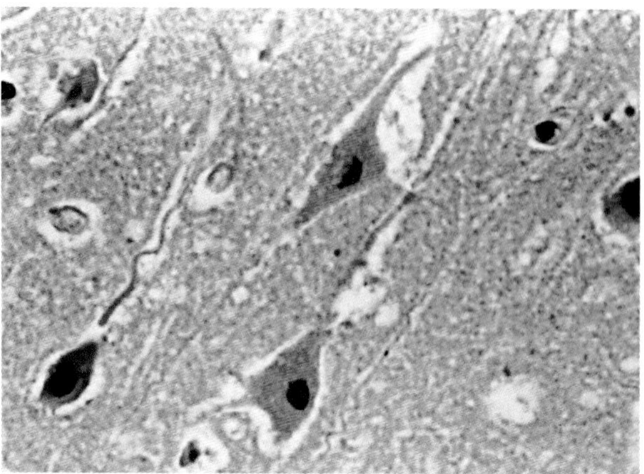

Fig. 4.22. Ischemic cell change. The neuron is shrunken, the nucleus is pyknotic, and the cytoplasm is diffusely eosinophilic ("red, dead neuron"). (H&E; ×400.)

Ischemic cell change may be triggered by any condition that deprives the neuron of sources for oxidative metabolism and energy production. These include abrupt interruption of blood flow (ischemia), lack of oxygen (hypoxemia) or glucose (hypoglycemia) in the blood, or the presence of a poison such as cyanide, which blocks oxidative metabolism. Approximately 2 to 5 minutes of complete oxygen deprivation results in irreversible neuronal damage, although under certain circumstances, such as extreme hypothermia, this time may be significantly increased. Neurons generally are more susceptible to energy deprivation than glial cells or endothelial cells. Some neurons are particularly vulnerable, particularly certain pyramidal neurons of the hippocampus.

Central Chromatolysis

Central chromatolysis is a change in the neuron cell body after severe injury to the axon (Fig. 4.23). In human pathology, this change is usually recognized only in large motor neurons of the ventral horn of the spinal cord and cranial nerve nuclei when the axons are injured close to the central nervous system. The reaction consists of swelling of the cell body and dissolution of the Nissl granules. This process begins near the nucleus and spreads to the periphery of the cell, where a rim of Nissl granules may remain intact. The nucleus migrates to the periphery of the cell body. These changes usually begin 2 to 3 days after injury and peak in 2 to 3 weeks. Unlike ischemic cell change, central chromatolysis is reversible and the normal appearance of the neuron may be restored in a few months.

- Ischemic cell change reflects irreversible neuronal injury due to acute severe deprivation of energy.
- Central chromatolysis is a reversible neuronal change that occurs after injury to the axon.

Neuronal Inclusions

The term *inclusion body formation* refers to abnormal, discrete deposits in neurons, glial cells, or the extracellular compartment that often identifies the type of disease and sometimes the specific disease. Inclusion bodies can be divided into intracytoplasmic and intranuclear types. Two important groups of cytoplasmic inclusions are filamentous inclusions and membrane-bound inclusions.

Filamentous inclusions are an important feature of several neurodegenerative diseases (Table 4.2). These inclusions consist of abnormal deposits of self-aggregating misfolded proteins that are normally present in the nervous system. They result from mutations or environmental factors that alter the structure, cellular distribution, kinetics of aggregation, or proteolytic processing

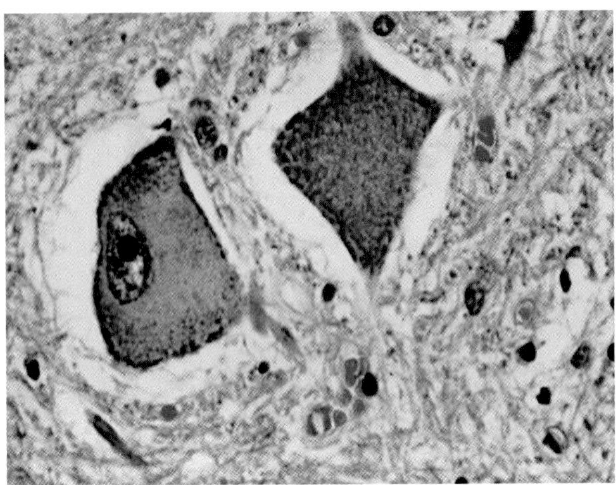

Fig. 4.23. Central chromatolysis. The neuron is swollen, the nucleus is eccentric, and the Nissl granules have disappeared except at the periphery. (H&E; ×400.)

of the proteins. These aggregates contain the abnormal protein as well as *ubiquitin*, which is normally involved in the mechanism of degradation of abnormal proteins. There are several important examples of filamentous cytoplasmic inclusions. One example is *neurofibrillary tangles*, which are clumped masses of neurofibrils within the cytoplasm, best seen with silver impregnation stains (Fig. 4.24). They are typically seen in *Alzheimer disease*, the most common degenerative dementia, but can also occur in other degenerative disorders, including some forms of *frontotemporal dementia.*

Alzheimer disease is also characterized by the accumulation of *neuritic plaques*, which have a central core composed by aggregates of *amyloid β peptide* (the result of abnormal processing of the amyloid precursor protein), surrounded by a halo of degenerated nerve processes, astrocytic fibers, and microglia (Fig. 4.24). Amyloid plaques are deposited extracellularly in the brain parenchyma and around cerebral vessel walls.

Spherical inclusions called *Lewy bodies* are identified, in routine preparations, by their eosinophilic core surrounded by a pale "halo" (Fig. 4.25). They are the characteristic feature of *Parkinson disease*, but they may also occur in other disorders, including *dementia with Lewy bodies*. Some hereditary neurodegenerative diseases, such as *Huntington disease*, are characterized by filamentous *intranuclear inclusions*, which are visible with electron microscopy.

Table 4.2. Examples of Inclusions in Neurodegenerative Diseases

Inclusion	Location	Characteristic	Composition	Disease association
Neurofibrillary tangle	Cytoplasm	Argyrophilic	Tau	Alzheimer disease
Pick body	Cytoplasm	Argyrophilic	Tau	Pick disease
Lewy body	Cytoplasm	Eosinophilic, with concentric lamination	α-Synuclein	Parkinson disease Dementia with Lewy bodies
Intranuclear filamentous inclusion	Nucleus	Visible with electron microscopy	Protein with polyglutamine repeats	Huntington disease
Neuritic plaque	Extracellular	Amyloid	β-Amyloid peptide	Alzheimer disease
Kuru plaque	Extracellular	Amyloid	Prion protein	Prion disorders
Negri body	Cytoplasm	Eosinophil	Viral particles	Rabies
Cowdry type A inclusion	Nucleus	Eosinophil	Viral particles	Herpes simplex and other DNA viral infections

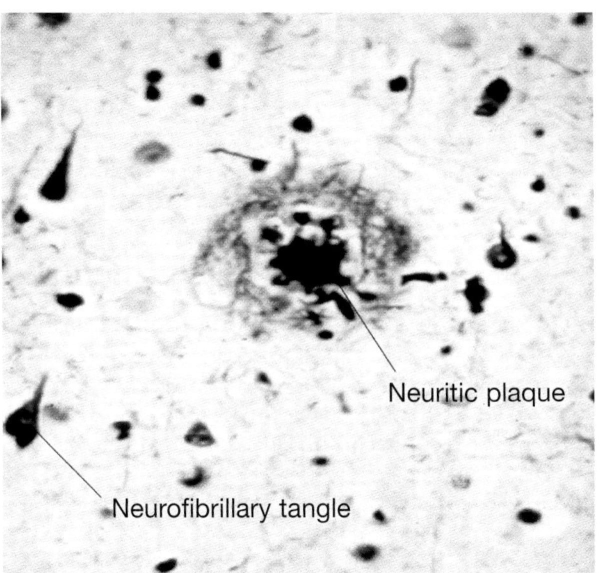

Fig. 4.24. Section of the brain of a patient with Alzheimer disease. Neurons have neurofibrillary tangles consisting of an accumulation of hyperphosphorylated tau proteins. Note also the neuritic plaque, which consists of extracellular accumulation of β-amyloid peptide surrounded by dystrophic neurites. (Bodian stain; ×400.)

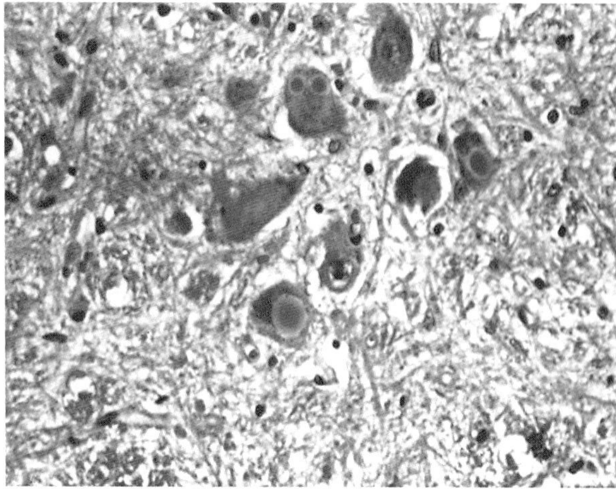

Fig. 4.25. Lewy bodies in pigmented dopaminergic neurons of the substantia nigra pars compacta in Parkinson disease. These cytoplasmic inclusions consist of accumulations of α-synuclein. (H&E; ×400.)

Neurofibrillary tangles are composed of hyperphosphorylated tau protein, a microtubule-associated protein. Tau hyperphosphorylation affects microtubule polymerization required for intracellular transport. Lewy bodies are composed of α-synuclein, a protein normally present in synaptic terminals (its function is poorly defined). Both types of proteins may be affected by mutations, which produce familial forms of dementia or parkinsonism. Mutations that affect the amyloid precursor protein or proteins called presenilins that are involved in its processing produce familial forms of Alzheimer disease. Mutations due to an increased number of trinucleotide repeats in genes that encode several proteins normally present in the nervous system lead to the accumulation of intranuclear inclusions. The most common example is expansion of the CAG (cytosine-adenine-guanine) repeat encoding for glutamine. In Huntington disease, the CAG expansion affects a protein called huntingtin, which has multiple functions in the nervous system.

- Filamentous inclusions consist of abnormal deposits of self-aggregating misfolded proteins and are an important feature of several neurodegenerative diseases.
- Neurofibrillary tangles and neuritic (amyloid) plaques are typical of Alzheimer disease.
- Cell loss and the accumulation of Lewy bodies in dopaminergic neurons are characteristic of Parkinson disease.

Cytoplasmic inclusions may also result from the accumulation of material in lysosomes. For example, *lipofuscin* is produced by oxidation of lipids and proteins within these organelles and accumulates in neurons and glial cells with aging and in some neurodegenerative disorders. Because of the deficiency of lysosomal enzymes, substances normally degraded in these organelles, including complex lipids such as glycogen or gangliosides, accumulate. In lysosomal storage disorders, the distended lysosomes appear as vacuoles and, as the substance accumulates, the cell body swells so much that it is called a *balloon cell* (Fig. 4.26). Identification of the specific disease requires identifying the stored material biochemically.

Viral particles may produce cytoplasmic or nuclear

inclusions. For example, rabies virus forms an eosinophilic cytoplasmic inclusion called the *Negri body*. Viruses containing DNA, such as the herpes simplex virus, produce nuclear eosinophilic inclusions called *Cowdry type A* inclusions (Fig. 4.27).

- Lysosomal storage diseases are characterized by distended cells that contain vacuoles consisting of enlarged lysosomes with incompletely digested material.
- Viral particles can produce cytoplasmic or intranuclear inclusions.

Vacuolar Change

Some disorders are characterized by the formation of small vacuoles that represent swollen dendritic and axonal processes, associated with loss of synaptic organelles and the accumulation of abnormal membranes, as visualized with electron microscopy. In cerebral gray matter, the resulting vacuolization is termed *spongiform change*, which is characteristic of *prion diseases* (e.g., Creutzfeldt-Jakob disease).

Prions (proteinaceous infection agents) consist of abnormal forms of a normal membrane protein called PrP protein. Abnormal prion proteins may result from mutations of the gene encoding the PrP protein or from conformational changes occurring either spontaneously or as a consequence of an infection with an abnormal prion protein.

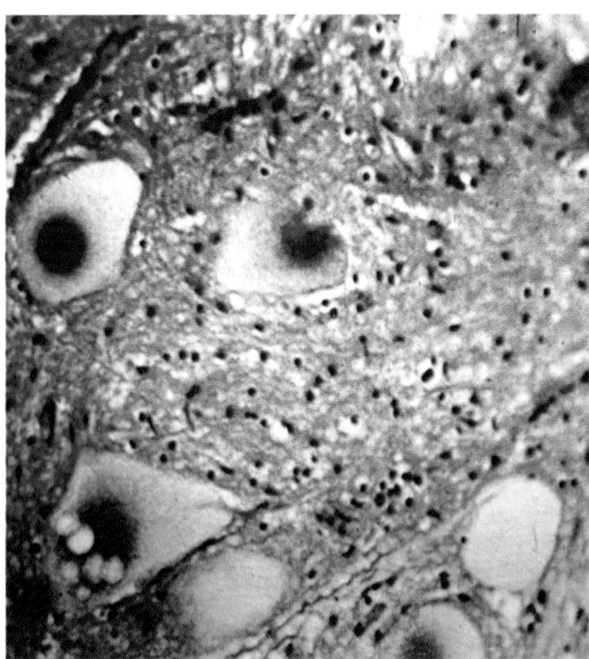

Fig. 4.26. Neurons in Tay-Sachs disease. Note ballooning of the cytoplasm with stored material, forcing the nucleus and Nissl granules to one corner of the cell body. (H&E; ×400.)

Pathologic Reactions of the Axon

Wallerian Degeneration

The process of degeneration of the axon and its myelin sheath is called *wallerian degeneration* (after Waller, who first described it in peripheral nerves in 1850). Wallerian degeneration occurs in the distal part of an axon after the parent cell body has been destroyed or separated from the axon by disease or injury along the axon (Fig. 4.28). The changes reflect the interruption of axonal transport and include the rapid disappearance of neurofibrils, followed by the axon breaking up into short fragments that eventually disappear completely. As axonal fragmentation proceeds, the myelin sheath begins to fragment in a similar manner into oval segments (*ovoids*). The myelin

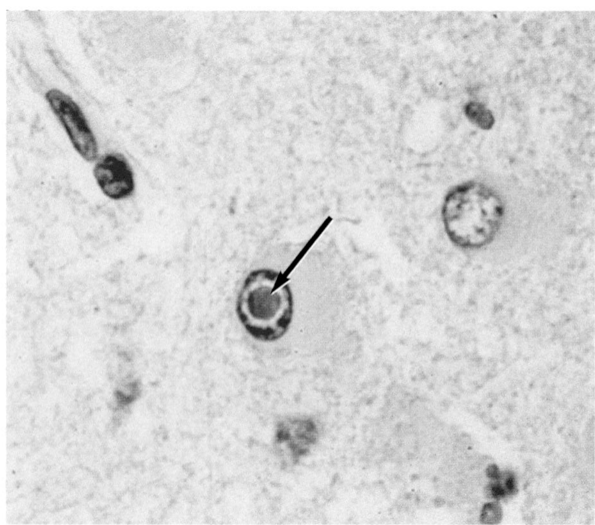

Fig. 4.27. Cowdry type A intranuclear inclusion (*arrow*) in herpes simplex encephalitis. (H&E; ×400.)

is broken down into its component lipids, which are eventually removed by phagocytosis. Wallerian degeneration proceeds more rapidly in peripheral nerves, where degenerative changes are completed in a few weeks. In the central nervous system, the degeneration proceeds over several months.

> Injury of an axon generally does not cause any change in the postsynaptic cell. However, when the motor innervation of a muscle is destroyed, the muscle becomes atrophic. A similar phenomenon, transneuronal degeneration, may occur in certain pathways in the central nervous system. In the past, the processes of chromatolysis and wallerian degeneration were used to trace neuroanatomical pathways. Tracing techniques that include the anterograde and retrograde transport of tracers such as horseradish peroxidase and transneuronal transport of viruses have replaced the "lesion techniques."

The term *axonal spheroids* refers to axonal swellings composed of neurofilaments and other organelles that accumulate focally when anterograde transport is impaired. Spheroids are a feature of axonal damage in response to several external insults, particularly trauma and ischemia. Axonal swellings that occur after interruption of axonal transport due to inherited or acquired metabolic disorders are called *dystrophic swellings*.

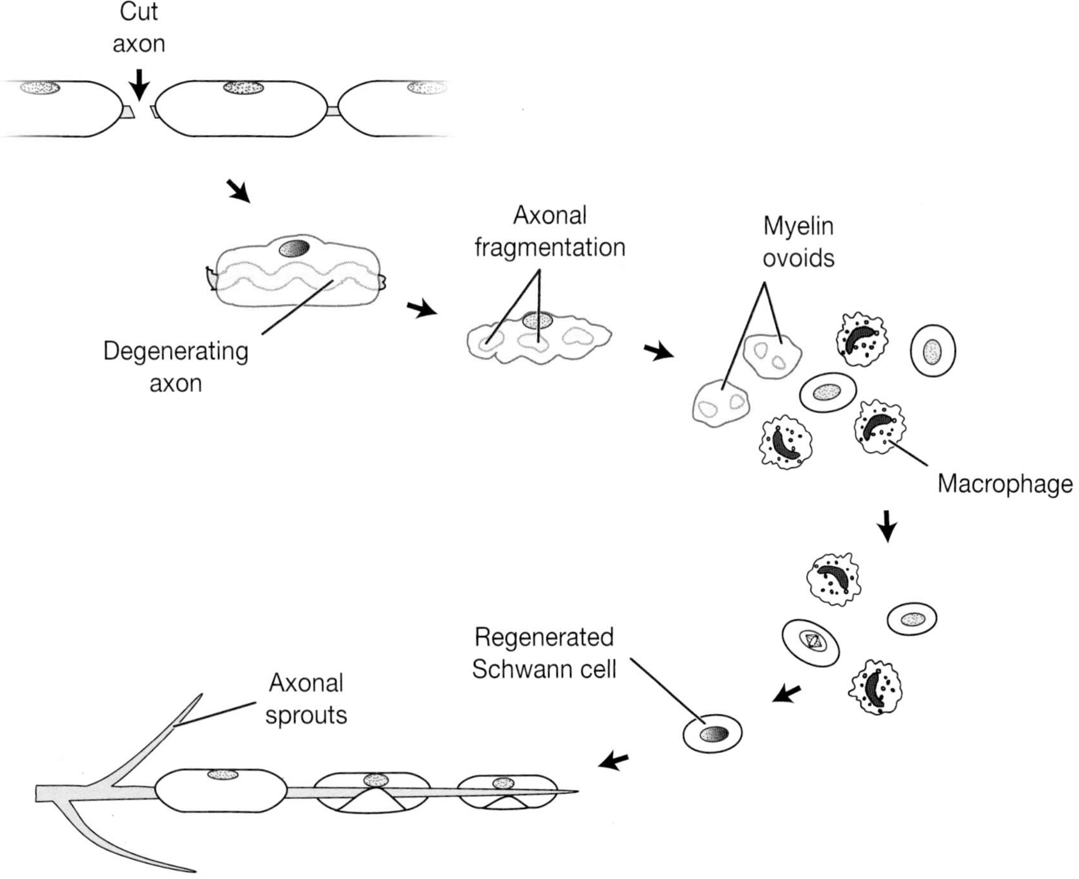

Fig. 4.28. Sequence of events in wallerian degeneration and early peripheral nerve regeneration. After degeneration and removal of myelin and axon debris, sprouts from the severed ends of an axon may find their way into a tube of regenerated Schwann cells.

Axonal Regeneration

An important difference between axons in the peripheral and central nervous systems is the potential for regeneration after injury. Axonal regeneration is possible in peripheral nerves if the parent cell body survives. In contrast, axonal regeneration does not occur in the central nervous system.

The regeneration of peripheral axons depends on trophic influences of the Schwann cells and trophic and structural support from the basement membrane.

Peripheral nerve injury disrupts the intimate axon-Schwann cell contact and leads to Schwann cell proliferation and dedifferentiation distal to the injury. Schwann cells provide a permissive environment for axon growth by secreting adhesion molecules and growth factors. These cells also regenerate the peripheral myelin. Thus, the distal portion of a damaged nerve provides a tubular superstructure that is ready to receive and myelinate new axonal sprouts growing from the proximal portion of the nerve. If these axonal sprouts find their way into one of these "tubes," they continue to grow at a rate of about 3 mm/day, and function may eventually be restored.

In contrast, multiple factors contribute to the lack of spontaneous axonal regeneration in the central nervous system, where neither basement membranes nor collagen sheaths surround nerve fibers and oligodendroglia are incapable of proliferation. Thus, functionally significant regeneration of tracts does not occur after damage to the central nervous system. However, central neurons do not intrinsically lack the ability to regenerate. When provided with the appropriate environment, adult central nervous system axons may be able to regrow and even form synaptic contacts. The two main obstacles to the regeneration of central axons after injury are the presence of a glial scar and the activity of inhibitory myelin proteins.

The glial scar is formed by astrocytes; changes in their morphology present a physical barrier to axonal growth. Several constituents of myelin, including a myelin-associated glycoprotein, and a molecule called Nogo, inhibit axonal growth. Thus, inhibiting the action of these proteins is an important therapeutic target to allow axonal regeneration in the central nervous system.

The process by which neurons form additional branches is called *collateral sprouting*. It constitutes an important compensatory mechanism in response to injury and axonal loss in the central and peripheral nervous systems. Sprouting usually occurs as a response to trophic factors secreted by microglia, macrophages, Schwann cells, or astrocytes at a site of injury.

- An axon separated from its cell body undergoes wallerian degeneration.
- Peripheral axons are able to regenerate because of the influence of Schwann cells and basement membrane.
- Central axons do not lack the intrinsic ability to regenerate after injury but fail to do so because of the presence of glial scarring and the effects of inhibitory myelin proteins.
- Collateral sprouting is a process by which surviving axons form additional branches to innervate the targets deprived of axonal inputs.

Pathologic Reactions of Supporting Cells

Oligodendrocytes

Oligodendrocytes and central myelin are extremely sensitive to injury, including ischemia and metabolic disorders. Oligodendrocytes have a range of responses to injury that vary according to the type of lesion. When affected by a pathologic process, oligodendrocytic nuclei shrink or break up and dissolve. Demyelination is the loss of normal myelin with relative preservation of axons. Demyelination in the central nervous system may be secondary to damage of the oligodendrocyte cell body or destruction of the myelin sheath. Partial or complete loss of myelin in an area of injury is demonstrated with myelin stains such as Luxol fast blue (Fig. 4.29). Demyelination may be a nonspecific manifestation of ischemic, infectious, toxic, or metabolic injury to oligodendrocytes, but it is often immune mediated. The most common immune-related demyelinating disease is *multiple sclerosis*.

More than one pathogenic mechanism contributes to injury in multiple sclerosis, including cellular- and antibody-mediated injury to the myelin sheath and primary involvement of oligodendrocytes. There is also axonal involvement. Remyelination occurs in multiple sclerosis and other demyelinating diseases and contributes to recovery of function.

A second group of disorders, called dysmyelinating disorders, or *leukodystrophies*, result from the failure to form and maintain normal myelin sheaths. Leukodystrophies are genetically determined disorders that are commonly due to defects of lysosomal or peroxisomal metabolism. Often, the type of metabolic defect can be determined with histochemical staining reactions and biochemical analysis of the tissue.

- Demyelination in the central nervous system may be secondary to damage of the oligodendrocyte cell body or destruction of the myelin sheath.
- Multiple sclerosis is the most common immune-mediated demyelinating disease in the central nervous system.
- Leukodystrophies are genetically determined disorders that affect the formation or maintenance of myelin sheaths.

Schwann Cells

Disease processes of Schwann cells affect peripheral axons. These diseases may be acquired or inherited. Immune-mediated disorders, such as acute or chronic inflammatory neuropathies, may produce segmental loss of myelin (*segmental demyelination*) (Fig. 4.30). Mutations of genes encoding for peripheral myelin proteins produce *hereditary demyelinating neuropathies*. In some of these disorders, there is repeated demyelination and remyelination of nerve fibers. Each episode leaves a layer of Schwann cells and collagen, forming concentric layers around the axon (*onion bulb* formation) (Fig. 4.31). Such nerves become large and firm; the axons may finally be lost, leaving only the stroma of the connective tissue.

- Immune disorders affecting Schwann cells produce segmental demyelination.
- Genetic disorders may result in onion bulb formation around the axon.
- Disorders affecting the myelin, if severe, cause secondary degeneration of the axon.

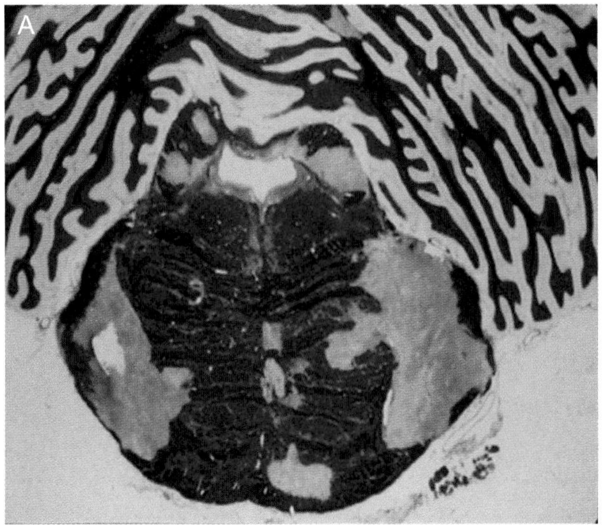

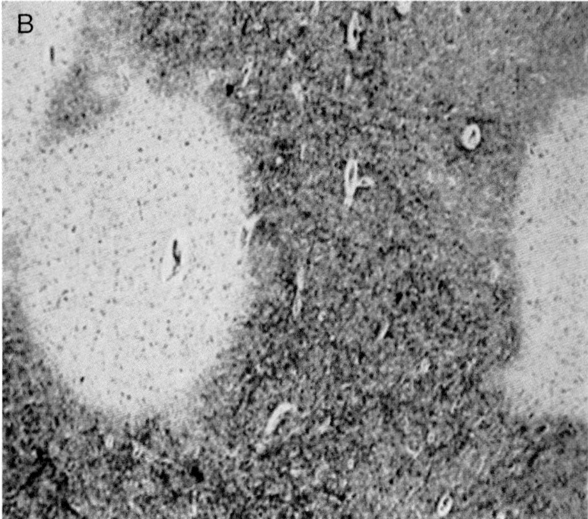

Fig. 4.29. Transverse section of the pons of a patient with multiple sclerosis. *A*, Myelin stain showing plaques of demyelination (light areas). (Luxol fast blue; ×4.) *B*, Glial fiber stain showing gliosis of demyelinated areas (dark areas). (Holzer stain; ×4.)

Astrocytes

Almost any injury to central nervous system tissue can produce a reaction of astrocytes. The swelling of astrocytes is a relatively rapid response to a wide range of stimuli. Acutely reactive astrocytes have a swollen eosinophilic cytoplasm and enlarged vesicular nuclei and are referred to as *gemistocytic* astrocytes (Fig. 4.32). With time, reactive astrocytes proliferate, a process that is called *astrocytosis*, and form progressively longer and thicker cytoplasmic processes that create a dense network in the adjacent damaged brain parenchyma. This reaction, called *fibrillary gliosis*, leads to the formation of glial scar tissue, which is equivalent to a scar formed by fibroblasts in other body organs.

The fibers of reactive astrocytes, although visible in hematoxylin- and eosin-stained sections, are seen more clearly with immunostaining for glial fibrillary acidic protein, the intermediate filament of astrocytes. In gliosis that occurs with destructive lesions, astrocytic processes are arranged haphazardly, whereas in neurodegenerative diseases, the processes are aligned according to the architecture of previously normal local tissue. Astrocytes also may react in more specific ways to certain injuries. For example, in hepatic failure and other disorders leading to the accumulation of ammonia, the astrocytes, which are normally involved in the detoxification of ammonia, enlarge and their nuclei swell (Alzheimer type 2 astrocytes). Astrocytes may also form intranuclear inclusion bodies in certain viral infections.

Fig. 4.30. Teased fiber preparation showing segmental demyelination.

- The proliferation of reactive astrocytes forms a glial scar at the site of injury or cell loss.
- Astrocytes may be affected by metabolic and viral disorders.

Ependymal Cells

Ependymal cells line the ventricular cavities of the brain and the central canal of the spinal cord. Their proliferative potential and repertoire of response to injury are limited. Atrophy, stretching, or tearing of the ependyma may occur as a consequence of ventricular enlargement

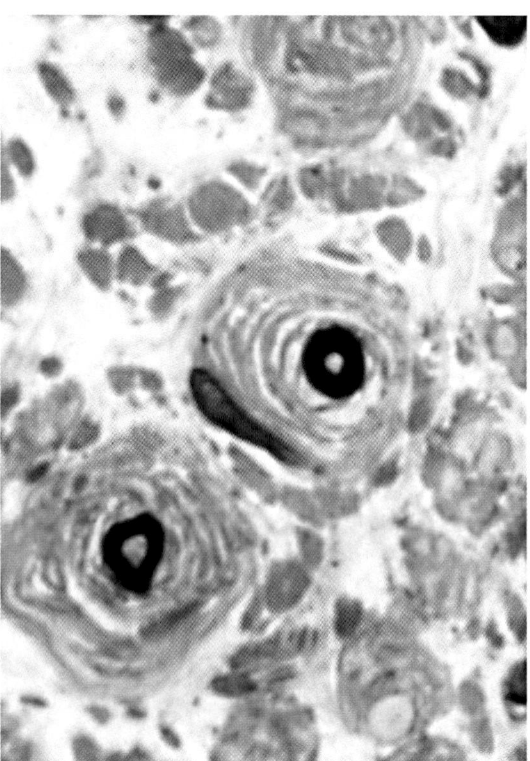

Fig. 4.31. Onion bulb formation reflecting cycles of degeneration and regeneration of the myelin sheath in a patient with hereditary sensory and motor peripheral neuropathy. (H&E; ×400.)

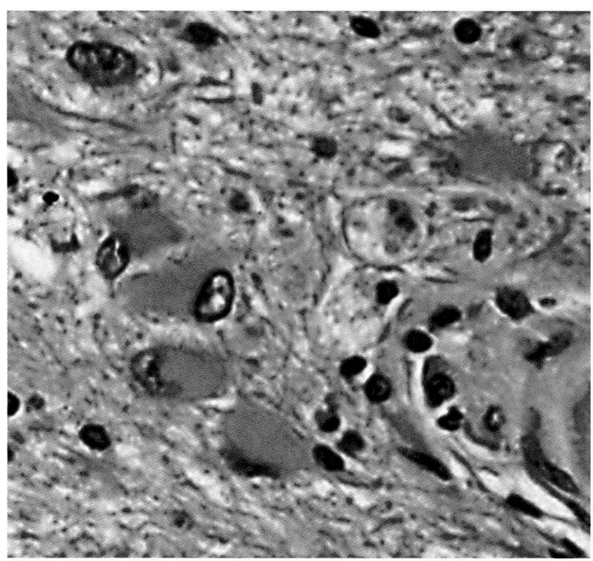

Fig. 4.32. Reactive astrocytes at the border of an infarct. Note the expansion of the cytoplasm producing a plump appearance (gemistocyte) and the dense tangle of fibers in the background. (H&E; ×250.)

(hydrocephalus). Viral infections, trauma, or toxins can interrupt the ependyma lining. This is followed by proliferation of astrocytes in the subventricular region. The astrocytic processes project to the denuded ventricular lining and form glial nodules that protrude into the ventricular system.

Inflammatory Response

Pathologic Reactions of the Microglia

Microglial cells react in a stereotyped way to most diseases that affect the central nervous system. Reactive microglial cells are recognized by their elongated rod-shaped nuclei, hence, the name *rod cells*. These cells are prominent in chronic infections. At times, microglia cells attack isolated, damaged neurons, a process called *neuronophagia*. After the neuron has been engulfed, the cluster of microglia remaining in its place forms a *microglial nodule* (Fig. 4.33). Enzymes and other toxic substances secreted by the microglia and monocytes may alter neuronal function and cause neuronal injury and loss. In regions where necrosis occurs, hematogenous monocytes infiltrate the central nervous system and microglial cells proliferate and their nuclei become rounded. Monocytes and microglia cells phagocytose dead cells and debris of the necrotic tissue. The accumulation of lipid material by these phagocytic cells gives their cytoplasm a foamy appearance, for which reason they are described as foam cells, or *foamy macrophages* (Fig. 4.34). Most of these cells eventually are reabsorbed into the blood stream.

Microglial activation involves increased entry of hematogenous monocytes into the central nervous system, proliferation of resident glia, and microglial cell secretion of proteins involved with antigen presentation and inflammation. In response to injury, microglial cells proliferate, become hypertrophic, express several marker molecules, including major histocompatibly complex antigens and costimulatory molecules for T lymphocytes, and release proinflammatory cytokines, proteolytic enzymes, complement, glutamate, nitric oxide, superoxide, and other mediators of inflammation and substances toxic to neurons. An important example is the case of central nervous system involvement by the human immunodeficiency virus. This virus infects the peripheral monocytes and lymphocytes, penetrates the brain, and infects microglia and perivascular macrophages, which

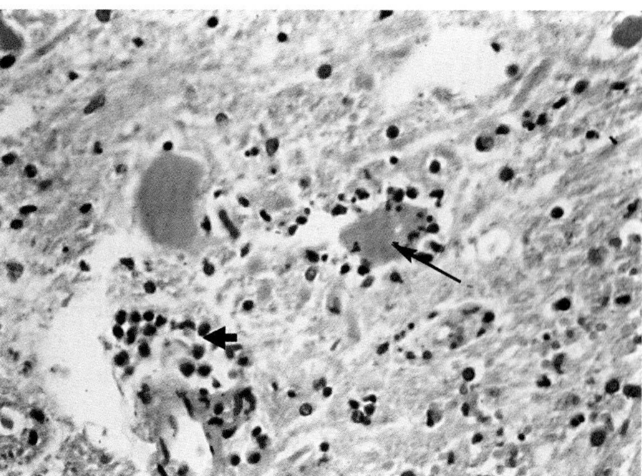

Fig. 4.33. Section of the ventral horn of a patient with poliomyelitis. Note the damaged neurons undergoing neuronophagia by microglial cells (*thin arrow*) and the formation of a microglial nodule (*thick arrow*). (H&E; ×250.)

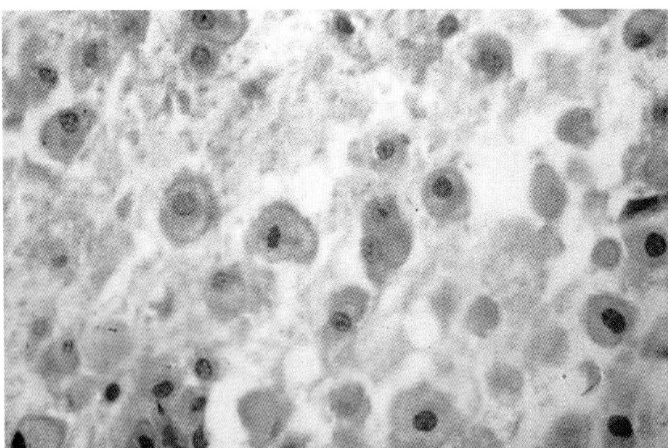

Fig. 4.34. Lipid-laden macrophages in an area of necrosis. Note the small eccentric nuclei and foamy cytoplasm. (H&E; ×250.)

form multinucleated giant cells that produce a substance toxic to neurons, even though these neurons are not directly infected by the virus.

- In response to injury, microglia cells proliferate, become hypertrophic, express antigen-presenting molecules, and secrete inflammatory mediators.
- Morphologic changes in microglia cells include formation of rod cells, neuronophagia, formation of microglial nodules, and transformation into foamy macrophages.

Mechanisms of Inflammation in the Central Nervous System

Inflammation and immune attacks on the nervous system are important mechanisms of neurologic disease, including infections, demyelinating diseases, systemic autoimmune disorders, and paraneoplastic disorders. Inflammation also occurs as a reaction to tissue necrosis, as in ischemic lesions. All these disorders are characterized by the presence of leukocyte infiltrates in the brain, spinal cord, peripheral ganglia, and nerves, in various combinations. Many of the interactions related to immune and inflammatory responses are mediated by proteins called *cytokines*, secreted by astrocytes, microglia cells, macrophages, and T lymphocytes. T lymphocytes have a crucial role in immune-mediated neurologic disorders. These responses may be mediated by humoral or cellular mechanisms or by both. The humoral mechanism involves the activation of B lymphocytes and the production of antibodies. Cellular mechanisms involve the activation of cytotoxic T cells that may bind to the antigen-presenting target cell and destroy it.

The passage of circulating leukocytes across the blood-brain barrier involves interactions with capillary endothelial cells, mediated by adhesion molecules. Leukocytes, microglial cells, and astrocytes secrete cytokines that initiate and amplify the inflammatory responses. Helper T cells produce proinflammatory cytokines, such as interleukin-1 and tumor necrosis factor, that activate macrophages and cytotoxic T cells and induce B cell growth and differentiation, leading to antibody production. Cytotoxic T cells produce granules containing enzymes and other toxic substances that directly damage neurons and other cells.

Neoplastic Transformation

Mechanisms of Oncogenesis in the Nervous System

Uncontrolled cellular proliferation of any of the cellular elements of the nervous system produces a *neoplasm*. The majority of neoplasms reflect sequential genetic alterations and somatic mutations that cause the cell to disregard the normal control of cell proliferation. The tendency of cells to enter the cell cycle, that is, to duplicate their DNA and undergo mitotic division, is under strong regulation at specific checkpoints of the cell cycle. Normally, progression through the cell cycle is determined by the balanced antagonist influences of *oncogenes*, which promote cell proliferation and survival, and *tumor suppressor genes*, which inhibit abnormal progression through the cell cycle.

Oncogenes are derived from normal cellular genes, called proto-oncogenes, which encode for growth factors, their receptors (e.g., epidermal growth factor receptor), or transduction molecules that promote cell proliferation or prevent apoptosis or do both. Tumor suppressor genes encode proteins that act as cyclin kinase inhibitors, promote cell death, or inhibit growth or survival pathways. Important examples include *p53*, which promotes cell cycle arrest and apoptosis of cells with abnormal DNA, the retinoblastoma protein, which controls DNA duplication, and neurofibromin-1, which inactivates the transduction cascades of several growth factors.

Neoplasms in the Nervous System

The type of neoplasm is named according to the predominant cell type (e.g., astrocytoma, oligodendroglioma, schwannoma, and meningioma). Cells of the nervous system vary greatly in their apparent potential to form a neoplasm. There is a general correlation between the normal capacity of a cell to undergo cell division and its tendency to undergo neoplasia. Astrocytes are the most reactive cells of the central nervous system, and *astrocytomas* are the most common primary tumors of the central nervous system. Except in extremely rare instances, tumors of the central nervous system do not metastasize outside the central nervous system. Their degree of malignancy is graded by considering the degree of pleomorphism of the tumor cells (lack of uniformity of appearance and nuclear-cytoplasmic ratio), frequency of mitotic figures, proliferation of tumor vessels, and necrosis of tumor tissue (Fig. 4.35). These factors, together with specific chromosomal abnormalities and gene mutation patterns in tumor cells, predict tumor severity, in terms of rapidity of growth, the likelihood of recurrence after surgical resection, and the length of patient survival. For example, astrocytic neoplasms

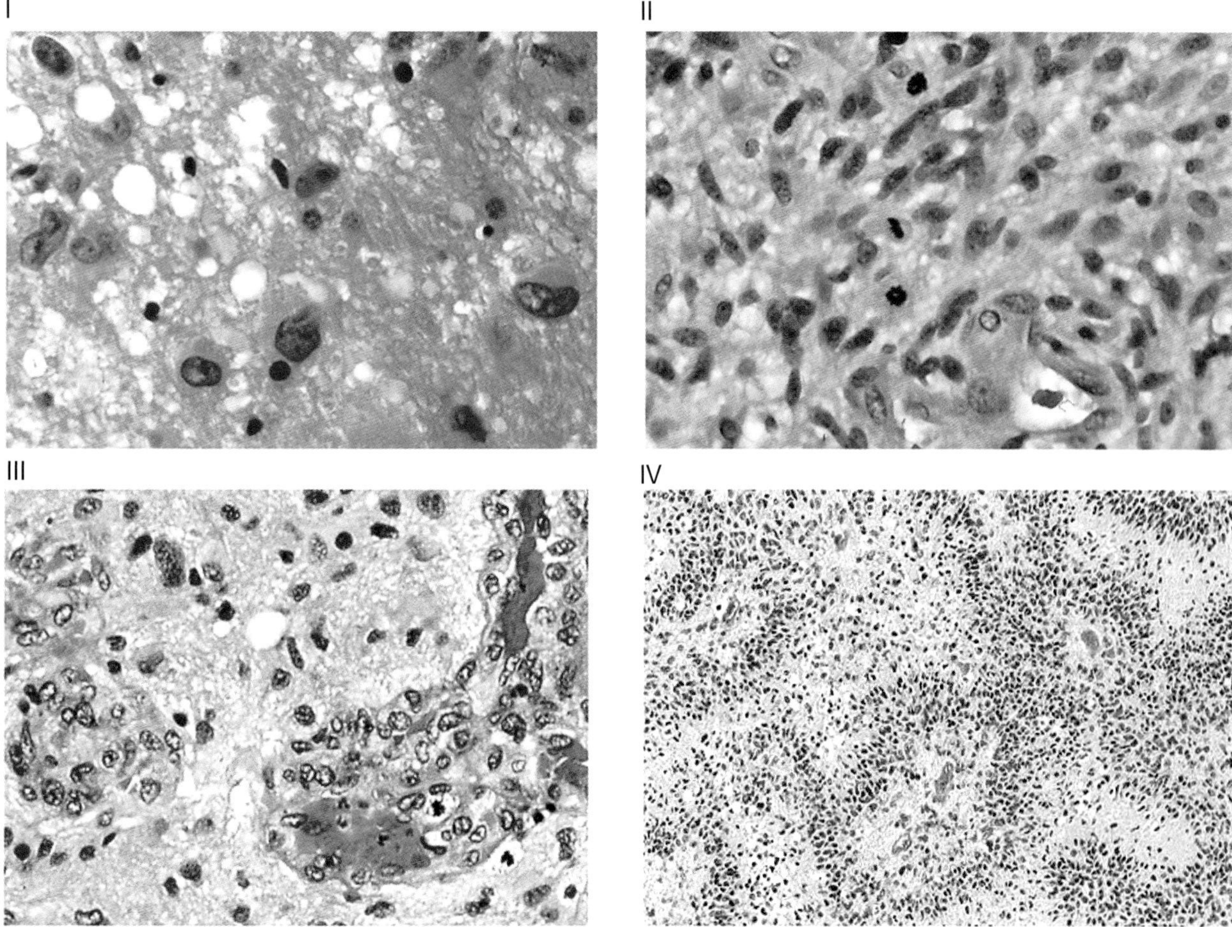

Fig. 4.35. Morphologic changes associated with progressively increased grades of malignancy in an astrocytoma. Grade I is characterized by cellular atypia only; the presence of mitosis defines grade II; vascular proliferation, grade III; and necrosis, grade IV (glioblastoma multiforme).

are subdivided into diffuse astrocytoma, anaplastic astrocytoma, and glioblastoma, which have increased degrees of severity. Diffuse astrocytoma is characterized by cells with mild atypia (nuclear pleomorphism and hyperchromasia); anaplastic astrocytoma, by more pronounced atypia and the presence of mitotic figures; and glioblastoma, by the additional presence of necrosis and microvascular proliferation. Astrocytomas generally arise in the white matter and infiltrate the adjacent parenchyma.

> The neoplastic progression from a normal astrocyte to astrocytoma then to anaplastic astrocytoma and finally to glioblastoma depends on the progressive acquisition of genetic abnormalities. Mutation of the *p53* tumor suppressor gene is an early event in neoplastic progression, whereas mutations that impair the expression of other tumor suppressor genes or produce amplification of oncogenes, such as the epidermal growth factor receptor, lead to glioblastoma. In other cases, glioblastoma may arise de novo, for example, as a consequence of mutations affecting the epidermal growth factor receptor.

Tumors of oligodendrocyte lineage, called *oligodendrogliomas*, arise primarily from the gray matter and are less frequent than astrocytomas; *ependymomas* occur even less frequently. An important neoplasm in the central nervous system is *primary central nervous system lymphoma*, which more commonly arises from B cells and often occurs in patients with an underlying immune deficiency, such as those receiving immunosuppressive therapy after organ transplantation or those with acquired immunodeficiency syndrome. The most common extra-axial tumors in the central nervous system are *meningiomas*, which originate from cells of the leptomeninges. Schwann cells give rise to *schwannomas*. The distribution and histologic type of brain neoplasms in children differs from that in adults. For example, children have a higher incidence of neoplasms in the brainstem, cerebellum, optic nerve, and hypothalamus than adults. Embryonal neuroepithelial neoplasms occur predominantly in children. They include cerebellar *medulloblastomas* and supratentorial *primitive neuroectodermal tumors*.

> Some hereditary syndromes due to mutations of tumor suppressor genes are associated with an increased risk of brain tumors. For example, neurofibromatosis type I is an autosomal dominant disorder caused by a mutation of the *NF-1* gene that encodes for neurofibromin, a protein that inhibits growth factor transduction pathways. These patients are at increased risk for the development of optic nerve astrocytomas, meningiomas, and neurofibromas (a tumor of the peripheral nerve sheath).

- Neoplasia results from activation of oncogenes, inactivation of tumor suppressor genes, or both.
- Astrocytomas and meningiomas are the most common primary nervous system tumors.
- The histologic degree of malignancy, specific chromosomal abnormalities, and gene mutation patterns predict the rapidity of growth, response to therapy, recurrence, and length of patient survival.

Cerebral Edema

An increase in tissue water content leading to increased brain volume is called *cerebral edema*. It is subdivided into two main types: vasogenic and cytotoxic.

Vasogenic Edema

The consequence of increased permeability of the blood-brain barrier to solutes and proteins is *vasogenic edema*. It occurs in the vicinity of brain neoplasms and other mass lesions (such as an abscess or hematoma), demyelinating plaques, and as a consequence of cerebral contusion or necrosis due to cerebral infarction. These conditions disrupt the tight junctions between endothelial cells, which results in edema. Vasogenic edema occurs predominantly in the white matter. It spreads from the site of irreversible injury through extracellular routes, causing expansion of the interstitial fluid space, increased interstitial pressure, and compromise of the regional microcirculation.

Cytotoxic Edema

The accumulation of fluid containing solutes, but no proteins, within glial cells and neurons is called *cytotoxic edema*. It reflects an impairment of intracellular solute homeostasis due to either energy failure to maintain pump mechanisms or osmotic disturbances. Cytotoxic edema affects predominantly astrocytes but also neurons and occurs primarily in the gray matter. Causes of cytotoxic edema include cerebral hypoxia or ischemia, head trauma, metabolic disorders (e.g., hepatic failure), and osmotic disturbances (e.g., hyponatremia).

The two types of cerebral edema are not mutually exclusive and often occur together in pathologic processes such as head trauma or cerebral infarction, which affect both the blood-brain barrier and neuronal and glial cell membranes. Except in infancy, the skull is nondistensible; thus, an increase in brain volume results in an increase in intracranial pressure, which compromises cerebral blood flow.

- Vasogenic edema reflects increased permeability of the blood-brain barrier and occurs with mass lesions or inflammatory disease.
- Cytotoxic edema is due to increased intracellular water in astrocytes or neurons and occurs with hypoxia and other metabolic disorders.
- Cytotoxic and vasogenic edema may coexist in ischemic or traumatic lesions.
- Cerebral edema leads to an increase in intracranial pressure, a decrease in cerebral blood flow, and secondary brain damage.

Clinicopathologic Correlations

Clinical diagnosis in neurology requires the analysis of two types of data. The first type is obtained from both the history and the neurologic examination and allows physicians to localize the disease process within the nervous system. On this basis, neurologic disease may be classified as *focal*, involving a single circumscribed area or group of contiguous structures in the nervous system; *multifocal*, involving more than one circumscribed area or several noncontiguous structures; and *diffuse*, involving portions of the nervous system in a bilateral, symmetrical fashion.

Different types of pathologic processes located in the same anatomical structure may produce similar symptoms and signs. Thus, the pathologic diagnosis must use information obtained from the patient's history that relates to the onset and evolution (temporal profile) of the disease (Fig. 4.35). The development of symptoms can be classified as *acute* (within minutes), *subacute* (within days), and *chronic* (within weeks or months). The evolution (course of symptoms after the onset) may be categorized as *transient*, when symptoms have resolved completely after onset; *improving*, when symptoms have decreased from their maximum but have not completely resolved; *progressive*, when symptoms continue to increase in severity or when new symptoms make their appearance; and *stationary*, when symptoms remain unchanged after reaching maximal severity and show no significant change during a period of observation.

Combining the above terms allows mass and nonmass lesions to be differentiated clinically. The presence of a *mass lesion* should be considered when the signs and symptoms, whether acute, subacute, or chronic in onset, suggest progression of a focal lesion. A *nonmass lesion* should be considered when the lesion is diffuse in location or when the signs and symptoms suggest a nonprogressive focal abnormality.

Interpretation of the temporal profile of disease depends on an understanding of the way in which pathologic processes affect neural tissue and the rates at which various destructive and reparative processes proceed. Although the final pathologic diagnosis can be established only by examination of the tissue by biopsy or at autopsy, it can be suspected on the basis of the topography and temporal profile of the lesion, established by the history and physical examination, and supported by neuroimaging studies, particularly *magnetic resonance imaging* (Table 4.3 and Fig. 4.36 and 4. 37).

- Localization of the neurologic deficit allows determination of whether the lesion is focal, multifocal, or diffuse.
- The temporal profile of the deficit allows determination of whether the lesion is acute, subacute, or chronic and whether it is transient, improving, stationary, or progressive in nature.
- Focal and progressive signs and symptoms, whether acute, subacute, or chronic in onset, suggest the presence of a mass lesion.

Table 4.3. Summary of the Most Important Spatial and Temporal Features of the Major Disease Categories

Type of lesion	Progression	Temporal profile	Pathology/etiology
Focal	Nonprogressive (nonmass)	Acute	Infarct
			Trauma
	Progressive (mass)	Acute	Hematoma
		Subacute	Abscess
			Granuloma
			Demyelinating plaque
		Chronic	Neoplasm
Diffuse (nonmass)	Nonprogressive	Acute	Hypoxia-ischemia
			Trauma
	Progressive	Acute	Subarachnoid hemorrhage
		Subacute	Encephalitis
			Meningitis
			Toxic-metabolic
		Chronic	Degenerative
			Toxic-metabolic

- Diffuse signs and symptoms, whether progressive or not, or nonprogressive signs or symptoms suggest a nonmass lesion.
- Neuroimaging, particularly magnetic resonance imaging, confirms the localization of the lesion determined by the history and clinical examination and provides insight into its possible pathologic basis.

Vascular Diseases

Neurons deprived of metabolic support from the blood, in the form of oxygen and glucose, cease functioning in seconds and undergo pathologic change in minutes. Therefore, the hallmark of a vascular disease process is its *sudden onset*. Neurologic function is altered abruptly and usually maximally within minutes after the initial insult or progresses within the first 24 hours. The two main categories of vascular lesions are ischemic and hemorrhagic.

Ischemia

Ischemic lesions can be diffuse or focal. Diffuse ischemic lesions are due to an abrupt global cessation of cerebral blood flow, as in cardiac arrest. Focal ischemic lesions occur as a consequence of the interruption of blood flow to a specific brain region from occlusion of a vessel that supplies that region. This focal ischemic lesion, called *cerebral infarction*, is the most common type of vascular lesion (Fig. 4.38). Ischemic neuronal change is the hallmark of ischemic lesions. When ischemia is prolonged or severe, all structural elements of the brain parenchyma are lost. The events that follow the acute insult are primarily attempts at repair; thus, the course of a patient's symptoms is generally that of stabilization or improvement. Clinical progression of symptoms, when it occurs, usually indicates cerebral edema or involvement of neurons in surrounding areas by the ischemic process.

The chronologic, microscopic events that occur in the region of an infarct are as follows: Within 6 to 12 hours after cessation of blood flow, neurons show acute swelling and pallor, and as the process progresses, they show typical ischemic change. After 24 to 48 hours, leukocytes begin migrating from the blood vessels into the brain substance. At 48 to 72 hours, microglia proliferate and macrophages begin to appear and steadily increase

Clinical Problem 4.1.

Identify the level, lateralization, presence of mass, and presumed pathologic basis of the following neurologic problem: A 68-year-old, right-handed man noted heaviness in his left arm while reading a newspaper. He tried to stand up but could not support his weight on his left leg. He was able to call for help. When his wife came into the room, she noted that the left side of his face was sagging. The neurologic symptoms had not changed by the time he was evaluated 1 hour later and were the same the next day.

in number up to the third week, after which their number gradually diminishes. The early stage corresponds only to the gross softening of the lesion (encephalomalacia) and, later, to cyst formation. After 4 to 5 days, in the region of astrocyte survival, astrocytes begin to proliferate and extend fibrillary processes; this peaks at about 6 weeks and results in the formation of a glial scar. During the second week, surviving capillaries also proliferate as part of the repair process.

Hemorrhage

The second type of vascular disorder is hemorrhage, which is due to rupture of a blood vessel either within the brain or in a surrounding structure. Intraparenchymal hemorrhage is the localized accumulation of a blood clot (*hematoma*) in neural tissue (Fig. 4.38). In this situation, both the symptoms and the pathologic changes appear abruptly and are focal. Because of the continuing pathologic changes that occur in response to a localized hemorrhage compressing neighboring tissue, the focal symptoms

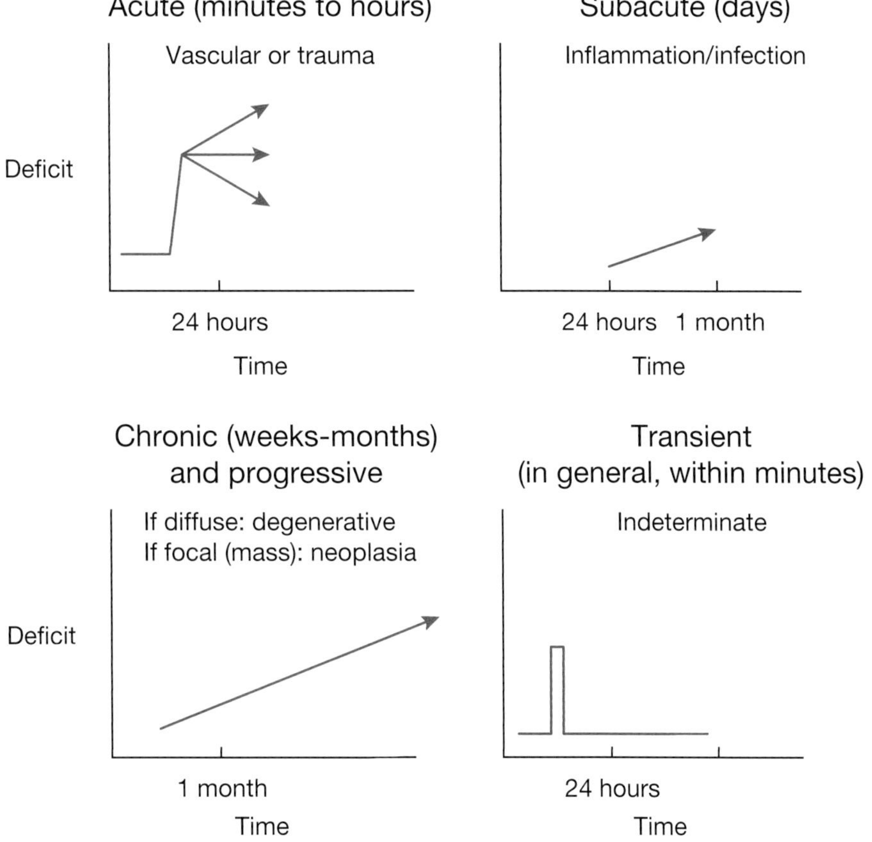

Fig. 4.36. Temporal profiles of neurologic deficits that point to the underlying pathologic cause.

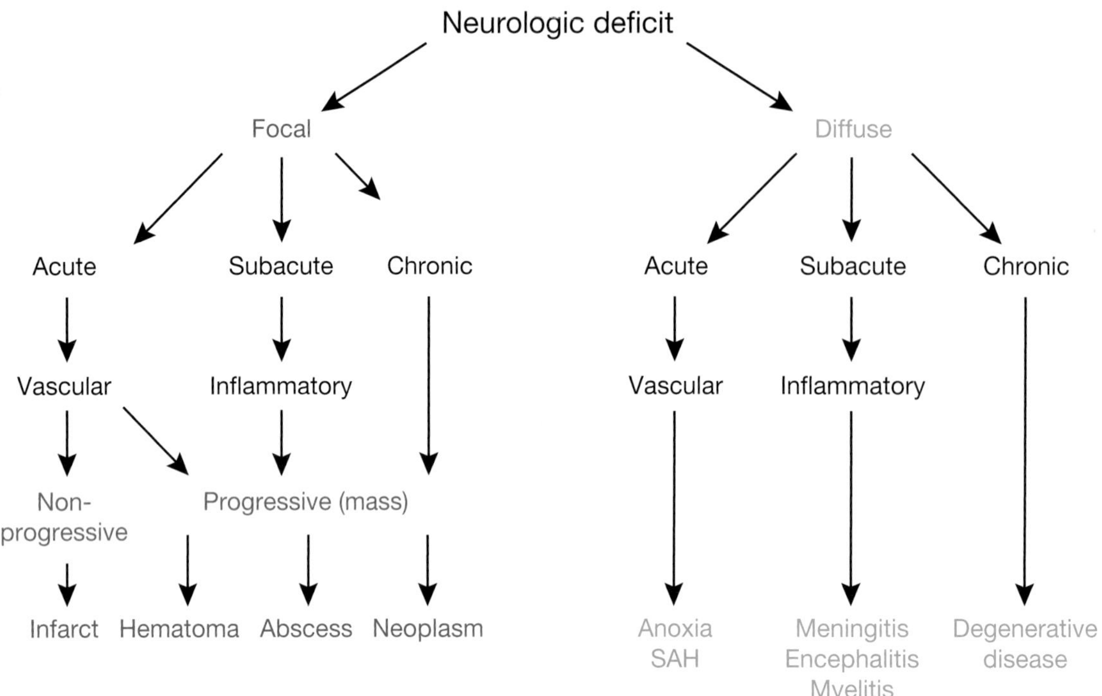

Fig. 4.37. Clues from the history and physical examination defining the spatial localization (focal vs. diffuse) and temporal profile (acute, subacute, or chronic, and nonprogressive or progressive) that lead to the presumptive pathologic diagnosis of neurologic disease. SAH, subarachnoid hemorrhage.

are progressive within 24 hours from onset, indicating a mass lesion. Thus, an acute, focal, and progressive neurologic deficit suggests a cerebral hematoma (a mass of vascular origin).

Subarachnoid hemorrhage occurs as a consequence of rupture of a vessel on the surface of the brain, commonly due to focal weakening and expansion of the vessel wall (aneurysm). In this situation, the symptoms and pathologic

Clinical Problem 4.2.

Identify the level, lateralization, presence of mass, and presumed pathologic basis of the following neurologic problem: A 74-year-old woman, with a past history of hypertension, suddenly developed a severe, right-sided headache, followed by progressing weakness of the left face, arm, and leg over 2 hours. On admission to the hospital 4 hours later, she was found to have severe weakness of the left face, arm, and leg, increased muscle stretch reflexes on the left, and decreased sensation on the left side.

Clinical Problem 4.3.

Identify the level, lateralization, presence of mass, and presumed pathologic basis of the following neurologic problem: A 46-year-old, left-handed woman suddenly noted the onset of a severe occipital headache. On lying down, she became violently ill, with nausea and vomiting. She complained of a stiff neck. She was taken immediately to the hospital, where she was noted to be somnolent but to respond appropriately when stimulated. She could move all four extremities with equal facility. Her level of consciousness deteriorated, and she became comatose.

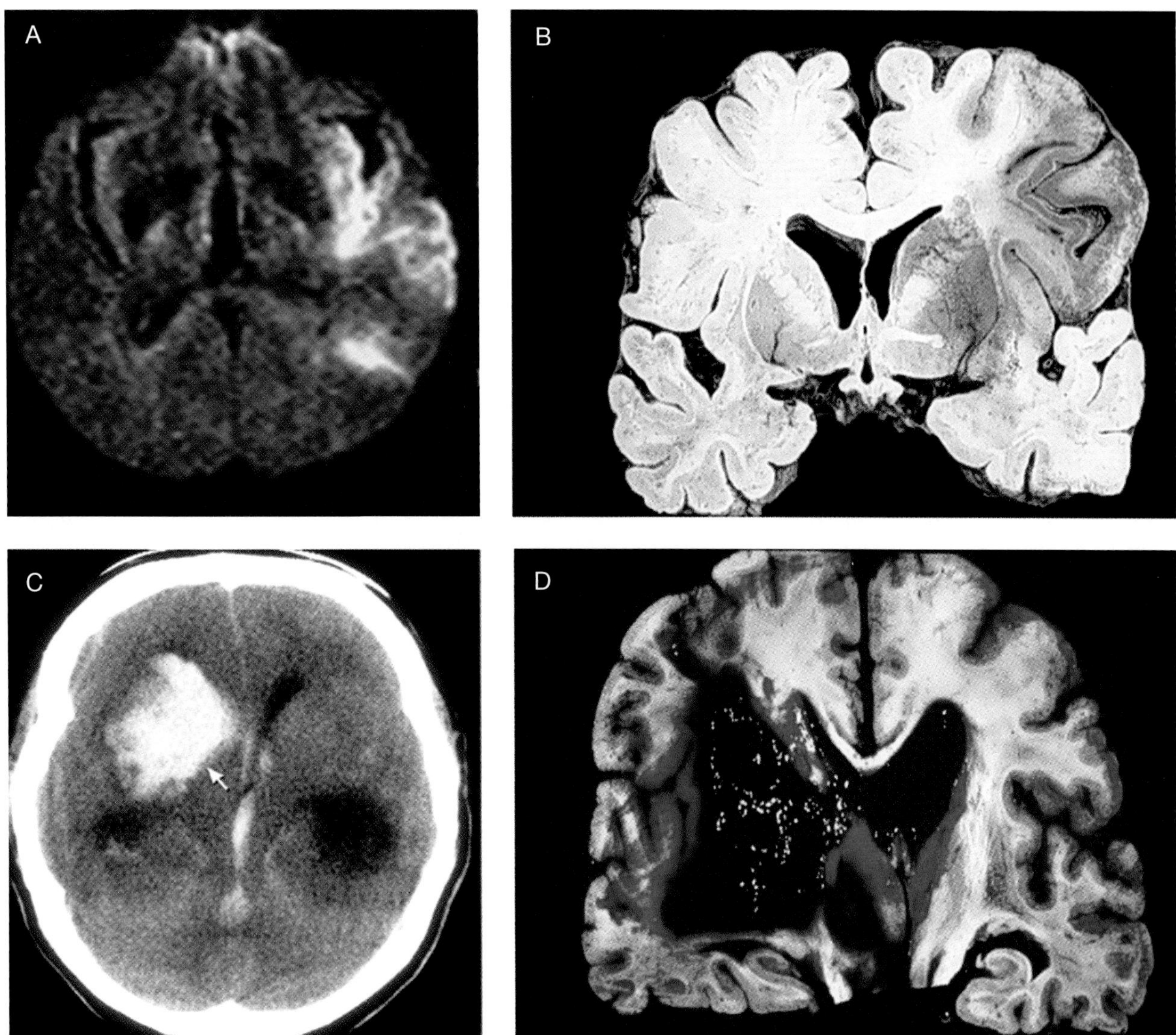

Fig. 4.38. Focal vascular lesions. *A*, Diffusion weighted magnetic resonance image showing an area of impaired water diffusion (indicative of impaired neuronal and glial metabolism) in the territory of the middle cerebral artery, consistent with a cerebral infarction. *B*, Pathology specimen showing a typical infarction in the distribution of the middle cerebral artery. *C*, Noncontrast computed tomographic scan of the brain showing a focal hyperintense lesion (*arrow*) consistent with an intracerebral hematoma. *D*, Pathology specimen showing a massive cerebral hematoma centered on the basal ganglia, with mass effect.

changes are abrupt in onset but diffusely distributed in the nervous system.

- Vascular disease is acute in onset.
- Vascular lesions may be ischemic or hemorrhagic and focal or diffuse in distribution.
- Acute, focal, nonprogressive clinical manifestations suggest a cerebral infarction.
- Acute, focal, progressive manifestations suggest an intraparenchymal hematoma.
- Acute, diffuse manifestations indicate global anoxia-ischemia or subarachnoid hemorrhage.

Inflammatory Diseases

The inflammatory response occurs in response to microorganisms (infections), immunologic reactions, or toxins. This response usually occurs rapidly but not suddenly; thus, its temporal profile is frequently subacute, developing from days to a few weeks. The pathologic hallmark of the inflammatory response is the outpouring of white blood cells. Inflammatory and immune processes may affect every component of the central or peripheral nervous system. Targets include the meninges, parenchyma of the brain, spinal cord, peripheral nerves, and blood vessels, in several combinations. Infections may be caused by viruses, bacteria, mycobacteria, fungi, or parasites. Immune reactions may occur against antigens present in the nervous system, including myelin (demyelinating disease), neurons, axons, or synaptic terminals, or as a manifestation of an autoimmune attack triggered by antigens present outside the nervous system (e.g., neoplastic cells in the lung). The type of cell infiltrate generally varies with the cause of the inflammatory diseases. In bacterial infections, the major component of the exudate is polymorphonuclear leukocytes, whereas in viral infections, indolent infections (e.g., tuberculosis), or fungal infections or in immunologic disorders, the predominant cells are mononuclear cells, especially lymphocytes. Inflammatory disorders may be diffuse, focal, or multifocal. Their evolution is progressive, but some may have a relapsing and remitting course.

Infections

In general, infections of the central nervous system are diffusely distributed either in the leptomeninges and cerebrospinal fluid (*meningitis*) or in the parenchyma of the brain (*encephalitis*) or spinal cord (*myelitis*).

Other central nervous system infections are more likely to be focal or multifocal. For example, bacterial infections may produce focal progressive lesions called *abscesses* (Fig. 4.39). Other infectious agents, such as mycobacteria (e.g., tuberculosis) or fungi, elicit a reaction characterized by macrophage infiltrates, called *granuloma*.

In response to a localized area of inflammation, astrocytes proliferate in the surrounding tissue and a wall of glial fibers is formed that limits the spread of the infection. The inflamed brain becomes softened and liquefied, and eventually a cavity may form. This process is called abscess formation. Unlike the cavity produced by an infarct, the wall of an abscess is surrounded by a collagenous capsule formed by fibroblasts. A brain abscess can exert a mass effect and progressively expand and compress neighboring structures.

Clinical Problem 4.4.

Identify the level, lateralization, presence of mass, and presumed pathologic basis of the following neurologic problem: A 4-year-old, right-handed boy complained of a sore throat, chills, and fever. He was put to bed and given acetaminophen and fluids. The next morning, he complained of headache and an increasingly stiff neck. His temperature was 105°F (40.5°C). When evaluated at a physician's office later that afternoon, he was difficult to arouse. He was confused and delirious when stimulated. He held his neck stiff but moved his extremities on command.

Immune Disorders

Whereas immune responses mediated by antibodies or cytotoxic T lymphocytes are normally directed against agents foreign to the body, such as microorganisms or tumor cells, faulty recognition mechanisms or abnormal immune regulation may result in an immune attack

Clinical Problem 4.5.

Identify the level, lateralization, presence of mass, and presumed pathologic basis of the following neurologic problem: A 6-year-old, right-handed girl had fever and ear pain for 2 days. She then started complaining of severe headaches that progressed over the next day and were associated with vomiting. Examination showed incoordination of the left arm and leg.

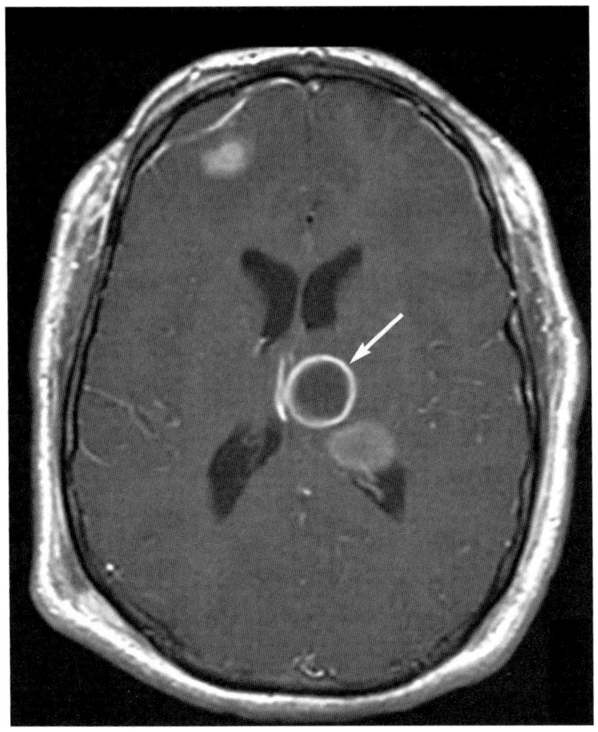

Fig. 4.39. Magnetic resonance image of the head with gadolinium showing the typical appearance of cerebral abscesses, which produce focal, inflammatory mass lesions. The ring of gadolinium enhancement indicates disruption of the blood-brain barrier (*arrow*).

Clinical Problem 4.6.

Identify the level, lateralization, presence of mass, and presumed pathologic basis of the following neurologic problem: A 23-year-old woman started experiencing pain and decrease of vision in the right eye over the course of 3 days. Examination showed decreased visual acuity and color vision in the right eye. Her vision slowly improved spontaneously over the course of 2 weeks. One year before, she had experienced an episode of numbness and weakness in the right leg and incoordination of the left arm, which developed over 2 days and resolved, with minimal residual deficit, over the course of 3 weeks.

on normal constituents of the nervous system. An immune attack on the myelin sheath (demyelinating disease), as in multiple sclerosis, may produce a focal lesion (such as transverse myelitis or optic neuritis) or multifocal lesions (Fig. 4.40). Unlike infectious disorders, which are always progressive without specific treatment, focal neurologic deficits due to immune demyelinating disease may remit spontaneously (because of remyelination) or follow a relapsing or secondary progressive course.

An immune attack also causes inflammatory demyelination of peripheral nerves, as in *Guillain-Barré syndrome*. Some immune demyelinating reactions are triggered by previous infections, particularly viral. Another important group of immune-mediated disorders is the *paraneoplastic diseases*. They are a consequence of an autoimmune response to antigens present in tumor cells outside the nervous system. Paraneoplastic disorders can affect specific areas of the cerebral cortex or basal ganglia, brainstem, cerebellum, spinal cord, or dorsal root ganglia, in various combinations. Immune deficiency may predispose to both infectious and neoplastic disorders of the nervous system. An important cause is human immunodeficiency virus, which infects monocytes and lymphocytes and impairs their function.

- Inflammatory and immune disorders are generally of subacute onset.
- Inflammatory disorders may be diffuse, focal, or multifocal.
- Abscesses, granulomas, and large demyelinating lesions may produce mass lesions.
- Whereas infectious disorders are always progressive without treatment, demyelinating and other immune disorders may remit and recur spontaneously.

Neoplastic Diseases

A neoplasm in the nervous system may be primary or metastatic from another organ. Primary neoplasms of the nervous system can be subdivided into intra-axial and extra-axial. Intra-axial neoplasms arise from elements of the brain parenchyma; the most common types are astrocytomas and oligodendrogliomas and, in

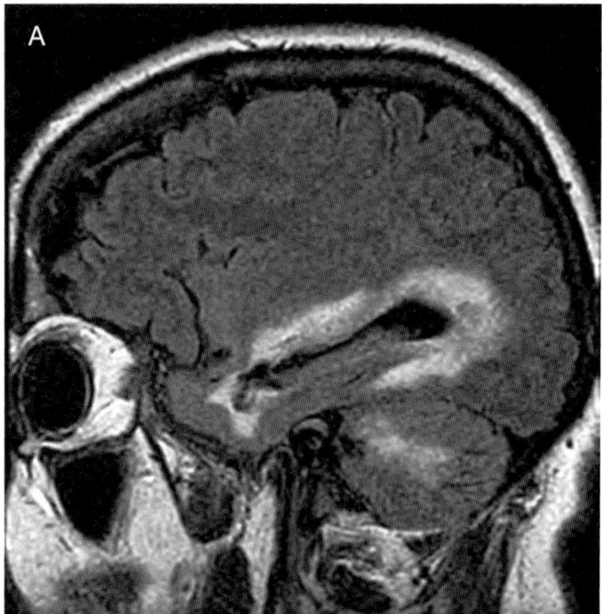

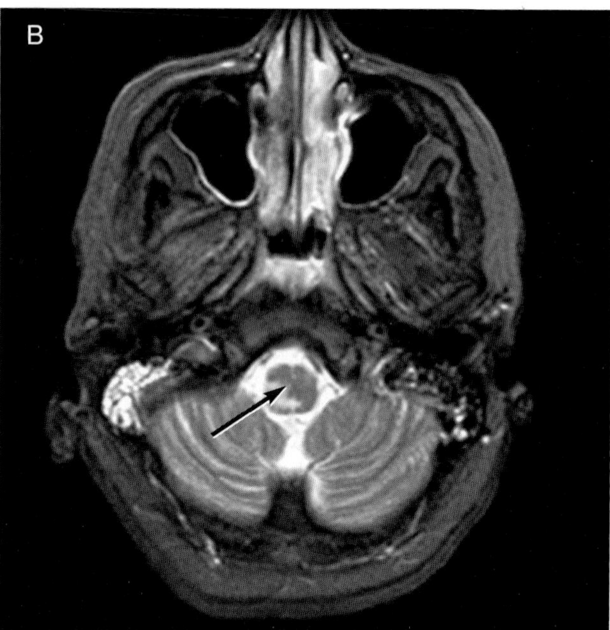

Fig. 4.40. Typical images of multiple sclerosis, the prototype inflammatory demyelinating disorder of the central nervous system. *A*, Sagittal magnetic resonance image with a fluid-attenuated inversion-recovery (FLAIR) sequence showing the distribution of demyelinating lesions in the periventricular white matter and cerebellum. *B*, Axial T2-weighted image showing a focal demyelinating lesion in the right medulla (*arrow*).

immunocompromised patients, lymphomas. Extra-axial tumors are derived from the meninges, cranial or peripheral nerves, pituitary gland, or pineal gland. The most common are meningiomas and pituitary adenomas. Lesions metastatic to the nervous system may arise from neoplasia in any organ, most commonly carcinoma of the lung, breast, or colon, as well as from melanoma of the skin. The metastasis may occur in the parenchyma, meninges, or bone (particularly the spinal column). A neoplastic mass progressively increases in size and alters the function of the region in which it lies. It may also alter the function of adjacent structures by compression or formation of edema around the primary mass (Fig. 4.41).

The clinical correlate of neoplastic disease is the presence of focal, progressive manifestations typical of a mass lesion, which are generally chronic in evolution.

It can be appreciated from the description of vascular and inflammatory lesions that not all focal and progressive (mass) lesions in the nervous system are composed of neoplastic cells. A vascular mass (hematoma) and inflammatory mass (abscess, granuloma, or large demyelinating lesion) may also produce focal progressive deficits, although their temporal profile is usually acute (intracerebral hematoma) or subacute (inflammatory disease). However, some nonneoplastic masses, such as

Clinical Problem 4.7.

Identify the level, lateralization, presence of mass, and presumed pathologic basis of the following neurologic problem: A 54-year-old, right-handed woman noted some difficulty in expressing her thoughts. This difficulty was mild, and she paid little attention to it. Two weeks later, she complained of clumsiness and weakness in her right arm and leg, but the results of an examination by her physician were considered normal. Headaches appeared several months later, along with increasing right-sided weakness. She also became aware of an inability to see the right half of the visual field with either eye.

chronic subdural hematoma, may have a chronic temporal profile, thus mimicking a neoplasm.

- Focal, progressive, and chronic neurologic deficits suggest the presence of neoplasia.
- Vascular or inflammatory disorders may produce mass lesions that resemble a neoplasm.

Degenerative Disease

Degenerative diseases have varied clinical manifestations that reflect progressive cell loss in specific regions of the nervous system. Despite their diversity, degenerative diseases share many features. They are all characterized by chronic, progressive, bilateral, and symmetrical involvement of specific neuronal groups in the nervous system. The pathology of this group of diseases is characterized by selective neuronal loss and synaptic alterations, associated with reactive astrocytosis and activated microglia, in specific regions of the nervous system. They are all characterized by abnormal deposits (inclusions) of self-aggregating misfolded proteins, as described above (Table 4.2).

The clinical differences among these diseases are related to the neuronal populations involved, the order in which cell death occurs, and the pace at which it proceeds.

Clinical Problem 4.8.

Identify the level, lateralization, presence of mass, and presumed pathologic basis of the following neurologic problem: A 50-year-old, right-handed woman, formerly an executive secretary for a local banker, had a neurologic evaluation because of a marked personality change that had occurred during the last several months. Her memory was poor. She could no longer do even simple calculations, and she had difficulty in following commands. She seemed ill informed about current events and no longer seemed interested in her personal appearance. Results of the rest of the examination were unremarkable.

For example, involvement of neurons in the cerebral cortex produces dementia (e.g., Alzheimer disease) (Fig. 4.42); involvement of neurons in basal ganglia circuits produces slowness of movement (e.g., Parkinson disease) or excessive movement (e.g., Huntington disease), and involvement of motor neurons produces muscle weakness and atrophy (e.g., amyotrophic lateral sclerosis). Also,

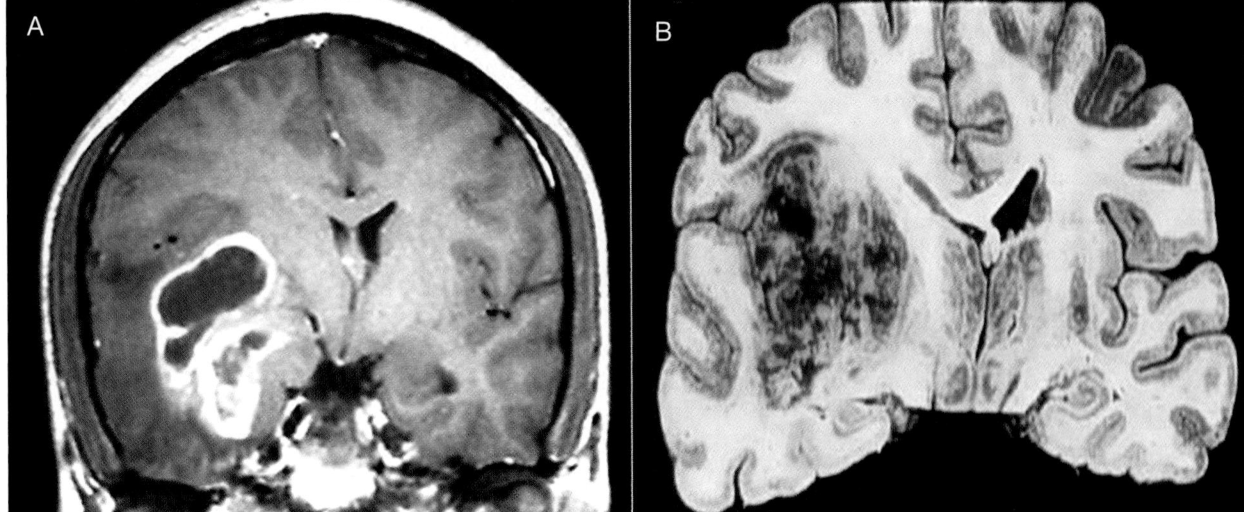

Fig. 4.41. *A*, Magnetic resonance imaging of the head with gadolinium showing a heterogeneous, contrast-enhancing mass in the white matter of the left temporal lobe, consistent with a high-grade astrocytoma (glioblastoma multiforme). *B*, Pathology specimen showing the macroscopic features (hemorrhage and necrosis) typical of this lesion.

degenerative disorders usually have both sporadic and familiar forms.

- Degenerative disorders produce chronic, progressive neurologic deficits that reflect bilateral loss of specific populations of neurons.
- The mechanisms of abnormal cell inclusions and neuronal loss in neurodegenerative disorders are an active area of research and provide potential targets for treatment.

Metabolic or Toxic Diseases

Metabolic disorders and toxic chemical agents, either exogenous or endogenous, may alter the function of neurons and supporting cells throughout the nervous system. These disorders may affect intermediate metabolism, synthesis, transport or degradation of macromolecules, formation and maintenance of myelin, astrocyte function and the neuronal microenvironment, or permeability of the blood-brain barrier. Thus, the hallmark of these disorders is the development of diffuse neurologic signs and symptoms. The temporal profile of these disorders may be acute, subacute, or chronic. The diagnosis of a metabolic or toxic disorder depends on the demonstration of a biochemical abnormality in the blood, cerebrospinal fluid, or cells obtained by biopsy of peripheral tissues.

Acute metabolic and toxic disorders produce a condition called *metabolic encephalopathy*, which results primarily from impaired energy metabolism, ionic homeostasis, or neurotransmitter function in the nervous system. Important examples are hypoxia, hypoglycemia, deficiency of vitamin B_1 (thiamine), which is critical for aerobic metabolism of glucose, and electrolyte abnormalities such as hyponatremia. Endogenous toxins may accumulate in the setting of hepatic or renal failure. The rapid recognition of all these disorders is vital for preventing neuronal death.

Some metabolic and toxic disorders produce chronic progressive neurologic deficits, thus resembling a neurodegenerative disease. A search for a potentially metabolic cause of a chronic progressive neurologic disease is important, because in some cases correction of the metabolic abnormality may prevent progression or even ameliorate some of the deficits. Important examples are vitamin B_{12} deficiency, thyroid hormone deficiency, and disorders of copper or amino acid metabolism.

Clinical Problem 4.9.

Identify the level, lateralization, presence of mass, and cause of the following neurologic problem: A 56-year-old man with diabetes became confused and less responsive over a period of several hours. He had self-injected the usual dose of insulin upon awakening, but because of an upset stomach, he failed to eat anything during the day. He was observed to have a generalized seizure. When brought to the emergency department, he was comatose. Lateral head movement to either side produced nystagmus. There were no other localizing neurologic signs. The fasting plasma glucose level was 15 mg/100 mL.

Genetic disorders that affect cell organelles may also produce chronic, progressive, and bilaterally symmetrical involvement of the gray matter, white matter, or both, thus manifesting as a neurodegenerative disorder. Important examples are *mitochondrial disorders*, due to mutations that affect nuclear or mitochondrial DNA and the respiratory chain. These disorders may affect the gray matter, white matter, peripheral nerve, and muscles, in various combinations. Mitochondrial DNA disorders are transmitted exclusively by the mother. Disorders affecting lysosomal enzymes or peroxisomes may produce leukodystrophy or gray matter disease.

- Metabolic and toxic disorders produce deficits that reflect bilateral and symmetrical involvement of the nervous system.
- The temporal profile of metabolic or toxic disorders may be acute, subacute, or chronic.
- Metabolic or toxic disorders may produce acute or subacute encephalopathy.
- Some metabolic disorders produce chronic progressive neurologic deficits and, thus, resemble a neurodegenerative disease.
- Diagnosis of a metabolic or toxic disorder requires identifying a specific chemical abnormality in the blood, urine, cerebrospinal fluid, or peripheral tissues.

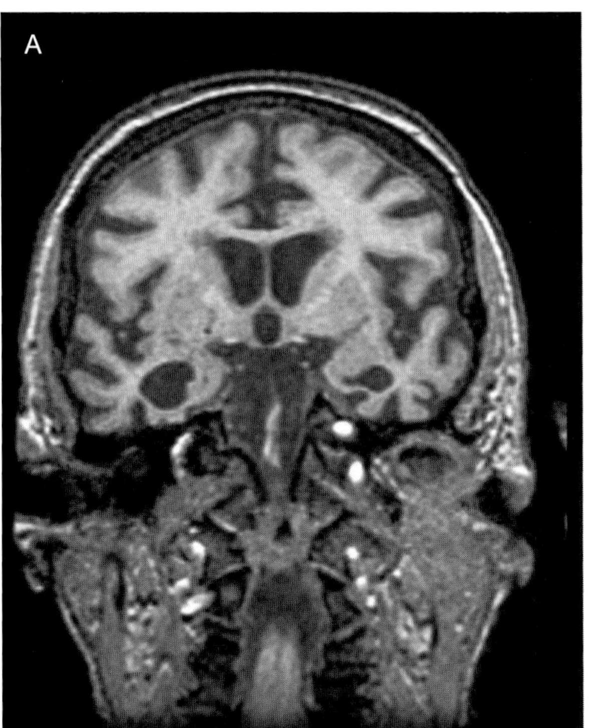

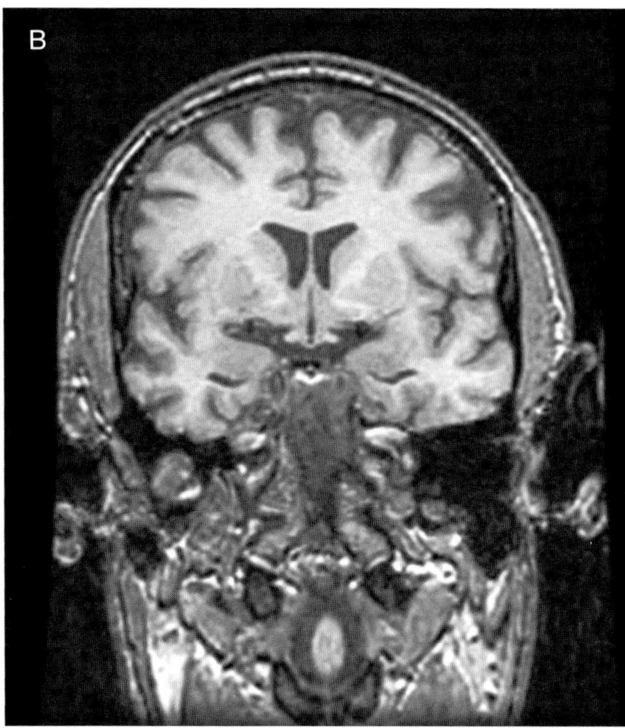

Fig. 4.42. Magnetic resonance imaging of the brain of a patient with Alzheimer disease (*A*) compared with that of an age-matched patient with normal cognitive function (*B*). Note the diffuse atrophy affecting predominantly the medial portion of the temporal lobe, consistent with a degenerative (diffuse, chronic progressive) disease.

- Recognition of a toxic or treatable metabolic cause of neurologic disease is critical for early treatment and prevention of irreversible damage in the nervous system.

Traumatic Disease

Trauma to the nervous system is always acute in onset, with a clearly identifiable precipitating event (e.g., automobile accident, fall, or missile wound). Traumatic lesions may produce maximal deficits from the onset or progressive deficits from vascular or other complications. Trauma in the central nervous system may produce diffuse or focal damage. The syndrome of *concussion* is a transient loss of consciousness that reflects acute functional impairment of axonal function that is maximal at onset and is followed by spontaneous resolution. *Contusions* are superficial bruises of the brain that are associated with hemorrhage in the leptomeninges and variable brain edema and are manifested as focal deficits. Patients who experience sustained *diffuse axonal injury* have multiple small contusions along the corpus callosum and brainstem. These patients typically are unconscious from the onset and remain so or at least severely disabled until death.

Bleeding in and around the brain is a common feature of head trauma and manifests as the development of progressive focal neurologic deficits. *Extradural hematoma* results from torn arteries in the leptomeninges and is usually associated with skull fractures. *Subdural hematoma* usually results from tearing of bridging veins in the subdural space. These hemorrhagic lesions produce focal and progressive neurologic deterioration typical of a mass lesion. This may occur over a period hours in the cases of epidural hematoma (because of the rapid accumulation of arterial blood) to several days, weeks, or even months in the case of subdural hematomas (because of the slower accumulation of venous blood). Thus, chronic subdural hematomas may manifest with focal, progressive, and chronic deficits, resembling a neoplasm.

Repeated exposure of the head to a large number of blows (as in boxing) may lead to progressive neurologic deterioration due to neuronal loss and cell inclusions that resemble some neurodegenerative disease (punch-drunk syndrome, or *dementia pugilistica*).

Injuries to the spinal cord produce neurologic deficits that are maximal from the onset and reflect spinal cord compression, laceration, contusion, or hemorrhage and secondary damage initiated by the trauma. The secondary damage is due to hypoxia, ischemia, and delayed deterioration that result from the formation of a cavity in the spinal cord (syringomyelia), continued compression, meningeal fibrosis, or atrophy of the spinal cord. Lesions affecting the peripheral nervous system produce focal deficits in the distribution of the nerve or nerves affected.

- Traumatic injury of the brain may produce sudden diffuse impairment of neuronal function (loss of consciousness), which may resolve spontaneously or persist until death.
- Focal deficits due to concussion tend to improve or stabilize.
- Traumatic hematoma produces focal, progressive deficits consistent with a mass lesion.
- Chronic subdural hematoma mimics a brain neoplasm.
- Spinal cord injury produces acute neurologic deficits, which may be followed by partial recovery, stabilization, or late deterioration.
- Traumatic injury to a peripheral nerve causes a focal deficit that is maximal from the onset and is followed by stabilization or recovery.

Additional Clinical Problems

For each of the following problems, identify the level, lateralization, presence of mass, and presumed pathologic basis.

Clinical Problem 4.10.

Identify the level, lateralization, presence of mass, and cause of the following neurologic problem: A 23-year-old man was stabbed in the mid back and developed severe pain in the back and chest. Almost immediately after the pain, he became weak and unable to support any weight on his right leg, but it did not worsen. Examination showed marked weakness of the right lower extremity, with a decrease in the perception of pinprick in the left leg to about the level of the umbilicus.

Clinical Problem 4.11.

A 54-year-old right-handed woman suddenly became dizzy, with nausea and vomiting. Examination showed dysarthria, difficulty in swallowing (with weakness of the left palate), loss of pinprick sensation over the left side of the face and right side of the body, and marked ataxia with use of the left extremities.

Clinical Problem 4.12.

A 47-year-old man became aware of loss of hearing in his left ear. These symptoms gradually progressed. Several months later, his wife noted a droop on the left side of his face. He began to complain of unsteadiness. On examination, hearing was absent on the left. There also was facial paralysis on the left, left-sided incoorrdination, and decreased sensation on the left side of the face.

Clinical Problem 4.13.

A 62-year-old right-handed man began to note generalized muscle cramps. In the ensuing months, he became aware of weakness in his arms and legs and some difficulty in speaking and swallowing. Examination showed weakness and atrophy and fasciculations of nearly all muscle groups, with no sensory changes. The sign of Babinski was present bilaterally.

Clinical Problem 4.14.

A 46-year-old right-handed woman noted gradually increasing pain and numbness extending down her right leg. She had no back pain. After these symptoms had been present for 12 months, she consulted her physician, who found slight weakness of the plantar flexor muscles, absence of the ankle reflex, and decreased sensation in the posterior aspect of the calf, all on the right side.

Additional Reading

Beal MF. Energetics in the pathogenesis of neurodegenerative diseases. Trends Neurosci. 2000;23:298-304.

Hardy J, Gwinn-Hardy K. Genetic classification of primary neurodegenerative disease. Science. 1998;282:1075-1079.

Lipton P. Ischemic cell death in brain neurons. Physiol Rev. 1999;79:1431-1568.

McDonald ES, Windebank AJ. Mechanisms of neurotoxic injury and cell death. Neurol Clin. 2000;18:525-540.

Noseworthy JH, Lucchinetti C, Rodriguez M, Weinshenker BG. Multiple sclerosis. N Engl J Med. 2000;343:938-952.

Chapter 5

Diagnosis of Neurologic Disorders: Transient Disorders and Neurophysiology

Objectives

1. Describe the structure of the cell membrane and ion channels.
2. Name the variables that determine the membrane potential.
3. Define equilibrium potential.
4. Describe the effects of increased permeability to sodium (Na^+), potassium (K^+), calcium (Ca^{2+}), and chloride (Cl^-) on the membrane potential and cell excitability.
5. Describe the mechanisms by which the resting potential is generated and maintained.
6. List the characteristics of a local potential, and name three examples.
7. Describe the features of an action potential and the associated ionic changes.
8. Define the threshold, afterpotential, accommodation, and refractory period.
9. Describe the effects of the myelin sheath on conduction of the action potential.
10. Define excitatory and inhibitory postsynaptic potentials and describe their ionic basis.
11. Define spatial summation, temporal summation, and presynaptic inhibition.
12. Describe the effect of anoxia and other causes of energy failure on membrane potential and neuronal excitability.
13. Describe the effects of an alteration in extracellular Na^+, K^+, or Ca^{2+} on the resting and action potentials.
14. List conditions that could result in excessive discharge of action potentials.

Introduction

Knowing the location and function of the structural components of the nervous system, as presented in Chapter 3, permits localization of the site of a lesion. The temporal profile of the major types of disease, as presented in Chapter 4, assists in identifying the cause of the disorder. However, the temporal profile that has not been considered is the *transient,* or rapidly reversible, abnormality. Many diseases that produce signs or symptoms of brief duration may not produce destructive changes in cells and may occur without demonstrable histologic abnormality of the involved structures. To understand transient manifestations of disease, it is necessary to understand the physiology of the cells of the nervous system and the mechanism by which they process information. Cells in the nervous system and muscle communicate by electrical signals. Neurons have the ability to generate, conduct, transmit, and respond to electrical activity. Information is transmitted between cells by neurochemical agents that convey the signals from one cell to the next. Information is integrated by the interaction of electrical activity in single cells and in groups of cells.

Although this chapter discusses only the physiology of single cells, it must be remembered that the activity of the central and peripheral nervous systems never depends on the activity of a single neuron or axon but is always mediated by a group of cells or nerve fibers. Information is represented in the nervous system by a change in activity in a group of cells or fibers as they respond to some change in input. The interactions of neurons in large groups are considered in later sections. Transient alterations in the electrophysiology of neurons or muscle cells cause transient symptoms and signs. This chapter provides an introduction to the physiology of neurons, axons, and muscle fibers, which is the basis for information transmission in the central and peripheral neural structures and for the transient symptoms and signs that accompany disease states.

Overview

The major functions of the nervous system are the transmission, storage, and processing of information. This function is accomplished by the generation, conduction, and integration of electrical activity and by the synthesis and release of chemical agents. The electrical activity in neurons and muscle cells is manifested as electrical potentials called *membrane potentials*. The membrane potential is the difference in electrical potential between the inside and outside of a cell. All neurons (including their cell bodies, dendrites, and axons), astrocytes, and muscle cells have a membrane potential. All membrane potentials result from the flow of ions through channels in the membrane. The ions involved include potassium (K^+), sodium (Na^+), calcium (Ca^{2+}), and chloride (Cl^-).

Cell membranes separate ions into different concentrations in the exterior and interior of the cell. The concentration of Na^+, Ca^{2+}, and Cl^- is higher extracellularly and that of K^+ and impermeable anions (A^-) is higher intracellularly (Table 5.1). These concentration gradients are maintained by the cell membrane, a lipid bilayer that is relatively impermeable to Na^+, K^+, Cl^-, and Ca^{2+} ions and by active transport of these ions across the membrane by adenosine triphosphate (ATP)-dependent ion pumps. The concentration differences produce a tendency of ions to move across the membrane, and this generates a change in electrical potential across the membrane. The *equilibrium potential* of each ion is the voltage difference across the membrane that exactly offsets the tendency of the ion to move down its concentration gradient.

Ions move across the cell membrane passively through *ion channels*. Ion channels are transmembrane proteins that provide aqueous pores which allow the movement of ions according to the transmembrane concentration gradient. The ability of each ion to move across the cell membrane depends on the *permeability* (or open probability) of the respective ion channel at a given time. Some ion channels are open at rest, but most open (or close) in response to specific stimuli. These stimuli include changes in membrane potential (voltage-gated ion channels), binding of a neurotransmitter to a postsynaptic receptor (ligand-gated channels), chemical changes in the cytoplasm (chemical-gated ion channels), or activation of a sensory receptor cell. The opening (increased permeability) of a channel for a particular ion shifts the membrane potential toward the equilibrium potential of that ion. Thus, the influence of a particular ion on the membrane potential depends on how permeable the membrane is to the ion. At a given time, the membrane potential is determined by both the concentration gradient of the ions (which determines their respective equilibrium potentials) and any changes in the permeability to individual ions across the membrane (Fig. 5.1).

- The membrane potential depends on the transmembrane ion concentration gradient and the membrane permeability to individual ions.

Table 5.1. Relative Ion Concentrations, Equilibrium Potential, and Resting Permeability

Ion	Na^+	K^+	Cl^-	Ca^{2+}
Internal concentration	Low	High	Low	Low
External concentration	High	Low	High	High
Equilibrium potential, mV	+40	−100	−75	>120
Resting permeability	Low	High	High	Low

Membrane potentials include resting potentials, action potentials, and local potentials such as synaptic potentials, generator (or receptor) potentials, and electrotonic potentials. The *resting membrane potential* is the membrane potential when the cell is at rest and not processing incoming information. This potential depends primarily on the transmembrane concentration of K^+ because the membrane at rest is highly permeable to this ion. Because the membrane at rest is also slightly permeable to Na^+, the resting potential is maintained at a steady state despite the tendency of K^+ ions to leak out of the cell and of Na^+ ions to leak into the cell. This steady state depends on the activity of the ATP-dependent Na^+-K^+ pump, which pumps K^+ into and Na^+ out of the cell. The maintenance of the transmembrane ion concentration critical for survival and excitability of the cell thus depends on energy metabolism. When a cell is active in processing information, the membrane potential varies. These variations are either local potentials or action potentials (Table 5.2).

The electrical signals, or nerve impulses, by which information is conducted from one area to another within a single cell are called *action potentials*. The action potential is an all-or-none change in membrane potential in the body or axon of a neuron or within a muscle fiber. It either occurs fully or not at all and depends on a transient increase in permeability of a voltage-gated Na^+ channel. The amplitude of the action potentials does not depend on the intensity of the stimulus. In general, action potentials are generated in neuronal cell bodies or axons and conducted by axons. The ability of a neuron or muscle cell to generate an action potential is called *excitability*, which depends on the ability of the membrane to reach a *threshold* to open the voltage-gated Na^+ channel. This threshold is approximately 10 mV positive from the resting potential.

Several stimuli produce local changes in membrane potential, called *local potentials*, that determine the ability of the membrane to reach the threshold to trigger an action potential. Unlike action potentials, local potentials are localized and graded signals whose size varies in proportion to the size of the stimulus. Local potentials can be summated and integrated by single cells and, thus, are an integral part of the processing of information by the nervous system. Local potentials include receptor, or generator, potentials, synaptic potentials, and electrotonic potentials (Fig. 5.2). The potentials that occur in receptor cells are

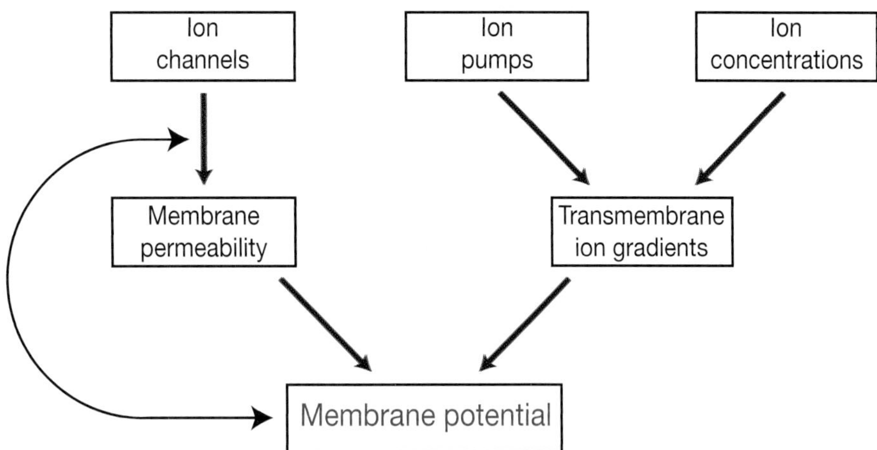

Fig. 5.1. Variables that determine the equilibrium potential of a particular ion. The transmembrane gradients depend on the activity of adenosine triphosphate (ATP)-driven ion pumps and the buffering effects of the astrocytes on the composition of extracellular fluid. Membrane permeability to a particular ion depends on the opening of specific ion channels. This opening can be triggered by voltage (voltage-gated channels), neurotransmitters (ligand-gated channels), or intracellular chemicals such as Ca^{2+}, ATP, or cyclic nucleotides (chemically gated channels). Increased membrane permeability to a given ion (the opening of an ion channel) brings the membrane potential toward the equilibrium potential of that ion.

Table 5.2. Comparison of Local Potentials and Action Potentials

Feature	Local potentials	Action potentials
Response to stimuli	Graded (proportional to intensity)	All-or-none
Amplitude	Decremental	Nondecremental
Propagation	Remain localized	Propagate at a distance
Ion channels involved	Na^+, K^+, Cl^-, Ca^{2+}	Na^+, K^+, sometimes Ca^{2+}
Function	Sensory transduction (receptor potential) Neurotransmitter effect (synaptic potential) Passive propagation of other potentials (electrotonic potentials[a])	Conduction of electrical signals at a distance along axons

[a]Electrotonic potentials are passive local changes in current flow and do not involve ion channels directly.

called *generator*, or *receptor*, *potentials*. (Receptor cells are neural structures in the body, such as the touch receptors in the skin and light receptors in the eye, that respond to specific stimuli.) The potentials that occur at synapses, specialized areas where adjacent neurons are in functional contact, are called *synaptic potentials*. These potentials are elicited by the binding of a neurotransmitter to a receptor molecule. Any localized change in membrane potential, such as the receptor potential or the synaptic potential, elicits a current flow to surrounding areas of membrane. This current flow produces a small change in the membrane potential of adjacent areas. This change is called an *electrotonic potential*.

Local potentials result from transient changes in permeability of ion channels, which may either increase or decrease the ability of the cell membrane to reach the threshold to trigger an action potential. Stimuli that increase permeability (open the channel) to sodium or calcium produce local potentials that make the membrane potential positive with respect to the resting potential. This is called

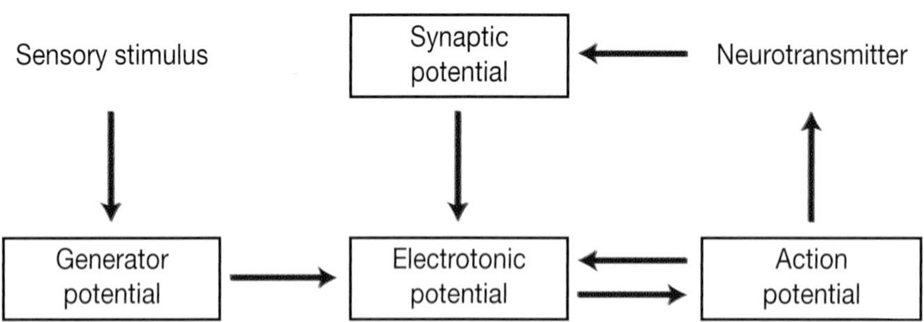

Fig. 5.2. Local potentials and triggering of the action potential. Three types of local potentials are 1) receptor (or generator) potential, triggered by the action of a sensory stimulus on a sensory receptor; 2) synaptic potential, triggered by the action of a neurotransmitter; and 3) electrotonic potential, which consists of the passive movement of charges according to the cable properties of a membrane. Both generator and synaptic potentials give rise to electrotonic potentials, which depolarize the membrane to threshold for triggering an action potential. The action potential is a regenerating depolarizing stimulus that, via electrotonic potentials, propagates over a distance without decrement of its amplitude.

depolarization, and, within certain values, it makes the cell more excitable (i.e., it increases the ability of the cell to trigger an action potential). Local depolarizing potentials may summate and reach threshold to trigger an action potential. In contrast, stimuli that increase permeability to K^+ or Cl^- produce local potentials that make the membrane potential negative with respect to the resting potential. This is called *hyperpolarization*, which makes the cell less excitable.

Once the local potential reaches threshold, an action potential is generated. The more intense the stimulus, the larger the local potential and the higher the frequency of discharge of action potentials. Action potentials are conducted along axons, and conduction velocity depends on the diameter of the axon and the presence of a myelin sheath. On reaching the presynaptic axon terminal, the action potential elicits a membrane depolarization that results in the opening of voltage-gated Ca^{2+} channels. The influx of Ca^{2+} into the presynaptic terminal triggers the release of neurotransmitter. This neurotransmitter binds to a receptor molecule in the postsynaptic cell membrane, triggering a local potential (synaptic potential) that, according to the type of neurotransmitter and receptor, may increase or decrease the excitability of the postsynaptic neuron by eliciting depolarization or hyperpolarization of its membrane. Thus, neurotransmitters transmit information from one cell to another by converting the electrical signal (action potential) into a chemical signal (neurotransmitter release) and then back into an electrical signal (synaptic potential). In turn, synaptic potentials produce electrotonic potentials, which can then initiate another action potential.

By acting on different receptors, neurotransmitters may evoke two types of postsynaptic effect. One is fast excitation (excitatory postsynaptic potential) or inhibition (inhibitory postsynaptic potential); this is referred to as *classic neurotransmission*. The second is a change in the ability of the postsynaptic cell to respond to other neurotransmitters. This is called *neuromodulation*.

The synaptic information is integrated in neurons by the interaction of local potentials generated in response to the different neurotransmitters that act on the cell. In the nervous system, information can be coded either as the rate of discharge in individual cells or axons or as the number and combination of active cells. Both of these are important mechanisms. Although the activity of the nervous system can be described conveniently in terms of the electrical activity of single cells, the combined activity of a large number of cells and axons determines the behavior of the organism. Transient alterations in function are the result of reversible disturbances in neuronal excitability, the ability to propagate action potentials, or communication by chemical synapses. Transient disorders reflect abnormalities in resting, local, or action potentials that are due to the failure of ion pumps to maintain electrochemical gradients, to impaired function of ion channels, or to alterations in the ionic composition of the extracellular fluid. Transient disorders may be generalized or focal and be manifested by excessive activity, decreased activity, or both.

Each type of alteration in neuronal or muscle cell physiology can produce symptoms or signs of short duration-transient disorders. The particular findings in a patient depend on which cells are altered. If the changes are in neurons that subserve sensation, there may be a loss of sensation or an abnormal sensation such as tingling, loss of vision, or "seeing stars." In other systems, there might be loss of strength, twitching in muscles, loss of intellect, or abnormal behavior. In all these cases, the physiologic alterations are not specific and may be the result of any one of several diseases. Transient disorders do not permit a pathologic or etiologic diagnosis. Any type of disease (vascular, neoplastic, inflammatory) may be associated with transient changes. Therefore, the pathologic mechanism of a disorder cannot be deduced when its temporal profile is solely that of transient episodes.

Plasma Membrane

Biochemical Composition

Lipid Bilayer

The plasma membrane is a lipid bilayer, with the polar (hydrophilic) heads facing outward and the nonpolar (hydrophobic) tails extending to the middle of the bilayer. Embedded in this lipid bilayer are protein macromolecules, including ion channels, receptors, and ionic pumps, that are in contact with both the extracellular fluid and the cytoplasm. The lipid bilayer is relatively impermeable to water-soluble molecules, including ions such as Na^+, K^+, Cl^-, and Ca^{2+}. These ions are involved in electrophysiologic activity and signal transmission. The concentrations of Na^+, Cl^-, and Ca^{2+} are higher extracellularly, and the concentrations of K^+ and impermeable anions (A^-) are higher intracellularly (Fig. 5.3). The maintenance of transmembrane ion concentration depends on the balance between 1) the passive diffusion of ions across ion channels, or pores, of the membrane and 2) active, energy (ATP)-dependent transport of ions against their concentration gradient by ATP-driven ion pumps. Both ion channels and ion pumps are membrane proteins with multiple transmembrane domains. In the central nervous system, astrocytes provide a buffer system to prevent excessive accumulation of extracellular K^+ ions.

- Transmembrane ion concentration gradients depend on the permeability of membrane ion channels and activity of ATP-driven ion pumps.

Ion Channels

Ion channels are intrinsic membrane proteins that form hydrophilic pores (aqueous pathways) through the lipid bilayer membrane. They allow the passive flow of selected ions across the membrane on the basis of the electrochemical gradients of the ion and the physical properties of the ion channel. Most channels belong to one of several superfamilies of homologous proteins with great heterogeneity in amino acid sequence. Ion channels vary in their selectivity; some are permeable to cations (Na^+, K^+, and Ca^{2+}) and others to anions (primarily Cl^-). The open state predominates in the resting membrane for a few channels; these are mostly the K^+ channels responsible for the

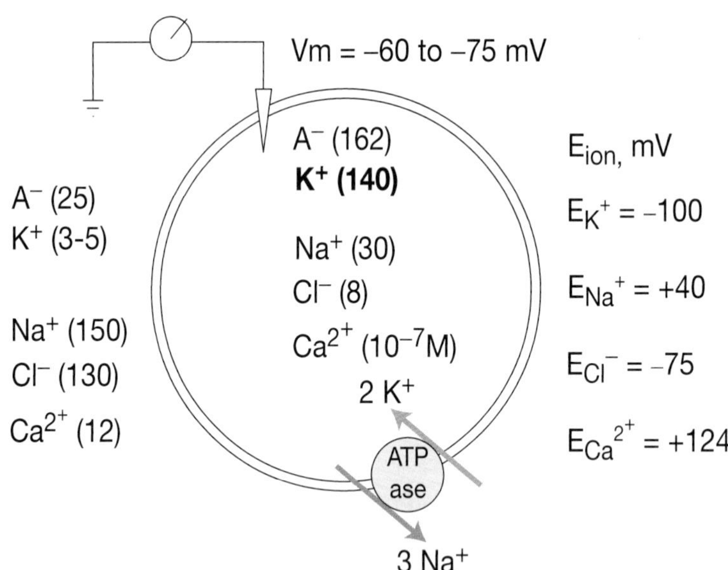

Fig. 5.3. Transmembrane ion concentrations, equilibrium potential, and resting membrane potential. The semipermeable cell membrane determines a differential distribution of ions in the intracellular and extracellular compartments. Sodium (Na^+) and chloride (Cl^-) ions predominate extracellularly and potassium (K^+) and nondiffusible (A^-) ions predominate intracellularly. The transmembrane ion composition is maintained by the activity of adenosine triphosphate-dependent pumps, particularly Na^+-K^+ adenosine triphosphatase (ATPase). The different transmembrane concentrations of diffusible ions determine the equilibrium potential of each ion (E_{ion}). The contribution of each ion to the membrane potential depends on the permeability of the membrane to that particular ion. Increased permeability to an ion brings the membrane potential toward the equilibrium potential of that ion. At rest, the membrane is predominantly, but not exclusively, permeable to K^+. Vm, resting membrane potential.

resting membrane potential (see below). Most ion channels are gated; that is, they open in response to specific stimuli. According to their gating stimuli, ion channels can be subdivided into 1) voltage-gated channels, which respond to changes in membrane potential; 2) ligand-gated channels, which respond to the binding of a neurotransmitter to the channel molecular complex; and 3) chemically gated channels, which respond to intracellular molecules such as ATP, ions (particularly Ca^{2+}), and cyclic nucleotides (Table 5.3). Other channels are gated by mechanical or other physical stimuli. Each type of ion channel is defined by the selectivity to a particular ion, gating stimulus, permeability (electrical conductance), kinetics of opening (activation) and closing (inactivation), and its sensitivity to drugs or toxins.

Generally, the transmembrane portion of the protein forms the "pore," and the specific amino acids in the region of the pore determine the ion selectivity, conductance, and voltage sensitivity of the channel. Amino acids in the extracellular or intracellular portion of the channel protein determine the gating mechanism and kinetics of inactivation.

- Ion channels are transmembrane proteins that provide an aqueous pore for the passive movement of ions.
- Different ion channels are selectively permeable to Na^+, Ca^{2+}, K^+, or Cl^-.
- Ion channels may be opened (gated) by voltage, binding of a neurotransmitter, or other signal.

Voltage-gated ion channels are critical for several electrophysiologic properties of neurons and muscle cells. Voltage-gated Na^+ channels are involved in the generation and transmission of the action potential (nerve impulse) in neurons and muscle cells. In neurons, Na^+ channels are concentrated in the initial segment of the axon (the site of generation of action potentials) and in the nodes of Ranvier (involved in rapid conduction of action potentials). There are several types of voltage-gated Ca^{2+} channels (Table 5.3). The influx of Ca^{2+} through voltage-gated channels in neurons is critical for the release of neurotransmitters from presynaptic terminals. Calcium channels mediate slow action potentials and are necessary for the rhythmic firing of some neurons. There are several types of K^+ channels, which are responsible for the resting membrane potential, repolarization of the action potential, and control of the probability of the generation of repetitive action potentials.

Table 5.3. Location and Function of Ion Channels

Ion channel	Location	Function
Voltage-gated		
Na^+	Axon hillock	Initiation of action potential
	Nodes of Ranvier	Conduction of action potential
K^+	Diffuse throughout neurons	Repolarization of action potential
		Decrease neuronal excitability and rate of discharge of action potentials
Ca^{2+}	Dendrites and soma	Slow depolarization (L channels)
		Rhythmic firing (T channel)
	Synaptic terminal	Neurotransmitter release (N and P/Q channels)
Ligand (neurotransmitter)-gated		
Cation (Na^+, Ca^{2+})	Dendrites, dentritic spines, soma	Fast synaptic excitation
Anion (Cl^-)	Dendrites, soma, axon hillock, presynaptic terminal	Fast synaptic inhibition

Voltage-gated cation channels are part of a superfamily of proteins that share a basic structure (Fig. 5.4). They consist of pore-forming subunits, generally referred to as α-subunits and a variable number of accessory subunits (β, γ, or δ). The α-subunits determine ion selectivity, mediate the voltage sensing of the channel, and are sufficient for the function of the channel. Voltage-gated K^+ channels are made up of four homologous α-subunits, each consisting of a polypeptide with six helical transmembrane segments (S1-S6) linked by intracellular and extracellular loops; its N- and C-terminal regions face the cytoplasm. The S4 segment acts as the voltage sensor, and the P loop, located between the S5 and S6 helices of each domain, forms the mouth of the pore and acts as a selectivity filter, regulating ion permeability.

The α-subunits of the voltage-gated Na^+ and Ca^{2+} channels contain four highly homologous domains in tandem (TM I-IV), each of which resembles the elementary α-subunits of the voltage-gated K^+ channel. The auxiliary subunits profoundly affect the time course and voltage dependence of channel activation or inactivation and influence the assembly and expression of voltage-gated channel α-subunits.

- The amino acid composition of the channel subunits forming the hydrophilic pores determines the ionic selectivity of the channel.
- Voltage-gated channels for Na^+, K^+, and Ca^{2+} control almost all the signals for rapid communication in the nervous system.

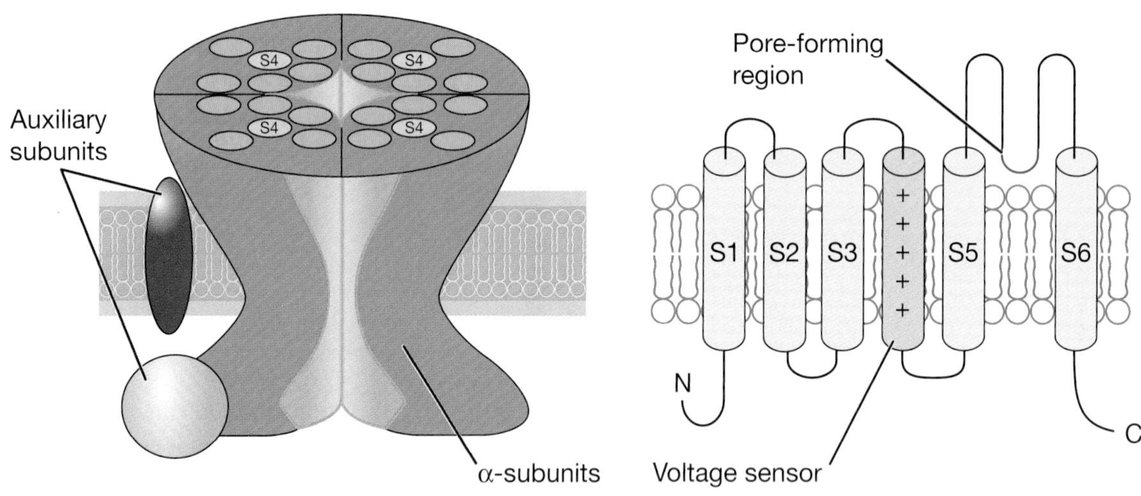

Fig. 5.4. General structure of voltage-gated cation channels. They are part of a superfamily of proteins with a common basic structure consisting of pore-forming subunits, generally referred to as α-subunits, and a variable number of accessory subunits. Voltage-gated K^+ channels are made up of four homologous α-subunits, each consisting of a polypeptide with six helical transmembrane segments (S1-S6) linked by intracellular and extracellular loops, and its N- and C-terminal regions face the cytoplasm. The S4 segment acts as the voltage sensor, and the P loop, located between the S5 and S6 helices of each domain, forms the mouth of the pore and acts as a selectivity filter, regulating ion permeability. The α-subunits of voltage-gated Na^+ and Ca^{2+} channels contain four highly homologous domains, with each resembling the elementary α-subunits of voltage-gated K^+ channels. (Modified from Benarroch EE. Basic neurosciences with clinical applications. Philadelphia: Elsevier; 2006. Used with permission of Mayo Foundation for Medical Education and Research.)

Ligand-gated channels open in response to the binding of neurotransmitters (Fig. 5.5). They include cation channels, permeable to Na^{+} or Ca^{2+} (or both), and anion channels permeable to Cl^{-}. These channels are discussed in relation to synaptic transmission. Other types of ion channels are present in sensory receptors. These include mechanically sensitive channels and channels gated by cyclic nucleotides, hydrogen ions, or thermal stimuli.

The influx of Ca^{2+} into neurons occurs through voltage-gated, ligand-gated, and sensory receptor channels. Also, Ca^{2+} may be released from intracellular stores in the endoplasmic reticulum, through channels activated by molecules generated in response to activation of some neurotransmitter receptors. Several cell processes, including neurotransmitter release and activation, are regulated by Ca^{2+}.

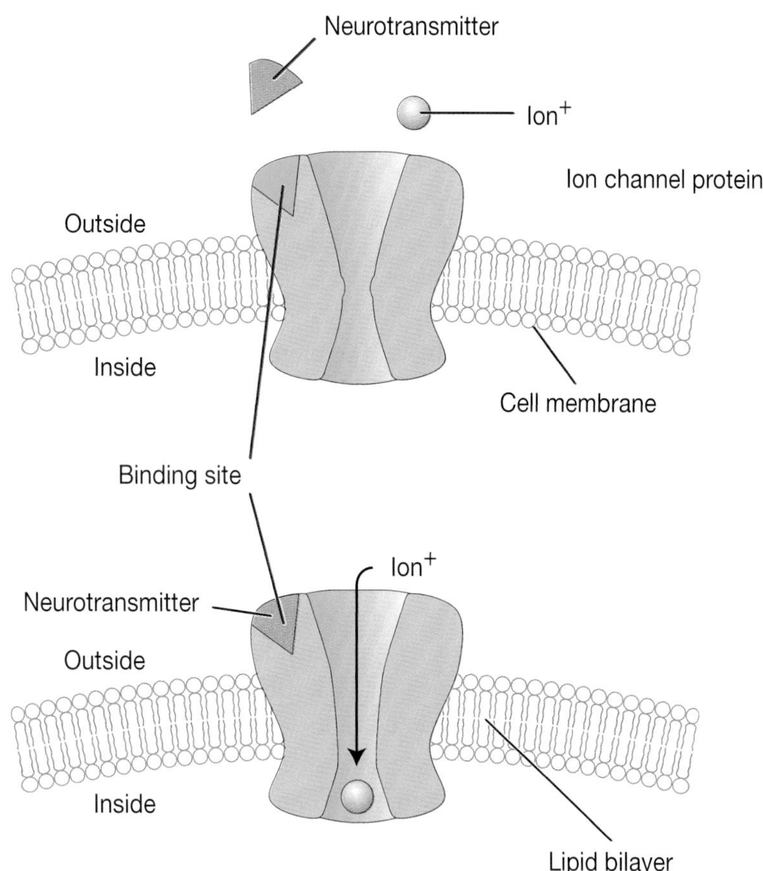

Fig. 5.5. The plasma membrane consists of a phospholipid bilayer that provides a barrier to the passage of water-soluble molecules, including ions. Passage of ions across the membrane depends on the presence of transmembrane proteins, including ion channels and ion pumps. Ion channels provide an aqueous pore for the passage of ions across the membrane, according to their concentration gradients. The opening of an ion channel, or pore, may be triggered, or gated, by several stimuli, such as voltage (voltage-gated channel) or neurotransmitters (ligand-gated channel). In the example shown here, a neurotransmitter (such as glutamate) binds to a specific ligand-gated cation channel, and this produces a change in the spatial configuration of the channel protein, allowing the pore to open and the cation to pass through the membrane. Changes in the amino acid composition of the ion channel protein affects its ion selectivity, gating mechanism, and kinetics of channel opening (activation) and closing (inactivation).

Calcium signals also control several enzymatic cascades, intracellular transport, energy metabolism, and gene expression. Also, Ca^{2+} is necessary for muscle contraction and glandular secretion.

Ion Pumps

Ion channels are transmembrane proteins that allow the passive movement of ions across the membrane driven by their concentration gradient. In contrast, *ion pumps* are transmembrane proteins that transport ions across the membrane against their concentration gradient, with the consumption of ATP. Active ion transport by ion pumps is critical for maintenance of the transmembrane ion concentration gradient. For example, there is continuous leakage of K^+ out of the cell and of Na^+ into the cell, driven by both the concentration gradient and electrical gradient. The ion gradient is restored by the activity of *Na^+-K^+ ATPase*. In nerve cells, glial cells, and muscle cells, the main source of ATP is the oxidative metabolism of glucose (aerobic glycolysis) involving the Krebs cycle and respiratory chain in mitochondria. The main consumption of ATP in the nervous system is to fuel Na^+-K^+ ATPase. Calcium ATPases, located in the plasma membrane and endoplasmic reticulum, are important for maintaining the cytosolic levels of Ca^{2+} within a narrow range. Sodium-potassium ATPase is critical for maintenance of the transmembrane concentration gradients of K^+ and Na^+.

Determinants of the Membrane Potential

The potential across the cell membrane at a given time depends on two variables: the transmembrane ion concentration gradient and the permeability of the membrane to each ion. The transmembrane concentration gradient and charge of each ion determines the *equilibrium potential* of that ion (Fig. 5.3). The permeability of the membrane to this individual ion at a given time determines the extent to which the equilibrium potential of the ion contributes to the membrane potential at that time.

Equilibrium Potential of Ions

The diffusible ions (Na^+, K^+, and Cl^-, but not Ca^{2+}) tend to move spontaneously across the cell membrane according to their concentration gradient. The molecular motion of ions is a source of energy known as the diffusion pressure. For example, the intracellular concentration of K^+ is 30 times greater than the extracellular concentration; therefore, K^+ tends to diffuse from intracellular to extracellular fluid. The opposite occurs with Na^+. As ions diffuse across the cell membrane, a separation of charges develops because the nondiffusible negatively charged intracellular ions (principally proteins) have a charge opposite that of the diffusible ions. Two regions that accumulate different charges have an electrical potential difference. The voltage that develops as a diffusible ion moves across the membrane and produces an electrical pressure that opposes the movement of the ion. The net ionic movement continues until the electrical pressure equals the diffusion pressure. At this time, the system is in equilibrium. At equilibrium, random ionic movement continues, but no net movement of ions occurs.

The electrical potential that develops across the membrane at equilibrium is called the *equilibrium potential*, and this potential is different for each ion. The equilibrium potential of an ion (E_{ion}) is the voltage difference across the membrane that exactly offsets the diffusion pressure of an ion to move down its concentration gradient. Therefore, the equilibrium potential is proportional to the difference between the concentration of the ion in the extracellular fluid and its concentration in the intracellular fluid. An algebraic representation of the equilibrium potential can be derived because the physical determinants of the diffusion pressure and electrical pressure are known. The final equation is the *Nernst equation*. The Nernst equation is an important relationship that defines the equilibrium potential inside the cell for any ion in terms of its concentration on the two sides of a membrane.

Electrical pressure is defined by

$$We = Em \times Zi \times F$$

in which We = electrical pressure (work required to move an ion against a voltage); Em = absolute membrane potential; Zi = valence (number of charges on the ion); and F = Faraday (number of coulombs per mol of ion).

Diffusion pressure is defined

$$Wd = R \times T \times (\ln[C]hi - \ln[C]lo)$$

in which Wd = diffusion pressure (work required to move an ion against a concentration gradient); R = universal gas constant; T = absolute temperature; ln = natural logarithm; [C]hi = ion concentration on the more concentrated side of the membrane; and [C]lo = ion concentration on the less concentrated side.

At equilibrium, We= Wd. Therefore,

$$Em \times Zi \times F = RT (\ln[C]hi - \ln[C]lo)$$

By rearrangement, the equilibrium potential is

$$Em = R \times T/F \times Zi \times \ln([C]hi/[C]lo)$$

By substituting for the constants at room temperature, converting to a base 10 logarithm, and converting to millivolts a useful form of the equation is obtained:

$$Em = 58 \log_{10} [C]hi/[C]lo$$

For example, $E_{Na} = 58 \log_{10} [140] / [25] = 43.3$ mV

The Nernst equation can be used to calculate the equilibrium potential for any ion if the concentrations are known for that ion on the two sides of the membrane. The approximate neuronal equilibrium potentials of the major ions are $K^+ = -100$ mV, $Na^+ = +40$ mV, $Cl^- = -75$ mV, and $Ca^{2+} = +124$ mV (Fig. 5.3).

- The equilibrium potential of an ion is the value of transmembrane potential that exactly counteracts the tendency of the ion to move across the membrane driven by its concentration gradient when the membrane is permeable to that ion.

Effect of Ion Channel Permeability on the Membrane Potential

The contribution of a given ion to the actual voltage developed across the membrane (i.e., membrane potential) depends not only on its concentration gradient but also on the permeability (P) of the membrane to that ion. Permeability is the ease with which an ion diffuses across the membrane. It is a reflection of the probability that the membrane channel that conducts the ion will open. For example, an ion with a high concentration gradient that has very low permeability (e.g., Ca^{2+}) does not contribute to the resting membrane potential. In contrast, the high permeability of K^+ at rest determines that this ion contributes significantly to the resting potential.

Algebraically, for K^+ in which P_K = potassium permeability: $E_K = R \times T/F \times Zi \times \ln P_K \times [K^+]_o / P_K \times [K^+]_o$.

Therefore, if a membrane is permeable to multiple ions that are present in different concentrations on either side of the membrane, the resultant membrane potential is a function of the concentrations of each of the ions and their relative permeabilities. The *Goldman equation* combines these factors for the major ions that influence the membrane potential in nerve and muscle cells:

$$Vm = R \times T/F \times Zi \times \ln(P_K \times [K^+]_o + P_{Na} [Na^+]_o + P_{Cl} [Cl^-]_i / P_K \times [K^+]_I + P_{Na} [Na^+]_I + P_{Cl} [Cl^-]_o)$$

On the basis of the actual ionic concentrations and ionic permeabilities, such calculations agree with measurements of these values in living cells. These equations also show that a change in either ionic permeability or ionic concentrations can alter membrane potential. If the concentration gradient of an ion is reduced, that ion will have a lower equilibrium potential. Therefore, if the resting membrane potential is determined by the equilibrium potential of that ion, this potential will decrease. In contrast, if the permeability for an ion is increased by the opening of channels for the ion, the membrane potential will approach the equilibrium potential of that ion.

An important corollary is that the opening of a channel (increase in membrane permeability) for a particular ion moves the membrane potential *toward* the equilibrium potential of that ion. In contrast, the closing of an ion channel moves the membrane potential *away from* the equilibrium potential of that ion. The movements of ions that occur with normal cellular activity are not sufficient to produce significant concentration changes; therefore, membrane potential fluctuations normally are due to permeability changes caused by channel opening and closing.

In an electrical model of the membrane, the concentration ratios of the different ions are represented by their respective equilibrium potentials (E_{Na}, E_K, E_{Cl}) and their ionic permeabilities are represented by their respective conductances (G). The conductance (i.e., the reciprocal of the resistance) for a particular ion is the sum of the conductances of all the open channels permeable to that ion. The movement of ions across the membrane is expressed as an ion current. By Ohm's law, this current depends on two factors: the conductance of the ion and the driving force for the ion. The driving force is the difference between the membrane potential and the equilibrium potential of that ion. When the membrane potential equals the equilibrium potential, the net ion current is zero.

- The membrane potential is a function of the concentrations of the ions on each side of the membrane and their relative permeabilities. The concentration gradient of an ion determines the equilibrium potential of that ion.
- The ease with which an ion diffuses across the membrane (conductance or permeability) depends on the ion channel.
- The greater the permeability of the membrane to a particular ion, the stronger the influence of the equilibrium potential of that ion on the membrane potential.
- The opening of a channel for a particular ion moves the membrane potential toward the equilibrium potential of that ion.
- The difference between the membrane potential and the equilibrium potential of a particular ion (driving force) and the membrane permeability (conductance) of that ion determine the ion current.

Resting Membrane Potential

The resting potential is the absolute difference in electrical potential between the inside and the outside of an inactive neuron, axon, or muscle cell. If an electrical connection is made between the inside and the outside of a neuron, the cell acts as a battery and an electrical current will flow. The potential is generally between 60 and 80 mV, with the inside of the cell negative to the outside. The resting potential can be measured directly with a microelectrode. The tip of the electrode must be less than 1 micrometer in diameter to be inserted into a nerve or muscle cell. By connecting the microelectrode with an appropriate amplifier, the membrane potential can be recorded and displayed on an oscilloscope (Fig. 5.6).

Steady State

The resting membrane potential is the transmembrane voltage at which there is no net flow of current across the membrane. Its value determines spontaneous neuronal activity and neuronal activity in response to extrinsic input. Because the resting potential is the absolute difference in potential between the inside and the outside of the cell, it represents transmembrane polarity. A decrease in the value of the resting membrane potential means less negativity inside the cell and the membrane potential moves toward zero; this constitutes *depolarization*. When the membrane potential becomes more negative than the value of the resting potential, the potential moves away from zero; this is *hyperpolarization*. The resting membrane potential depends on two main factors: 1) the presence of leak ion channels open at rest with markedly different permeabilities to K^+ and Na^+, making the cell membrane a semipermeable membrane, and 2) the presence of energy-dependent pumps, particularly the Na^+-K^+ pump. At rest, there is a continuous "leak" of K^+ outward and of Na^+ inward across the membrane. Potassium diffuses through the membrane most readily because of the presence of "leak" K^+ channels open at rest, so that K^+ conductance is much higher than that of other ions. Therefore, K^+ is the largest source of separation of positive and negative charges (voltage) as it diffuses out and leaves the large anions behind. This is illustrated in Figure 5.7. Thus, in the absence of synaptic activity, the membrane potential is dominated by its high permeability to K^+, and the membrane potential is drawn toward the equilibrium potential of this ion (–100 mV). Cells at rest have a much lower permeability to Na^+ than to K^+. However, because the membrane at rest is also permeable to Na^+, the membrane potential is pulled slightly toward the equilibrium potential of this ion. Thus, the resting potential varies among different types of neurons, but it is typically –60 to –80 mV. At rest, small amounts of Na^+ entering the cell, driven by both electrical and

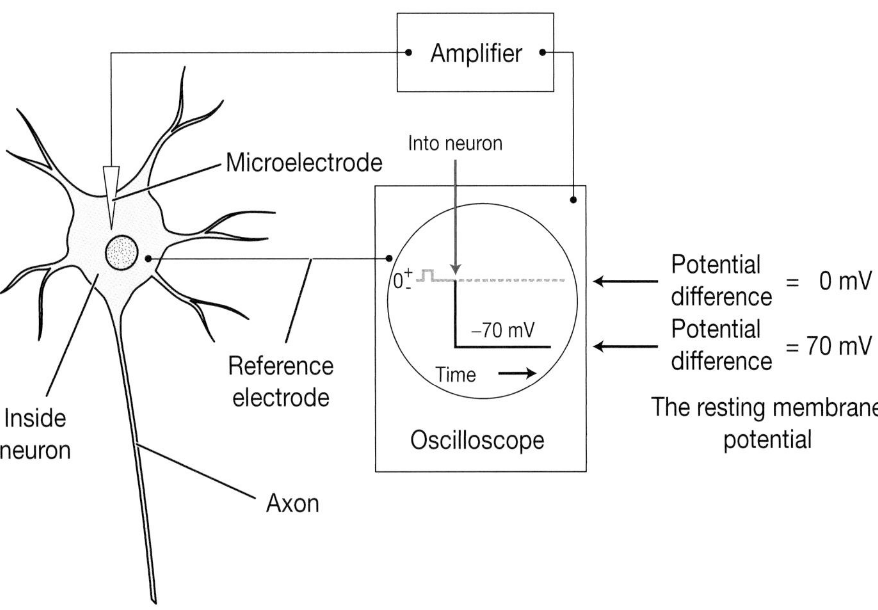

Fig. 5.6. Oscilloscopic recording of a membrane potential from a neuron. The oscilloscope registers the potential difference between the two electrical inputs and displays it as a vertical deflection of a spot of light that moves continuously from left to right across the cathode ray tube of the oscilloscope. A negative membrane potential is registered as a downward deflection; thus, when a microelectrode enters a neuron or muscle fiber, the oscilloscope beam moves down to a new position.

chemical forces, tend to depolarize the membrane. The membrane potential is not equal to the equilibrium potential of K^+; therefore, K^+ flows out of the cell. This small outward K^+ leak must be exactly equal in magnitude to the rate at which K^+ is transported into the cell. The same is true also for Na^+. Thus, the cell is not in equilibrium but in a steady state, in which the net movement of each ion across the membrane is zero. This constitutes the resting membrane potential.

Clinical Problem 5.1.

A man named Nernst has a wooden boat with a hole in its bottom which he uses on Lake Sodium. When he wants to sit and fish, he lets the boat fill with water until no more comes in, and he keeps his feet up. This condition is one of ____(a)____.

If he wants to go elsewhere, he must lower the water level in the boat, so he turns on his Lake Sodium pump, which pumps water out. He then achieves a condition in which inflow equals outflow, with little water in the boat. This he calls ____(b)____.

The process requires energy, so the pumping process is called ____(c)____.

Sodium-Potassium ATPase

The Na^+-K^+ pump (Na^+-K^+ ATPase) maintains the intracellular concentrations of Na^+ and K^+ despite their constant leaking through the membrane. The Na^+-K^+ pump transports three Na^+ ions out of the cell for every two K^+ ions carried into the cell. Because the pump is not electrically neutral, it contributes directly to the resting potential; that is, it is electrogenic. The contribution of the Na^+-K^+ pump steady state to the resting potential is approximately −11 mV. The cell membrane at rest is permeable also to Cl^- ions. In most membranes, Cl^- reaches equilibrium simply by adjustment of its internal concentration to maintain electroneutrality, without affecting the steady-state membrane potential.

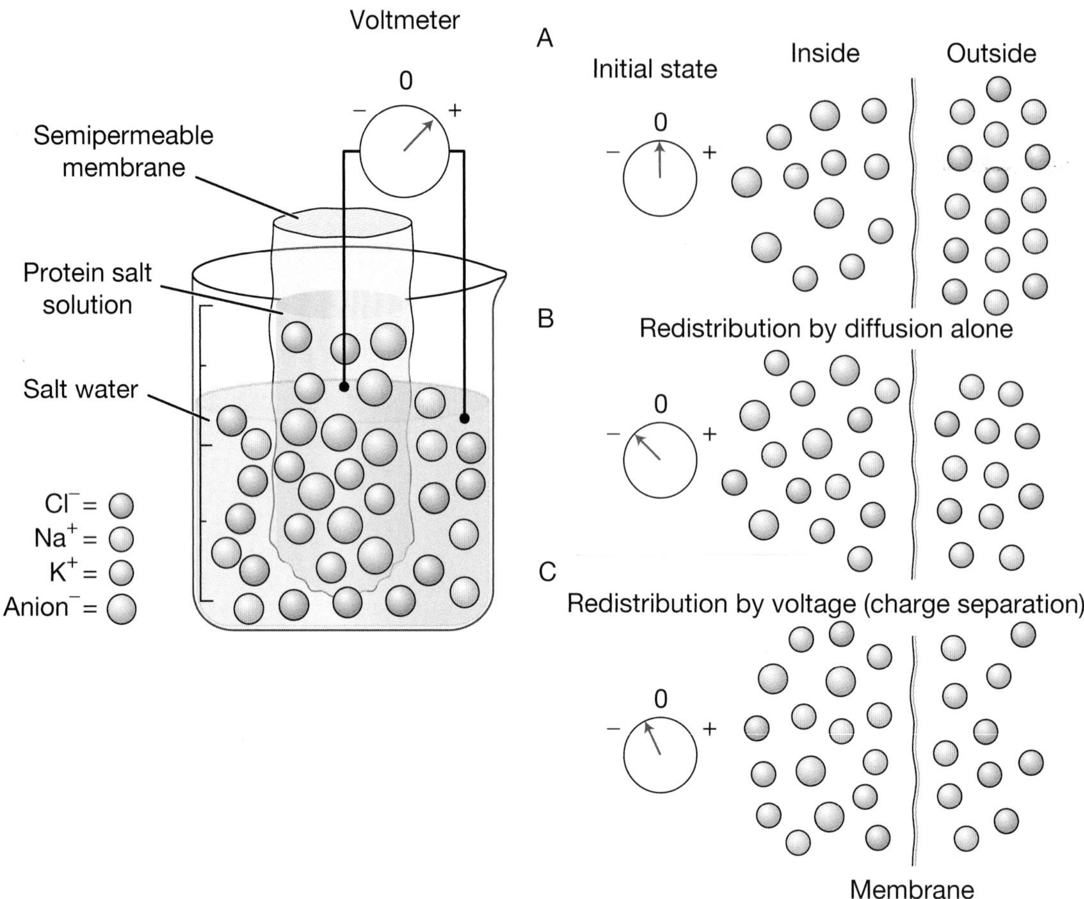

Fig. 5.7. A theoretical model of the generation of a membrane potential by diffusion of ions across a semipermeable membrane. *A*, Equal amounts of anions and cations are dissolved on each side of the membrane; thus, no voltage gradient. The membrane is permeable to all ions except large anions. *B*, K^+, Na^+, and Cl^- redistribute themselves solely by diffusion; this results in a charge separation, with greater negativity inside. *C*, Electrical pressure due to charge separation and diffusion pressure due to concentration differences are balanced at the resting membrane potential.

Depolarization and Hyperpolarization

In a normal nerve cell or muscle cell with adequate sources of oxygen and glucose, the resting potential is maintained at a stable, relatively unchanging level. However, the membrane potential changes readily in response to stimuli. It can change from the resting state in only two ways. It can become either more negative, called hyperpolarization, or less negative, called depolarization. Even if the membrane potential reverses so that the inside becomes positive with respect to the outside, it is still referred to as depolarization, because the potential is less negative than the resting potential.

Long-lasting (minutes to hours) changes in the membrane potential may occur in the absence of external stimuli in some pathologic conditions. In general, these changes occur in three settings: 1) energy failure producing impairment of the Na^+-K^+ ATPase; 2) changes in transmembrane concentrations of ions, particularly K^+ (given the high permeability of the membrane to this ion at rest); and 3) genetic or acquired disorders that affect the kinetics of activation (opening) or inactivation (closing) of channels.

Failure of the Na^+-K^+ ATPase leads to an inability to pump Na^+ out of and K^+ into the cells to oppose the leak flow of these ions driven by their concentration gradients. This leads to membrane depolarization. Changes in transmembrane concentrations of K^+ may also have a profound effect on the resting membrane potential, which is determined primarily (although not solely) by the equilibrium potential of this ion. Thus, an increase in the extracellular concentration of K^+ results in a decrease in the transmembrane concentration gradient and, thus, the value of the equilibrium potential of this ion (for example, from –100 to –80 mV). This leads to membrane depolarization. In contrast, a decrease in the extracellular concentration of K^+ leads to membrane hyperpolarization.

In physiologic conditions, changes in the membrane potential are rapid and transient (seconds or less). They can occur in response to electrical, mechanical, or chemical stimuli that produce transient activation or inactivation of ion channels, resulting in current flow through the membrane.

Membrane Excitability

The excitability of a neuron, axon, or muscle cell is defined as the probability that the neuron or muscle cell will generate or transmit (or both) an action potential (Fig. 5.8). Because triggering of an action potential depends on the opening of a voltage-gated Na^+ channel, the membrane potential needs to reach a value that activates (gates) the channel. This is called *threshold*. For a neuron with a resting membrane potential of –60 to –80 mV, the threshold for opening of voltage-gated Na^+ channels is approximately 10 mV positive from the resting potential (approximately –55 mV). Therefore, influences that depolarize the membrane toward threshold make the neuron more excitable, whereas influences that hyperpolarize the membrane make the cell less excitable. However, because the voltage-gated Na^+ channel closes (inactivates) rapidly at membrane potentials more positive than threshold, the membrane has to return to its resting value (repolarize) before the channel can be activated again. Thus, whereas small membrane depolarizations toward threshold increase neuronal (or muscle cell) excitability, a large depolarization above threshold renders the cell inexcitable because of inactivation of voltage-gated Na^+ channels.

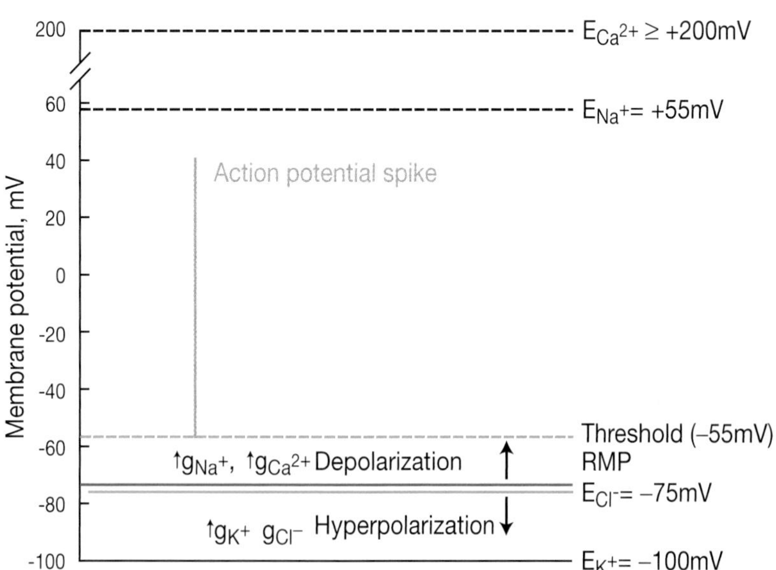

Fig. 5.8. Changes in membrane conductance (g) resulting in depolarization or hyperpolarization affect the probability of the neuron reaching threshold to trigger an action potential (neuronal excitability). RMP, resting membrane potential. (Modified from Benarroch EE. Basic neurosciences with clinical applications. Philadelphia: Elsevier; 2006. Used with permission of Mayo Foundation for Medical Education and Research.)

This is referred to as *depolarization block.* This has important clinical implications. Failure of the Na^+-K^+ pump, by allowing accumulation of intracellular Na^+ and extracellular K^+, leads to depolarization of the cell membrane. This may result in a transient increase in neuronal excitability (by moving the membrane potential toward threshold), but if the depolarization is more marked and persistent, it would render the cell inexcitable (from inactivation of voltage-gated Na^+ channels).

Role of Extracellular Calcium

The external surface of the cell membrane contains a high density of negative charges because of the presence of glycoprotein residues in membrane proteins. This produces a negative potential difference that contributes to the resting membrane potential. By binding to the negative charges of the surface membrane, extracellular Ca^{2+} neutralizes this negative surface potential. This increases the contribution of the transmembrane potential to the resting potential and thus increases the threshold for opening voltage-gated Na^+ channels. This explains the stabilizing effect of extracellular Ca^{2+} on membrane excitability and the increased spontaneous activity (tetany) that occurs in patients with hypocalcemia or alkalosis.

Role of Glial Cells

Astrocytes are important in controlling the extracellular concentration of K^+. Astrocytes are highly permeable to K^+ and are interconnected with each other by gap junctions. When the extracellular concentration of K^+ increases from neuronal activity, astrocytes incorporate K^+ and transfer it from one cell to another through gap junctions. This prevents the extracellular accumulation of K^+ and maintains neuronal excitability. This is referred to as *spatial buffering* of extracellular K^+.

- No net flow of current occurs at the resting potential, that is, the absolute difference in electrical potential between the inside and the outside of an inactive neuron, axon, or muscle cell.
- Hyperpolarization moves the resting potential away from zero; depolarization moves it toward zero.
- The resting potential is determined primarily by the high permeability of the membrane to K^+.
- In the resting state, the outward leakage of K^+ and inward leakage of Na^+ are exactly balanced by the reverse action of the Na^+-K^+ pump.
- Calcium stabilizes the membrane potential.
- Glial cells buffer the extracellular concentration of K^+.
- The value of the membrane potentials determines nerve cell excitability, which is the probability that voltage-gated Na^+ channels will open and trigger an action potential.

Local Potentials

A local potential is a transient depolarizing or hyperpolarizing shift of the membrane potential in a localized area of the cell. Local potentials result from current flow due to localized change in ion channel permeability to one or more ions. Ion channel opening or closing may result from 1) a chemical neurotransmitter released at the level of the synapse, a synaptic potential; 2) activation of a sensory receptor channel by a stimulus, a receptor potential; or 3) current from an externally applied voltage, an electrotonic potential (Table 5.4).

Ionic Basis

Synaptic Potentials

Synaptically released neurotransmitters elicit local changes in membrane potential by two main mechanisms mediated by two different types of neurotransmitter receptor. When a neurotransmitter binds to a ligand-gated ion channel receptor, it increases the permeability of the ion channel. Neurotransmitter binding to a cation channel receptor leads to increased permeability to Na^+ or Ca^{2+}, eliciting depolarization (fast excitatory postsynaptic potential). In contrast, neurotransmitters that bind to a Cl^- channel receptor elicit fast inhibitory postsynaptic potentials. Neurotransmitters may also increase or decrease the permeability to K^+ channels. Accordingly, they may elicit either the opening of K^+ channels (leading to hyperpolarization of the membrane and decreased cell excitability) or the closing of K^+ channels (leading to membrane depolarization and increased cell excitability).

Table 5.4. Ionic Basis of Local Potentials

Ion	Equilibrium potential, mV	Effect of ion channel opening on membrane potential	Example
Na^+	+40	Depolarization	Receptor potential Fast excitatory postsynaptic potential
Ca^{2+}	+124	Depolarization	Receptor potential Fast excitatory postsynaptic potential
K^+	–100	Hyperpolarization	Slow inhibitory postsynaptic potential
Cl^-	–75	Depolarization, hyperpolarization, or no change	Fast inhibitory postsynaptic potential

Receptor Potentials

Stimulation of sensory receptors, including mechanoreceptors (such as those involved in the sensation of touch or hearing) and receptors involved in the sensations of pain, temperature, smell, and taste, results in the opening of a cation channel, leading to membrane depolarization. The only exception is the case of photoreceptors, in which light triggers a biochemical cascade that results in the closing of a cation channel that is open during darkness. Thus, with the exception of photoreceptors, receptor (generator) potentials are depolarizing, leading to the triggering of action potentials.

Electrotonic Potentials

Electrotonic potentials participate in the transfer of information throughout a cell. These potentials occur in one of two ways: 1) the opening of Na^+ channels by a current arising from a voltage in an adjacent area of membrane, producing depolarization, and 2) the opening or closing of several different ion channels by an externally applied negative voltage. The application of a negative voltage to the outside of the membrane causes outward current flow and depolarization of the membrane. When voltage is applied to the outside of the axonal membrane, the negative pole is commonly referred to as the cathode and the positive pole is called the anode. The cathode depolarizes and the anode hyperpolarizes a membrane.

Characteristics of Local Potentials

All local potentials have certain characteristics in common (Table 5.2). Importantly, the local potential is a graded potential; that is, its amplitude is proportional to the size of the stimulus (Fig. 5.9). Measurement of a local potential uses the resting potential as its baseline. If the membrane's resting potential is depolarized from −80 to −70 mV during the local potential, the local potential has an amplitude of 10 mV. This potential change is one of decreasing negativity (or of depolarization), but it could also be one of increasing negativity (or of hyperpolarization).

Summation

Because the local potential is a graded response proportional to the size of the stimulus, the occurrence of a second stimulus before the first one subsides results in a larger local potential. Therefore, local potentials can be summated. They are summated algebraically, so that similar potentials are additive and hyperpolarizing and depolarizing potentials tend to cancel one another. Summated potentials may reach threshold and produce an action potential when single potentials individually are subthreshold. When a stimulus is applied to a localized area of the membrane, the change in membrane potential has both a temporal and spatial distribution. A study of the temporal course of the local potential shows that the increase in the potential is not instantaneous but develops over a few milliseconds (Fig. 5.9). After the stimulus ends, the potential then subsides over a few milliseconds. Therefore, local potentials have a temporal course that out lasts the stimulus. The occurrence of a second stimulus at the same site shortly after the first produces another local potential, which summates with any residual of the earlier one that has not yet subsided (Fig. 5.10). The summation of local potentials occurring near each other in time is called *temporal summation*. Different synaptic potentials have different time courses. Most synaptic potentials range from 10 to 15 milliseconds in duration; however, some are very brief, lasting less than 1 millisecond, but others may last several seconds or several minutes. The longer the duration of the synaptic potential, the greater the chance for temporal summation to occur. By means of temporal summation, the cell can integrate signals that arrive at different times. Study of the spatial distribution of local potentials reveals another characteristic. As their name implies, they remain localized in the region where the stimulus is applied; they do not spread throughout the entire cell. However, because of local current flow, the locally applied stimulus has an effect on the nearby membrane. The potential change is not confined sharply to the area of the stimulus but falls off over a finite distance along the membrane, usually a few millimeters. The application of a simultaneous second stimulus near the first (but not at the same site) results in summation of the potentials in the border zones; this is called *spatial summation*.

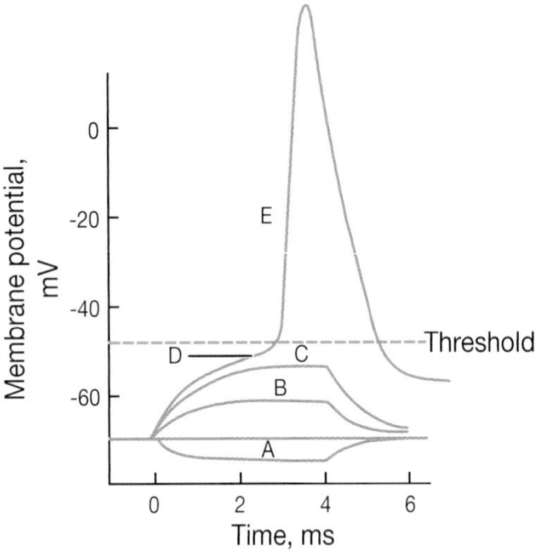

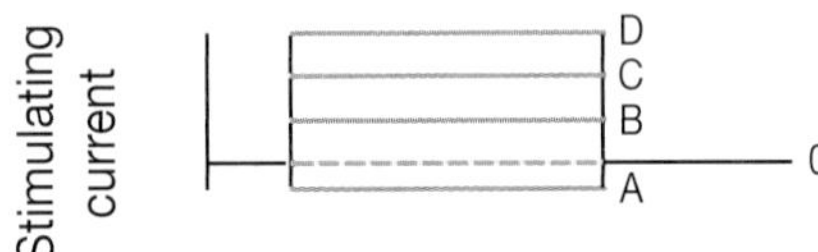

Fig. 5.9. Local potentials. These potentials are shown as an upward deflection if they are depolarizing and as a downward deflection if they are hyperpolarizing. The resting potential is –70 mV. At time zero, electrical currents of varied polarities and voltage are applied to the membrane (bottom). A is an anodal current; B, C, and D are cathodal currents. A produces a transient hyperpolarization; B, C, and D produce a transient depolarization that is graded and proportional to the size of the stimulus. All of these are local potentials. D produces an action potential, E.

Thus, the membrane of the cell can act as an integrator of stimuli that arrive from different sources and impinge on areas of membrane near one another. Spatial and temporal summation are important mechanisms in the processing of information by single neurons; when summated local potentials reach threshold, they initiate an action potential.

Accommodation

If a current or voltage is applied to a membrane for more than a few milliseconds, the ion channels revert to their resting state, changing ionic conductances of the membrane in a direction to restore the resting potential to baseline value. This phenomenon is known as *accommodation* (Fig. 5.11). Therefore, if an electrical stimulus is increased slowly, accommodation can occur and no change will be seen in the membrane potential. The changes in conductance during accommodation require several milliseconds, both to develop and to subside. As a result, if an electrical stimulus is applied gradually so that accommodation prevents a change in resting potential, then when the stimulus is turned off suddenly, the residual change in conductance will produce a transient change in resting potential. Thus, accommodation can result in a cell responding to the cessation of a stimulus.

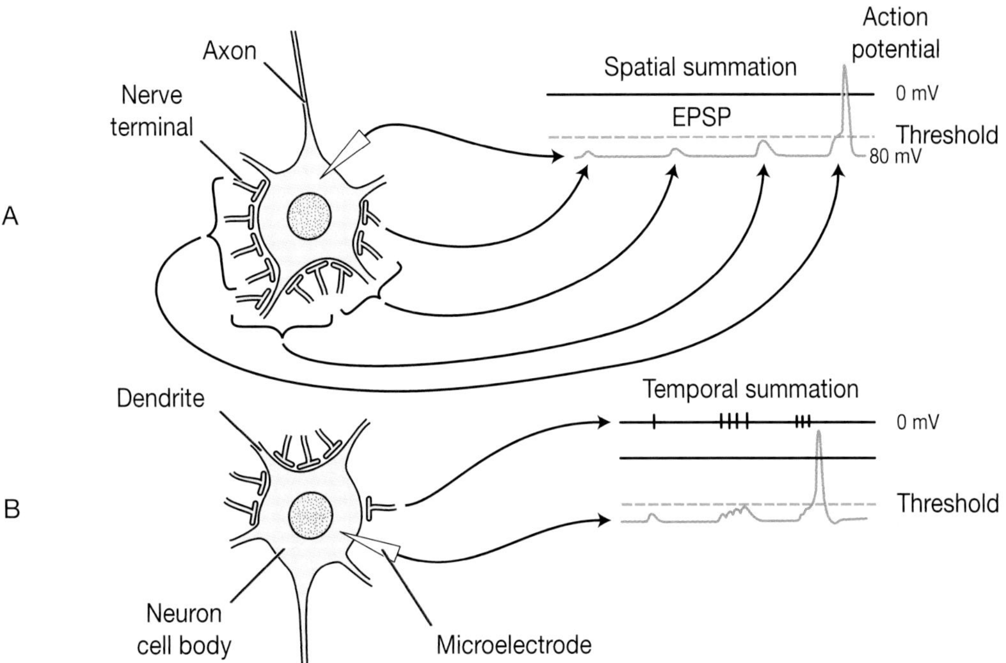

Fig. 5.10. Summation of local potentials in a neuron. *A*, Spatial summation occurs when an increasing number of nerve terminals release more neurotransmitter to produce larger excitatory postsynaptic potentials (EPSPs). *B*, Temporal summation occurs when a single terminal discharges repetitively more rapidly to produce larger EPSPs.

- Local potentials are local changes in membrane potential that are triggered by synaptic neurotransmitters, sensory stimuli, or voltage changes.
- Local potentials may be depolarizing or hyperpolarizing, and their amplitude depends on stimulus intensity.
- Local potentials can be summated spatially and temporally.

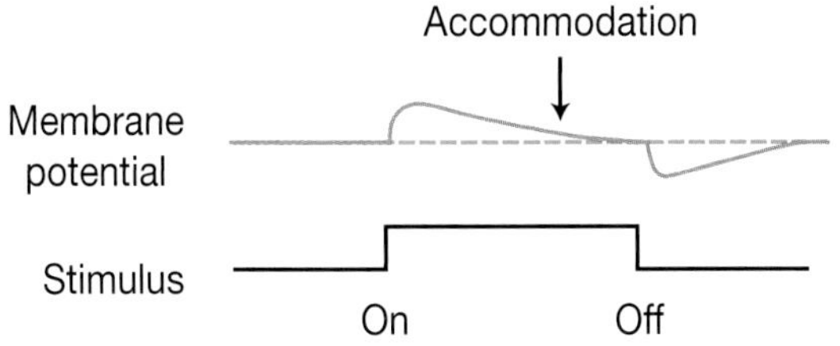

Fig. 5.11. Accomodation of the membrane potential to an applied stimulus of constant strength. Note the response to sudden cessation of the stimulus.

Action Potentials

Action potentials have several advantages for the rapid transfer of information in the nervous system. Because action potentials are all-or-none (they either occur or do not occur), they can transfer information without loss over relatively long distances. The all-or-none feature also allows information to be coded as frequency rather than as the less stable measure of amplitude. Also, the threshold of action potentials eliminates the effects of small, random changes in membrane potential.

Ionic Basis

In the resting state, many more K^+ channels are open, the conductance of Na^+ is much less than that of K^+, and the resting potential is near the equilibrium potential of K^+. At threshold, the voltage-gated Na^+ channels open so that the conductance of Na^+ suddenly becomes greater than that of K^+, and the membrane potential shifts toward the equilibrium potential of Na^+, approximately +40 mV. This depolarization reverses the polarity of the membrane, with the inside becoming positive with respect to the outside. With the opening of the Na^+ channels and increased Na^+ conductance, current flows inward with movement of Na^+ ions. In most cases, voltage-gated Na^+ channels inactivate rapidly after depolarization, so that the increase in Na^+ conductance is usually transient, lasting only a few milliseconds. Depolarization triggers the opening of slowly activating K^+ channels, leading to an increase in K^+ conductance and an outward movement of K^+ ions, bringing the membrane potential back toward the equilibrium potential of K^+. This is called *repolarization*. These three changes overlap, and the potential of the membrane during these changes is a function of the ratios of the conductances (Fig. 5.12). Sodium conductance increases several thousandfold early in the process, whereas K^+ conductance increases less, does so later, and persists longer. The conductance changes for these two ions result in ionic shifts and current flows that are associated with a membrane potential change, namely, the action potential (Fig. 5.13). Thus, the duration of the action potential depends on the speed of inactivation of the voltage-gated Na^+ channel and the increase in K^+ conductance.

The return of the membrane potential to baseline slows after Na^+ conductance has returned to baseline (Fig. 5.13). This produces a small residual component that is positive with respect to the resting potential when recorded with an intracellular microelectrode. However, it is named the negative afterpotential on the basis of its polarity when recorded with an extracellular electrode. The persistent increase in K^+ conductance results in hyperpolarization after the spike component of the action potential. This is called afterhyperpolarization because it consists of a transient shift

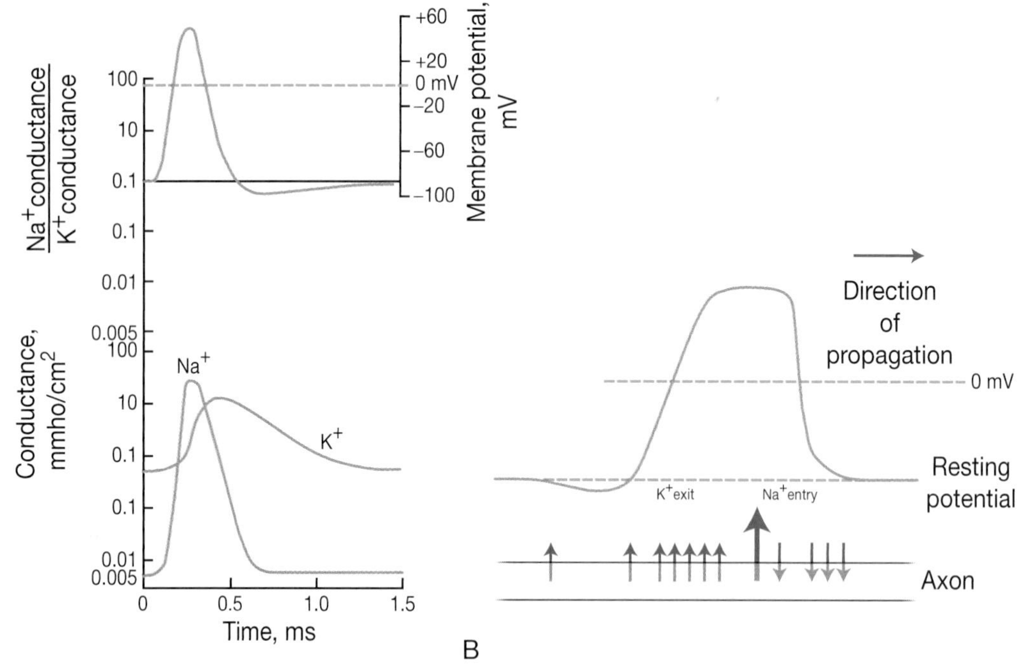

Fig. 5.12. Conductance changes during an action potential. *A*, Temporal sequence at a single site along an axon. Changes in conductances (permeabilities) of Na^+ and K^+ are plotted against time as they change with associated changes in membrane potential. Note that Na^+ conductance changes several thousandfold early in the process, whereas K^+ conductance changes only about 30-fold during later stages and persists longer than Na^+ conductance changes. *B*, Spatial distribution of an action potential over a length of axon at a single instant.

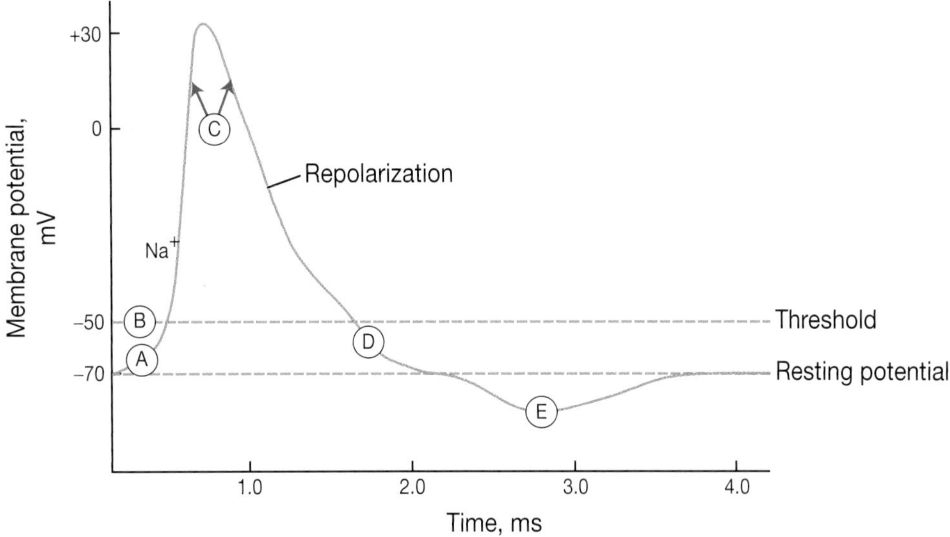

Fig. 5.13. Component of an action potential with a resting potential of −70 mV. A, Local electronic potential; B, threshold level; C, spike; D, negative (depolarizing) afterpotential; E, positive (hyperpolarizing) afterpotential.

of the membrane potential near the equilibrium potential of K^+, which is negative with respect to the membrane potential. However, this after-hyperpolarization is called a positive afterpotential, on the basis of its polarity when recorded with an extracellular electrode. During the positive afterpotential, the membrane potential is near the K^+ equilibrium potential, and oxygen consumption is increased with increased activity of the Na^+ pump.

The amounts of Na^+ and K^+ that move across the membrane during the action potential are small, buffered by surrounding astrocytes, and do not change the concentration enough to affect the resting potential. In addition, the Na^+ that moves into the cell during the action potential is continually removed by the Na^+ pump during the relatively long intervals between action potentials.

Dendrites also have voltage-gated Na^+ and Ca^{2+} channels. Calcium-mediated action potentials generally are of longer duration and smaller amplitude than typical Na^+ potentials. In many cases, the voltage-dependent opening of Ca^{2+} channels elicits a depolarization that brings the membrane to threshold for opening voltage-gated Na^+ channels. The action potential consists of a Ca^{2+} component with superimposed repetitive Na^+-mediated spikes. In these cases, the increased concentration of Ca^{2+} opens Ca^{2+}-dependent K^+ channels, which leads to progressive repolarization of the cell membrane and interruption of the firing of action potentials.

Threshold

Another characteristic that the membranes of neurons, axons, and muscle cells have that is basic to their ability to transmit information from one area to another is *excitability*. If a membrane is depolarized by a stimulus, there is a point at which many voltage-gated Na^+ channels open suddenly. This point is known as the threshold for excitation (Fig. 5.9). If the depolarization does not reach threshold, the evoked activity is a local potential. Threshold may be reached by a single local potential or by summated local potentials. When threshold is reached, the membrane's permeability to Na^+ suddenly increases. This change in conductance results in the action potential. Action potentials usually are generated at the initial segment of the axon or axon hillock, because it contains a high concentration of voltage-gated Na^+ channels. The action potentials are conducted along the axon, which also contains voltage-gated Na^+ channels. In myelinated axons, these Na^+ channels are concentrated at the nodes of Ranvier.

Refractory Period

The excitability of a membrane is the ease with which an action potential can be generated; it depends on the probability of the opening of voltage-gated Na^+ channels. As mentioned, voltage-gated Na^+ channels responsible for the action potential in most cells open when membrane depolarization is about 10 to 15 mV positive from the resting potential. This constitutes the threshold. However, voltage-gated Na^+ channels are rapidly inactivated at more positive potentials; therefore, the membrane potential has to return to baseline for the channels to open again. In electrophysiologic studies, membrane excitability usually is measured in terms of the voltage required to initiate an action potential. During increased Na^+ conductance, the membrane cannot be stimulated to discharge again. A second stimulus at this time is without effect; therefore, action potentials, unlike local potentials, cannot summate. This period of unresponsiveness is the *absolute refractory period* (Fig. 5.14). As Na^+ conductance returns to normal because of progressive inactivation of the voltage-gated channel, the membrane again becomes excitable; however, for a short period, it requires a larger stimulus to produce a smaller action potential. This is called the *relative refractory period*. After the relative refractory period, while the negative afterpotential is subsiding, the membrane is partially depolarized, is closer to threshold, and has increased excitability. This is the *supernormal period*. Finally, during the positive afterpotential, the membrane is hyperpolarized and stronger stimuli are required. This is the *subnormal period*. Up to this point, the term threshold has been used to refer to the membrane potential at which Na^+ channels open and an action potential is generated. The threshold of a membrane remains relatively constant. If the membrane potential becomes hyperpolarized, the membrane potential moves away from threshold and the membrane is less

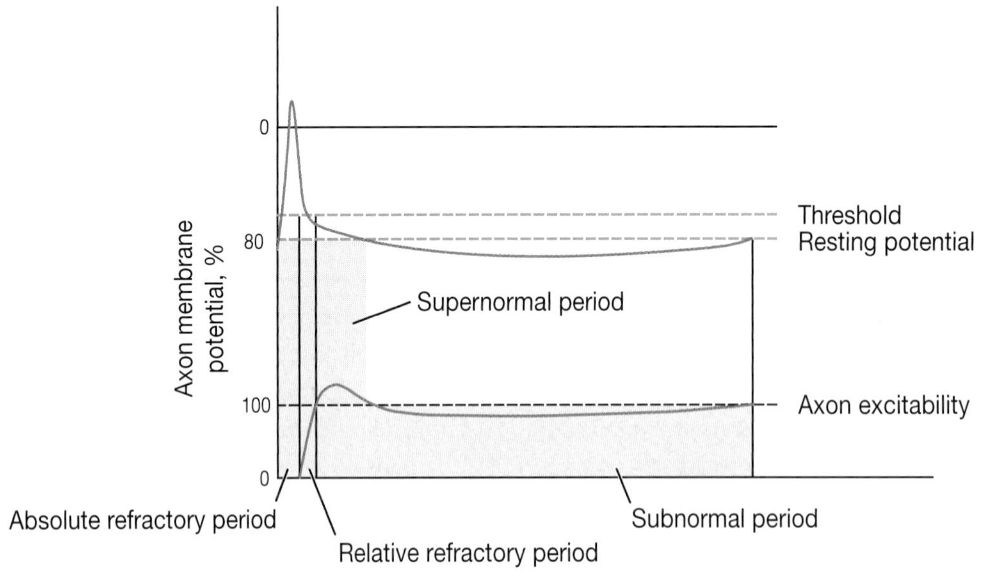

Fig. 5.14. Excitability changes during an action potential. The lower portion of the diagram shows the ease with which another action potential can be elicited (change in threshold). During absolute and relative refractory periods, the amplitude of the action potential evoked is low. Subsequently, it is normal.

excitable. If the membrane potential moves closer to threshold, the membrane becomes more excitable and will generate an action potential with a smaller stimulus. If the membrane potential is very near threshold, the cell may fire spontaneously. If the membrane potential remains more depolarized than threshold, however, the membrane cannot be stimulated to fire another action potential (Fig. 5.15).

The threshold of the membrane differs in different parts of the neuron, and this depends on the density of voltage-gated Na^+ channels. The threshold is high in dendrites and cell bodies and lowest at the initial segment of the axon. Thus, an action potential is usually generated in the initial segment.

The term threshold is also used to describe the voltage required to excite an action potential with an externally applied stimulus. When threshold is used in this sense, an axon with increased excitability due to partial depolarization may be said to have a lower threshold for stimulation, even though the actual threshold is unchanged. The first meaning of threshold is used when intracellular recordings are considered, and the second is used in reference to extracellular stimulation and recording.

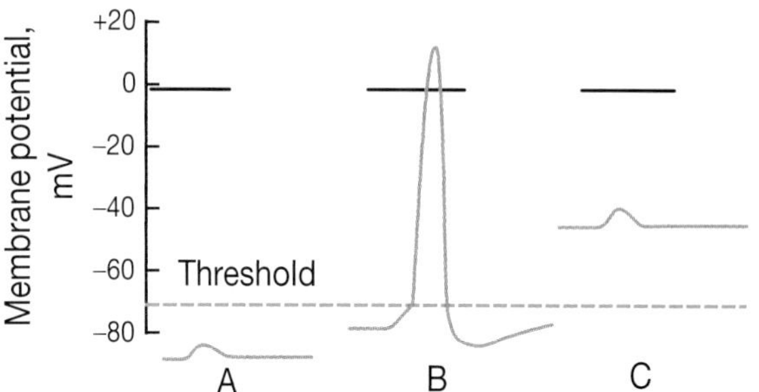

Fig. 5.15. The effect of stimulation of a neuron at different resting potentials as recorded with a microelectrode. *A*, The membrane is hyperpolarized, and a stimulus produces a subthreshold local potential. *B*, The membrane is normally polarized at –65 mV, and a stimulus produces a local potential that reaches threshold and results in an action potential. *C*, The membrane is depolarized beyond threshold, and a stimulus produces only a small local potential.

- The action potential consists of a fast membrane depolarization due to the opening of rapidly inactivating voltage-gated Na^+ channels, followed by a repolarization due to delayed opening of voltage-gated K^+ channels.
- The excitability of the membrane is the probability of its reaching threshold to trigger an action potential.
- The threshold to trigger an action potential depends on the density of voltage-gated Na^+ channels.
- Membrane depolarization toward threshold increases excitability, depolarization above threshold inactivates voltage-gated Na^+ channels and elicits a refractory period.

Frequency and Population Coding

As discussed above, the amplitude of local potentials increases with the intensity of the stimulus. In contrast, the generation of an action potential is an all-or-none event, and above threshold the amplitude of the action potential is the same regardless of the intensity of the stimulus. However, the more intense the stimulus, the shorter the time needed to reach threshold, and the higher the frequency of discharge of action potentials. This strength-latency relationship allows the encoding of information about the intensity of the stimulus as a *frequency code*. Even at rest, many neurons exhibit intrinsic rhythmic fluctuations of the membrane potential. These fluctuations create subthreshold activation of the membrane, bringing it closer to threshold for the opening of voltage-gated Na^+ channels. Thus, neurons have an active role in determining not only *whether* but also *when* a given input will trigger an action potential. Thus, information could be conveyed by specific patterns of firing of individual neurons, including their firing frequency (*rate code*) or the intervals in between individual action potentials (*temporal code*) or both. However, the response of single neurons varies even to identical stimuli. Simultaneous recordings of the activity of different neurons indicate that information in the nervous system is encoded by the synchronized firing of networks or populations of neurons that may be widely distributed in the brain (*population code*). These networks may constitute the basic "encoding units" in the nervous system.

Patterns of Activity

The electrophysiologic properties of neurons vary according to the magnitude, cellular distribution, and pharmacologic sensitivity of ionic currents through voltage-gated Na^+, Ca^{2+}, and K^+ channels. The heterogeneous repertoire and distribution of these channels result in a wide variety of patterns of neuronal activity in the brain. Neuronal firing of action potentials may occur spontaneously or in response to external stimulation. Beating, or pacing, neurons fire repetitively at a constant frequency; their intrinsic firing rate may be increased or decreased by external stimulation. Bursting neurons generate regular bursts of action potentials separated by hyperpolarization of the membrane. Such neurons are important for rhythmic behavior such as breathing, walking, and chewing. Neurons that fire in response to external stimulation may do so in one of three ways. A sustained response neuron shows repeated action potentials with a constant firing frequency that reflects the strength of the stimulus. A delayed response neuron fires action potentials only after stimulation of sufficient intensity. An accommodation response neuron fires only a single potential at the onset of stimulation and remains silent thereafter.

> Neurons can generate both fast Na^+ spikes and slow Ca^{2+} spikes. Some neurons may exhibit sustained firing of action potentials from prolonged baseline depolarizations mediated by non-inactivating Na^+ or Ca^{2+} currents. Some neurons (e.g., in the thalamus) are able to discharge either in rhythmic bursts or with typical action potentials. The firing pattern depends on the level of the resting membrane potential. An important property of this type of neuron is the presence of a particular class of Ca^{2+} channel, the T channel. This channel can be activated only if the membrane potential is relatively hyperpolarized (e.g., –80 mV). Under this condition, a stimulus opens the T channel and Ca^{2+} enters the cell and produces a small, brief Ca^{2+}-based depolarizing potential change called the low-threshold Ca^{2+} spike. This spike triggers the opening of Na^+ channels, which produces a burst of repetitive action potentials. As Ca^{2+} accumulates in the cell, it opens Ca^{2+}-activated K^+ channels that allow the efflux of K^+. The resulting hyperpolarization allows reactivation of the T channel, the entry of Na^+, and recurrence of the cycle. This sequence generates rhythmic burst firing of the neuron.

Propagation of the Action Potential

Another important characteristic of action potentials is propagation. If an action potential is initiated in an axon in the tip of the finger, for instance, the potential spreads along the entire length of that axon to its cell body in the dorsal root ganglion, and then along the central axon, ascending in the spinal cord to the brainstem. The propagation of action potentials permits the nervous system to transmit information from one area to another. The velocity of propagation depends on the distribution of ion channels, the diameter of the axon, and the presence or not of a myelin sheath.

Distribution of Ion Channels in the Axons

In unmyelinated axons (such as those involved in the sensation of pain or temperature), axons of autonomic ganglion neurons, and many central axons, the voltage-gated Na^+ and K^+ channels responsible for the action potential are evenly distributed along the membrane of the axon. In myelinated axons, however, the distribution of ion channels is more complicated. Voltage-gated Na^+ channels are concentrated at the nodes of Ranvier, whereas several types of K^+ channels are distributed in the paranodal region and along the internode. Therefore, repolarization at the node of Ranvier depends primarily on inactivation of Na^+ channels.

Cable Properties

When an area of membrane is depolarized during an action potential, there is flow of ionic currents (Fig. 5.16). In the area of depolarization, Na^+ ions carry positive charges inward. There is also a longitudinal flow of current both inside and outside the membrane. This flow of positive charges (current) toward nondepolarized regions internally and toward depolarized regions externally tends to depolarize the membrane in the areas that surround the region of the action potential. This depolarization is an electrotonic potential. In normal

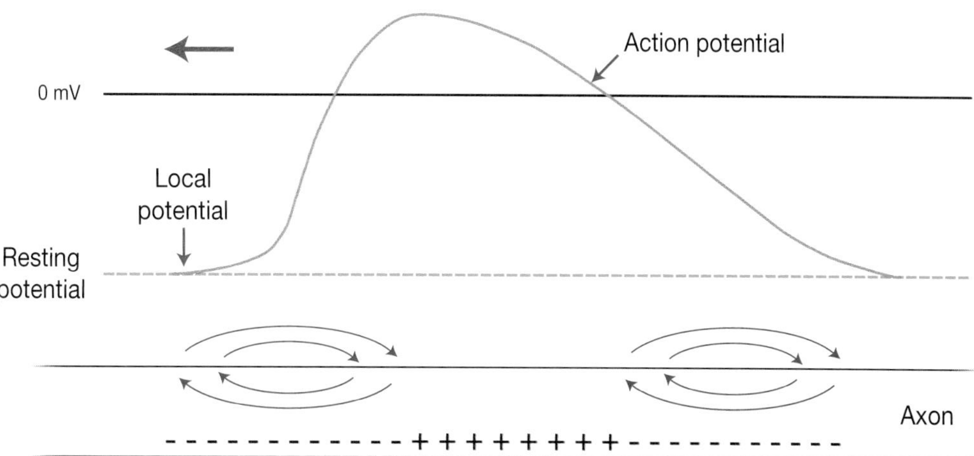

Fig. 5.16. Current flow and voltage changes in an axon in the region of an action potential. The voltage changes along the membrane are shown in the upper part of the diagram, and the spatial distribution of current flow is shown in the lower part as arrows through the axon membrane.

tissue, this depolarization is sufficient to shift the membrane potential to threshold and thereby generate an action potential in the immediately adjacent membrane. Thus, the action potential spreads away from its site of initiation along an axon or muscle fiber. Because of the refractory period, the potential cannot reverse and spread back into an area just depolarized. The rate of conduction of the action potential along the membrane depends on the amount of longitudinal current flow in the form of electrotonic potentials and on the amount of current needed to produce depolarization in the adjacent membrane in order to reach the threshold for opening of voltage-gated Na^+ channels. Spread of electrical currents along axons depends on the passive electrical properties of the membrane, referred to as *cable properties*. Spread of electrotonic potentials along the axon is decremental and limited by two factors: the high resistance of the axoplasm to longitudinal current flow and the outward leakage of current through the axon membrane (axolemma) because of a relatively low membrane resistance and a relatively high membrane capacitance. The distance over which the local potential spreads depends on the ratio between the transverse membrane resistance and the longitudinal axoplasm resistance. This ratio is proportional to the radius of the axon. Therefore, conduction velocity is higher in large-diameter than in small-diameter fibers. The longitudinal current flow can be increased by increasing the diameter of an axon or muscle fiber, because this increase reduces the internal resistance, just as a larger electrical wire has a lower electrical resistance.

However, the most important determinant of the increase in conduction velocity in large-diameter axons is the presence of a myelin sheath, which serves as an electrical insulator. The myelin sheath consists of tightly packed membrane wrapped around the axon, resulting in an increase in membrane resistance and decrease in membrane capacitance that are proportional to the number of wrappings. These two changes prevent the transverse dissipation of current across the membrane resistance and capacitance; thus, myelin provides an effective insulation to the axon. In a myelinated axon, the membrane is bare only at the nodes of Ranvier; consequently, transmembrane current flow occurs almost exclusively at the nodal area.

When current flow opens enough Na^+ channels to reach threshold in the nodal area, it results in many more Na^+ channels opening and an influx of Na^+ ions and, thus, the generation of an action potential. The nodal area in the mammalian nervous system is unique in that it consists almost exclusively of Na^+ channels, with an almost complete absence of K^+ channels. The action potential generated at the node consists predominantly of inward Na^+ currents, with little outward K^+ currents. Repolarization is achieved by the inactivation of Na^+ channels. An action potential at one node of Ranvier produces sufficient longitudinal current flow to depolarize adjacent nodes to threshold, thereby propagating the action potential along the nerve in a skipping manner called *saltatory conduction* (Fig. 5.17).

- The action potential is an all-or-none signal that is transmitted without decrement along the axon.
- The amplitude of the stimulus is encoded by the frequency of discharge of action potentials.
- The velocity of conduction of the action potential depends on axon diameter and the insulating effect of the myelin sheath.
- In myelinated axons, the voltage-gated Na^+ channels are clustered at the nodes of Ranvier, whereas the K^+ channels are covered by the myelin sheath.

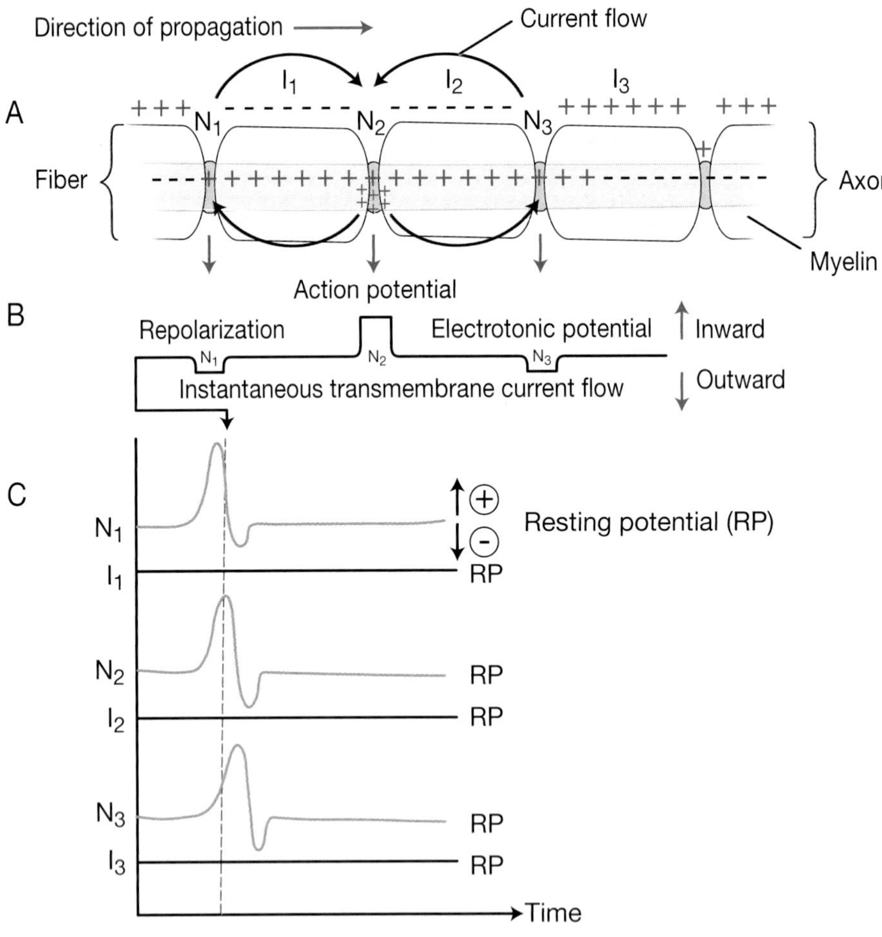

Fig. 5.17. Saltatory conduction along an axon from left to right. *A*, The charge distribution along the axon is shown with an action potential (depolarization) at the second node of Ranvier (N_2). Current flow spreads to the next node (N_3). I_1-I_3, internodes. *B*, Membrane current flow along the axon. *C*, The portion of the action potential found at each node is indicated by the red dashed line.

Synaptic Transmission

A *synapse* is a specialized contact zone where one neuron communicates with another neuron. The contact zone between an axon terminal and a muscle fiber or other nonneural target is referred to as a *neuroeffector junction*. There are two types of synapses: chemical and electrical. Chemical synapses are the more common form of communication in the nervous system.

Chemical Synapses

A chemical synapse consists of a presynaptic component (containing synaptic vesicles), a postsynaptic component (dendrite, soma, or axon), and an intervening space called the *synaptic cleft* (Fig. 5.18). Many drugs used in clinical medicine have their pharmacologic site of action at chemical synapses.

General Properties

The mechanisms underlying chemical synaptic transmission should make it apparent that this process has four unique characteristics. First, conduction at a synapse is delayed because of the brief time required for the chemical events to occur. Second, because the two sides of the synapse are specialized to perform one function, transmission of chemical signals generally occurs in only one direction across the synapse. Thus, neurons are polarized with respect to the direction of impulse transmission. However, retrograde signals from the target may affect the function of the presynaptic neuron. Third, because nerve impulses from many sources impinge on single cells in the central and peripheral nervous systems, synaptic potentials summate both temporally and spatially. Fourth, each synaptic input may be mediated by different neurotransmitters with different effects on the neuron (Table 5.5). Thus, a single neuron can integrate activity from many sources. When the membrane potential reaches threshold, an action potential is generated. A summary of the electrical events in a single cell underlying the transmission, integration, and conduction of information is shown in Figure 5.19.

The membrane of a cell is continually bombarded with chemical signals from a large number of neurotransmitters released from presynaptic vesicles. These include amino acids (glutamate, γ-aminobutyric acid [GABA], and glycine), acetylcholine, monoamines (dopamine, norepinephrine, serotonin, histamine), neuropeptides, and purines, including ATP. The mechanisms of synthesis, storage, and release of these neurotransmitters, their effects on target neurons, and their function are discussed in more detail in Chapter 6. Only general concepts about the synaptic effects of neurotransmitters are discussed in this chapter.

Presynaptic Events

Amino acid neurotransmitters (glutamate, GABA, and glycine) and acetylcholine are synthesized from intermediates of the Krebs cycle, but the different monoamines are synthesized from essential amino acid precursors by the action of specific enzymes. Amino acid and monoamine neurotransmitters are incorporated into synaptic vesicles at the level of the presynaptic terminal. In contrast, neuropeptides are synthesized in the cell body and transported in secretory vesicles along the axon to the synaptic terminal. Neurotransmitter release is triggered by the influx of Ca^{2+} through voltage-gated channels that open in response to the arrival of an action potential in the presynaptic terminal. These channels are clustered in specific regions of the presynaptic membrane called *active zones* (Fig. 5.18).

> The presynaptic voltage-gated Ca^{2+} channels are the N and P/Q type channels, which form complexes with presynaptic proteins that also allow the synaptic vesicles to cluster at the active zones.

Classic Neurotransmission

Neurotransmitters act through two main classes of receptors: ligand-gated receptors and G (guanine nucleotide binding) protein-coupled receptors. Ion channels that open in response to the chemical transmitter, allowing the rapid influx of cations (Na^+, Ca^{2+}) or Cl^-, are called *ligand-gated receptors*. The influx of cations elicits rapid depolarization of the membrane, called *fast excitatory postsynaptic potentials* (EPSPs) because they allow the membrane to reach threshold to trigger the action potential. Important examples of excitatory neurotransmitters that activate cation channels are glutamate, acting through different

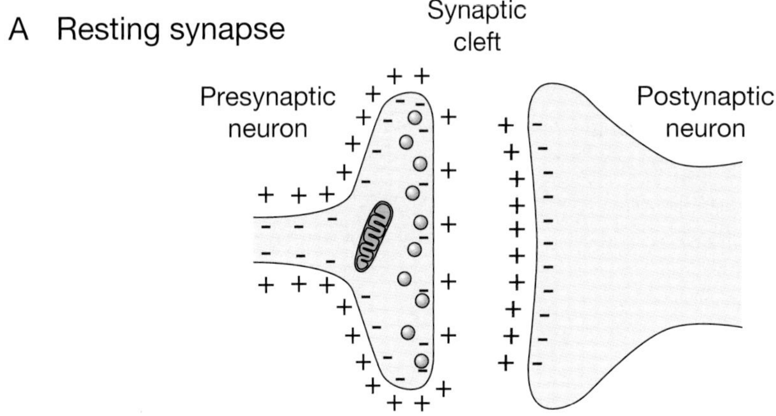

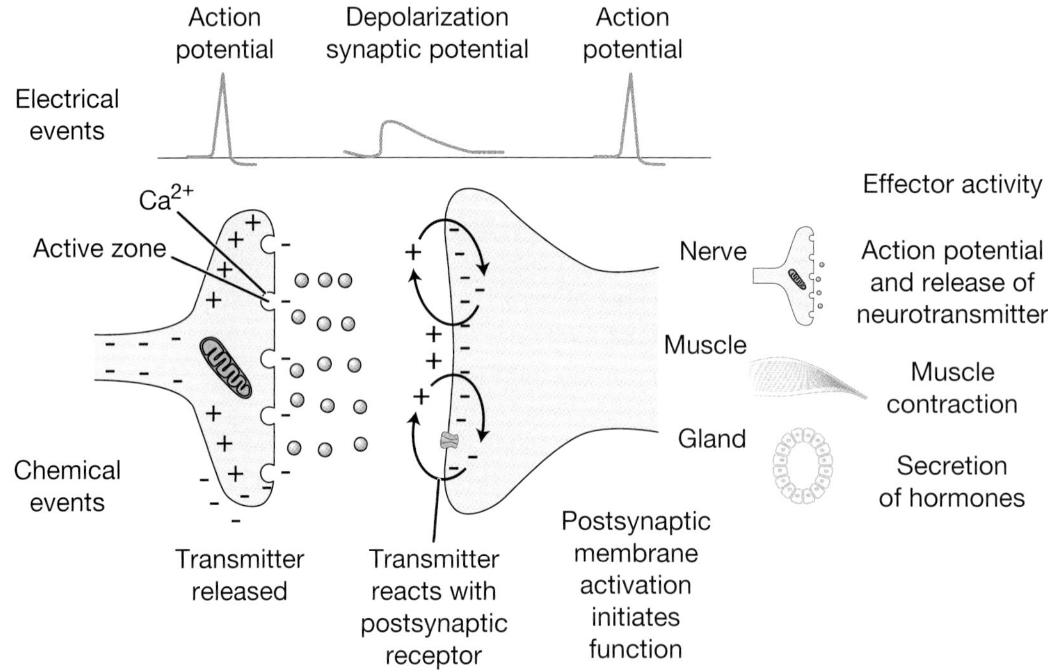

Fig. 5.18. Synaptic transmission. *A*, In a resting synapse, both the presynaptic axon terminal and the postsynaptic membrane are normally polarized. *B*, In an active synapse, an action potential invades the axon terminal (from left in the diagram) and depolarizes it. Depolarization of the axon terminal of a presynaptic neuron results in the release of neurotransmitter from the terminal. The neurotransmitter diffuses across the synaptic cleft and produces local current flow and a synaptic potential in the postsynaptic membrane, which initiates the effector activity (neuronal transmission, neurotransmitter release, hormonal secretion, or muscle contraction).

ionotropic receptors, and acetylcholine, acting through nicotinic receptors. In contrast, the influx of Cl^- rapidly brings the membrane potential toward the equilibrium potential of this ion (–75 mV). This results in a *fast inhibitory postsynaptic potential* (IPSP) that prevents the membrane from reaching the threshold for action potentials. The inhibitory neurotransmitters that activate Cl^- channels include GABA and glycine.

Table 5.5. Postsynaptic Potentials

Receptor (example)	Ionic mechanism	Effect
Nicotinic Ionotropic glutamate	Increased Na^+ or Ca^{2+} conductance	Fast excitation
$GABA_A$ Glycine	Increased Cl^- conductance	Fast inhibition
G protein-coupled receptors	Decreased K^+ conductance Increased K^+ conductance	Slow excitation Slow inhibition

Fast excitatory or inhibitory potentials allow rapid, point-to-point transfer of excitatory or inhibitory information between the cells. This is called *classic neurotransmission* (Table 5.6).

Neuromodulation

The second class of neurotransmitter receptors, *G protein-coupled receptors*, mediates the effects of monoamines and neuropeptides and some of the effects of acetylcholine, glutamate, and GABA. There are many types of G protein-coupled receptors, and unlike ligand-gated receptors, they indirectly affect the function of ion channels. The activation of G protein-coupled receptors increases or decreases the permeability of voltage-gated ion channels either through interactions of G protein subunits with the channel or phosphorylation of the channel triggered by molecules generated in response to activation of the G protein-coupled receptor. The main targets of regulation by G protein-coupled receptors are the several types of K^+ channels and the voltage-gated Ca^{2+} channels. The permeability of these channels may be increased or decreased in response to different G

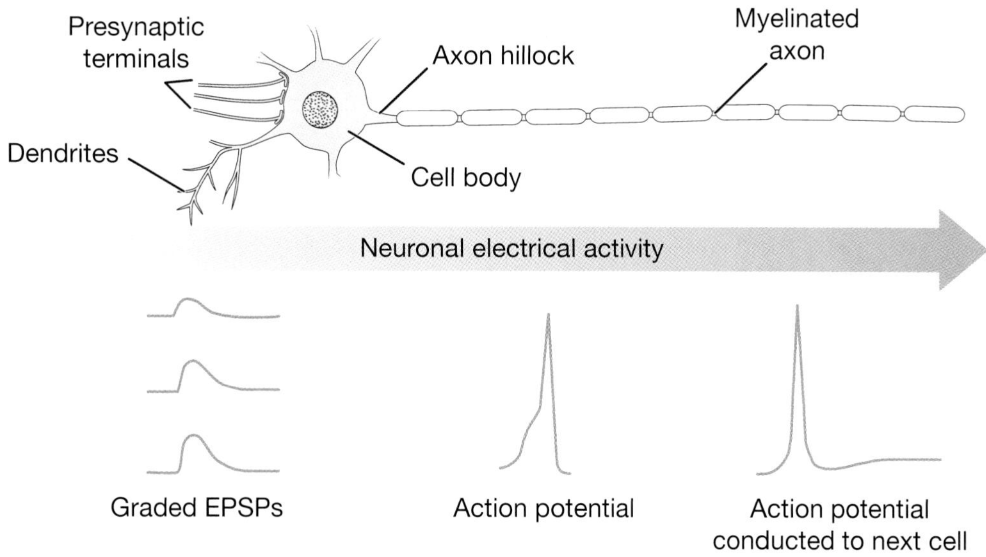

Fig. 5.19. Neuronal electrical activity from its initiation by excitatory postsynaptic potentials (EPSPs) to its transmission as an action potential to another area.

Table 5.6. Comparison of Classic Neurotransmission and Neuromodulation

Feature	Classic neurotransmission	Neuromodulation
Function	Rapid synaptic excitation or inhibition	Regulation of neuronal excitability and neurotransmitter release
Receptor mechanisms	Ion channel receptors (ligand-gated ion channels)	G protein-coupled receptors
Ionic mechanism	Opening of Na^+ or Ca^{2+} channels (fast EPSP) or Cl^- channels (fast IPSP)	Opening or closing of voltage-gated K^+ or Ca^{2+} channels

EPSP, excitatory postsynaptic potential; IPSP, inhibitory postsynaptic potential.

proteins. Activation of these G protein-coupled receptors does not elicit fast excitatory or inhibitory postsynaptic responses (as in the case of classic neurotransmission) but rather elicits a change in neuronal excitability. This is called *neuromodulation*. Potassium channels are the main target for neuromodulatory signals. Signals that lead to closure of K^+ channels (thus moving the membrane potential away from the equilibrium potential of this ion) elicit slow membrane depolarization toward threshold, thus increasing excitability and the probability of triggering an action potential. In contrast, G protein-coupled mechanisms that lead to the opening of K^+ channels (thus moving the membrane potential toward the equilibrium potential) elicits slow membrane hyperpolarization (away from threshold), which decreases neuronal excitability and responsiveness to other stimuli (Table 5.6).

A neurotransmitter may also act through ion channel receptors or G protein-coupled receptors located in the *presynaptic* membrane. Through these presynaptic receptors, neurotransmitters may regulate their own release or the release of other neurotransmitters. Most presynaptic receptors are G protein-coupled receptors that trigger the closure of voltage-gated Ca^{2+} channels, thus inhibiting the release of neurotransmitters. In fact, as a feedback mechanism, many neurotransmitters inhibit their own release by acting on presynaptic inhibitory *autoreceptors*.

Synaptic Interactions

There are several patterns of synaptic interactions. One pattern of synaptic microcircuit is that of synaptic *divergence*, by which a single excitatory or inhibitory axon terminal synapses with multiple dendrites. If the synapse is excitatory, this pattern provides an amplification of activity of a single axon into simultaneous excitation in many postsynaptic neurons. Another example of divergence occurs in many relay nuclei of the sensory and motor systems. In these nuclei, the basic synaptic circuit is a *triad* consisting of an excitatory afferent axon, the cell body and dendrites of an excitatory projection neuron, and a local inhibitory interneuron that synapses with the projection neuron. Another pattern of synaptic interaction is the *convergence* of inputs on a single neuron. When several stimuli are excitatory, the resulting excitatory postsynaptic potentials may undergo temporal or spatial summation. Synaptic convergence also provides the basis for algebraic summation of excitatory and inhibitory postsynaptic potentials.

The inhibitory effects of a neurotransmitter on the target neuron is called *postsynaptic* inhibition (Fig. 5.20). This involves an increase in permeability to either Cl^- (fast IPSP) or K^+ (slow IPSP). However, some neurotransmitters may also inhibit neurotransmitter release from the presynaptic axon terminal. This is called *presynaptic inhibition* (Fig. 5.21). The mechanism for this is decreased opening of presynaptic voltage-gated Ca^{2+}

channels. In addition to the effects of neurotransmitters on presynaptic receptors, described above, presynaptic inhibition may occur through axoaxonic synapses. The inhibitory axon elicits a partial depolarization that decreases the magnitude of the action potential in the presynaptic axon, thus reducing the number of voltage-gated channels that open and the number of synaptic vesicles that release neurotransmitter.

Electrical Synapses

Although most synapses in the nervous system use chemical neurotransmitters, neurons may also interact through gap junctions adjoining the membrane of two adjacent neurons. Each membrane contributes a hemichannel, composed of a protein called connexin, which forms a gap junction channel that allows bidirectional flow of ion current. Transmission across the electrical synapse is rapid, without the synaptic delay of chemical synapses. Also, electrical synapses are bidirectional, in contrast to chemical synapses, which transmit signals primarily in only one direction. Typically, gap junctions occur between astrocytes. Astrocytes connected by gap junctions form a functional syncytium that provides a pathway for the transmission of electrical and chemical information over large distances in the central nervous system.

Synaptic activity affects the function of astrocytes, which are an integral component of the synaptic unit. For example, synaptic release of the excitatory neurotransmitter glutamate not only elicits depolarization of the postsynaptic neuron but also provides a signal to the astrocytes surrounding the synapse. This signal results in part from the extracellular K^+ that accumulates from action potentials in the postsynaptic neuron, by the effects of glutamate on astrocytes, and by the active reuptake of glutamate by astrocytes. Synaptic activity results in depolarization, increased intracellular Ca^{2+}, and increased energy metabolism in astrocytes. All these signals are transmitted through gap junctions within the astrocytic network. Most communication in the nervous system occurs through chemical synapses.

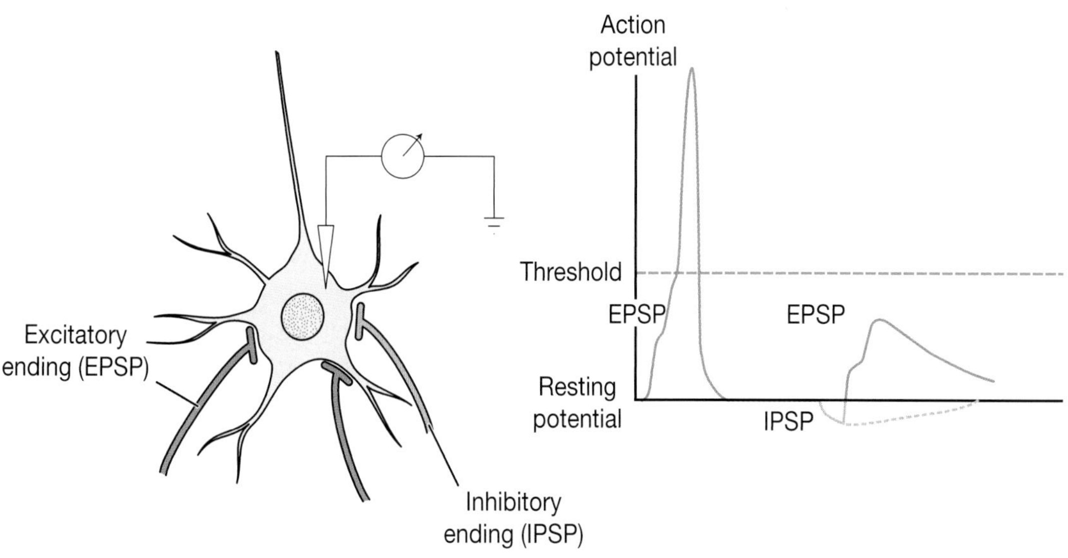

Fig. 5.20. Postsynaptic inhibition in the neuron on the left occurs when the inhibitory and excitatory endings are active simultaneously. On the right, a microelectrode recording shows two excitatory postsynaptic potentials (EPSPs) summating to initiate an action potential. If an inhibitory postsynaptic potential (IPSP) occurs simultaneously with an EPSP, depolarization is too low to reach threshold and no action potential occurs.

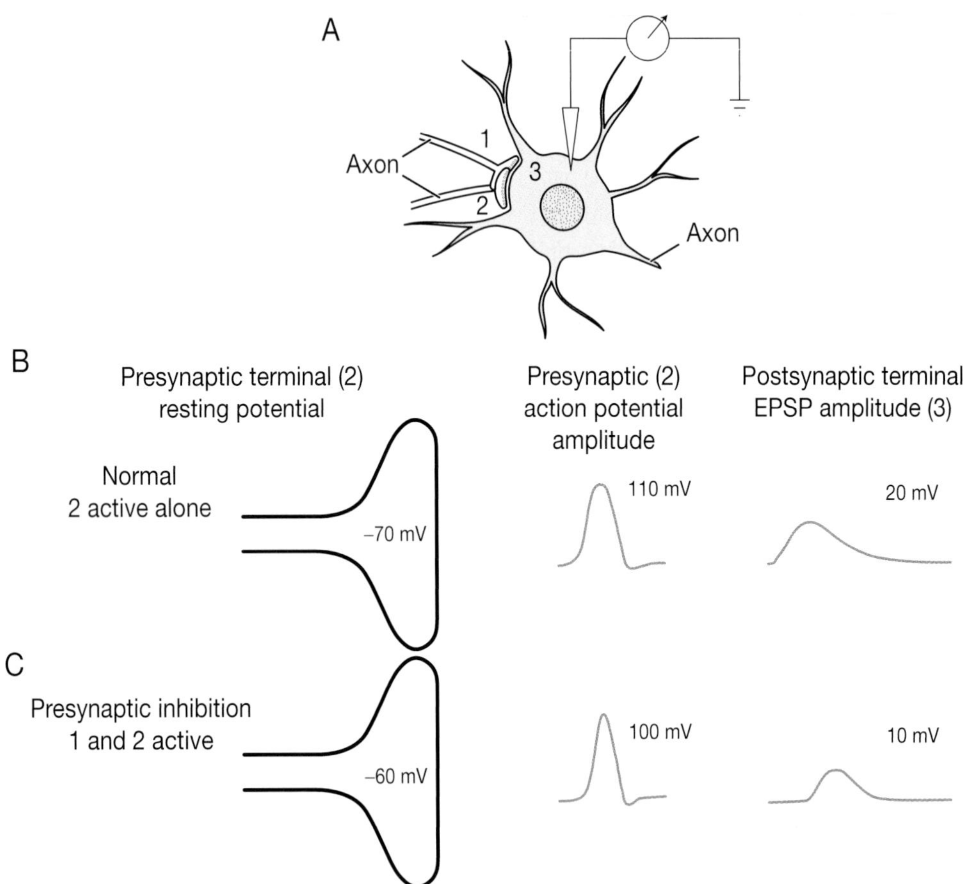

Fig. 5.21. *A*, Presynaptic inhibition of neuron 3 when axon 1 partially depolarizes axon 2. *B*, Response to axon 2 acting alone. *C*, Response to axon 2 after depolarization of axon 1. In the latter case, there is less neurotransmitter and a smaller excitatory postsynaptic potential (EPSP).

- Presynaptic events include the synthesis and storage of neurotransmitters in synaptic vesicles, vesicle mobilization, and neurotransmitter release by exocytosis.
- Exocytosis is triggered by the opening of voltage-gated Ca^{2+} channels in the presynaptic active zones, triggered by the arrival of action potentials.
- Neurotransmitters act through ligand-gated cation or Cl^- channels to elicit fast excitatory or inhibitory postsynaptic potentials (classic neurotransmission).
- Neurotransmitters act through G protein-coupled receptors to elicit, by transduction cascades, changes in the permeability of voltage-gated K^+ or Ca^{2+} channels, resulting in changes in neuronal excitability (neuromodulation).

Clinical Correlations

Pathophysiologic Mechanisms

The mechanisms responsible for neuronal excitability, impulse conduction, and synaptic transmission in the central and peripheral nervous systems may be altered transiently to produce either a loss of activity or overactivity of neurons. A loss of activity results in a clinical deficit of relatively short duration (seconds to hours); overactivity results in extra movements or sensations. Both types of transient alteration are usually reversible. Transient disorders may be focal or generalized (Table 5.7) and may be due to many mechanisms (Table 5.8). Transient disorders reflect disturbances in neuronal excitability due to abnormalities in membrane potential.

Table 5.7. Transient Disorders

Neuronal excitability	Focal disorders	Generalized disorder
Increased	Focal seizure Tonic spasm Muscle cramp Paresthesia Paroxysmal pain	Generalized seizure Tetany
Decreased	Transient ischemic attack Migraine aura Transient mononeuropathy	Syncope Concussion Cataplexy Periodic paralysis

Table 5.8. Mechanisms of Transient Disorders

Energy failure
- Hypoxia-ischemia
- Hypoglycemia
- Seizures
- Spreading cortical depression
- Trauma

Ion channel disorders
- Mutation of channel protein (channelopathies)
- Immune blockade
- Drugs
- Toxins

Electrolyte disorders

Demyelination

Energy Failure

Energy metabolism is necessary for maintenance of the membrane potential by the ATP-coupled Na^+-K^+ pump. Most of the ATP produced in the nervous system by aerobic metabolism of glucose is used to maintain the activity of the Na^+ pump. Conditions such as hypoxia, ischemia, hypoglycemia, or seizures affect the balance between energy production and energy consumption of neurons and cause energy failure and thus impaired activity of Na^+-K^+ ATPase. If the active transport process stops, the cell accumulates Na^+ and loses K^+ and the membrane potential progressively decreases. This depolarization has two consequences. First, there may be a transient increase in neuronal excitability as the membrane potential moves closer to threshold for opening voltage-gated Na^+ channels and triggering action potentials. This may produce a paroxysmal discharge of the neuron or axon. Second, if depolarization persists, Na^+ channels remain inactivated and the neuron becomes inexcitable. This is known as *depolarization blockade* and results in a focal deficit, such as focal paralysis or anesthesia, or a generalized deficit, such as paralysis or loss of consciousness (Fig. 5.22).

The neuron also uses ATP to maintain ion gradients that allow active presynaptic reuptake of neurotransmitters, such as the excitatory amino acid L-glutamate. Under conditions of energy failure, glutamate accumulates in the synapse and produces prolonged activation of its postsynaptic receptors, leading to neuronal depolarization and the accumulation of Ca^{2+} in the cytosol. Because the lack of ATP also impairs active transport of Ca^{2+} into the endoplasmic reticulum or toward the extracellular fluid, Ca^{2+} accumulates, which leads to cell injury.

Clinical Problem 5.2.

A 64-year-old man had sudden occlusion of a blood vessel in an area of the brain that controls speech and was unable to speak for 10 minutes. His speech gradually returned to normal over a 15-minute period.

a. How could anoxia of the involved cells result in loss of function?
b. By what mechanism could recovery occur?

Electrolyte Disorders

Disorders affecting serum electrolyte levels may produce transient changes in the excitability of nerve and muscle. Changes in extracellular ionic concentration produce concomitant changes in the transmembrane ion gradient and, thus, the equilibrium potential of the ion. The effect of this change depends on the state of membrane permeability. An alteration in extracellular K^+ affects mainly the resting membrane potential, whereas changes in extracellular Na^+ affect predominantly the magnitude of the action potential. Changes in the serum concentration of K^+ affect mainly excitability in the periphery (peripheral axons and skeletal or cardiac muscle). A decrease in extracellular K^+, for example, when this ion is lost because of disease (vomiting or diarrhea) or medication (diuretics), increases the concentration gradient and equilibrium potential of K^+, hyperpolarizing the cell at rest. This makes the cell less excitable and may produce severe weakness. An increase in extracellular K^+, as in renal or adrenal failure, decreases the concentration gradient and equilibrium potential of K^+, lowering the resting potential. The effects vary with the degree and duration of the increase in K^+. Small increases produce an initial depolarization that moves the resting membrane potential closer to the threshold for opening Na^+ channels and generating action potentials. The cell is more excitable and fires action potentials in response to weaker stimuli or even spontaneously. A large increase in

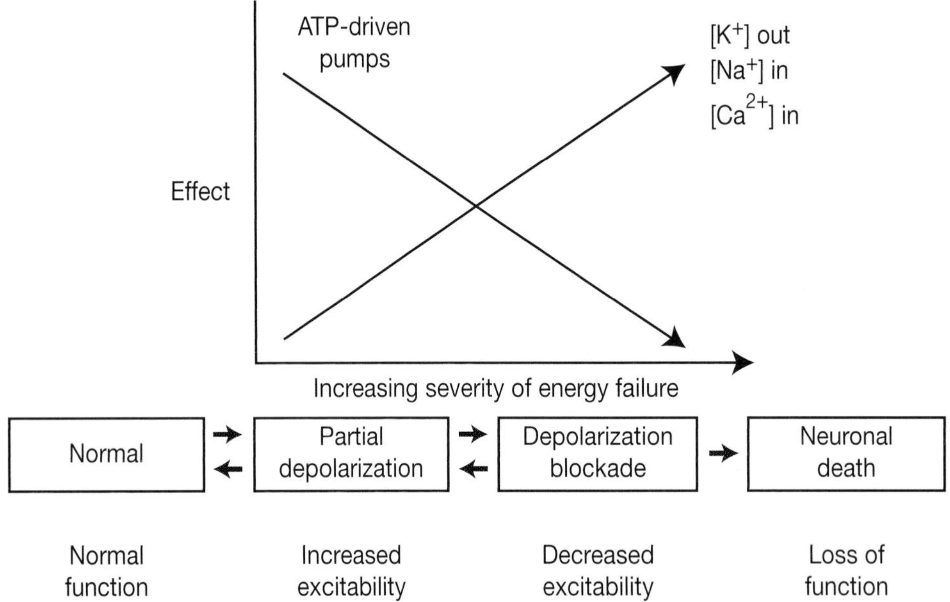

Fig. 5.22. Effects of increasing severity of energy failure (and adenosine triphosphate [ATP] depletion) on activity of ATP-driven pumps, ionic concentrations in the intracellular and extracellular fluids, and neuronal electrical activity. With progressive failure of ATP-driven pumps, K^+ accumulates in the extracellular fluid and Na^+ and Ca^{2+} accumulate inside the neuron. This produces progressive neuronal depolarization. With partial depolarization, the resting potential moves closer to the threshold for triggering an action potential; this results in a transient increase in neuronal excitability, which may be manifested by paresthesias or seizures. With further depolarization, the membrane potential is at a level that maintains inactivation of Na^+ channels, preventing further generation of action potentials and, thus, reducing neuronal excitability. This constitutes a depolarization block, which is manifested by transient and reversible deficits such as paralysis or loss of consciousness. If the energy failure is severe and prolonged, the excessive accumulation of intracellular Ca^{2+} triggers various enzymatic cascades that lead eventually to neuronal death and irreversible loss of function.

extracellular K^+ produces a persistently low resting membrane potential. This leads to persistent inactivation of voltage-gated Na^+ channels, rendering the membrane inexcitable (depolarization block). Therefore, an excess of extracellular K^+ may produce either excessive activity or a loss of activity of neurons or muscle cells.

An increase in extracellular Na^+ increases the Na^+ equilibrium potential, the size of the action potential, and the rate of rise of the action potential. Such increases do not have significant clinical effects. A decrease in extracellular Na^+ has the reverse effect; that is, it may lower the amplitude of the action potential and slow its rate of increase. If the action potential is low enough, it may not generate sufficient local current to discharge adjacent membrane, and action potential conduction may be blocked. Calcium acts primarily as a membrane stabilizer. Thus, hypocalcemia increases excitability and may produce spontaneous activity. In addition, because the entry of Ca^{2+} into the axon terminal is necessary for the release of neurotransmitter, a low level of Ca^{2+} may block synaptic transmission. Therefore, hypocalcemia may have opposite effects; that is, it may impair synaptic transmission but produce spontaneous firing of a neuron or axon. An excess of Ca^{2+} tends to block action potentials and to enhance synaptic transmission. Hypercalcemia does not produce demonstrable changes, except at very high concentrations of Ca^{2+}, whereas even moderate hypocalcemia may produce muscle twitching or tingling.

Clinical Problem 5.3.

A 10-year-old boy has severe kidney disease, which has resulted in a marked increase in the serum level of K^+. He has cardiac abnormalities and generalized muscle weakness. How could the altered K^+ concentration produce these signs of striated muscle dysfunction?

Ion Channel Blockade

The electrical activity of neurons can be altered transiently by drugs, toxins, or autoantibodies that act on the cell membrane. Blockade of Na^+ channels at the node of Ranvier slows conduction velocity or causes conduction block; this produces a reversible focal deficit. For example, the blockade of Na^+ channels in sensory axons by local anesthetic agents produces anesthesia. Ion channels are an important target of drugs used to treat disorders associated with excessive neuronal excitability.

Clinical Problem 5.4.

For each of the following features, what will be the effect of a drug that blocks voltage-gated Na^+ channels?

a. Neuronal excitability
b. Axon conduction velocity
c. Neurotransmitter release
d. What will be the potential therapeutic uses of this drug?

Synaptic transmission is particularly susceptible to drugs or autoantibodies that may act on presynaptic or postsynaptic membranes. Examples of the types of transmission block are illustrated in Figure 5.23. There may be presynaptic block of neurotransmitter release or postsynaptic block by competitive or noncompetitive inhibition of postsynaptic receptors or by depolarizing substances.

Several drugs that act on ion channels or affect synaptic transmission have therapeutic applications. Drugs that block Na^+ channels (phenytoin, carbamazepine) or increase inhibitory synaptic transmission (benzodiazepines) are used in the treatment of seizures and pain. Several biologic toxins exert their actions by altering ion channels or synaptic transmission or both. For example, tetrodotoxin, a poison occurring in certain fish, blocks Na^+ channels and causes paralysis. Clostridial toxins, such as tetanus and botulinum toxin, prevent the release of neurotransmitter by destroying protein essential for the docking of synaptic vesicles at the active zone.

Clinical Problem 5.5.

A patient is brought to the emergency department because of rapid onset of generalized muscle weakness that developed 3 hours after the patient ate sushi. You suspect intoxication with saxitoxin, a toxin that blocks voltage-gated Na^+ channels. By what mechanism would the toxin cause muscle weakness?

Several neuroimmunologic disorders produce abnormalities in voltage-gated or ligand-gated ion channels. Autoantibodies may also block ion channels involved in neuromuscular transmission and produce reversible muscle fatigue or paralysis. For example, antibodies against gangliosides produce conduction block in motor axons by affecting the function of voltage-gated Na^+ channels at nodes of Ranvier. Antibodies may affect neuromuscular transmission and cause transient and reversible muscle fatigue or weakness. Antibodies against voltage-gated Ca^{2+} channels interfere with the release of acetylcholine from motor nerve endings, as in

Clinical Problem 5.6.

A 44-year-old man with a 30-year history of cigarette smoking is evaluated for progressive muscle weakness and erectile dysfunction over the past 2 months. Neurologic examination shows symmetric weakness in the proximal upper and lower limb muscles, which transiently improves with sustained effort, and absence of muscle stretch reflexes in the four limbs. Laboratory testing shows antibodies directed against presynaptic voltage-gated Ca^{2+} channels. What mechanism is most likely to explain the patient's symptoms and findings on the neurologic examination?

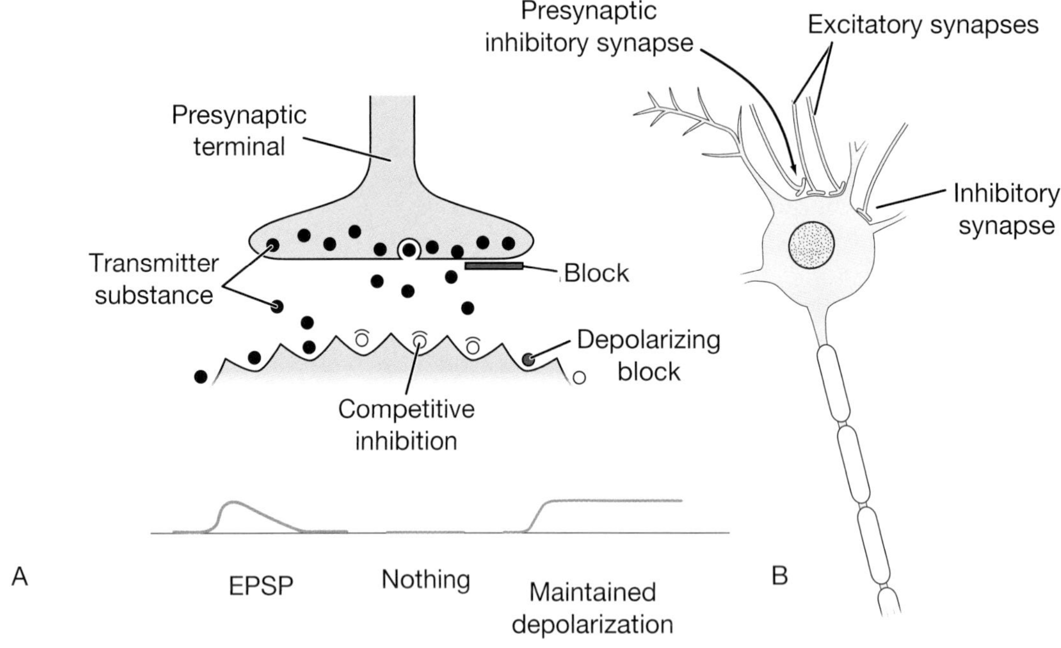

Fig. 5.23. *A*, Abnormalities of synaptic transmission. Types of transmission block include block of transmitter release (block), block of transmitter binding to postsynaptic membrane (competitive inhibition), and binding of another depolarizing agent to the membrane (depolarizing block). EPSP, excitatory postsynaptic potential. *B*, These types of abnormalities may occur at each neuronal synapse shown.

Lambert-Eaton myasthenic syndrome. Antibodies against nicotinic acetylcholine receptors in muscle membrane at motor end plates are the hallmark of myasthenia gravis.

Channelopathies

Genetic disorders that alter the amino acid composition of ion channel subunits produce changes in the function of the channel. These disorders are called *channelopathies*. Several genetic disorders that affect voltage- or neurotransmitter-gated Na^+, K^+, or Ca^{2+} channels have been described. Muscle channelopathies affecting the voltage-gated ion channels may be manifested as episodic weakness (called periodic paralysis) or increased muscle excitability producing impaired muscle relaxation (myotonia) or both. Neuronal channelopathies may be manifested by increased neuronal excitability leading to seizures or episodic cerebellar ataxia.

Seizures

Seizures are transient episodes of supratentorial origin in which there is abrupt and temporary alteration of cerebral function (see Chapter 11). They are produced by spontaneous, excessive discharge of cortical neurons caused by several pathophysiologic mechanisms. Excessive excitation or abnormal rhythmic synchronized activity may occur in focal areas of the cerebral cortex (focal seizures) or over the entire cerebral cortex (generalized seizures). A focal or generalized increase in neuronal excitability may result from energy failure producing transient depolarization or lack of local inhibition.

Cortical Spreading Depression

Cortical spreading depression has been associated with the induction of focal neurologic deficits during attacks of migraine (the migraine aura) and the progression of neurologic deficits during focal brain ischemia. It consists of a short-lasting depolarization wave that moves across the cortex at a rate of 3 to 5 mm/min and produces a brief phase of excitation, followed by prolonged neuronal depression. During spreading depression, there is an abrupt increase in the brain of extracellular K^+ and release of excitatory amino acids. The spread of the depolarization may occur partly through the gap junctions of astrocytes.

Clinical Problem 5.7.

A 25-year-old man is evaluated for spells. He experienced three stereotyped episodes in which he felt a prickling numbness spreading rapidly from the left corner of his mouth, to his thumb and fingers, and up the arm, followed by involuntary jerking of the arm. The episodes lasted about 2 minutes. The findings on neurologic examination are normal. The electroencephalogram shows an epileptic focus in the right frontal cortex.

1. Which of the following mechanisms may increase neuronal excitability leading to seizures?
    a. Increased K^+ conductance
    b. Increased Na^+ conductance
2. Which of the following drug effects may be helpful in preventing the onset and generalization of seizures?
    a. Blockade of voltage-gated K^+ channels
    b. Blockade of voltage-gated Na^+ channels
    c. Increased Cl^- permeability
    d. Increased Ca^{2+} permeability

Consequences of Demyelination

Demyelination is an important mechanism of neurologic disease. Myelin disorders may be caused by genetic defects in myelin composition or, more commonly, by acquired disorders of myelin. Acquired disorders of myelin are frequently due to immune-mediated mechanisms. In the peripheral nervous system, these disorders include acute and chronic inflammatory demyelinating neuropathies. In the central nervous system, the most important example is multiple sclerosis. In demyelinating diseases, there is not only loss of myelin but also a redistribution of Na^+ and K^+ channels. The loss of myelin means that the insulation of the axon is lost and the electrical current is dissipated because of increased capacitance and decreased resistance of the membrane. The loss of myelin around the internodes and the loss of the concentration of Na^+ channels at the nodes of Ranvier interfere with saltatory conduction by slowing nerve conduction or, in severe cases, by causing conduction block. Conduction block produces such deficits as paralysis and loss of sensation.

Transient conduction block may be caused by drugs (e.g., local anesthetics) that block Na^+ channels or by nerve compression.

Clinical Problem 5.8.

A 36-year-old woman with multiple sclerosis (with focal areas of loss of myelin in the central nervous system) had a 2-week loss of vision in one eye.

How could loss of myelin in the optic nerve have affected her vision?

Clinical Problem 5.9.

After sitting in a biochemistry lecture for 1.5 hours and sleeping with your arm over a chair for 10 minutes, you awaken to find the back of your hand numb. As you rub it, it begins to tingle.

1. What is the level of the lesion?
2. Which of the following changes could account for the tingling?
   a. Hyperpolarization of the internode
   b. Partial axonal depolarization of the node of Ranvier

Additional Reading

Ackerman MJ, Clapham DE. Ion channels: basic science and clinical disease. N Engl J Med. 1997;336:1575-86. Erratum in: N Engl J Med. 1997;337:579.

Benarroch EE. Ion channels and channelopathies. In: Basic neurosciences with clinical applications. Philadelphia: Elsevier; 2006. pp. 173-211.

Cannon SC. Voltage-gated ion channelopathies of the nervous sysem. Clin Neurosci Res. 2001;1:104-17.

Kleopa KA, Barchi RL. Genetic disorders of neuromuscular ion channels. Muscle Nerve. 2002;26:299-325.

Llinas RR. The intrinsic electrophysiological properties of mammalian neurons: insights into central nervous system function. Science. 1988;242:1654-64.

McCormick DA. Membrane properties and neurotransmitter actions. In: Shepherd GM, editor. The synaptic organization of the brain. 4th ed. New York: Oxford University Press; 1998. pp. 37-75.

Waxman SG. Acquired channelopathies in nerve injury and MS. Neurology, 2001;56:1621-7.

Chapter 6

Synaptic Transmission and Neurochemical Systems

Objectives

1. Name the molecules involved in chemical synaptic transmission.
2. Name the two types of receptors involved in synaptic transmission.
3. Describe the mechanisms of synthesis, storage, release, and reuptake of neurotransmitters.
4. Describe the differences between classic neurotransmission and neuromodulation.
5. Describe the general organization of relay, diffuse, and local circuit systems.
6. Describe the distribution and functions of L-glutamate in the brain.
7. Define long-term potentiation.
8. Describe the distribution, neurochemistry, and functions of γ-aminobutyric acid (GABA).
9. Describe the distribution, neurochemistry, and functions of acetylcholine.
10. Describe the distribution, neurochemistry, and functions of dopamine.
11. Describe the distribution, neurochemistry, and functions of norepinephrine, serotonin, and histamine.
12. Name the general features of neuropeptides as neurochemical transmitters.
13. Name the mechanisms of production and function of nitric oxide.
14. Name the involvement of glutamate in neuronal injury, GABA in seizures, acetylcholine in memory and autonomic disorders, and dopamine in motor and psychiatric disorders.

Introduction

Communication between neurons occurs primarily at the level of synapses. The most common form of communication in the nervous system is through *chemical synapses* (Fig. 6.1). They consist of presynaptic and postsynaptic components that are separated by a synaptic cleft. The presynaptic terminals contain *synaptic vesicles*, which are involved in the storage and release of *neurotransmitters* by the process of *exocytosis*. Complex mechanisms control the synthesis, vesicular storage, and release of neurotransmitters and regulate the availability of neurotransmitter at the level of the synaptic cleft. The effects of the neurochemical transmitter on its target are mediated by *neurotransmitter receptors*. Specific neurotransmitter systems are responsible for fast neuronal excitation or inhibition, and other neurotransmitter systems regulate the excitability of neurons in the nervous system. Abnormalities in neurochemical transmission are responsible for many disorders, causing acute neuronal death, seizures, neurodegenerative disorders, and psychiatric diseases. Most importantly, neurochemical systems provide the target for pharmacologic treatment of these disorders. The aims of this chapter are to review the basis of neurochemical transmission and the distribution, biochemistry, and function of specific neurotransmitter systems.

Overview

Molecules involved in chemical neurotransmission include amino acids (such as L-glutamate, γ-aminobutyric acid

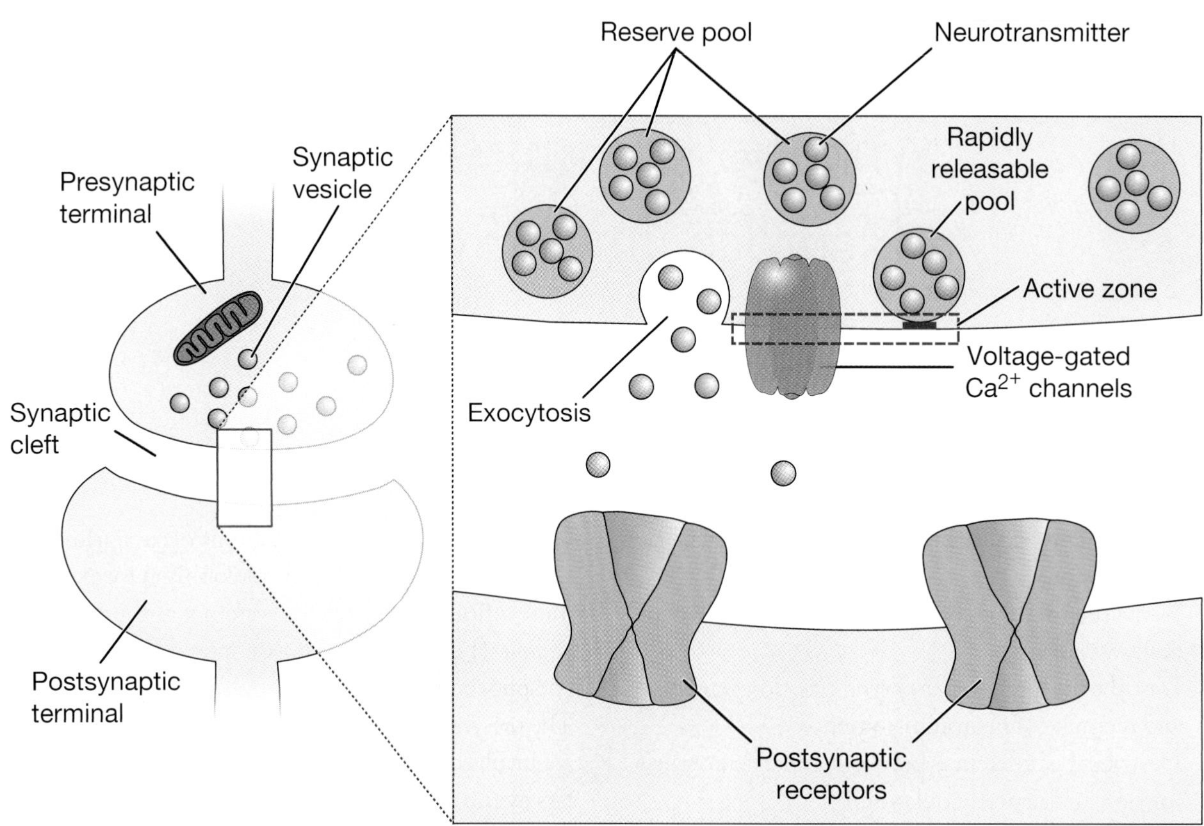

Fig. 6.1. Diagram of a synapse in the central nervous system. The synaptic vesicles in the presynaptic terminal form two pools: a reserve pool and a rapidly releasable pool that consists of vesicles docked close to the voltage-gated Ca^{2+} channels at the active zone. The clustering of postsynaptic receptors facing these active zones allows rapid and secure transmission of synaptic signals.

[GABA], and glycine), acetylcholine, monoamines (dopamine, norepinephrine, serotonin, and histamine), neuropeptides, and purines such as adenosine triphosphate (ATP) (Table 6.1). These chemical signals act through two main classes of receptors located on the soma and dendrites of the postsynaptic neuron (Table 6.2). The *ligand-gated receptors* are ion channels that open in response to the chemical transmitter and allow the rapid influx of cations (sodium [Na^+] and calcium [Ca^{2+}]) or chloride (Cl^-). This results in fast excitatory or inhibitory postsynaptic responses, respectively. This rapid point-to-point transfer of information is referred to as *classic neurotransmission*. In contrast, *G protein-coupled receptors* mediate slower changes in neuronal excitability through activation or inhibition of potassium (K^+) or Ca^{2+} channels, either directly or through transduction pathways

Table 6.1. Neurochemical Transmitters

Amino acids
L-Glutamate
γ-Aminobutyric acid
Glycine
Acetylcholine
Catecholamines
Dopamine
Norepinephrine
Epinephrine
Serotonin
Histamine
Neuropeptides
Purines (adenosine triphosphate, adenosine)
Nitric oxide

Table 6.2. Functions of Neurochemical Transmitters

Function	Classic neurotransmission	Neuromodulation
Receptor	Ion channel receptors	G protein-coupled receptors
Effect	Rapid excitation or inhibition	Modulation of excitability
Ionic mechanism	Opening of either a cation channel or Cl^- channel	Opening or closing of voltage-gated K^+ or Ca^{2+} channels
Examples	Ionotropic glutamate receptor $GABA_A$ receptor Nicotinic receptor	Metabotropic glutamate receptor $GABA_B$ receptor Muscarinic receptor Receptors for monoamines Receptors for neuropeptides

GABA, γ-aminobutyric acid.

involving several second messengers. These effects are referred to as *neuromodulation*. The synaptic effects of the chemical transmitters are terminated by different mechanisms, including presynaptic or glial *reuptake*, enzymatic metabolism, or a combination of these, according to the type of neurotransmitter.

L-Glutamate mediates most excitatory neurotransmission in the central nervous system, and GABA mediates most inhibitory effects. Acetylcholine, dopamine, norepinephrine, serotonin, histamine, and neuropeptides predominantly have a neuromodulatory function. Because a single neuron receives multiple types of synapses, the neurochemical control of neuronal function is complex. In addition to rapid changes in neuronal excitability, neurochemical systems may produce long-term effects on neuronal activity critical for neural development, learning, and response to injury. Thus, neurochemical systems are important for *plasticity* in the nervous system.

- The most important form of communication in the nervous system is chemical synapses.
- Neurotransmitters are stored in synaptic vesicles and released by exocytosis triggered by Ca^{2+}.
- Ligand-gated receptors mediate the fast excitatory or inhibitory effects of neurotransmitters.
- G protein-coupled receptors mediate modulatory effects on neuronal excitability.
- Glutamate is the main excitatory neurotransmitter and GABA is the main inhibitory neurotransmitter in the central nervous system.
- Acetylcholine, monoamines, and neuropeptides are involved primarily in neuromodulation.
- Chemical signals not only affect neuronal excitability but also exert long-term effects important for synaptic plasticity.

Principles of Neurochemical Transmission

Chemical synapses are sites of bidirectional communication (Fig. 6.2). The presynaptic terminal, synaptic cleft, and postsynaptic target membrane have a complex morphologic and molecular organization that provides the basis for the multiple presynaptic and postsynaptic events that underlie chemical neurotransmission.

Presynaptic Events

Presynaptic events include the synthesis and vesicular storage of the neurotransmitter; trafficking, docking, and priming of the synaptic vesicles in the presynaptic terminal; Ca^{2+}-dependent neurotransmitter release by exocytosis; endocytotic recycling of synaptic vesicles; and presynaptic reuptake and inactivation of the neurotransmitter (Fig. 6.3) (Table 6.3).

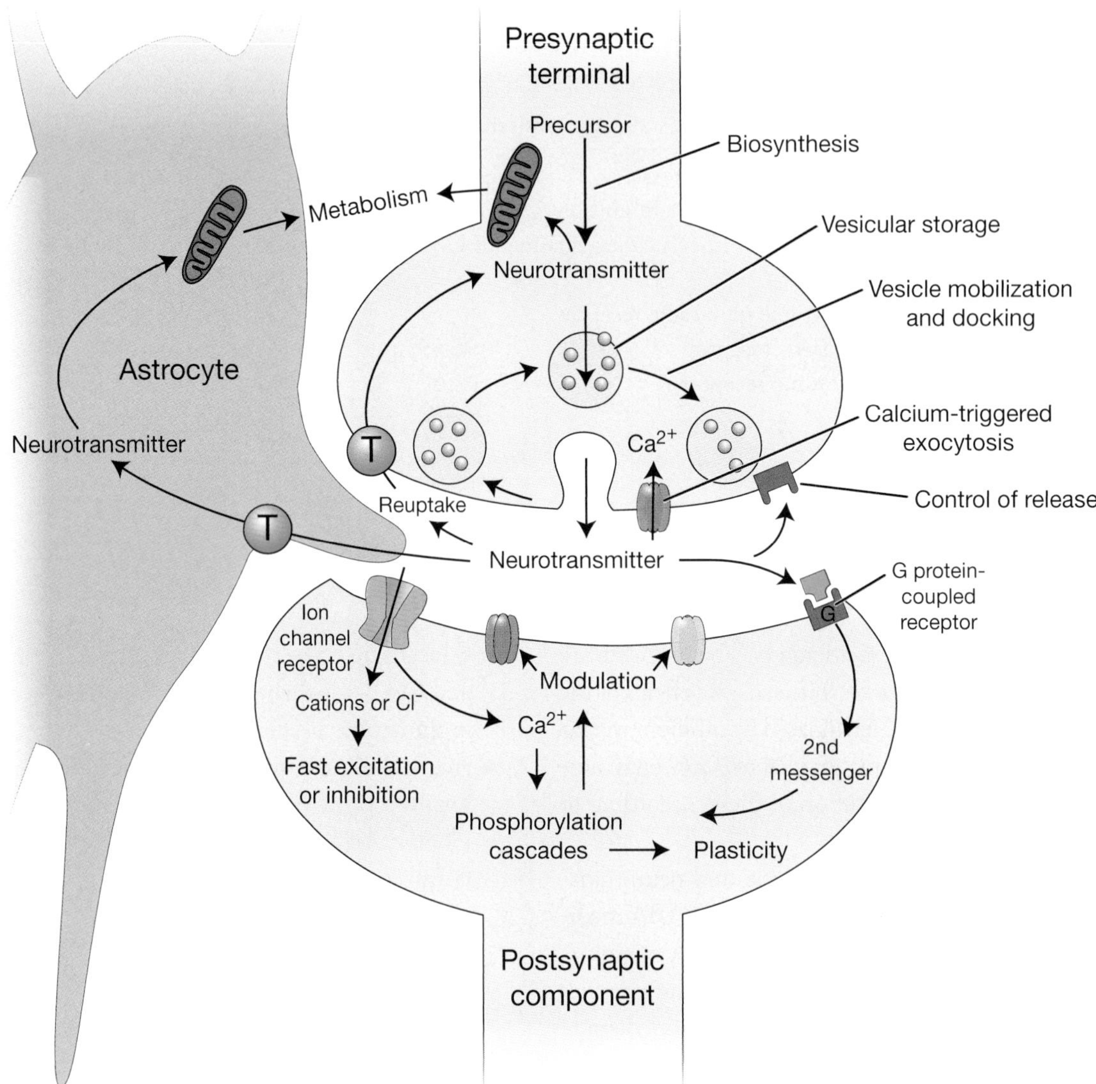

Fig. 6.2. Overview of the presynaptic and postsynaptic events involved in chemical synaptic transmission. G, guanine nucleotide-binding protein; T, neurotransmitter reuptake transporter. (Modified from Benarroch EE. Basic neurosciences with clinical applications. Philadelphia: Elsevier; 2006. Used with permission of Mayo Foundation for Medical Education and Research.)

Synthesis of Neurotransmitters

The excitatory amino acid L-glutamate and the inhibitory amino acids GABA and glycine are derived from substrates of the intermediate metabolism of glucose. The synthesis of acetylcholine is indirectly related to the oxidative metabolism of glucose. The biosynthetic pathways for dopamine, norepinephrine, serotonin, and histamine have many features in common. They are all derived from essential amino acid precursors provided by the diet, and their synthesis involves a specific, rate-limiting enzymatic step that is regulated by such factors as the state of enzyme phosphorylation and feedback mechanisms. Unlike other neurotransmitters, which are synthesized in the nerve terminal, neuropeptides are synthesized in the cell body as a large precursor that undergoes cleavage and posttranslational modifications as it travels through the secretory granule pathway, and they reach the synaptic terminal by fast anterograde transport.

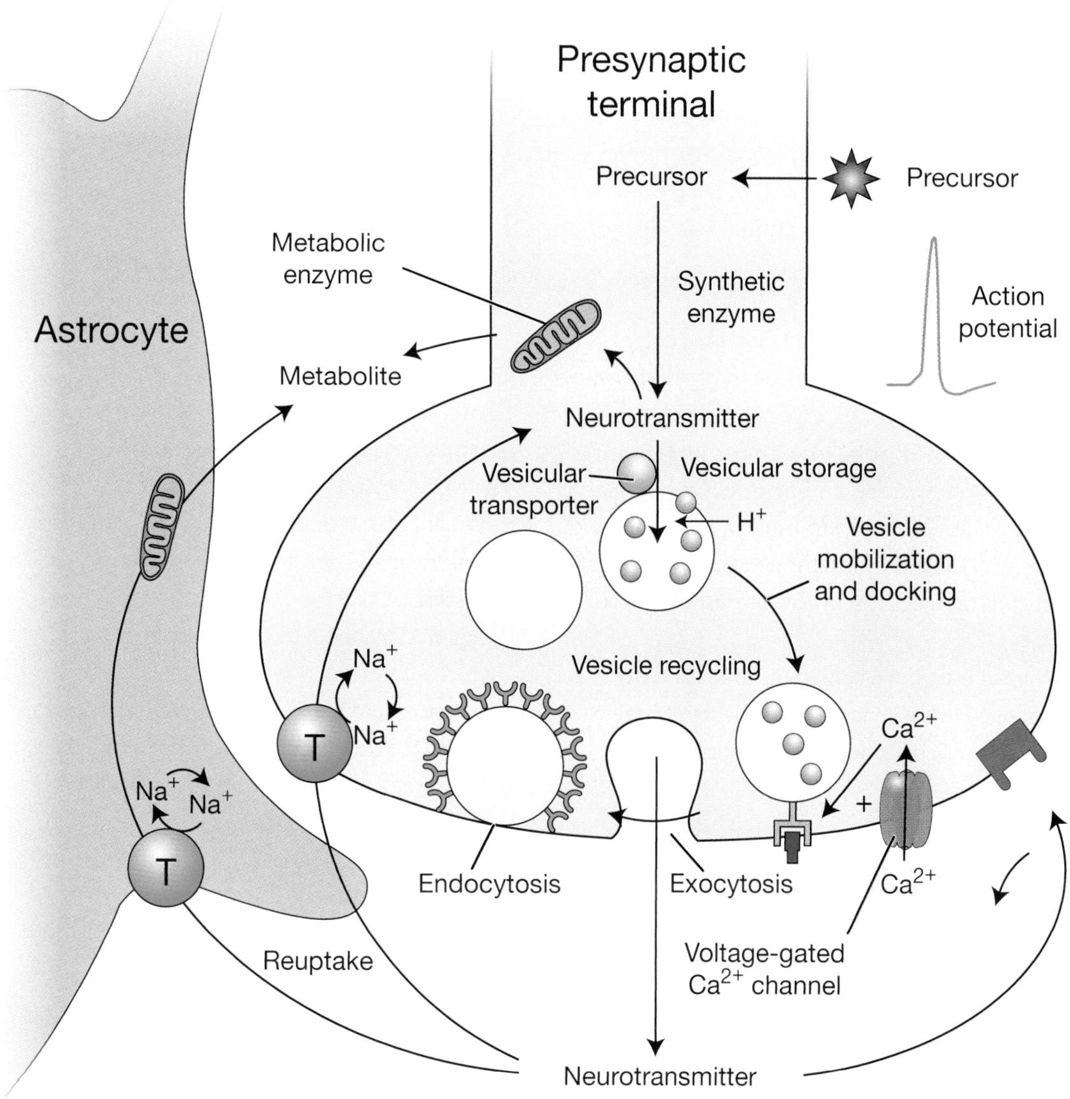

Fig. 6.3. Overview of the presynaptic events involved in chemical neurotransmission. Neurotransmitters are synthesized from specific precursors by action of specific enzymes; they are stored in synaptic vesicles by action of a vesicular transporter coupled to a proton ATPase; they are released by exocytosis in response to Ca^{2+} influx through voltage-gated channels opened by the depolarization elicited by the axon action potential; and many undergo reuptake by the presynaptic terminals and astrocytes by specific transporters (T), followed by metabolism. Neurotransmitters may regulate (in general, inhibit) their own release by acting on presynaptic autoreceptors coupled to G (guanine nucleotide-binding) proteins. The synaptic vesicle cycle includes vesicle mobilization from the reserve pool, docking at the presynatic active zone, fusion with the presynaptic membrane for exocytosis, and retrieval from presynaptic membrane by endocytosis. (Modified from Benarroch EE. Basic neurosciences with clinical applications. Philadelphia: Elsevier; 2006. Used with permission of Mayo Foundation for Medical Education and Research.)

- Glutamate, GABA, glycine, and acetylcholine are derived from intermediates of the oxidative metabolism of glucose.
- Monoamines are derived from essential amino acids by the action of rate-limiting enzymes.
- Neuropeptides are synthesized in the cell body and transported to the synaptic terminal by fast axonal transport.

Storage of Neurotransmitters in Synaptic Vesicles

Neurotransmitters are stored in different types of synaptic vesicles. Glutamate, GABA, glycine, and acetylcholine are stored in small clear vesicles, monoamines in intermediate dense-core vesicles, and neuropeptides in large dense-core vesicles (secretory granules). The storage of amino acids, acetylcholine, and monoamines in synaptic vesicles depends on specific *vesicular transporters* (Fig. 6.3).

There are at least three families of vesicular transporters: one family includes the vesicular acetylcholine and vesicular monoamine transporters, a second family includes the GABA and glycine transporter, and a third family includes the glutamate vesicular transporter. Vesicular storage of neurotransmitter is driven by an electrochemical gradient of H^+ across the vesicle membrane. This gradient is generated by the vacuolar ATP-dependent proton pump. Within the vesicle, neurotransmitters may be costored with ATP, synthetic enzymes, or ions such as zinc (Zn^{2+}).

Calcium-Triggered Exocytosis

After a synaptic vesicle is loaded with neurotransmitter, it undergoes mobilization and docking at a presynaptic active zone, followed by priming for Ca^{2+}-triggered exocytosis. The synaptic vesicles that are ready for release dock near the presynaptic active zones, which contain clusters of voltage-gated Ca^{2+} channels. Exocytosis is triggered by depolarization of the presynaptic terminals, which allows a massive and transient Ca^{2+} influx through voltage-gated Ca^{2+} channels in response to each action potential. After the synaptic vesicles fuse with the synaptic

Table 6.3. Main Mechanism of Synthesis and Inactivation of Neurochemical Transmitters

Neurotransmitter	Precursor	Key enzyme	Inactivation
L-Glutamate	α-Ketoglutarate Glutamine	Dehydrogenase Glutaminase	Reuptake by astrocytes
GABA	L-Glutamate	Glutamic acid decarboxylase	Reuptake by neurons and astrocytes
Acetylcholine	Acetylcoenzyme A and choline	Choline acetyltransferase	Acetylcholinesterase
Dopamine	Tyrosine	Tyrosine hydroxylase	Presynaptic reuptake, followed by MAO and COMT
Norepinephrine	Tyrosine	Tyrosine hydroxylase and dopamine β-hydroxylase	Presynaptic reuptake, followed by MAO and COMT
Serotonin (5-hydroxytryptamine)	Tryptophan	Tryptophan hydroxylase	Presynaptic reuptake, followed by MAO
Histamine	Histidine	Histidine decarboxylase	Methyltransferase
Neuropeptides	Prepropeptide	Convertases	Peptidases
Nitric oxide	Arginine	Nitric oxide synthase	Spontaneous short half-life

COMT, catechol-*O*-methyltransferase; GABA, γ-aminobutyric acid; MAO, monoamine oxidase.

membrane and release the neurotransmitter, the vesicular membrane proteins are retrieved by *endocytosis* and recycled (Fig. 6.3).

All these processes involve complex interactions between synaptic vesicle and presynaptic membrane proteins. The synaptic vesicle synapsin links the vesicle to the cytoskeleton and undergoes phosphorylation to facilitate vesicle mobilization for exocytosis. Membrane docking, priming, and fusion depend on interactions of synaptobrevin, located in the synaptic vesicle, and two proteins, syntaxin and SNAP-25, located in the presynaptic membrane. These three proteins are the targets of cleavage by botulinum toxin, and this explains why botulinum toxin impairs neurotransmitter release. Calcium-induced exocytosis requires interactions with the synaptic vesicle protein synaptotagmin. Vesicle endocytosis and recycling involve vesicle coating by clathrin and fission by action of dynamin; these processes are regulated by adaptor proteins such as amphiphysin.

- Vesicular storage of amino acids, acetylcholine, and monoamines involves specific transporters.
- Vesicular mobilization, docking, and exocytosis involve complex interactions between vesicular and presynaptic membrane proteins.
- Exocytosis requires a large and localized influx of Ca^{2+} through voltage-gated channels clustered at the active zones.
- Following neurotransmitter release, the synaptic vesicle membrane and proteins are retrieved by endocytosis.

Termination of the Action of Neurotransmitters

The synaptic effects of a neurotransmitter are terminated by three mechanisms: uptake by presynaptic terminals or astrocytes, enzymatic metabolism, and diffusion out of the synaptic cleft (Table 6.3). Uptake by astrocytes and presynaptic terminals is the sole mechanism for rapid termination of the synaptic action of glutamate, GABA, and glycine and the initial mechanism of inactivation of catecholamines and serotonin. Uptake involves Na^+/ATP-dependent *uptake transporters* (Fig. 6.3). The activity of these specific carriers depends on the concurrent movement of Na^+ into the terminals. This is determined by a concentration gradient, which is maintained by the Na^+,K^+-ATPase. Thus, decreased levels of ATP impair neurotransmitter reuptake.

In the case of dopamine, norepinephrine, and serotonin, reuptake is followed by enzymatic degradation to inactive metabolites by action of *monoamine oxidases*. Catecholamines are also metabolized by *catechol-O-methyltransferase*. Enzymatic degradation is the sole mechanism for termination of the action of acetylcholine (by action of acetylcholinesterase) and neuropeptides (peptidases).

- Neurotransmitter uptake by astrocytes and presynaptic terminals is mediated by energy-dependent transporters.
- Astrocyte and presynaptic uptake terminate the synaptic effects of glutamate and GABA.
- After presynaptic reuptake, catecholamines and serotonin are metabolized.
- Acetylcholine and neuropeptides are degraded by specific enzymes in the synaptic space.

Synaptic Effects of Neurotransmitters

Classic Neurotransmission

Classic neurotransmission is responsible for phasic postsynaptic excitatory or inhibitory effects, which are rapid in onset, short in duration, and spatially restricted. The receptors mediating classic neurotransmission are ligand-gated ion channels, also called *ionotropic receptors* (Fig. 6.4). Binding of the neurotransmitter to the receptor produces a change in the tridimensional conformation of the receptor protein, which opens the ion channel. Neurotransmitter-gated ion channel receptors can be subdivided into cation channels and Cl^- channels. The cation channels include *nicotinic* acetylcholine receptors, *ionotropic* glutamate receptors, and P_{2X} receptors for ATP. With the opening of these channels, there is a rapid influx of Na^+ or Ca^{2+} (or both), which results in local neuronal depolarization. This is referred to as an *excitatory postsynaptic potential* because it increases the probability of an action potential being generated. The neurotransmitter-

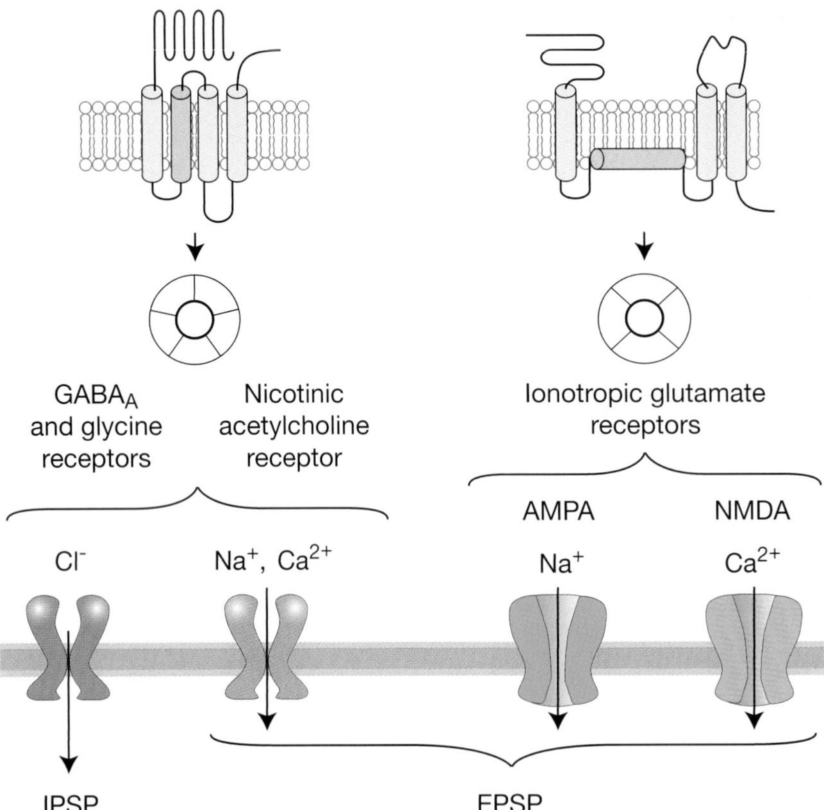

Fig. 6.4. General structure, ion permeability, and synaptic effects of the most abundant ion channel receptors. Most of these receptors belong to two families. Nicotinic acetylcholine receptors, γ-aminobutyric acid A ($GABA_A$) receptors, and glycine receptors belong to a family consisting of pentamers of subunits with four transmembrane domains, with a second domain (blue) of each subunit forming the walls of the channel pore. The ionotropic glutamate receptor family, including AMPA (α-amino-3-hydroxy-5-methyl-4-isoxazole propionate) and NMDA (*N*-methyl-D-aspartate) receptors are tetramers of subunits with four domains; the second domain, which forms the walls of the channel pore, occupies the cytoplasmic face of the membrane. Activation of nicotinic, AMPA, or NMDA receptors allows influx of cations, leading to an excitatory postsynaptic potential (EPSP), whereas the $GABA_A$ or glycine receptors allow influx of Cl^-, leading to an inhibitory postsynaptic potential (IPSP). (Modified from Benarroch EE. Basic neurosciences with clinical applications. Philadelphia: Elsevier; 2006. Used with permission of Mayo Foundation for Medical Education and Research.)

gated Cl^- channels include $GABA_A$ and glycine receptors. Opening of these channels allows rapid influx of Cl^-, which results in an *inhibitory postsynaptic potential*, because it prevents the membrane from reaching threshold to trigger an action potential (Table 6.4).

There are two main families of inotropic receptors (Fig. 6.4). One family includes nicotinic, $GABA_A$, and glycine receptors. They consist of pentamers of subunits with four transmembrane domains, in which the second domain forms the pore of the channel. The second family includes different ionotropic glutamate receptors. These are tetramers of subunits containing three transmembrane domains, with a domain located on the cytoplasmic side of the membrane forming the channel pore. The subunits of each ionotropic receptor include different subtypes, which vary in amino acid composition and distribution in the nervous system. The amino acid composition of the channel

Table 6.4. Fast Synaptic Effects of Neurotransmitters (Classic Neurotransmission)

Receptor	Ionic mechanism	Effect
Cholinergic nicotinic Glutamate ionotropic (AMPA, NMDA) Serotonin 5-HT_3 P_{2X} (ATP)	Increased cation (Na^+, Ca^{2+}) conductance	Fast excitatory postsynaptic potential
$GABA_A$ Glycine	Increased Cl^- conductance	Fast inhibitory postsynaptic potential

AMPA, α-amino-3-hydroxy-5-methyl-4-isoxazole propionate; ATP, adenosine triphosphate; NMDA, *N*-methyl-D-aspartate.

subunits determines the function of the receptor. Neurotransmitter-gated ion channel receptors cluster at specialized postsynaptic sites that are closely apposed to the presynaptic active zones, which ensures rapid and precise intercellular signal transmission. These receptors are part of macromolecular complexes and interact through specific adapter proteins with other transduction molecules and submembrane cytoskeletal proteins.

- Classic neurotransmission is mediated by ligand-gated ion channels.
- Opening of cation channels, such as nicotinic and inotropic glutamate receptors, elicits fast excitatory postsynaptic potentials.
- Opening of Cl^- channels, such as $GABA_A$ and glycine receptors, elicits fast inhibitory postsynaptic potentials.

Neuromodulation

Neuromodulation refers to the regulation of neuronal excitability. Neuromodulatory signals affect the response of ion channels to other signals. Neuromodulation involves the binding of a neurochemical transmitter to G protein-coupled receptors (Fig. 6.5). These include the metabotropic glutamate receptors, $GABA_B$ receptors, *muscarinic* cholinergic receptors, and receptors for monoamines and neuropeptides (Table 6.2). The binding of neurotransmitters to G protein-coupled receptors results in activation or inhibition of ion channels, particularly voltage-gated K^+ channels and Ca^{2+} channels, directly or by activating enzymes that lead to the production of several *second messenger* molecules, such as *cyclic adenosine monophosphate* (cAMP), *diacylglycerol*, and *inositol triphosphate* (IP_3). These second messengers activate specific *protein kinases*, either directly or, in the case of IP_3, by the release of Ca^{2+} from the smooth endoplasmic reticulum. Protein kinases phosphorylate ion channels, which affects the permeability (also called *conductance*) of these channels. This, in turn, results in changes in neuronal excitability and the ability to release neurotransmitter. For example, activation of one group of G protein-coupled receptors leads to increased K^+ permeability, which decreases neuronal excitability. Generally, the same type of receptor that increases K^+ permeability decreases the permeability of presynaptic Ca^{2+} channels, thus reducing neurotransmitter release. In contrast, activation of G protein-coupled receptors that decrease K^+ permeability increase neuronal excitability (Table 6.5).

- Neuromodulation is mediated by G protein-coupled receptors.
- G protein-coupled receptors include the metabotropic glutamate, $GABA_B$, muscarinic monoamine, and neuropeptide receptors.
- G protein-coupled receptors affect neuronal excitability and neurotransmitter release by increasing or decreasing the permeability of voltage-gated K^+ or Ca^{2+} channels.

Multiple Effects of Neurochemical Transmitters

Chemical synapses allow for complex effects on neuronal function. A single neurotransmitter may act on different receptor subtypes and thus produce different effects in the target neuron. For example, acetylcholine, GABA, or glutamate activate both ion channel and G protein-coupled receptors, whereas monoamines may activate different subtypes of G protein-coupled receptors. In addition, neurotransmitters may act through *presynaptic receptors*. These receptors regulate the release of neurotransmitters from presynaptic terminals. Presynaptic receptors may be activated by the neurotransmitter released from the same terminal (these are called *autoreceptors*) or by other neurotransmitters. Generally, neurotransmitters act through presynaptic autoreceptors to inhibit their own release, providing a negative feedback mechanism.

Persistent activation of neurotransmitter receptors produces receptor *desensitization*. The mechanisms of desensitization vary for ion channel receptors and G protein-coupled receptors. They include phosphorylation and internalization of the neurotransmitter-bound receptor, reducing the availability of receptors in the membrane. In contrast, decreased exposure of G protein-coupled receptors to their ligand causes *upregulation* of the receptors, which increases synaptic responses to the neurotransmitter.

- A single neurotransmitter may exert different effects by acting on different receptor subtypes.
- Different neurotransmitters may produce the same final synaptic effect.
- Neurotransmitters may inhibit their own release by acting on presynaptic autoreceptors.

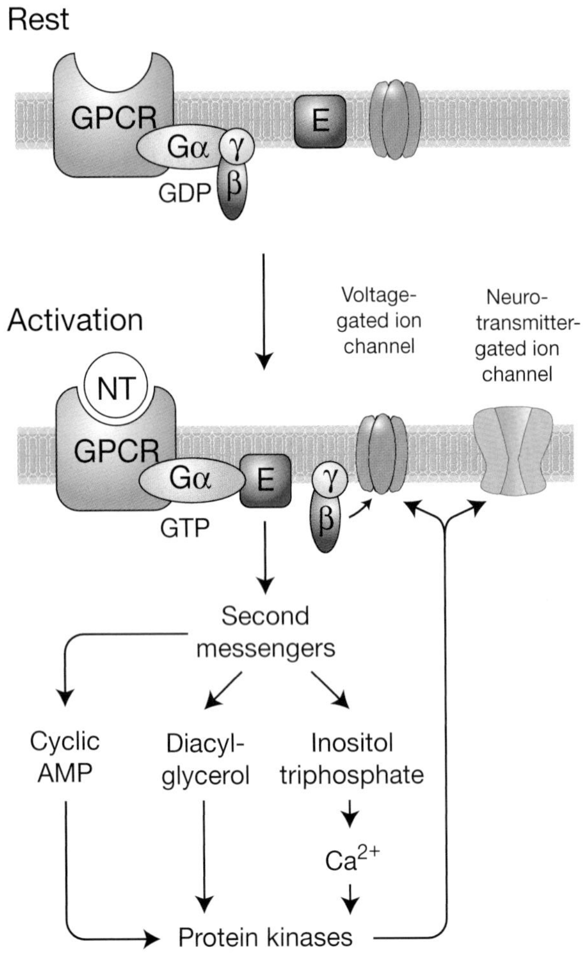

Fig. 6.5. G protein-coupled receptors (GPCR) mediate the modulatory effects of chemical transmitters on neuronal excitability and neurotransmitter release. G proteins are heterotrimers composed of three distinct subunits: α, β, and γ. The Gα subunit acts as a molecular switch by reversibly changing from an inactive guanosine diphosphate (GDP)-bound state to an active guanosine triphosphate (GTP)-bound state. In the inactive state, the Gα-GDP forms a tightly associated complex with the β/γ subunits. With neurotransmitter (NT) binding, the Gα subunit binds GTP, becomes activated, and dissociates from the β/γ complex. In many cases, the α subunit triggers downstream transduction cascades via effector enzymes (E) activating various second-messenger molecules. These include adenylate cyclase, leading to the production of cyclic adenosine monophosphate (AMP) and phospholipase C, which acts on membrane phosphatidyl inositol biphosphate, leading to the production of diacylglycerol and inositol triphosphate. In turn, inositol triphosphate triggers the release of Ca^{2+} from intracellular stores in the endoplasmic reticulum. The final effectors of these cascades are protein kinases, which phosphorylate several effector proteins, including voltage- and neurotransmitter-gated ion channels. (Modified from Benarroch EE. Basic neurosciences with clinical applications. Phildelphia: Elsevier; 2006. Used with permission of Mayo Foundation for Medical Education and Research.)

Table 6.5. Neuromodulatory Effects of G Protein-Coupled Receptors

Receptor (example)	G protein-coupled transduction mechanism	Effect
Metabotropic glutamate type 1 Muscarinic M_1 Adrenergic α_1 Serotonin 5-HT_2 Histamine H_1 Substance P (neurokinin-1) Hypocretin (orexin 1 and 2)	$G_{q/11}$ protein-coupled: activation of phospholipase C Decrease K^+ conductance Release intracellular Ca^{2+}	Increase neuronal excitability
Metabotropic glutamate type 2 $GABA_B$ Muscarinic M_2 Dopamine D_2 Adrenergic α_2 Serotonin 5-HT_1 Histamine H_3 Opioid Adenosine A_1	$G_{i/o}$ protein-coupled: inhibition of adenylate cyclase Increase K^+ conductance Decrease presynaptic Ca^{2+} conductance	Decrease neuronal excitability Presynaptic inhibition of neurotransmitter release
Dopamine D_1 Adrenergic β Histamine H_2 VIP CGRP	G_s protein-coupled: activation of adenylate cyclase	Cyclic AMP-mediated ion channel phosphorylation leading to increased or decreased neuronal excitability

AMP, adenosine monophosphate; CGRP, calcitonin gene-related peptide; GABA, γ-aminobutyric acid; VIP, vasoactive intestinal polypeptide.

- Prolonged exposure of the receptor to a chemical transmitter causes receptor desensitization.
- Lack of exposure to the neurotransmitter causes upregulation of the receptors.

There are many other forms of communication between neurons and glial cells. One mechanism is volume transmission, by which a chemical signal released from a neuron diffuses through the extracellular space to affect receptors located at a distance to affect other neurons or nonneuronal elements. Postsynaptic target neurons may release a chemical signal that provides a retrograde message affecting the release of neurotransmitter from the presynaptic terminal. Molecules that affect neural activity by these nonsynaptic mechanisms include nitric oxide (NO), arachidonic acid and prostaglandins, growth factors, cytokines, and steroids.

Long-Term Effects of Neurochemical Transmitters and Synaptic Plasticity

An important consequence of activation of ligand-gated ion channels and G protein-coupled receptors is an increased level of Ca^{2+} in the cytosol. This results primarily from Ca^{2+} influx through glutamate receptors, the opening of voltage-gated channels by neuronal depolarization, and the release of Ca^{2+} from intracellular stores triggered by IP_3. Cytosolic Ca^{2+}, cAMP, and other messenger molecules activate protein kinases that phosphorylate many proteins, including nuclear transcription factors. One important target is the *cAMP-responsive element binding protein* (CREB), which is a transcription factor that binds to specific promoter sequences of DNA and activates transcription of several synaptic proteins. This produces long-term changes critical for synaptic plasticity (Fig. 6.6). These phosphorylation cascades also regulate other important functions, including the assembly and disassembly of cytoskeletal proteins, which results in a use-dependent change in the morphology of dendritic spines.

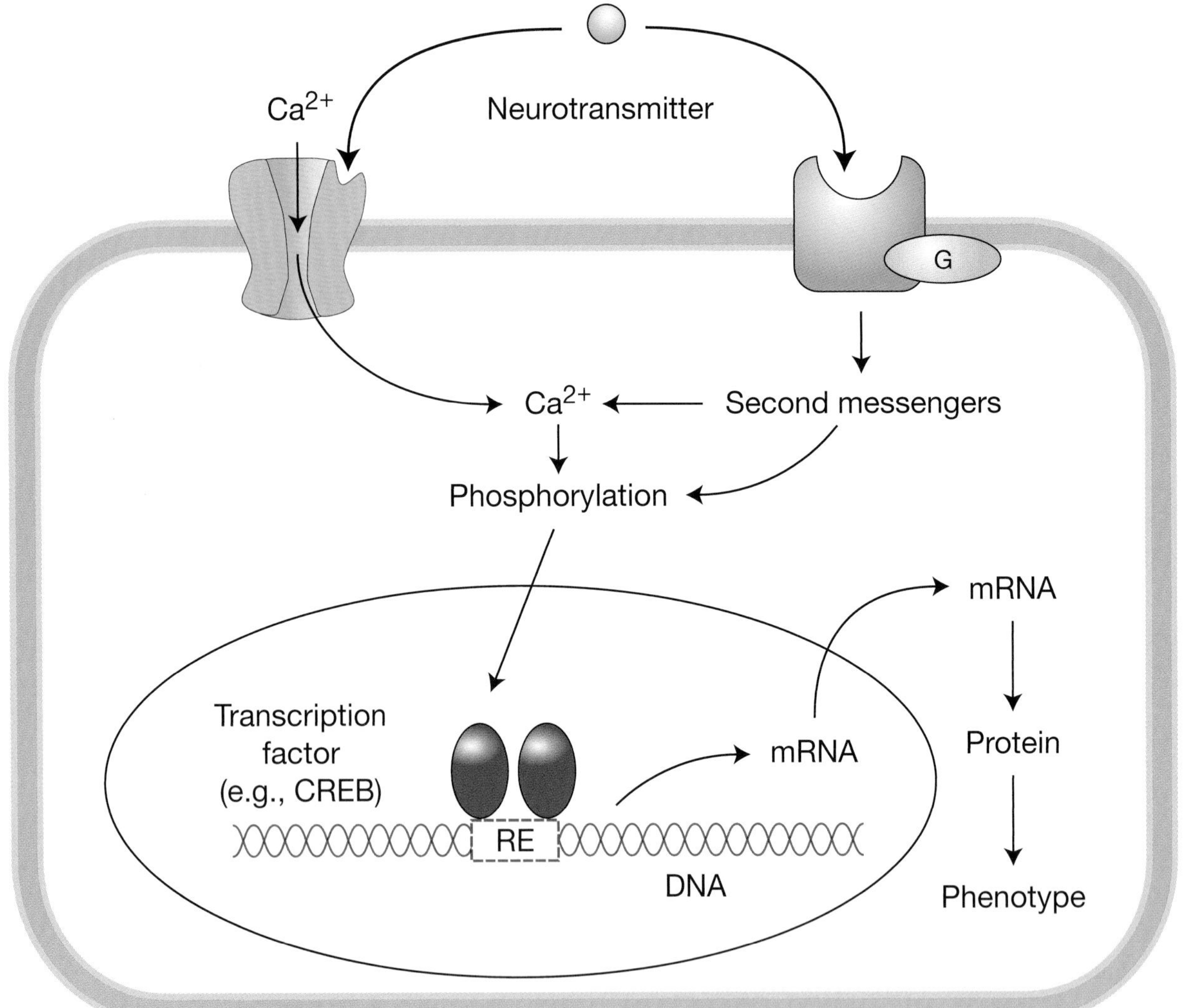

Fig. 6.6. Neurochemical signals may elicit long-term changes in postsynaptic neurons that underlie synaptic plasticity. Activation of ionotropic glutamate receptors and several G protein-coupled receptors leads to an increase in intracellular Ca^{2+}, which together with other second messengers such as cyclic AMP activates several protein kinases that phosphorylate transcription factors, particularly the Ca^{2+} and cyclic adenosine monophosphate (AMP)-responsive element binding protein (CREB). CREB binds to specific sequences (response element [RE]) of the promotor region of the DNA encoding for several target proteins involved in synaptic regulation and activates transcription. Through this mechanism, neurochemical signals acting on membrane receptors may trigger long-term effects in synaptic efficacy and neuronal function. (Modified from Benarroch EE. Basic neurosciences with clinical applications. Philadelphia: Elsevier; 2006. Used with permission of Mayo Foundation for Medical Education and Research.)

- Many neurochemical signals lead to increased intracellular Ca^{2+} and activation of phosphorylation cascades.
- Phosphorylation of transcription factors, particularly CREB, regulates the transcription of several proteins involved in synaptic plasticity.

Specific Neurochemical Systems

The different neurochemical systems vary in distribution, mechanism of action, and function. Amino acids are the most abundant neurotransmitters in the central nervous system and are used for fast neurotransmission in most clinically relevant pathways. Monoamines are less abundant and produce more prolonged effects that are important in modifying neural responses to amino acid neurotransmitters. Neuropeptides are the least abundant, but they are potent and produce responses that have a long latency and long duration.

Organization of Neurochemical Pathways in the Nervous System

The patterns of distribution of neurochemical transmitters in the central nervous system can be organized into three general systems: relay systems, diffuse systems, and local circuits (Fig. 6.7).

Relay Systems

Relay systems include the central pathways of the sensory and motor systems. These pathways generally consist of excitatory projection neurons that use L-glutamate as a neurotransmitter and have myelinated axons that form clearly defined fiber tracts. Relay systems provide fast, precise, point-to-point information along the central nervous system. They mediate both serial and parallel processing of sensory and motor information. This involves transmission of information through several *relay nuclei* or *stations* interconnected by projection neurons. A lesion at any point within a relay system produces a specific neurologic deficit, which allows precise localization of the lesion. An important exception is the relay circuits that interconnect the basal ganglia. The neurotransmitter of these circuits is GABA.

Diffuse Projection Systems

Diffuse projection systems arise from a few neuronal groups that are localized in restricted areas of the brainstem, hypothalamus, or basal forebrain and have axons that arborize extensively within the central nervous system. These neurons use acetylcholine or monoamines (norepinephrine, serotonin, or histamine) as neurotransmitters and modulate the spontaneous activity and excitability of neurons throughout the brain and spinal cord. These diffuse cholinergic and monoaminergic projection systems are part of the consciousness and internal regulation systems. They are involved in global functions such as regulation of the sleep-wake cycle, attention, emotion, and responses to stress as well as visceral, hormonal, sexual, adaptive, and immune functions.

Local Circuit Neurons

The activity of neurons of the relay and diffuse systems is regulated by local neurons, which usually have GABA or neuropeptides as neurotransmitters. Inhibitory neurons in the brainstem and spinal cord also use glycine.

- Relay systems are involved in fast, serial transmission of sensory and motor information.
- Diffuse systems modulate excitability of the central nervous system.
- Local neurons regulate the excitability of neurons of the relay and diffuse systems.

Excitatory Amino Acid Systems

L-Glutamate is the primary neurotransmitter of all excitatory neurons in the central nervous system. This includes all pyramidal neurons of the cerebral cortex and neurons in the relay nuclei of all sensory and motor pathways.

Biosynthesis and Reuptake of L-Glutamate

L-Glutamate is the most abundant amino acid in the brain. It is derived from *α-ketoglutarate*, an intermediate metabolite of the Krebs cycle in neurons, and from *glutamine*, which is synthesized in astrocytes. Through the action of a specific vesicular transporter, L-glutamate

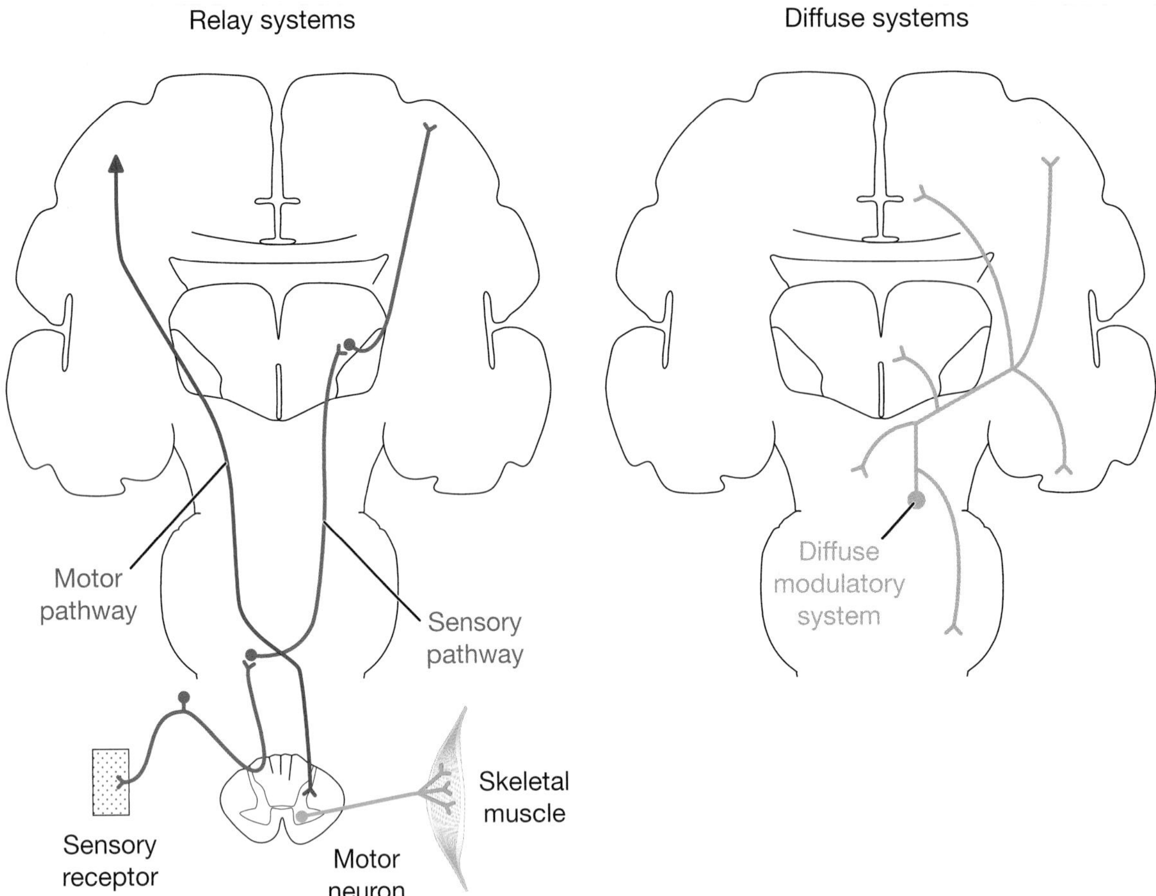

Fig. 6.7. Overview of the organization of neurochemical pathways in the nervous system. Relay systems generally consist of pathways that interconnect relay nuclei containing excitatory projection neurons that use L-glutamate. These pathways are topographically organized and constitute the sensory and the motor systems. In contrast, diffuse systems arise from a restricted group of neurons in the brainstem, hypothalamus, or basal forebrain, use acetylcholine or monoamines, and project to several portions of the central nervous system. These pathways participate in global functions such as arousal, attention, and emotion and are components of the consciousness and internal regulation systems. (Modified from Benarroch EE. Basic neurosciences with clinical applications. Philadelphia: Elsevier; 2006. Used with permission of Mayo Foundation for Medical Education and Research.)

is stored in small clear vesicles and released by exocytosis. The synaptic effects of L-glutamate are terminated by its uptake by the astrocytes via several specific excitatory amino acid transporters.

Glutamate uptake is associated with the uptake of Na^+ and depends on the maintenance of a Na^+ gradient by action of the Na^+,K^+ ATPase. In conditions of energy failure leading to ATP depletion, the Na^+ gradient cannot be maintained and glutamate transport may be decreased or even reversed. This leads to the release of glutamate from astrocytes and excessive accumulation of glutamate in the synaptic space.

Receptor Mechanisms

Glutamate acts through two main families of receptors: ionotropic receptors and metabotropic receptors. Ionotropic glutamate receptors are cation channels that mediate fast excitatory transmission. These include the *AMPA* (α-amino-3-hydroxy-5-methyl-4-isoxazole propionate) receptor, *kainate* receptors, and the *NMDA* (*N*-methyl-D-aspartate) receptor (Fig. 6.4). Metabotropic glutamate receptors are G protein-coupled receptors that are involved in the modulation of excitatory and inhibitory synapses. An important result of the activation of glutamate receptors is increased levels of cytosolic Ca^{2+}.

Most AMPA receptors are permeable only to Na^+ and are present in essentially all excitatory glutamatergic synapses. NMDA receptors are ligand-gated Ca^{2+} channels that are blocked by magnesium (Mg^{2+}) ions at normal resting. The influx of Ca^{2+} through an NMDA receptor requires removal of this Mg^{2+} blockade by membrane depolarization, in general triggered by Na^+ influx via the AMPA receptors. The activation NMDA receptors also requires binding of glycine to an allosteric site of the receptor molecule.

Role of Glutamate in Synaptic Plasticity

In several areas of the central nervous system, the strength of the excitatory connection between presynaptic and postsynaptic neurons exhibits a high degree of *use-dependent plasticity*. Synaptic transmission may be either enhanced or depressed over time, ranging from milliseconds to days or weeks or even longer. The long-term increase in the strength of an excitatory synapse is called *long-term potentiation*, and the converse phenomenon is *long-term depression*. Both long-term potentiation and long-term depression are critical for the establishment and refinement of connections during brain development, for memory functions, and for adaptive changes after injury of the nervous system.

The mechanisms of long-term potentiation and long-term depression vary for different excitatory synapses and may occur at both presynaptic and postsynaptic levels. In most synapses, long-term potentiation and long-term depression involve activation of glutamate receptors, increase in intracellular Ca^{2+}, and activation of protein kinases or phosphatases that affect the state of phosphorylation of AMPA and NMDA receptors, other synaptic proteins, or transcription factors, particularly CREB (Fig. 6.6).

- Glutamate is the primary excitatory neurotransmitter in the central nervous system.
- Glutamate originates from either α-ketoglutarate or astrocyte-derived glutamine.
- The synaptic effects of glutamate are terminated by ATP-dependent uptake by astrocytes.
- Glutamate produces fast excitation through AMPA and NMDA receptors.
- Glutamatergic synapses undergo a use-dependent long-term increase or decrease of efficacy.

Inhibitory Amino Acid Systems

The two main inhibitory amino acid neurotransmitters are GABA and glycine. GABA occurs in local inhibitory neurons throughout the central nervous system, including the cerebral cortex, thalamus, and all sensory and motor relay nuclei. GABA is also the primary neurotransmitter in circuits of the basal ganglia and cerebellum involved in motor control. Glycine mediates inhibitory transmission in the brainstem and spinal cord.

Biosynthesis, Reuptake, and Metabolism of GABA

The synthesis and metabolism of GABA are intimately linked with those of L-glutamate and involve interactions between GABAergic neurons and astrocytes. In GABAergic terminals, GABA is synthesized from L-glutamate by the action of glutamic acid decarboxylase. This enzyme requires pyridoxal phosphate, a derivative of vitamin B_6 (pyridoxine). GABA is incorporated into the synaptic vesicles by a vesicular GABA transporter and released by exocytosis. After release, GABA is taken up by astrocytes and presynaptic GABAergic terminals.

Following reuptake, GABA is metabolized by GABA transaminase to an intermediate that is metabolized through the Krebs cycle to reconstitute α-ketoglutarate, the precursor of glutamate. In GABAergic neurons, glutamate is the source of GABA. In contrast, astrocytes lack glutamic acid decarboxylase and thus cannot reconstitute GABA. Astrocytes contain glutamine synthetase and use glutamate as a substrate for the biosynthesis of glutamine. This is a critical mechanism for ammonia detoxification in the central nervous system.

Receptor Mechanisms

The inhibitory actions of GABA are mediated by two classes of receptor: *$GABA_A$* receptors, which are ligand-gated Cl^- channels, and *$GABA_B$* receptors, which are G protein-coupled receptors. Activation of $GABA_A$ receptors triggers rapid influx of Cl^-, which brings the membrane potential close to the equilibrium potential of that ion (–75 mV). In most neurons, this produces hyperpolarization, but in some cases it may cause depolarization. Activation of $GABA_A$ receptors elicits fast inhibition because the membrane is unable to reach threshold to trigger an action potential.

$GABA_A$ receptors contain several allosteric modulatory sites. One site binds benzodiazepines, which facilitate the $GABA_A$ receptor-mediated inhibitory effects. Benzodiazepines are used to treat various neurologic and psychiatric disorders, including seizures, insomnia, and anxiety. Barbiturates and ethanol also potentiate the inhibitory effect of GABA.

Activation of postsynaptic $GABA_B$ receptors increases the permeability of voltage-gated K^+ channels, which results in slow hyperpolarization and synaptic inhibition. Activation of presynaptic $GABA_B$ receptors inhibits the release of neurotransmitter.

In the brainstem and spinal cord, glycine contributes to fast inhibitory postsynaptic transmission by acting on specific glycine receptors that, like $GABA_A$ receptors, allow rapid influx of Cl^-. These inhibitory glycine receptors are blocked by strychnine, a toxin that produces severe hyperexcitability.

Functions of GABAergic Neurons in the Central Nervous System

Local GABAergic inhibitory neurons act as interneurons in feed-forward and feedback circuits in all motor and sensory pathways. The basic microcircuit in these regions is a triad consisting of an excitatory axon that synapses on both an excitatory projection (relay) neuron and a local GABAergic interneuron (Fig. 6.8). In response to the excitatory afferent input, there is monosynaptic excitation of the projection neuron and disynaptic GABAergic inhibition of the same neuron, which restricts the duration of activation. In addition, local GABAergic neurons inhibit other projection neurons that surround the active neuron. This mechanism, called *lateral inhibition*, is important for mechanisms of sensory discrimination and fine motor control. In the cerebral cortex and hippocampus, GABAergic interneurons prevent the propagation of recurrent excitatory influences among pyramidal neurons. Impairment of this inhibitory activity may result in paroxysmal synchronized discharge of populations of cortical pyramidal neurons and cause a seizure. Some GABAergic neurons form interconnected networks in the cerebral cortex, thalamus, and brainstem. These networks are important for the synchronization of activity across widely distributed but functionally related populations of neurons, for example, during sleep. GABA is also the primary neurotransmitter of neurons in the striatum and basal ganglia and of Purkinje cells in the cerebellum. All these neurons are critical in motor control circuits.

- GABA is the main inhibitory neurotransmitter in the central nervous system.
- GABA is synthesized by the action of glutamic acid decarboxylase.
- The inhibitory effects of GABA are mediated by $GABA_A$ and $GABA_B$ receptors.
- The $GABA_A$ receptor is a Cl^- channel that is allosterically activated by benzodiazepines, barbiturates, and ethanol.
- Glycine mediates fast inhibitory transmission in the brainstem and spinal cord.
- GABAergic interneurons are critical for sensory discrimination and fine motor control.
- Cortical GABAergic neurons prevent seizure activity.
- Networks of cortical GABAergic neurons allow synchronization of thalamocortical activity.
- GABA is the neurotransmitter of neurons in the striatum and globus pallidus and of Purkinje cells.

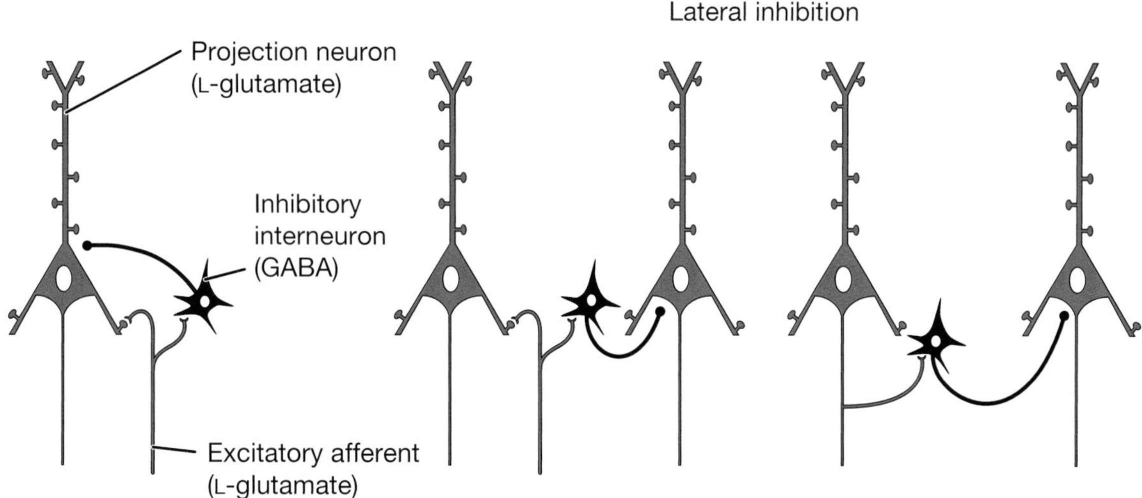

Fig. 6.8. Local circuit neurons (interneurons), using γ-aminobutyric acid (GABA), control the transfer of information at each relay station of the motor and sensory systems and in nuclei of the diffuse systems. In the relay systems, an excitatory afferent not only activates the next-order projection neuron but also a local GABAergic neuron, which then inhibits the projection neuron, thus restricting the duration of excitation. GABAergic neurons mediate lateral inhibition of surrounding projection neurons, thus spatially restricting the relay of the excitatory signal. This is critical for sensory discrimination and fine motor control; it also prevents synchronization of excitatory signals that may lead to seizures.

Cholinergic Systems

Acetylcholine is an important neurotransmitter in both the central and peripheral nervous systems. Cholinergic systems include 1) spinal and brainstem somatic motor neurons innervating skeletal muscle, 2) spinal and brainstem preganglionic neurons innervating autonomic ganglia, 3) parasympathetic ganglion neurons innervating the viscera, 4) neurons in the basal forebrain (*septal area* and *nucleus basalis*) innervating the cerebral cortex, 5) neurons in the tegmentum of the pons and midbrain innervating the thalamus and medulla, and 6) local neurons in the striatum.

Biosynthesis and Metabolism of Acetylcholine

Acetylcholine is synthesized from acetylcoenzyme A and choline by action of choline acetyltransferase. Acetylcholine is incorporated into synaptic vesicles by a specific vesicular transporter and released by exocytosis. The synaptic actions of acetylcholine are rapidly terminated through hydrolysis by acetylcholinesterase. Drugs that inhibit this enzyme (*anticholinesterase agents*) markedly potentiate cholinergic transmission.

Receptor Mechanisms

Acetylcholine acts through two classes of receptors: *nicotinic* and *muscarinic*. Nicotinic receptors are cation channel receptors that allow the influx of Na^+ or Ca^{2+} (or both), producing fast excitatory postsynaptic potentials in the target cells. Muscarinic receptors are G protein-coupled receptors that mediate the slow excitatory (M_1-type receptors) or inhibitory (M_2-type receptors) synaptic effects of acetylcholine.

Functions of Acetylcholine

Acetylcholine mediates important synaptic effects in the peripheral and central nervous systems. It is released at the synapse between the motor neuron and skeletal muscle (neuromuscular junction) and acts through muscle-type nicotinic receptors to elicit muscle depolarization that leads to muscle contraction (*neuromuscular transmission*). Preganglionic neurons in the brainstem and spinal cord release acetylcholine in the autonomic ganglia, where acetylcholine acts on ganglion-type nicotinic receptors to activate sympathetic and parasympathetic postganglionic neurons. Acetylcholine is the neurotransmitter of parasympathetic ganglia neurons innervating all visceral organs and sympathetic ganglia neurons innervating the sweat glands. It acts on different subtypes of muscarinic receptors to control the function of exocrine glands, visceral smooth muscle, and the heart.

In the central nervous system, acetylcholine has a major role in the mechanisms of arousal, attention, and memory. It is a critical neurotransmitter of neurons of the consciousness system. Most of the central effects of acetylcholine are mediated by muscarinic receptors. However, activation of presynaptic nicotinic receptors regulates the release of many neurotransmitters. Cholinergic neurons in the tegmentum of the pons and midbrain project to the thalamus and other regions of the brainstem and are critical for arousal and regulation of the sleep-wake cycle. Cholinergic input to the cerebral cortex arises from neurons in the basal forebrain and is important in mechanisms of attention and memory. These effects are mediated by muscarinic M_1 receptors, which increase the responses of cortical neurons to excitatory inputs containing glutamate, thus facilitating long-term potentiation.

- Acetylcholine is synthesized by choline acetyltransferase and hydrolyzed by acetylcholinesterase.
- Acetylcholine acts through nicotinic and muscarinic receptors.
- Nicotinic receptors mediate fast postsynaptic or presynaptic excitation.
- Different subtypes of muscarinic receptors differentially affect neuronal excitability.
- Acetylcholine is the neurotransmitter at the neuromuscular junction, in autonomic ganglia, and in parasympathetically innervated target organs.
- Basal forebrain cholinergic projections to the cerebral cortex facilitate attention and memory.
- Brainstem cholinergic mechanisms are critical for arousal and the sleep-wake cycle.

Dopaminergic Systems

Dopamine is the neurotransmitter of two main groups of neurons in the central nervous system. The mesencephalic dopaminergic group includes the *substantia nigra pars compacta* and the *ventral tegmental area*. The substantia nigra pars compacta innervates the striatum, and the ventral tegmental area innervates the frontal lobes and limbic system. The hypothalamic dopaminergic group controls the function of the anterior pituitary.

Biosynthesis, Reuptake, and Metabolism of Dopamine

Similar to other catecholamines, dopamine is synthesized from the amino acid L-tyrosine by the action of tyrosine hydroxylase. This is the rate-limiting step in the biosynthesis of all catecholamines and results in the production of L-dihydroxyphenylalanine (*L-dopa*). L-Dopa is metabolized by L-amino acid decarboxylase to dopamine. Dopamine is incorporated into synaptic vesicles by a *vesicular monoamine transporter* coupled to the proton ATPase and released by exocytosis. The synaptic effects of dopamine are terminated by its reuptake by a *dopamine transporter* located in the presynaptic dopaminergic terminal. Once inside the terminal, dopamine is metabolized by monoamine oxidase B to its final metabolite, homovanillic acid.

Receptor Mechanisms

Dopamine receptors are G protein-coupled receptors and can be subdivided into two main subfamilies: D_1 and D_2. D_1-type receptors activate adenylate cyclase and trigger cAMP-dependent phosphorylation of different types of ion channels and other proteins. D_2-type receptors inhibit adenylate cyclase, activate K^+ channels, inhibit Ca^{2+} channels, and mediate the postsynaptic and presynaptic inhibitory effects of dopamine.

Functions of Dopamine in the Central Nervous System

Dopamine is critical for motor control. It has a major role in the initiation of voluntary motor behavior triggered by a novel or rewarding stimulus. Dopaminergic inputs from the substantia nigra pars compacta and ventral tegmental area to the striatum provide a reward signal to the basal ganglia that initiates a specific motor act at the expense of all other motor acts. Dopaminergic input from the ventral tegmental area to the frontal lobe is important for attention to novel stimuli. Dopamine is also important for endocrine function. For example, hypothalamic dopaminergic influence on the anterior pituitary tonically inhibits the secretion of prolactin. Dopaminergic neurons in the medulla are involved in the mechanism of vomiting.

- Dopamine is the neurotransmitter of neurons of the substantia nigra and ventral tegmental area of the midbrain; these dopaminergic neurons project to the striatum, limbic system, and frontal lobe.
- Dopamine is synthesized from L-tyrosine by tyrosine hydroxylase.
- Dopamine undergoes presynaptic reuptake by a dopamine transporter and is metabolized by monoamine oxidase.
- Dopamine acts through D_1- and D_2-type receptors.
- Dopaminergic inputs to the striatum provide a reward signal to initiate a specific motor act.
- Dopaminergic input to the frontal cortex is important for attention to novel stimuli.

Noradrenergic, Serotonergic, and Histaminergic Systems

Norepinephrine, serotonin, and histamine are the neurotransmitters of diffuse projection systems in the brain. Diffuse projection systems consist of neurons located in restricted regions of the brainstem or hypothalamus and whose axons provide collaterals to widespread regions of the central nervous system. The main source of noradrenergic innervation in the central nervous system is the *locus ceruleus*, located in the dorsal portion of the pons. Neurons in this nucleus project to the cerebral cortex, basal ganglia, thalamus, cerebellum, and sensory and motor nuclei. The *lateral tegmental system* consists of neurons containing norepinephrine or epinephrine that are located mainly in the reticular formation of the ventrolateral medulla and innervate the hypothalamus and autonomic nuclei of the brainstem and spinal cord. In the periphery, norepinephrine is the neurotransmitter of sympathetic ganglion neurons that innervate all effector organs except sweat glands.

Serotonin (5-hydroxytryptamine [5-HT]) is the neurotransmitter of neurons in the *raphe nuclei*, which are located in the midline along the length of the brainstem. Rostral and caudal groups of raphe nuclei send ascending or descending projections diffusely throughout the central nervous system. The histamine-containing neurons are located in the *tuberomammillary nucleus* of the hypothalamus, and their axons innervate all areas of the central nervous system.

Biosynthesis, Reuptake, and Metabolism of Norepinephrine, Serotonin, and Histamine

Norepinephrine is synthesized from L-tyrosine by action of tyrosine hydroxylase, and this leads to the formation of L-dopa, followed by decarboxylation by L-amino acid decarboxylase to dopamine. In noradrenergic neurons, dopamine is transformed into norepinephrine by the action of dopamine β-hydroxylase, present in the synaptic vesicle. In some neurons in the lateral tegmental system, and adrenal medulla, norepinephrine is transformed into epinephrine by the action of phenylalanine N-methyltransferase. Serotonin is synthesized from L-tryptophan by the action of tryptophan hydroxylase, followed by decarboxylation by L-amino acid decarboxylase. Histamine is synthesized from histidine by the action of histidine decarboxylase.

Norepinephrine, serotonin, and histamine are incorporated into synaptic vesicles by a vesicular monoamine transporter. After release, norepinephrine undergoes presynaptic reuptake by the *norepinephrine transporter*, and serotonin, by the *serotonin transporter*. In contrast, histamine does not appear to undergo reuptake. Norepinephrine, serotonin, and histamine are metabolized by monoamine oxidases and methyltransferases. The metabolite of norepinephrine in the central nervous system is 3-methoxy-4-hydroxyphenylglycol, the metabolite of serotonin is 5-hydroxyindoleacetic acid, and the metabolite of histamine is methylimidazoleacetic acid.

Receptor Mechanisms

The synaptic effects of norepinephrine, serotonin, and histamine are complex and mediated by different types of receptors. Norepinephrine acts on α_1, α_2, and β receptors (including β_1 and β_2 receptor subtypes). Serotonin acts on many receptors, including 5-HT_1, 5-HT_2, 5-HT_3, and 5-HT_4 receptors. Histamine acts through H_1, H_2, and H_3 receptors. Except for 5-HT_3 receptors, which are ligand-gated cation channels, all monoaminergic receptors are G protein-coupled receptors that have complex postsynaptic and presynaptic effects.

In general, activation of α_1-adrenergic, 5-HT_2-serotonergic, and H_1-histaminergic receptors increases neuronal excitability; α_2-adrenergic, 5-HT_1-serotonergic, and H_3-histaminergic receptors elicit postsynaptic and presynaptic inhibition; and β-adrenergic, 5-HT_4-serotonergic, and H_2-histaminergic receptors activate adenylyl cyclase and several cAMP-dependent phosphorylation cascades.

Functions of the Diffuse Monoaminergic Systems

Through widespread projections and complex receptor mechanisms, the central norepinephrine, serotonin, and histamine systems as well as the acetylcholine and dopamine systems modulate the activity of neuronal groups distributed throughout the brain and spinal cord (Fig. 6.9). These systems are involved in the mechanisms of arousal, attention, and response to stress, including control of autonomic and hypothalamic functions, pain suppression, and motor responses. The activity of the monoaminergic systems depends on the behavioral state of the organism. For example, all these systems are active during wakefulness and inactive during sleep. The noradrenergic neurons in the locus ceruleus are specifically activated in response to novel, potentially challenging environmental stimuli. In the periphery, norepinephrine is released from sympathetic terminals

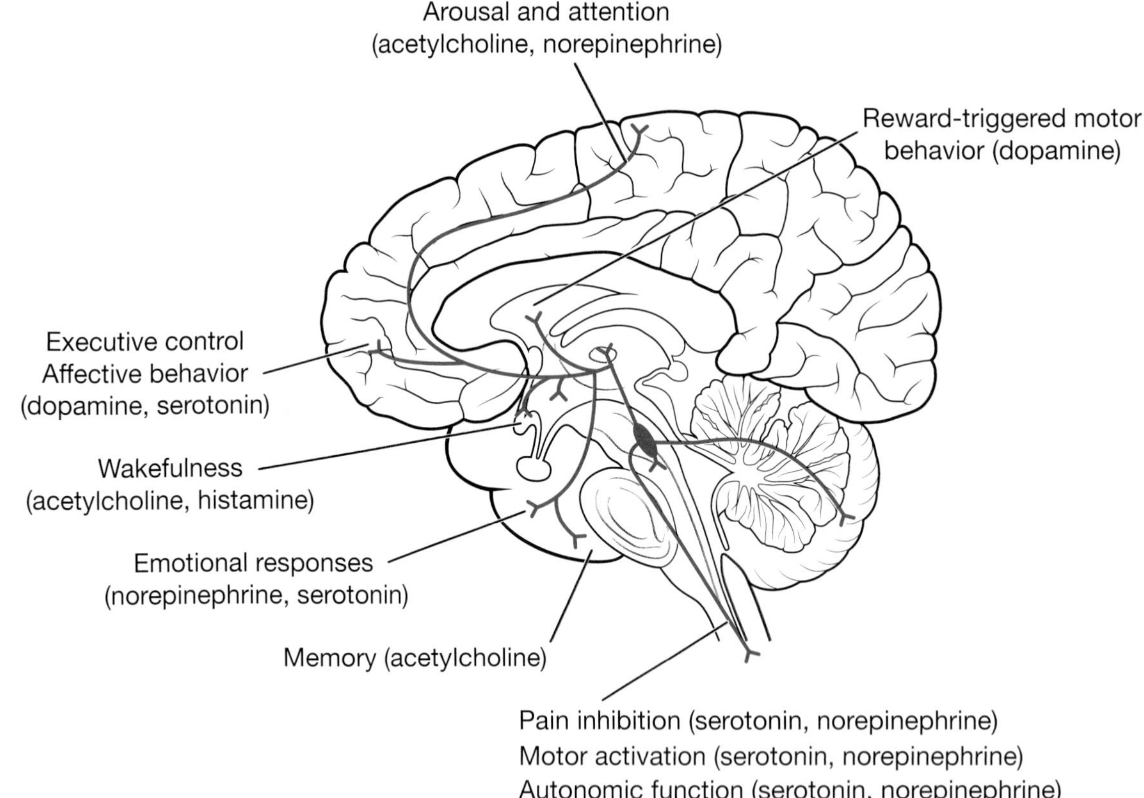

Fig. 6.9. General functions of the diffuse cholinergic and monoaminergic systems. Through widespread projections, these systems affect multiple functions. Acetylcholine is important for memory, arousal, and attention; dopamine for reward-triggered motor behavior; norepinephrine for attention and responses to novel, challenging stimuli; and serotonin and norepinephrine for control of emotion and affect. Both acetylcholine and monoamines control the sleep-wake cycle. For example, histamine is critical for maintaining wakefulness. Norepinephrine and serotonin modulate pain sensation as well as motor and autonomic functions. (Modified from Benarroch EE. Basic neurosciences with clinical applications. Philadelphia: Elsevier; 2006. Used with permission of Mayo Foundation for Medical Education and Research.)

and elicits numerous effects, including vasoconstriction (via α_1 receptors), stimulation of the heart (by β_1 receptors), and relaxation of visceral smooth muscle (by β_2 receptors).

- Norepinephrine is the neurotransmitter of neurons in the locus ceruleus, lateral tegmental system, and sympathetic ganglia.
- Norepinephrine is synthesized by the action of tyrosine hydroxylase and dopamine β-hydroxylase.
- Serotonin is the neurotransmitter of the raphe nuclei.
- Serotonin is synthesized by the action of tryptophan hydroxylase.
- Histamine is the neurotransmitter of neurons in the tuberomammillary nucleus.
- Histamine is synthesized by histidine decarboxylase and does not undergo presynaptic reuptake.
- Norepinephrine and serotonin, but not histamine, undergo presynaptic reuptake.
- Norepinephrine, serotonin, and histamine exert complex synaptic actions through different G protein-coupled receptor subtypes; 5-HT_3 receptors are cation channels.
- The diffusely projecting monoaminergic systems are involved in arousal, attention to environmental stimuli, and responses to stress.
- In the periphery, norepinephrine is the primary neurotransmitter of sympathetic neurons innervating the heart, blood vessels, and visceral organs.

Neuropeptide Systems

Neuropeptides are abundant in the central and peripheral nervous systems. In the central nervous system, the highest concentration is in the hypothalamus, followed by the amygdala, autonomic nuclei, and the pain-modulating circuits of the brainstem and spinal cord. Thus, neuropeptides are important neurochemical transmitters in the consciousness and internal regulation systems. Important examples of neuropeptides include *corticotropin-releasing hormone* (CRH), *arginine vasopressin* (AVP), *substance P*, *calcitonin gene-related peptide* (CGRP), *vasoactive intestinal polypeptide* (VIP), *neuropeptide Y* (NPY), *opioid* peptides (including enkephalins, endorphins, and dynorphins), and *hypocretins* (also called *orexins*).

Central peptidergic neurons are organized into two main systems: 1) diffuse projection systems arising from the hypothalamus, amygdala, and brainstem, and 2) local or short projection neurons located throughout the central nervous system. Neuropeptides frequently coexist with other neurotransmitters, including other neuropeptides, acetylcholine, monoamines, or GABA.

Biosynthesis, Release, and Processing

Neuropeptides form several families, and members of each family have common gene precursors, structural homologies, and functional similarities. Unlike other neurotransmitters, neuropeptides are not synthesized in nerve terminals but in the cell bodies from messenger RNA. They undergo posttranslational modification within the endoplasmic reticulum and Golgi apparatus and are transported in large vesicles to the synaptic terminal by fast anterograde axonal transport. The release of neuropeptides is not restricted to presynaptic active zones but occurs at voltage-gated Ca^{2+} channels distributed throughout the presynaptic terminal. In neurons that contain both monoamines and neuropeptides, continuous low-frequency firing releases the monoamine and high-frequency burst firing releases the neuropeptide. Neuropeptides do not undergo presynaptic reuptake. Their action is terminated by hydrolysis by extracellular *peptidases*.

Receptor Mechanisms

Neuropeptides act mainly as synaptic modulators and have potent presynaptic and postsynaptic effects of slow onset and long duration. These effects are mediated by G protein-coupled receptors. For example, CRH, VIP, and CGRP activate adenylyl cyclase; substance P and hypocretins inhibit K^+ channels and increase neuronal excitability; and opioids activate K^+ channels, reducing neuronal excitability, and inhibit presynaptic Ca^{2+} channels, reducing neurotransmitter release. These prolonged modulatory effects occur not only at postsynaptic sites but also in a paracrine fashion by volume transmission. Neuropeptides may act at a distance from the site of release and thus affect neighboring neurons, glial cells, and blood vessels. Some hypothalamic neuropeptides are released into the bloodstream (neuroendocrine effect). Neuropeptides have not only neuromodulatory but also trophic and vasomotor effects. For example, VIP, CGRP, and substance P produce vasodilatation, and AVP and NPY cause vasoconstriction.

Functions of Neuropeptides

Neuropeptides exert a potent effect on endocrine, autonomic, sensory, motor, and behavioral functions, in many cases by interacting with other neurotransmitter systems. Many neuropeptides are critical for specific homeostatic functions. For example, CRH is critical for responses to stress, AVP for fluid homeostasis, opioid peptides for central pain control mechanisms, and hypocretin for control of the sleep cycle and food intake. Substance P and CGRP are neurotransmitters in nociceptive afferents; NPY participates in sympathetic neurotransmission and VIP in parasympathetic neurotransmission.

- Neuropeptides are most abundant in the hypothalamus and amygdala and in autonomic and pain circuits.
- Neuropeptides are synthesized in the cell body from messenger RNA and are transported to the synaptic terminal by fast anterograde axonal transport.
- Neuropeptides exert potent and prolonged modulatory influences through G protein-coupled receptors and may act by both synaptic and volume conduction mechanisms.
- Neuropeptides are critical for the control of homeostasis, including responses to stress and the sleep-wake cycle, food intake, autonomic functions, and pain mechanisms.

Other Neurochemical Messengers

Purines

The purines, ATP and *adenosine*, may act both as neurotransmitters and neuromodulators in the central and peripheral nervous systems. ATP acts through P_2-purinoreceptors and has important functions in the nociceptive and autonomic systems. ATP is also important in communication between astrocytes. Adenosine acts through P_1 (or adenosine) receptors. Activation of adenosine receptors inhibits the presynaptic release of other neurotransmitters and produces vasodilatation.

Nitric Oxide

Nitric oxide is an important intercellular messenger synthesized from arginine by nitric oxide synthase. Constitutive forms of the enzyme are present in neurons and endothelial cells and are activated by an increase in intracellular Ca^{2+} in response to activation of glutamate and other neurotransmitter receptors. The inducible form is present in macrophages and mononuclear cells and is activated during inflammation. Nitric oxide rapidly crosses membranes and reacts with the iron contained in the heme molecule and in several key enzymes, including those in the mitochondrial respiratory chain. Nitric oxide is an important synaptic modulator in the central and autonomic nervous systems and is a potent vasodilator.

- ATP and adenosine act as neurochemical transmitters.
- Nitric oxide is synthesized from arginine by nitric oxide synthase.
- Nitric oxide regulates neuronal excitability and promotes vasodilatation.

Clinical Correlations

The neurochemical systems are involved in the pathophysiology of various neurologic and psychiatric disorders and are the target for pharmacologic treatment of these conditions. Although a discussion of this topic is beyond the aims of this chapter, important examples are mentioned below (Table 6.6).

Neurologic Disorders

Excitotoxicity and Neuronal Injury

Excessive activation of glutamate receptors can kill neurons and oligodendrocytes; this is referred to as *excitotoxicity*. Rapid glutamate-induced excitotoxicity is responsible for neuronal death in conditions such as cerebral hypoxia or ischemia, hypoglycemia, epilepsy, and traumatic injury of the brain or spinal cord. Slow excitotoxic injury leading to oxidative stress and

Table 6.6. Examples of Involvement of Neurochemical Systems in Neurologic and Psychiatric Disorders

Neurotransmitter	Disorder (examples)
Glutamate	Cell death in hypoxia-ischemia, hypoglycemia, seizures, head trauma Neurodegenerative disease
GABA	Seizures
Acetylcholine	Alzheimer disease Myasthenia gravis
Dopamine	Parkinson disease Schizophrenia Drug addition
Norepinephrine, serotonin	Anxiety Depression

GABA, γ-aminobutyric acid.

apoptosis has been implicated in the mechanisms of cell death in many neurodegenerative diseases, including Alzheimer disease and amyotrophic lateral sclerosis. Cells become more vulnerable to acute excitotoxic injury during energy deprivation because this impairs their ability to pump out excess Na^+ and Ca^{2+} entering through AMPA and NMDA receptors and prevents the uptake of glutamate by astrocytes. Rapid glutamate-induced cell death, as in energy failure, involves a massive influx of Na^+ and Cl^- and cell swelling, followed by massive influx of Ca^{2+}.

Calcium activates several potentially damaging cascades, involving phospholipase A_2, calpain, and nitric oxide. Many of these pathways lead to oxidative stress and disrupt plasma and mitochondrial membranes and the cytoskeleton, which produces cell death by necrosis. In addition, glutamate-induced injury may follow a slow pathway, involving a mechanism of apoptosis, triggered by the release of cytochrome *c* and other proapoptotic molecules from Ca^{2+}-loaded mitochondria.

Clinical Problem 6.1.

A 55-year-old man had a cardiorespiratory arrest. After resuscitation, he remained comatose, with impaired pupil and corneal reflexes. The electroencephalogram showed persistent slowing, indicative of hypoxic neuronal injury.

a. Where is the lesion?
b. What central neurochemical system is most likely to cause this type of neuronal injury?
c. What are the general mechanisms of injury?
d. Name possible pharmacologic approaches for neural protection in this and similar cases.

Seizures

Impaired GABAergic inhibition in the cerebral cortex may lead to a paroxysmal and synchronized discharge of populations of pyramidal neurons and result in seizures. Many drugs used to treat seizures act either by increasing the availability of GABA or by facilitating $GABA_A$ receptor-mediated mechanisms that increase Cl^- permeability. Other drugs act by blocking Na^+ or

Clinical Problem 6.2.

A 44-year-old bartender with a history of alcohol abuse had been taking "sleeping pills" to control his anxiety and insomnia. Because of a flulike illness, with vomiting and diarrhea, he abruptly discontinued taking the medication and drinking alcohol, and 2 days later he had a generalized tonic-clonic seizure.

a. What is the location of the disorder?
b. What neurochemical system mediates the depressing effects of alcohol and sedative agents?
c. What mechanism is involved that explains the patient's symptoms?
d. What drug may help control the disorder?

Ca^{2+} channels in pyramidal neurons or by inhibiting the release of glutamate. Chronic exposure to depressant drugs that facilitate $GABA_A$ receptor mechanisms, such as alcohol, benzodiazepines, or barbiturates, desensitizes the receptor. Therefore, abrupt cessation of these drugs causes rebound hyperexcitability of the central nervous system, leading to a withdrawal syndrome, including anxiety, insomnia, tremor, and seizures, that may be life-threatening.

Dementia and Delirium

The most common cause of dementia is *Alzheimer disease*, a degenerative disorder of the brain. An important feature of this disease is the loss of cholinergic neurons in the basal forebrain that innervate the cerebral cortex. Impairment of cholinergic input may contribute to memory loss in this disease. The central cholinergic system is also severely affected in patients with *dementia with Lewy bodies*. Drugs that inhibit acetylcholinesterase (anticholinesterase agents) increase the availability of acetylcholine in the cerebral cortex and produce some improvement in cognitive function in these two disorders. In contrast, many drugs, including some used to treat neurologic and psychiatric disorders, may block central muscarinic receptors. This may impair alertness, attention, and perception, referred to as *confusional state* or *delirium*, particularly in elderly persons.

Clinical Problem 6.3.

A 65-year-old man with a 1-year history of progressive memory loss was given a drug for treatment of depression and sleep disturbance. After the dose of medication was increased, there was relatively rapid onset of disorientation, agitated behavior, and visual hallucinations. Dry hot skin, dry mouth, tachycardia, and pupil dilatation were noted on physical examination.

a. Involvement of what area of the brain most likely explains the progressive memory loss?
b. What type of lesion accounts for the memory loss?
c. Impairment of what neurochemical system is most likely responsible for the development of the patient's symptoms?
d. What treatment may help improve memory function in this condition?

Parkinson Disease

Parkinson disease is a neurodegenerative disorder characterized by the loss of dopaminergic neurons in the substantia nigra pars compacta. Decreased dopaminergic activity in the striatum results in reduced spontaneous motor activity, or akinesia, rigidity, and other manifestations of the disease. Similar effects are produced by the intake of drugs that block dopamine receptors.

> Akinesia and other manifestations of Parkinson disease may also result from the loss of dopaminergic neurons after exposure to toxins or from blockade of dopaminergic receptors in the striatum by drugs used to treat psychosis or vomiting. Antiparkinsonian drugs include L-dopa (a precursor of dopamine) in combination with carbidopa (an inhibitor of peripheral decarboxylation of L-dopa) and direct dopamine receptor agonists.

Disorders of Neuromuscular Transmission

Impaired neurotransmission at the level of the neuromuscular junction produces a use-dependent muscle weakness that improves with rest. Presynaptic disorders include the *Lambert-Eaton myasthenic syndrome*, which is due to autoantibodies against voltage-gated Ca^{2+} channels in the active zones of the motor nerve terminal. The most important postsynaptic disorder is *myasthenia gravis*, which is due to autoantibodies against muscle nicotinic acetylcholine receptors.

Psychiatric Disorders

Schizophrenia

Schizophrenia is a brain disorder that affects cognition and behavior. The cognitive, emotional, and motivational manifestations of schizophrenia resemble those that occur with damage to the frontal lobe, whereas the perceptual disorders, including hallucinations,

Clinical Problem 6.4.

A 55-year-old woman in a psychiatric ward received a drug treatment for her bizarre behavior and auditory hallucinations. After the treatment was initiated, she had decreased facial expression and an absence of arm swing while walking.

a. Involvement of what level of the brain explains the underlying psychiatric disorder?
b. Impairment of what neurochemical system is the most likely cause of the motor symptoms?
c. What is the most common neurodegenerative disorder characterized by these manifestations?
d. What is the anatomical substrate of this disorder?

may in part reflect dysfunction of the temporal lobe. These areas receive abundant dopaminergic and serotonergic innervation. Drugs used to treat this disorder act on the dopaminergic and serotonergic systems.

Classic antipsychotic drugs block the D_2-receptors and control the hallucinations in schizophrenia. Because they also potently block these receptors in the striatum, they commonly cause motor side effects. Newer antipsychotic drugs block both D_2 and 5-HT_2 serotonergic receptors.

Drug Addiction

Dopaminergic inputs from the ventral tegmental area to the limbic striatum and frontal cortex have a major role in mechanisms of reward and reinforcement associated with drug addiction. An increase in dopamine levels in the striatum is considered the critical mechanism for the reinforcing and addictive effects of cocaine, amphetamine, and nicotine and an important component of opioid and alcohol abuse.

Cocaine and amphetamine increase dopamine levels by interfering with the function of the presynaptic dopamine transporter, thus reducing dopamine reuptake. Nicotine acts through presynaptic cholinergic nicotinic receptors to increase the release of dopamine. Opiates inhibit GABAergic neurons in the ventral tegmental area, thus disinhibiting the dopaminergic neurons.

Anxiety and Depression

Abnormal function of central noradrenergic and serotonergic circuits has been implicated in disorders of arousal, attention, and affect, including anxiety and depression. Excessive activity of locus ceruleus noradrenergic neurons has been implicated in the manifestations of anxiety disorders, including panic disorder and posttraumatic stress disorder. Several drugs that reduce firing of the locus ceruleus neurons have antianxiety effects. Serotonin is thought to have a major role in depression and in manic-depressive (bipolar) and obsessive-compulsive disorders.

Antianxiety drugs include benzodiazepines, which act through $GABA_A$-receptor mechanisms, drugs that activate presynaptic α_2 inhibitory autoreceptors; drugs that increase norepinephrine levels and thus lead to activation of inhibitory autoreceptors and down-regulation of β-receptors; and selective serotonin reuptake inhibitors that inhibit locus ceruleus neurons by increasing levels of serotonin. Antidepressant drugs include drugs that decrease the presynaptic reuptake of monoamines, including selective serotonin reuptake inhibitors, norepinephrine reuptake inhibitors, 5-HT_2 receptor blockers, and monoamine oxidase inhibitors.

- Glutamate-induced excitotoxicity results in cell death in acute chronic neurologic diseases.
- Impaired GABAergic mechanisms may result in seizures.
- Decreased cholinergic input to the cerebral cortex produces memory loss and confusional state.
- Decreased dopaminergic innervation of the striatum produces parkinsonism.
- Dopaminergic circuits in the striatum and frontal lobe mediate reinforcing effects of addictive drugs.
- The central norepinephrine and serotonin systems are involved in anxiety and depression.

Additional Reading

Benarroch EE. Basic neurosciences with clinical applications. Philadelphia: Elsevier; 2006. (Chapter 8, pp 213-240; Chapter 10, pp 275-300; Chapter 11, pp 301-318; Chapter 23, pp 807-866.)

Hyman SE, Malenka RC. Addiction and the brain: the neurobiology of compulsion and its persistence. Nat Rev Neurosci. 2001;2:695-703.

Lipton P. Ischemic cell death in brain neurons. Physiol Rev. 1999;79:1431-1568.

Malenka RC, Nicoll RA. Long-term potentiation: a decade of progress? Science. 1999;285:1870-1874.

PART II

Longitudinal Systems

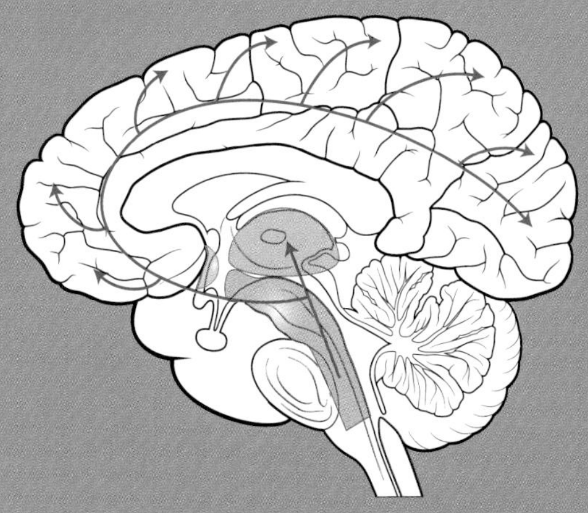

Chapter 7

The Sensory System

Objectives

1. Define receptor, sensory unit, and receptive field.
2. Define receptor potential, frequency and population coding, receptor adaptation, and receptor specificity.
3. Define in physiologic terms the differences between rapidly adapting (phasic) and slowly adapting (tonic) receptors.
4. List the types of somatic receptors.
5. Describe the main features of wide dynamic range neurons in the dorsal horn.
6. Describe the two main types of primary nociceptive units.
7. Name the main components of the central pain regulation system.
8. Name the function of the following pathways and trace their paths:
   a. Direct dorsal column–lemniscal tract
   b. Direct spinothalamic (neospinothalamic) tract
   c. Indirect spinothalamic (paleospinothalamic) tract
   d. Dorsal spinocerebellar tract
   e. Ventral spinocerebellar tract
9. Describe the clinical manifestations of lesions involving the five pathways listed in objective 8, and list the differences that may be encountered when the lesion is located at the peripheral, spinal, posterior fossa, or supratentorial level.
10. Describe sacral sparing, cortical sensory loss, and Brown-Sequard syndrome, and describe the anatomical basis of these conditions.
11. Describe the mechanisms of sensory dissociation in syringomyelia and in selective lesions of large compared with small dorsal root ganglion neurons and fibers.
12. Distinguish between sensory and motor ataxia.
13. Given a patient problem, list the aspects of the history and physical examination that point to a disturbance in the sensory system, localize the area of disturbance to a particular portion of the neuraxis, and state the pathologic nature of the lesion responsible.

Introduction

The function of the sensory system is to provide information to the central nervous system about the external world, the internal environment, and the position of the body in space. Impulses traveling toward the central nervous system are called *afferent* impulses. Afferent information may be transmitted 1) as conscious data that are perceived by the organism and then used to modify behavior; 2) as unconscious data that, although used to modify behavior, remain unperceived by the organism; and 3) as both conscious and unconscious data. Afferent impulses are functionally subdivided into the following:

1. General somatic afferent—sensory information from skin, striated muscles, and joints
2. General visceral afferent—sensory information, largely unconscious, from serosal and mucosal surfaces, smooth muscle of the viscera, and baroreceptors

3. Special somatic afferent—sensory information relating to vision, audition, and equilibrium
4. Special visceral afferent—sensory information relating to taste and smell

Although introductory comments are made in relation to each of these afferent subdivisions, this chapter is concerned primarily with the organization and function of the general somatic afferent system.

Overview

The translation of information from the environment is the function of the *receptor organs*. The function of these specialized portions of the peripheral nervous system is to convert mechanical, chemical, photic, and other forms of energy into electrical potentials, one of the forms of information used by the nervous system. Action potentials are then transmitted by specific sensory pathways to regions of the central nervous system where the information is integrated and perception occurs. The peripheral region from which a stimulus affects a central sensory neuron is the *receptive field* of that neuron.

The pathways involved in conscious perception have both a hierarchical and a parallel organization. *Hierarchical organization* means that sensory information is transmitted sequentially by several orders of neurons located in relay nuclei and processed at each relay station under the control of higher stations in the pathway. *Parallel organization* implies that different submodalities within tactile, visual, and other sensations are transmitted by separate, parallel channels and a given sensory modality, such as simple touch, is transmitted by different ascending pathways.

Somatosensory pathways from the trunk and extremities course in the spinal cord, and those transmitting information from the face form the trigeminal system. The trigeminal system is discussed further in Chapter 15A.

Somatosensory pathways can be subdivided according to three different functions: 1) transmission of precise information about the type, intensity, and localization of a sensory stimulus; 2) initiation of arousal, affective, and adaptive responses to the stimulus; and 3) continuous unconscious monitoring and control of motor performance.

The first group of pathways is referred to as *direct*, or discriminative, pathways. These pathways are commonly tested clinically because they allow localization of lesions in the nervous system. The two most important direct pathways are the direct *dorsal column pathway*, involved in transmission of tactile-discriminative and conscious proprioceptive information, and the *spinothalamic tract*, involved in transmission of pain and temperature sensation (Table 7.1). These direct pathways consist of three orders of neurons.

The *first-order neurons* are the receptor neurons; they are derivatives of the neural crest. Their cell bodies lie outside the central nervous system in *dorsal root ganglia* of the spinal nerves or in sensory ganglia of cranial nerves, and their axons bifurcate into a peripheral branch and a central branch. The peripheral branch contributes to a sensory nerve and innervates receptor organs. The central branch enters the spinal cord or the brainstem through a dorsal, or sensory, root.

The *second-order neurons* have cell bodies in regions of the embryonic alar plate, that is, in the gray matter of the dorsal horn of the spinal cord or in relay nuclei of the medulla and pons. The axons of these second-order neurons decussate (cross the midline) and continue cephalad. As the axons of first- or second-order neurons ascend in the spinal cord, they are grouped into tracts (fasciculi) located primarily in the white matter (funiculi) of the spinal cord (Fig. 7.1). In the brainstem, the axons of second-order neurons continue to ascend in tracts (in this region, some are referred to as lemnisci) to reach the thalamus, where they terminate in specific sensory nuclei. Along their ascending course, these sensory pathways maintain a somatotopic organization, so that the surface of the body is represented in a topographic manner both in the pathways and in the relay stations.

The *third-order neurons* have cell bodies in the sensory relay nuclei of the thalamus. Somatosensory thalamic neurons are located in the ventral posterior complex of the thalamus, which includes the ventral posterolateral nucleus for sensory input from the trunk and extremities and the ventral posteromedial nucleus for sensory input from the face (the trigeminal system).

Table 7.1. Direct Pathways Commonly Tested Clinically

	Direct dorsal column pathway	Spinothalamic tract
Receptors	Proprioceptors Tactile receptors	High-threshold mechanoreceptors Polymodal nociceptors Tactile and thermoreceptors
First-order neuron	Dorsal root ganglion	Dorsal root ganglion
Second-order neuron	Medulla (dorsal column nucleus)	Dorsal horn
Third-order neuron	Ventral posterolateral nucleus of thalamus	Ventral posterolateral and posterior nuclei of thalamus
Decussation	Medulla	Spinal cord
Localization	Ipsilateral dorsal column	Contralateral anterolateral quadrant
Function	Spatiotemporal discrimination (e.g., stereognosis) Two-point touch, vibration, proprioception	Discriminative pain and temperature Simple touch

Like other relay stations, thalamic relay nuclei have a somatotopic and submodality-specific organization. Axons of somatosensory thalamic neurons project through the thalamocortical radiation to the primary somatosensory cortex of the parietal lobe (Fig. 7.2).

The primary somatosensory cortex is located in the postcentral gyrus of the parietal lobe and is concerned with discriminative aspects of reception and appreciation of somatic sensory impulses. It consists of at least four functionally distinct areas, each containing a complete somatotopic map. Fibers terminate in the postcentral gyrus in an organized fashion, with the lower extremity

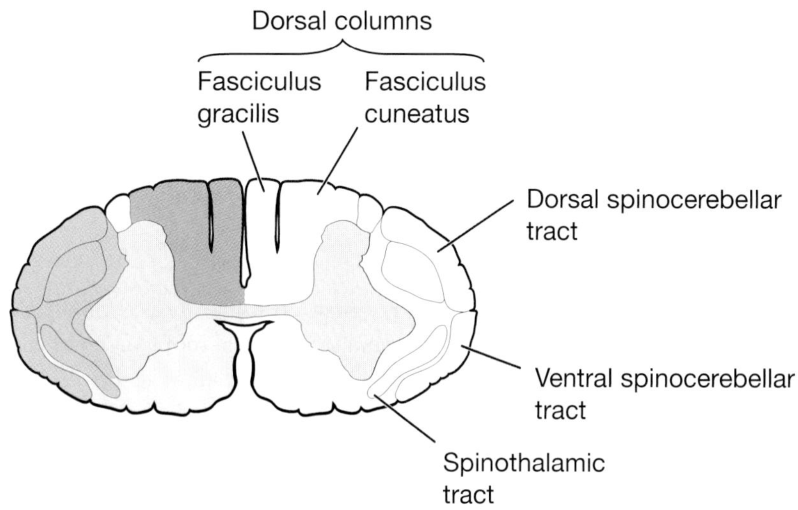

Fig. 7.1. Cross section of upper cervical spinal cord illustrating the location of the major ascending sensory pathways and their relation to the posterior (pink), lateral (blue), and anterior (yellow) funiculi.

represented on the medial surface of the hemisphere and the arm and hand represented on the lateral surface. The face, mouth, and tongue are represented in the suprasylvian region (Fig. 7.3). The cortical representation of pain is not only in the parietal cortex but also in the insular cortex and cingulate gyrus.

An important feature of the somatosensory and other sensory cortices is that the representation of the body map is dynamic, *use-dependent cortical plasticity*. The shape and size of the representation of a particular body part may be modified in response to peripheral injury or training.

A second group of somatosensory pathways, referred

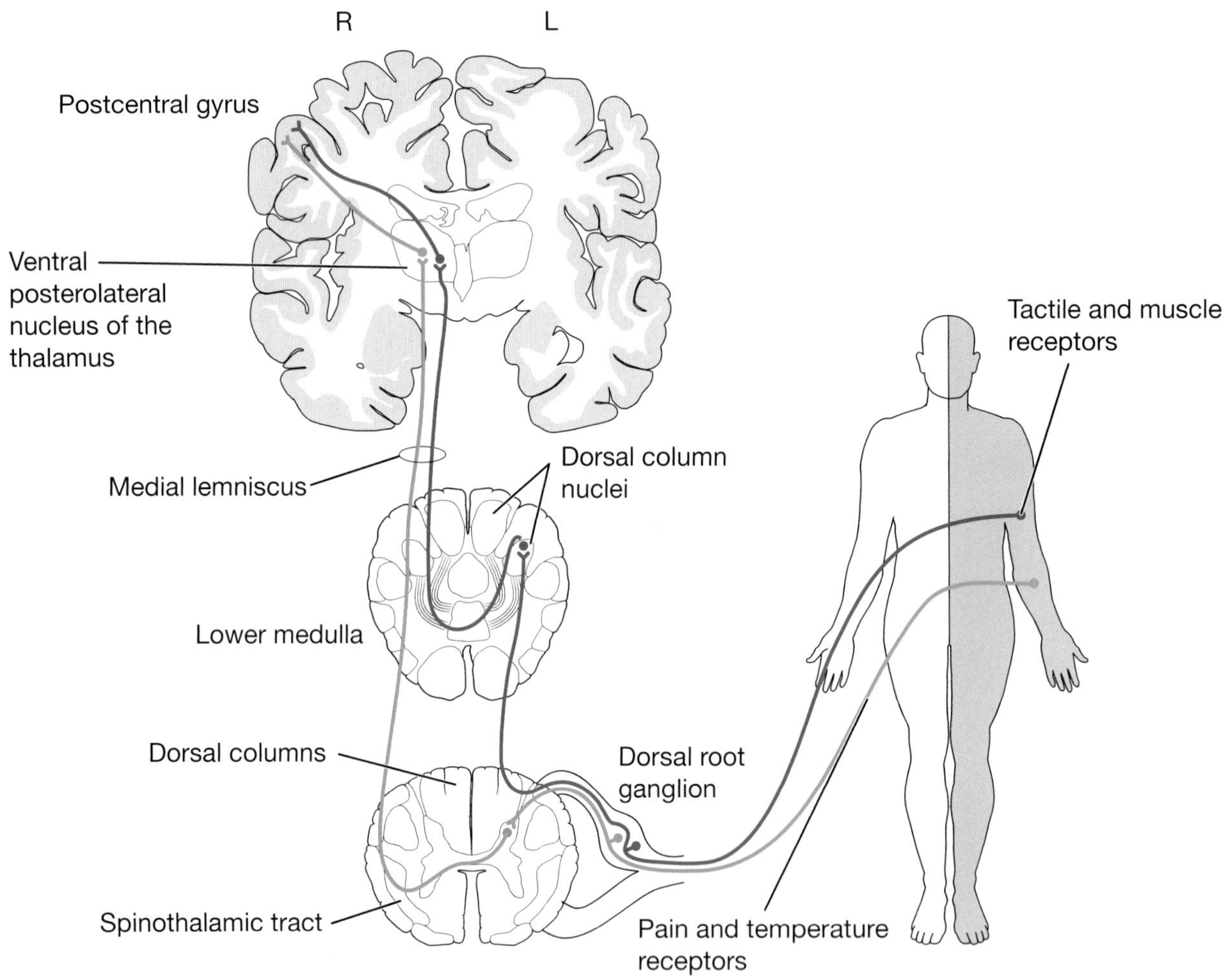

Fig. 7.2. Diagram of the pathway for discriminative touch, vibration, and proprioception (red) and for pain and temperature (green) of the left arm. First-order neurons are large and small dorsal root ganglion neurons. Large-diameter afferents for touch and proprioception ascend ipsilaterally in the left dorsal column at the cervical level (fasciculus cuneatus) and synapse on second-order neurons in the lower medulla (nucleus cuneatus). Axons from second-order neurons decussate and ascend in the right (contralateral) medial lemniscus to synapse in the ventral posterolateral nucleus of the thalamus, which projects to the primary sensory area in the postcentral gyrus. Small-diameter afferents for pain and temperature synapse on second-order neurons in the dorsal horn of the spinal cord. Axons of these second-order neurons decussate in the ventral white commissure and ascend as the spinothalamic tract in the contralateral ventrolateral quadrant. This tract joins the medial lemniscus and terminates in the ventral posterolateral nucleus and other nuclei in the thalamus.

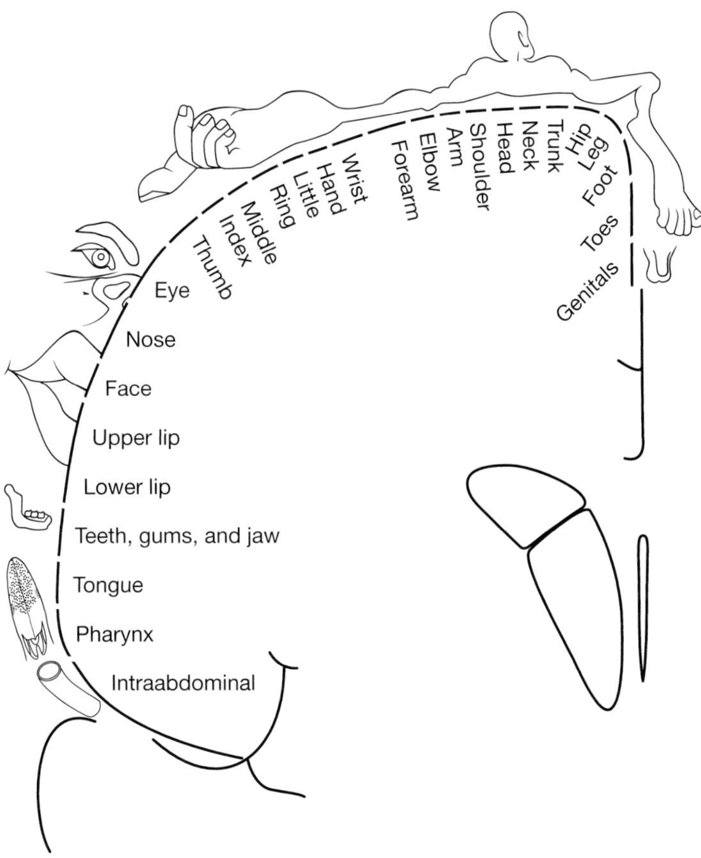

Fig. 7.3. Coronal section of cerebral hemisphere showing the distribution of third-order sensory fibers in the postcentral gyrus (sensory homunculus). (Modified from Penfield W, Rasmussen T. The cerebral cortex of man: a clinical study of localization of function. New York: Macmillan; 1950. Used with permission.)

to as *indirect pathways*, mediate arousal-affective aspects of somatic sensation (particularly pain) and visceral sensation (Table 7.2). Unlike direct pathways, indirect pathways are not helpful in the localization of lesions in the central nervous system because they have poor somatotopy, ascend bilaterally, and terminate diffusely in the reticular formation, intralaminar thalamic nuclei, and other subcortical and cortical regions. Indirect pathways are important for mechanisms of pain and analgesia and for visceral and sexual sensation. They include the *paleospinothalamic*, *spinoreticular*, and *spinomesencephalic tracts* and the *propriospinal multisynaptic system*. Propriospinal neurons interconnect several segments of the spinal cord.

A third group of somatosensory pathways, the *dorsal* and *ventral spinocerebellar tracts*, transmit information for unconscious control of posture and movement. These are two-neuron pathways that do not relay in the thalamus but terminate in the ipsilateral cerebellum.

The direct somatosensory pathways are of major importance in understanding and interpreting neurologic disease. Lesions at different levels of the neuraxis alter sensory function in different ways; by correlating the patient's signs and symptoms with the anatomical distribution of these pathways, neurologic disorders can be localized. Abnormalities in the peripheral nerves or spinal roots are distributed in a segmental fashion, often involve all sensory modalities, and may be associated with the sensation of pain. Lesions involving the spinal cord may be associated with segmental sensory loss at the level of the lesion and varied sensory loss at all levels below the

Table 7.2. Comparison of Direct and Indirect Somatosensory Pathways

Feature	Direct (lemniscal)	Indirect (extralemniscal)
Location in the neuraxis	Outer tube	Inner tube (core)
Number of synapses in the central nervous system	2 or 3	Multiple
Receptive fields	Small	Large
Body representation	Contralateral	Bilateral
Somatotopy	Yes	No
Thalamic station	Ventral posterior complex	Midline nuclei
Cortical station	Parietal cortex	Cingulate gyrus
Function	Discriminative	Affective-arousal
Pathways	Dorsal column pathways, spinothalamic pathway, dorsolateral quadrant pathways	Spinoreticulothalamic, spinoreticular, propriospinal pathways

lesion. Lesions in the posterior fossa produce contralateral sensory loss over the trunk and extremities and may be associated with ipsilateral sensory disturbance in the face at the level of the pons and medulla. Supratentorial lesions produce entirely contralateral sensory deficits. Because each somatosensory pathway subserves different functions, loss of a particular sensory modality with preservation of others allows the anatomical localization of lesions in the nervous system. Lesions of the direct dorsal column pathway affect tactile discrimination, whereas lesions of the spinothalamic system predominantly affect pain and temperature sensation. Because of overlap, or redundancy, of parallel somatosensory pathways, some somatosensory modalities, particularly touch, can still be perceived in cases of interruption of an individual pathway.

Other sensory pathways, such as the visual pathway, are also important for localization in clinical neurology. Similar to the somatosensory pathways, the visual pathway has a topographic organization (called *retinotopy*), a hierarchical organization (with synaptic relays in the thalamus and primary visual cortex), and parallel organization (with submodality-specific channels transmitting information about object movement or shape and color).

Receptors: General Organization and Mechanisms

Sensory receptors are highly specialized structures that respond to environmental changes by producing action potentials that are transmitted to the central nervous system. This process is called *transduction*. There are many types of receptors subserving different sensory functions.

Receptor Specificity

Generally, each receptor type is specialized in that it is more sensitive (i.e., has the lowest threshold) to one particular kind of stimulus. Receptors can be classified according to their sensory modality as *mechanoreceptors*, *chemoreceptors*, *thermoreceptors*, and *photoreceptors* (Table 7.3). Receptors also can be classified according to the origin of the stimulus as *exteroceptors* (skin mechanoreceptors for touch and pain, skin thermoreceptors, labyrinthine mechanoreceptors for hearing, retinal photoreceptors, and chemoreceptors for taste and smell), *proprioceptors* (mechanoreceptors in muscles, tendons, and joints and vestibular mechanoreceptors), and *visceral receptors* (mechanoreceptors and chemoreceptors encoding signals related to internal body functions).

Impulse Initiation in Sensory Receptors

Although the mechanism by which receptor potentials are produced varies with the receptor organ, certain principles of receptor physiology are common to all of them. The process starts with the application of a specific stimulus, that is, the stimulus for which the receptor has the lowest threshold. The minimal intensity of stimulus necessary to produce excitation in the appropriate class of first-order neuron is called *threshold*.

The major steps in sensory processing are transduction, receptor potential generation, electrotonic spread, and impulse generation. In most cases, transduction of sensory stimuli occurs in a specialized site in the membrane of the receptor cell and leads to gating of an ion current in the membrane channel.

Somatic receptors, including skin and muscle receptors and hair cells of the inner ear, contain mechanically sensitive cation channels that open in response to deformations of the cell membrane. Transduction in photoreceptors, odor receptors, and some taste receptors involves cyclic nucleotide-gated channels that constitute a large gene family of related proteins which are either nonselective cation or selective K^+ channels. Some are particularly permeable to Ca^{2+}.

In all sensory receptors, the common result of transduction is the production of a change in conductance of a membrane ion channel. This change constitutes the receptor potential, also called the generator potential. In most receptors, the receptor potential is depolarizing, either by the opening of a Na^+ or Ca^{2+} channel or the closing of a K^+ channel. In photoreceptors, however, the receptor potential is hyperpolarizing, because light causes a cyclic nucleotide-gated cation channel to close.

Receptor potentials affect the primary sensory neuron either directly or indirectly, according to the type of receptor. Skin and muscle mechanoreceptors are innervated by the axon of the first neuron of the sensory pathway. The exceptions are nociceptors and thermoreceptors, that consist of free nerve endings. Olfactory receptors constitute the first neuron of the olfactory pathway. In contrast, photoreceptors, hair cells, and taste receptors are specialized cells that tonically release an excitatory transmitter, L-glutamate, which maintains a basal level of activity in the first-order neuron. In

Table 7.3. Classification and Comparison of Receptor Types

Receptor type	Receptor	Modality
Mechanoreceptors		
Somatosensory system	Low-threshold mechanoreceptors	Light touch, vibration
	Muscle spindles	Proprioception
	Tendon organs	Proprioception
	Free nerve endings	Pain, temperature
Vestibular system	Hair cells	Head position and motion
Auditory system	Hair cells	Audition
Internal regulation system	Free nerve endings	Visceral distention, pain
Chemoreceptors		
Taste system	Taste buds	Taste
Olfactory system	Olfactory receptor cells	Olfaction
Internal regulation system	Visceral chemoreceptors	Pain
Photoreceptors	Rods and cones	Vision

response to the specific stimulus, the receptor cell may generate a depolarizing receptor potential, which results in increased release of glutamate and, thus, increased activity in the primary afferent. The exception is photoreceptors, which are depolarized at rest and undergo transient hyperpolarization in response to light; this produces a transient decrease in the tonic release of glutamate.

Like synaptic potentials, receptor potentials do not give rise directly to an impulse discharge; frequently, the site where receptor potentials are generated is separate from the site where impulses are generated. In somatosensory receptors, receptor potentials and impulses are generated on axons. In other systems, the sites are on different cells, requiring synaptic relay (e.g., vision, hearing, and taste). The spread of receptor potentials, like that of synaptic potentials, is accomplished by means of electrotonic potentials.

Encoding of Sensory Information

The final step is the encoding of the electrotonically transmitted receptor impulse into an impulse discharge in the primary afferent that conducts the information to the central nervous system. The receptor potential is graded smoothly and continuously in relation to the intensity of the stimuli. Sensory reception involves the transformation of this graded response into a pattern of *all-or-none* impulses. The frequency of discharges varies continuously in relation to the underlying level of depolarization of the receptor potential and its rate of change.

Cell ensembles are needed to encode spatial and temporal information about the stimulus that cannot be encoded by a single cell. Stimulus location is encoded by the firing of a specific population of neurons located at particular points in each relay nucleus. Stimulus intensity is encoded in the somatosensory system through both the frequency of firing of specific neuronal populations (*frequency coding*, or temporal summation) and the size of the active population (*population coding*, or spatial summation).

Receptor Adaptation

Receptor adaptation is a function of the intrinsic properties of the receptor. It is the mechanism by which the amplitude of the generator potential, and thus the firing of action potentials, progressively decreases in response to a continuous stimulus (Fig. 7.4). Receptors can be subdivided into *rapidly adapting*, or *phasic*, and *slowly adapting*, or *tonic*, receptors. They transmit different types of information to the central nervous system. Rapidly adapting receptors detect transient and rapidly changing stimuli. They fire a few impulses on application of a sustained stimulus but are silent during its steady continuation; they may discharge again when the stimulus is removed. The number of action potentials initiated in their axon is related to the rate of change of the stimulus. Rapidly adapting receptors serve to alert the nervous system to any change in the environment and are particularly suitable for spatiotemporal discrimination. Slowly adapting receptors respond to a sustained stimulus with fairly sustained firing. The time course and peak frequency of discharge of rapidly adapting receptors may reflect the final intensity as well as the rate of application of the stimulus. Slowly adapting receptors keep the nervous system constantly apprised of the status of the body and of its relation with its surroundings.

The transient abolition of the excitability of a sensory receptor in response to repetitive stimulation is *receptor fatigue*. Repetitive stimuli produce generator potentials with successively smaller amplitude to the point that the receptor no longer responds either to the stimulus or to a change in the stimulus.

Functional Organization of the Sensory Pathways

Serial and Parallel Processing of Sensory Input

After the stimulus is transformed into a frequency code, it is transmitted to the central nervous system by a primary afferent neuron. In the central nervous system, sensory information is relayed through a series of relay centers, and at each center the signal is processed and integrated with other signals. A sensory pathway is the series of modality-specific neurons connected by synapses.

The pathways of different sensory systems share some characteristics. A pathway consists of connections in series that determine the temporal sequence of events. In addition, sensory circuits are organized in parallel, so that

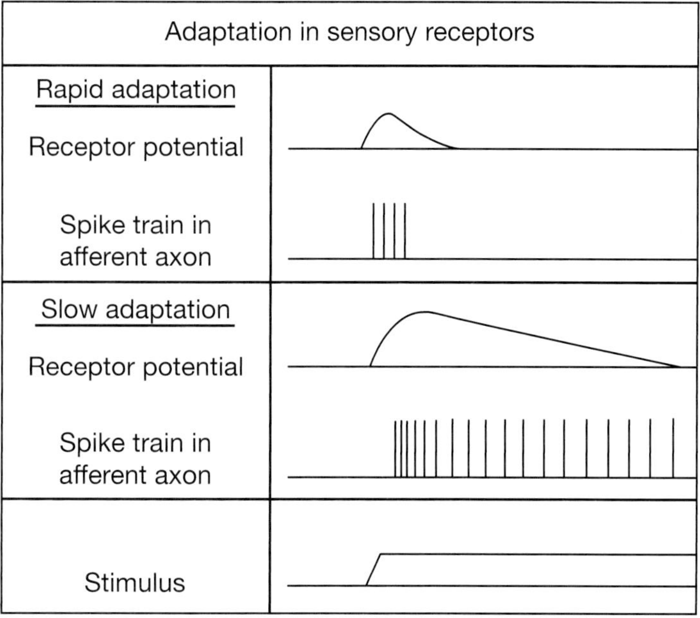

Fig. 7.4. Rate of adaptation in sensory receptors to a prolonged stimulus. Adaptation of receptor potentials and spike trains in primary afferent axons in rapidly and slowly adapting receptors is shown.

different forms of information are transferred and combined at the same time. The axon of a primary afferent neuron divides and synapses on more than one central neuron (this is called *divergence*), and a single central sensory neuron may be contacted synaptically by more than one axon (this is called *convergence*).

Some central pathways transmit the input from one type of receptor and are referred to as *specific sensory pathways*; they provide for precise transmission of sensory information. Other pathways, through convergence and divergence, become *multimodal*, or nonspecific; they are involved in sensory integration and behavioral adjustments of the organism.

Sensory Unit and Receptive Field

The *receptive field* of a neuron consists of all the sensory receptors that can influence its activity. The connections with a cell may be excitatory (through a projection relay neuron) or inhibitory (through interneurons). Receptive fields are organized topographically. For example, in the somatosensory system, each point of the body surface is topographically represented at each level of the sensory pathway; this is known as *somatotopy*. In the visual system, the visual field of each eye is represented topographically at each relay station, *retinotopy*.

The somatosensory and visual representations of the receptive fields, or maps, are primarily contralateral (contralateral hemibody or contralateral visual field). In the auditory system, the representation is mainly contralateral, but bilateral representation is also prominent. The somatotopic and retinotopic maps are distorted in that the size of the population of central neurons with a particular receptive field is proportional to the density of innervation. Areas of high sensory discrimination (fingertips in the somatosensory system, macula in the visual system) have a large number of receptors per unit area and are innervated by a large number of neurons, each with a small receptive field. The size of a receptive field is not fixed. It may vary in response to denervation and other factors (Fig. 7.5).

Receptive fields have a *center-surround* organization. In the somatosensory system, the discharge of a receptor or central sensory neuron is greatest when the stimulus is applied to the center of the receptive field, and the discharge decreases gradually as the stimulus moves toward

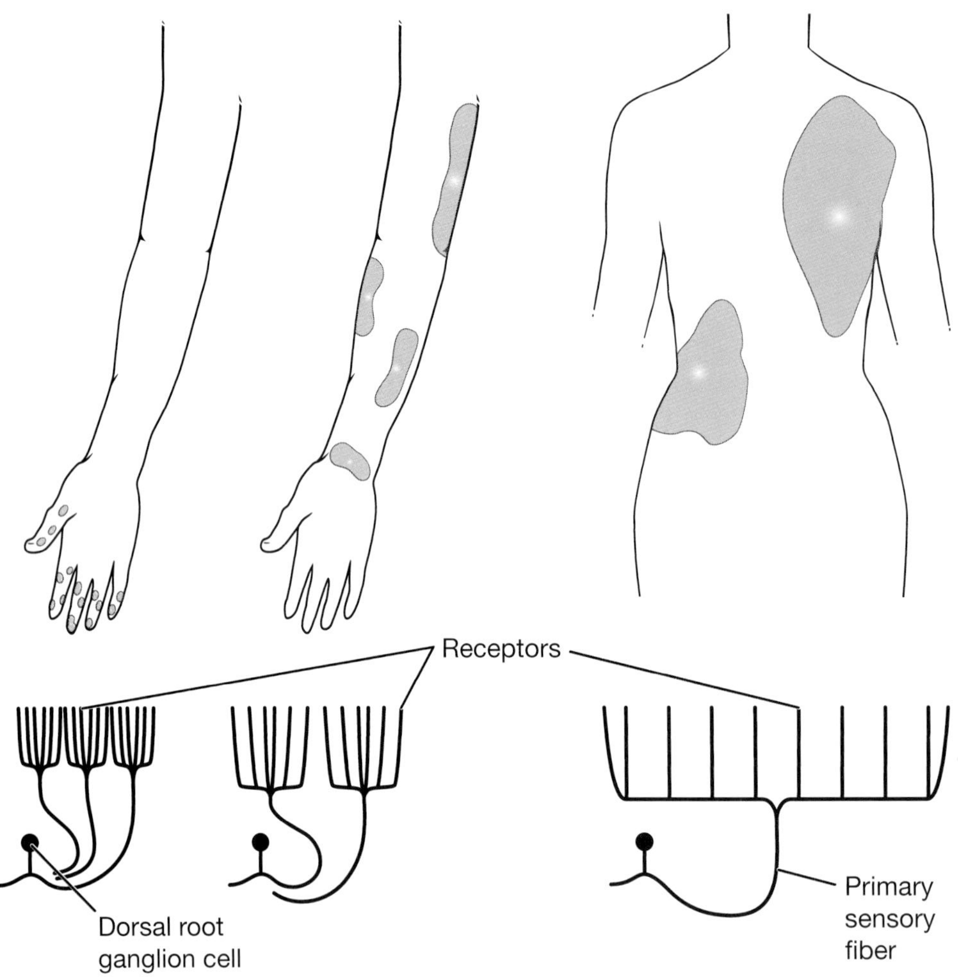

Fig. 7.5. Variation in the size of receptive fields as a function of peripheral innervation density. The greater the density of receptors, the smaller the receptive fields of individual afferent fibers. (Modified from Warren S, Capra NF, Yezierski RP. The somatosensory system I: tactile discrimination and position sense. In: Haines DE, editor. Fundamental neuroscience. 2nd ed. New York: Churchill Livingstone; 2002. pp. 255-272. Used with permission.)

the periphery of the receptive field. Stimulation of the area immediately surrounding the receptive field may inhibit the central neuron. This is the *inhibitory surround.*

The organization of a sensory relay station is characterized by a synaptic arrangement that includes three elements: an afferent fiber, a projection neuron, and local inhibitory interneurons. The afferent axon excites both the projection neuron and inhibitory interneurons. This excitation is thought to be mediated by L-glutamate. The projection neuron (also called a relay neuron) sends its axon to the next relay station. This neuron also has L-glutamate as a neurotransmitter agent.

Thalamic Station

All sensory modalities, except olfaction, relay in specific relay nuclei of the thalamus. The thalamus is not only the relay station for most sensory channels, but it also is important in gating sensory transmission to the cerebral cortex.

Each thalamic relay nucleus contains excitatory neurons that project to a specific area of the cerebral cortex. The activity of these thalamocortical neurons is controlled by interneurons in the relay nucleus.

Primary Sensory Areas of the Cerebral Cortex

Axons from each specific relay nucleus in the thalamus terminate in a specific area of cerebral cortex known as a *primary sensory area*. Each of these areas contains neurons that respond selectively to specific characteristics of stimuli; for example, certain neurons in primary somatosensory cortex respond to texture and certain neurons in primary visual cortex respond to color. Each primary sensory area projects to *association areas* of the cerebral cortex. Neurons in cortical association areas often respond selectively to a specific combination of features. For example, neurons in one association area respond selectively to faces or images of faces. Mature brains retain the capacity to undergo reorganization, which allows dynamic changes in sensory maps in response to peripheral injury or experience. This is referred to as *plasticity* of the cortical sensory field.

- Receptors are specialized structures that respond to environmental changes by producing action potentials and are often classified by sensory modality.
- When the stimulus reaches threshold, the receptor generates a receptor potential.
- Receptor potentials are graded. However, the information of this graded response is transformed into an all-or-none action potential.
- Receptor adaptation is the mechanism by which the amplitude of the generator potential, and thus firing of action potentials, progressively decreases in response to a continuous stimulus.
- A sensory pathway is a series of modality-specific neurons connected by synapses.
- The receptive field of a neuron consists of all sensory receptors that can influence the neuron's activity.
- The thalamus is a relay center for all sensory modalities except olfaction.
- Thalamic relay nuclei project to the primary sensory cortical area corresponding to the sensory modality.

General Organization of the Somatosensory Systems

Somatosensory Receptors

Somatosensory receptors include cutaneous receptors, joint receptors, and muscle receptors (Table 7.4). Cutaneous receptors consist of low-threshold mechanoreceptors, which are innervated by large myelinated fibers and transmit touch sensation, and high-threshold mechanoreceptors, chemoreceptors, and thermoreceptors, which are innervated by small myelinated or

Table 7.4. Receptors of the Somatosensory System

Receptor	Innervation	Function
Encapsulated superficial skin receptors (Meissner corpuscles, Merkel disks)	Large myelinated fibers	Detection of edges, texture
Paccinian corpuscle	Large myelinated fibers	Vibration
Muscle spindles	Large myelinated fibers	Muscle length (proprioception)
Golgi tendon organs	Large myelinated fibers	Muscle tension (proprioception)
Free endings in skin, muscles, and joints	Small myelinated or unmyelinated fibers	Pain
Free endings in skin (thermoreceptors)	Small myelinated or unmyelinated fibers	Cold or warmth

unmyelinated fibers and mediate pain and temperature sensation. Joint and muscle receptors are innervated mainly by large, rapidly conducting myelinated fibers. Muscle receptors include muscle spindles, which signal muscle length and rate of change in length, Golgi tendon organs, which respond to changes in muscle tension, and free nerve endings, which respond to muscle pressure and pain.

Dorsal Root Ganglion Neurons

Information from somatic receptors is transmitted to the spinal cord by first-order neurons. The cell bodies of these neurons are located in the *dorsal root ganglia* (spinal ganglia). Each of these neurons has a single nerve process that divides into two branches. The distal, or peripheral, branch corresponds to the sensory afferent that innervates the receptor, and the proximal, or central, branch enters the spinal cord through the dorsal root. The area of the skin innervated by a single dorsal root is called a *dermatome* (Fig. 7.6). Dermatomes are arranged in a highly ordered way on the body surface. The sensory field of each dorsal root is continuous and tends to form a strip perpendicular to the spinal cord. Each spinal nerve receives afferents from several peripheral nerves; therefore, the area innervated by an individual dorsal root is less well defined than the area innervated by a single peripheral nerve (Fig. 7.7). Furthermore, the areas innervated by different dorsal roots overlap considerably. Whereas damage of a peripheral cutaneous nerve produces a circumscribed area of sensory loss in the skin, damage to the spinal nerve or dorsal root often results in only a moderate sensory deficit.

The two main types of neurons in a dorsal root ganglion are *large neurons*, with large myelinated axons that innervate low-threshold mechanoreceptors (touch) and proprioceptors, and *small neurons*, with small myelinated or unmyelinated axons that innervate nociceptors, thermoreceptors, and visceral receptors (Table 7.5). This subdivision is relevant clinically because diseases that selectively affect large sensory fibers or large dorsal root ganglion neurons produce severe loss of all tactile modalities and proprioception but spare pain and temperature sensations. Diseases of small sensory fibers or small dorsal root ganglion neurons affect pain and temperature but spare touch and proprioceptive sensations.

Dorsal Root Entry Zone and Termination in the Spinal Cord

Primary afferent fibers from the dorsal root ganglion cells enter the spinal cord mainly in the posterolateral sulcus at the *dorsal root entry zone*. In this zone, the larger and most heavily myelinated proprioceptive and tactile fibers are located medially (medial division), and the finely myelinated and unmyelinated fibers mediating pain and temperature sensations are located laterally (lateral division) (Fig. 7.8). From this common entry zone, the dorsal root fibers branch to ascend and descend in the white matter and to arborize in the gray matter. The pathways for the different sensory modalities diverge as they ascend in the spinal cord to higher centers.

The medially located large myelinated fibers bifurcate into branches that may 1) ascend directly in the ipsilateral dorsal columns, without synapsing in the spinal cord, as the *direct dorsal column pathway*; 2) synapse on dorsal horn neurons that in turn contribute axons to the dorsal column (the *postsynaptic dorsal column pathway*), dorsolateral funiculus, and spinothalamic tract; 3) synapse in the intermediate gray matter on neurons that give rise to the spinocerebellar tract; 4) synapse on interneurons and motor neurons in the ventral horn for segmental, or myotatic, reflexes; and 5) synapse in the dorsal horn on interneurons that provide segmental modulation of pain transmission.

The laterally located small myelinated and unmyelinated fibers bifurcate into ascending and descending branches that run longitudinally in *Lissauer tract*, part of the dorsolateral funiculus (Fig. 7.8). Within several segments, these axons leave Lissauer tract to enter the dorsal horn and the intermediate gray matter of the spinal cord. In the gray matter, they may 1) synapse on different groups of dorsal horn and intermediate gray matter neurons that form the spinothalamic and other tracts ascending in the contralateral ventrolateral quadrant, 2) synapse on dorsal horn interneurons involved in segmental modulation of pain and in intrinsic (propriospinal) intersegmental pathways, and 3) synapse on interneurons and activate somatic and preganglionic autonomic motor neurons to initiate segmental visceral and somatic reflexes.

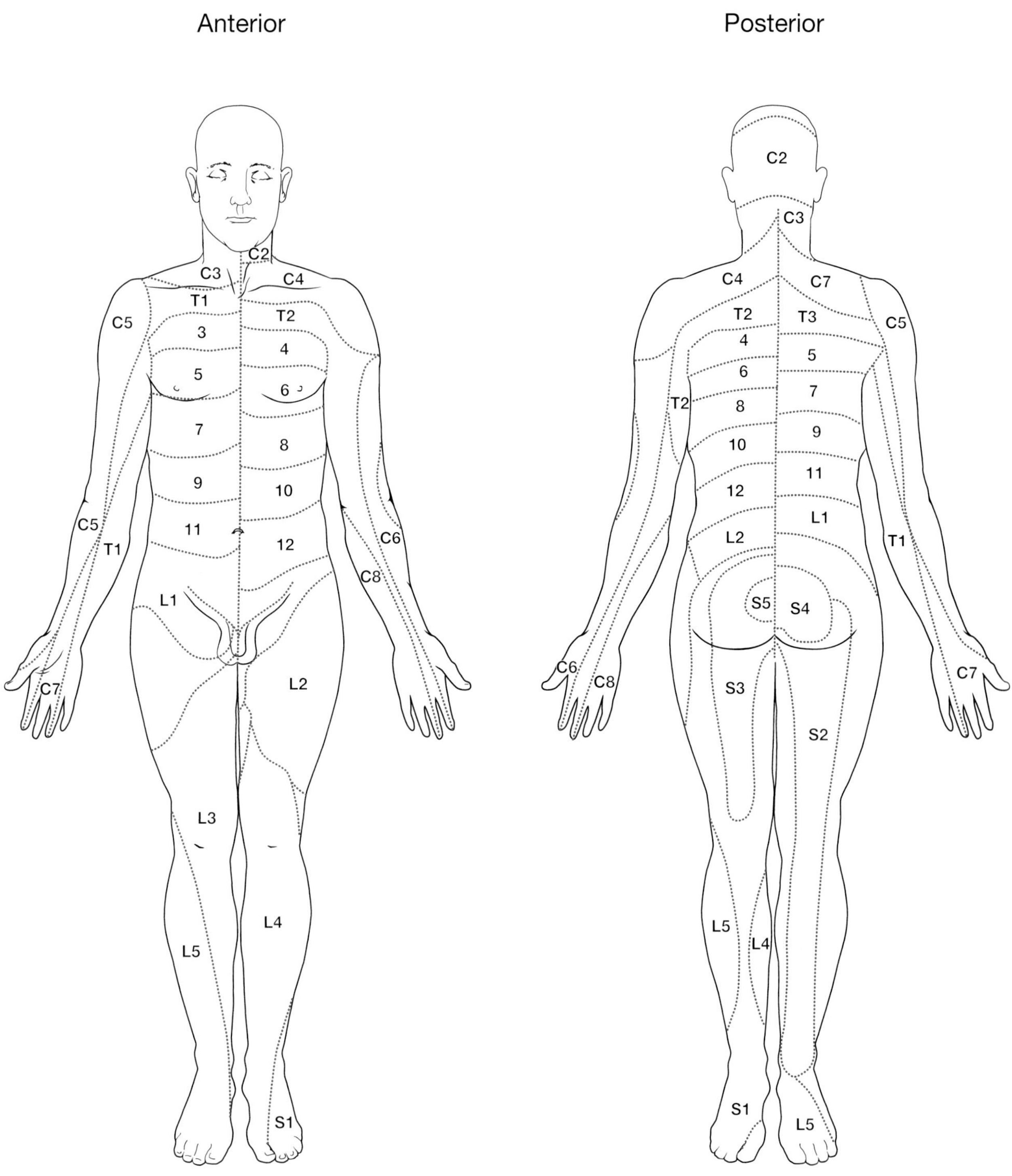

Fig. 7.6. Cutaneous, or dermatomal, distribution of spinal nerve roots. Note that the overlap between segments is considerable and the distribution differs from that of peripheral nerves.

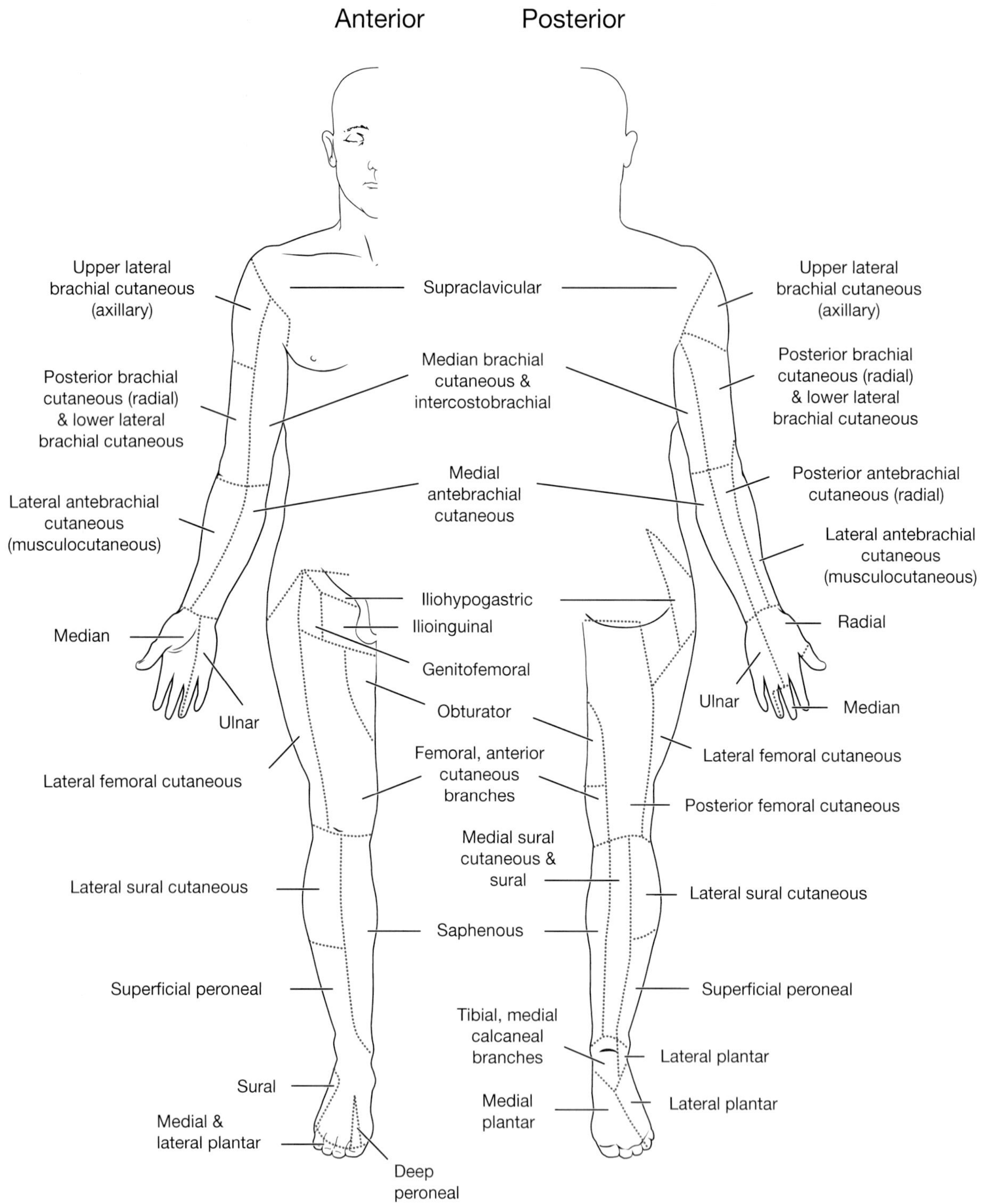

Fig. 7.7. Cutaneous distribution of the major peripheral nerves.

Table 7.5. Comparison of Large Neurons and Small Neurons in Dorsal Root Ganglia

	Type	
Feature	**Large**	**Small**
Sensory function	Touch Vibration Joint position Proprioception	Pain Temperature Visceral sensation
Axon	Large myelinated	Small myelinated Unmyelinated
Receptor	Low-threshold mechanoreceptors Muscle and joint proprioceptors	High-threshold mechanoreceptors Polymodal nociceptors Chemoreceptors Thermoreceptors
Conduction of stimuli	Orthodromic	Orthodromic and antidromic (axon reflex)
Neurotransmitter	L-Glutamate	L-Glutamate and neuropeptides (e.g., substance P)

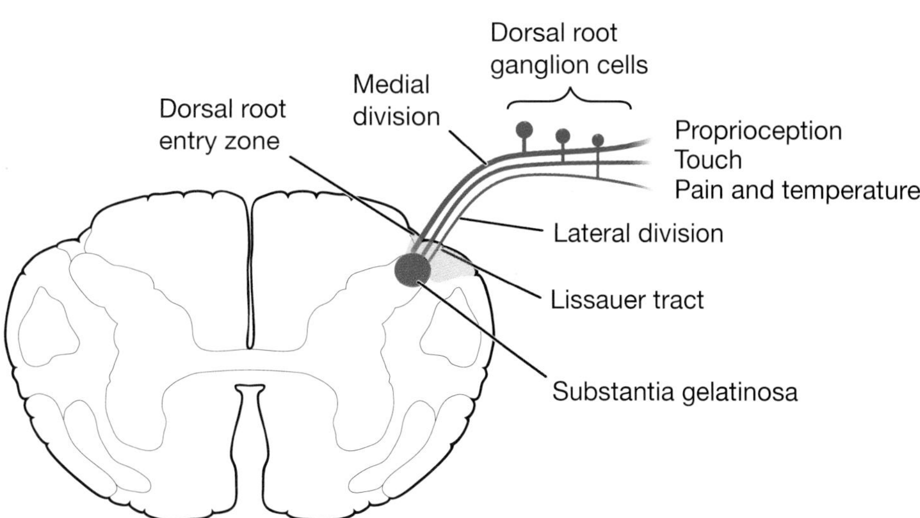

Fig. 7.8. Dorsal root entry zone. The largest, most heavily myelinated fibers mediating proprioception occupy the medial division. Medium-sized myelinated fibers mediating touch are located centrally, and finely myelinated fibers carrying pain and temperature sensation occupy the lateral division.

Spinal Somatosensory Neurons

Second-order spinal somatosensory neurons occupy the dorsal horn and intermediate gray matter of the spinal cord. These neurons contribute to all somatosensory pathways except the direct dorsal column pathway. Spinal neurons, similar to other central somatosensory neurons, can be subdivided into several types on the basis of their response characteristics: nociceptive-specific neurons, low-threshold mechanoreceptive neurons, and wide dynamic range neurons (Table 7.6). Wide dynamic range neurons are the most abundant and contribute to all ascending pathways that relay in the spinal cord. An important feature is that the response characteristics of an individual type of neuron may change according to segmental and suprasegmental control mechanisms. This is relevant for mechanisms of central pain.

Somatosensory Pathways

From the standpoint of anatomical organization, somatosensory pathways can be subdivided into three groups. The *direct*, or *lemniscal*, pathways are contralateral, somatotopically organized pathways that synapse in the ventral posterior complex of the thalamus, which in turn sends axons to primary sensory cortex. These pathways are involved in sensory discrimination and are useful clinically for localizing central lesions. They are in the outer tube of the neuraxis and include the following: 1) pathways for tactile discrimination and conscious proprioception: the *direct dorsal column–lemniscal pathway* and parallel pathways in the dorsal column and dorsolateral quadrant; and 2) pathways for discriminative aspects of pain and temperature sensation: the *direct spinothalamic*, or *neospinothalamic*, *tract*. Note that simple touch and spatial discrimination are transmitted by the dorsal column, the neospinothalamic tract, and other parallel pathways. Therefore, abnormalities of simple touch are less helpful than other sensory modalities in localizing lesions in the central nervous system.

The *indirect pathways* have poor somatotopy, ascend bilaterally, have multiple interconnections with the reticular formation and other subcortical regions, relay in midline thalamic nuclei, and affect limbic and paralimbic cortical areas. The indirect pathways are not helpful for localization, but they are important for the transmission of affective-arousal components of pain and visceral sensation and for the initiation of reflex somatic, autonomic, and hormonal responses to external stimuli. These pathways are part of the inner tube of the neuraxis and include the following: 1) the *paleospinothalamic*, *spinoreticular*, and *spinomesencephalic tracts*, which ascend

Table 7.6. Functional Classification of Dorsal Horn Neurons

Type of neuron	Primary afferent input	Pathway	Function
Nociceptive-specific	Small myelinated Unmyelinated	Spinothalamic Spinoreticular Spinomesencephalic	Pain
Low-threshold mechanoreceptive	Large myelinated	Postsynaptic dorsal column Spinothalamic Dorsolateral funiculus	Touch Proprioception
Wide dynamic range	Large myelinated Small myelinated Unmyelinated	Spinothalamic Spinoreticular Spinomesencephalic Postsynaptic dorsal column Dorsolateral funiculus	Pain Temperature Touch Visceral sensation
Thermoreceptive	Small myelinated Unmyelinated	Spinothalamic	Temperature

predominantly in the anterolateral quadrant of the spinal cord; and 2) the *propriospinal multisynaptic pathway* (Table 7.2).

The *spinocerebellar tracts* are two-neuron pathways that transmit unconscious proprioceptive information to the ipsilateral cerebellum.

- Information from somatosensory receptors are transmitted to the spinal cord by first-order neurons with cell bodies in a dorsal root ganglion.
- A dermatome is the area of skin innervated by a single dorsal root.
- Large-fiber neurons typically carry information about conscious and unconscious proprioception, touch, and vibration. Small-fiber neurons typically carry pain, temperature, and visceral sensory information.
- Sensory information enters the spinal cord in the posterolateral sulcus at the dorsal root entry zone.
- Second-order spinal somatosensory neurons are in the dorsal horn and intermediate gray matter of the spinal cord.
- Somatosensory pathways can be divided into the direct (dorsal column and spinothalamic tracts), indirect (paleospinothalamic, spinoreticular, spinomesencephalic, and propiospinal tracts), and spinocerebellar pathways.

Specific Somatosensory Pathways

Pathways for Tactile Discrimination and Conscious Proprioception: the Direct Dorsal Column–Lemniscal Pathway

The direct dorsal column–lemniscal pathway is important in humans and is critical for highly discriminative tactile sensation, called *stereognosis*, and for fine motor control. The dorsal columns also provide the most important pathway for transmission of conscious proprioception (e.g., joint position sense), static tactile discrimination (e.g., two-point discrimination), and vibration. These last three modalities are also transmitted in parallel pathways. This pathway contributes to the *medial lemniscus* located in the brainstem.

Primary Afferents

Tactile discrimination involves an active process with multiple contacts on the skin and integration of low-threshold mechanoreceptive cutaneous and proprioceptive information (Table 7.6). The skin contains four main types of low-threshold mechanoreceptors. Proprioception involves activity of low-threshold mechanoreceptors in the joints, tendons, and muscles. Muscle spindles have an important role in position sense of the fingers, which is essential for the ability to recognize the form of objects. In humans, the hand, particularly the fingertips, has the highest innervation density and tactile acuity of any body surface and is the most important tactile organ for identifying objects. This involves the process of active exploration.

Low-threshold tactile and proprioceptive information is transmitted by large myelinated, fast-conducting axons of large dorsal horn neurons. Large primary afferents ascend directly in the ipsilateral dorsal column and synapse on second-order neurons in the medulla (the direct dorsal column pathway). Some of these primary afferents also synapse on second-order neurons in the dorsal horn or intermediate gray matter, which have axons that ascend ipsilaterally in the dorsal columns and the dorsolateral funiculus. All these pathways relay in the lower medulla and then decussate to ascend with the contralateral medial lemniscus.

Dorsal Column–Lemniscal System

The direct dorsal column pathway is the most important component of the lemniscal system and consists of large myelinated, primary dorsal root axons that ascend ipsilaterally to the dorsal column nuclei in the medulla (Fig. 7.9). This pathway is important for spatiotemporal tactile discrimination and fine motor control.

The two major anatomical divisions of the dorsal columns are the fasciculus gracilis, which is medial and transmits information from the lower extremities and lower trunk (spinal cord segment T7 and lower), and the fasciculus cuneatus, which is lateral and carries input from the upper extremities and the upper trunk (spinal cord segment T6 and higher). The cutaneous and muscle afferents from the upper and lower limbs are segregated anatomically in the dorsal columns.

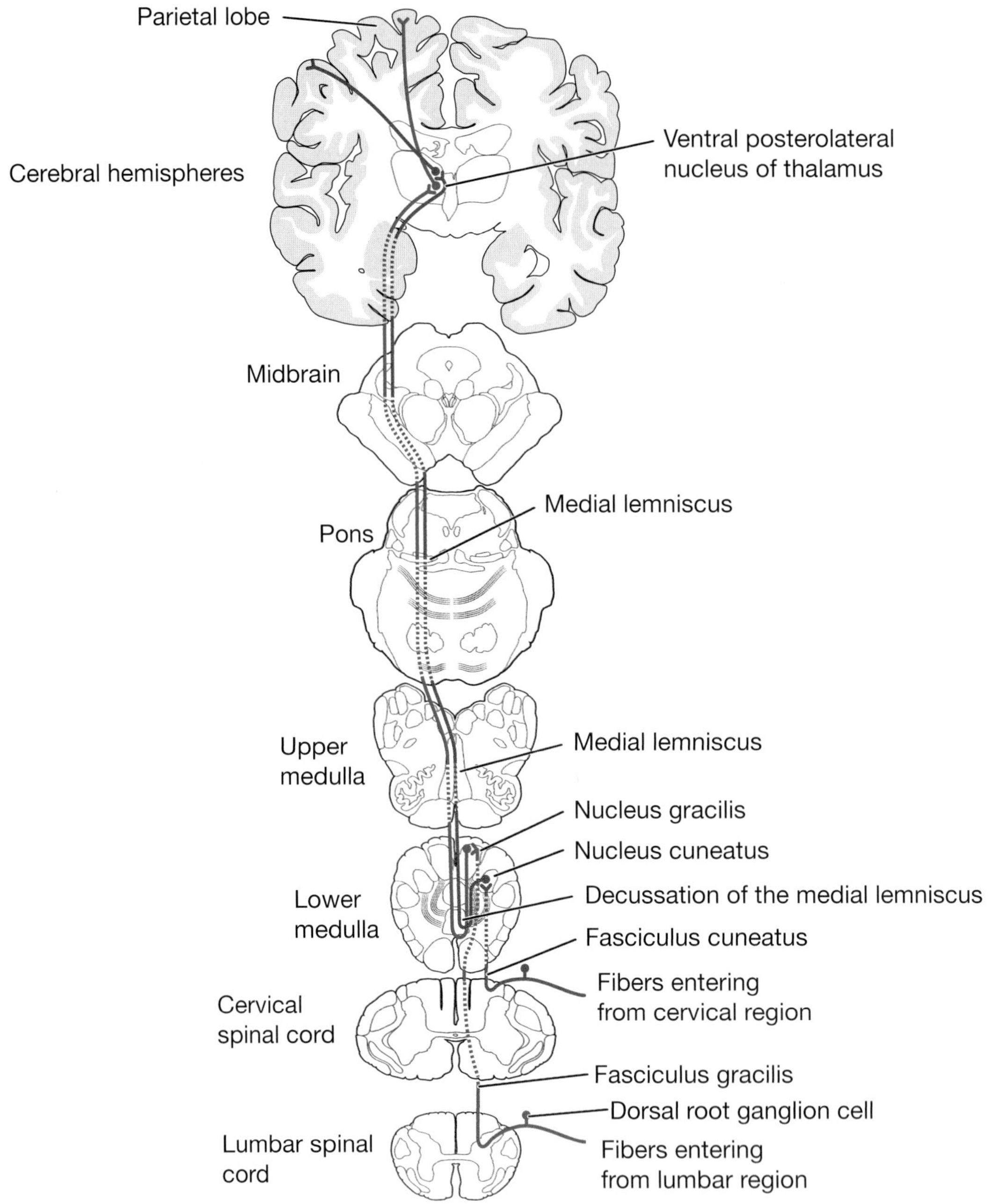

Fig. 7.9. Dorsal column–lemniscal pathway. Conscious proprioception and discriminative sensation.

The dorsal columns are functionally heterogeneous and carry mostly cutaneous and some proprioceptive input to the dorsal column nuclei (direct dorsal column–lemniscal pathway), but also proprioceptive input to cerebellar relay nuclei (spinocerebellar pathway). The latter is discussed below in this chapter.

Second-order neurons of the direct dorsal column pathway are located in the dorsal column nuclei of the lower medulla. These nuclei are the *nucleus gracilis*, which receives cutaneous input from the lower extremity by way of the fasciculus gracilis, and the *nucleus cuneatus*, which receives cutaneous and some proprioceptive input from the upper extremities by way of the fasciculus cuneatus. The dorsal column nuclei are not simple relay stations but sites of modulation of sensory transmission necessary for sensory discrimination. Second-order axons from the dorsal column nuclei cross to the opposite side in the lower medulla as the *internal arcuate fibers* (the decussation of the medial lemniscus) and form the *medial lemniscus*, which ascends to the thalamus.

The medial lemniscus maintains a somatotopic organization, but its position varies at different levels of the brainstem (Fig. 7.10). In the upper medulla, the medial lemniscus is arranged dorsoventrally on either side of the midline, with the cervical segments represented dorsally and the sacral segments ventrally. In the pons,

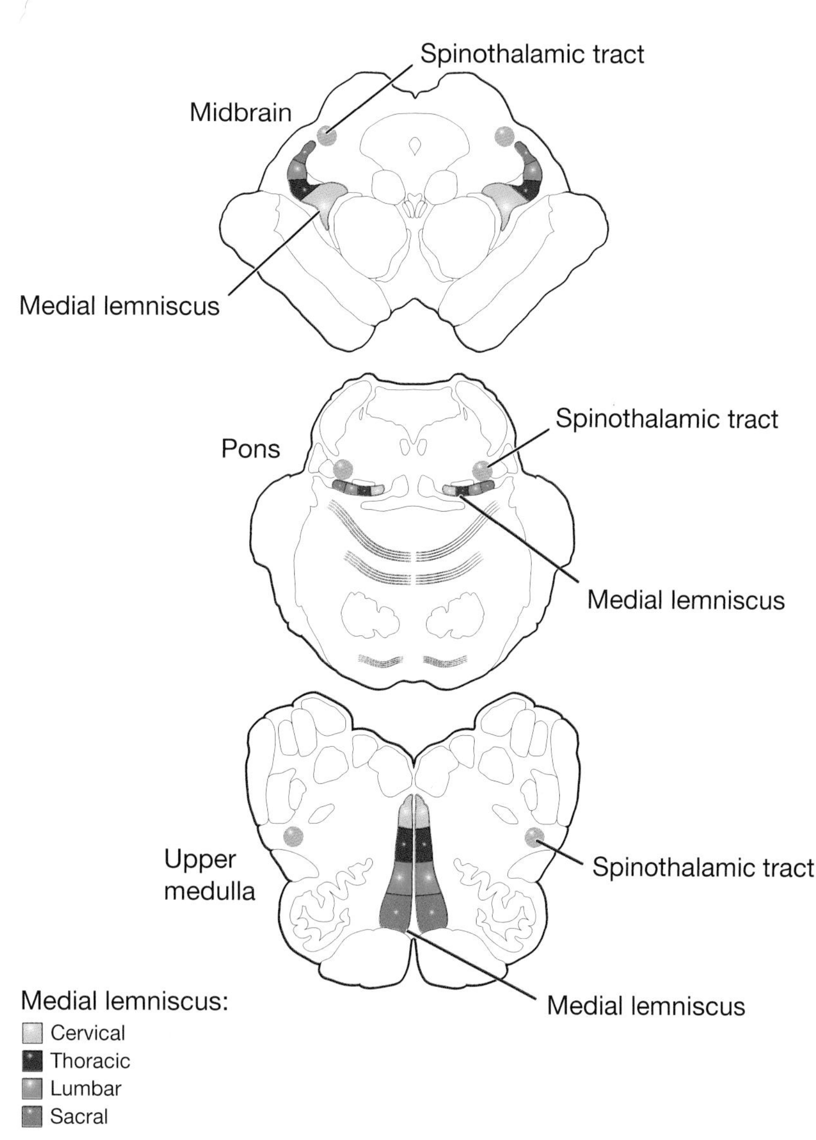

Fig. 7.10. Somatotopic organization of the medial lemniscus and location of the spinothalamic pathway in the brainstem.

it is arranged mediolaterally, with the cervical segments represented medially and the sacral segments laterally.

The medial lemniscus terminates in the ventral posterolateral nucleus and other subdivisions of the ventral posterior complex of the thalamus. The *ventral posterolateral nucleus* receives rapidly adapting cutaneous input from the upper and lower extremities and forms a functional unit with the ventral posteromedial nucleus, which receives similar input from the face through the trigeminal system. Other subdivisions of the ventral posterior complex receive muscle spindle and slowly adapting mechanoreceptive input. Thus, the thalamus contains somatotopically organized, modality-specific maps of the body surface, with the head represented medially, the hand centrally, and the leg laterally in the ventral posterior complex. Somatosensory thalamic neurons project through the posterior limb of the internal capsule to primary somatosensory cortex located in the postcentral gyrus of the parietal lobe.

Primary somatosensory cortex consists of at least four functionally distinct areas. Each of these areas contains a separate somatotopic representation of body receptors, with specific representation of cutaneous or proprioceptive inputs. In each area, the lower extremity is represented on the medial surface of the hemisphere and the upper extremity and the head are represented on the lateral surface (Fig. 7.3). Neurons in primary somatosensory cortex have a high degree of submodality specificity and are organized into separate submodality-specific columns. Processing of somatosensory information also occurs in the secondary and supplementary sensory cortices and in the somatosensory association cortex in the posterior parietal lobe.

Mechanisms of Sensory Discrimination in the Direct Dorsal Column–Lemniscal System

Features of the dorsal column–lemniscal system crucial for sensory discrimination include small receptive fields, mechanisms of contrast sharpening, and parallel modality-specific channels.

The fingertips have the smallest receptive fields and the largest cortical representation (larger than the trunk and legs together). The density of innervation of the fingertips is four times that of the palm, and the threshold for discrimination of two points in these areas is 1 mm and 10 mm, respectively. The dorsal column nuclei and the ventral posterolateral nucleus of the thalamus are not only relay stations but also sites of information processing necessary for spatial and temporal discrimination. This involves a process of *contrast sharpening*, which depends on *lateral inhibition* (Fig. 7.11). Long ascending dorsal column afferents contain the neurotransmitter L-glutamate and excite both the relay cells in the nucleus and the local interneurons containing γ-aminobutyric acid (GABA). These inhibitory GABAergic interneurons also receive excitatory input from somatosensory cortex, and they make presynaptic and postsynaptic inhibitory synapses with both afferent terminals and relay projection cells. Thus, input to a given projection neuron produces, through inhibitory interneurons, lateral inhibition of surrounding projection neurons. This prevents the fusion of the excitatory zones when two stimuli are brought close together and, thus, allows spatial discrimination.

> At all relay stations of the dorsal column–lemniscal pathway, there are specific and spatially segregated sensory channels for the various submodalities. In the dorsal column nuclei, thalamus, and primary somatosensory cortex, a single neuron responds to only one sensory submodality (e.g., touch or muscle spindles). All cells responding to one submodality are located together and segregated from cells responding to other submodalities. In the cerebral cortex, each neuron in a vertical column is activated by the same sensory submodality; thus, neurons in a vertical column form the elementary topographic and modality-specific unit of function.

Parallel Pathways for Proprioceptive and Tactile Discriminative Function

In addition to the direct dorsal column–lemniscal pathway, other parallel pathways contribute to the lemniscal system and transmit tactile discriminative and proprioceptive information. All these spinal pathways consist of second-order axons from low-threshold mechanoreceptive or wide dynamic range neurons in the dorsal horn. These pathways include 1) the *postsynaptic dorsal column pathway*, which contributes to the ipsilateral gracile and cuneate fasciculi; 2) two pathways that ascend ipsilaterally

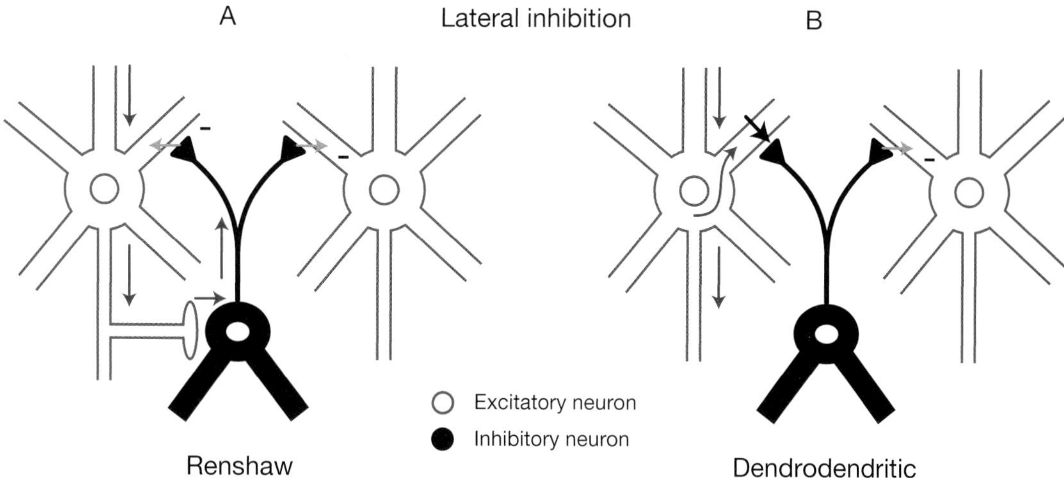

Fig. 7.11. There are two patterns of lateral inhibition. *A*, Renshaw inhibition involves forward input from the axon hillock to axon collaterals (red) that synapse on an interneuron and this interneuron inhibits (green) other neurons through lateral axon connections. *B*, Back propagation of excitatory input (red) from axon hillock to the dendrites activate the inhibitory (black) interneuron via dendroaxonic interaction.

in the dorsolateral funiculus, namely, the *spinocervical tract*, which relays in the lateral cervical nucleus in the upper cervical cord, and the *spinomedullary tract*, which relays in a nucleus of the lower medulla; third-order axons from these two pathways and the postsynaptic dorsal column pathway decussate and join the contralateral medial lemniscus; and 3) the spinothalamic tract, which joins the medial lemniscus before reaching the thalamus.

Effects of Lesions in the Dorsal Column–Lemniscal System

The clinical signs of injury to the dorsal column–lemniscal pathway vary according to the site of involvement. Diffuse involvement of large dorsal root ganglion neurons or large myelinated fibers causes loss of tactile discrimination and inability to detect joint position and vibration. With these lesions, objects cannot be manipulated without visual guidance and movements of the fingers are erratic in the absence of visual clues (pseudoathetosis). These lesions also cause *sensory ataxia*, which is loss of muscle coordination and severe disturbance of gait from the lack of proprioceptive information. Unless the patients can watch the movements of their limbs and correct the errors, they stumble, stagger, and fall. Central lesions of the dorsal column system produce similar but less severe or partial abnormalities because of the redundancy of ascending pathways for the transmission of tactile and proprioceptive information transmitted by large afferents.

Lesions of the dorsal columns in humans produce major defects in vibration sense and in spatiotemporal discrimination, or stereognosis; the deficit is called *astereognosia*. Stereognosis includes graphesthesia (recognition of numbers drawn on the skin), detection of speed and direction of moving cutaneous stimuli, detection of shapes and patterns, and detection of other stimuli that require object manipulation and active exploration with the digits (active touch). These highly discriminative functions are also affected by lesions in primary somatosensory cortex, thalamus, medial lemniscus, and dorsal column nuclei. In addition to astereognosia, lesions of the fasciculus cuneatus may produce deficits similar to those produced by corticospinal lesions, including loss of dexterity of the fingers and disruption of spatiotemporal motor precision.

Spatial discrimination of static stimuli, such as two-point discrimination, stimulus localization, and joint position sense, is relayed not only by the dorsal column–lemniscal pathways but also by several parallel channels. Thus, this ability may not be permanently impaired after lesions restricted to the dorsal columns. Gross touch-pressure sensation may also travel in parallel pathways, particularly the spinothalamic pathway. Only lesions that involve both the dorsal column and the dorsolateral funiculus produce a severe deficit of conscious proprioception. Sensory ataxia may require the associated involvement of the spinocerebellar pathways.

- The dorsal column–lemniscal pathway transmits conscious proprioception, static tactile discrimination, and vibration sense.
- Receptors for this pathway include cutaneous and joint mechanoreceptors.
- First-order neurons are located in dorsal root ganglia and information is carried by large-fiber axons to the dorsal horn of the spinal cord and ascend ipsilaterally to the medulla.
- Fibers carrying lemniscal information from the lower extremities and lower trunk (spinal cord segment T7 and below) travel to the medulla in the fasciculus gracilis; fibers carrying information from the upper extremities and upper trunk (spinal cord segment T6 and above) travel to the medulla in the fasciculus cuneatus.
- Second-order neurons for the upper extremities and lower extremities are located in nucleus cuneatus and nucleus gracilis, respectively.
- Fibers from nuclei cuneatus and gracilis sweep ventrally as the internal arcuate fibers and cross the midline to form the medial lemniscus.
- The medial lemniscus ascends in the mediolateral aspect of the pons and midbrain to synapse in the ventral posterolateral nucleus of thalamus.
- Third-order neurons from the thalamus project to the primary somatosensory cortex.

Clinical Problem 7.1.

A 65-year-old woman has reduced appetite and has lost weight because of poor nutritional intake. She has noticed a subacute, progressive decline in her gait. She also has noticed a mild reduction in her memory. Neurologic examination shows decreased joint position sense and vibration sense in her upper and lower extremities and a vibratory level at approximately C5. Laboratory studies disclose macrocytic anemia.

a. What is the anatomicopathologic diagnosis?
b. What sensory structure(s) is (are) involved by the lesion?
c. What is the most likely pathologic lesion responsible for this clinical syndrome?

Pathways for Pain and Temperature: Ventrolateral Quadrant System

The mechanisms and pathways for pain sensation have been studied more extensively than those for temperature sensation. On the basis of clinical data, it is likely that these two pathways have a similar course through the nervous system; therefore, these two modalities are considered together. The sensation of pain has two components: a *sensory-discriminative* component that informs about quality, intensity, and location of the stimulus, and an *arousal-affective* component that is involved in the emotional, behavioral, and autonomic responses to pain. These two components are carried in a direct pathway and several indirect pathways, respectively, which are intermingled and ascend mainly in the *spinothalamic tract* in the anterolateral quadrant of the spinal cord.

Primary Afferents

Specific low-threshold *thermoreceptive* fibers are excited by either warming or cooling but not by tactile stimulation. The peripheral receptors for pain are free nerve endings. The two main types of *nociceptive units* are high-threshold mechanoreceptive units innervated by small myelinated axons and polymodal nociceptive units innervated by unmyelinated axons (Table 7.7). High-threshold mechanoreceptive units respond to noxious mechanical stimuli (pressure) and mediate *first*, or fast, *pain*, which

Table 7.7. Types of Nociceptive Fibers

Feature	High-threshold mechanoreceptive type	Polymodal nociceptive type
Axon	Small myelinated	Unmyelinated
Stimulus	Noxious pressure	Noxious pressure, pinch Noxious thermal Chemicals (K^+, histamine)
Neurotransmitter	L-Glutamate	Substance P Calcitonin gene-related peptide
Sensation	First, or fast, pain Well-localized Sharp Prickling	Second, or slow, pain Diffuse Dull Aching Burning

is the well-localized, sharp sensation (prickling pain) induced by pinprick or laceration. Polymodal units respond not only to noxious mechanical but also to noxious thermal and chemical (substances released during inflammation) stimuli and mediate *second*, or slow, *pain*, which is a diffuse, dull-aching or burning discomfort that may outlast the stimulus.

The first-order nociceptive neurons include 1) medium-sized dorsal root ganglion neurons with small myelinated fibers that have L-glutamate as a neurotransmitter and correspond to high-threshold mechanoreceptors, and 2) small dorsal root ganglion neurons with unmyelinated axons that contain not only glutamate but also various neuropeptides, including substance P and calcitonin gene-related peptide, and correspond to polymodal nociceptors. Axons of small nociceptive dorsal root neurons branch extensively and innervate several sensory fields; some of their proximal projections enter the spinal cord through ventral roots instead of dorsal roots (ventral root afferents) to reach the dorsal horn.

Small dorsal root ganglion neurons may release neuropeptides antidromically from their peripheral branches at the site of stimulation. Antidromic release of neurotransmitters by peripheral branches is called the axon reflex. Nociceptive axon reflexes are the basis of neurogenic inflammation, or the flare response. Stimulation of nociceptive endings by mechanical damage or local substances released during inflammation (histamine, prostaglandins, and potassium ions) not only produces pain but also causes the antidromic release of substance P and other vasoactive neuropeptides, which produce vasodilatation and increase vascular permeability at the site of injury.

Pain fibers, together with fibers involved in temperature and visceral sensation, enter the spinal cord in the lateral division of the dorsal root entry zone and divide into short ascending and descending branches that run longitudinally in the dorsolateral funiculus (Lissauer tract). Within several segments, they leave the tract to form excitatory synapses on second-order neurons in the dorsal horn. The excitatory neurotransmitters include L-glutamate and several neuropeptides, particularly substance P.

Dorsal Horn Neurons

Second-order nociceptive neurons include 1) *nociceptive-specific* neurons, which predominantly are located superficially in the dorsal horn and receive input solely from small myelinated and unmyelinated fibers; and 2) *wide dynamic range*, or multiceptive, neurons, which predominantly are located deep in the dorsal horn and in the intermediate gray matter and receive input not only from small myelinated and unmyelinated fibers but also from visceral afferents and large myelinated fibers. Wide dynamic range neurons are functionally important because they contribute most of the axons to the spinothalamic system. Also, these neurons transmit both nociceptive and nonnociceptive information, are the site of viscerosomatic convergence for *referred visceral pain*, and can change their functional properties according to local modulatory influences by central pain-modulating mechanisms.

Second-order axons from both nociceptive-specific and wide dynamic range neurons, together with axons from thermoreceptive neurons, cross to the opposite side and continue rostrally in the anterolateral quadrant of the spinal cord, primarily in the spinothalamic pathways.

Spinothalamic Tract

The sensations of pain and temperature are transmitted primarily in the spinothalamic tract, which ascends in the ventrolateral quadrant of the spinal cord contralateral to the side of entry of the primary afferents (Fig. 7.12). The spinothalamic tract is complex and functionally heterogeneous. It mediates the discriminative and arousal-emotional components of pain sensation as well as thermal, visceral, and simple tactile information. The different components of the spinothalamic tract include 1) a direct pathway, the neospinothalamic pathway, which mediates the discriminative aspect of pain and temperature and is important for localization; and 2) several indirect pathways, including the paleospinothalamic, spinoreticular, and spinomesencephalic tracts, for the affective-arousal components of pain; they form part of the core, or inner tube, of the neuraxis (Table 7.8).

The *neospinothalamic tract* consists of second-order axons from both nociceptive-specific and wide dynamic range neurons. The axons cross the midline through the ventral white commissure and ascend strictly contralaterally in the anterolateral quadrant of the spinal cord. The neospinothalamic tract is somatotopically organized in the spinal cord, with the sacral component represented dorsolaterally and the cervical component ventromedially.

The spinothalamic tract ascends in the lateral portion of the brainstem. In the medulla, it is dorsal to the lateral aspect of the inferior olivary nucleus, and in the pons and midbrain, it is lateral to the medial lemniscus. At the mesodiencephalic junction, the spinothalamic tract and medial lemniscus join (Fig. 7.10). Throughout its course, the spinothalamic tract maintains a somatotopic organization, with cervical segments represented medially and sacral segments laterally.

Spinothalamic tract axons synapse on third-order neurons in several thalamic nuclei, particularly the ventral posterolateral nucleus that, in turn, projects to the primary sensory cortex in the postcentral gyrus. Other spinothalamic tract axons terminate in thalamic relay nuclei that project to either the insular cortex or anterior cingulate gyrus.

The spinothalamic tract is involved in the rapid transmission of nociceptive and thermal information for localization and intensity of pain and temperature sensations. Thus, this pathway is important clinically for localizing lesions in the central nervous system. Another important function is to provide a parallel channel for transmission of tactile information, including simple touch and static discriminative touch modalities.

The spinothalamic pathway transmits information about pain and temperature sensations from the contralateral upper and lower extremities and trunk. Pain and temperature sensations from the face and cranium are transmitted by the trigeminal system. Pain fibers from the face travel primarily in the trigeminal nerve (cranial nerve V). The cell bodies of these primary sensory neurons are located in the *gasserian*, or *semilunar*, *ganglion* (Fig. 7.13). On entering the brainstem at the pons, these fibers descend in the ipsilateral descending, or *spinal tract of the trigeminal nerve*, to the upper cervical cord. Axons of this tract synapse with second-order neurons in the adjacent *nucleus of the spinal tract of the trigeminal nerve*. Axons of the second-order neurons cross to the opposite side of the brainstem and ascend to the ventral posteromedial nucleus of the thalamus. Third-order neurons in this thalamic nucleus project to the parietal lobe through the posterior limb of the internal capsule.

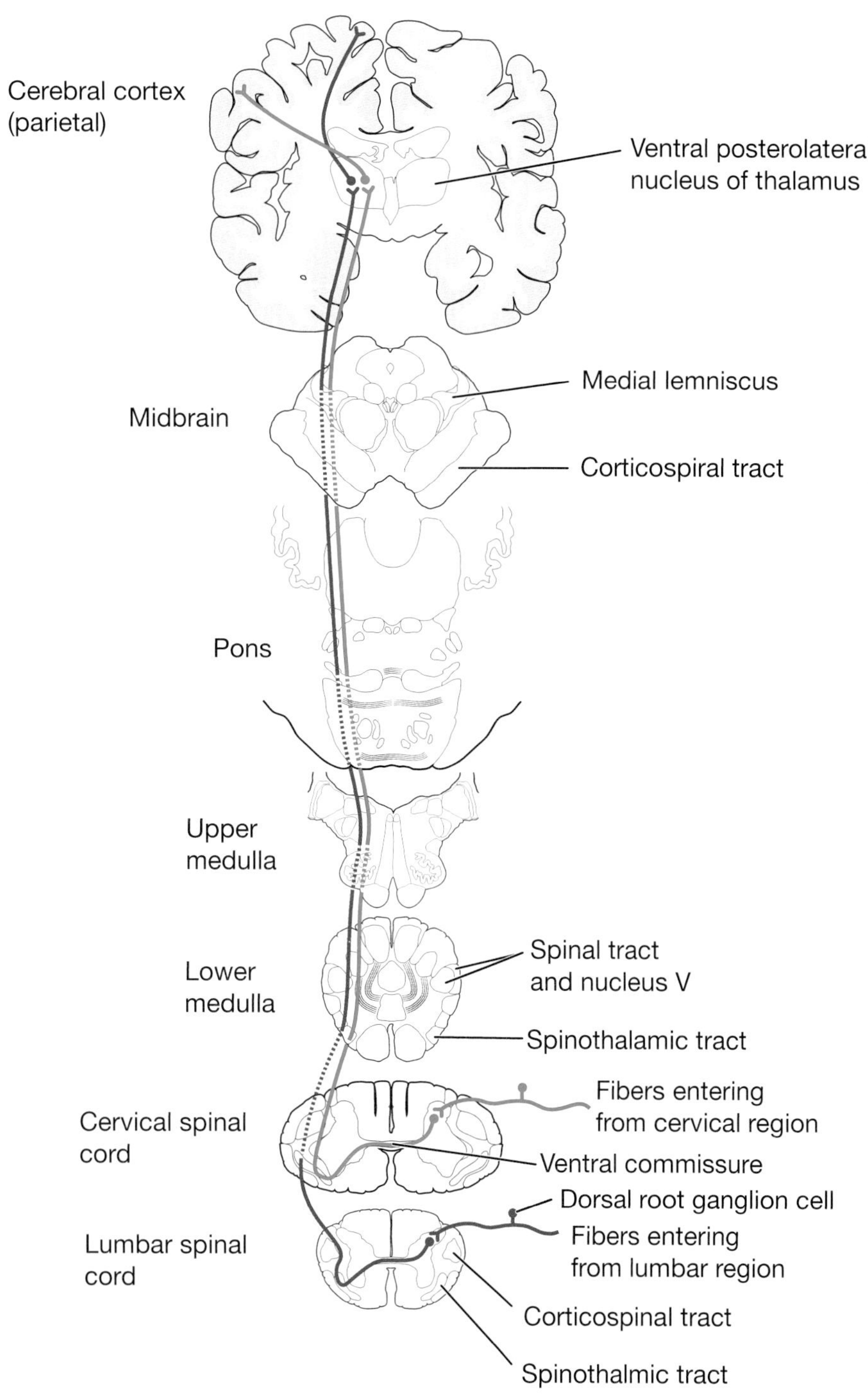

Fig. 7.12. Spinothalamic (neospinothalamic) tract. Pathway for pain and temperature sensation.

Table 7.8. Pathways for Pain Transmission

Feature	Direct or lateral (outer tube)	Indirect or medial (inner tube)
Pathway	Neospinothalamic	Paleospinothalamic Spinoreticular Spinomesencephalic Propriospinal
Somatotopy	Yes	No
Body representation	Contralateral	Bilateral
Synapse in reticular formation	No	Yes
Subcortical targets	None	Hypothalamus Limbic system Autonomic centers
Thalamic nucleus	Ventral posterolateral nucleus	Intralaminar nuclei Midline nuclei
Cortical region	Parietal lobe, insular cortex	Cingulate gyrus
Role	Discriminative pain	Affective-arousal component of pain
Other function	Temperature Touch	

Pathways for the Affective-Arousal Components of Pain
The indirect pathways involved in the affective and arousal aspects of pain sensation originate mainly from wide dynamic range neurons in the deep dorsal horn and intermediate gray matter. Their second-order axons ascend bilaterally in the spinal cord, have poor somatotopy, and make multiple synapses in the reticular formation. These pathways are components of the inner tube system. Collaterals of these pathways reach the hypothalamus and other areas of the limbic system. Neurons involved in these complex, multisynaptic pathways have large bilateral receptive fields and receive convergent input from not only cutaneous but also visceral and other receptors. These pathways initiate arousal, autonomic, endocrine, and motor responses to pain stimulation. The two main groups of these pathways are 1) ventrolateral quadrant pathways, which include the paleospinothalamic, spinoreticular, and spinomesencephalic tracts (Fig. 7.14); and 2) the propriospinal multisynaptic ascending system.

In the spinal cord, second-order axons that contribute to these pathways ascend contralaterally and ipsilaterally in the ventrolateral quadrant (they intermingle with those of the neospinothalamic pathway), the dorsolateral quadrant, and the propriospinal system. The paleospinothalamic tract provides multiple input to the reticular formation and terminates in the *midline* and *intralaminar thalamic nuclei*, which project diffusely to the cerebral cortex, particularly to the anterior cingulate gyrus. The spinoreticular tract terminates in sensory, motor, autonomic, and endocrine relay areas of the medullary and pontine reticular formation. The spinomesencephalic tract synapses in the periaqueductal gray matter.

The *multisynaptic ascending propriospinal system* originates from neurons in the substantia gelatinosa of the dorsal horn and in the intermediate gray matter. This system forms a functional continuum with the reticular formation of the brainstem.

In addition to transmitting affective-arousal components of pain sensation, all these indirect pathways are important for activation of central antinociceptive (pain inhibition) mechanisms (discussed below).

Effect of Lesions of the Spinothalamic System

Lesions that involve the peripheral level may cause either the sensation of pain or some loss of pain and temperature in the distribution of the affected nerves. Lesions of the central nervous system seldom produce pain unless pain-sensitive structures are involved or central pain-controlling pathways are interrupted. A central lesion that interrupts the spinothalamic tract results in the inability to perceive painful stimuli and to discriminate between hot and cold in the areas below the level of the lesion. A lesion

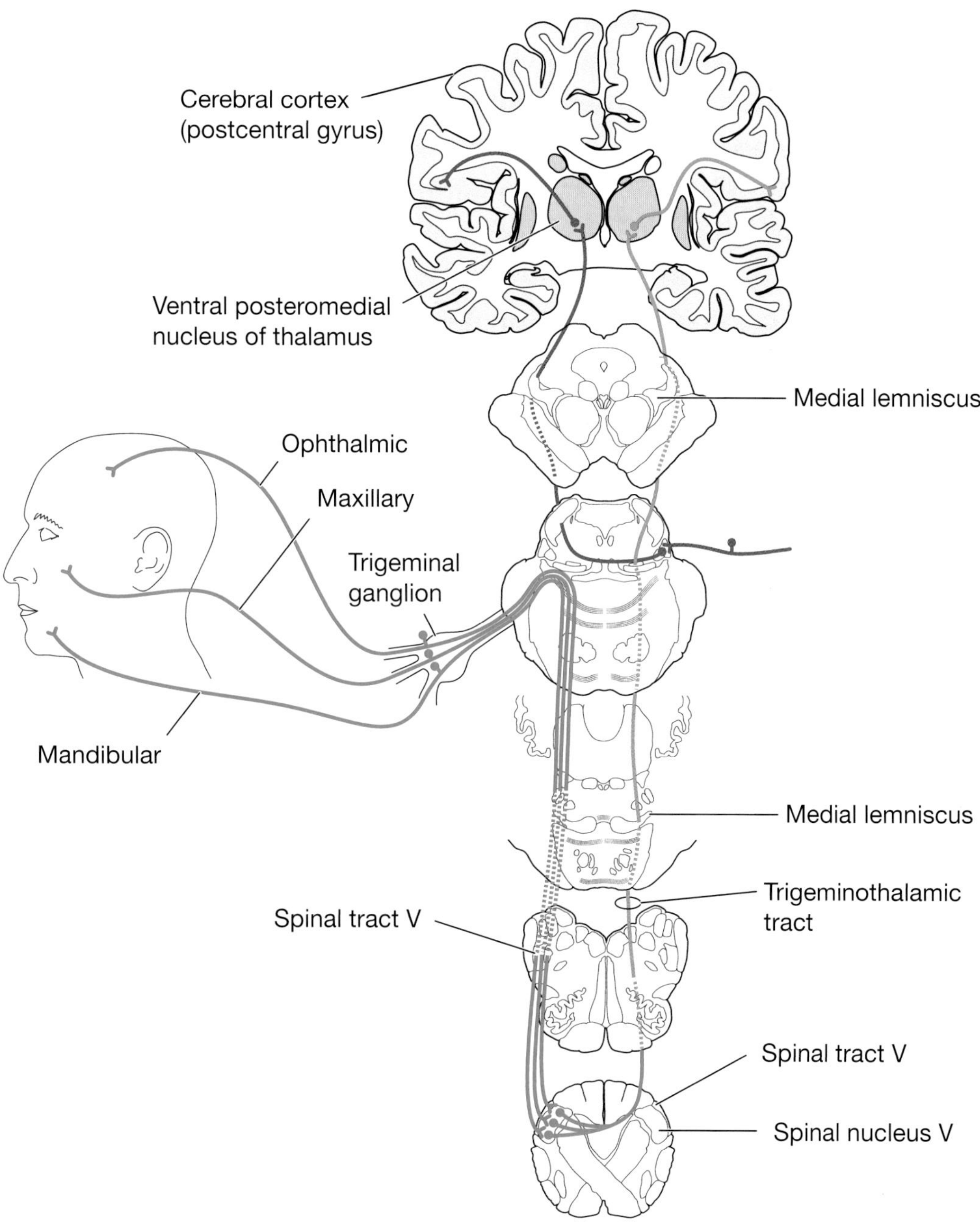

Fig. 7.13. Pathway of pain fibers of the face.

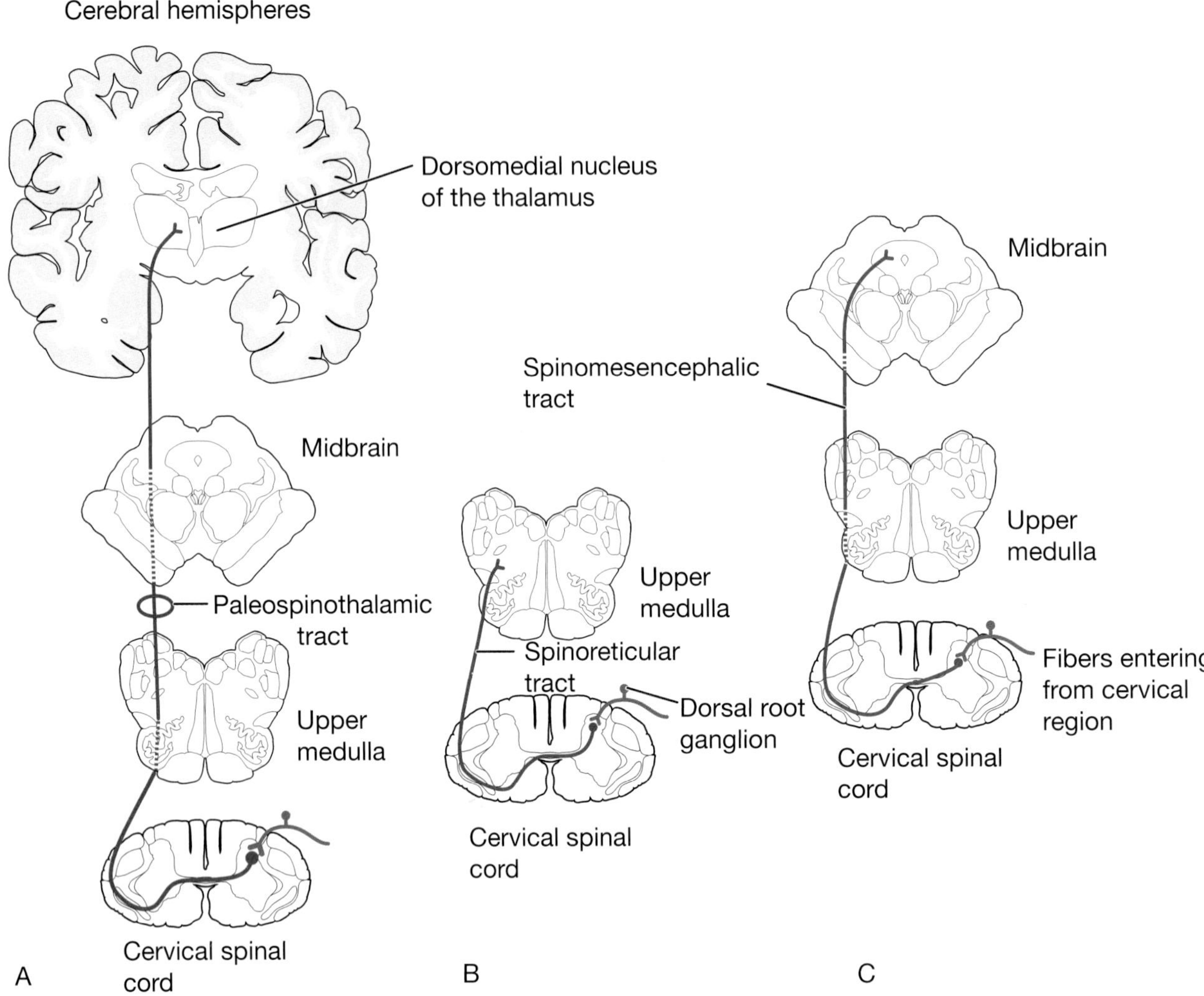

Fig. 7.14. The three individual pain pathways of the inner tube that transmit affective and arousal components of pain. *A*, Paleospinothalamic tract. *B*, Spinoreticular tract. *C*, Spinomesencephalic tract.

at the spinal level involving the spinothalamic tract results in contralateral loss of pain and temperature sensations below the level of the lesion. A lesion at the posterior fossa level results in *contralateral* loss of pain and temperature sensations in the trunk and extremities, but if the same lesion also involves the pain fibers in the descending tract of the trigeminal nerve, there is *ipsilateral* loss of pain and temperature sensation of the face. The separate pathways for body and limb pain and for facial pain are the neuroanatomical basis for this clinical observation. Thus, lesions at the level of the medulla produce *crossed anesthesia*, whereas those rostral to the medulla produce *complete contralateral hemianesthesia*, which includes the face. Lesions at the supratentorial level produce contralateral loss of pain and temperature sensations. With suprathalamic lesions, crude pain perception may remain intact, but precise localization of painful stimuli is impaired.

- Receptors that transmit temperature and pain are called thermoreceptors and nociceptors, respectively.
- The direct spinothalamic tract transmits pain and temperature information to the cortex over a three-neuron pathway.
- First-order neurons for the spinothalamic pathway

Clinical Problem 7.2.

A 48-year-old woman experienced the abrupt onset of pain, followed by paresthesia and loss of feeling in a rather circumscribed area along the lateral aspect of her right thigh. Neurologic examination showed a localized area of decreased perception of pinprick, temperature, and touch. The results of the rest of the examination were normal.

a. What is the anatomicopathologic diagnosis?
b. What specific anatomical structure is involved?
c. How would the distribution of symptoms be different if the lesion involved the median nerve at the wrist?

are located in dorsal root ganglion and are small-fiber neurons.

- Second-order neurons are located in the dorsal horn of the spinal cord. Their axons cross the midline in the ventral white commissure and ascend contralaterally in the anterolateral quadrant of the spinal cord and lateral portion of the brainstem.
- Spinothalamic tract axons synapse on third-order neurons in the ventral posterolateral nucleus of the thalamus, which projects to primary somatosensory cortex.
- The indirect pathways involved in the affective and arousal aspects of pain sensation are complex, multisynaptic pathways and include two main groups: 1) ventrolateral quadrant pathways and 2) the propriospinal multisynaptic ascending system.

Pathways for Transmission of Simple Touch

Tactile sensation is initiated by the stimulation of low-threshold mechanoreceptors in the skin. These receptors vary in degree of adaptation and size of receptive field. The axons of primary, large dorsal root ganglion neurons are in the medial division of the dorsal root entry zone. These large myelinated fibers either ascend directly in the dorsal columns or stimulate low-threshold mechanoreceptive and wide dynamic range neurons in the deep dorsal horn. Thus, simple tactile information is carried rostrally by several parallel pathways, including the direct and postsynaptic dorsal column pathways, the spinocervical tract in the dorsolateral funiculus, and the neospinothalamic tract in the anterolateral quadrant.

All these pathways are part of the outer tube system. They contribute to the lemniscal system, terminate in the contralateral ventral posterolateral nucleus of the thalamus, and activate low-threshold cutaneous mechanoreceptive neurons in the primary somatosensory cortex. These pathways overlap with the ones that mediate discriminative touch and proprioception (dorsal columns) and discriminative pain and temperature (neospinothalamic tract).

The transmission of simple tactile modalities (detection, localization, and, to some extent, two-point discrimination) over several parallel pathways explains the preservation of the sensation of touch despite lesions affecting other sensory modalities. Thus, touch is not very useful clinically for localizing lesions in the central nervous system.

- Simple touch sensation may be carried by both the dorsal column–lemniscal system and the spinothalamic tract.
- Touch is not clinically useful for localizing lesions in the central nervous system.

Mechanisms of Pain and Analgesia

Pain is a frequent manifestation of neurologic and nonneurologic disease. Organic pain can be subdivided into *nociceptive pain* and *neurogenic pain*. Nociceptive pain is related to the activation of normal pain mechanisms in response to tissue injury or inflammation; neurogenic pain is due to peripheral or central nervous system lesions that affect processing of information in the pain transmission pathway. Transmission of nociceptive information is regulated by a balance between excitatory and inhibitory influences acting on spinothalamic and other neurons of the pain pathways. Endogenous antinociceptive mechanisms are activated by stress, exercise, sexual activity, and previous nociceptive stimulation of peripheral tissues.

Nociceptive Afferents

As mentioned above, the two types of nociceptive afferents are the small myelinated high-threshold mechanoreceptors and the unmyelinated polymodal nociceptors (Table 7.7). Primary nociceptive afferents contain L-glutamate and various neuropeptides, the most abundant of which are calcitonin gene-related peptide and substance P. Neuropeptides are released in the dorsal horn from the central process of the first-order neuron and in the periphery from the peripheral process. The release of neuropeptides from the peripheral process occurs through an axon reflex. The release from the end of the peripheral process triggers vasomotor and other phenomena referred to as *neurogenic inflammation*, or the *flare response*. Neuropeptides are released in response to many different stimuli, including potassium and hydrogen ions, histamine, serotonin, cytokines, and nerve growth factor.

Dorsal Horn

The dorsal horn is not only a station for pain transmission. It also contains many complex, dynamic circuits that support the transmission of sensory input and a high degree of sensory processing. One of the important aspects of this sensory processing is the central modulation of pain transmission.

The transmission of pain is modulated by both segmental mechanisms and descending suprasegmental mechanisms through complex circuits at the spinal or medullary level. These regulatory circuits involve primary afferents, descending pathways, and local interneurons.

Interneurons in the Dorsal Horn

Interneurons in the dorsal horn are located primarily in the *substantia gelatinosa*, or lamina II. They may be excitatory or inhibitory. Inhibitory interneurons contain GABA, enkephalins, or neuropeptides and are important for local processing and modulation of pain transmission. They receive input from segmental large and small primary afferent fibers and from descending supraspinal fibers.

Segmental Mechanisms

There are two important segmental mechanisms for the modulation of pain transmission. The first involves inhibition of pain transmission by activation of large-diameter afferents; that is, stimulation of low-threshold, large myelinated mechanoreceptive afferents inhibits pain transmission in the dorsal horn, probably by the activation of local inhibitory interneurons. This is the basis for the *gate control theory of pain modulation*. A second mechanism involves exaggeration of pain transmission after repetitive activation of small nociceptive fibers; that is, repetitive firing of nociceptive fibers results in increased activity of dorsal horn nociceptive neurons (Fig. 7.15). This mechanism, known as the *windup phenomenon*, may explain the pain that occurs with nerve injury and during nerve regeneration.

Several reciprocally connected brain regions form a central pain-control network. The nuclei and pathways of this endogenous analgesia system are part of the internal regulation system of the inner tube and are diffusely distributed. They include the cerebral cortex, thalamus,

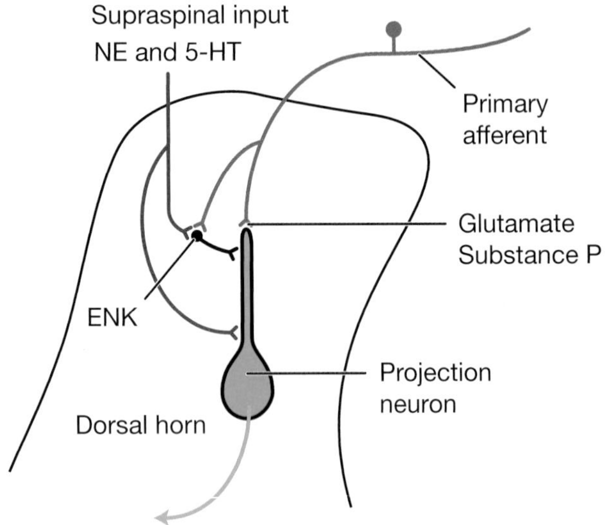

Fig. 7.15. Local circuit in the dorsal horn involved in transmission and modulation of pain sensation at the spinal level. Primary afferents release L-glutamate and substance P to excite second-order relay neurons (projection neuron) of the spinothalamic system. This transmission is inhibited by local interneurons containing enkephalin (ENK) or other transmitters and by descending brainstem pathways containing serotonin (5-HT) and norepinephrine (NE).

hypothalamus, brainstem, and dorsal horn. Important components of this system are the *periaqueductal gray matter* of the midbrain; the *rostral ventromedial medulla*, particularly the *raphe nucleus*, which produces serotonin; and the *locus ceruleus* and adjacent medullary neurons that produce norepinephrine (Fig. 7.16). All these central structures have several properties in common: 1) they contain endogenous opioid neurons and receptors; 2) they are stimulated by opioids and mediate the analgesic effects of morphine-like drugs; 3) they receive input from the indirect ascending nociceptive pathways and thus provide feedback inhibition of pain transmission; 4) when stimulated, they produce analgesia, and they selectively affect pain transmission and do not affect the transmission of *nonnociceptive* information in the dorsal horn.

Opioids disinhibit antinociceptive neurons in the periaqueductal gray matter. These neurons, in turn, activate the serotoninergic and noradrenergic bulbospinal neurons that project to the dorsal horn through the dorsolateral funiculus of the spinal cord. Noradrenergic and serotoninergic inputs inhibit pain transmission either directly or through inhibitory GABA-containing or opioid-containing interneurons in the dorsal horn.

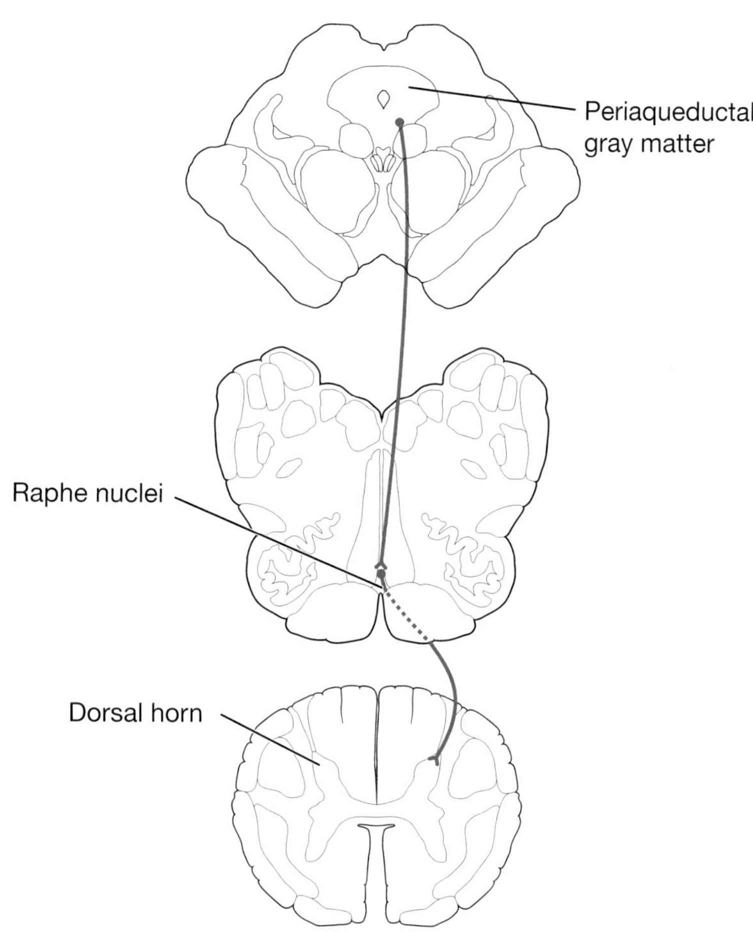

Fig. 7.16. Brainstem components of the central pain-controlling network (endogenous analgesic system). The periaqueductal gray matter stimulates serotoninergic neurons in the raphe nuclei and norepinephrine-synthesizing cell groups of the reticular formation in the ventral medulla. Descending serotoninergic and noradrenergic pathways inhibit pain transmission in the dorsal horn. The periaqueductal gray matter and ventral medulla are sites for analgesic action of opioids.

The symptom of nociceptive pain is most important in calling attention to pathologic processes that occur in many organ systems. Lesions located outside the nervous system frequently stimulate pain-sensitive free nerve endings and produce the subjective sensation of pain. Acute nociceptive pain is initiated through the stimulation of nociceptive fibers by several chemical mediators of inflammation (e.g., K^+ ions, histamine, bradykinin, and prostaglandins) and is potentiated by the antidromic release of substance P and other neuropeptides from nociceptive axon terminals (neurogenic inflammation, or flare response). The parenchyma of internal organs, including the brain, is not supplied with pain receptors. However, the wall of arteries, the dura mater, mesothelial surfaces (e.g., synovial surfaces, pleura, pericardium, and peritoneum), the wall of hollow viscera, and muscle are subject to inflammation or mechanical traction. Unlike somatic pain, visceral pain is poorly localized and the sensation generally is felt in an area of skin remote from the actual source of stimulation. This is the phenomenon of *referred pain* (Fig. 7.17).

An important example of nociceptive pain is headache. The pain-sensitive structures in the cranium include the wall of blood vessels, the dura mater, and the periostium. Migraine is a typical example of vascular headache. The pain in migraine headache is thought to reflect inflammation and antidromic vasodilatation at trigeminovascular junctions. The extracranial blood vessels receive sensory innervation from the trigeminal nerve. Several triggering factors may activate trigeminal afferents that innervate these blood vessels; these afferents antidromically release substance P and calcitonin gene-related peptide, which are potent vasodilators and elicit the release of inflammatory mediators. Stretching of the blood vessel wall and inflammation increase impulse conduction in trigeminal afferents and increase the antidromic release of vasodilator neuropeptides. This mechanism may contribute to headache that occurs in association with meningeal irritation or mechanical distortion of pain-sensitive structures during an increase in intracranial pressure.

Neurogenic pain includes *neuropathic pain*, *deafferentation pain*, and *sympathetically maintained pain*. Neuropathic pain occurs in cases of painful nerve compression or after

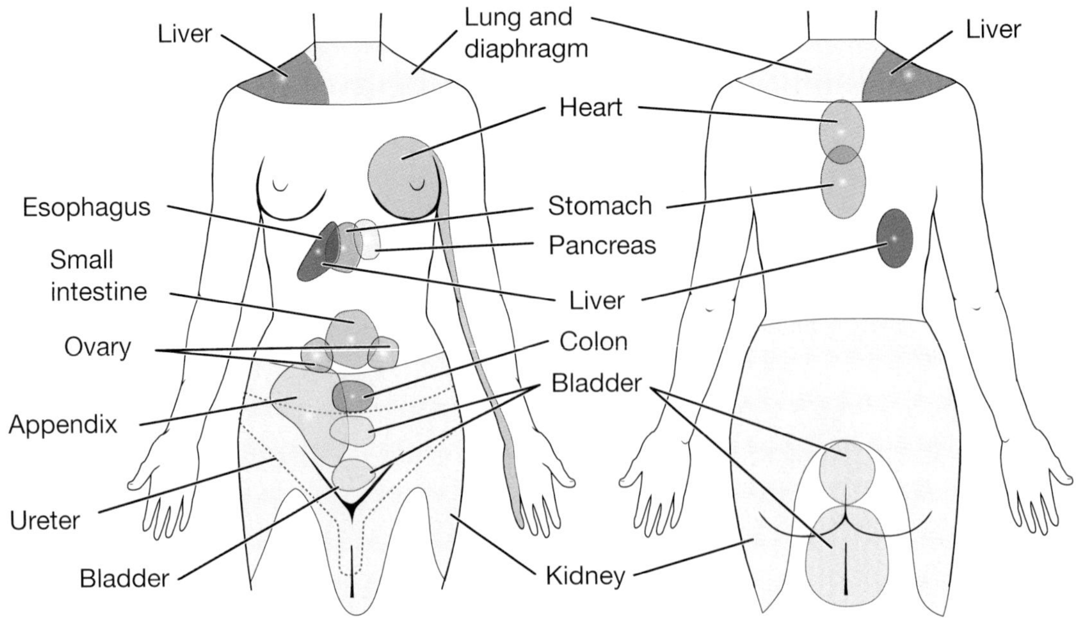

Fig. 7.17. Referred pain. (Modified from Timby BK. Instructor's resource CD-ROM to accompany *Fundamental Nursing Skills and Concepts*, 8th ed. Philadelphia: Lippincott Williams & Wilkins; 2004. Used with permission.)

formation of posttraumatic neuroma following a nerve lesion. This may produce abnormal discharges in the areas of demyelination, selective loss of large fiber–mediated segmental inhibition, and increased activity of small nociceptive fibers.

Deafferentation pain may complicate any type of injury along the course of the somatosensory pathways. This can occur at the peripheral level (e.g., phantom pain after limb amputation), along the ascending pathways (e.g., demyelinating spinal cord lesions in multiple sclerosis), or at the level of the thalamus (thalamic syndrome). In these conditions, pain occurs in the area of sensory loss. It is due to perturbation of the central processing of pain information that results from interference with normal pain-control mechanisms.

Sympathetically maintained pain is characterized by the simultaneous occurrence of pain, local autonomic dysregulation (edema, vasomotor disturbances, and sweat abnormalities), and trophic changes in the skin, soft tissues, and bone. It occurs mainly with lesions of peripheral nerves or roots.

Neurogenic pain involves plastic changes (called *sensitization*) at the level of the nociceptors, dorsal root ganglia, and dorsal horn. Normally, polymodal nociceptors have no spontaneous activity. In response to injury, the nociceptors are sensitized by cytokines and other products of inflammation. This sensitization is characterized by increased spontaneous (background) activity, decreased threshold and supernormal discharge in response to noxious stimulation, increased size of receptive fields, increased sensitivity to heat or cold stimuli, increased discharge in response to sympathetic stimulation, and antidromic release of neuropeptides. One mechanism that contributes to the development of neuropathic pain is the activation of *silent nociceptors* through the products of inflammation.

Increased activity of nociceptive afferents produces the phenomenon of *central sensitization* at the level of the dorsal horn. The mechanism is similar to that of the windup phenomenon. The result is increased discharge, decreased threshold, and enlarged receptive fields of spinothalamic neurons. The mechanisms include increased release of L-glutamate and neuropeptides and triggering of different Ca^{2+}-dependent biochemical cascades in spinothalamic neurons (see Chapter 14).

Neurogenic pain has several clinical characteristics: 1) spontaneous pain (burning,aching, shock-like), 2) increased sensitivity to noxious stimulation (called *hyperalgesia*), and 3) pain caused by innocuous (e.g., tactile) stimulation (called *allodynia*). Spontaneous pain and hyperalgesia involve the small myelinated and unmyelinated nociceptive fibers. Allodynia is mediated by myelinated, nonnociceptive fibers. These fibers normally evoke nonnociceptive responses in spinothalamic neurons and trigger segmental inhibition of nociceptive neurons by local GABAergic mechanisms. In central sensitization, the increased excitability of spinothalamic neurons and impaired local inhibition cause a normally innocuous stimulus to provoke increased firing of spinothalamic neurons, resulting in pain sensation.

Another positive manifestation of nerve injury is *paresthesia* (pins-and-needles sensation), which reflects increased spontaneous activity in large myelinated fibers and can be elicited in normal subjects by nerve compression, hyperventilation, or repetitive nerve stimulation. The mechanism is ectopic discharge of the nerve produced by sustained depolarization, which is the result of increased permeability to Na^+ (e.g., with decreased extracellular ionized Ca^{2+} after hyperventilation) or accumulation of extracellular K^+ (e.g., after a period of nerve ischemia). The positive sensory symptoms of spontaneous pain and paresthesia typically occur with lesions that affect a peripheral sensory nerve or nerve root. However, these symptoms can occur with lesions that involve any part of the somatosensory pathways, including the spinal cord, thalamus, and parietal cortex.

Lancinating pain in the head or face that occurs spontaneously or in response to minimal stimuli is referred to as *neuralgia*. A typical example is *trigeminal neuralgia*, which consists of paroxysmal, electric shocklike facial pain in the distribution of the trigeminal nerve.

- Nociceptive pain is related to activation of normal pain mechanisms in response to tissue injury or inflammation.
- Neurogenic pain is due to peripheral or central nervous system lesions that affect processing of information in the pain transmission pathway.

- Two types of nociceptive afferents are the small myelinated high-threshold mechanoreceptors and the unmyelinated polymodal nociceptors.
- The transmission of pain is modulated by both segmental mechanisms in the dorsal horn and descending suprasegmental mechanisms involving contributions from the cerebral cortex, thalamus, hypothalamus, and specific structures in the brainstem such as the periaqueductal gray matter, raphe nuclei, locus ceruleus, and rostral ventrolateral medulla.
- Migraine headache is nociceptive pain thought to reflect inflammation and antidromic vasodilatation at trigeminovascular junctions.
- Neurogenic pain includes neuropathic pain, deafferentation pain, and sympathetically maintained pain.

Somatosensory Pathways and Control of Motor Function

Input from muscle spindles, Golgi tendon organs, joint proprioceptors, and low-threshold mechanoreceptors are processed not only centrally for conscious sensation but also for unconscious reflex adjustments of posture and muscle tone and for continuous monitoring of motor performance. Input from the muscles, joints, and skin provide continuous information about the position and movement of the limbs and trunk. This information is fed back to all components of the motor system, including the motor cortex, cerebellum, brainstem, and motor neurons in the spinal cord.

The main sources of the somatosensory information that acts as feedback to the motor system are the muscle spindles, Golgi tendon organs, and low-threshold mechanoreceptors of the skin and tendons. Joint and muscle receptors are innervated by rapidly conducting, large myelinated peripheral axons of large dorsal root ganglion neurons (first-order neurons). Their proximal axons are primary afferent fibers that enter the spinal cord in the medial division of the dorsal root entry zone. These proprioceptive fibers may 1) course directly through the dorsal gray matter to the ventral gray matter; 2) ascend directly in the dorsal columns or synapse on second-order neurons in the spinal cord to form the lemniscal system; and 3) synapse on second-order neurons in the intermediate gray matter, which contribute to the spinocerebellar tracts.

Primary afferent fibers that synapse directly on ventral horn motor neurons initiate a two-neuron muscle stretch reflex that is the anatomical basis for the muscle stretch, or deep tendon, reflexes commonly tested in clinical neurology. Sudden stretching of a muscle, as elicited by tapping a tendon with a reflex hammer, stimulates muscle spindle receptors. This, in turn, produces action potentials in the afferent fibers that enter the spinal cord and synapse on motor neurons in the ventral horn. These ventral horn cells initiate action potentials that travel back to the muscle of origin, causing the muscle to contract. This is a *local segmental reflex* (see Chapter 14). This reflex is lost whenever disease affects the primary proprioceptive axon or other component of the reflex arc at that segment.

More important is the role of primary afferent input to the *interneuronal pool* in the ventral horn. These interneurons integrate primary afferent, supraspinal, and local circuit information to control motor neuron activity for the maintenance of muscle tone (degree of stiffness) and the execution of coordinated motor acts.

Motor Function of the Dorsal Column–Lemniscal System

The dorsal column system has extensive interconnections with the corticospinal motor system. Afferent input from the dorsal column–lemniscal system affects the firing of corticospinal neurons through thalamocortical and corticocortical connections. Fibers from somatosensory cortex travel in the corticospinal tract to modulate sensory processing in the thalamus and dorsal column nuclei. The lemniscal and corticospinal systems are the afferent and efferent components, respectively, of transcortical *long loop reflexes*, which complement the segmental myotatic reflexes in the control of motor neuron activity (see Chapter 8).

Spinocerebellar Tracts

The spinocerebellar tracts transmit information about the activity of the effector muscles or motor neuron pools to the cerebellum, where it is integrated and processed. The cerebellum is capable of modifying the action of different muscle groups so that movements are performed smoothly and accurately. Because the information carried by these pathways does not reach consciousness directly, it is referred to as *unconscious proprioception*.

The two spinal cord pathways that convey unconscious proprioceptive information to the cerebellum are the *dorsal* and *ventral spinocerebellar tracts*. They are part of the outer tube system and have some features in common, but they also have important anatomical and functional differences. Both tracts 1) originate from neurons in the intermediate gray matter; 2) contain large-diameter, rapidly conducting secondary axons (they are among the fastest conducting pathways in the central nervous system); 3) are located in the periphery of the lateral white matter of the spinal cord; 4) transmit information from the lower extremities; and 5) provide input predominantly to the ipsilateral cerebellum.

Dorsal Spinocerebellar Tract

The *dorsal spinocerebellar tract* originates in neurons of the nucleus dorsalis of Clarke (*Clarke column*) (Fig. 7.18). These neurons are potently excited by first-order proprioceptive fibers from muscle spindles of a single muscle or few agonists and from low-threshold cutaneous mechanoreceptors. Second-order axons from Clarke column enter the *ipsilateral* lateral funiculus to form the dorsal spinocerebellar tract. Fibers ascend near the lateral margin of the spinal cord. At the level of the medulla, they enter the cerebellum through the inferior cerebellar peduncle, or restiform body.

Because Clarke column is found only between spinal cord segments T1 and L1, two modifications of the basic organization of this pathway occur above and below these levels:

1. Fibers carrying proprioceptive information from the lower extremities and entering *below* L1 course in the dorsal column (fasciculus gracilis) until they reach segment L1. Thus, the lumbosacral spinal cord has no dorsal spinocerebellar tract.
2. Proprioceptive fibers entering *above* T1 (carrying information from the upper extremities to the cervical cord) do not have access to Clarke column or the dorsal spinocerebellar tract. Proprioceptive input from the upper extremities ascends in the dorsal column (fasciculus cuneatus) to synapse in the lower medulla in the *lateral*, or *accessory*, *nucleus cuneatus*, which is homologous to Clarke column.

Second-order neurons in the lateral nucleus cuneatus give rise to axons that form the *cuneocerebellar tract* (Fig. 7.18), which joins the dorsal spinocerebellar tract in the ipsilateral restiform body.

The dorsal spinocerebellar tract and cuneocerebellar tract are important in the rapid, efficient transmission of proprioceptive and exteroceptive signals from a single muscle or a few muscles to the cerebellum. This allows *feedback control* of motor performance through cerebellar influences on neurons in motor cortex and subcortical motor nuclei.

Ventral Spinocerebellar Tract

The *ventral spinocerebellar tract* originates in spinal border neurons in the lateral region of the ventral horn of the lumbar spinal cord. These neurons receive information simultaneously from primary proprioceptive and exteroceptive afferents and descending supraspinal pathways affecting ventral horn motor neurons and interneurons. Axons of the spinal border cells cross the midline to form the ventral spinocerebellar tract. This tract is lateral in the ventrolateral quadrant and ascends through the spinal cord, medulla, and pons to enter the cerebellum by a circuitous route through the superior cerebellar peduncle, or brachium conjunctivum. Within the posterior fossa, most of these fibers again cross so that the ventral spinocerebellar tract provides the cerebellum with bilateral but predominantly ipsilateral input about activity in the lower extremities. Input from the upper extremities relays on interneurons at spinal cord level C7 and C8. Axons of these interneurons ascend as the *rostral spinocerebellar tract*, entering predominantly the ipsilateral cerebellum through either the superior or inferior cerebellar peduncle.

The ventral spinocerebellar tract neurons act as comparators between the action of inhibitory and excitatory inputs to spinal motor neurons and interneurons. Thus, this tract provides the cerebellum with information about the state of excitation of these spinal cord neurons. The ventral spinocerebellar tract provides feed-forward information to the cerebellum about the activity of motor neuron pools, whereas the dorsal spinocerebellar

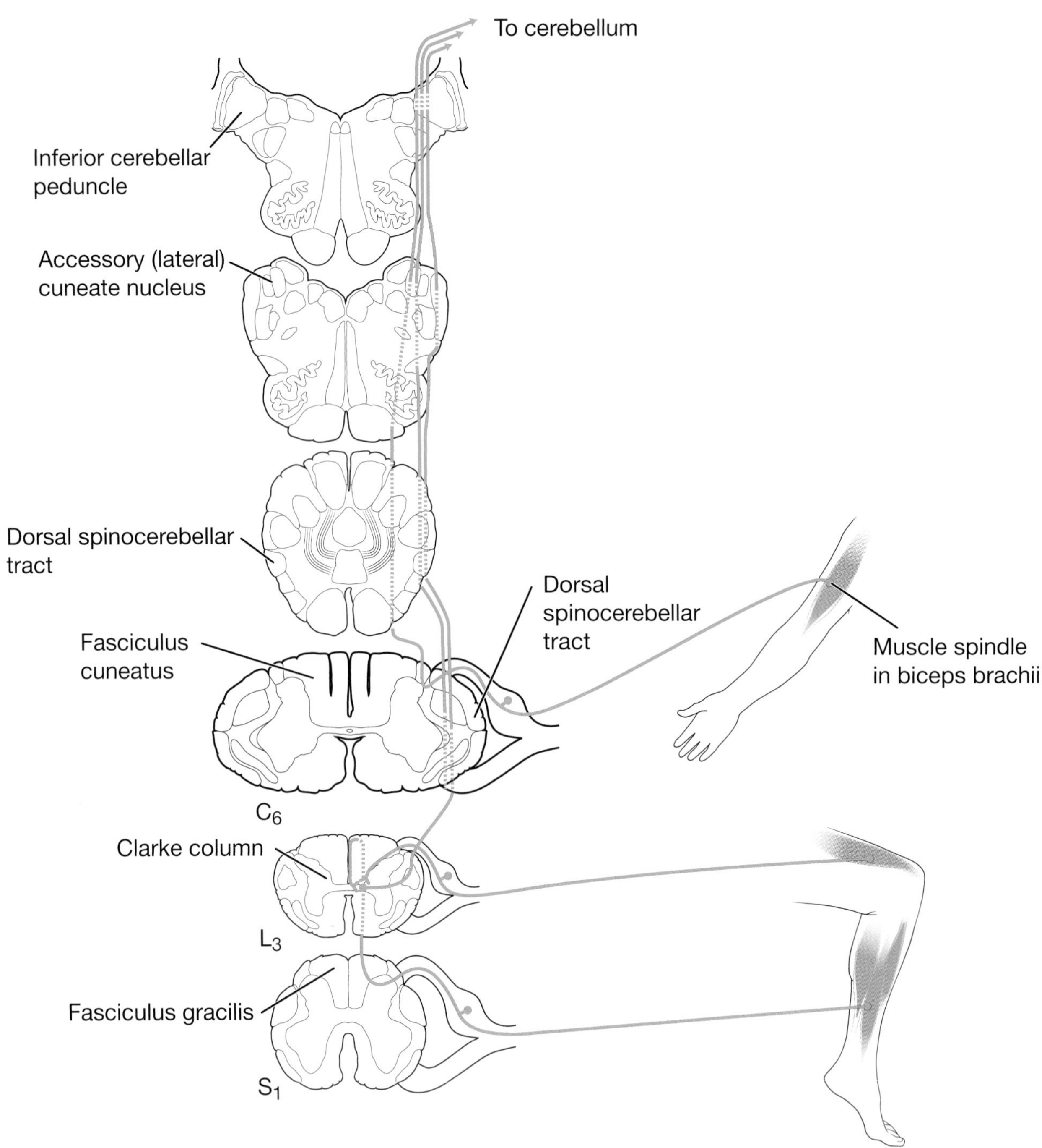

Fig. 7.18. Spinocerebellar pathways.

tract conveys feedback information about the resulting movement.

Effect of Lesions

The clinical manifestation of disease involving these pathways is motor incoordination, or ataxia, of the extremities. Although these pathways are physiologically important, it is extremely difficult clinically to identify abnormalities from damage of these pathways, which are commonly involved together with the dorsal columns.

The Differential Diagnosis of Ataxia

Definition

Sensory information is essential for the smooth, harmonious production of motor activity. A failure to produce normally smooth motor acts is referred to as *ataxia*. Ataxia may be manifested in the motion of a single limb but is more commonly evident during walking. With ataxia, movements become jerky and uncoordinated. The central nervous system must constantly be apprised of the position, tone, and movement of the limbs and trunk. This is accomplished by the integration (primarily in the cerebellum) of proprioceptive input and information from the receptors for equilibrium, which are located in the labyrinths of the inner ear, and by the transmission of these data back to the motor neurons. Visual input may be used in part to compensate for a defect in this integrating mechanism.

Types of Ataxia

Conditions in which motor performance is faulty when the motor pathways and the cerebellum are intact are examples of *sensory ataxia*. This occurs because of a defect in the transmission of proprioceptive or equilibratory information to higher centers. Frequently, sensory ataxia can be compensated for by using visual input to guide limb position; hence, the ataxia is often worse in the dark or when the eyes are closed. Conditions in which the sensory pathways are intact but motor performance is faulty are examples of *motor ataxia*. This occurs because of a defect in the integration and processing of proprioceptive information. Motor ataxia is usually due to disease of the cerebellum. This type of ataxia is often poorly compensated for by visual input.

The Romberg test is a quick and convenient method of distinguishing between sensory and motor ataxias. A patient who shows no unsteadiness when standing with the feet together and eyes open but who is unsteady with the eyes closed has a *Romberg sign*, which indicates that the patient has a sensory ataxia. Patients with a motor (cerebellar) ataxia may or may not be unsteady in the Romberg position but show little or no increase in unsteadiness when they close their eyes; thus, they do not have a Romberg sign.

Patients who have sensory ataxia generally have difficulty with either vestibular function or proprioception as a result of peripheral nerve or spinal cord disease. Ataxic patients without a Romberg sign often show abnormalities in cerebellar function.

- Sensory input from the muscles, joints, and skin provide continuous information about the conscious and unconscious position and movement of the limbs and trunk by large-fiber input to the spinal cord.
- The dorsal column–lemniscal system provides information about conscious proprioception.
- The dorsal and ventral spinocerebellar tracts transmit information about unconscious proprioception.
- The dorsal spinocerebellar and cuneocerebellar tracts are important in the rapid, efficient transmission of proprioceptive and exteroceptive signals from a single muscle or a few muscles to the cerebellum.
- The ventral spinocerebellar and rostral spinocerebellar tracts act as comparators between the action of inhibitory and excitatory inputs to spinal motor neurons and interneurons and thus provide the cerebellum with information about the state of excitation of these spinal cord neurons.
- Sensory ataxias include conditions in which motor performance is faulty when the motor pathways and the cerebellum are intact. Sensory ataxia is due to a defect in the transmission of proprioceptive information to higher centers.
- The Romberg test is used to distinguish between sensory and motor ataxias.

Other Sensory Systems

The pathways discussed above mediate the major general somatic sensations. Sensation from visceral structures (general visceral sensations), including visceral pain and sexual sensations, are mediated primarily by the spinothalamic and other anterolateral quadrant pathways, as discussed in Chapter 9. The special visceral afferent sensations of taste and smell and the special somatic sensations of hearing and balance are discussed in association with the posterior fossa (see Chapter 15B) and supratentorial (see Chapter 16A) levels. Because of the importance of the special somatic sensation of vision in clinical neurologic diagnosis and in localizing lesions, an overview of this pathway is warranted.

Visual Pathway

The visual pathway has many features typical of the lemniscal pathways, including a precise contralateral topographic representation of the sensory field (in this case, the visual field). Therefore, like the dorsal column and spinothalamic pathways, the visual pathway is commonly tested clinically to localize lesions in the nervous system. In contrast, the central organization of the pathways for audition, taste, and smell is largely bilateral and of limited value in the precise localization of a lesion to one side of the neuraxis.

The visual pathway is located entirely at the supratentorial level and is discussed in detail in Chapter 16A. Some of its features are considered here to emphasize important differences with the somatosensory pathways (Table 7.9). The receptor for light stimuli, the photoreceptor, is a specialized cell that responds to light stimuli by closing a cyclic nucleotide-gated channel. Thus, unlike the response of other receptors, the response to light stimuli is hyperpolarization. This results in a decrease in the tonic release of L-glutamate and its effects on the first-order neurons of the visual pathway, bipolar cells. Bipolar cells synapse on the second-order neurons of the visual pathway, ganglion cells. The axons of ganglion cells form the optic nerve (Fig. 7.19). The receptor, first-order neurons, and second-order neurons of the visual pathway are located in the retina, a derivative of the diencephalon, and the optic nerve is a tract of the central nervous system. The visual field is represented topographically (retinotopy) in the visual pathway. The nasal portion of the visual field is projected onto the temporal portion of the retina and the temporal portion of the visual field onto the nasal portion of the retina. The axons of ganglion cells in the nasal retina (which relay information from the temporal portion of the visual field) decussate in the optic chiasm, and the axons of ganglion cells in the temporal retina (which relay information from the nasal portion of the visual field) remain uncrossed. Crossed (contralateral) nasal and uncrossed (ipsilateral) fibers join at the optic chiasm and form the optic tracts. Thus, axons related to the right visual field travel in the left optic tract, and axons related to the left visual field travel in the right optic tract. Like other second-order axons, the right

Table 7.9. Comparison of the Somatosensory and Visual Pathways

Feature	Somatosensory pathways	Visual pathway
Stimulus	Mechanical or thermal	Light
Receptor	Specialized mechanoreceptors (touch, proprioception) or free nerve endings (nociceptors, thermoreceptors)	Photoreceptor
Ionic mechanism	Opening of a mechanosensitive cation channel	Closing of a cyclic nucleotide-gated cation channel
Response to stimulus	Depolarization of the axon of the first-order neuron	Hyperpolarization and decreased tonic release of glutamate at the synapse with the first-order neuron
First-order neuron	Dorsal root ganglion cell	Bipolar cell of the retina
Second-order neuron	Dorsal horn or dorsal column nuclei	Ganglion cell of the retina
Third-order neuron (thalamus)	Ventral posterolateral nucleus	Lateral geniculate nucleus
Cortical termination	Postcentral gyrus of the parietal lobe	Calcarine cortex of the occipital lobe

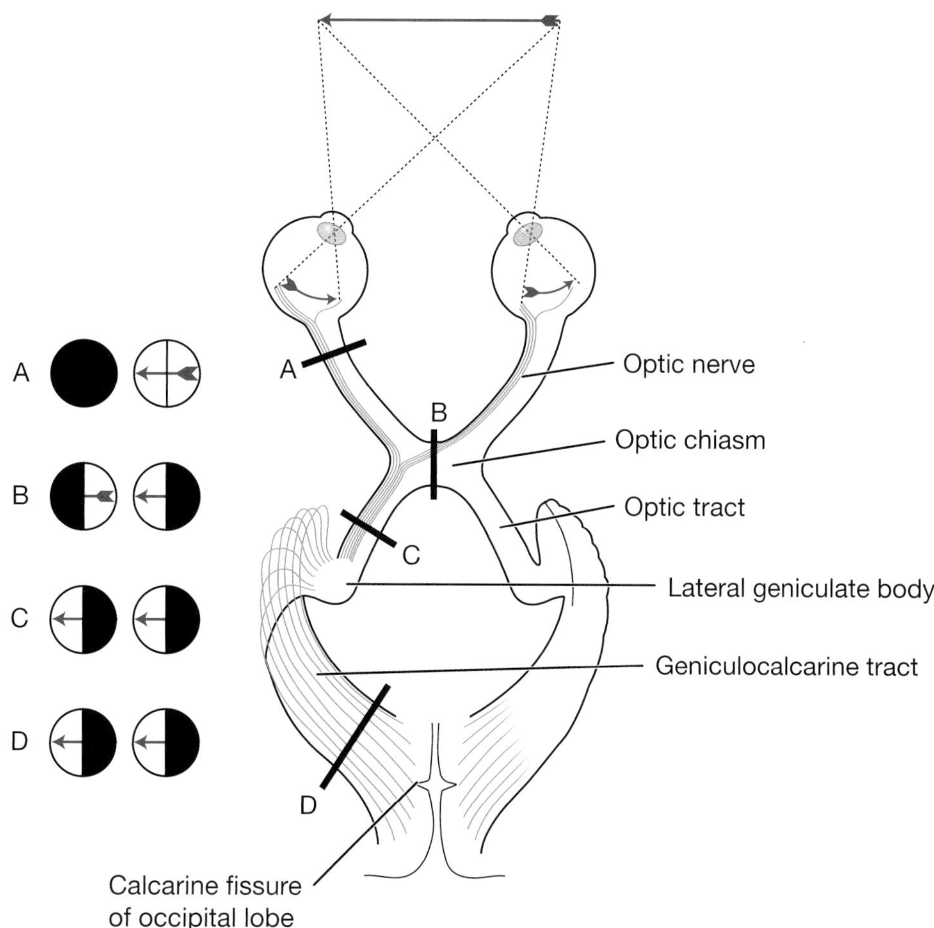

Fig. 7.19. The visual pathway. Visual field defects produced by lesions in this pathway are shown at the left. The visual field of the left eye is shown in the left circle, that of the right eye in the right circle. Lesions anterior to the optic chiasm (*A*) produce monocular loss of vision. Lesions at the optic chiasm (*B*) produce bitemporal hemianopia because of involvement of nasal-retinal crossing fibers. Unilateral lesions posterior to the optic chiasm affecting the optic tract (*C*), lateral geniculate body, optic radiations (*D*), or occipital cortex produce contralateral homonymous hemianopia.

and left optic tracts project to the thalamus and synapse in the ipsilateral lateral geniculate body. Neurons of the lateral geniculate body project through the optic radiations to the primary visual area, located in the calcarine cortex of the occipital lobe. Thus, the visual images of the right half of the visual field project to the left occipital cortex, and the images of the left visual field project to the right occipital cortex.

Lesions located anterior to the optic chiasm in the optic nerves interfere with vision only in the ipsilateral eye (monocular visual loss). Lesions in the center of the optic chiasm interfere only with the nasal crossing fibers, producing a loss of function of the nasal retina and of temporal vision in both eyes (*bitemporal hemianopia*). Lesions located posterior to the optic chiasm, that is, in the optic tracts, lateral geniculate body, optic radiations, or occipital cortex, produce a loss of vision in the contralateral visual fields of both eyes (*homonymous hemianopia*).

- The visual pathway is located entirely at the supratentorial level.
- The receptor for light stimuli is the photoreceptor.
- Bipolar cells synapse on the second-order neurons of the pathway, the ganglion cells, some of which

project to the contralateral lateral geniculate body and others to the ipsilateral lateral geniculate body.

- Third-order neurons arise from the lateral geniculate body and project to the primary visual cortex in the occipital lobe.
- Visual images of the right half of the visual field project to the left occipital cortex, and the images of the left visual field project to the right occipital cortex.

Clinical Correlations

Disease processes affecting the sensory system produce various symptoms, including pain, *hypesthesia* (reduced sensation), *anesthesia* (complete loss of cutaneous sensibility), *dysesthesia* (altered or perverted interpretation of sensation, such as a burning, tingling, or painful feeling in response to touch), and *paresthesia* (spontaneous sensation of prickling or tingling). In some instances, sensory stimuli are felt more keenly than normal (*hyperesthesia*). It is extremely important in every case of pain or sensory loss to determine its exact distribution.

Lesions at the Peripheral Level

The distal axons of the primary sensory neurons mediating all types of afferent input are gathered together, along with motor and autonomic fibers, in peripheral nerves. Thus, a lesion that affects peripheral nerves would be expected to produce a variable sensory loss for all modalities and a loss of muscle stretch reflexes in the anatomical distribution of that nerve. Some motor or autonomic deficit usually can be found if such fibers are present in the involved nerve. This type of deficit may occur in a focal distribution when only a single peripheral nerve is involved (as might occur from trauma) and is called *mononeuropathy*. When these symptoms and signs occur in a diffuse distribution, the deficit is called *polyneuropathy*. Pain, paresthesias, or dysesthesias are common accompaniments of peripheral nerve lesions. The cutaneous distribution of the major peripheral nerves is shown in Figure 7.7.

Lesions at the Spinal Level

Disease processes located within the spinal canal typically produce 1) a segmental neurologic deficit limited to one level of the body and usually caused by involvement of the nerve roots or spinal nerves, and 2) an intersegmental sensory deficit involving all the body below a particular level and caused by the interruption of the major ascending sensory pathways. Mechanical compression or local inflammation of a dorsal root or spinal nerve produces pain along the anatomical distribution of the affected root. Pain due to nerve root involvement and located in the distribution of one or more dermatomes (Fig. 7.6) is known as *radicular pain*. This type of pain, which may vary in intensity, is often lancinating (a sharp, darting type of pain). Maneuvers that increase intraspinal pressure (and presumably increase the traction on irritated nerve roots), such as coughing, sneezing, and straining, produce a characteristic increase in this type of pain. In addition

Clinical Problem 7.3.

A 40-year-old man had onset of neck pain and paresthesias over the occipital region of the head 6 months earlier. These symptoms were aggravated by coughing and sneezing. Three months ago, his symptoms became worse, and he noted a tingling sensation up and down his spinal column whenever he bent his neck. One month ago, he noted progressive difficulty in walking in the dark. On examination, he was found to have decreased perception to touch and pinprick sensation over the posterior scalp region, reduced position sense in his arms and legs bilaterally, decreased vibratory sensation in both upper and lower extremities, and decreased ability to perceive discriminative tactile sensation bilaterally.

a. What is the anatomicopathologic diagnosis?
b. What segmental structures provide sensory innervation to the posterior scalp region?
c. What sensory structures are involved by the lesion?
d. What is the precise level of lesion responsible?
e. How would the symptoms and signs differ if the lesion were located at the T6 spinal level?

to producing radicular pain, lesions of the dorsal root or spinal nerve produce areas of paresthesia, hyperesthesia, or loss of cutaneous sensation in a dermatomal distribution. At appropriate levels, segmental loss of muscle stretch reflexes, weakness, and autonomic disturbances can be seen.

Commissural Syndrome

A special type of segmental deficit can result from a lesion involving the central regions of the spinal cord, usually over several segments. This deficit is characterized by a loss of pain and temperature sensation from interruption of the second-order axons as they decussate to form the spinothalamic tracts (Fig. 7.20). The sensory loss is bilateral because fibers from both sides are interrupted by the lesion, and it involves the crossing fibers of several adjacent segments. Thus, a lesion involving the central regions of segments T2 through T5 produces loss of pain and temperature sensation only in those segments. The commissural syndrome can be produced only by a lesion in the substance of the spinal cord.

As the lesion enlarges, adjacent sensory tracts become involved. This type of lesion may result from trauma (*hematomyelia*), neoplasm, or other conditions, including *syringomyelia*.

Clinical Problem 7.4.

A 41-year-old woman noted a painless, slowly progressive loss of sensation in an area involving the back of her head, neck, shoulders, and both upper extremities. Neurologic examination showed a sensory loss involving only pain and temperature in this area. Specific testing of all other modalities of sensation in the affected areas and elsewhere showed no abnormalities. There was no change in motor performance, strength, or muscle stretch reflexes.

a. What is the anatomicopathologic diagnosis?
b. What sensory structure(s) is (are) involved by the lesion?
c. What is the most likely pathologic lesion responsible for this clinical syndrome?

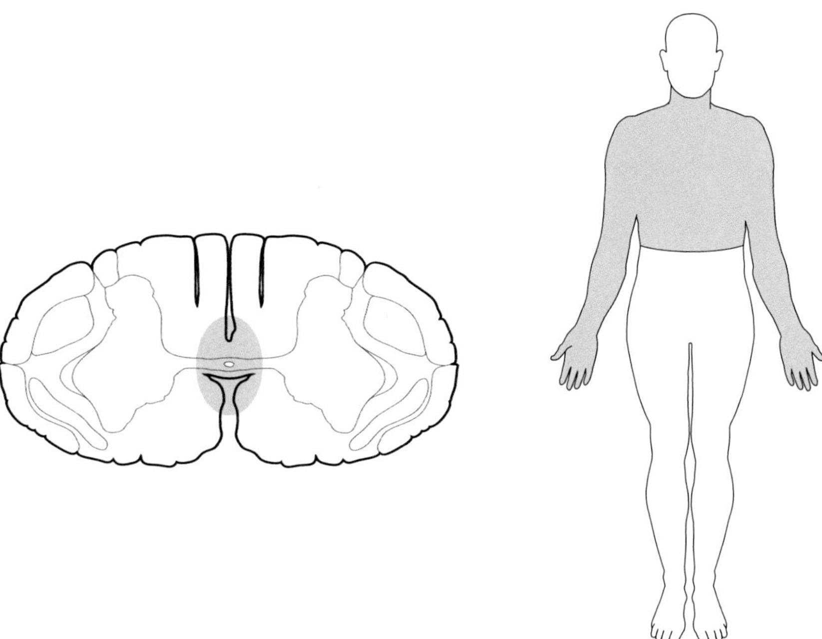

Fig. 7.20. Commissural syndrome. Distribution of loss of pain and temperature sensation with a lesion in the location shown on the left.

Syringomyelia is a common cause of the commissural syndrome and consists of cavitation occurring within the central area of the spinal cord (Fig. 7.21). Whether the cavity develops as a result of dilatation of the primitive central canal (hydromyelia) or from some other destructive process in the central region of the cord, such as an intramedullary neoplasm, is not always clear. Although initially the cavity is centrally located, its expansion and the surrounding gliosis tend to extend the syrinx irregularly throughout the gray matter and, at times, into the spinothalamic tract neurons.

Spinothalamic Tract Syndrome

A lesion involving the spinothalamic tract causes a loss of pain and temperature sensation on the opposite side of the body, involving all segments below the level of the lesion. Pain and temperature fibers enter through the dorsal root and extend rostrally in Lissauer tract for up to two segments above their entry zone before synapsing with the spinothalamic tract neurons of the dorsal horn.

Therefore, the sensory level on the side opposite a spinothalamic tract lesion is usually at least two segments below the level of the actual lesion. Within the spinothalamic tract, the fibers are arranged in a laminar fashion, with the sacral fibers near the periphery and fibers from higher levels toward the center. Hence, lesions arising within the substance of the spinal cord (intramedullary lesions) may involve only the central portions of the tract and spare the peripheral fibers and produce a loss of pain and temperature sensation at all levels below the lesion except the sacral level. This is referred to as sacral sparing. When present, sacral sparing is an important clue to an intramedullary spinal cord lesion (Fig. 7.22).

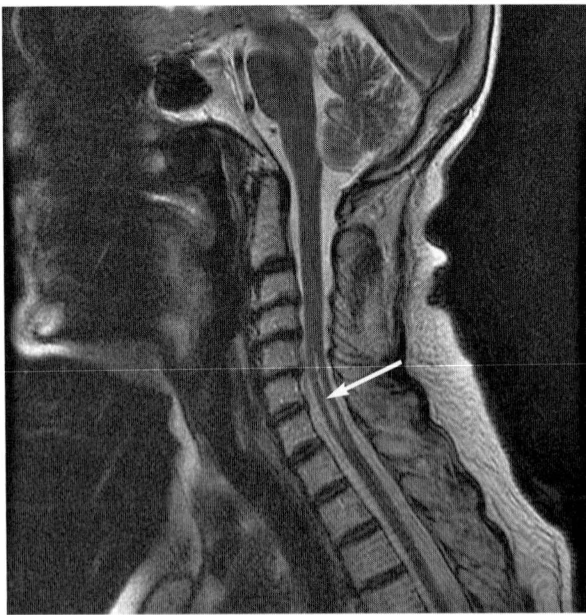

Fig. 7.21. Syringomyelia. Magnetic resonance image of syringomyelia at the level of the cervical spinal cord (*arrow*).

In certain instances of intractable pain involving the lower extremity, pain may be relieved by placing a lesion in the spinothalamic tract (spinothalamic tractotomy). It is usually done by surgically cutting the ventral portion of the lateral funiculus in the cervical area, although there is probably some damage to the dorsal and lateral columns. The lesion most commonly occurs in the cervical area.

Brown-Séquard Syndrome

This syndrome occurs in pure form with hemisection of the spinal cord. In clinical practice, the syndrome is often partial and incomplete; however, the findings of ipsilateral motor deficit, ipsilateral dorsal column deficit, and contralateral loss of pain and temperature sensation usually are present and are characteristic of a unilateral spinal cord lesion (Fig. 7.23).

Lesions at the Posterior Fossa Level

Disease processes affecting the posterior fossa level are characterized by a contralateral intersegmental loss of sensory function in the trunk and limbs because of interruption of the major ascending pathways. However, frequently sensory function (primarily pain and temperature sensation) is also lost over the ipsilateral face because of segmental involvement of the trigeminal nerve or its descending tract and nucleus (Fig. 7.24).

Lesions at the Supratentorial Level

At this level, all major sensory pathways have crossed to the contralateral side; therefore, lesions at this level alter sensory function over the entire contralateral side of the body. Two important variations of sensory loss may be

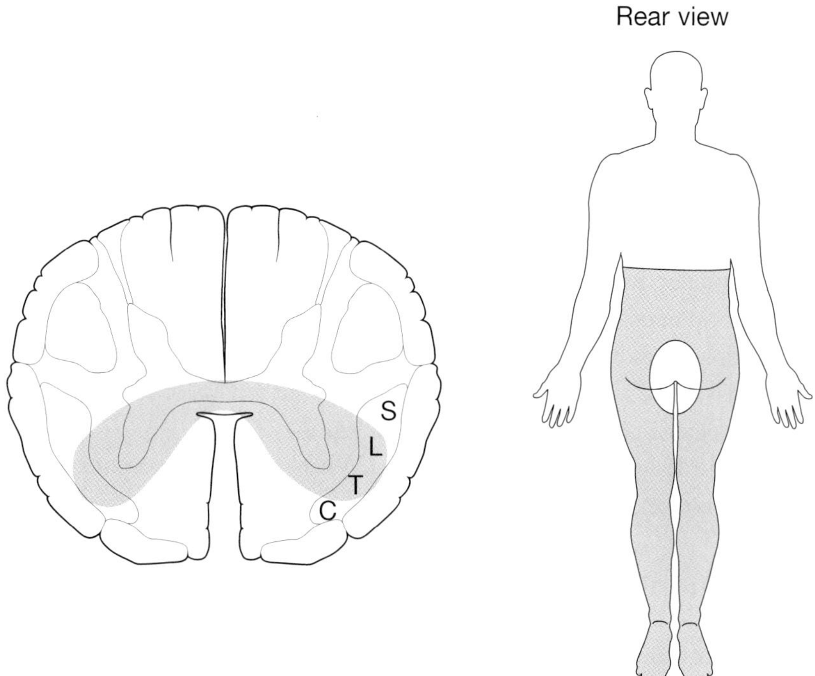

Fig. 7.22. Sensory loss with sacral sparing due to the intramedullary lesion shown on the left. The lesion involves the spinothalamic tracts bilaterally. (Note that the figure in the diagram is viewed from behind.) C, cervical; T, thoracic; L, lumbar; S, sacral.

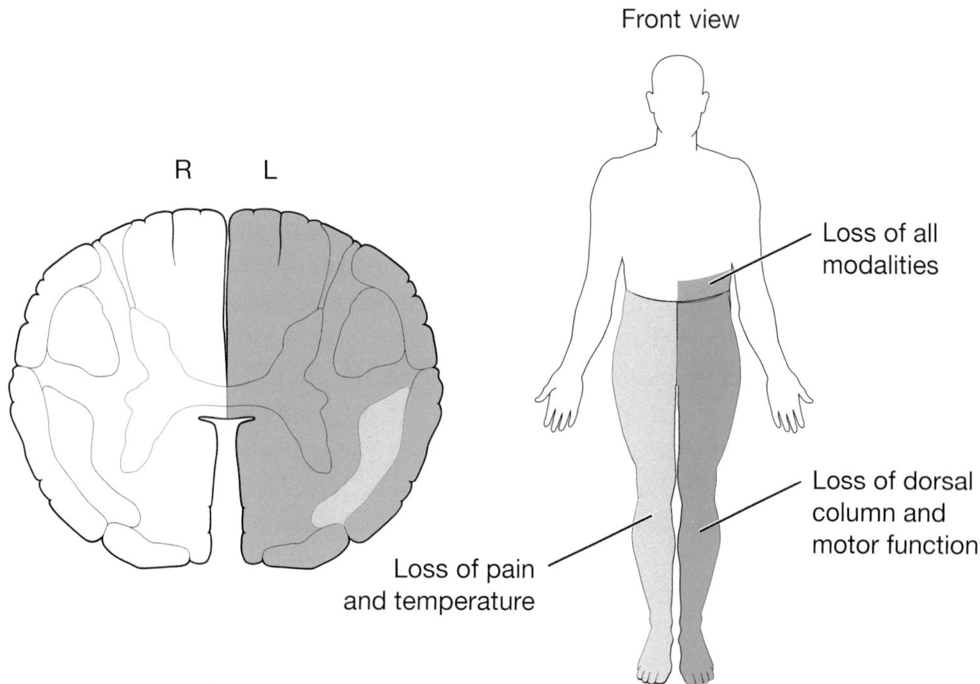

Fig. 7.23. Brown-Séquard syndrome. Sensory loss produced by damage to one-half of the spinal cord by the lesion shown on the left. An ipsilateral motor deficit would also be present (see Chapter 8).

Clinical Problem 7.5.

A 21-year-old soldier returned from battle after sustaining a gunshot wound in his spinal column. On neurologic examination, you note that he has weakness of the left lower extremity. In addition, he has loss of pain and temperature perception on the right side from about the level of his navel downward. Vibration, joint position sense, and discriminatory function are reduced in the left leg. Touch sensation is normal.

a. What is the anatomicopathologic diagnosis?
b. What is the precise level of the lesion?
c. What is the name given to this type of syndrome?
d. Why is the sensation of touch preserved in this patient?
e. Where in the nervous system would you expect to find evidence of wallerian degeneration?

Clinical Problem 7.6.

A 68-year-old woman with hypertension awoke one morning and noticed that she was unable to feel anything over the entire left side of her body. On neurologic examination, motor strength and reflexes were normal, as were the visual fields; however, she did not respond to pinprick, temperature, or touch stimuli over the left side of her face, trunk, and extremities, and she could not perceive joint motion or vibration in her left arm and leg.

a. What is the anatomicopathologic diagnosis?
b. What specific sensory system structure(s) is (are) most likely involved?
c. Where in the nervous system would you expect to find evidence of wallerian degeneration?

encountered with lesions at this level: the thalamic syndrome and suprathalamic syndrome.

Thalamic Syndrome

The thalamus is an important integrating and relay station for sensory perception. A lesion affecting the specific sensory nuclei of the thalamus causes a relatively complete loss of all forms of general somatic afferent sensation in the contralateral face, trunk, and limbs (Fig. 7.25). If the portion of the thalamus related to vision is also involved, a contralateral homonymous hemianopia is produced. After a localized lesion of the thalamus, a severe burning (dysesthetic) pain is sometimes produced in the area of sensory loss, perhaps from faulty integration of sensory information.

Suprathalamic Syndrome

Lesions that involve sensory pathways from the thalamus to the cerebral cortex or in the cerebral cortex itself also alter all forms of general somatic afferent sensation on the contralateral side of the body. However, in contrast to the dense loss of sensation found with thalamic lesions, suprathalamic involvement is characterized by only minimal involvement of pain, temperature, touch, and vibratory sensibility and by a severe deficit in the discriminative sensations that require cortical participation (Fig. 7.26). These sensations are joint position sense, two-point discrimination, touch localization, and the recognition of objects placed in the hand (*stereognosis*), suggesting that discriminative sensations require intact thalamocortical pathways for their full appreciation, whereas the primary modalities of superficial sensation are perceived and integrated at the thalamic level. This type of discriminative sensory loss is often found with lesions of the parietal lobe and is commonly referred to as a *cortical sensory deficit*. If the optic radiations are also involved, a contralateral visual field defect is produced. In the absence of a visual field defect or other signs of supratentorial involvement, this type of sensory deficit may be confused with the findings of dorsal column disease. A severe deficit in conscious proprioception, bilateral involvement, and associated alteration in vibratory sense

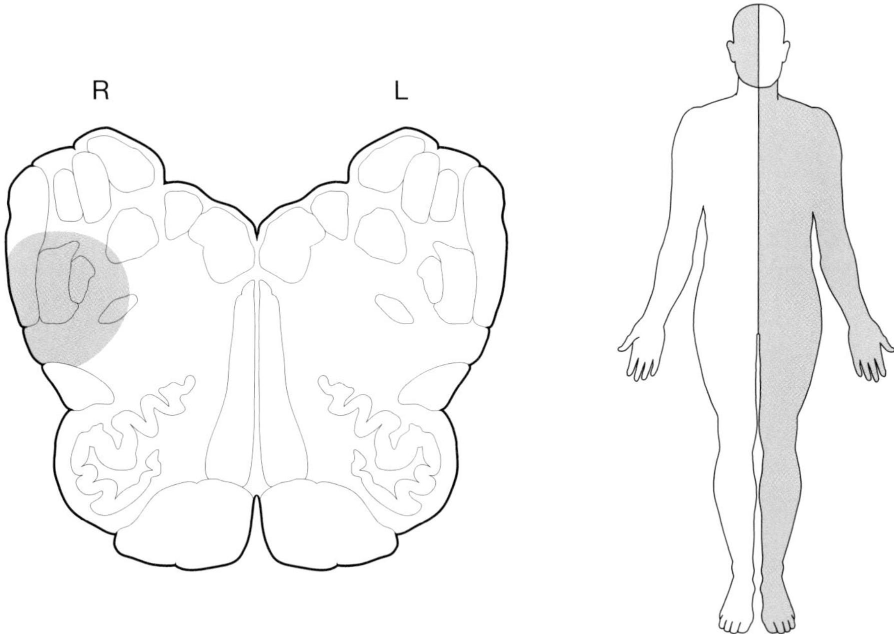

Fig. 7.24. Distribution of pain and temperature sensation loss characteristic of lesions at the posterior fossa level, as shown on the left.

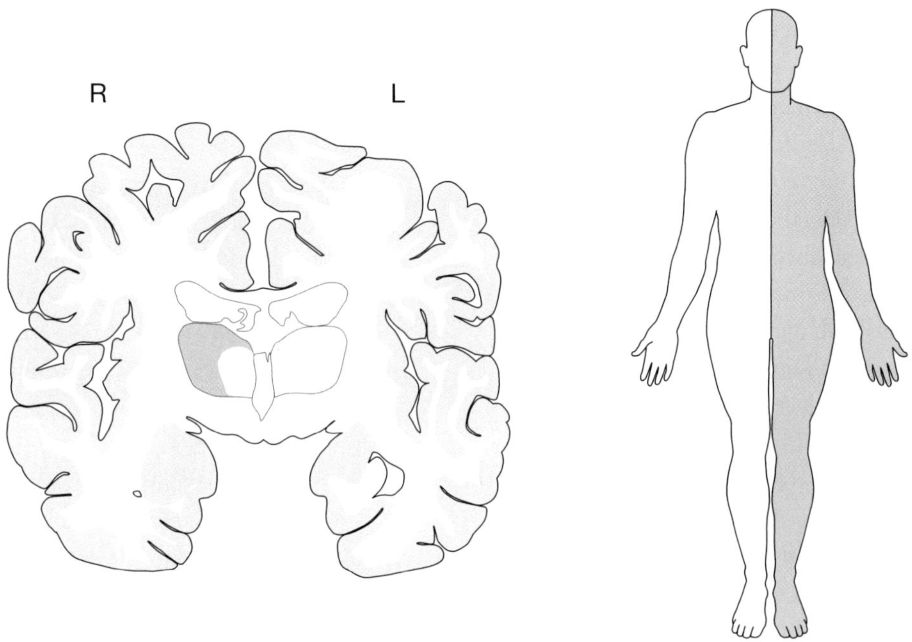

Fig. 7.25. Thalamic syndrome. Loss of all sensory modalities contralateral to the lesion.

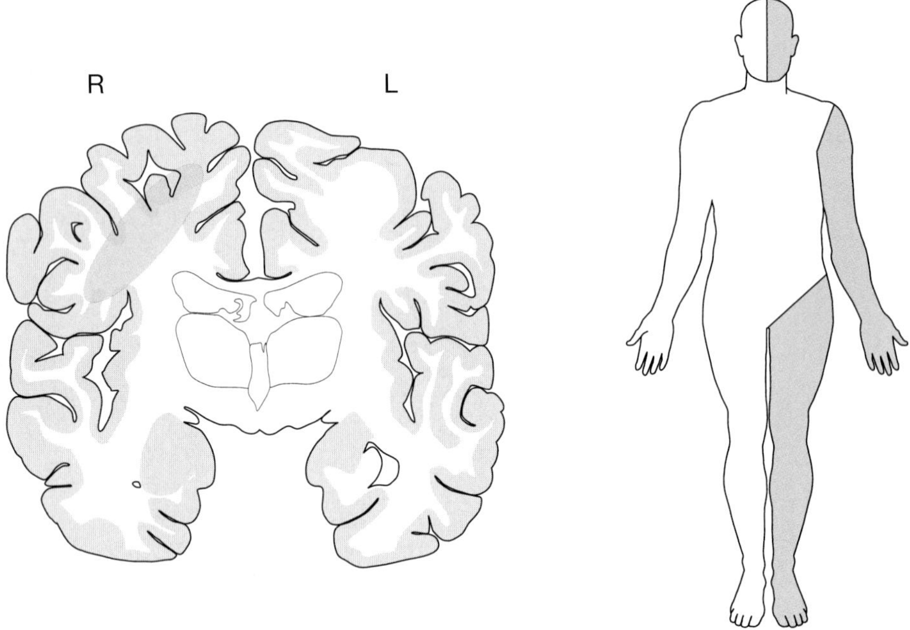

Fig. 7.26. Suprathalamic syndrome. Loss of cortical sensory functions contralateral to the lesion.

all favor a lesion of the dorsal columns. When the deficit is unilateral, the distinction between a suprathalamic and a high cervical spinal cord lesion can be extremely difficult unless other signs and symptoms are present to aid with localization.

Irritative lesions located in the region of the postcentral gyrus may initiate seizures. The clinical manifestations of seizures in this area consist primarily of a feeling of tingling (paresthesias) on the opposite side of the body. As the localized neuronal discharge spreads from its focus of origin, these sensations may be experienced as moving in an orderly fashion dictated by the topographic organization of the gyrus. Further spread to the adjacent precentral gyrus may produce associated motor activity, and spread to subcortical structures may produce a loss of consciousness.

Somatosensory Evoked Response

The somatosensory evoked response is an electrodiagnostic test used to evaluate the sensory system (Fig. 7.27). Evoked responses are electrical potentials that occur with a fixed latency in response to a stimulus.

Clinical Problem 7.7.

A 31-year-old man noticed the gradual onset of headaches. On several occasions during the last month, he experienced spells consisting of a curious tingling, burning sensation that began in the left thumb and the left corner of his mouth. This gradually became more intense and spread to involve his left hand and the left side of his face and then extended up his arm, trunk, and leg. In 5 minutes, the spell would cease and he would feel sleepy. Neurologic examination shows a striking inability to perceive joint position, motion, and other discriminative testing over the left side. Touch, pain, temperature, and vibratory sensations are preserved.

a. What is the anatomicopathologic diagnosis?
b. What is the nature of the spell experienced by the patient?
c. Why were some forms of sensation involved and not others?

Because these potentials are very small, many successive responses need to be averaged and amplified to be seen. Somatosensory evoked responses are potentials that occur in response to stimulation of a peripheral nerve and can be recorded from the nerve, the plexus, the sensory pathways within the spinal cord and brainstem, the thalamocortical pathways, and the somatosensory cortex. Abnormalities of the somatosensory evoked responses occur with lesions or disease processes involving the sensory pathways at any of these levels and are manifested either by an increase in latency or by a decrease in amplitude or an absence of response. Somatosensory evoked responses are used to document or diagnose multiple sclerosis, degenerative processes, traumatic lesions, and other structural lesions affecting the peripheral or central sensory system.

- Lesions at the peripheral level typically result in variable sensory loss for all modalities and a loss of muscle stretch reflexes in the anatomical distribution of that nerve.
- Lesions at the spinal level cause a segmental neurologic deficit limited to one level of the body (usually caused by involvement of the nerve roots or spinal nerves) and an intersegmental sensory deficit involving all the body below a particular level.
- Lesions at the posterior fossa level are characterized by a contralateral intersegmental loss of sensory function in the trunk and limbs because of interruption of the major ascending pathways. However, frequently sensory function (primarily pain and temperature sensation) is also lost over the ipsilateral face because of segmental involvement of the trigeminal nerve or its descending tract and nucleus.
- Lesions at the supratentorial level alter sensory function over the entire contralateral side of the body.

Neurologic Examination: Sensory System

A complete sensory examination includes the evaluation of touch, pain, temperature, joint position, and vibratory sensations as well as various discriminatory modalities. Comparison of one side of the body with the other and with the examiner's own sensory abilities is useful for establishing "normal" and "abnormal." Much of the sensory examination is best performed with the patient's eyes closed to eliminate visual cues. Examination of sensation consists of three portions: 1) qualitative, to determine the elements of sensation that are affected; 2) quantitative, to determine the degree of involvement when sensation is impaired; and 3) anatomical, to map the areas of sensory impairment.

Sensation is tested in the following ways:

1. Touch—Lightly place a piece of cotton on the face, trunk, and extremities, and ask the patient to respond when it is felt.
2. Pain—Gently prick the patient with a pin. A more

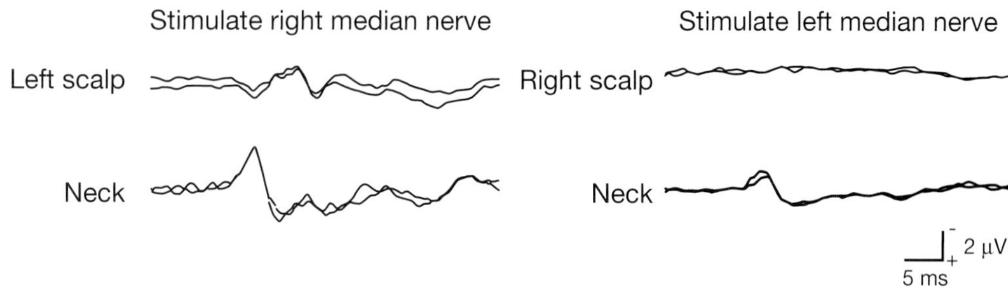

Fig. 7.27. Somatosensory evoked responses recorded from the neck and scalp in a patient with multiple sclerosis. Note the decrease in the amplitude of the potential recorded from the right neck and scalp compared with those recorded from the left side.

accurate determination can be made by randomly touching the patient with the point or head of a pin and noting whether the patient can appreciate sharp and dull sensations.

3. Temperature—Randomly apply warm and cool objects to the skin, and note the patient's ability to distinguish between them.
4. Vibration sense—Place a vibrating tuning fork over bony prominences, and note whether the patient can detect the sensation and determine when the vibration ceases. (In patients older than 50 years, vibratory sense is often reduced in the feet.)
5. Joint position sense—Firmly grasp the sides of the great toe or a finger, and ask the patient to detect and respond to movements in an upward or downward direction.
6. Two-point discrimination—A two-point caliper is used. This sensation is normally examined only on the fingertips by asking the patient to respond to the tactile stimulus of one or two points. The threshold (minimal recognizable separation) is determined and compared on the two sides of the body.
7. Tactile localization—Touch the patient, and request that the point of contact be identified.
8. Graphesthesia—Ask the patient to identify numbers or letters traced on the palm of his or her hand with a blunt object.
9. Stereognosis—Ask the patient to close his or her eyes and identify objects of different sizes, shapes, and textures (such as a coin, key, clip, or safety pin) placed in the hand.

In the absence of any sensory symptoms or the patient's subjective sensation of pain, a brief screening examination consisting of a test of touch, pain, joint position, and vibratory sense in both hands and both feet and of a test of pain and touch perception on the face is all that is required. When a sensory deficit is suspected or identified, the examiner must determine the modality of sensation involved and map its distribution to discover if it conforms to that found with lesions of a peripheral nerve, a spinal nerve or dorsal root, the spinal cord, the posterior fossa, or the supratentorial region.

Additional Reading

Almeida TF, Roizenblatt S, Tufik S. Afferent pain pathways: a neuroanatomical review. Brain Res. 2004;1000:40-56.

Davidoff RA. The dorsal columns. Neurology. 1989;39:1377-1385.

Fields HL, Heinricher MM, Mason P. Neurotransmitters in nociceptive modulatory circuits. Annu Rev Neurosci. 1991;14:219-245.

Freund HJ. Somatosensory and motor disturbances in patients with parietal lobe lesions. Adv Neurol. 2003;93:179-193.

Sewards TV, Sewards M. Separate, parallel sensory and hedonic pathways in the mammalian somatosensory system. Brain Res Bull. 2002;58:243-260.

Willis WD, Westlund KN. Neuroanatomy of the pain system and of the pathways that modulate pain. J Clin Neurophysiol. 1997;14:2-31.

Chapter 8

The Motor System

Objectives

1. Define lower motor neuron, motor unit, and size principle.
2. Describe the receptors, afferents, central connections, and functions of the muscle stretch reflex and Golgi tendon organ reflex.
3. Describe the function of the gamma motor neuron, Ia inhibitory interneuron, presynaptic Ia inhibitory interneuron, Ib inhibitory interneuron, and Renshaw cell.
4. Describe the importance of interneurons in motor control.
5. Describe the consequences of lesions involving the final common pathway.
6. Describe the cortical motor areas and the composition, course, termination, and function of the corticospinal tract.
7. Name the location and functions of the brainstem nuclei that project to the motor neurons and interneurons.
8. Describe the manifestations of the upper motor neuron syndrome. Compare these manifestations with those of the lower motor neuron syndrome.
9. Describe the pathophysiologic mechanisms of spasticity and the location of lesions producing decorticate and decerebrate postures.
10. Describe the gross anatomy and basic circuit of the cerebellum.
11. Describe the main connections and functions of the cerebellar flocculonodular lobe, vermis, and hemispheres.
12. Name the manifestations of lesions involving the cerebellar flocculonodular lobe, vermis, or hemisphere.
13. Name the components, main neurotransmitters, and principal connections of the basal ganglia circuits.
14. Describe how the basal ganglia control the execution of motor programs.
15. Describe the source and effects of dopamine on the basal ganglia.
16. Name the features of parkinsonism and hyperkinetic movement disorders.
17. Diagram the connections of the major components of the motor system: motor cortex, thalamus, basal ganglia, cerebellum, brainstem, spinal cord, and final common pathway.

Introduction

The entire range of human activity—from walking and talking to gymnastics to control of the space shuttle—depends on the motor system. On the basis of external sensory information and centrally determined goals, this system initiates and coordinates the actions of muscles moving the joints. The unique capacities of the motor system cannot be duplicated by even the most sophisticated robots, especially the ability to learn new patterns and to adapt to unexpected changes. The inability to duplicate the capabilities of the motor system is a reflection of its complexity and our incomplete understanding of how it works.

All bodily movements, including those of internal organs, are the result of muscle contraction, which is under neural control. The muscles of the limbs, trunk, neck, and eyes are derived from somites. The muscles involved in facial expression, mastication, phonation, and swallowing are derived from the branchial arches. Somatic and limbic motor pathways arising from the cerebral cortex and brainstem control the activity of the motor neurons innervating all these muscles. The internal organs are part of the internal regulation system. The general visceral efferent structures that control smooth muscle are described in Chapter 9.

The motor system, like the sensory system, includes a complex network of structures and pathways at all levels of the nervous system. This network is organized to mediate many types of motor activity. An understanding of this organization and the integration of the motor system with the sensory system is necessary for accurate localization and diagnosis of neurologic disease. Weakness, paralysis, twitching, jerking, staggering, wasting, shaking, stiffness, spasticity, and incoordination involving the arms, legs, eyes, or muscles of speech are all due to impairment of the motor system. This chapter describes and discusses an organization of the motor system that can help in the identification of disorders of the system.

Overview

The general organization of the motor system is depicted in Figure 8.1. The final output from the central nervous system to the effector muscles arises from alpha motor neurons (also called lower motor neurons) located in the ventral horn of the spinal cord and motor cranial nerve nuclei of the brainstem. This output is referred to as the

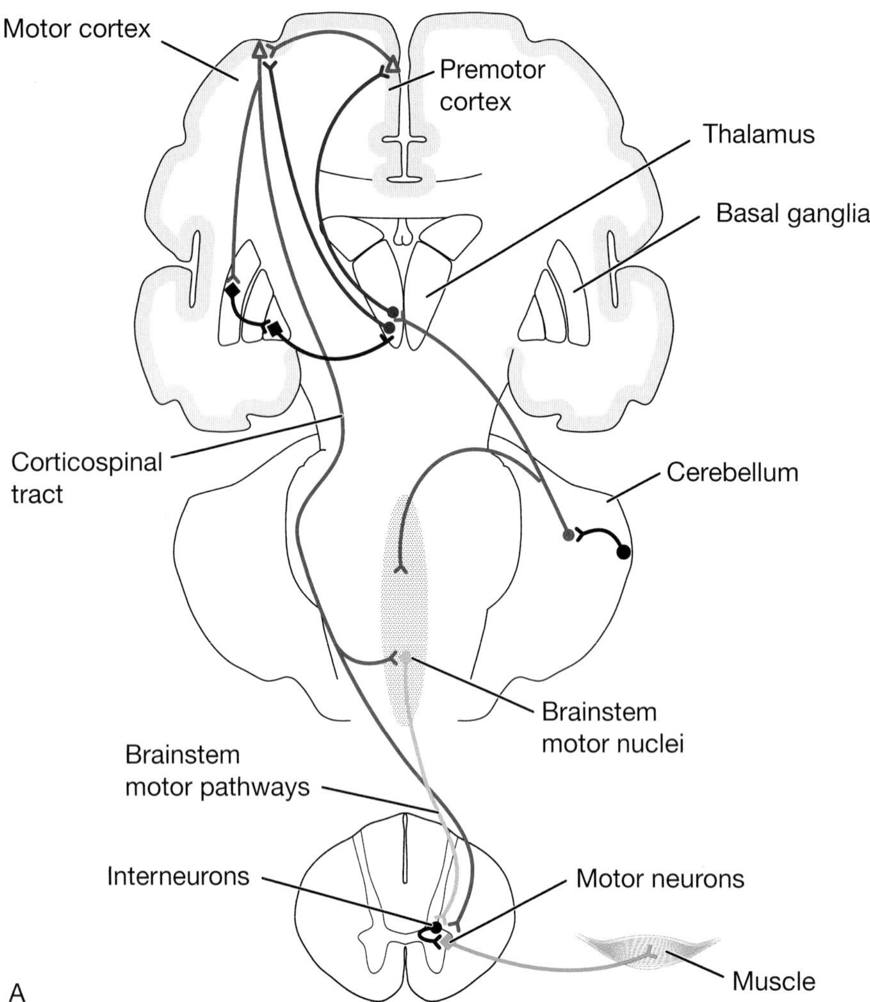

Fig. 8.1. *A*, Outline of the motor system. *B*, Basic connections of the motor system. Motor neurons in the ventral horn of the spinal cord and the motor nuclei of the brainstem are the final common pathway that innervate skeletal muscles. Motor neurons receive input from the contralateral motor cortex through the corticospinal tract and from several brainstem nuclei. The cerebellum coordinates ipsilateral movements of the limbs by its connections with the spinal cord, brainstem, and contralateral motor cortex. The basal ganglia participate in motor planning and initiation of motor programs through connections with ipsilateral motor cortex. Afferents from muscle receptors and other receptors initiate segmental reflexes and provide sensory feedback to the cerebellum, brainstem, and cerebral cortex.

final common pathway because it mediates all types of movement. The alpha motor neuron, its axon (traveling peripherally in a nerve), its terminal arborizations, and all the muscle fibers it innervates constitute a *motor unit*. The alpha motor neuron excites muscle fibers by the release of acetylcholine and exerts a trophic influence on the muscle by the release of other chemical signals.

The activity of alpha motor neurons is controlled by segmental inputs (primary afferents) from the limbs and by descending inputs from supraspinal structures. With few important exceptions, these segmental and supraspinal inputs affect motor neurons indirectly through excitatory or inhibitory *interneurons*. The segmental inputs arise from receptors in muscles, joints, and skin and trigger several reflexes that activate or inhibit specific populations of alpha motor neurons. An important example is the *muscle stretch* (or myotatic) reflex. In this reflex, stimulation of muscle spindles activates large myelinated afferents that stimulate the alpha motor neurons innervating the corresponding muscle. This reflex provides a feedback mechanism for maintenance of muscle length and excitability of alpha motor neurons and contributes to the maintenance of muscle tone.

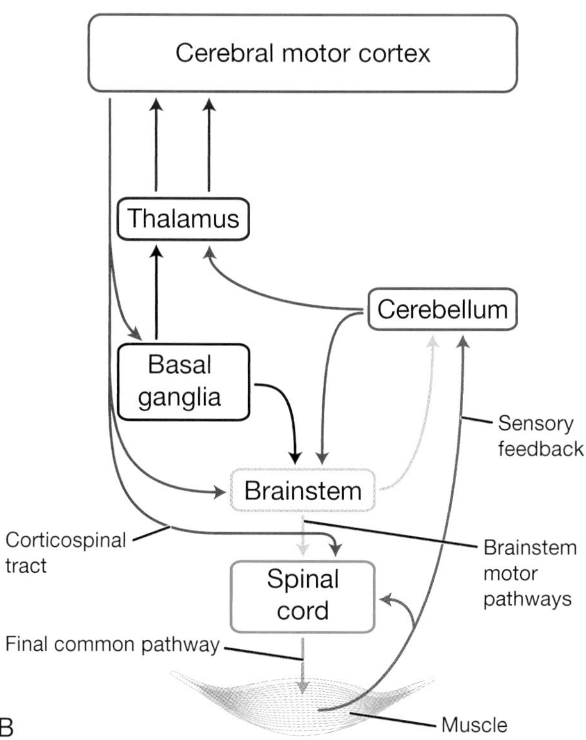

Disease processes that impair the function of a motor unit prevent the normal activation and maintenance of the muscle fibers of that motor unit. This is manifested by the inability of the muscle to contract fully (weakness or paralysis) and by muscle atrophy, loss of muscle stretch reflexes and muscle tone, and abnormal spontaneous activity of the motor axon leading to contraction of all the fibers of the motor unit (fasciculation). These effects constitute the *lower motor neuron syndrome*. Because intact muscle stretch reflexes involve both afferents from the muscle and motor output to the muscle, the loss of these reflexes may be due to damage to either the final common pathway or the sensory input pathway to the motor neuron.

The descending pathways that control motor neurons originate from motor areas of the cerebral cortex and the brainstem. These pathways control the activity of motor neurons either directly or, more commonly, indirectly through interneurons and mediate all voluntary movements and postural and segmental reflexes. The largest, best-defined descending motor pathway is the *corticospinal tract* (or pyramidal tract), which arises from several motor areas in the frontal cortex and provides a direct activation pathway to contralateral motor neurons. These cortical motor neurons are referred to as *upper motor neurons*. Damage restricted to the corticospinal tracts produces contralateral weakness, with loss of voluntary movements, especially fine, skilled movements.

The descending indirect pathways from the brainstem originate from several nuclei, including the red nucleus, vestibular nuclei, and nuclei of the pontine and medullary reticular formation. The vestibular nuclei are critical for maintenance of the erect posture against gravity. The medullary reticular formation, which receives input from the motor cortex, suppresses segmental and postural reflexes that may interfere with the execution of voluntary motor acts. Lesions of the central nervous system generally affect both the direct corticospinal and the indirect cortical pathway through the medullary reticular formation. Therefore, the *upper motor neuron syndrome* includes both weakness and loss of dexterity (from involvement of the corticospinal pathway), but also exaggeration of segmental reflexes (from impaired function of the corticoreticulospinal system) and increased muscle tone, called *spasticity*. A typical feature of the upper motor neuron syndrome is the abnormal extensor response of the toe evoked by stimulation of the sole of the foot, called the *Babinski sign*.

The cortical and brainstem motor areas are regulated by cortical motor association areas called *premotor* areas. These areas are involved in learning and programming of motor acts. Lesions that affect the premotor cortex produce *apraxia*, which is the inability to perform learned motor acts without the person having weakness or other motor disorder.

The motor system includes two control circuits that center on the *cerebellum* and *basal ganglia*. Both the cerebellum and basal ganglia receive input from the motor cortex and project back to the premotor and motor cortices by way of the thalamus and also project to motor areas of the brainstem. The cerebellum controls the execution of individual movements and postures, including the timing, coordination, and correction of errors of movements. Abnormalities of the cerebellar circuits result in disorders of coordination, such as *ataxia* of eye movements, speech, gait, and ipsilateral limbs. The basal ganglia are concerned primarily with the initiation of specific, behaviorally relevant automatic motor programs. Damage of the basal ganglia circuits may impair the initiation of voluntary and automatic motor acts (*hypokinesia*) and increase muscle tone (*rigidity*) or cause inappropriate involuntary movements (*hyperkinesia*). Therefore, unlike lesions affecting lower or upper motor neurons, lesions affecting the premotor cortex, basal ganglia, or cerebellar circuits do not produce weakness, but rather impair the planning, selection, and execution of movements, respectively.

Motor control also depends critically on feedback proprioceptive input from muscle spindles and joint receptors. This input to motor neurons initiates segmental reflexes, provides information to the cerebral cortex (lemniscal system) for fine control of the digits, and provides input to the cerebellum (spinocerebellar pathway) to control posture and gait. Impairment of this proprioceptive system produces sensory ataxia, as described in Chapter 7. The functions of the different components of the motor system and the clinical manifestations of their involvement by disease are summarized in Table 8.1.

Final Common Pathway

The final common pathway is the effector mechanism that mediates all motor activity. It includes the motor neurons in the ventral horn of the spinal cord and in the cranial nerve motor nuclei of the brainstem and their axons that extend peripherally through motor nerves to innervate muscles. These motor neurons are called alpha motor neurons, or alpha efferents, and they innervate the muscle fibers which, when stimulated, produce skeletal muscle contraction. The basic functional component of the final common pathway is the *motor unit* (Fig. 8.2). The motor unit is a physiologic concept, developed largely from the work of Sir Charles Sherrington and his colleagues. A motor unit consists of the cell body of a motor neuron, its axon, and all the muscle fibers innervated by the terminal arborization of the axon (Fig. 8.2).

- A motor neuron, its axon, and all the muscle fibers innervated by it constitute a motor unit.

Anatomy

Ventral Horn and Cranial Nerve Motor Nuclei

The ventral horn (also called the anterior horn) of the spinal cord is derived from the basal plate and contains the motor neurons (also called *motoneurons*) and interneurons involved in control of the neck, trunk, and limb muscles. Similar neurons located in the cranial nerve motor nuclei control the craniofacial muscles. Alpha motor neurons are relatively large (50–80 mm in diameter) and are arranged in the ventral horn in well-defined columns that innervate individual skeletal muscles. A second type of motor neuron, gamma motor neurons, innervates muscle spindles, as described below. All motor neurons have acetylcholine as their neurotransmitter.

Motor Axons

Motor axons are large myelinated fibers (6–20 μm in diameter) located in peripheral nerves. Nearly one-half of these fibers are the large alpha motor neuron axons, which innervate the muscle fibers (extrafusal fibers) that produce muscle contraction; the other fibers are gamma motor neuron axons that innervate muscle spindles (intrafusal fibers). Motor nerve fibers branch along the course of nerves, at the nodes of Ranvier. Most of the branching occurs distally in the muscle. Each terminal ramification of a nerve fiber ends as a motor end plate on a single muscle fiber, forming a neuromuscular junction. The nerves innervating the muscle also contain many sensory fibers that arise mainly from muscle spindles.

Neuromuscular Junction

The points of contact between the terminal ramifications of motor axons and the muscle fibers innervated by them are known as *motor end plates*, or *neuromuscular junctions*. The terminal axon lies in a hollow indentation on the surface of the muscle fiber, the synaptic gutter. The membrane of the nerve terminal and that of the muscle fiber are separated by a narrow space, the synaptic cleft. The nerve terminal holds many vesicles that contain and release *acetylcholine*. The muscle membrane contains postjunctional folds that harbor clusters of *nicotinic acetylcholine receptors*.

Organization of Muscle Fibers in a Motor Unit

The nerve terminals of a single motor axon innervate muscle fibers that may be distributed widely throughout

Table 8.1. Components of the Motor System and Clinical Correlations

Component	Function	Clinical manifestation
Alpha motor neuron (lower motor neuron)	Final common pathway for voluntary, postural, and reflex movements, including those involved in muscle tone Trophic influence on muscle fiber Maintenance of electrical stability of the axon and muscle membrane	Weakness Hyporeflexia or areflexia Hypotonia or atonia Muscle atrophy Fasciculations Fibrillation potentials
Descending motor pathways (upper motor neuron)		
Corticospinal tract (direct pathway)	Control of skilled voluntary movements, particularly those of the fingers Control of muscle force	Weakness Loss of dexterity Inability to increase force
Corticoreticulospinal system (indirect pathway)	Inhibition of segmental reflexes that interfere with voluntary action Posture and locomotion	Hyperreflexia and clonus Spasticity Babinski sign
Cortical motor association areas	Planning and programming of movements	Apraxia
Cerebellar control circuits	Control of execution of individual movements (timing, intensity, duration)	Nystagmus Gait ataxia Limb ataxia Intention tremor
Basal ganglia control circuit	Selection of a specifc motor program and inhibition of other motor programs	Rigidity Akinesia Rest tremor Hyperkinesia (dystonia, chorea, ballismus)
Proprioceptive system	Sensory feedback to spinal cord, motor cortex, and cerebellum	Sensory ataxia Romberg sign Areflexia

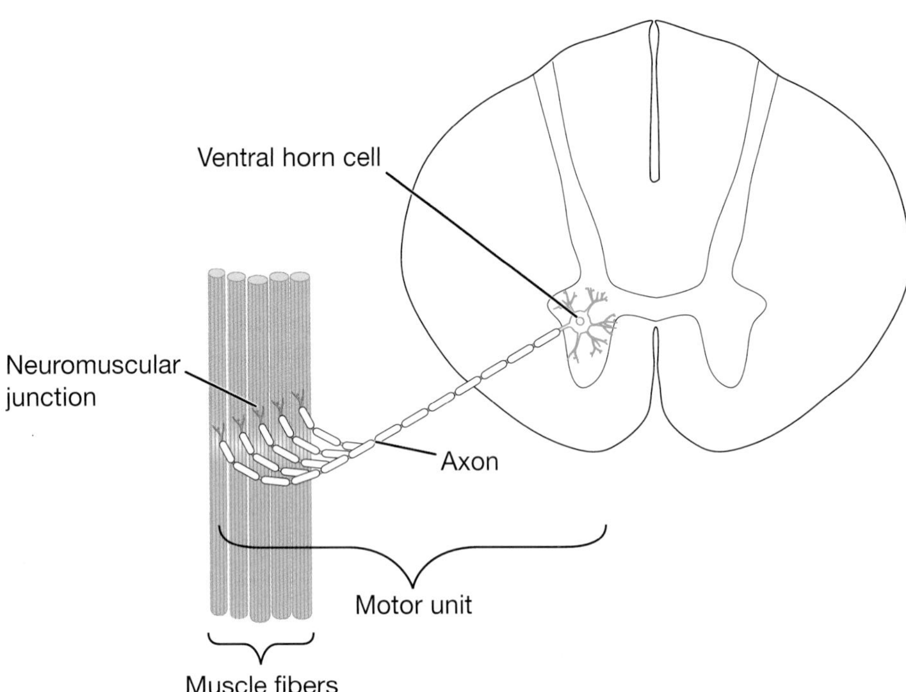

Fig. 8.2. A single motor unit and its components: the lower motor neuron and muscle fibers innervated by it.

the muscle and intermingle with muscle fibers innervated by other neurons. A muscle may contain from 50 to 2,000 motor units. The size of a motor unit, expressed as the *innervation ratio*, is determined by the number of extrafusal fibers innervated by the axon of a single motor neuron. Muscles that produce fine movements have smaller innervation ratios than those that perform cruder movements. Motor units in intrinsic hand muscles have innervation ratios of only 50 to 400, and eye muscles have ratios of 3 to 10. In contrast, the motor units of the powerful limb muscles each contain from 500 to 2,000 muscle fibers.

Muscle

Skeletal muscle fibers are long cylindrical structures, each of which is a syncytium containing hundreds of nuclei. The cytoplasm of the muscle fiber contains mitochondria, sarcoplasmic reticulum, and myofibrils, which are the contractile elements of the muscle. The myofibrils have a banded structure that subdivides them into units called *sarcomeres*. The fine structure of muscle is described in more detail in Chapter 13.

Physiology

The motor unit is the physiologic unit of all reflex, postural, and voluntary movements. Under normal conditions, the motor unit behaves in an all-or-none manner, so that the action potential in a motor nerve axon produces an action potential in and synchronous contraction of all the muscle fibers the axon supplies. Thus, the resulting contraction of the motor unit is the sum of the mechanical responses of the component muscle fibers. An alpha motor neuron not only excites but also exerts a trophic effect on the muscle fibers it innervates.

Motor Neurons

The motor neurons that innervate extensor muscles are called extensor motor neurons and those innervating flexor muscles are flexor motor neurons. Muscles that functionally aid one another are called *synergists*, and those that functionally oppose one another are *antagonists*. Any movement of a joint requires the balanced interaction between antagonist muscle groups acting on that joint.

The activity of alpha motor neurons depends on their

intrinsic electrophysiologic properties and on the spatial and temporal summation of multiple excitatory and inhibitory synaptic potentials triggered by inputs from segmental afferents and descending cortical and brainstem pathways (Fig. 8.3). The neurotransmitter of most of these inputs is the excitatory amino acid L-glutamate. In addition to motor neurons, the ventral horn contains several types of *interneurons* that integrate the activity of segmental afferents and descending motor pathways. In fact, with few exceptions, the segmental and descending inputs influence motor neurons indirectly through excitatory or inhibitory interneurons. Excitatory interneurons have L-glutamate as a neurotransmitter, and inhibitory interneurons have γ-aminobutyric acid (GABA), glycine, or both. Motor neurons also receive modulatory inputs from descending pathways that have norepinephrine or serotonin as a neurotransmitter.

Neuromuscular Transmission

Activation of alpha motor neurons produces an action potential that spreads to each of the terminal branches of the motor axon in the muscle, triggering the release of acetylcholine from the presynaptic active zones. Acetylcholine diffuses rapidly across the synaptic cleft and acts on nicotinic receptors clustered along the junctional folds in the postsynaptic membrane of the muscle fiber. These receptors are cation channels, and their activation by acetylcholine causes fast local depolarization of the muscle fiber. This is called the *endplate potential*; it initiates an action potential in the muscle fiber.

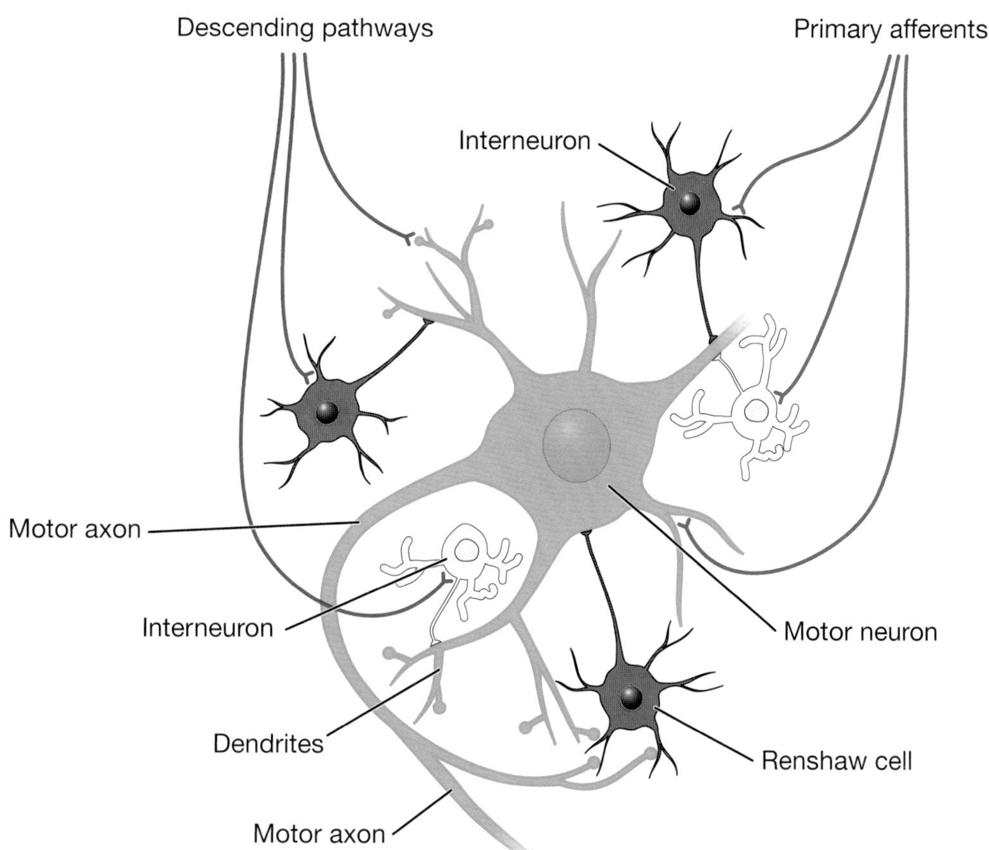

Fig. 8.3. Influences on motor neurons. Alpha motor neurons receive segmental and suprasegmental inputs. The segmental input arises from primary afferents of muscle receptors and skin receptors that initiate segmental reflexes. Suprasegmental input includes descending pathways from the motor cortex (direct activation pathway) and brainstem. With few exceptions, segmental and suprasegmental inputs affect motor neurons through excitatory (white) or inhibitory (dark) interneurons.

This action potential spreads along the entire length of the muscle fiber through voltage-gated sodium (Na^+) channels located at clefts between the junctional folds. The electrical currents generated by the muscle action potential invade the depths of the muscle fiber through a tubular system to turn on the contractile mechanism that produces the actual twitch of the muscle. This sequence of steps converts the activation of motor neurons into muscle contraction.

The precise apposition of the nicotinic acetylcholine receptors with the presynaptic active zones affords highly efficient neuromuscular transmission. The amplitude of the end plate potential is much higher than the threshold required to open the voltage-gated Na^+ channels of the muscle membrane. The difference between the amplitude of depolarization caused by the end plate potential and the depolarization required to activate these voltage-gated Na^+ channels is called the *safety margin* of neuromuscular transmission. This important concept is discussed further in Chapter 13.

Motor Unit

Normal movements involve the coordinated activity of hundreds to thousands of motor units in many muscles. The speed and strength of a movement are controlled by the number of motor units active, their rate of firing, and the characteristics of the motor units activated. The size of the motor unit depends on the number of muscle fibers innervated by its axon, that is, the innervation ratio. Units with a low innervation ratio produce fine movements, such as those controlling eye movements. The number of muscle fibers in a motor unit is also related to the load that it must move. For example, to move the mass of the lower limb even slightly requires the simultaneous action of many muscle fibers, and the muscles responsible for such movements have high innervation ratios.

Because activation of a normal alpha motor neuron causes all the muscle fibers in the motor unit to contract, gradation of contraction is accomplished by varying the frequency of firing of single motor units and the number of motor units activated. With increased effort, more motor units are activated. The physiologic properties of the muscle fibers of the motor units depend on the alpha motor neuron that innervates them. All the muscle fibers within a motor unit have the same biochemical and physiologic characteristics. The motor units in limb muscles generally may be divided into two groups according to the speed of contraction: fast twitch and slow twitch.

> The distinction between fast and slow twitch motor units is based on the differences in time from the start of the contraction to the time at which the motor unit develops peak tension in response to a single stimulus. For a typical fast twitch motor unit, this contraction time is approximately 25 milliseconds, and for a slow twitch unit, it is approximately 75 milliseconds. The physiologic properties of the motor neurons determine the twitch time and biochemical characteristics of the muscle fiber. Small alpha motor neurons innervate slow muscle fibers that are able to generate small but sustained tension, are resistant to fatigue, and are rich in oxidative enzymes. Larger alpha motor neurons innervate fast muscle fibers that generate large but short-lasting tension, fatigue rapidly, and are rich in glycolytic enzymes (see Chapter 13).

Slow twitch motor units tend to be found in certain muscles (called slow muscles), for example, the soleus muscle. Other muscles containing predominantly fast twitch motor units are designated fast muscles. The segregation of more motor units of a particular speed into certain muscles is of functional significance. Slow limb muscles, such as the soleus muscle, subserve a predominantly postural role, whereas fast limb muscles are concerned more with phasic, voluntary movements. However, fast and slow twitch motor units are intermingled in most muscles.

The force of muscle contraction is increased by two mechanisms: increased firing rates of individual motor units (temporal summation) and recruitment of other motor units (spatial summation). With normal activation of lower motor neurons, the neurons discharge repetitively at rates of 5 to 20 per second. At these rates, the twitch of slow muscles is not completed before the next action potential arrives, so that smooth movements or steady contractions can be obtained from repetitive action potentials. During muscle contractions of increasing force, alpha motor neurons are recruited according to the *size principle*: small motor neurons, which innervate slow twitch muscle fibers (slow twitch units), are recruited earlier, and large motor neurons, which innervate fast twitch muscles (fast twitch units), are recruited later.

- Alpha motor neurons elicit rapid activation of the muscle fibers of the motor unit and have trophic effects on these muscle fibers.
- Neuromuscular transmission is a fast, efficient mechanism of communication that is mediated by acetylcholine acting on nicotinic receptors in the muscle end plate.
- Alpha motor neurons determine the properties of the muscle fibers of the motor unit.
- During increased force of contraction, slow twitch units are recruited earlier, and fast twitch units are recruited later.

Segmental Control of the Motor Neurons

Segmental inputs to motor neurons and interneurons arise from muscle receptors and trigger various reflexes. These include the muscle stretch reflex, Golgi tendon organ reflex, and flexion reflex. Of these, the stretch reflex is the most important clinically because it is the main basis for neurologic testing of tendon reflexes.

Muscle Stretch Reflex

The muscle stretch reflex, also called the *myotatic reflex*, provides a length servomechanism that controls the activity of the motor neuron in response to a change in length of the muscle the motor neuron innervates (Fig. 8.4). An increase in muscle length activates specific muscle receptors, called *muscle spindles*. Activation of the muscle spindles triggers, through fast-conducting afferents, reflex activation of alpha motor neurons innervating the muscle, leading to muscle contraction. Muscle spindles are proprioceptive organs that consist of specialized muscle fibers, called *intrafusal fibers*, which lie in parallel with the contractile (extrafusal) fibers of the muscle (Fig. 8.5).

Muscle spindles contain one of two main types of receptors: nuclear bag receptors located in the center of the fiber and nuclear chain receptors distributed along its middle portion. Muscle spindles are innervated by two types of afferents. Primary, or type Ia, afferents innervate nuclear bag receptors and discharge vigorously to changes in length over time, and secondary, or type II, afferent endings innervate nuclear chain receptors and respond in proportion to the maintained length or stretch (Fig. 8.6).

The classic muscle stretch reflex is a simple two-neuron reflex elicited by stimulation of the muscle spindles and mediated by type Ia afferents. Activation of these Ia afferents in response to lengthening (stretch) of the spindle elicits a powerful monosynaptic excitation of the alpha motor neuron innervating the corresponding muscle (*homonymous* connection). This strong monosynaptic excitatory input provides a length servomechanism and is critical for maintaining the excitability of the alpha motor neuron, which is necessary to attain maximal strength of contraction.

For a muscle spindle to respond appropriately to a stretch or change in muscle length, spindle length must be adjusted to changes in muscle length during contraction. This is accomplished through a separate motor innervation of the intrafusal fibers of muscle spindles. The motor neurons that innervate intrafusal fibers are called *gamma motor neurons* (fusimotor system). During muscle contraction, type Ia fiber discharge would be suppressed completely by unloading if the gamma motor neuron were not simultaneously active. For most movements, gamma motor neurons are coactivated with the alpha motor neurons innervating the muscle, thus maintaining the sensitivity of the spindle receptor during muscle shortening (Fig. 8.7 and 8.8).

The fusimotor system produces an internal change in length and local stiffening of the intrafusal fiber, so that more stretch is transmitted to the regions innervated by the Ia and II afferent terminals. Different classes of gamma motor neurons can preferentially increase either the phasic (changing) discharge from the muscle spindle or the tonic (maintained) discharge. Dynamic gamma motor neurons innervate the nuclear bag receptors and increase the sensitivity and responsiveness of primary Ia endings to small, rapid changes in muscle length. In contrast, static gamma motor neurons innervate bag 2 and nuclear chain receptors and increase the sensitivity of type II afferents to static position responses.

The response of the endings in the muscle spindle to a quick stretch is the primary basis of muscle stretch reflexes tested during a neurologic examination. A physician taps a tendon with a reflex hammer, which causes the muscle to stretch. The brief stretch stimulates muscle spindles in the muscle, thus activating Ia afferents. These afferents excite the corresponding alpha motor neurons, which cause the muscle to twitch. The resulting discharge of a large number of Ia afferents is sufficient to activate the corresponding motor neurons and to cause a muscle twitch. Therefore, with the loss of either the afferent fibers or the lower motor neuron, the myotatic reflex is reduced or lost, referred to as *hyporeflexia* and *areflexia*, respectively.

A critical mechanism for motor control is the activation of synergistic muscles and reciprocal inhibitory control of antagonist muscles that act on a particular joint. In addition to the monosynaptic stretch reflex, the Ia afferents activate the alpha motor neurons that innervate the synergistic muscles. A second important consequence of activation of Ia afferents is the disynaptic inhibition of alpha motor neurons that innervate the antagonist muscles. This process, called *reciprocal*

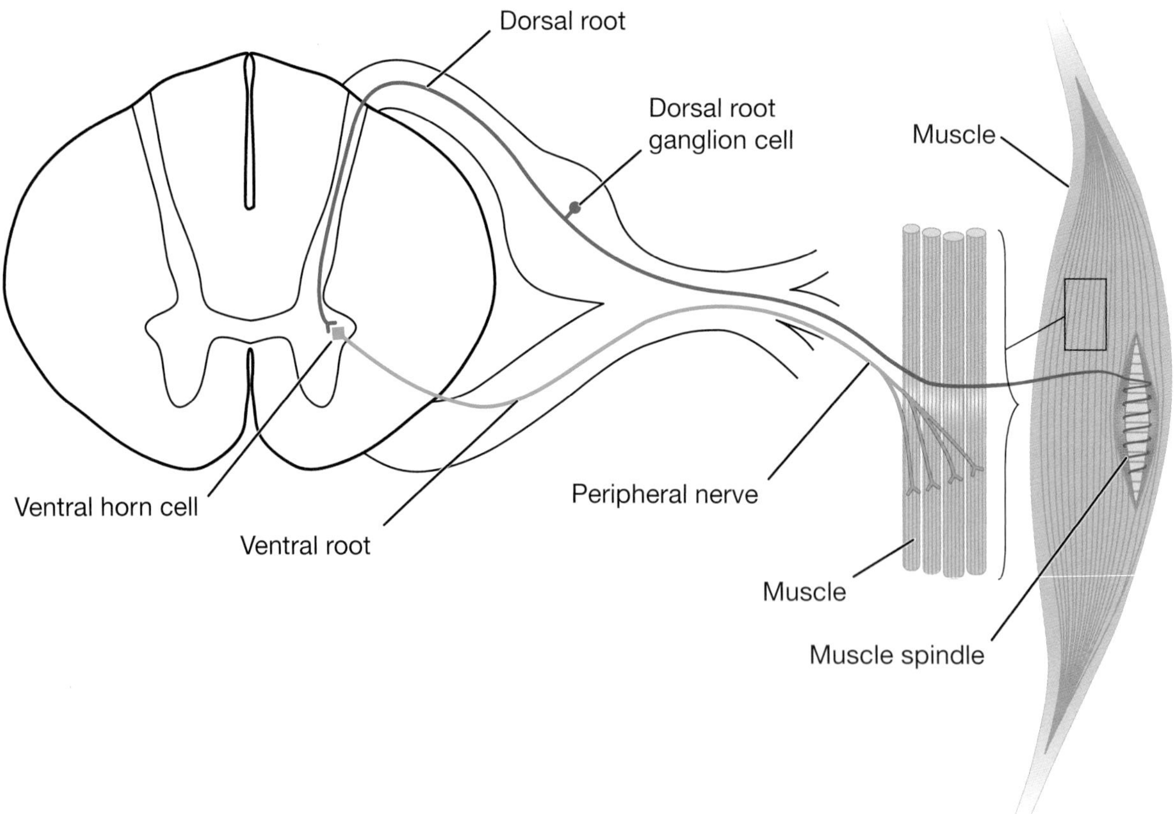

Fig. 8.4. Anatomical basis of the classic monosynaptic muscle stretch reflex. This reflex is triggered by activation of stretch receptors in the muscle spindle, which through Ia afferents elicit monosynaptic excitation of the alpha motor neuron innervating the corresponding muscle, resulting in muscle contraction. This provides a length servomechanism.

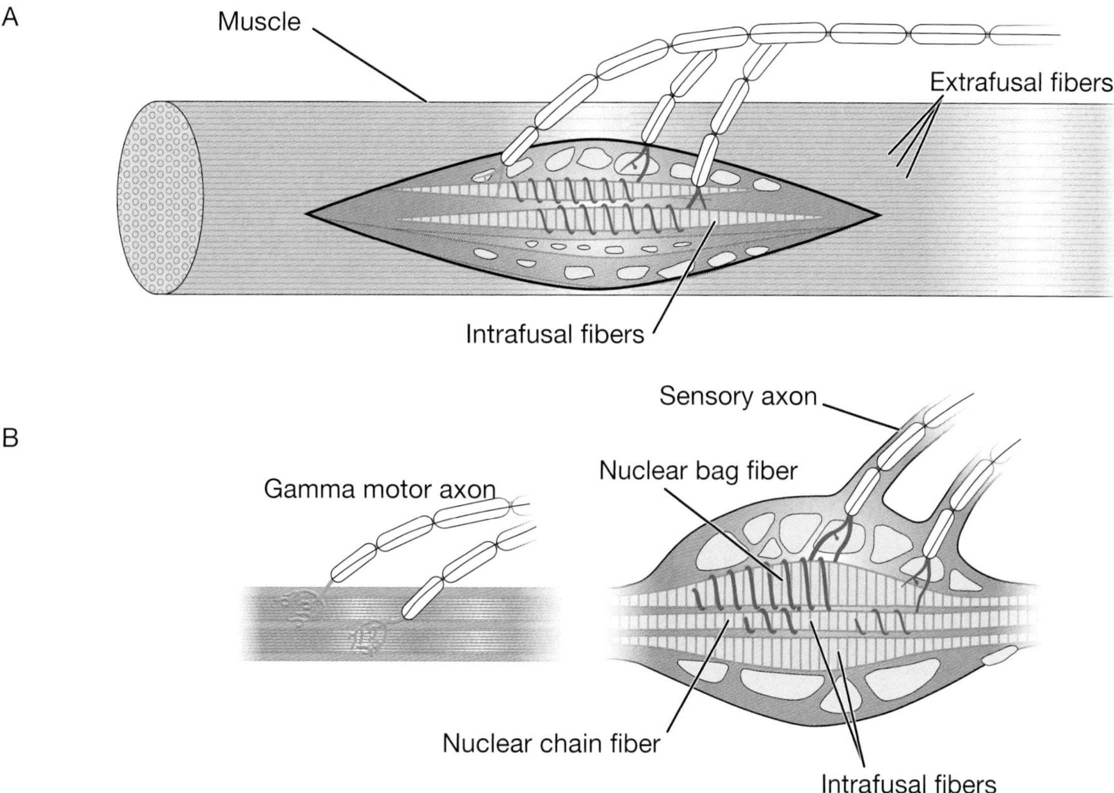

Fig. 8.5. Muscle spindle. *A*, Entire spindle and the axons innervating it. *B*, Detailed longitudinal view of one end and the center of a muscle spindle.

inhibition, is mediated by *Ia inhibitory interneurons* (Fig. 8.9).

Muscle spindles are not distributed equally among the muscles. More are present in slow muscles, such as the soleus, than in fast muscles, such as the gastrocnemius. Within the spinal cord, monosynaptic spindle afferents are concentrated on the synergistic slow motor neurons. Thus, the spindle mechanism is of greater importance in the control of the tonic activity of slow muscles. The central connections of the type II axons from the secondary spindle endings are more complex than those of the primary endings. Like the type Ia endings, type II endings have excitatory connections with synergistic muscles and have inhibitory connections with antagonistic muscles; thus, they also participate in myotatic reflexes. However, they also have more widespread disynaptic and polysynaptic connections that have a longer duration of action, which may be part of flexion reflexes.

- A muscle stretch reflex is triggered by activation of muscle spindles innervated by Ia afferents and results in monosynaptic excitation of alpha motor neurons innervating the corresponding muscle.
- Muscle stretch reflexes provide a length servomechanism that maintains motor neuron excitability.
- Gamma motor neurons, which are coactivated with alpha motor neurons, maintain Ia afferent input during muscle contraction.
- Ia inhibitory interneurons mediate reciprocal inhibition of antagonist muscles.
- Lesions that affect either the large myelinated afferents (i.e., Ia afferents) or the final common pathway (i.e., alpha motor neuron) interrupt the muscle stretch reflex.

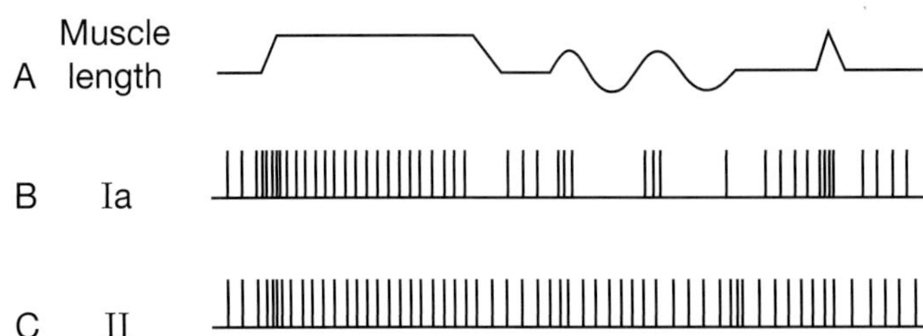

Fig. 8.6. Responses of afferent fibers from a muscle spindle. *A*, Length of muscle containing muscle spindle. Muscle length is changed with various waveforms of stretch. *B*, Response of type Ia afferent fibers from a primary ending of the muscle spindle. *C*, Response of type II afferent fibers from a secondary ending of the muscle spindle. Type Ia afferents respond to rapid stretch; type II afferents respond to length.

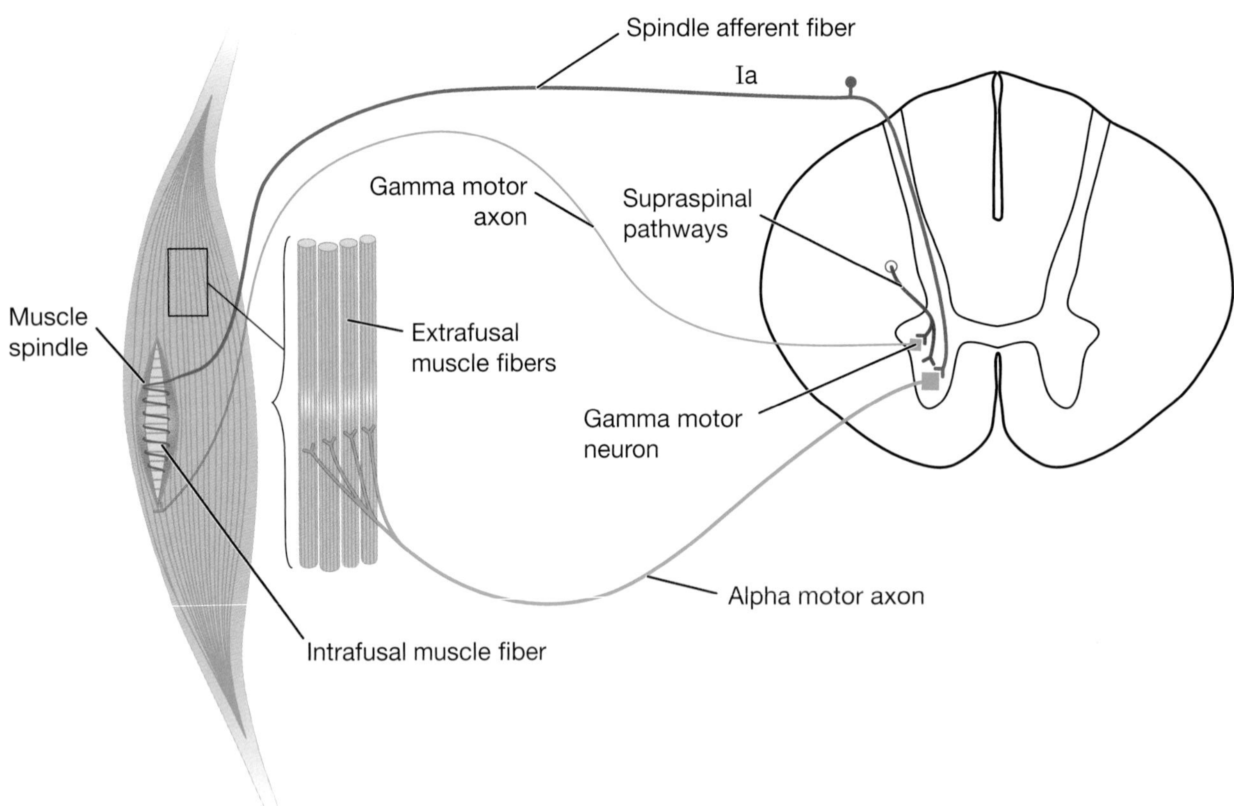

Fig. 8.7. Gamma motor system. Contraction of intrafusal fibers by gamma motor neurons can maintain a muscle spindle at the proper length to respond to muscle stretch even though muscle length changes. Descending pathways elicit coactivation of gamma and alpha motor neurons during most motor tasks.

Golgi Tendon Organ Reflex

The Golgi tendon organ reflex provides a tension servomechanism that inhibits the discharge of a motor neuron in response to an increase in muscle tension. Golgi tendon organs are mechanoreceptors that are located in series with the ends of muscle fibers and innervated by Ib afferents. They are generally silent in relaxed muscles and in response to passive stretch, but their discharge increases with the strength of muscle contraction (Fig. 8.10). Activation of Ib afferents triggers a reflex inhibition of the corresponding alpha motor neurons and synergistic motor neurons. This is mediated by *Ib inhibitory interneurons* (Fig. 8.11).

> However, during locomotion, activation of Ib afferents from extensor muscles facilitates the homonymous extensor motor neuron. This is important for maintaining extension of the lower extremity during the stance phase of locomotion.

Together, muscle spindles (length servomechanism) and Golgi tendon organs (tension servomechanism) provide the nervous system with the information necessary to control muscle stiffness (Fig. 8.12).

Flexion Reflexes

Flexion reflex afferents consist of group II muscle spindle afferents, group III and group IV muscle afferents, and skin afferents. Although this term reflects the role of these afferents in the generation of flexion reflexes, flexion reflex afferents are functionally heterogeneous and participate in multiple polysynaptic reflexes. *Polysynaptic proprioceptive reflexes* are the basis for the integration of inputs from muscle, joint, and skin and the convergence of supraspinal commands on common spinal interneurons that provide excitatory or inhibitory connections to flexor and extensor motor neurons. This reflex system is activated by contact of the foot with the ground and triggers polysynaptic pathways that determine the direction, velocity, and amplitude needed to maintain equilibrium and generate a pattern of activation of leg muscles during locomotion.

The nociceptive flexion reflex is triggered by activation of nociceptive cutaneous flexion reflex afferents, and it results in the withdrawal of the limb from the noxious stimulus. Stimulation of skin afferents provokes a polysynaptic reflex that activates ipsilateral flexor motor neurons and reciprocally inhibits ipsilateral extensor motor neurons. Activation of flexor motor neurons is typically widespread so that flexor muscles at the ankle, knee, and hip contract to withdraw the whole limb.

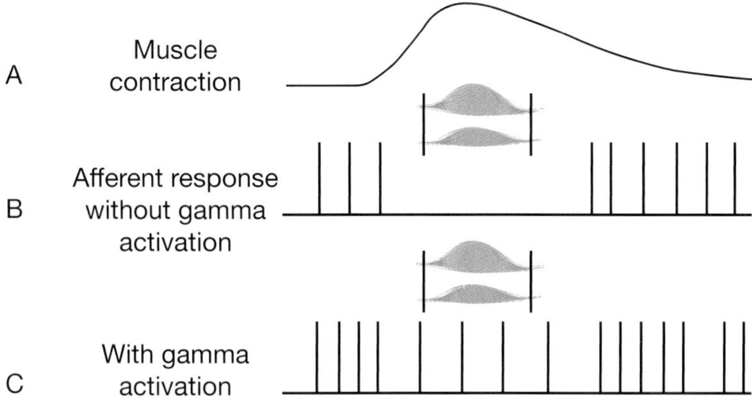

Fig. 8.8. Effect of gamma motor neuron activation. *A*, Muscle contraction. *B*, In the absence of gamma efferent activity, contraction reduces the length of the muscle spindle receptor, interrupting Ia afferent activity. *C*, Gamma efferent input to the intrafusal fiber maintains the length of the muscle spindle recceptor, allowing continuous Ia activity despite shortening of the muscle.

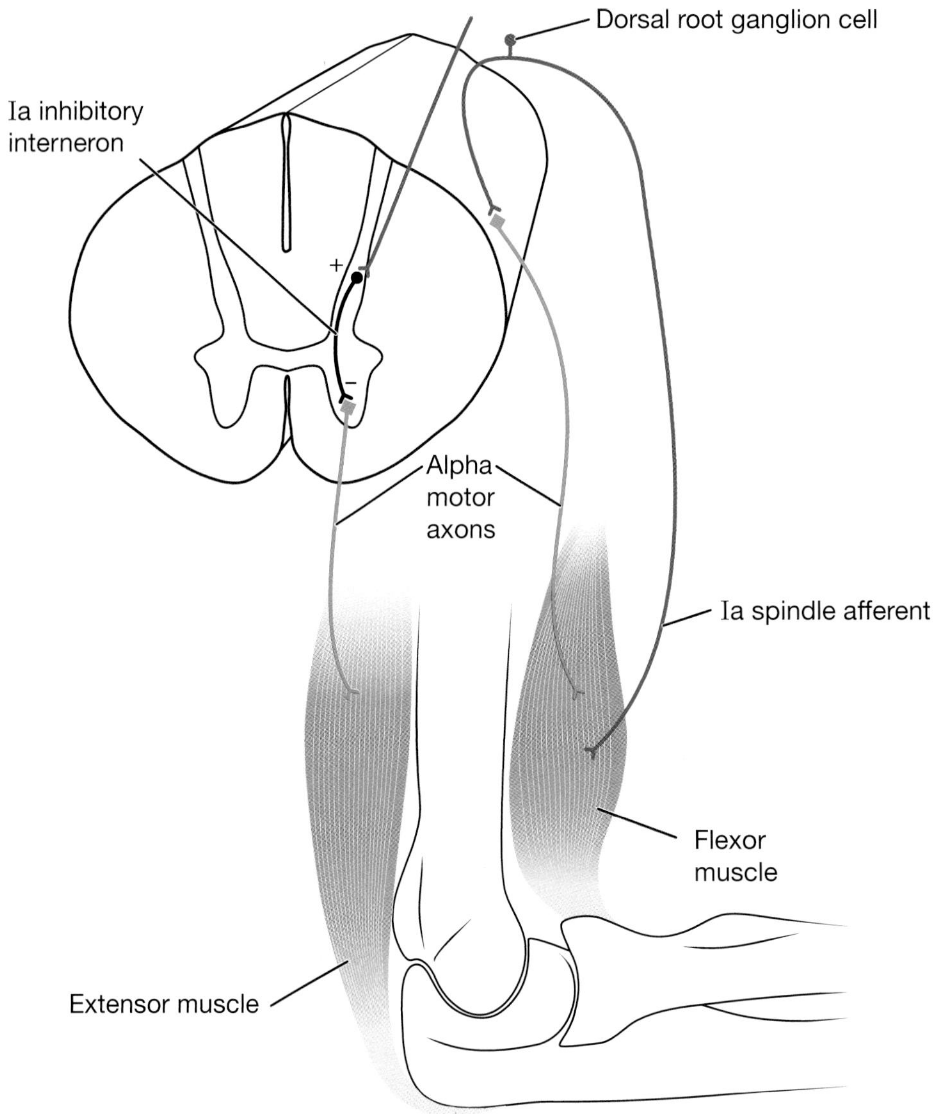

Fig. 8.9. Pathway for the monosynaptic stretch reflex and reciprocal inhibition. Ia afferents act on Ia inhibitory interneurons, thus inhibiting the motor neurons that innervate the antagonist muscle.

Contralateral to the side of stimulation, flexor motor neurons are inhibited and extensor motor neurons are excited, a process called *double reciprocal inhibition*. This crossed extension reflex stabilizes the body while the limb ipsilateral to the stimulus is flexed (Fig. 8.13).

- The Golgi tendon organ reflex, mediated by Ib inhibitory interneurons, provides a tension servomechanism.
- Flexion reflex afferents initiate polysynaptic reflexes that are involved in locomotion and withdrawal from noxious stimuli.

The main components of segmental reflexes affecting motor neurons are summarized in Table 8.2.

Interneurons and Integration of Inputs to Motor Neurons
The control of the activity of motor neurons by segmental reflexes and descending inputs occurs primarily through excitatory or inhibitory interneurons and propriospinal

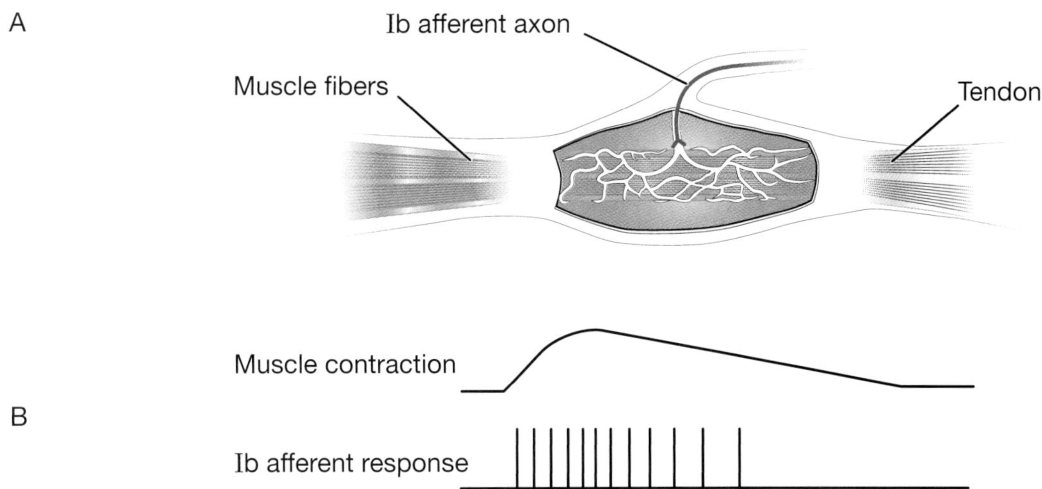

Fig. 8.10. Golgi tendon organ. *A*, Diagram of a Golgi tendon organ. *B*, Afferent activity with active muscle contraction.

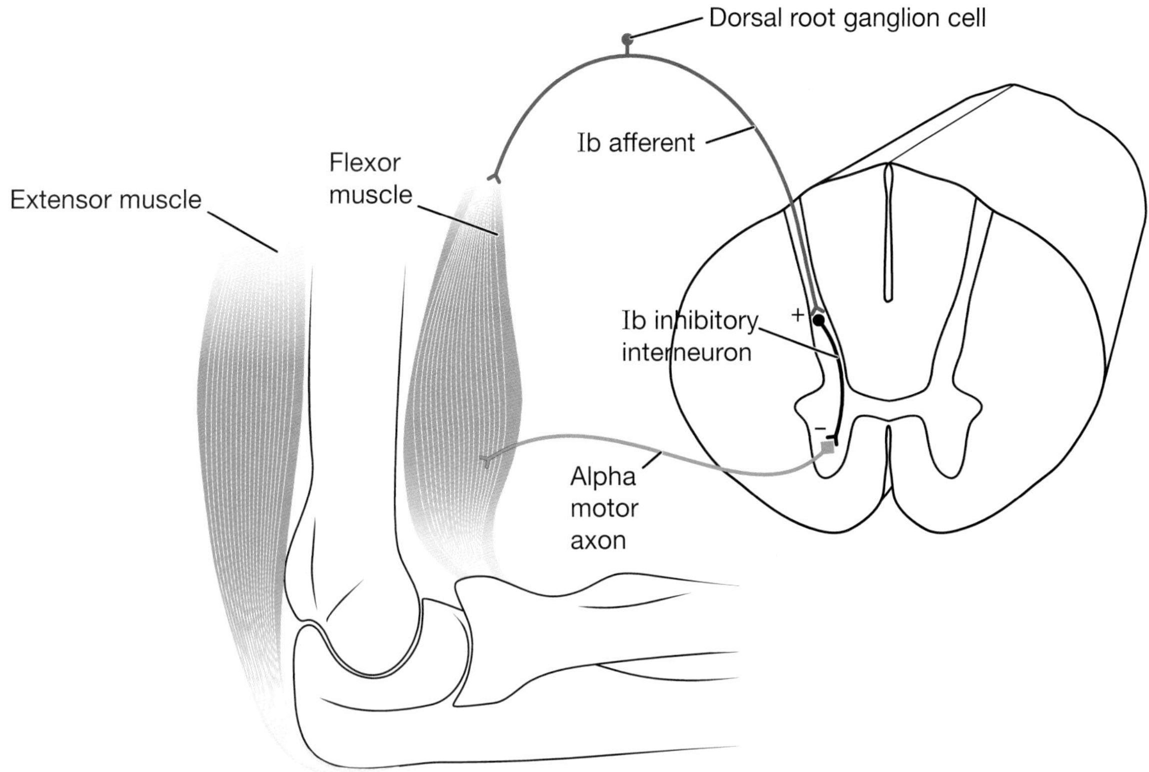

Fig. 8.11. Golgi tendon organ reflex. Activation of Ib afferents of the Golgi tendon organ during active muscle contraction leads to a disynaptic inhibition of alpha motor neurons innervating the corresponding muscle. This is mediated by the Ib inhibitory interneuron.

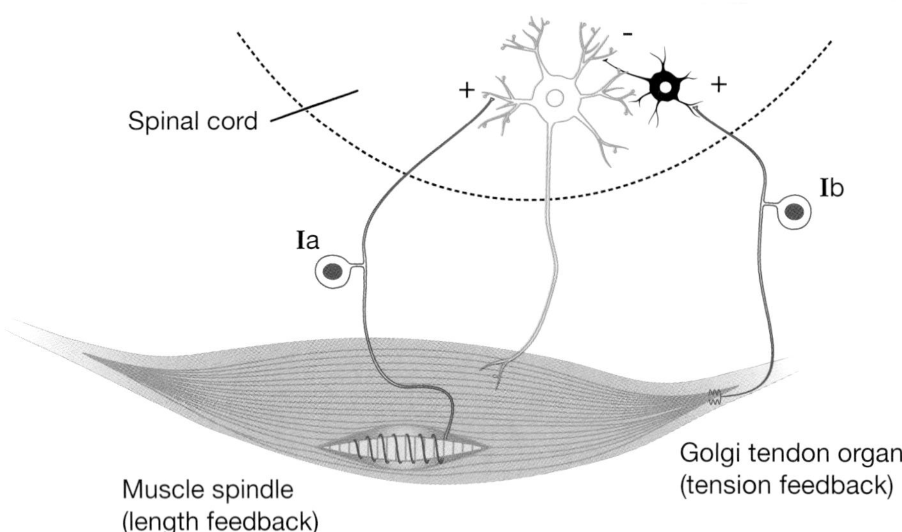

Fig. 8.12. Control of muscle stiffness by interaction of a length feedback (muscle spindle) producing Ia afferent-mediated monosynaptic excitation and a tension feedback (Golgi tendon organ) producing a Ib afferent-mediated disynaptic inhibition of the alpha motor neurons innervating the muscle.

neurons. Interneurons are interposed between the afferent and efferent components of the reflex pathway, whereas propriospinal neurons provide longitudinal connections between different segments of the spinal cord.

Interneurons and Control of Segmental Reflexes

Spinal inhibitory interneurons have a critical role in regulating the excitability of segmental reflexes. They include Ia and Ib inhibitory interneurons, described above, as well as presynaptic Ia inhibitory neurons and Renshaw cells. Presynaptic Ia inhibitory neurons form GABAergic axoaxonic synapses on primary Ia afferents and, thus, inhibit the release of neurotransmitters from these afferents (Fig. 8.14). Collaterals of motor axons excite *Renshaw cells*, which in turn inhibit alpha motor neurons, a mechanism referred to as *recurrent inhibition*, which is mediated by glycine and GABA (Fig. 8.15). The individual spinal reflexes triggered by muscle spindles, Golgi tendon organs, or flexion reflex afferents are not distinct entities resulting from the operation of distinct circuits, rather the spinal cord integrates the incoming sensory information from different primary afferents with motor commands descending from supraspinal centers. This integration depends on the spinal interneurons. The normal activity of spinal inhibitory neurons depends on input from the medullary reticular formation.

Interneuronal Networks and Central Pattern Generation

Interneurons in the spinal cord and brainstem form interconnected networks that control complex patterns of motor activity, including locomotion, swallowing, and respiration. These networks are called *central pattern generators*. The generation of motor patterns depends both on the intrinsic ionic conductance properties of individual neurons and reciprocal excitatory and inhibitory synaptic interactions.

Locomotion in mammals depends on a central pattern generator distributed in the intermediate gray matter across lower thoracic and all lumbar segments. These interneurons can generate rhythmic bursts of reciprocal activity in flexor and extensor motoneurons, even in the absence of sensory input or descending influences. However, normal patterns of locomotion depend on descending input from the cerebral cortex and brainstem reticular formation and are modulated by afferent input from Golgi tendon organs and flexion reflex afferents.

- Spinal interneurons integrate inputs from multiple primary afferents and descending motor pathways and coordinate the activity of multiple motor neuron pools in a flexible manner, according to the specific motor task.

Muscle Tone

A common clinical test is to gauge the resistance of a muscle to passive movement. Normally, when a limb is moved by an examiner and a muscle is stretched, there is mild resistance to the passive movement referred

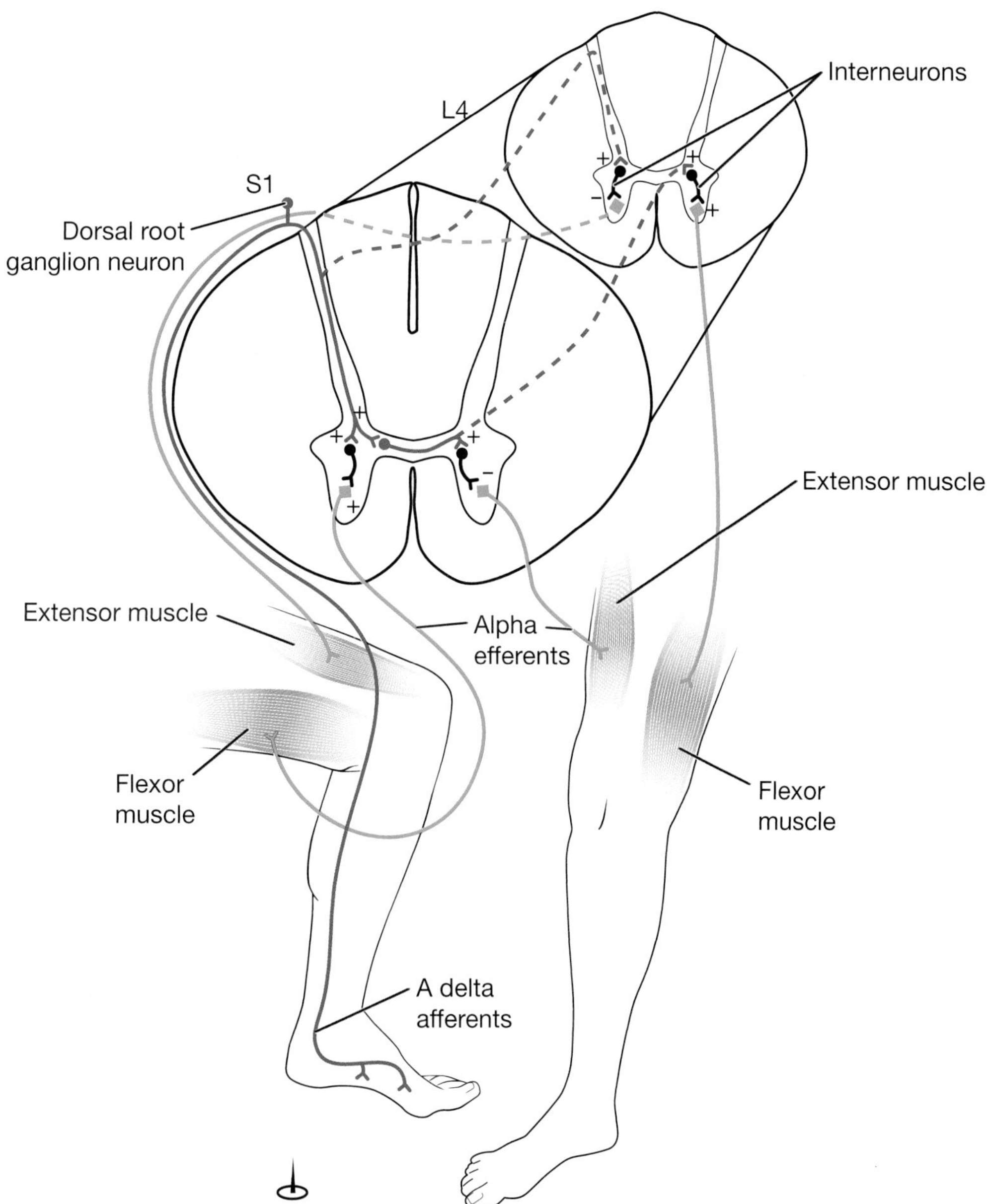

Fig. 8.13. Nociceptive flexion reflex pathways. Type II muscle spindle, muscle mechanoreceptors types III and IV, and cutaneous nociceptive afferents (A delta) activate polysnaptic reflexes mediated by excitatory and inhibitory interneurons. The nociceptive flexion reflex pathway triggers an ipsilateral flexion (withdrawal) response. If the stimulus intensity is sufficiently high, there is also reflex extension of the contralateral limb (crossed extension reflex).

Table 8.2. Segmental Reflexes

	Stretch reflex	Golgi tendon reflex	Multisynaptic Proprioceptive	Multisynaptic Nociceptive
Receptor	Muscle spindle	Golgi tendon organ	Muscle spindle Joint receptors	Skin and muscle nociceptors
Stimulus	Change in muscle length	Tension generated by active contraction	Various mechanical inputs	Noxious input
Afferents	Ia	Ib	II, III-IV, FRAs	Nociceptive III-IV muscle FRAs
Interneuron	Ia inhibitory	Ib inhibitory	Multiple excitatory or inhibitory	Multiple excitatory or inhibitory
Effect on agonist motor neurons	Monosynaptic excitation	Disynaptic inhibition	Polysynaptic excitation or inhibition	Polysynaptic excitation of ipsilateral flexors and contralateral extensors
Effect on antagonist	Disynaptic (reciprocal) inhibition	Excitation or inhibition	Excitation or inhibition	Polysynaptic inhibition of ipsilateral extensors and contralateral extensors
Function	Length servomechanism	Tension servomechanism	Locomotion	Withdrawal

FRA, flexion reflex afferent.

to as *muscle tone*. Muscle tone depends on several variables, including the intrinsic elasticity of the tissue and state of excitability of the motor neurons innervating the muscle. One component of muscle tone arises from activation of motor units through stretching of muscle spindles. However, this reflex does not appear to contribute to muscle tone in deeply relaxed subjects. Tone depends critically on the level of arousal and increases when stretch reflexes are reinforced through mental concentration or muscle contraction. Therefore, although tonically active motor neurons excited by Ia efferents contribute to muscle tone, their optimal activity requires facilitatory support from descending supraspinal inputs. Afferents from muscle spindles, projecting through the lemniscal system, may activate corticospinal input to motor neurons. These *long loop reflexes* contribute to muscle tone.

An increase in the excitability of alpha or gamma motor neurons either from the interruption of descending pathways that activate inhibitory Ia or Ib interneurons or from an abnormal increase in central excitation through long loop reflexes increases muscle tone, called *hypertonia*. When hypertonia is the consequence of the interruption of descending inputs to inhibitory interneurons, it is the manifestation of exaggerated muscle stretch reflexes. In contrast, a decrease in the afferent input from muscle spindles or in the excitation of lower motor neurons decreases muscle tone, called *hypotonia*. This is typically associated with hyporeflexia.

Clinical Correlations

Diseases may affect the final common pathway at the level of the ventral horn cell, the axon, or the muscle fiber. Damage to any of these sites has common clinical features that permit the clinician to identify disease of the motor unit. These include weakness, atrophy, loss of reflexes, and loss of tone. Other features that may indicate abnormal function of the motor unit include fasciculations, cramps, and excessive contraction. All these features characterize the *lower motor neuron syndrome*.

Weakness

Destruction of an alpha motor neuron results in degeneration of the axon and loss of innervation of the muscle fibers of the motor unit. In final common pathway disease, the muscle becomes weak or paralyzed and voluntary and reflex contractions of the muscle are lost. The weakness occurs either because the action potentials cannot be transmitted to the muscle owing to disease of the lower motor neuron or because diseased muscle fibers cannot respond to the input from the lower motor neuron. Mild damage to the motor axons in a peripheral nerve can block the conduction of action potentials to the muscle, and severe damage can cause wallerian degeneration of the axon distal to the site of the lesion. In either instance, muscle function is lost.

Atrophy

The loss of muscle bulk in disease is referred to as *atrophy*. Two types of atrophy must be differentiated. The first type, *neurogenic atrophy*, occurs with the loss of innervation from disease affecting the final common pathway. In this case, the muscle that atrophies is weak (out of proportion to size). Atrophy may also occur in muscle disease. The second type is *disuse atrophy*. In this type of atrophy, strength is appropriate to the size of the muscle. Unlike neurogenic atrophy, disuse atrophy is not a sign of disease of the neuromuscular system.

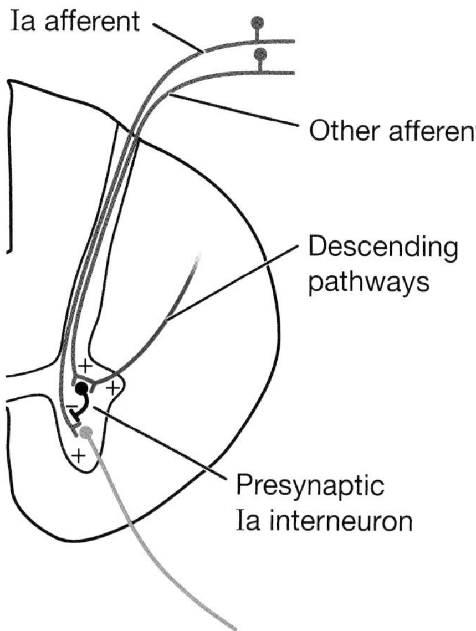

Fig. 8.14. Presynaptic inhibition. Presynaptic inhibitory neurons make GABAergic axoaxonic synapses with Ia or other primary afferents, decreasing neurotransmitter (L-glutamate) release. Presynaptic inhibition of Ia afferents decreases the gain of a muscle stretch reflex. Presynaptic Ia inhibitory interneurons may be activated by other segmental afferents or descending pathways.

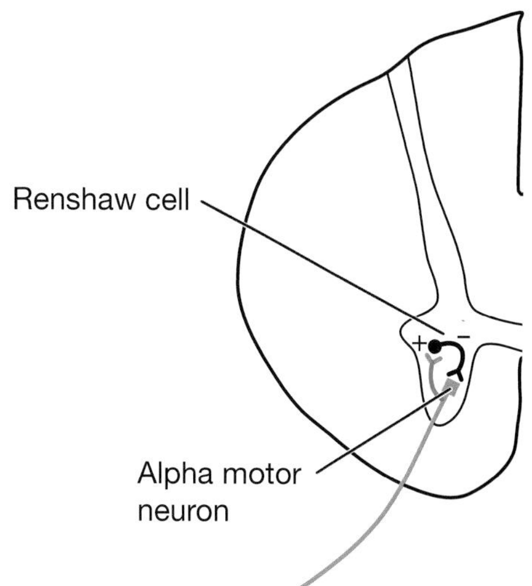

Fig. 8.15. Recurrent inhibition. A recurrent collateral of the axon of an alpha motor neuron makes excitatory synaptic content (mediated by acetylcholine acting on nicotinic receptors) with a Renshaw cell, which uses GABA or glycine to inhibit the alpha motor neuron.

After destruction of an alpha motor neuron or motor axon, some of the denervated muscle fibers may be reinnervated by collaterals from the remaining motor nerve fibers. This process, referred to as collateral sprouting, depends on signals arising from the denervated muscle fibers, Schwann cells, and extracellular matrix. The new collateral sprouts of intact axons form new motor end plates on the denervated muscle fibers, incorporating these muscle fibers into the motor unit of the neuron supplying the axon collaterals. Thus, although the number of motor units decreases because of the loss of motor neurons or motor axons, the size of the surviving motor units (the innervations ratio) increases; this helps maintain strength.

Loss of Muscle Stretch Reflexes and Muscle Tone

Generally, if lower motor neurons are lost, reflexes, particularly stretch reflexes, are reduced or lost (*hyporeflexia or areflexia*). Reflexes are most consistently lost if the disease process also damages the afferent fibers of the reflex arc. With disruption of the reflex arc, normal tone—the response to passive movement—is lost. This state is called *flaccidity*, and the weakness caused by disease of the final common pathway is *flaccid paralysis*. Weakness, flaccidity, and atrophy also occur in the face, tongue, and pharyngeal muscles with disease of the lower motor neurons in the brainstem. This produces a characteristic breathy, imprecise, nasal speech called *flaccid dysarthria* (dysarthria means abnormal utterances).

Spontaneous Activity of the Motor Unit and Muscle Fibers

Diseases of the motor unit also may be associated with excessive activity or spontaneous firing due to a low threshold for discharge. This may take the form of a single spontaneous discharge of a motor unit, a *fasciculation*. A fasciculation can be seen on the surface of the skin as a brief localized twitch. A continuous high-frequency discharge of fascicles of muscle fibers is a cramp. Fasciculations and cramps may be manifestations of disease or may be due simply to physiologic irritability, as can occur after excessive exertion.

After destruction of the lower motor neuron, the individual muscle fibers that have lost their innervation generate slow repetitive action potentials and contract regularly, a process called fibrillation. Fibrillations are not visible through the skin but are detectable with electromyography (see Chapter 13).

- Lower motor neuron lesions produce weakness, atrophy, loss of muscle stretch reflexes, decreased muscle tone, and fasciculations.
- Lower motor neuron findings localize the lesion to the corresponding spinal cord segment, root, or peripheral nerve.

Clinical Problem 8.1.

A 9-year-old boy had a mild cold, and a day later, fever and severe aching muscle pains, predominantly in the back, developed. By the fourth day, he was unable to move his right leg and the fingers of his left hand. His generalized symptoms cleared over the next week. Three weeks after the onset of symptoms, neurologic examination showed that the boy had almost complete paralysis of the right leg, moderate weakness of the left arm, and mild weakness of other muscles, including facial muscles. Reflexes were absent in the right leg, which was flaccid, and in the left arm. There was atrophy of all muscles, most strikingly in the right leg and left arm.

a. Identify the level, side, and type of disease.
b. Which component of the motor system is involved?
c. What are the signs of disease of this component?
d. What are important infectious causes of this disorder?
e. List the main components of this portion of the motor system.

Cortical Motor Control: Direct Activation Pathway

The activity of the motor unit and the segmental reflexes are controlled by supraspinal inputs arising from motor cortex and brainstem nuclei. These supraspinal influences control the activity of motor neurons primarily through interneurons. In humans, the three main functions of these descending motor pathways are 1) to facilitate extension reflexes to keep the body in an erect posture against gravity, 2) to transiently inhibit these postural reflexes to allow independent, flexion movements of the extremities for voluntary movements and locomotion, and 3) to provide for independent movements of the fingers. Whereas the first function occurs independently of cortical control, the other two functions require activity of the motor cortex.

The motor cortex provides the most important descending control to motor neurons. Cortical motor neurons are referred to as *upper motor neurons*. The direct input from the cerebral cortex to the ventral horn and cranial nerve motor nuclei is referred to as the *direct activation pathway*. The descending motor pathways from the brainstem constitute the basic suprasegmental control system for regulation of posture and muscle tone. These pathways are referred to as *indirect pathways*, because they arise from nuclei that receive input from the motor cortex (Fig. 8.16). The contribution of the cortical and brainstem motor pathways to motor control are summarized in Table 8.3.

Anatomy

The motor areas of the cerebral cortex in each hemisphere control motor neurons in the ventral horn on the opposite side of the spinal cord and in the motor nuclei of the brainstem. Cortical projections to the spinal cord constitute the *corticospinal tract*. Those projecting to brainstem motor nuclei form the *corticobulbar tract*.

Cortical Motor Areas

The motor cortex comprises several areas in the frontal lobe. These include the *primary motor cortex* (M1), located in the anterior lip of the central sulcus (Brodmann area 4); the *lateral premotor cortex*, located on the lateral aspect of the hemisphere (lateral area 6 of Brodmann), and the *supplementary motor area*, *pre-supplementary motor area*, and *anterior cingulate motor area*, located on the medial aspect of the cerebral hemispheres (Fig. 8.17).

These areas have a basic pattern of connectivity (Fig. 8.18). The primary motor cortex, lateral premotor cortex, supplementary motor area, and anterior cingulate motor cortex all contribute to corticospinal and corticobulbar pathways. The lateral premotor cortex, supplementary motor area, and primary motor cortex receive input from the parietal lobe and participate in programming and executing movements in response to sensory stimuli. The supplementary motor area, through the pre-supplementary motor area, and the anterior cingulate motor cortex receive input from the prefrontal cortex and are involved in planning and programming goal- or emotion-driven movements. By way of the thalamus, all cortical motor areas receive inputs from the ipsilateral basal ganglia and contralateral cerebellum.

The primary motor cortex has a somatotopic organization, with the contralateral body represented upside down, just as in the sensory cortex (Fig. 8.19). The head area is located above the fissure of Sylvius, the representation of the upper extremity is next (with the thumb and index finger in proximity to the face), the trunk is interposed between the shoulder and hip areas high on the convexity of the hemisphere, and the lower limb area extends onto the paracentral lobule in the longitudinal fissure. The size of the cortical representation varies with the functional importance and dexterity of the part represented. Thus, the lips, jaw, thumb, and index finger each have a large representation; the forehead, trunk, and proximal portions of the limbs have a small one. Input from different neurons within specific territories (face, arm, leg) of the primary motor cortex converge in the spinal cord to control individual motor units, and individual cortical neurons within each territory project to motor neurons that innervate different but functionally related muscles. An important feature of the motor (as well as the sensory) cortex is the *plasticity* of cortical representation: the area representing a given area of the body may be enlarged or reduced in response to injury or acquisition of specific motor skills.

The primary motor cortex provides monosynaptic

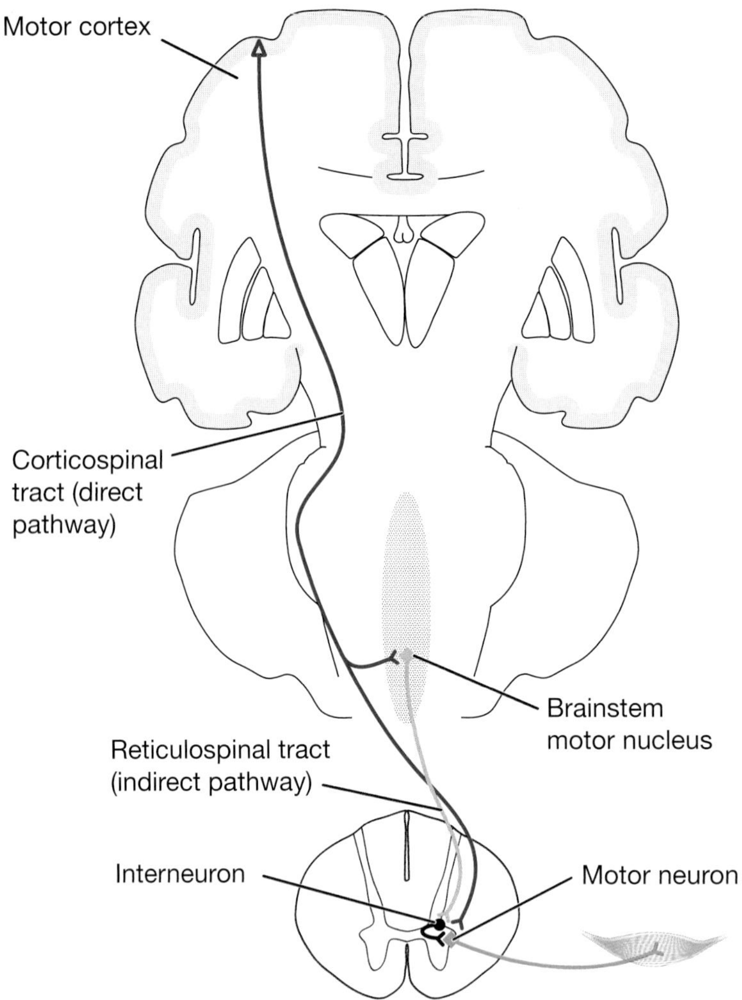

Fig. 8.16. Diagram of the direct and indirect pathways for cortical control of motor neurons. Except for the direct monosynaptic projection from primary motor cortex to motor neurons innervating the hand muscles, most cortical and brainstem effects are exerted through interneurons.

projections to the motor neurons that innervate the distal muscles of the limbs, particularly the fingers. Other spinal projections from primary motor cortex as well as projections from lateral premotor cortex, supplementary motor area, and anterior cingulate motor area terminate predominantly on spinal interneurons. These areas also provide input to the brainstem reticular formation, which projects to the spinal cord to control complex motor synergies and postural adjustments during voluntary movement.

Immediately rostral to the lateral premotor area is the frontal eye field (area 8), which contains neurons involved in the generation of spontaneous and visually guided rapid eye movements called saccades, directed toward the contralateral visual fields. The area of Broca is immediately ventral to the lateral premotor area, in the frontal operculum of the left cerebral hemisphere near the representation of the face. Neurons in the area of Broca participate in the motor programming necessary for speech. These functions are described in more detail in Chapter 16.

Corticospinal Tract

The corticospinal tract is the most important component of the *pyramidal tract* (Fig. 8.20). This name is from the medullary pyramids, which are large paired fiber tracts on the ventral surface of the medulla that contain the corticospinal tracts. In humans, approximately 80% of the pyramidal fibers arise from area 4 (primary motor cortex) and area 6 (including the lateral premotor cortex and supplementary motor area); some arise from the anterior cingulate motor area, and, to a lesser extent, from somatosensory areas 3, 2, 1, and 5 of the parietal lobe.

> Each corticospinal tract contains more than one million fibers. Only 3% to 4% of all the fibers originate from giant pyramidal cells of Betz in the primary motor cortex. Projections from the parietal lobe terminate in the dorsal horn and dorsal column nuclei for processing sensory information for motor control.

Axons from the motor cortex converge in the corona radiata toward the posterior limb of the internal capsule. Here, the compact fiber group is somatotopically organized (Fig. 8.21). The corticobulbar fibers, which innervate the cranial nerve motor nuclei, are located more anteriorly in the genu, between the anterior and posterior limbs of the internal capsule. In the posterior limb, the corticospinal fibers are located from anterior to posterior in the following order: face, arm, leg, bladder, and rectum.

The corticospinal fibers remain a compact group as they pass from the internal capsule into the cerebral peduncle in the midbrain. In the midbrain, the corticospinal and corticobulbar fibers occupy the middle two-thirds of each cerebral peduncle, with the corticobulbar fibers medial to the corticospinal fibers. In the pons, corticospinal fibers are separated into small bundles by the interspersed pontine nuclei. However, the topographic localization persists, with the face represented medially, the leg laterally, and the upper limb intermediately. The fibers reunite in the medulla to form the medullary pyramids.

The pyramidal decussation occurs mainly at the lower border of the medulla, where about 80% of the fibers cross to the opposite side to descend in the dorsolateral quadrant of the spinal cord as the lateral corticospinal tract. The somatotopic organization is maintained in the lateral corticospinal tract (Fig. 8.22). A smaller number of uncrossed pyramidal fibers descend in the ventral column as the ventral corticospinal tract to the cervical and

Table 8.3. Main Descending Motor Pathways and Their Functions

Pathway	Functions
Corticospinal	Fine motor control of finger movements Motor neuron recruitment to increase force Inhibition of postural reflexes
Corticobulbar	Control of muscles of facial expression, mastication, speech, and swallowing
Lateral vestibulospinal	Facilitation of extension reflexes against gravity
Pontine reticulospinal	Facilitation of postural reflexes in erect posture
Medullary reticulospinal	Inhibition (under cortical influence) of segmental muscle stretch and flexor reflexes
Medial vestibulospinal	Locomotion
Tectospinal, interstitiospinal	Coordination of head with eye movements
Rubrospinal	Facilitation of flexor movements of upper limb

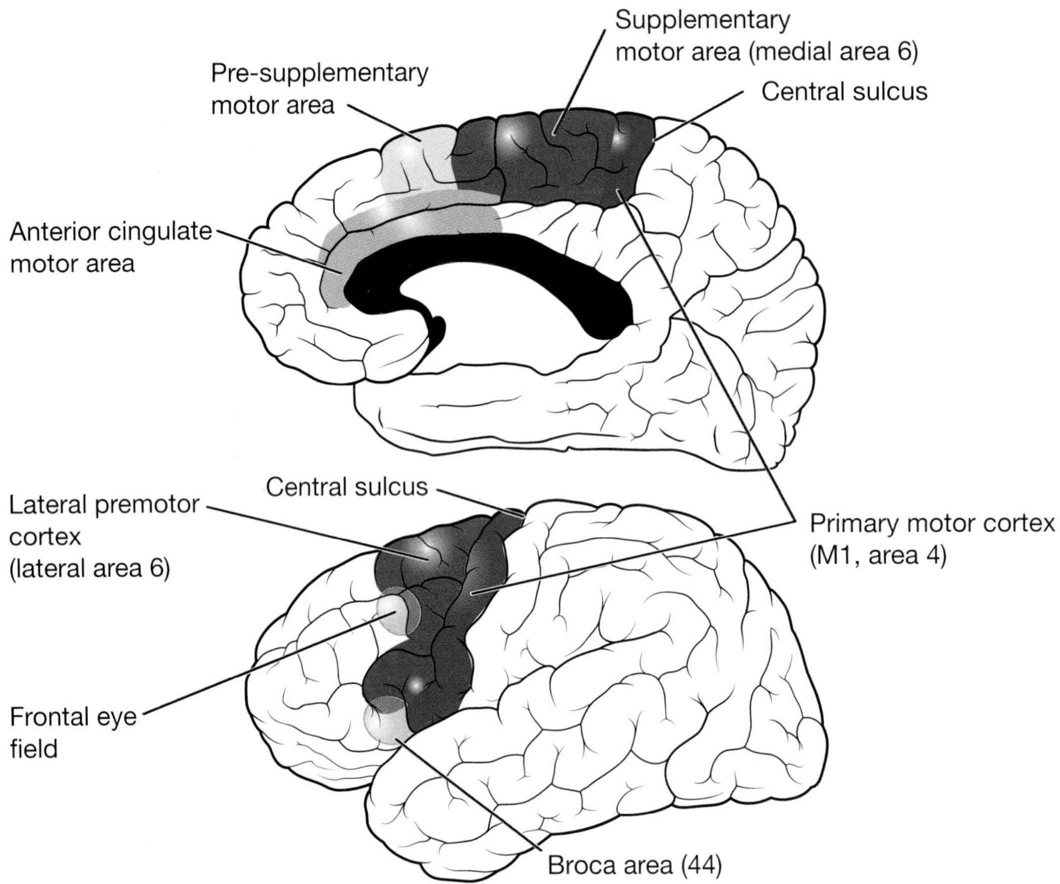

Fig. 8.17. Motor areas of the cerebral cortex. *Bottom*, Lateral view of the cerebral hemisphere showing primary motor cortex (area 4), lateral premotor cortex (lateral area 6), frontal eye fields (area 8), and the area of Broca (area 44). *Top*, Medial view of the cerebral hemisphere showing the supplementary motor area (medial area 6), pre-supplementary motor area, and anterior cingulate motor area. The numerals in parentheses refer to Brodmann areas.

thoracic levels. Some of them remain uncrossed and project to motor neurons that innervate ipsilateral muscle groups.

Individual corticospinal axons branch extensively to innervate several functionally related pools of motor neurons. Although axons arising from primary motor cortex synapse directly on motor neurons that control the distal muscles of the hand, most corticospinal axons influence motor neurons indirectly through interneurons.

- The corticospinal tract originates from primary and nonprimary motor cortical areas and descends in the corona radiata, posterior limb of the internal capsule, cerebral peduncle, and medullary pyramid.
- Most corticospinal axons decussate in the lower medulla and descend in the dorsolateral quadrant of the spinal cord.
- The corticospinal tract affects predominantly motor neurons that innervate distal muscles of the contralateral limbs.

Cortical Inputs to Brainstem Motor Nuclei

In the brainstem, corticobulbar fibers leave the pyramidal tract at several levels, with some fibers crossing the midline and others remaining uncrossed. These fibers synapse in nuclei of the cranial nerves (trigeminal, facial, vagus, spinal accessory, and hypoglossal nerves). Collateral axons from the corticospinal tract also terminate on several nuclei involved in motor control, including the red nucleus, reticular formation, pontine nuclei, and inferior olivary nucleus. The functions of these nuclei are described below in this chapter.

Because of the decussation of most of the fibers of the pyramidal tracts, the voluntary movements of one side of the body are under the control of the opposite cerebral hemisphere. However, some exceptions to this rule are important in clinical diagnosis. Generally, muscle groups of the two

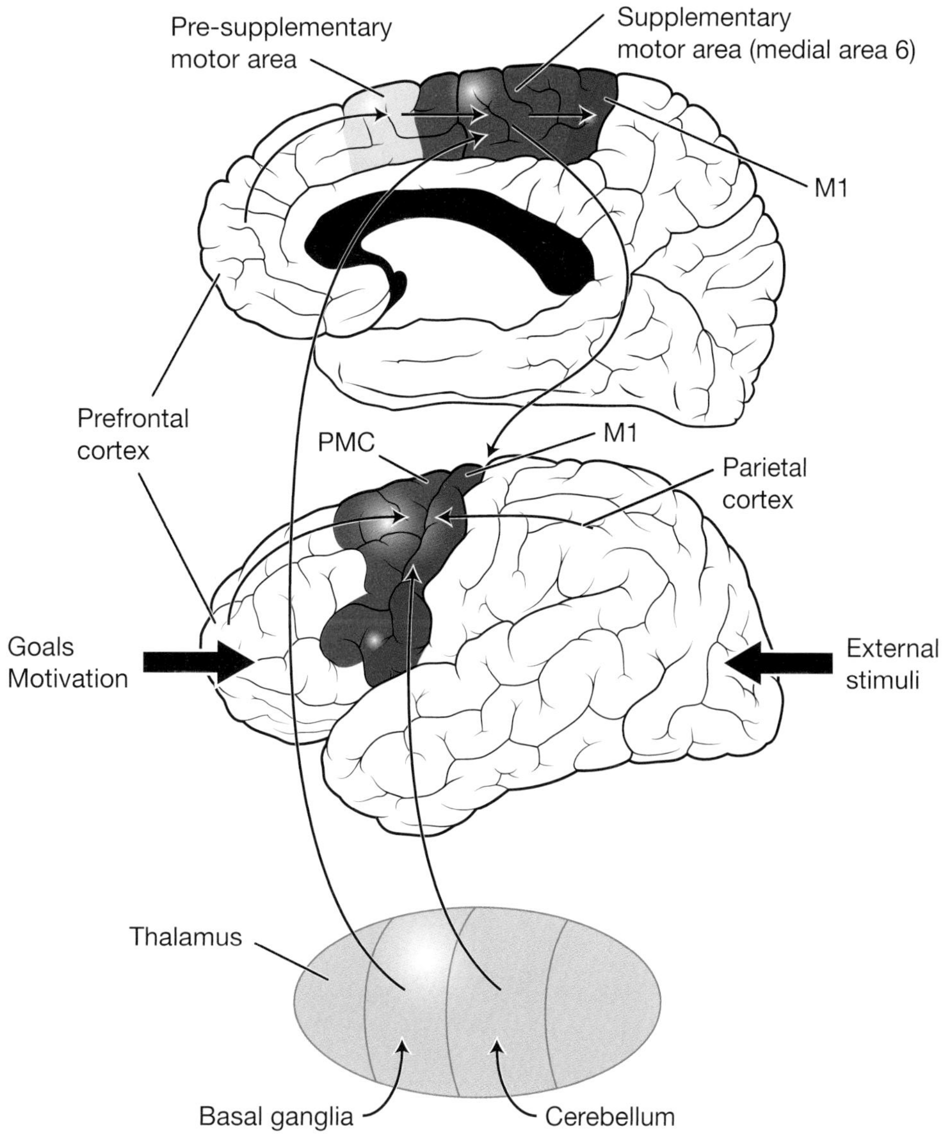

Fig. 8.18. Basic pattern of connectivity of cortical motor areas. Primary motor cortex (M1), lateral premotor cortex (PMC), supplementary motor area, and anterior cingulate motor area (not shown) all project to the spinal cord through the corticospinal tract and to brainstem nuclei controlling motor neurons. These cortical areas receive input from the parietal cortex (relaying integrated somatosensory and visual information for control of movement in response to external stimuli) and the prefrontal cortex (triggers movement according to goals and motivation). Cortical motor areas receive information from the ipsilateral basal ganglia and contralateral cerebellar circuits through the thalamus.

sides of the body that habitually act in unison tend to have bilateral cortical control, whereas muscle groups that act alone in isolated, delicate, and especially learned movements tend to have unilateral control from the opposite hemisphere. Thus, paraspinal muscles are controlled by both hemispheres, as are the muscles in the upper half of the face, pharynx, and larynx (Fig. 8.23). Because of this arrangement, a massive lesion of one hemisphere causes severe weakness of the opposite side of the body but not of upper facial or paraspinal muscles. These principles do not apply in all cases. Even for muscles such as those of the tongue and the palate, which might be expected to work in unison, there is a greater control from the contralateral hemisphere.

Physiology

The motor cortex is the site of convergence of input from a large number of cortical and subcortical areas. The main cortical inputs arise from the ipsilateral parietal, prefrontal, and anterior cingulate cortical areas. The subcortical inputs arise from the ipsilateral basal ganglia and the contralateral cerebellum through relays in the thalamus. The motor cortex controls the spinal motor neurons and segmental reflexes through both direct corticospinal projections (direct pathway) and projections to brainstem nuclei, which in turn project to the ventral horn (indirect pathway). The neurotransmitter of the corticospinal pathway is glutamate; thus, cortical

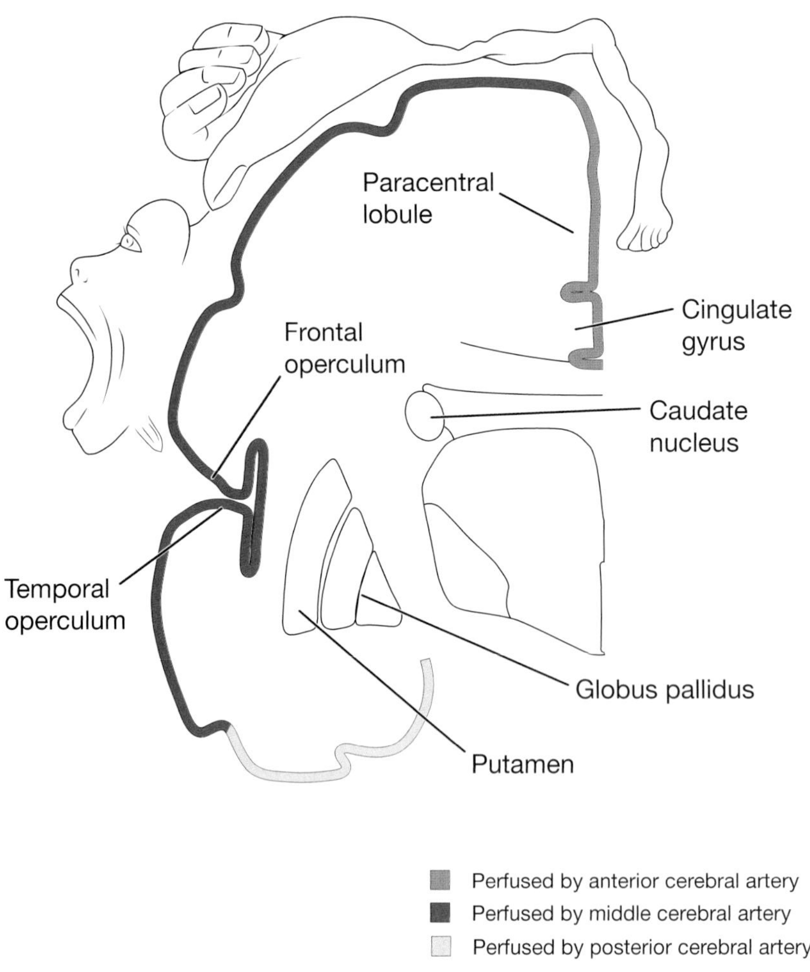

Fig. 8.19. Classic representation of the somatotopic organization of the motor cortex and its arterial supply.

input depolarizes motor neurons, bringing about both an increase in frequency of firing and the recruitment of additional motor units. Consequently, the corticospinal system is important in increasing the force of muscle contraction.

Primary Motor Cortex

The primary motor cortex is organized into functional columns containing neurons that control the same muscle and receive similar inputs from peripheral receptors activated by the resulting movement. Movement in

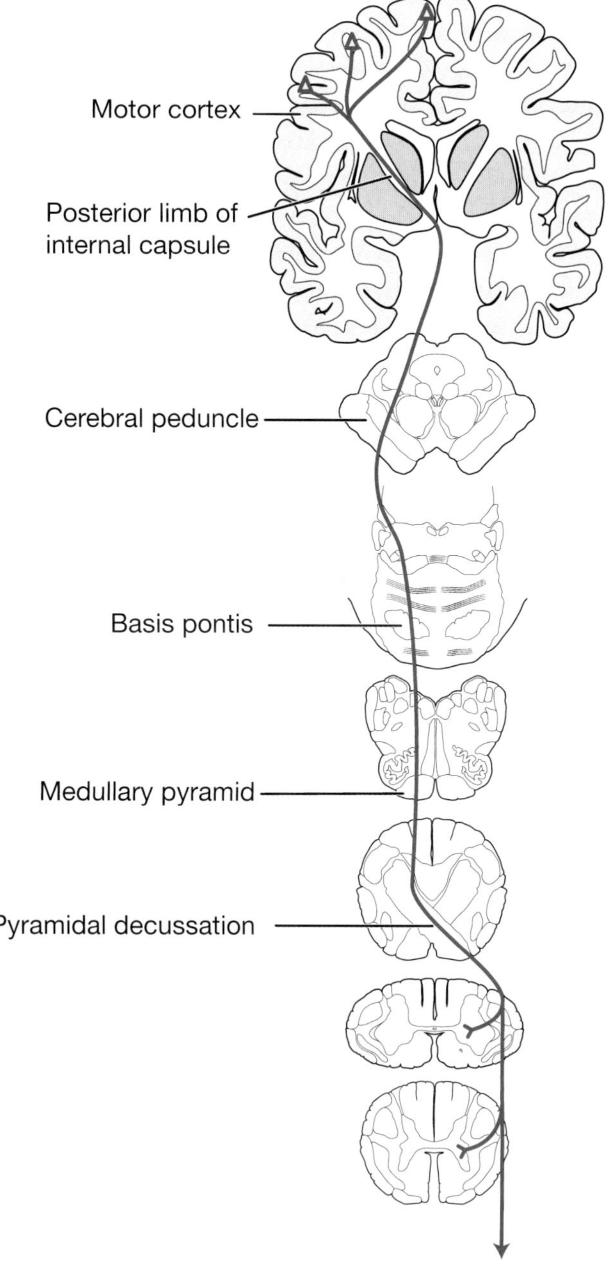

Fig. 8.20. Corticospinal tract. This tract descends through the cerebral hemispheres, brainstem, and spinal cord. Some of the axons in the tract extend the entire length of the spinal cord.

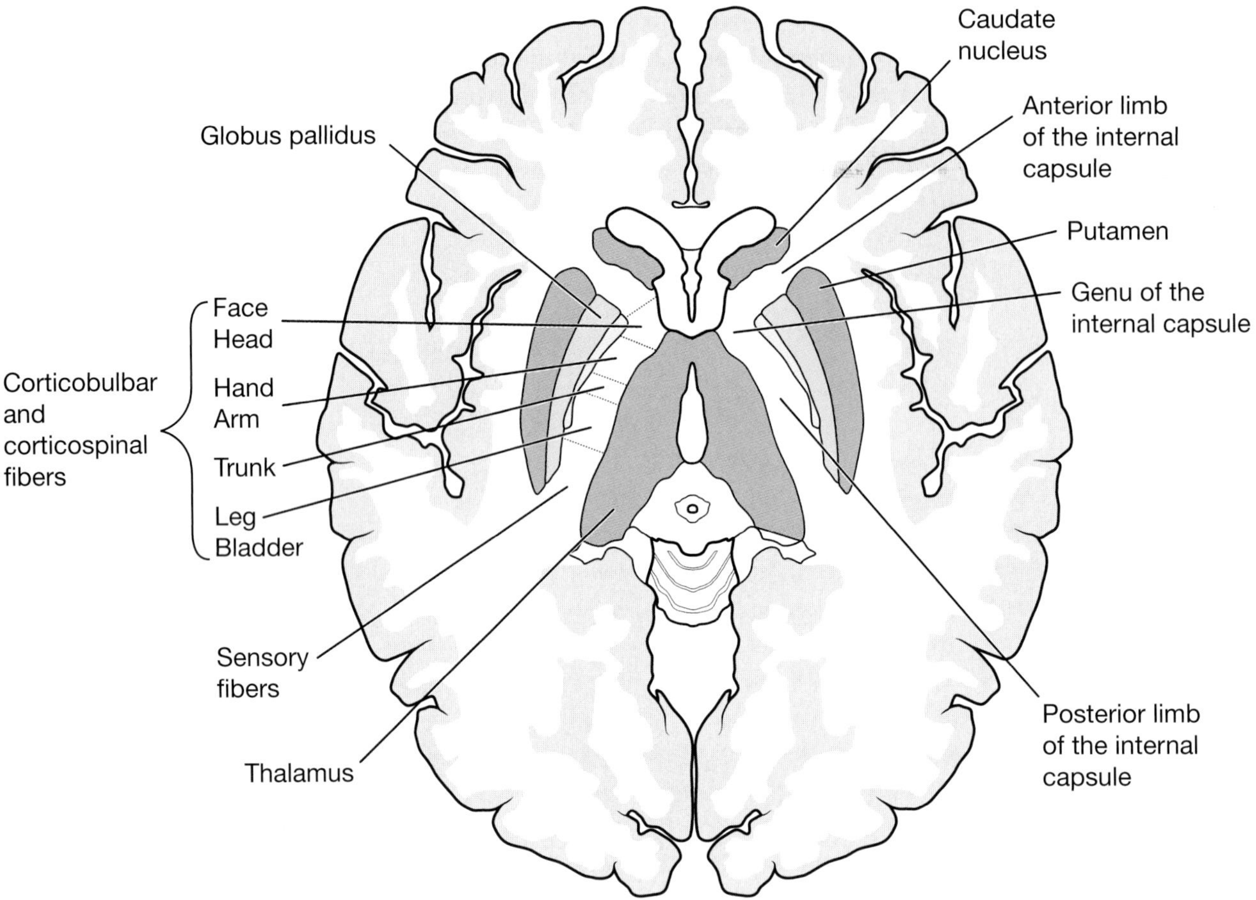

Fig. 8.21. Horizontal section through the cerebral hemispheres showing the somatotopic representation of motor function in the internal capsule.

a particular direction is determined by the net action of a large population of neurons in the primary motor cortex. The powerful direct cortical projections from the primary motor cortex to the motor neurons that innervate the distal muscles allow individual movements of the digits.

Nonprimary Motor Areas

The nonprimary motor areas, including the lateral premotor cortex and supplementary motor area, are involved in the planning and programming of movements. These areas project to the primary motor cortex, which is primarily responsible for the execution of movements.

The lateral premotor cortex receives input from neurons in the posterior parietal cortex that respond to both proprioceptive input from the limbs and visual input. These connections are involved in the control of reaching and grasping movements under visual guidance. The supplementary motor area is involved in the selection and preparation of movement and in the generation of motor sequences and bimanual coordination. The pre-supplementary motor area is implicated in the learning of sequential movements and in the decision to initiate a movement. These two areas receive input from the prefrontal cortex, which is critical for goal-directed motor control.

The cortical motor areas are activated well before the movement is executed. They also are activated when a movement is imagined but not actually performed. This cortical activity is recorded as different *movement-related cortical potentials*, which are used to assess motor reaction times, preparatory activity preceding self-paced movements, and potentials triggered by a warning stimulus.

For simple motor tasks, predominantly the contralateral primary motor cortex is activated, but for the performance of newly acquired complex tasks, the supplementary motor area and lateral premotor cortex are activated bilaterally. As the movement is learned and executed more efficiently, the area of motor cortex activated progressively decreases.

Plasticity of the motor cortex has been demonstrated after cortical lesions, motor training, and disconnection between the primary motor cortex and its peripheral targets. In patients who have recovered from lesions that involved the motor cortex or internal capsule, the activity in ipsilateral primary motor cortex and lateral premotor cortex and supplementary motor areas bilaterally is increased in comparison with that in normal control subjects during performance of motor tasks.

The anterior cingulate motor area is involved in motor responses initiated by emotional motivational cues. The anterior cingulate cortex receives important input from the prefrontal cortex, which is critical for executive control of voluntary motor acts, and dopaminergic input from the midbrain, which provides a reward signal to the motor system, as described below.

- The primary motor cortex is critical for the control of fractionated movements of the fingers and the recruitment of motor neurons for increasing force.
- The lateral premotor cortex is involved in visually guided movements, such as reaching and grasping.
- The supplementary and pre-supplementary motor areas are involved in motor learning and programming.
- The primary motor cortex has a somatotopic organization that changes in response to injury and practice of learned movements.

Clinical Correlations

Knowledge of the clinical manifestations of disease of the corticospinal pathway comes equally from experimental studies and observation of clinical disorders. Disturbances of the corticospinal system may be irritative (positive) or paralytic (negative). These two types of disturbance are exemplified clinically by seizures and paralysis and exemplified experimentally by the results of stimulation and ablation.

Motor Seizures

John Hughlings Jackson, from his study of the attacks that now bear his name (jacksonian seizures), surmised

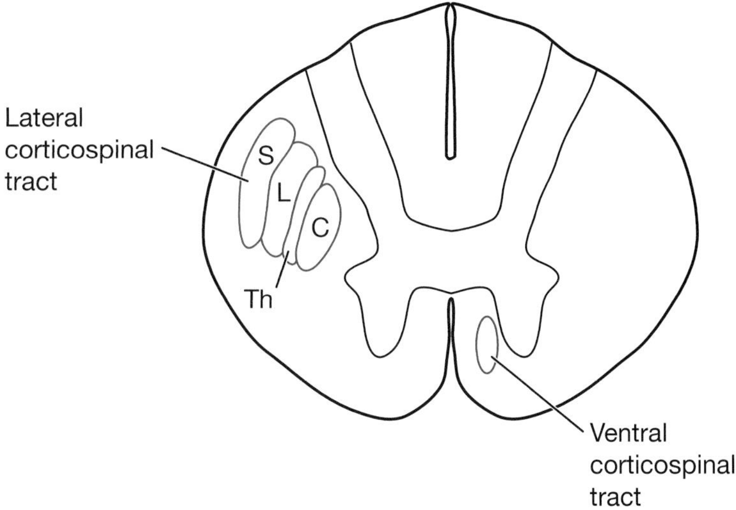

Fig. 8.22. Somatotopic organization of the lateral corticospinal tract. C, cervical; L, lumbar; S, sacral; Th, thoracic.

that there must be a somatotopic representation of motor function in the brain. Focal motor seizures are likely to start in the cortical areas governing the thumb and index finger, the corner of the mouth, or the great toe, because of the relatively large extent of these areas. The spread (march) of the attack is determined by the pattern of cortical localization. Thus, a seizure starting in the thumb and index finger may spread to involve the wrist, elbow, shoulder, trunk, and lower limb, spreading from hip to foot. Seizures arising from the lateral premotor cortex or supplementary motor area can cause complex motor actions, such as raising of the contralateral hand and turning of the head and eyes toward the hand.

Weakness and Lack of Dexterity

Although the corticospinal pathway innervates (either directly or through interneurons) all motor neurons of the ventral horn, it has a major influence on the motor neurons that control the distal movements of the extremities. Therefore, lesions limited to the corticospinal pathways produce a characteristic clinical pattern. There is weakness or paralysis, especially affecting the distal limb muscles of the extremities. The impairment is greatest for fine, skilled movements and movements under voluntary control.

The distribution of the weakness is a function of the site of the lesion. Widespread cortical lesions may affect

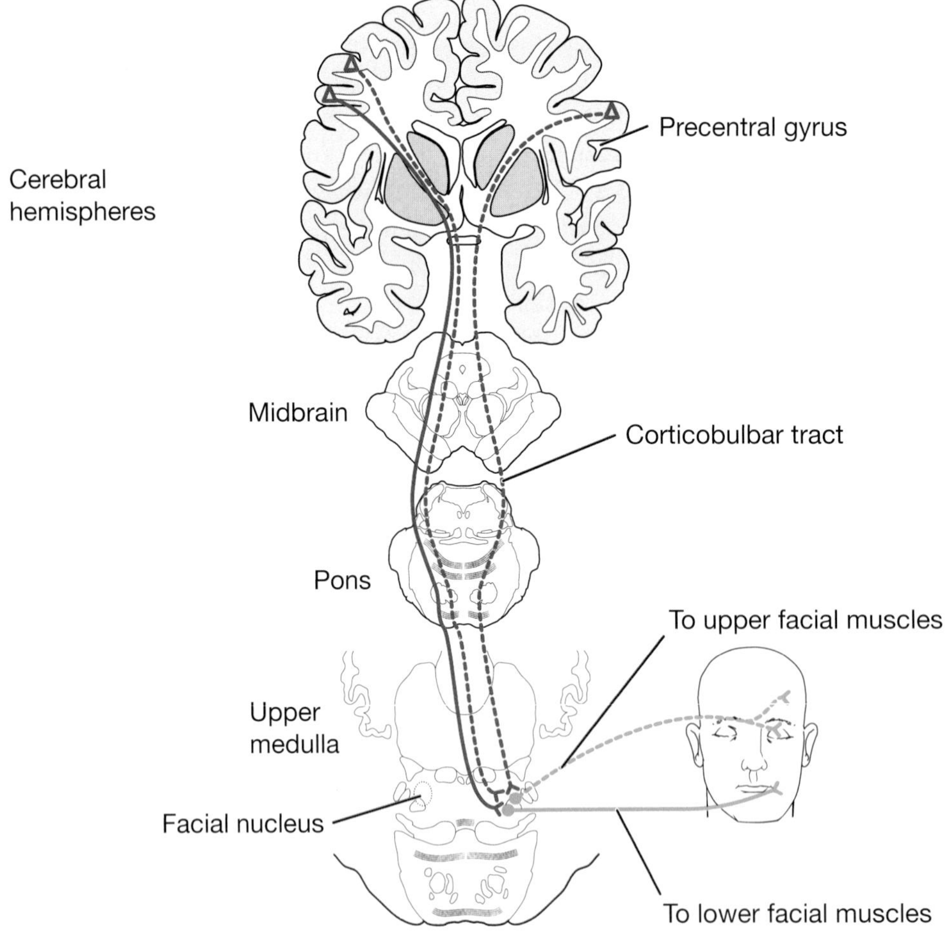

Fig. 8.23. Crossed cortical innervation of motor neurons to the facial muscles on one side. Motor neurons that innervate upper facial muscles have bilateral input from motor cortex, but motor neurons that innervate lower facial muscles have input from only contralateral motor cortex.

all of one side of the body, but a facial, arm, or leg monoplegia is more likely with a lesion of the cerebral cortex. Occasionally, the arm and face are involved together because of the proximity of their cortical representations. Lesions in the internal capsule or cerebral peduncles typically produce weakness of the opposite side of the face and opposite arm and leg. If the lesion involves only the pyramidal tract fibers in the pyramids of the medulla or the spinal cord, one side of the body below the level of the lesion is affected. The distribution also depends on whether the innervation is unilateral or bilateral. For example, the upper part of the face is spared when corticobulbar lesions involve upper motor neurons projecting to the facial nucleus. Unlike the weakness due to lower motor neuron lesions, the paralysis is not associated with atrophy.

With pure corticospinal lesions (which are rare), muscle stretch reflexes may be preserved, although they are often mildly decreased. The corticospinal pathway provides background excitation to motor neurons. After acute interruption of the corticospinal input, spinal motor neurons become unresponsive to segmental stimuli for a period of time. Therefore, acute interruption of the corticospinal input produces not only immediate weakness but also a decrease in reflexes and muscle tone. With recovery of excitability, alpha motor neurons regain the ability to respond to afferent stimuli from the muscle. Reflexes may then become exaggerated because of the loss of inhibition through the concomitant involvement of the indirect activation pathways (see below).

Babinski Sign

The cortical motor input inhibits, through the medullary reticular formation (indirect pathway), the antigravity muscle stretch reflexes, but it facilitates the ipsilateral segmental reflexes elicited by cutaneous stimulation. These include the *abdominal reflexes*, elicited by stimulation of the skin of the abdomen, and the *cremasteric reflex*, elicited by stimulation of the skin of the inner thigh.

Some abnormal reflexes become manifest after a corticospinal tract lesion. The plantar response to noxious stimulation of the sole of the foot is part of a reflex that involves all muscles that shorten the leg. In the newborn, this response is referred to as the *triple flexion reflex*. It is brisk and includes the toe extensors, which also shorten the leg on contraction and thus are flexors from the physiologic standpoint. As the corticospinal tract myelinates and controls alpha motor neurons, the triple flexion reflex becomes less brisk, and in normal subjects, the toe extensors are no longer part of it after age 2 years. The toes curl down in response to noxious stimulation of the sole that elicits a segmental reflex involving the small foot muscles, comparable to the abdominal and cremasteric reflexes. When the corticospinal tract is damaged, noxious stimulation of the sole of the foot elicits extension (dorsiflexion) of the great toe and spreading of the other toes. This is the *extensor plantar response*, or *Babinski sign*.

The occurrence of pure distal flaccid paralysis with the Babinski sign is rarely seen clinically and occurs only with small lesions in the primary motor cortex or medullary pyramids or lesions that selectively involve the direct corticospinal system.

The cerebral cortex, both directly and through collaterals of the corticospinal tract, innervates areas of the brainstem that project to the spinal cord (indirect pathway) and control the segmental and postural reflexes. Because the direct corticospinal and indirect pathways are intermingled at the level of the internal capsule, cerebral peduncles, basis pontis, and spinal cord, a lesion at any of these levels produces a combined effect that accounts for the typical clinical manifestations of the upper motor neuron syndrome, as described below.

- Corticospinal tract lesions produce predominantly distal limb weakness, loss of finger dexterity, and the Babinski sign.

Apraxia

Lesions involving the lateral premotor cortex, supplementary motor area, or posterior parietal cortex, particularly of the left hemisphere, may spare the primary motor cortex and produce no weakness. However, such lesions can result in loss of the ability to perform skilled learned motor acts voluntarily, even though these motor acts can still be elicited automatically or reflexly. This is called *apraxia*. Apraxia may involve any of the motor activities. Patients with limb apraxia are

Clinical Problem 8.2.

A 58-year-old banker suddenly lost the ability to speak and move his right arm. Neurologic examination later in the day showed no progression in his symptoms. He appeared to understand what he was told, but he could not answer questions. In attempting to speak, he uttered nonsense or garbled words. A very few words were uttered correctly, such as "hello." His right arm was paralyzed, and the right cheek and right side of his mouth drooped. Forehead movements were normal. Leg strength was normal. Myotatic reflexes were hypoactive in his right arm but normal elsewhere. He seemed to recognize sensations everywhere. The results of coordination tests were normal, except in the right arm. His gait was normal. Optic fundi were normal.

a. Identify the level, side, and type of lesion.
b. Specifically, what component of and what site in the motor system are involved?
c. How do plantar responses and abdominal reflexes change with lesions in this division?
d. What is the most prominent motor deficit likely to result from this lesion?
e. What term is used to describe this speech disorder?
f. Why is forehead movement on the right normal?

unable to pantomime or imitate a particular gesture or the use of simple objects, such as a hammer. Apraxia of speech is characterized by an inability to say a word at will, but still be able to think of it and to utter it correctly automatically or reflexly.

Patients with lesions affecting the prefrontal cortex, lateral premotor cortex, or supplemental motor area may exhibit primitive motor reflexes that are present in the newborn but suppressed with maturation of the cerebral cortex. In these patients, gently touching the corner of the mouth elicits a *snout reflex* and gentle stroking of the palm elicits an abnormal grasping response, the *grasp reflex.*

Brainstem Motor Pathways

Anatomy

In addition to direct input to the ventral horn and cranial motor nuclei, the motor cortex projects to several regions of the brainstem with neurons whose axons contribute to pathways that project in parallel with the corticospinal system to the spinal and brainstem motor neurons and interneurons. These indirect pathways originate from the red nucleus, superior colliculus, and reticular formation of the pons and medulla (Fig. 8.24). The vestibular nuclei, which also project to the spinal cord, do not receive direct cortical input; they instead receive input from the vestibular organs. Like the cerebral cortex, all these brainstem motor regions receive input from sensory pathways and the cerebellum.

Red Nucleus

The red nucleus is located in the midbrain and contains a group of large (magnicellular) neurons with axons that cross the midline at the level of the midbrain and form the *rubrospinal tract* (Fig. 8.25). This pathway descends in the brainstem and dorsolateral quadrant of the spinal cord to terminate in the ventral horn of cervical segments, where it synapses on mainly the motor neurons that control the flexor muscles of the upper limb. Rubrospinal neurons receive both direct excitatory and indirect inhibitory (via interneurons) inputs from the motor cortex.

Superior Colliculus

The superior colliculus, located in the tectum of the midbrain, receives input from the frontal eye fields and visual and motor cortices and participates in orienting responses. It is involved with conjugated movements of the head, eyes, and limbs toward contralateral space. The superior colliculus is the source of the crossed *tectospinal tract*, which projects primarily to the cervical segments, synapsing on motor neurons that control neck movements (Fig. 8.25), and to areas of the reticular formation that control eye movements (see Chapter 15).

Vestibular Nuclei

The vestibular nuclei form a complex of several nuclei located in the dorsolateral portion of the medulla and pons (see Chapter 15). They receive input from the vestibular organs in the inner ear, which signal changes in the position and movement of the head, and from neck proprioceptors and the cerebellum. The function of the vestibular nuclei is to initiate the reflex movements of the eyes, neck, trunk, and limbs that maintain normal erect posture and equilibrium. The *lateral vestibular nucleus* gives rise to the *lateral vestibulospinal tract*, which descends to all segments of the spinal cord to activate the motor neurons and interneurons that facilitate extensor reflexes of the trunk and limbs (Fig. 8.26). These vestibulospinal extensor reflexes are critical for the maintenance of erect posture. The *medial* and *inferior vestibular nuclei* give rise to the *medial vestibulospinal tract*, which descends together with the tectospinal tract in the ventral quadrant of the spinal cord to synapse on motor neurons that control the neck muscles.

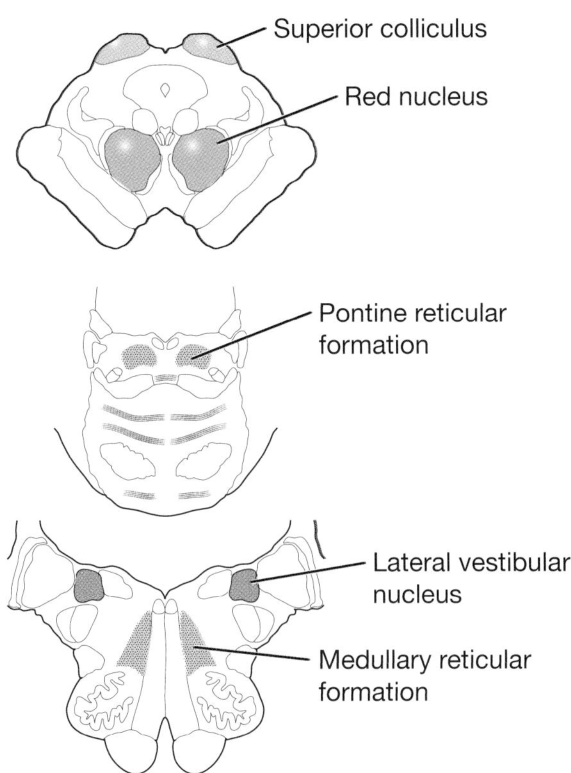

Fig. 8.24. Brainstem nuclei that project to the ventral horn and contribute to the indirect activation pathways.

Reticular Formation

The reticular formation consists of diffuse groups of neurons located throughout the brainstem. These neurons are intimately interconnected, receive input from most motor and sensory pathways, and are critical for sensorimotor integration. Neurons of the reticular formation of the midbrain and rostral pons are the origin of ascending projections and are a major component of the consciousness system (see Chapter 10). Neurons of the reticular formation of the medial dorsal tegmentum of the lower pons and medulla project to the spinal cord through the *reticulospinal tracts* (Fig. 8.27). These are heterogeneous tracts that control all spinal reflexes and are critical for the control of muscle tone, posture, and locomotion. Reticulo-spinal tracts reach all segments of the spinal cord, either directly or through propriospinal neurons. Reticulospinal axons synapse primarily on interneurons that control the function of alpha and gamma motor neurons. According to their origin and course in the spinal cord, reticulospinal tracts have been divided into components that exert different influences on spinal reflexes. The pontine reticular formation gives rise to the *medial (pontine) reticulospinal tract*, which descends ipsilaterally in the ventral portion of the spinal cord. The medullary reticular formation gives rise to the *lateral reticulospinal tract* and *dorsolateral reticulospinal tract*, which occupy the lateral portions of the spinal cord.

The pontine reticulospinal neurons are in the nuclei reticularis pontis caudalis and pontis oralis, and the medullary reticulospinal neurons are in the ventromedial reticular formation, including the nucleus reticularis gigantocellularis.

Physiology

The brainstem motor pathways can be subdivided into two main groups: medial and lateral pathways. The medial pathways include the vestibulospinal, reticulospinal, and tectospinal tracts. They descend bilaterally in the ventral and ventrolateral portion of the spinal cord and synapse on ventral horn neurons that control the neck, trunk, and proximal limb muscles. These pathways control eye and head movements, posture, muscle tone, segmental reflexes, and locomotion. The lateral pathways

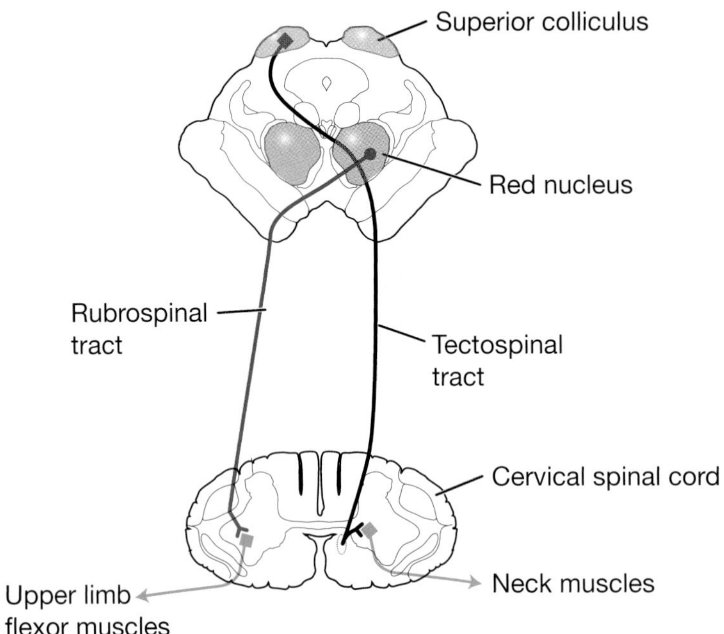

Fig. 8.25. Rubrospinal and tectospinal pathways (both are bilateral, but are shown unilaterally). The rubrospinal tract arises in the red nucleus on the opposite side and reaches the cervical spinal cord to activate flexor movements of the arm. The tectospinal tract arises in the contralateral superior colliculus and, together with the medial vestibulospinal tract (not shown), coordinates movements of the head with those of the eyes.

include the rubrospinal tract, which descends together with the corticospinal tract, in the dorsolateral quadrant of the spinal cord and synapses on motor neurons that innervate flexors of the upper limb.

Control of Posture

Posture is the ability to adjust the position of the body to the direction of gravity and parts of the body in relation to one another. Equilibrium is the capacity to assume an upright posture and maintain balance. The positions of the eyes, head, body, and limbs are all interdependent and signaled to the brain by the visual, vestibular, and proprioceptive systems. Postural adjustments are preprogrammed and aimed at keeping the center of mass of the body in line with the support base. Vestibular and neck postural reflexes are innate reflexes that contribute to the maintenance of postural stability. The most important pathway for maintaining posture against gravity is the lateral vestibulospinal tract. The primary function of this pathway is excitation of the alpha and gamma motor neurons that innervate the extensor axial and proximal limb muscles, which keep the body upright against the pull of gravity. The pontine reticulospinal tract also promotes antigravity reflexes in the standing position, including flexion of the upper limb and extension of the lower limb.

Under normal conditions, postural reflexes are controlled by motor cortex through the indirect motor pathway and integrated into the selected pattern of voluntary movement. In humans, these reflexes cannot be elicited normally in isolation but become obvious after bilateral interruption of descending cortical motor pathways (see below).

Control of Spinal Reflexes, Muscle Tone, and Locomotion

Medullary reticulospinal pathways mediate cortical control of segmental spinal reflexes. This is important for inhibiting postural or flexor reflexes that may interfere with the execution of voluntary motor acts. Neurons of the medullary reticular formation are activated by input from the motor cortex and generally inhibit segmental spinal reflexes by synapsing on inhibitory interneurons. Neurons of the ventromedial medullary reticular formation that project through the lateral reticulospinal tract inhibit the postural extensor reflexes triggered by gravity or head movement. This allows execution of voluntary motor acts by preventing the effects of muscle stretch reflexes of antagonist muscles, which would oppose the effects of the contraction of the desired muscle. Neurons projecting through the dorsolateral reticulospinal tract tonically inhibit polysynaptic reflexes triggered by flexor reflex afferents. The inhibitory effects of the medullary reticulospinal pathway (and thus the corticomedullary reticulospinal system) on spinal reflexes is mediated by inhibitory GABAergic and glycinergic interneurons in the spinal cord.

Medullary reticulospinal neurons also receive input from mesencephalic neurons involved in locomotion (mesencephalic locomotor center). Through reticulospinal input to propriospinal neurons and interneurons of the spinal locomotor pattern generator, the medullary reticular formation supports coordinated movements required for locomotion.

Coordinated Control of Head and Eye Movements

The coordinated control of the movements of the head and eyes is essential for maintaining equilibrium and visual acuity during head movement. This function depends on several brainstem areas that project to both ocular motor nuclei and spinal motor neurons that innervate the neck muscles. These areas include the medial vestibular nucleus, superior colliculus, and the *interstitial nucleus of Cajal.* Spinal projections from these areas descend together in the ventral part of the spinal cord as the descending component of the *medial longitudinal*

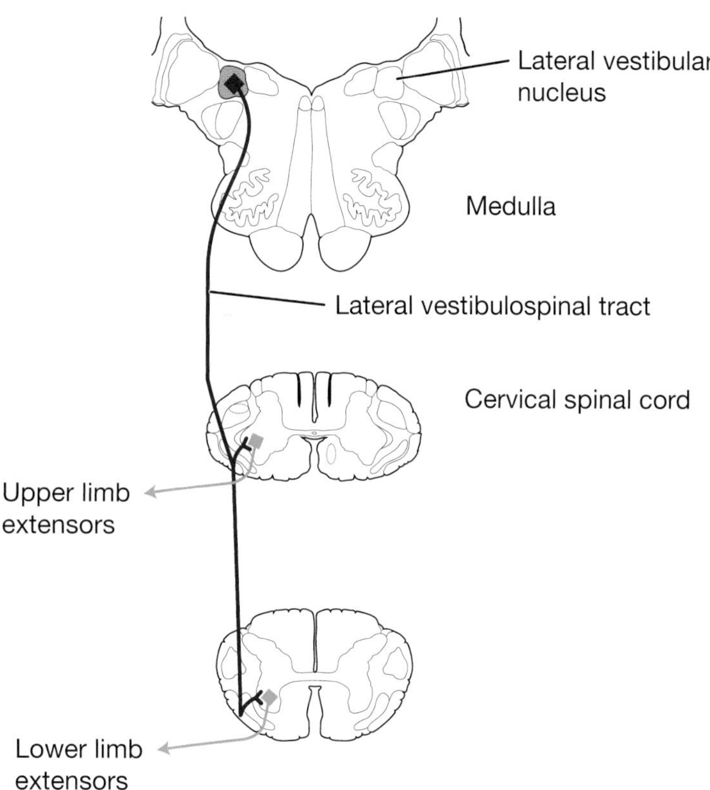

Fig. 8.26. The lateral vestibulospinal tract arises in the lateral vestibular nucleus, which receives inputs from the labyrinth, cerebellum, and neck proprioceptors, but not the cerebral cortex. This pathway descends in the anterior quadrant of the spinal cord and activates extensor reflexes necessary for maintaining posture.

fasciculus. The axons end in the cervical segments. The medial longitudinal fasciculus is also a major brainstem pathway that interconnects the vestibular nuclei and ocular motor nuclei (see Chapter 15).

Rubrospinal Tract and Ancillary Control of Upper Limb Flexion

Magnicellular neurons of the red nucleus receive cortical input from corticorubral fibers and from collaterals of corticospinal axons. The corticorubrospinal system may participate in the control of voluntary flexor movements of the forearm and hand, particularly those requiring simultaneous synergistic actions of the digits, such as gripping movements. However, the function of this system is only ancillary; under normal conditions, these are the functions of the corticospinal tract.

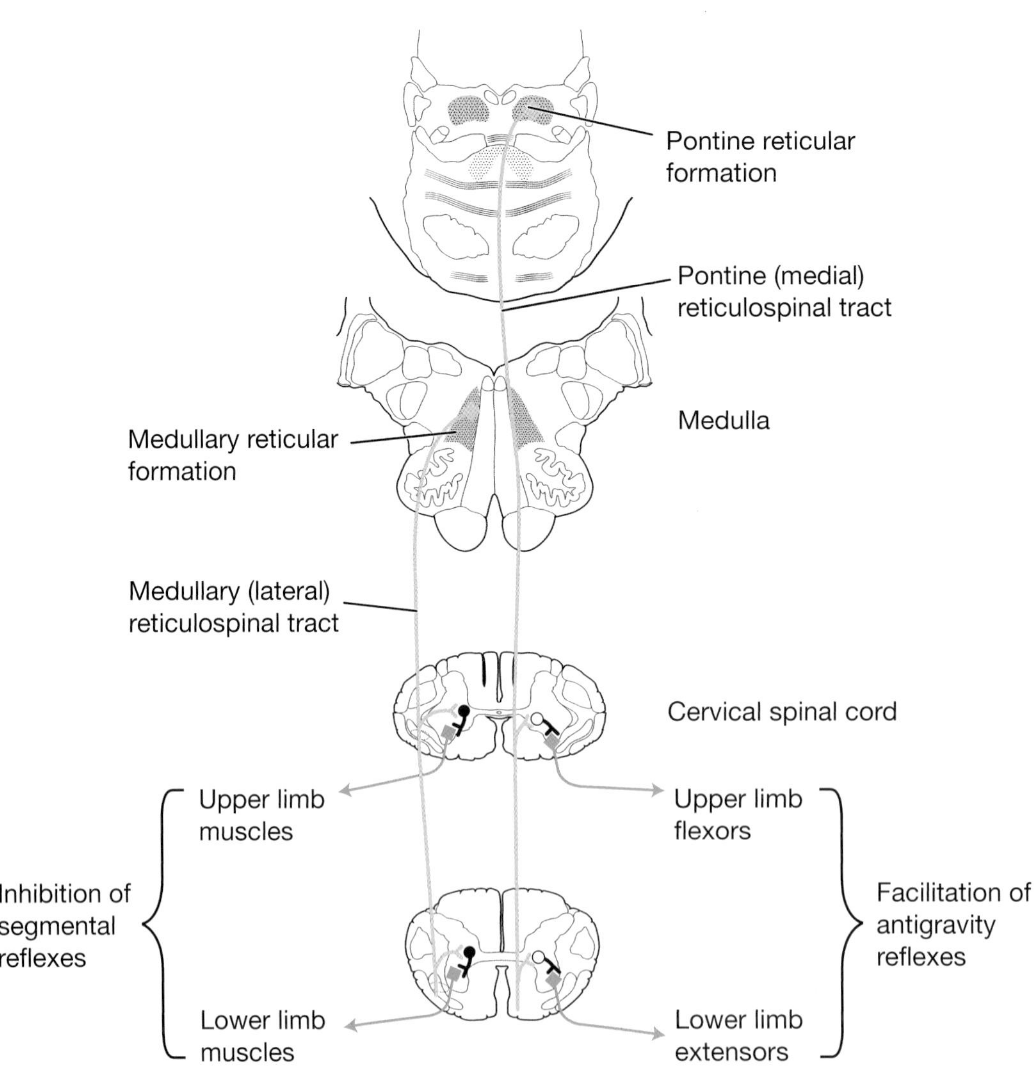

Fig. 8.27. Reticulospinal pathways arise from neurons in the medial tegmentum of the pons and medulla. Both tracts occur bilaterally but are shown here only on one side. The pontine reticulospinal tract activates antigravity reflexes in the erect position (flexion of the upper and extension of the lower limbs). The medullary reticular formation receives input from the cerebral cortex and projects through the lateral reticulospinal tract and inhibits segmental stretch reflexes and flexor reflexes to allow voluntary motor acts and locomotion.

- The lateral vestibulospinal and pontine reticulospinal tract facilitate postural antigravity reflexes.
- The medullary reticulospinal tract mediates cortical influences that inhibit segmental reflexes that interfere with the execution of voluntary movement.
- The medial vestibulospinal and tectospinal tracts coordinate head and eye movements.
- The rubrospinal tract has an ancillary role in facilitating flexion of the forearm and hand.

Clinical Correlations

Spasticity

The interruption of cortical input to the medullary reticular formation at the supratentorial or posterior fossa level or interruption of the medullary reticulospinal system at the spinal level interrupts the excitatory input to spinal inhibitory interneurons (including Ia, Ib, and other inhibitory interneurons) that is required to inhibit segmental reflexes. The result is an abnormal exaggeration of muscle stretch reflexes and flexor reflexes. Without medullary reticulospinal inhibition, the lateral vestibulospinal and pontine reticulospinal tracts increase motor neuron excitability.

The velocity-dependent increase in muscle tone due to exaggerated tonic stretch reflexes is called *spasticity*. This is associated with an exaggeration of muscle stretch reflexes (hyperreflexia). A common manifestation of hyperreflexia is *clonus* (i.e., repeated jerking of a muscle), which occurs when stretch reflexes occur in series and relaxation in one muscle initiates contraction in another muscle. Spasticity is commonly associated with other phenomena such as the *clasp-knife phenomenon*, which is a manifestation of uninhibited polysynaptic flexion reflexes. In the clasp-knife phenomenon, the increased resistance to passive movement with initial stretch subsides with continuous stretch. Spasticity may also be associated with flexor or extensor spasms of the affected limbs.

- Spasticity is a velocity-dependent increase in muscle tone associated with exaggerated muscle stretch reflexes.
- Spasticity is due to lack of inhibition of muscle stretch reflexes from interruption of descending cortical and medullary reticulospinal inputs to spinal inhibitory interneurons.

Postural Responses in Comatose Patients

Large bilateral lesions of the brainstem reticular formation produce *coma*, a state of loss of arousal due to impairment of the ascending reticular activation of the thalamus and cerebral cortex, which is a function of the consciousness system (see Chapter 10). These lesions also interrupt the cortical input to the neurons of the medullary reticular formation that mediate the cortical control of

Clinical Problem 8.3.

A 44-year-old woman began to notice problems with walking about 1 year ago. She felt that her gait was becoming stiff and slow. This problem has been progressive since that time. More recently, she has had episodes of urinary urgency and incontinence. On neurologic examination, she was noted to have a stiff gait. Mental status; cranial nerve function; and muscle strength, tone, reflexes, and sensation in the upper limbs were all normal. She had mild weakness in the iliopsoas and hamstring muscles and in foot and toe extensors bilaterally. Increased muscle tone, exaggerated knee and ankle reflexes, clonus, and Babinski signs were demonstrated bilaterally. Vibration sense was decreased in the toes bilaterally.

a. What are the manifestations of upper motor neuron involvement in this patient?
b. What is the mechanism of the increase in muscle stretch reflexes and tone in this patient?
c. What are the characteristics of spasticity as opposed to rigidity?
d. Why did the bladder develop symptoms?
e. What is the cause of decreased vibration sense in the toes?
f. What is the most likely cause of her symptoms?

postural reflexes. This interruption leads to disinhibition of stereotyped reflex posture response patterns that are normally suppressed or incorporated into the voluntary action. These postural reflexes are triggered by pain or other stimuli, including movement of the head and tracheal suctioning.

The pattern of posturing in comatose patients has localizing value. If the damage is rostral to the red nucleus, the response is characterized by flexion and pronation of the arms and extension of the legs. This is called *decorticate posture.* It reflects disinhibition of antigravity reflexes mediated by the pontine reticular formation, which consist of flexion of the upper limb and extension of the lower limb. The rubrospinal tract (upper limb flexion) and vestibulospinal tract (lower limb extension) may possibly contribute to this posture. If the lesion is in the midbrain or upper pons caudal to the red nucleus but rostral to the vestibular nuclei, the postural response is characterized by extension of all the extremities. This is called *decerebrate posture.* It reflects disinhibition of extensor postural reflexes mediated by the lateral vestibulospinal tract. Lesions caudal to the level of the vestibular nuclei interrupt all excitatory input to spinal motor neurons. In the acute state, this leads to inexcitability of these neurons and lack of response to segmental afferents. The result is loss of muscle tone (flaccidity) in all the limbs.

- In comatose patients, decorticate posture indicates a lesion rostral to the red nucleus; decerebrate posture indicates a lesion between the red nucleus and vestibular nuclei.

Upper Motor Neuron Syndrome

The consequence of an interruption of both the corticospinal input (direct pathway) and parallel corticoreticulospinal input (indirect pathway) to spinal interneurons and motor neurons is the *upper motor neuron syndrome.* Involvement of the corticospinal (direct) pathway produces the two negative phenomena of the syndrome, namely, weakness and loss of dexterity. Involvement of the corticoreticulospinal (indirect) pathways produces the three positive components of the syndrome, that is, enhanced muscle stretch reflexes, increased muscle tone (spasticity), and release of flexor reflexes. When function of the corticospinal tract is impaired, noxious stimulation of the sole elicits extension of the great toe (physiologic flexion); this extensor plantar response is the Babinski sign. This exaggeration of the intersegmental flexion reflex response is in sharp contrast to the inhibition of segmental nociceptive reflexes such as the abdominal and cremasteric reflexes.

The distribution of neurologic findings of the upper motor neuron syndrome varies with the localization of

Clinical Problem 8.4.

A 21-year-old single woman was found lying unresponsive in bed by her girlfriend, who had stopped by in the morning to drive the woman to work. The girlfriend called for an ambulance and went with the patient to the hospital. The following facts were obtained from the girlfriend on questioning. The patient had been in good health. She was well the evening before. She apparently was not taking any medications, and no empty or partially filled bottles were in evidence. There were no signs of a struggle or violence and no suicide note. The patient was in bed as though she had been asleep. There were no unusual findings about the patient: no blood, urine, feces, or injuries. However, her skin had a peculiar pink appearance. On neurologic examination, she was unresponsive to all but painful stimuli, to which she responded with a stiff extension of her neck, arms, and legs. Her eyes apparently did not respond to threatening stimuli but appeared to close randomly. Her jaw was tightly clenched. Bilateral extensor plantar responses were noted. Her respirations were irregular. Tone was generally increased, and muscle reflexes were hyperactive.

a. What is the pattern of postural response in this patient?
b. What is the most likely location of the lesion?
c. Why is the patient comatose?
d. What are possible causes of her condition?

the lesion. The combination of paralytic and release phenomena are typical of a lesion in the internal capsule. Such a lesion produces a characteristic pattern of impaired motor activity on one side of the body. If the paralysis is severe, the pattern is called *hemiplegia*. If the paralysis is mild, it is called *hemiparesis*. Another common pattern is the result of bilateral involvement of descending motor pathways in the spinal cord. When the lesion is at the cervical level, both the upper and lower limbs are affected (*quadriplegia* or *quadriparesis*); when the lesion affects the thoracic or lumbar spinal cord, both lower limbs are affected (paraplegia or paraparesis).

The typical findings of hemiparesis include slowed motor activity and weakness. The weakness has a characteristic distribution: the upper portion of the face is spared and the lower portion is weak contralateral to the lesion. Volitional facial movements are weak, but emotional and associated movements such as smiling are spared or exaggerated. There may be slight weakness of the palate contralateral to the lesion and a tendency for the tongue, on protrusion, to deviate to the side of the hemiplegia. In the upper extremity, the extensors are weaker than the flexors, but in the lower extremity, the flexors are weaker than the extensors. Chiefly affected are skilled, delicate, precision movements. Thus, the fingers are particularly affected. Movements tend to be massive and crude. The patient may not be able to perform selective movements; for instance, he or she may be able to flex and extend all the fingers together but not individually and, when attempting to dorsiflex the ankle, may also flex the knee. The patient walks with a characteristic circumduction of the affected leg. Movements that the patient is unable to perform voluntarily may occur reflexly; for example, when the patient yawns or is tickled, the paretic upper limb may elevate and the fingers extend and abduct. Involuntary associated movements also occur in the paralyzed limb when powerful movements occur on the nonparalyzed side.

With an upper motor neuron lesion, there is increased resistance to passive movement (spasticity) and overactivity of the spinal reflexes that maintain upright posture and a corresponding increase of tone in the antigravity muscles. In humans, the antigravity muscles are the flexors in the upper limb and the extensors in the lower limb. Upper motor neuron lesions produce a characteristic posture: the upper limb is adducted and flexed at the elbow, wrist, and fingers; the lower limb is adducted and extended at the hip and knee. The response to passive movement includes the clasp-knife phenomenon, in which the increased resistance to passive movement present with initial stretch subsides with continued stretch. Large, acute, supratentorial lesions may produce a transient flaccid paralysis. Speech also is impaired by upper motor neuron lesions. Because of the bilateral innervation of bulbar muscles, impaired speech is most common with bilateral disease. This speech impairment is referred to as spastic dysarthria, characterized by a harsh, labored, slow, monotonous, and weak speech with poor articulation.

Clinical Problem 8.5.

A 60-year-old housewife began 10 months ago to have infrequent, brief episodes of twitching of her left hand. These ceased 4 months ago, but she then noted clumsiness when using her left hand. This progressed to moderate weakness and a peculiar feeling in her hand. In the past month, she began to have headaches. On neurologic examination, she was lethargic but otherwise intact mentally. Both optic discs were mildly swollen. She had mild drooping of the lower part of her face on the left, moderate weakness, and slowing of rapid alternating movements of the left hand. Reflexes were hyperactive in the left arm and leg, and the Babinski sign was elicited on the left. Muscle tone was increased on the left. Sensation was normal except for the inability to recognize some objects placed in her left hand.

a. What are the level, site, and pathologic basis of the lesion?
b. What is the mechanism of motor impairment in this patient?
c. What is the term used for the inability to recognize an object by touch, and what is its localizing value?

In upper motor neuron disease, the stretch reflexes differ from normal in that the threshold is lowered, the response is exaggerated and more protracted (hyperreflexia), and they are associated with clonus (clonus must be distinguished from the clonic, jerking movements in a seizure). The abdominal and cremasteric reflexes are impaired or lost, but the Babinski sign appears. The main differences between lower motor neuron and upper motor neuron syndromes are summarized in Table 8.4.

- The upper motor neuron syndrome consists of negative phenomena (weakness, lack of dexterity, and impaired segmental cutaneous reflexes), positive phenomena (spasticity, hyperreflexia, and exaggerated multisynaptic flexion reflexes), and the Babinski sign.

Motor Neuron Disease

Many degenerative diseases selectively affect the motor system. One of these is *amyotrophic lateral sclerosis*, or motor neuron disease. This condition is characterized pathologically by degeneration of motor neurons in the spinal cord, brainstem, and cerebral cortex, which is associated with secondary axonal degeneration in the peripheral nerves and lateral funiculus of the spinal cord (corticospinal tract).

Motor neuron disease expresses itself with various degrees of involvement of the final common pathway and

Clinical Problem 8.6.

A 57-year-old woman began to notice problems with walking about 1 year ago. She felt that her gait was becoming stiff and slow. This problem has been progressive since that time. More recently, she has noted some weakness in the left hand, especially when trying to grip something with it. Neurologic examination showed atrophy and weakness in the left hand muscles. The triceps reflex is absent. Reflexes are increased in the left leg. There is mild weakness in the left leg, especially in hip and knee flexion and ankle dorsiflexion. Muscle tone is increased in the left leg. The Babinski sign is present on the left.

a. What are the manifestations of upper motor neuron involvement in this patient?
b. What is the mechanism of increased muscle stretch reflexes and tone in this patient?
c. What are the characteristics of spasticity as opposed to rigidity?
d. What are the lower motor neuron findings in this patient?
e. How do they help to localize the lesion?
f. What diagnostic study is indicated in this patient?

Table 8.4. Differences Between Lower and Upper Motor Neuron Syndromes

Feature	Lower motor neuron syndrome	Upper motor neuron syndrome
Weakness (distribution)	Yes (distribution of myotome or peripheral nerve)	Yes (predominantly distal, more severe in upper limb flexors and lower limb extensors)
Atrophy	Yes	No
Fasciculations	Yes	No
Muscle tone	Decreased	Increased (spasticity)
Muscle stretch reflexes	Decreased	Increased (with clonus)
Babinski sign	No	Yes

corticospinal and corticobulbar pathways. Initially after being damaged, lower motor neurons are irritable, which is expressed as frequent, widespread fasciculations. After death of the cell body and degeneration of the axon, there is a combination of flaccid weakness and muscle atrophy. The denervated muscle shows fibrillation potentials, which are not seen clinically but detected with electromyography (see Chapter 13). Involvement of the descending pathways may also produce the Babinski sign and hyperactive reflexes.

Involvement of corticobulbar pathways produces *spastic dysarthria* (slow, strained speech), and involvement of the motor nuclei that innervate the pharynx, larynx, or tongue produces *flaccid dysarthria* (see Chapter 15). In motor neuron disease, dysarthria is commonly associated with *dysphagia* (inability to swallow).

Clinical Problem 8.7.

A 72-year-old man had progressive difficulty walking for 1 year. He complained his legs were "stiff and clumsy." He also complained of trouble swallowing and slurred speech. Neurologic examination showed that the patient's speech was slow and strained, and atrophy and fasciculations were noted on both sides of the tongue. He had bilateral footdrop and a steppage gait. The weakness in the legs and arms was asymmetric. Atrophy and fasciculations were seen in both legs and arms. Reflexes were reduced in the arms and legs, and the Babinski sign was elicited bilaterally. Sensation was normal.

a. What are the manifestations of lower motor neuron involvement in this patient?
b. What are the manifestations of upper motor neuron involvement?
c. What term is used for this condition?
d. What is the most likely cause of this patient's condition?

Cerebellar Control Circuit

The cerebellum and its connections constitute one of the two major control circuits of the motor system. The cerebellum is essential for learning, planning, initiating, executing, and adapting movements and postures. It controls the initiation, speed, amplitude, and termination of movement by providing timing signals to the motor areas that control the contraction of agonist and antagonist muscles acting on one or multiple joints. The cerebellum acts as a comparator between the central motor commands and the sensory consequences of execution of the movement and provides signals to the motor center to correct the execution of movement when appropriate. The cerebellum controls eye movement, speech, posture, gait, and coordination of the ipsilateral limbs.

Anatomy

Gross Anatomy and Main Connections

The cerebellum is subdivided into two main components, the *flocculonodular lobe* and the body of the cerebellum (Fig. 8.28). The body of the cerebellum includes the midline *vermis* and the lateral *cerebellar hemispheres*. Both the vermis and the hemispheres are subdivided into anterior and posterior lobes. Each lobe is divided into several *lobules*, each consisting of several leaflet-like *folia*. The gray matter of the cerebellum consists of the *cerebellar cortex* and the *deep cerebellar nuclei*. Both the cerebellar cortex and deep cerebellar nuclei receive afferents to the cerebellum. The cerebellar cortex projects to the deep cerebellar nuclei, which are the source of the output of the cerebellum (Fig. 8.29).

On the basis of their connections and functions, the cerebellar vermis and hemispheres are subdivided into sagittal zones. The vermis includes a medial portion, which projects to the *fastigial nucleus*, and a lateral portion, which projects directly to the lateral vestibular nucleus. The cerebral hemispheres include the *paravermis*, which projects to the *globose* and *emboliform nuclei* (deep cerebellar nuclei), and the large lateral portion, which projects to the *dentate nucleus*, the largest deep cerebellar nucleus and the source of the main output of the cerebellum.

The inputs and outputs of the cerebellum travel through the *cerebellar peduncles*. The inputs reach the cerebellum primarily through the inferior and middle cerebellar peduncles and the outputs leave through the superior cerebellar peduncle. The *inferior cerebellar peduncle* (also called the restiform body) contains cerebellar inputs from the spinal cord and medulla, and the *middle cerebellar peduncle* (also called the brachium pontis) contains the massive input from the contralateral pons. The *superior cerebellar peduncle* (also called the brachium conjunctivum) contains the output of the deep cerebellar nuclei, including projections to the contralateral midbrain and thalamus and ones that descend to the pons and medulla.

The main connections of the cerebellar hemispheres, which are the most developed portion of the human cerebellum, are summarized in Figure 8.30. The cerebellum receives input from the contralateral cerebral cortex through the *pontine nuclei*, whose axons cross the midline and enter the middle cerebellar peduncle. This pathway between the cerebral cortex and the contralateral cerebellum is the *corticopontocerebellar pathway*. It provides

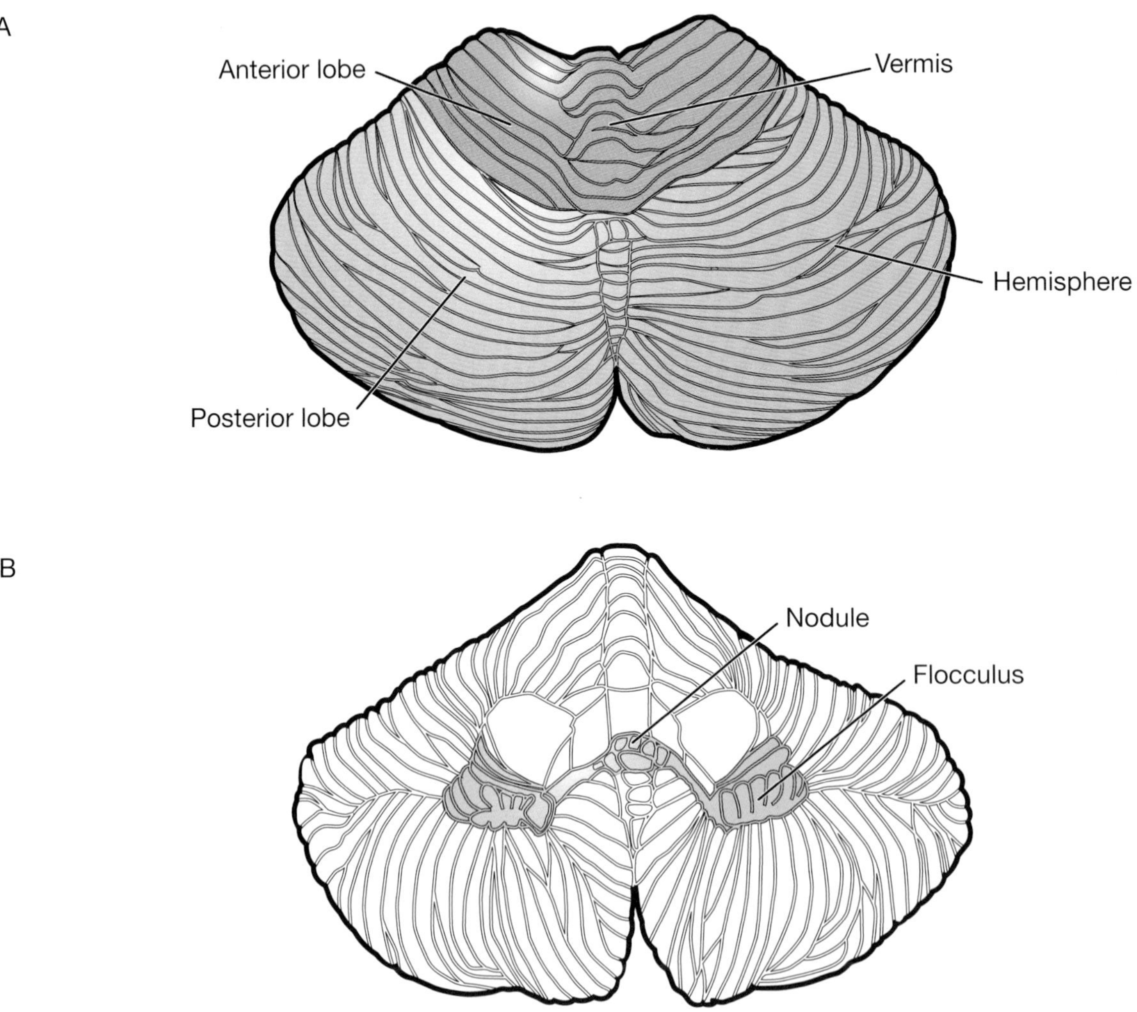

Fig. 8.28. Gross anatomy of the cerebellum. *A*, Superior (dorsal) view. The body of the cerebellum includes a medially located vermis and the expanded lateral hemispheres. The primary fissure divides the dorsal portion of the cerebellum into an anterior lobe and posterior lobe. *B*, Inferior (ventral) view. The cerebellum consists of a flocculonodular lobe and a body, which consists of the anterior and posterior lobes. Most of the body of the cerebellum corresponds to the cerebellar hemispheres (posterior lobe).

"feed-forward signals" to the cerebellum about cortical motor commands. The cerebellar hemispheres project to the deep cerebellar nuclei (particularly the dentate nucleus), which project through the superior cerebellar peduncle to the contralateral thalamus. The thalamus then relays the information to the cerebral cortex. This is the *cerebellothalamocortical pathway*. Thus, each cerebellar hemisphere controls the coordination of the *ipsilateral* limbs through interaction with the contralateral motor cortex. Feedback information about limb movement reaches the cerebellum from the ipsilateral spinal cord through the *spinocerebellar pathways*.

The cerebellum also receives input from the vestibular nuclei and reticular formation. The connections of the flocculonodular lobe and medial vermis with these brainstem areas are the basis of the cerebellar control of eye movements, balance, and gait.

The function of the cerebellum is regulated by "error signals" generated in the *inferior olivary nucleus*. This nucleus sends axons to the contralateral cerebellum through the inferior cerebellar peduncle. The functions of all these connections are described below.

Basic Intrinsic Cerebellar Circuit

The basic cerebellar circuit involves the cerebellar cortex and deep cerebellar nuclei. The cerebellar cortex consists of the granular layer, Purkinje cell layer, and molecular layer (Fig. 8.31). *Purkinje cells* are large GABAergic (hence, inhibitory) neurons whose axons form the output of the cerebellar cortex; these axons synapse in the

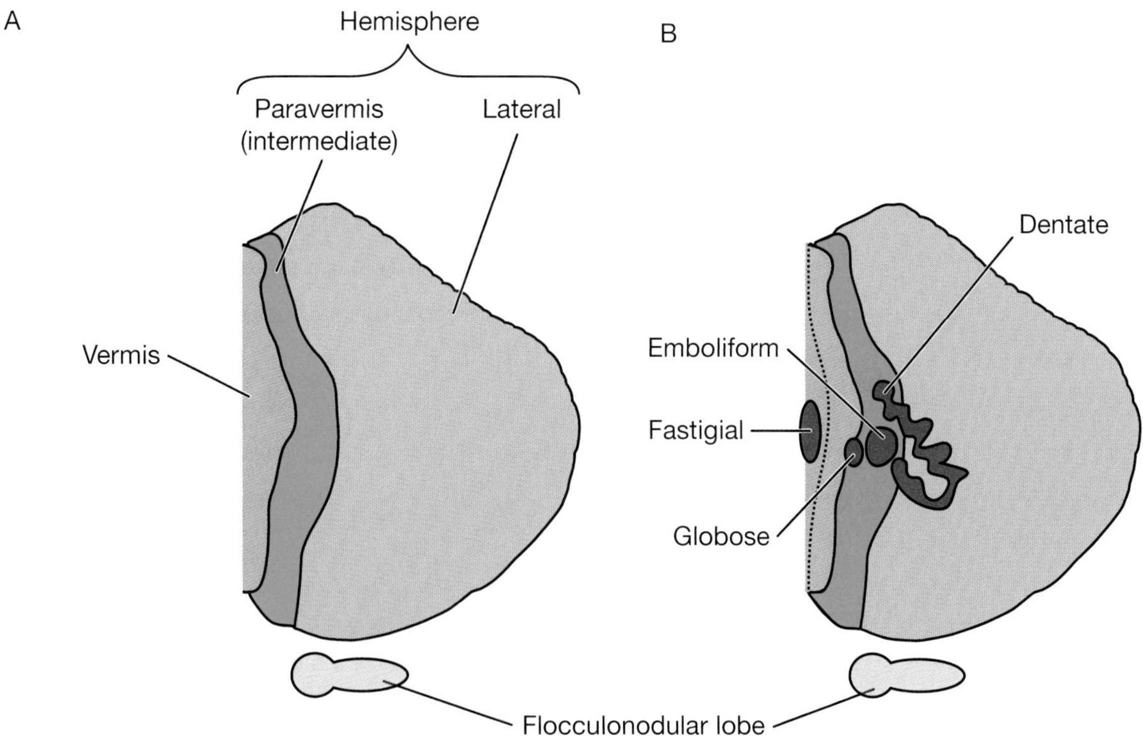

Fig. 8.29. Horizontal section showing the main functional subdivisions of the cerebellum and their output nuclei. *A*, Functional subdivisions of the cerebellar cortex. *B*, Cerebellar output nuclei. The flocculonodular lobe corresponds to the vestibulocerebellum and has direct reciprocal connections with the vestibular nuclei, controlling ocular movements. The vermis acts through the fastigial nucleus to control trunk movement and gait. The cerebellar hemispheres include an intermediate region (paravermis) that by way of the globose and emboliform nuclei controls movements of the ipsilateral limbs. The lateral portion of the hemispheres, through the dentate nucleus, controls ipsilateral limb movement and cognitive function.

deep cerebellar nuclei. The deep cerebellar nuclei send excitatory glutamatergic axons to all cerebellar targets except the inferior olivary nucleus (see below).

Both Purkinje cells and cells in the deep cerebellar nuclei receive two types of excitatory input: mossy fibers and climbing fibers. The *mossy fibers* are axons from the ipsilateral spinal cord (spinocerebellar pathway), contralateral pontine nuclei (pontocerebellar pathway), and

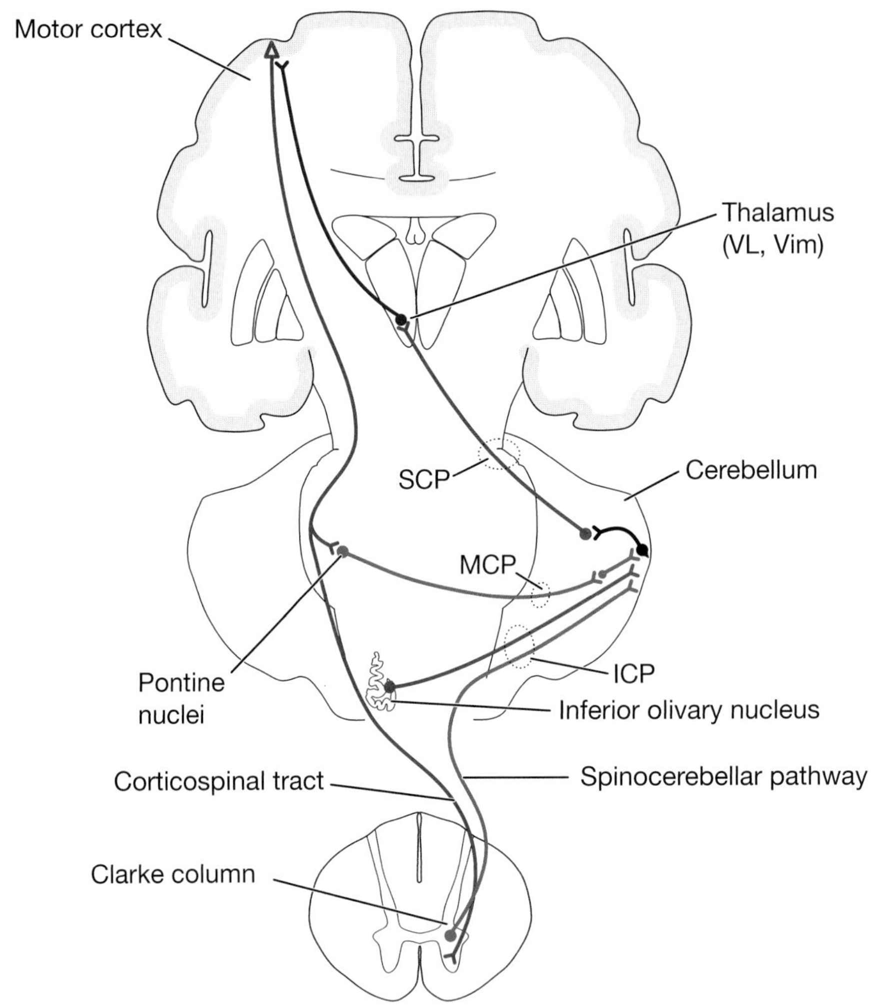

Fig. 8.30. The main connections of the cerebellum. The cerebellum receives input from the contralateral cerebral cortex via the pontine nuclei, which project to the cerebellum through the middle cerebellar peduncle (MCP). The cerebellum also receives input from the ipsilateral spinal cord via the spinocerebellar tracts and input from the vestibular nuclei and reticular formation. All these inputs end as mossy fibers. The cerebellum also receives input from the contralateral inferior olivary nucleus, whose axons end as climbing fibers. Dorsal spinocerebellar, vestibulocerebellar, reticulocerebellar, and olivocerebellar pathways reach the cerebellum through the inferior cerebellar peduncle (ICP). All cerebellar inputs are excitatory and reach the Purkinje cells of the cerebellar cortex and the cerebellar nuclei. The Purkinje cells inhibit the deep cerebellar nuclei, which are the source of the output of the cerebellum and project through the superior cerebellar peduncle (SCP). This peduncle decussates at the level of the lower midbrain and provides excitatory inputs, through a relay in contralateral thalamus, to motor areas of the cerebral cortex. Other cerebellar outputs (not shown) end in brainstem motor nuclei and inferior olivary nucleus. Vim, ventral intermedius thalamic nucleus; VL, ventral lateral thalamic nucleus.

ipsilateral labyrinth, vestibular nuclei (vestibulocerebellar pathway), and reticular formation (reticulocerebellar pathway). Mossy fibers are glutamatergic, send collaterals into the deep cerebellar nuclei, and synapse on the *granule cells* of the cerebellar cortex. The granule cells are also glutamatergic, and their unmyelinated axons ascend toward the superficial molecular layer, where they bifurcate and form the *parallel fibers* that synapse on dendritic spines of Purkinje cells.

The parallel fibers run for several millimeters in both directions along the folia, perpendicular to the plane of arborization of Purkinje cell dendrites. Each parallel fiber may synapse with one or two dendritic spines on 250 to 750 Purkinje cells. In humans, each Purkinje cell may collect information from as many as one million granule cells, and on average, the cell may be intersected by as many as 200,000 parallel fibers. Each Purkinje cell may receive a total of 150,000 to 175,000 granule cell synapses from parallel fibers. The parallel fibers also synapse on three types of local inhibitory GABAergic neurons in the cerebellar cortex. Golgi neurons inhibit the transmission of information between mossy fibers and granule cells. Stellate and basket cells, located in the molecular layer, mediate local and lateral inhibition of Purkinje cells.

The *climbing fibers* arise solely from the contralateral inferior olivary nucleus. They provide a powerful, direct excitatory glutamatergic input to both the deep cerebellar nuclei and Purkinje cells. Climbing fibers extend along the dendritic tree of only one or two Purkinje cells. This is unlike the parallel fiber system, which is a highly divergent system with each fiber exciting only one or a few dendritic spines.

Physiology

Control of Eye Movements

The cerebellum has a critical role in controlling the functions of the vestibular and oculomotor systems. This cerebellar control is mediated by the flocculonodular lobe and dorsal vermis (Fig. 8.32).

The flocculonodular lobe is the most primitive portion of the cerebellum and is referred to as the *vestibulocerebellum* because of its reciprocal connections with the vestibular system. The primary function of the flocculonodular lobe is the control, through the vestibular system, of eye movement. The flocculonodular lobe receives input from the labyrinth and vestibular nuclei and, through the pontine nuclei, from neurons in the parieto-occipital cortex activated by the visual perception of object movement. This lobe also receives input from brainstem areas involved in the control of eye movement. The main output of the flocculonodular lobe is to the medial and superior vestibular nuclei, which in turn project to brainstem ocular motor neurons. Through these connections, the flocculonodular lobe regulates the gain of *vestibulo-ocular reflexes* (which maintain visual fixation during movement of the head), allows smooth tracking of the object with the eyes (*smooth visual pursuit*), and contributes to the maintenance of gaze in the excentric position (see Chapter 15).

Through projections to the fastigial nucleus, the dorsal vermis controls the amplitude, direction, and velocity of fast (saccadic) eye movements to changes in target location. These cerebellar regions receive input from areas of the reticular formation that control eye movement and relay information from the frontal eye fields and the superior colliculus (see Chapter 15).

Control of Posture and Gait

The vermis and paravermis receive somatosensory information from the spinal cord through the spinocerebellar tracts, and together, they are referred to as the *spinocerebellum*. They also receive cortical input through the corticopontocerebellar pathway and input from the reticular formation and vestibular nuclei.

The dorsal spinocerebellar tract originates in Clarke column and provides proprioceptive and exteroceptive input from the ipsilateral lower extremity. Similar information from the upper extremities is transmitted by the cuneocerebellar tract, which originates from the lateral cuneate nucleus in the medulla. The ventral spinocerebellar tract originates from interneurons in the lateral portion of the

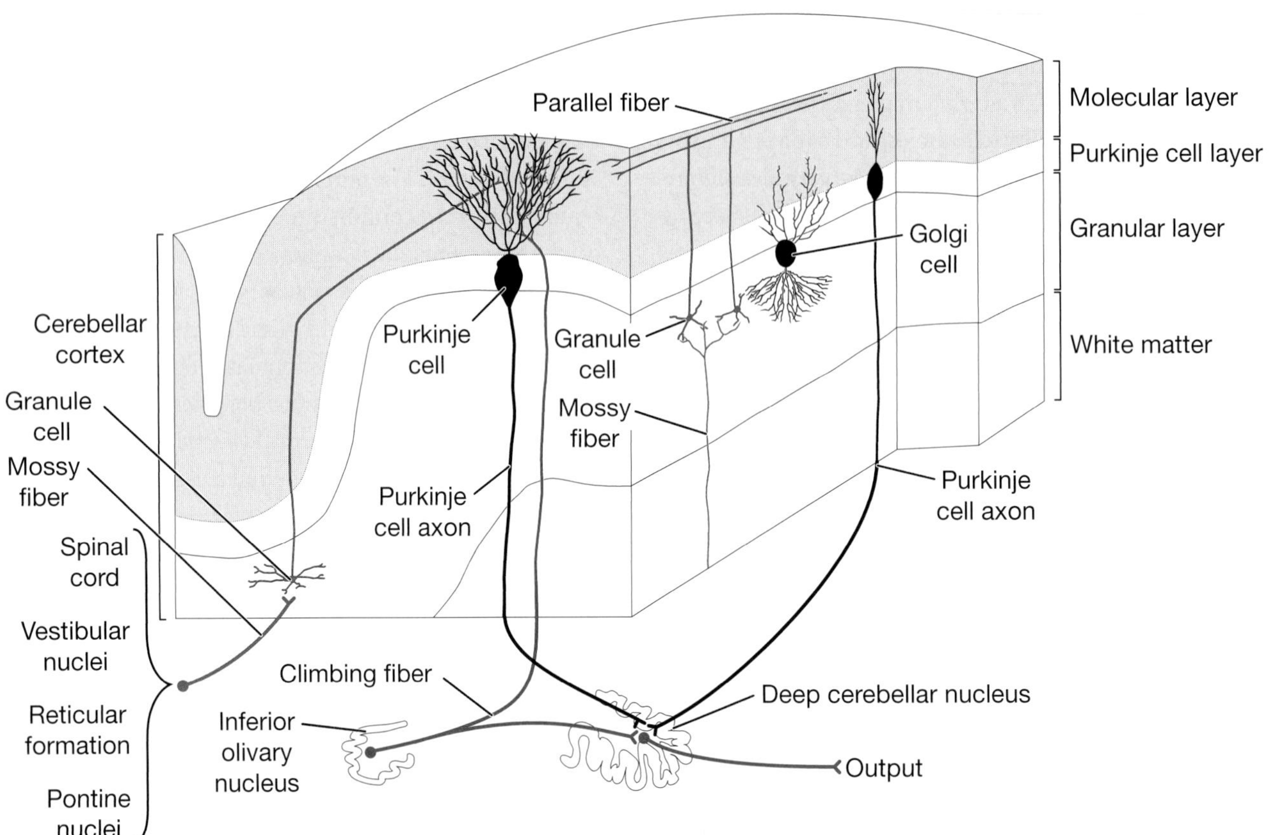

Fig. 8.31. The basic cerebellar circuit involves the cerebellar cortex and deep cerebellar nuclei. The cerebellar cortex consists of the granular layer, Purkinje cell layer, and molecular layer. Purkinje cells are large GABAergic neurons that form the output of the cerebellar cortex: an inhibitory projection to the deep cerebellar nuclei. Deep cerebellar nuclei send excitatory glutamatergic projections to all cerebellar targets, except for the inhibitory projection to the inferior olivary nucleus. Both Purkinje cells and cells of the deep cerebellar nuclei receive excitatory input from mossy fibers and climbing fibers. Mossy fibers are axons arising in the spinal cord, pontine nuclei, vestibular nuclei, and reticular formation. They synapse on granule cells, which send ascending axons to the molecular layer, where they bifurcate and form parallel fibers that synapse on dendritic spines of Purkinje cells and inhibitory interneurons, such as Golgi cells. Golgi cells inhibit synaptic transmission between mossy fibers and granule cells. Other inhibitory interneurons are stellate cells and basket cells (not shown) in the molecular layer; they inhibit Purkinje cells in adjacent folia. All climbing fibers are from the contralateral inferior olivary nucleus and provide a powerful, direct excitatory input to both the deep cerebellar nuclei and Purkinje cells.

ventral horn. The axons ascend contralaterally in the spinal cord and then cross again in the superior cerebellar peduncle to terminate in the ipsilateral vermis and paravermis. This pathway provides the cerebellum with information about the activity of the inhibitory interneurons and the descending motor pathways (see Chapter 7).

The vermis receives spinocerebellar input from the trunk and proximal portion of the extremities, particularly the lower limbs. It consists of a medial portion that projects, by way of the fastigial nucleus, to the reticular formation and vestibular nuclei and a lateral portion that projects directly to the lateral vestibular nucleus (Fig. 8.33). Through these projections, the vermis controls the neurons whose axons form the reticulospinal and vestibulospinal tracts that innervate the spinal motor neurons involved in postural reflexes of the head and trunk and proximal limb movements involved in locomotion.

Control of Limb Movements

The cerebellar hemispheres, including the intermediate (paravermis) and the large lateral portions, control movement of the ipsilateral arm and leg (Fig. 8.34). The paravermis receives input from the contralateral motor cortex (via the pontine nuclei) and the ipsilateral spinal cord (via the spinocerebellar tract). It projects to the globose and emboliform nuclei, which in turn send axons to the contralateral thalamus and the magnicellular portion of the red nucleus (the origin of the rubrospinal tract). The thalamus projects to the motor cortex. With these connections, the paravermis controls the activity of the crossed lateral motor pathways that control movement of the limbs, particularly the upper extremities. The cerebellum provides continuous feedback for monitoring and correcting motor commands that activate agonist and antagonist muscles of the ipsilateral arm and leg.

The large lateral portion of the cerebellar hemisphere receives, via the pontine nuclei, input from wide-

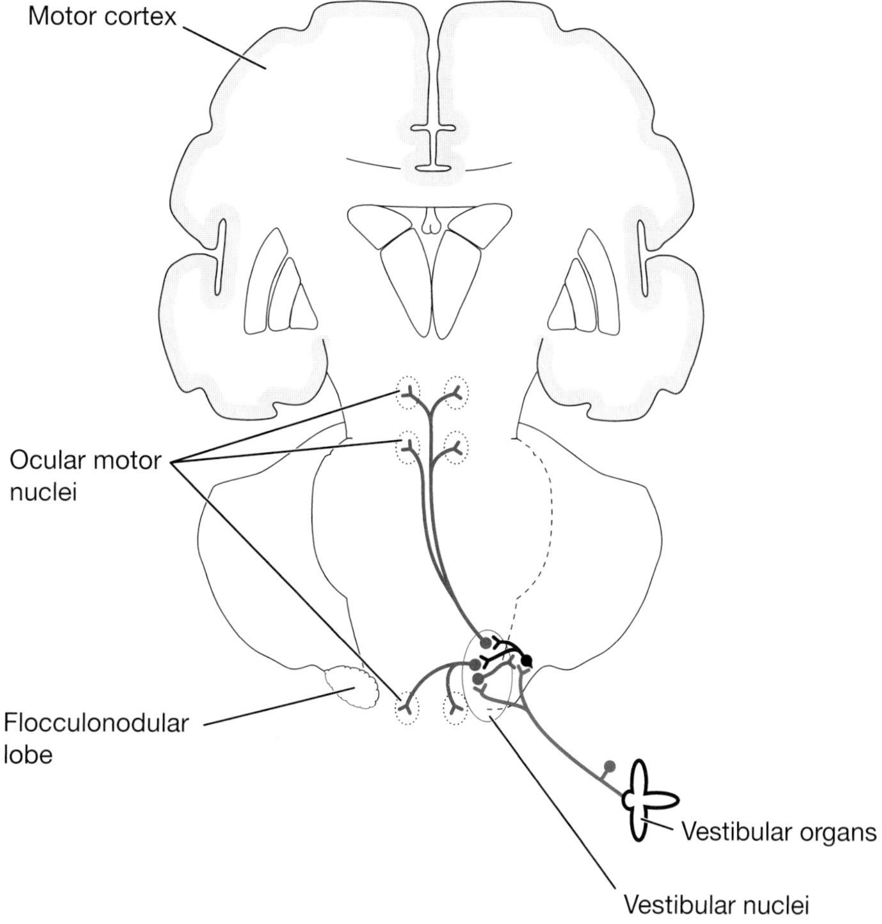

Fig. 8.32. Connections of the flocculonodular lobe involved in control of eye movement. Purkinje cells of the flocculonodular lobe receive vestibular input directly from first-order sensory neurons and from vestibular nuclei and send inhibitory projections to the vestibular nuclei. The vestibular nuclei innervate the ocular motor neurons mediating vestibulo-ocular reflexes and ocular smooth pursuit movements.

spread areas of the cerebral cortex. These cortical areas include not only motor and premotor cortices, but also association areas such as the prefrontal cortex. The lateral cerebellar hemisphere projects to the dentate nucleus, which sends axons to the contralateral thalamus, specifically to the *ventral lateral* or *ventral intermedius nucleus* (the "cerebellar territory" of the thalamus). This thalamic nucleus projects to primary motor cortex and lateral premotor cortex. Through these connections, the lateral cerebellar hemispheres control the initiation and timing of movements, motor learning, and creation of motor programs.

- **The flocculonodular lobe and vermis control eye movements.**
- **The cerebellar vermis controls the posture of the head and trunk and gait.**
- **The cerebellar hemispheres are involved in motor learning, and they control the initiation and coordination of ipsilateral limb movements.**

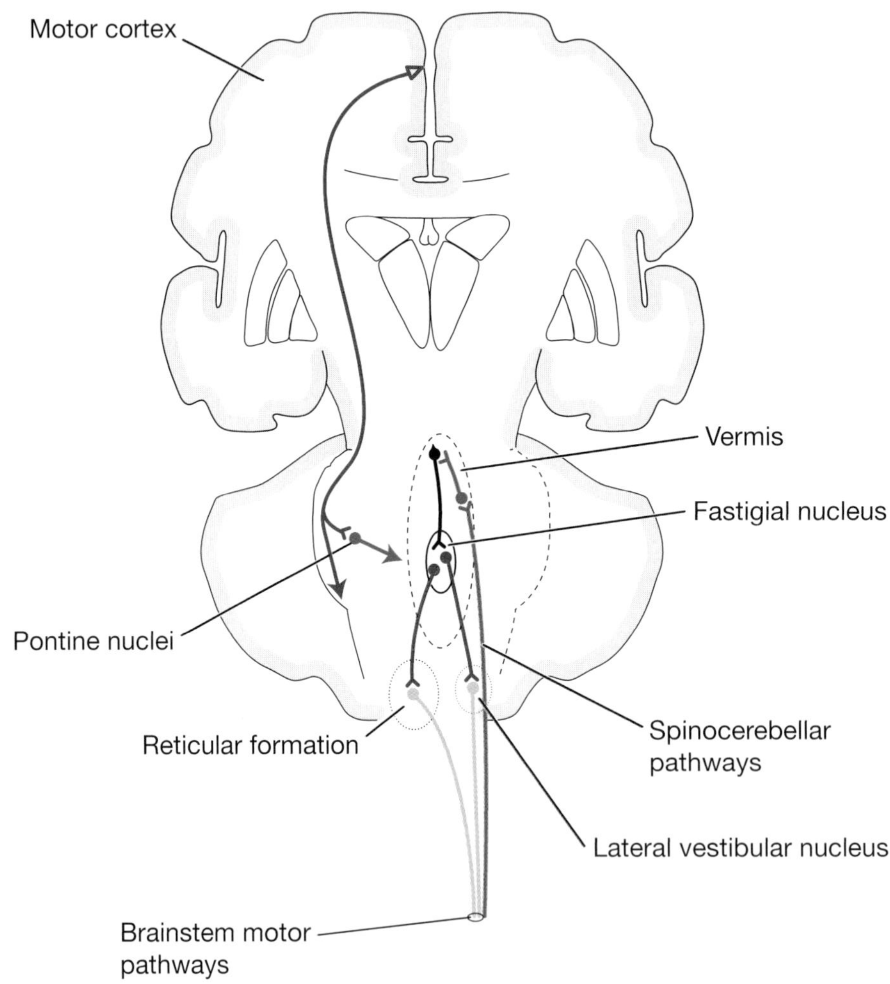

Fig. 8.33. Main connections of the vermis involved in control of posture and gait. The main input to the vermis is from spinocerebellar pathways as well as vestibular nuclei, reticular formation, and contralateral motor cortex. The medial vermis projects, via the fastigial nucleus, to the reticular formation. The lateral vermis projects directly to the lateral vestibular nucleus. With these connections, the vermis controls the activity of medial motor pathways regulating posture and gait. The black neuron represents a Purkinje cell.

Cerebello-Olivary Interactions, Error Correction, and Motor Learning

The inferior olivary nucleus receives projections from all brain regions that provide input to the cerebellum, including the cerebral cortex, reticular formation, vestibular nuclei, and spinal cord. Axons from the inferior olivary nucleus travel through the inferior cerebellar peduncle and terminate in the contralateral cerebellar cortex as climbing fibers (Fig. 8.35).

By acting as a comparator between motor commands and the results of their execution, the inferior olivary nucleus may generate an error signal when the inputs do not match. In response to an unexpected perturbation leading to an error in motor control, there is an increase in the discharge of inferior olivary neurons and, thus, an increase in the firing rate of climbing fibers. Thus, the motor program can be modified and the movement adapted to the circumstances, leading to progressive improvement in motor performance.

Neurons of the inferior olivary nucleus have a low-frequency discharge that is synchronized by gap junctions between the neurons. The activity of the inferior olivary nucleus is regulated by monosynaptic inhibitory input from the contralateral dentate nucleus, the direct GABA-ergic *dentato-olivary pathway*, and by disynaptic excitatory input from the *parvicellular portion* of the red nucleus (Fig. 8.35). These outputs from the dentate nucleus ascend in the superior cerebellar peduncle to the contralateral midbrain. The inhibitory pathway descends directly to the inferior olivary nucleus. The disynaptic excitatory pathway relays in the red nucleus, which sends an excitatory projection to the inferior olivary nucleus. Both the direct inhibitory and the indirect excitatory pathways descend in the brainstem as part of the *central tegmental tract*.

> The climbing fibers from the inferior olivary nucleus provide a powerful, rhythmic depolarizing input to both deep cerebellar nuclei and Purkinje cells. This depolarization, called complex spikes, decreases the ability of Purkinje cells to discharge action potentials (called simple spikes) in response to parallel fiber input. The long-term decrease in synaptic efficacy of the parallel fiber input to the Purkinje cells is called long-term depression and is an important mechanism for motor learning and adaptation.

- The inferior olivary nucleus, through its climbing fibers, provides an error signal to the cerebellum.

Cognitive Function of the Cerebellum

The cerebropontocerebellar path provides the cerebellum with information from the prefrontal cortex (involved in executive functions), anterior cingulate cortex (involved in the initiation of movement, motivation, and goal-oriented behaviors), posterior cingulate and medial temporal cortices (involved in spatial and declarative memory), and posterior parietal cortex (involved in visuospatial processing). The cerebellar output to these nonmotor areas of the cerebral cortex is from the ventral portion of the dentate nucleus, which projects to territories in the contralateral thalamus that send axons to these cortical areas. Brain imaging studies and the effects of lesions indicate that the cerebellum is involved in executive tasks and visuospatial, language, and affective functions.

Clinical Correlations

The functions, main connections, and manifestations of lesions affecting the main subdivisions of the cerebellum are summarized in Table 8.5.

Disturbance in Ocular Motor Control

Lesions that affect the flocculonodular lobe or its vestibular connections cause *nystagmus*. Nystagmus consists of repetitive to-and-fro eye movements initiated by a slow drift, or slow phase in one direction, followed by a fast corrective movement in the opposite direction. Nystagmus caused by flocculonodular lesions is due to an inability to hold the eyes in an eccentric position. On attempting to sustain the position of gaze toward the affected side, the eyes slowly drift back toward the primary position; this is followed by a corrective fast component toward the affected side. Another manifestation of flocculonodular lesions is the inability to perform smooth pursuit (tracking) eye movements.

Disturbance in Posture, Equilibrium, and Gait

Lesions of the caudal vermis cause postural ataxia of the head and trunk during sitting, standing, and walking. Gait ataxia is characterized by a broad-based gait, with the tendency of the person to veer toward either side. Tandem

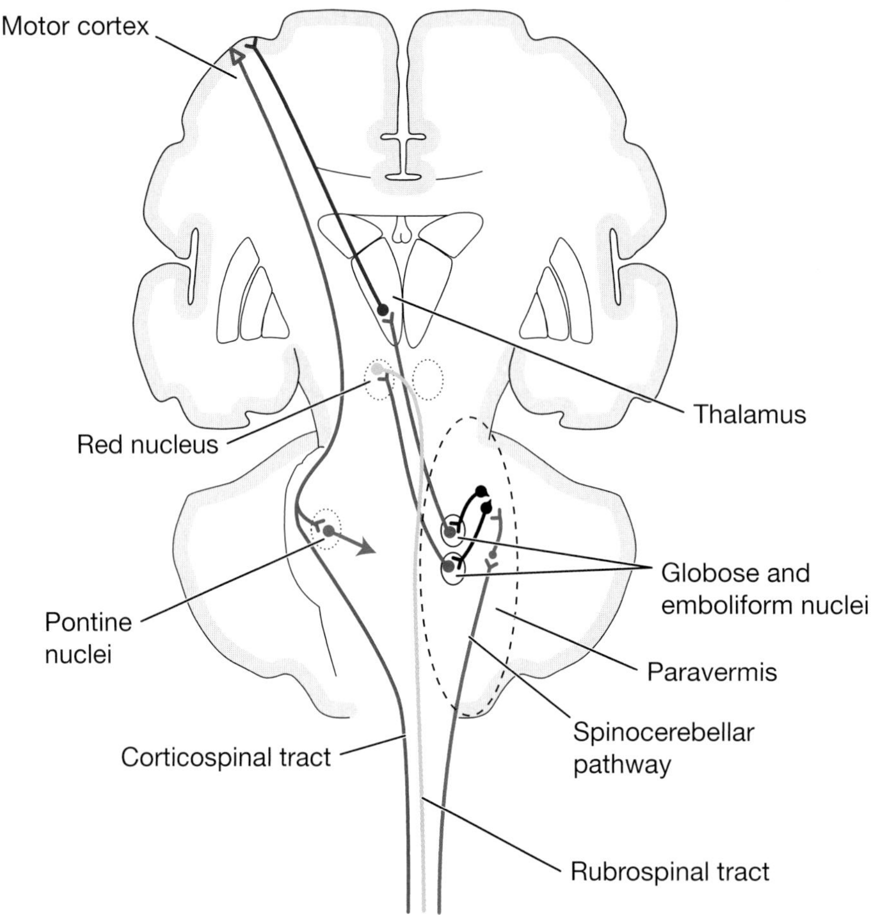

Fig. 8.34. The cerebellar hemispheres control movements of the ipsilateral limbs through reciprocal connections with contralateral motor cortex. *A*, The intermediate portion of the hemispheres (paravermis) receives cortical input via the contralateral pontine nuclei and spinocerebellar input from the ipsilateral spinal cord. The paravermis projects to the globose and emboliform nuclei, which project to the contralateral motor cortex (by way of the thalamus) and magnicellular portion of the red nucleus (origin of the rubrospinal tract). *B*, The lateral portion of the cerebral hemispheres receives, via the pontine nuclei, input from widespread areas of the cerebral cortex and projects to the dentate nucleus, which then projects to the contralateral thalamus. The cerebellar territory of the contralateral thalamus is the ventral lateral or ventral intermedius nucleus.

gait is particularly impaired. There is also instability of the trunk. Unlike ataxia due to proprioceptive or vestibular lesions, cerebellar ataxia is apparent with the eyes open and is not unmasked only after eye closure. Therefore, the Romberg sign is *not present* in cerebellar ataxia.

Limb Ataxia

Lesions of the cerebellar hemisphere lead to errors in the timing, direction, and the extent of movement of the ipsilateral limb. The inaccuracy and poor coordination of multijoint movements is called *limb ataxia* (irregular movements of the limb). Involvement of the paravermis of the hemisphere disrupts the accuracy of reaching movements, producing *dysmetria* (loss of the ability to measure the range of motion). The inability to coordinate the contraction of agonist and antagonist muscles that act on a particular joint produces cerebellar tremor, which is an *intention tremor*. The voluntary movement becomes an

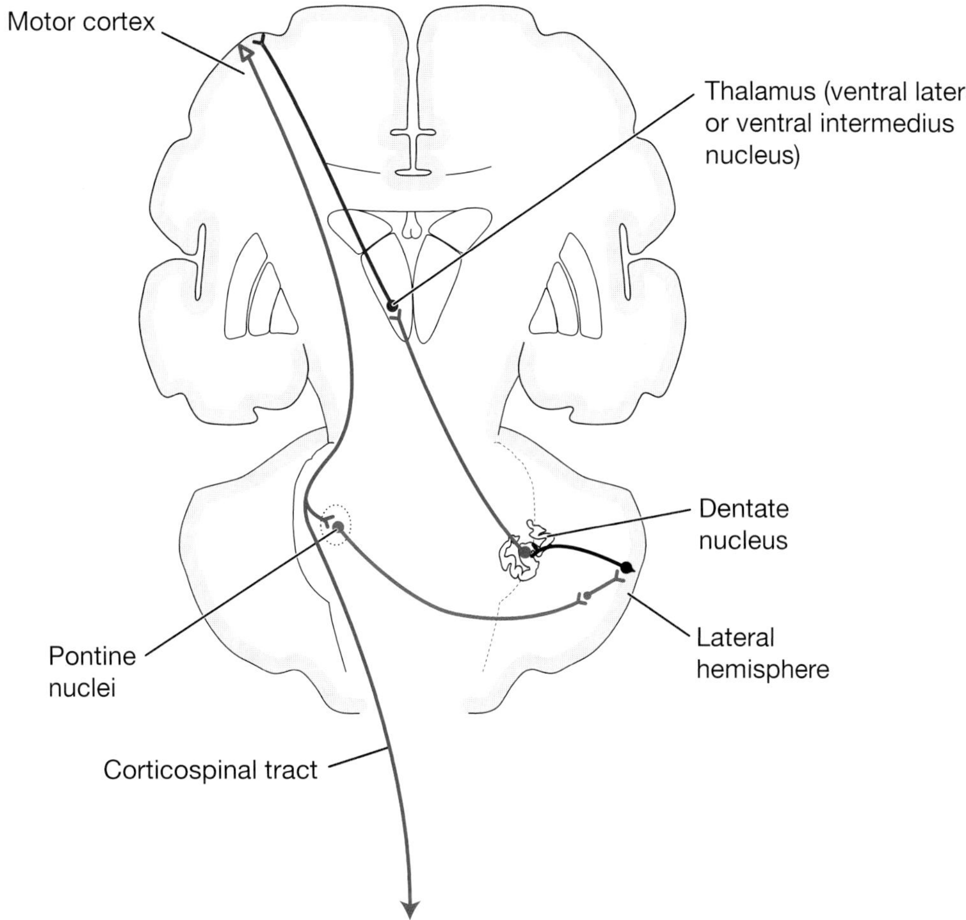

oscillatory movement during goal-related activity. Lesions of the lateral cerebellum and dentate nucleus result in delays in the initiation of movement and irregularities in the timing of the components of a movement. Movements occur sequentially instead of being coordinated smoothly; this decomposition of movement is known as *dyssynergy*. The combination of abnormalities in timing, velocity, and acceleration produces an irregularity in the rate of alternate movements called *dysdiadochokinesia*.

Ataxic Dysarthria

Dysarthria is a motor disorder that affects the production of speech. Cerebellar lesions are associated with irregularities in articulation, loudness, and rhythm of speech. Speech is slow, with excessive stress on some words or syllables and random breakdown of articulation (see Chapter 15).

- Lesions of the flocculonodular lobe produce nystagmus and other ocular motor abnormalities.
- Lesions of the vermis produce trunk and gait ataxia.
- Lesions of the cerebellar hemisphere produce ipsilateral limb ataxia.

Basal Ganglia Control Circuit

The *basal ganglia* (more appropriately, the basal nuclei) are essential subcortical components of circuits involved in motor, ocular motor, cognitive, and affective functions. Although the precise function of the basal ganglia in motor control is incompletely understood, they appear to have a triple role: 1) to facilitate the automatic execution of selected sequential motor programs while simultaneously suppressing all other potentially competing and interfering motor programs, 2) to interrupt ongoing motor behavior in favor of a response to a novel, behaviorally significant stimulus, and 3) to scale the amplitude and duration of postures and movements during the execution of a motor plan. The main input to the basal ganglia is from the ipsilateral frontal cortex; the basal ganglia project back to the frontal cortex through a relay in the thalamus.

Anatomy

The basal ganglia circuits include two core structures: the *striatum* and *globus pallidus*. Two other critical components of the basal ganglia are the *substantia nigra* and the *subthalamic nucleus*.

Gross Anatomy

The striatum includes the *putamen*, *caudate nucleus*, and *nucleus accumbens* (limbic striatum). These nuclei are structurally and functionally equivalent. The caudate nucleus forms the lateral wall of the lateral ventricle and is separated from the putamen by the anterior limb of the internal capsule. The globus pallidus has an *external segment* and an *internal segment* (external and internal pallidal segments). The main neurons of the striatum and globus pallidus are inhibitory GABAergic neurons. The substantia nigra consists of the *pars reticulata*, which is homologous to the internal segment of the globus pallidus, and the *pars compacta*, which contains dopaminergic neurons. The subthalamic nucleus contains glutamatergic excitatory neurons. The main components of the basal ganglia circuits are summarized in Figure 8.36.

Connectivity

The main connections of the basal ganglia circuits are shown in Figure 8.37. The cerebral cortex, particularly the frontal lobe, sends excitatory projections to the striatum, subthalamic nucleus, and substantia nigra pars compacta. The striatum contains GABAergic neurons (called medium spiny neurons) that send inhibitory projections to the external and internal pallidal segments. The internal pallidal segment (and substantia nigra pars reticulata) constitute the output nucleus of the basal ganglia and provide tonic GABAergic inhibition of the thalamic nuclei that project to different portions of the frontal lobe, including the prefrontal cortex and supplemental motor area, and to brainstem targets that control locomotion or eye movements.

In addition to inhibitory input from the striatum, the external and internal pallidal segments receive excitatory input from the subthalamic nucleus. The external pallidal segment, in turn, inhibits both the subthalamic nucleus and internal pallidal segment. The dopaminergic input from the substantia nigra pars compacta modulates the activity of all components of the basal ganglia circuit, particularly the striatum.

Clinical Problem 8.8.

An 8-year-old boy is evaluated for a 4-month history of progressive difficulty with gait, difficulty with coordination, and the recent onset of headache associated with morning vomiting. Neurologic examination showed an ataxic gait with veering to the right, irregular placement of the right foot, dysmetria of the right hand and right leg, and an intention tremor of the right arm. Performance of the finger-to-nose and heel-to-shin test was impaired on the right. Rapid alternating movements were slow and irregular on the right. Strength, reflexes, and sensation were normal.

a. What are the most likely location, side, and nature of the lesion?
b. What major division of the motor system is involved?
c. What is the major role of the involved structure in motor control?
d. How do these clinical manifestations help to localize the area most affected within this structure?
e. What would be the location of the lesion if the main manifestations were vertigo and nystagmus?
f. Lesions of what portion of this structure would produce bilateral leg ataxia?
g. What diagnostic tests may be helpful in evaluating this patient's condition?

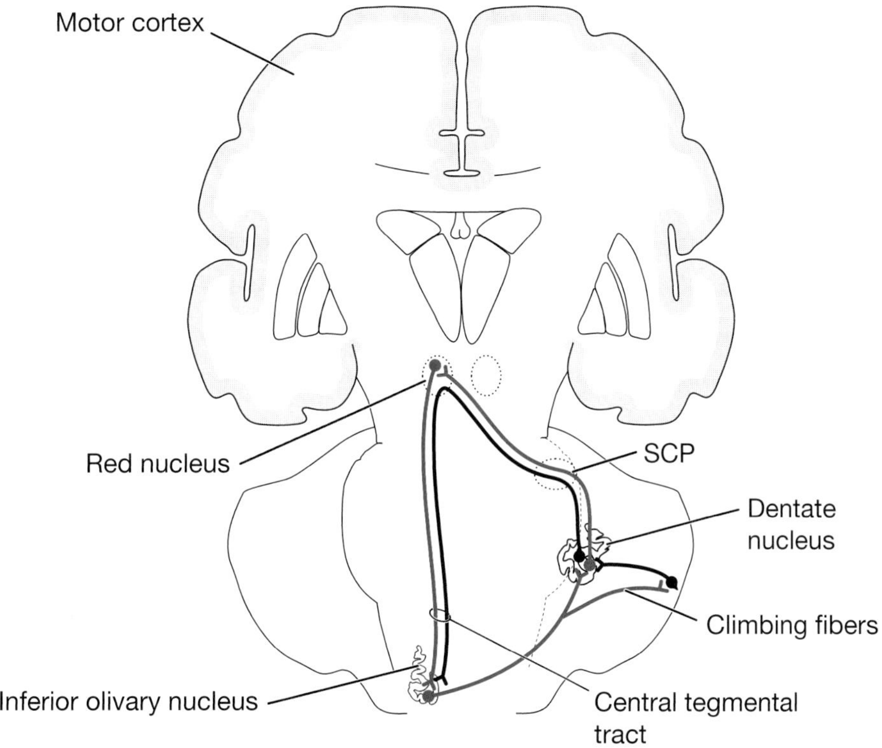

Fig. 8.35. Reciprocal cerebello-olivary connections. The inferior olivary nucleus receives input from the cerebral cortex, brainstem motor nuclei, and spinal cord (not shown) and sends climbing fibers to the cerebellar cortex. These fibers provide a signal to Purkinje cells about errors in motor execution and also synapse in contralateral cerebellar nuclei. The activity of the inferior olivary nucleus is regulated by dual input from the contralateral dentate nucleus: a direct monosynaptic inhibitory dentato-olivary pathway and a disynaptic excitatory input through the parvicellular portion of the red nucleus. The output from the dentate nucleus ascends in the superior cerebellar peduncle (SCP) to the contralateral midbrain. The direct dentato-olivary inhibitory and the excitatory rubrospinal input reach the inferior olivary nucleus through the central tegmental tract.

The basal ganglia form parallel fronto-striato-pallido-thalamocortical circuits that control motor, ocular motor, cognitive, and affective functions. The *motor circuit* of the basal ganglia involves excitatory inputs from motor cortex to the putamen, inhibitory projections from the putamen to the ventrolateral portion of the internal pallidal segment, and the inhibitory projection from this pallidal segment to the *ventral oralis* thalamic nucleus, which projects to the supplementary motor area, involved in the initiation of motor programs. This portion of the internal pallidal segment also sends inhibitory projections to the *pedunculopontine nucleus*, which is in the upper pons and lower midbrain and is involved with the control of muscle tone and locomotion.

The ocular motor circuit involves projections from the frontal eye fields, prefrontal cortex, and posterior parietal cortex to the body of the caudate, which sends an inhibitory projection to the substantia nigra pars reticulata. The nigra pars reticulata sends a tonic inhibitory projection to the area of the superior colliculus involved in the initiation of saccadic eye movements. The cognitive circuit of the basal ganglia involves the dorsolateral and orbital prefrontal cortices, head of the caudate nucleus, substantia nigra pars reticulata, and two thalamic nuclei, the ventral anterior and mediodorsal nuclei, which project back to the prefrontal cortex. The emotional (limbic) circuit

Table 8.5. Main Subdivisions of the Cerebellum and Their Connections, Functions, and Effect of Lesions

Subdivision (deep cerebellar nucleus)	Main connections	Main function	Main effect of lesions
Flocculonodular lobe	Vestibular nuclei	Control of smooth pursuit and gaze holding	Nystagmus
Vermis (fastigial)	Spinal cord, vestibular nuclei, reticular formation	Control of posture and gait	Gait ataxia
Hemisphere	Cerebral cortex		
Paravermis (globose and emboliform)		Coordination of ipsilateral limb movements	Limb ataxia Dysmetria Dyssynergy
Lateral (dentate)		Initiation and learning of movement	Intention tremor Dysdiadochokinesia

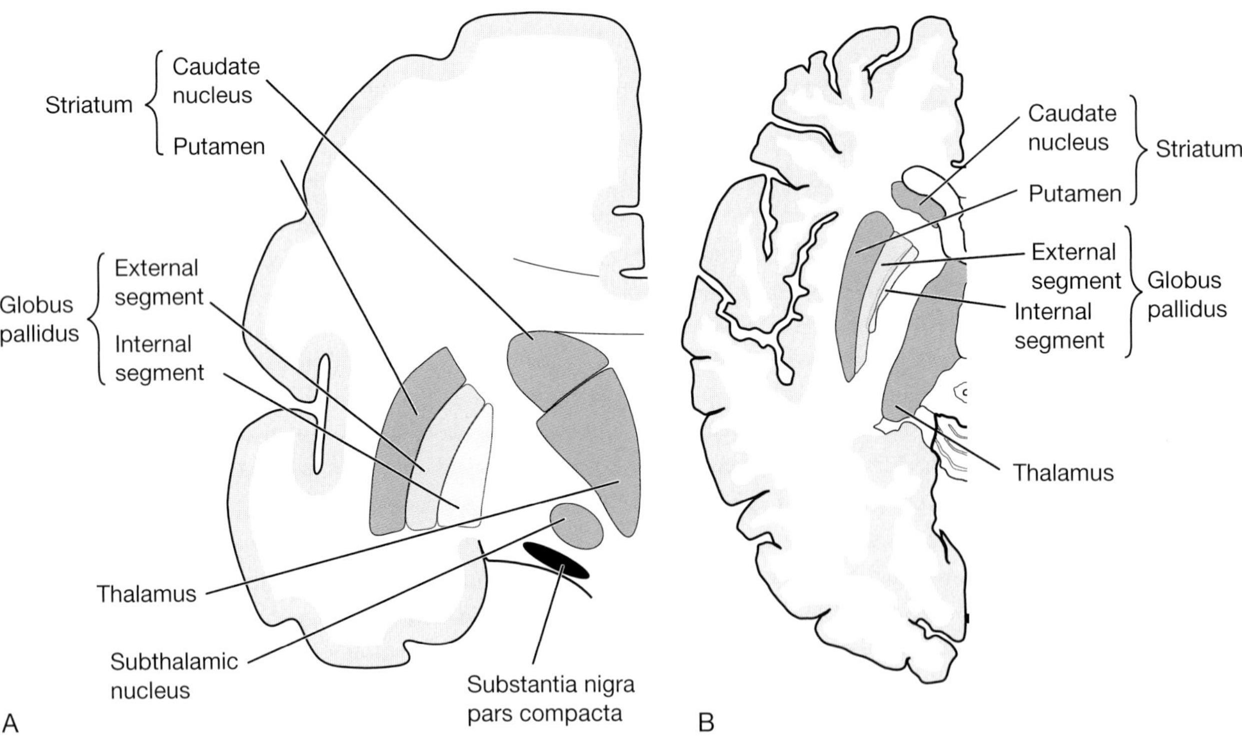

Fig. 8.36. The main nuclei and connections of the basal ganglia circuit. The basal ganglia include the striatum (putamen, caudate nucleus, and accumbens nucleus [not shown]), globus pallidus (including external and internal segments), subthalamic nucleus, and substantia nigra (including pars reticulata [not shown] and pars compacta). *A*, Coronal section. *B*, Horizontal section.

involves the anterior cingulate cortex, nucleus accumbens, ventral pallidum, and mediodorsal thalamic nucleus (see Chapter 16).

- The components of basal ganglia circuits include the striatum (putamen, caudate nucleus, and nucleus accumbens), globus pallidus (external and internal segments), substantia nigra (pars reticulata and pars compacta), and subthalamic nucleus.
- The cerebral cortex provides excitatory input to the striatum, subthalamic nucleus, and substantia nigra pars compacta.
- The striatum sends an inhibitory input to both segments of the globus pallidus.
- The internal segment of the globus pallidus and the substantia nigra pars reticulata provide the tonic

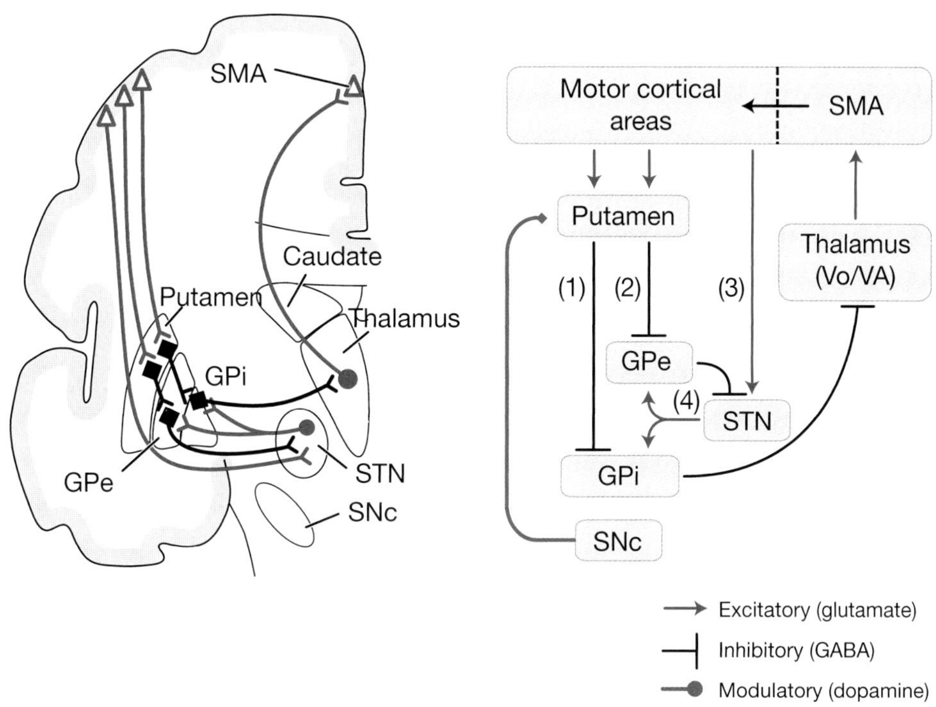

Fig. 8.37. Connectivity of the basal ganglia as exemplified in the motor circuit of the basal ganglia. The cerebral cortex provides input to the striatum and subthalamic nucleus (STN). The putamen is a component of the striatum. Neurons of the striatum contain GABA and project to both the external (GPe) and internal (GPi) segments of the globus pallidus and substantia nigra (projection not shown). The GPi (and the substantia nigra pars reticulata, not shown) contains GABAergic neurons that tonically inhibit basal ganglia targets, including the ventral oralis (Vo) and ventral anterior (VA) nuclei of the thalamus. These thalamic nuclei project to the supplementary motor area (SMA) and prefrontal cortex, respectively, to control initiation of motor programs. The GPi also sends an inhibitory projection to the pedunculopontine tegmental nucleus (not shown), which controls muscle tone and locomotion. The STN sends an excitatory projection to both the GPe and GPi. The STN receives direct excitatory input from the cerebral cortex and reciprocal inhibitory input from GPe. The substantia nigra pars compacta (SNc) sends dopaminergic axons to all components of these circuits, particularly the striatum. These basal ganglia connections are organized into three intrinsic pathways: (1) direct corticostriatopallidal pathway to the GPi, (2) indirect corticostriatopallidal (GPe) STN pathway, and (3) hyperdirect corticosubthalamic pathway. The direct pathway inhibits the GPi, whereas the indirect and hyperdirect pathways, via the STN, increases the activity in the GPi. Reciprocal connections between GPe and STN (4) sustain oscillatory activity in the basal ganglia circuits.

inhibitory output of the basal ganglia to the thalamus and brainstem.

- The subthalamic nucleus activates the globus pallidus.

Intrinsic Circuitry

There are several general principles of organization of the basal ganglia. One principle is that the basal ganglia output, mediated by the internal pallidal segment and substantia nigra pars reticulata, tonically inhibits targets involved in the initiation of motor programs, including those related to voluntary and automatic movements (the supplementary motor area through the thalamus), locomotion (pedunculopontine nucleus), and saccadic eye movements (superior colliculus). Another feature is that the basal ganglia exert a dual control on the initiation and execution of movement: 1) they facilitate the initiation of a particular motor program by transiently interrupting the output of the internal pallidal segment and substantia nigra pars reticulata to a target thalamic or brainstem neuron, and 2) they inhibit the initiation of competing motor programs by increasing the tonic inhibitory output of the internal pallidal segment and substantia nigra pars reticulata to all other targets. This dual effect of the basal ganglia circuit arises from the output of the internal pallidal segment and substantia nigra pars reticulata being regulated by two opposing influences: tonic excitation by the subthalamic nucleus and transient (phasic) inhibition by the striatum. Thus, the dual functions of the basal ganglia (facilitation of one motor program and inhibition of all others) are mediated by different pathways within the basal ganglia circuit. These pathways are triggered by inputs from the cerebral cortex and regulated by dopaminergic input to the striatum.

1. The *direct pathway* consists of excitatory input from the cerebral cortex to a group of neurons in the striatum that send GABAergic inhibitory input to the internal pallidal segment and substantia nigra pars reticulata. Thus, cortical activation of this direct pathway results in a net inhibition of the internal pallidal segment and *disinhibition* of its target, facilitating the initiation of a particular motor program.
2. The *indirect pathway* involves excitatory input from the cerebral cortex to a group of striatal neurons that send GABAergic inhibitory input to the external pallidal segment. Because this pallidal segment inhibits both the subthalamic nucleus (which excites the internal pallidal segment and substantia nigra pars reticulata) and the internal pallidal segment and substantia nigra pars reticulata, activation of the indirect pathway increases the activity of the internal pallidal segment and substantia nigra pars reticulata, thus *increased inhibition* of their target, preventing the initiation of a motor program.
3. The *hyperdirect pathway* consists of excitatory input from the cerebral cortex to the subthalamic nucleus. Because this nucleus activates the internal pallidal segment and substantia nigra pars reticulata, the hyperdirect pathway also increases the inhibitory output of the basal ganglia.

Physiology

Control of the Activity of the Striatum

Because of their intrinsic electrophysiologic properties, striatal output neurons (medium spiny GABAergic neurons) have very low activity at rest (inactive or "off-state"). Only when activated by powerful, converging excitatory glutamatergic input from the cerebral cortex, these neurons fire a burst of action potentials (active or "on-state") that phasically inhibit the internal or external pallidal segment.

The ability of the medium spiny striatal neurons to reach the "on" state is modulated by dopaminergic input from neurons in the substantia nigra pars compacta. These neurons specifically discharge in response to a reward signal from the environment or in anticipation of a reward signal and facilitate the initiation of a specific, behaviorally relevant motor program.

Dopamine has a dual role in the striatum, mediated by D_1 and D_2 receptors. When striatal cells are in the "off-state," dopamine maintains this state, thus preventing spurious activation by weak cortical stimuli. In contrast, if a behaviorally significant, powerful cortical input brings the striatal neurons to the "on-state," dopamine acts on D_1 receptors and facilitates firing of the neurons. Thus, dopamine increases the signal-to-noise ratio in the striatum.

The activity of the medium spiny GABAergic neurons is regulated also by acetylcholine released from tonically active local neurons in the striatum. In general, striatal acetylcholine, acting on muscarinic receptors, opposes the effects of dopamine.

Dual Control of the Basal Ganglia Output

The GABAergic neurons of the internal pallidal segment and substantia nigra pars reticulata fire tonically at high frequency because of tonic excitatory input from the subthalamic nucleus. Thus, in the resting state, the initiation of motor programs is tonically inhibited at the level of the cerebral cortex (supplementary motor area), superior colliculus, and pedunculopontine nucleus. The initiation of a specific motor program requires a powerful cortical input to the medium (spiny) striatal GABAergic neurons of the direct pathway, which transiently inhibits the internal pallidal segment and substantia nigra pars reticulata, and thus disinhibits its targets (Fig. 8.38 *A*).

At the same time, the cerebral cortex inhibits the initiation of potentially competing motor programs. These effects are mediated by the hyperdirect pathway to the subthalamic nucleus and by the indirect pathway from the striatum to the external pallidal segment. Through this indirect pathway, the cerebral cortex activates the neurons in the striatum that inhibit the external pallidal segment, and because this pallidal segment inhibits both the internal pallidal segment and subthalamic nucleus, the net effect is increased activity in the subthalamic nucleus and internal pallidal segment and substantia nigra pars reticulata. This increases the inhibitory effect of the basal ganglia on the effectors that may initiate the unwanted motor programs (Fig. 8.38 *B*).

The balance between the ability of the striatum to initiate or to block the initiation of individual motor programs depends critically on the dopaminergic input from the substantia nigra pars compacta. Dopamine has a net excitatory effect on the striatal neurons of the direct pathway (which contains more D_1 receptors than D_2 receptors) that disinhibit the motor programs and a net inhibitory effect on striatal neurons of the indirect pathway (which contain more D_2 receptors than D_1 receptors) that inhibit motor programs. Because the discharge of dopaminergic neurons provides a reward signal, these neurons allow the context-dependent initiation of selected motor programs in response to behaviorally significant stimuli.

Potential for Oscillatory Activity in the Basal Ganglia Circuits

The reciprocal interconnections between the excitatory glutamatergic neurons of the subthalamic nucleus and the GABAergic inhibitory neurons of the external pallidal segment form a network that supports the oscillatory activity in the basal ganglia circuits that influences the output of the internal pallidal segment and substantia nigra pars reticulata. The cerebral cortex influences this network by its direct monosynaptic projections to the subthalamic nucleus. By increasing the signal-to-noise ratio in the basal ganglia circuits, dopamine prevents synchronized oscillatory output of this circuit, which could degrade motor performance.

- Cortical activation of the direct pathway from the striatum to the internal segment of the globus pallidus transiently interrupts the tonic inhibition of the thalamus and other targets, allowing the initiation of selected motor programs.
- Cortical activation of the subthalamic nucleus and the indirect pathway from the striatum to the external segment of the globus pallidus exaggerates the tonic inhibition of the thalamus and other targets, preventing the initiation of unwanted motor programs.
- Dopaminergic input to the striatum facilitates the initiation of motor programs by relatively facilitating the direct pathway and inhibiting the indirect pathway.
- Dopaminergic inputs prevent abnormal oscillatory activity in basal ganglia circuits.

Clinical Correlations

Pathophysiology of Movement Disorders

According to the "dual model" of the basal ganglia circuits, shifts in the balance between the activity in the direct and indirect pathways underlies several movement

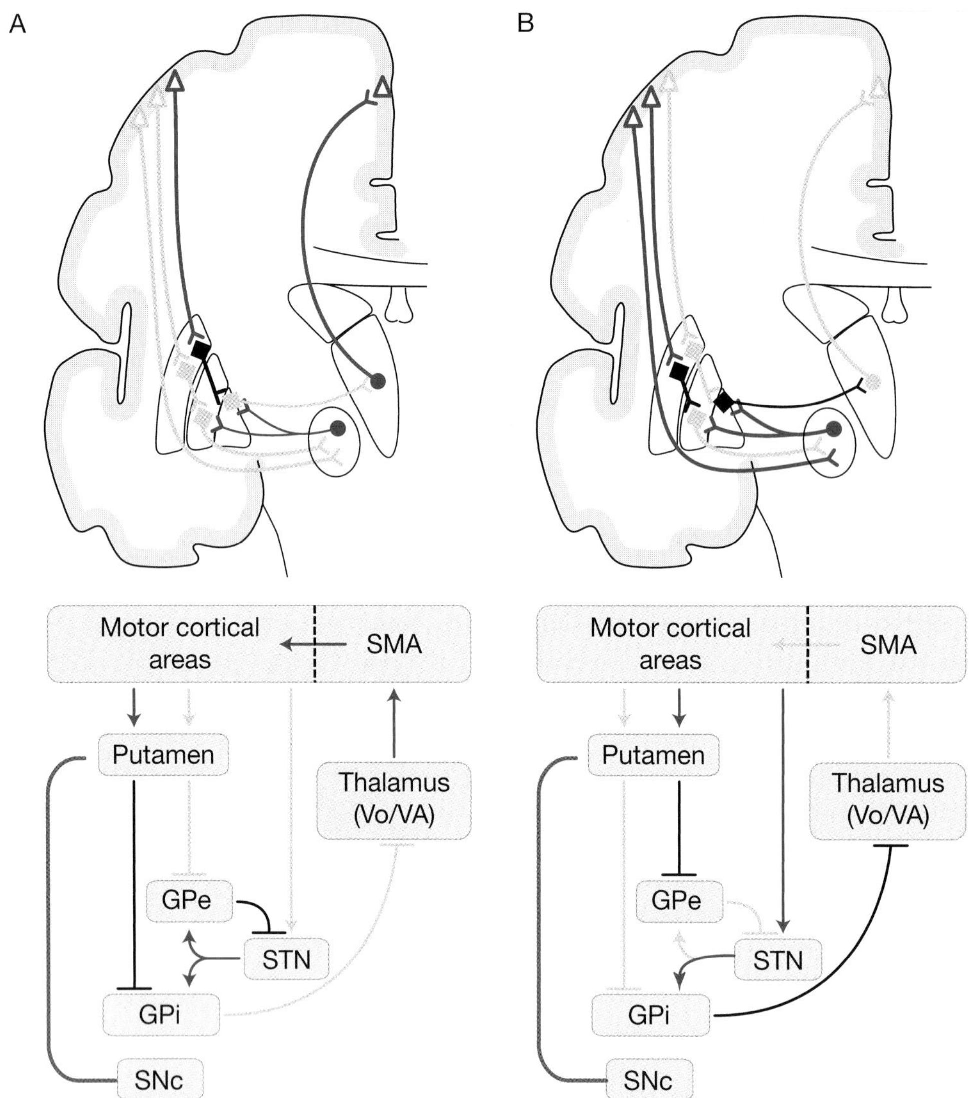

Fig. 8.38. The cerebral cortex, via the basal ganglia, exerts a dual control on motor programs, promoting the initiation of a behaviorally relevant motor program while simultaneously inhibiting or interrupting competing motor programs. The basal ganglia output, mediated by the internal segment of the globus pallidus (GPi) and substantia nigra pars reticulata (not shown), exerts a tonic inhibition on targets involved in initiation of motor programs, including the thalamic ventral oralis (Vo) and ventral anterior (VA) nuclei that project to supplementary motor area (SMA) and prefrontal cortex, respectively. *A*, Initiation of a selected motor act is triggered by a reward signal provided by dopaminergic input from the substantia nigra pars compacta (SNc) to the striatum (in this case, the putamen), which promotes activation of a direct inhibitory pathway from the striatum to GPi. This pathway, originating in the cerebral cortex, transiently interrupts the tonic inhibitory activity of the GPi on the thalamus and brainstem targets, facilitating initiation of the motor program. *B*, The cerebral cortex, through inputs to the striatum and subthalamic nucleus (STN), also inhibits the execution of competing motor programs and interrupts ongoing movement. This involves both a hyperdirect excitatory projection to the STN and an indirect pathway via a second group of neurons of the striatum that project to the external segment of the globus pallidus (GPe). Transient inhibition of the GPe reduces its inhibitory influence on STN. Increased activity in the STN exaggerates the inhibitory output of GPi.

disorders. A decrease in dopaminergic transmission in the striatum decreases the activity in the direct pathway and increases that in the indirect pathway. The net effect is excessive activity in the subthalamic nucleus and in the output from the internal pallidal segment and substantia nigra pars reticulata, leading to exaggerated inhibition of the thalamic neurons that project to the supplementary motor area and the inability to interrupt this inhibition when attempting to initiate a motor program. This results in the *akinetic/rigid* syndrome of *parkinsonism*. In contrast, decreased activity in the subthalamic nucleus (and thus the internal pallidal segment) gives rise to *hyperkinetic* movement disorders. These assumptions have been supported by electrophysiologic studies in experimental animals and intraoperative microelectrode recordings in patients. These studies have also demonstrated that a common feature in parkinsonism and various hyperkinetic disorders is an abnormal synchronized oscillatory discharge in the different components of the basal ganglia circuits. Regardless of whether the output of the internal pallidal segment is increased or decreased, this synchronized oscillatory activity is disruptive for the basal ganglia control of motor function. This explains why procedures such as ventrolateral pallidotomy (which destroys the motor region of the internal pallidal segment) or high-frequency deep brain stimulation of the subthalamic nucleus or internal pallidal segment are successful in the treatment of both hypokinetic and hyperkinetic movement disorders.

Hypokinetic-Rigid Syndromes

Hypokinetic-rigid syndromes (parkinsonism) are characterized by akinesia (or hypokinesia), bradykinesia, muscle rigidity, and postural instability. The typical example is *Parkinson disease*, in which these manifestations are associated with tremor at rest. Parkinson disease is a degenerative disorder due to loss of dopaminergic neurons in the substantia nigra pars compacta (Fig. 8.39). The same syndrome occurs with drugs that block dopamine receptors (such as antipsychotics or antiemetics) and with the ingestion of some toxins. The global paucity of spontaneous or associated movements (e.g., eye blinking and arm swing) is referred to as *hypokinesia* (or akinesia). It is associated with *bradykinesia*, which is slowness in the initiation and performance of voluntary or automatic acts (e.g., finishing a meal and getting dressed). The patient has difficulty rising from a chair, walks with a stooped posture and a short-stepped shuffling gait, and takes several steps to make a turn. The speech is low volume (*hypokinetic dysarthria*).

Hypokinesia commonly occurs in conjunction with an increase in muscle tone, referred to as *rigidity*. Rigidity is increased resistance to passive limb movement that, unlike spasticity, is independent of velocity and occurs throughout the range of motion of the limb. The patient has a stooped, flexed posture of the trunk and limbs, and movement is slow, stiff, and initiated or stopped with great difficulty. In parkinsonism, *tremor* typically occurs at rest and diminishes with voluntary activity.

> The primary treatment of Parkinson disease is dopamine replacement therapy. The most effective treatment is the administration of levodopa, a precursor of dopamine, together with carbidopa, a drug that prevents the peripheral decarboxylation of the precursor. In patients with severe disease or disease of long duration, levodopa may have a short-duration effect and cause excessive movements (levodopa-induced dyskinesias). In this situation, reducing the dose of levodopa and prescribing drugs that activate dopamine receptors (direct dopamine agonists) are beneficial.

Hyperkinetic Movement Disorders

There are several types of hyperkinetic movement disorders, and their pathologic substrate varies. Irregular, writhing, involuntary movements that flow from one part of the body to another and interfere with the execution of motor acts is called *chorea*. It generally, but not always, is associated with lesions in the caudate nucleus. A typical example is *Huntington disease*, an autosomal dominant neurodegenerative disorder characterized by chorea, cognitive deterioration, and affective and psychiatric symptoms from severe involvement of the caudate nucleus (Fig. 8.40). Slow writhing movements of the fingers is called *athetosis*. It is commonly associated with chorea.

Clinical Problem 8.9.

A 63-year-old man is evaluated for hand tremor and gait instability. Two years ago, he developed tremor at rest in his right hand and difficulty with handwriting. Two months later, tremor developed in the left hand and he became aware of increased "slowness and stiffness" when he tried to rise from a sitting position or to roll over in bed. Most recently, the tremor has worsened, and he has developed a "shuffling" gait and postural imbalance, with a tendency to fall forward. His wife complains that his speech has become unintelligible, and he is very slow getting dressed or finishing a meal.

Neurologic examination showed that he had a lack of spontaneous movements while giving the history, a masked facies, and a whispery voice. He had a pill-rolling tremor in both hands, most evident at rest. He walked with a short-stepped shuffling gait and took approximately 10 steps to make a turn. He had poor postural balance. Muscle tone was increased in both upper and lower limbs throughout the range of motion. Alternate motion rate was reduced in the fingers and feet, with progressive deterioration in amplitude. Muscle strength and reflexes were normal. There was no Babinski sign. Coordination and sensation were intact.

a. What is this clinical syndrome called? What are its features?
b. What is the most common cause of this syndrome? What is its pathologic basis?
c. What are other possible causes of this syndrome?
d. What major division of the motor system is involved in these manifestations?
e. What is the mechanism of decreased spontaneous movements in this condition?
f. What is the pharmacologic treatment of this condition?
g. What structures are targets for surgical treatment of this condition?

Sustained muscle contraction that leads to abnormal fixed postures and intermittent twisting movements characterizes *dystonia*. It may be focal (e.g., torticollis in the neck) or generalized. Although dystonia is a typical manifestation of basal ganglia disease, the pathophysiologic mechanism is heterogeneous. It may occur from a lesion involving the putamen or it may occur without a recognizable lesion.

Lesions in the subthalamic nucleus produce *hemiballismus*, which consists of involuntary, often violent, predominantly proximal movements of the contralateral limb. All these hyperkinetic movement disorders may also occur as a manifestation of overdosage of levodopa in patients with Parkinson disease or as a toxic manifestation of some drugs, including cocaine and amphetamine, that increase dopamine levels.

Other Movement Disorders

An oscillating movement that affects one or more body parts, particularly the limbs, is called *tremor*. It also affects the neck, orofacial muscles, and vocal cords. Tremor is usually rhythmic and regular and due to alternate or simultaneous contraction of agonist and antagonist muscles. There are different types of tremors. Tremor may occur when the muscle is at rest (resting tremor), which is typical of parkinsonism. Tremor during muscle contraction may occur with posture-holding against gravity (e.g., with the arms extended in front of the body), typical of *essential tremor*, or with intention maneuvers (e.g., bringing the finger to touch the nose), which is typical of *cerebellar (intention) tremor*.

Tics are abnormal movements (motor tics) or sounds (vocal tics) that are involuntary, paroxysmal movements that can be simple jerks (such as eye-blinking or shoulder shrug) or complex coordinated sequential movements. The combination of simple and complex motor and vocal tics is typical of *Tourette syndrome*. Motor jerks consisting of sudden, brief, shocklike muscle contractions that can be rhythmic or arrhythmic and may or may not be provoked by sensory stimuli are characteristic of *myoclonus*. It may occur with lesions of the cerebral cortex, brainstem, or spinal cord.

■ Parkinsonism is characterized by hypokinesia (or

Clinical Problem 8.10.

A 55-year-old man is evaluated for development of progressive changes in personality and behavior and recent onset of excessive movements. Neurologic examination showed that he had impaired concentration and rapid, irregular, involuntary movements that flowed from one part of the body to another, involving the face, tongue, and limbs. He has excessive facial grimacing and appears to be dancing when he walks. His 75-year-old mother has been in a nursing home for the past 5 years with severe dementia. His 25-year-old daughter has experienced irritability and difficulty concentrating at work.

a. What are the most likely location and nature of the lesion?
b. What type of movement disorder does this patient have?
c. What areas of the brain are most likely to be involved in producing the behavioral and motor symptoms?
d. What is the most likely diagnosis?
e. What would magnetic resonance imaging of the head likely show?

Clinical Problem 8.11.

A 56-year-old right-handed woman is evaluated for the sudden onset of uncontrollable movements of the left arm. Neurologic examination showed arrhythmic, large-amplitude, involuntary movements of the left upper limb.

a. What are the level, side, and cause of the lesion?
b. What is the name of the disorder?
c. What structure is most likely involved?
d. What are the main connections and functions of this structure?
e. What is the significance of this structure in the treatment of movement disorders?

akinesia), bradykinesia, rigidity, postural instability, and tremor at rest.

- Parkinson disease is due to loss of dopaminergic neurons in the susbtantia nigra pars compacta.
- Huntington disease is characterized by loss of neurons in the caudate nucleus and prefrontal cortex,

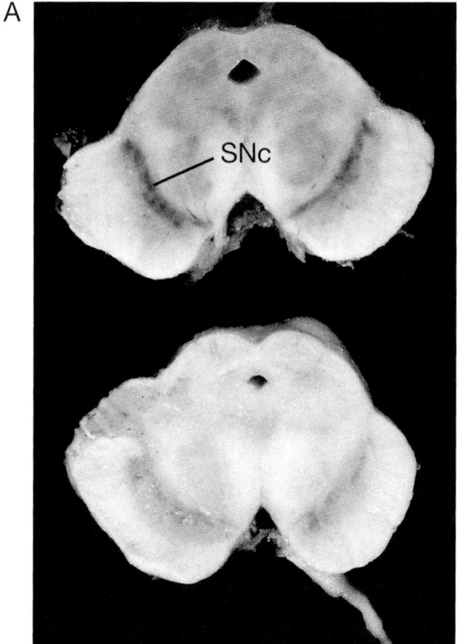

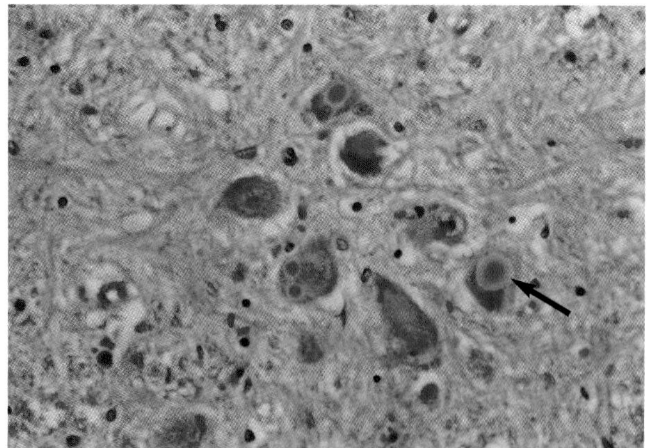

Fig. 8.39. *A*, Parkinson disease is characterized by loss of dopaminergic neurons from the substantia nigra pars compacta (SNc), resulting in loss of neuromelanin pigment normally visible on gross examination of the midbrain. *B*, Neuronal loss is associated with the accumulation of cytoplasmic Lewy bodies in the SNc (*black arrow*).

resulting in chorea, cognitive deterioration, and behavioral abnormalities.

- Lesion of the subthalamic nucleus produces contralateral hemiballismus.
- Deep brain stimulation of the subthalamic nucleus or internal segment of the globus pallidus improves the symptoms of parkinsonism and hyperkinetic movement disorders.

Motor System Examination

In a normal person, movement involves the simultaneous, coordinated activities of all the major divisions of the motor system. Therefore, these are tested together in the neurologic examination. The examination is best organized into separate evaluations of strength, reflexes, coordination, gait, tone, and muscle bulk and observation for abnormal movements. The typical findings in disorders of the motor system are summarized in Table 8.6.

Strength

Strength testing evaluates the power of muscle groups in performing specific actions. Strength depends on age, occupation, physical activity, and muscular development. It apparently may be decreased in patients with bone deformity, pain, or a lack of understanding of the test.

Clinical Problem 8.12.

A 23-year-old woman has a slowly progressive disorder that first began in high school when she was noted to be "fidgety." She did well in school and worked as a secretary for 3 years. During this time, she experienced gradually increasing jerking movements of her arms and face, and her speech became slurred to the point that she was no longer able to work. During the past 2 years, her gait has become unsteady and her movements have slowed. She also has had occasional, uncontrollable flailing movements of her arms. During the past year, her memory has been poor and her intellectual capabilities have deteriorated. On neurologic examination, she had occasional grimacing and coarse, asymmetric jerks of the upper extremities. Muscle tone was increased, with rigidity in all the extremities. She had severe dysmetria in finger-to-nose testing and coarse intention tremor of both arms. Strength, reflexes, and sensation were normal.

a. What major divisions of the motor system are involved?
b. What two general types of cause must be considered in this disorder?

A

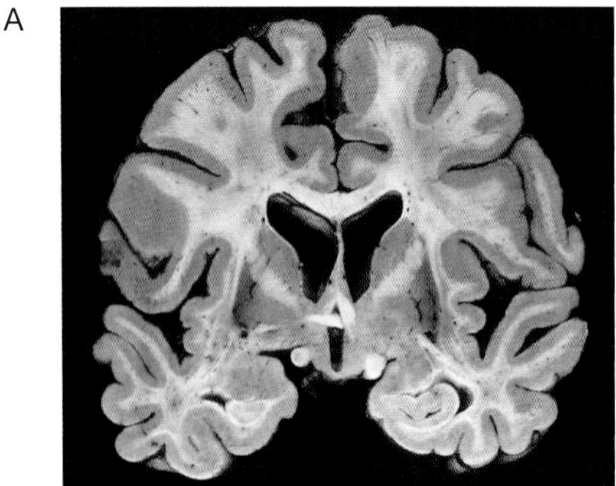

B

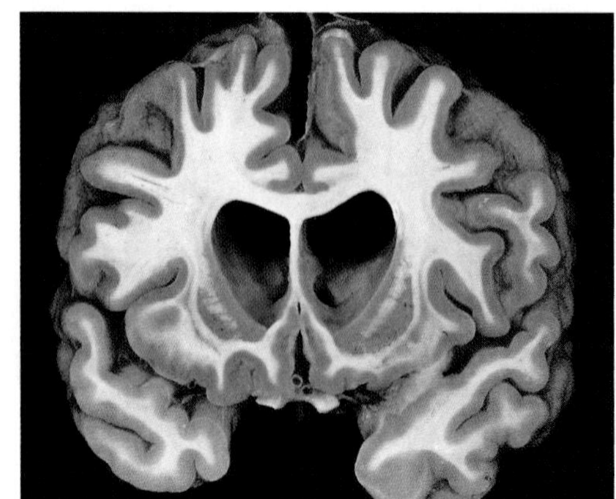

Fig. 8.40. Coronal section of the brain of a normal control (*A*) and an age-matched patient with Huntington disease (*B*). In the latter, note the severe atrophy of the caudate nucleus, which produces a bat-wing shape or ballooning of the lateral ventricles.

Because the object of strength testing is to detect disease of the neuromuscular system, these extraneous factors must be excluded. Strength cannot be graded as abnormal on the basis of an absolute measure of force. It must be judged for each person on the basis of age and all the other variables noted.

Strength is tested by having the patient resist pressure initiated by the examiner. The position of the extremity during testing is of great importance in isolating the action of specific muscle groups and in providing optimal leverage. Each muscle group should be tested in the position that best isolates its function and puts it at a relative mechanical disadvantage (partially contracted position). Force should not be applied suddenly but gradually to a maximum. The strength of a muscle is generally proportional to its size: an elderly lady has less strength than a young weight lifter, although both have normal muscle function. A physician must evaluate strength in proportion to size. There are several systems for grading strength (or weakness). A simple and universally understood one uses a verbal description:

Normal: level of strength expected for that person
Mild weakness: level of strength less than expected but not sufficient to impair any daily function
Severe weakness: strength sufficient to activate the muscle and move it against gravity but not against any added resistance
Complete paralysis: no detectable movement

The following muscle groups are tested as part of the general neurologic examination. The individual muscles participating in these functions are discussed in Chapters 13 and 15.

Facial muscles: upper and lower facial muscles are tested separately by having the patient wrinkle the forehead, squeeze the eyes shut, and show the teeth.
Neck muscles: the patient resists attempts by the examiner to flex and extend the neck by exerting pressure on the occiput and forehead, respectively.
Arm abductors: the patient holds the arms laterally at right angles to the body while the examiner pushes down on the elbows.
Elbow flexors and extensors: with the elbow bent at a right angle, the patient resists attempts to straighten it (flexing to prevent extension) and to bend it (extending to prevent flexion).
Wrist extensors: the patient holds the wrist straight with knuckles up while the examiner attempts to depress it.
Finger flexors: the patient resists attempts to straighten the fingers of a clenched fist (or squeezes two of the examiner's fingers in his or her hand).
Trunk flexors: the patient attempts to sit up from a supine position, with the legs extended.
Hip flexors: in a sitting position, the patient holds the knee up off the chair against resistance; supine, the patient keeps the knee pulled up to the chest.
Hip extensors: prone, the patient holds the bent knee off the examining table; supine, the patient resists attempts to lift the leg straight off the examining table; these are the major muscles used in arising from a squatting position (with knee extensors).
Knee flexors: the patient resists attempts to straighten the knee from a 90-degree angle position.
Knee extensors: the patient resists attempts to bend the knee from a 90-degree angle position; these are the major muscles used in arising from squatting.
Ankle plantar flexors: the patient's ability to rise onto the toes of one foot or to walk on the toes is assessed. This ability is too powerful to test by hand unless it has been severely weakened.
Ankle dorsiflexors: the patient holds the ankle in a resting 90-degree angle position against attempts to depress it.

Muscle Tone

The elbows, wrists, and knees are passively flexed and extended with the patient completely relaxed. There should be only minimal smooth resistance to the movement.

Muscle Bulk

All major muscle groups should be examined for signs of focal atrophy. The circumference of the extremities may be measured and compared with each other.

Table 8.6. Findings on Neurologic Examination of Motor Function Related to the Divisions of the Motor System at the Four Levels of the Nervous System

	Level of damage			
	Peripheral	Spinal	Posterior fossa	Supratentorial
Final common pathway	Weakness, atrophy, hyporeflexia, hypotonia, absent abdominal reflexes, cramp, and fasciculation	Weakness, atrophy, hyporeflexia, hypotonia, absent abdominal reflexes, cramp, and faciculation	Weakness, atrophy, and fasciculation	
Corticospinal tract		Weakness, loss of abdominal reflex, and Babinski sign	Weakness, loss of abdominal reflex, Babinski sign, hyporeflexia, and hypotonia	Weakness, loss of abdominal reflex, Babinski sign, seizure, apraxia, hyporeflexia, and hypotonia
Brainstem motor pathway		Hyperreflexia, clonus, spasticity, and clasp-knife phenomenon	Hyperreflexia, clonus, spasticity, clasp-knife phenomenon, and decerebrate posture	Hyperreflexia, clonus, spasticity, clasp-knife phenomenon, apraxia, decorticate posture
Cerebellar control circuit			Ataxia, dysmetria, dyssynergia, intention tremor, past pointing, rebound, hyporeflexia, and hypotonia	Ataxia
Basal ganglia control circuit				Rigidity, athetosis, dystonia, chorea, hemiballismus, hyperkinesia, and resting tremor

Reflexes

Two major types of reflexes are tested in the neurologic examination: muscle stretch reflexes and superficial (cutaneous) reflexes. The former depend on a rapid, brisk stretch of the muscle, and the latter depend on an uncomfortable stimulus to the skin. Correct positioning and application of the stimulus are extremely important in eliciting reflexes. Also, there are significant variations among patients and even of the same reflex in a single patient on repeated testing. Therefore, much experience with normal reflexes is required before the presence of abnormality can be assessed. The jaw, biceps, triceps, knee, and ankle reflexes are the most important stretch reflexes. In testing all these reflexes, the patient must be completely relaxed.

Jaw jerk: the examiner's index finger is placed lightly on the patient's mandible below the lower lip and then tapped briskly with the reflex hammer. The reflex is brisk jaw closure.
Biceps jerk: the patient's elbow is bent to a 90-degree angle position, with the forearm resting on the lap or on the examiner's arm. The examiner's thumb is placed on the patient's biceps tendon with slight pressure. The thumb is then tapped firmly and briskly with the reflex hammer. The reflex is a quick biceps muscle contraction with tendon (and forearm) movement.
Triceps jerk: the patient's elbow is bent to a 90-degree angle position, with the forearm hanging limply and supported at the elbow by the examiner's hand. A firm, brisk tap is applied directly to the tendon of the triceps 1 to 3 cm above the olecranon. The elbow extends in this reflex.
Knee jerk: the patient's knee is bent to 90 degrees in the sitting position. A firm, brisk tap is applied to the quadriceps tendon 0.5 to 1.0 cm below the patella. The knee extends in this reflex.
Ankle jerk: the patient's ankle is passively bent to 90 degrees and held by the examiner in that position. The examiner gives a firm, brisk tap to the Achilles tendon 2 to 3 cm above the heel. The foot plantar flexes.

The cutaneous reflexes include the abdominal reflexes, plantar response, cremasteric reflex, and anal reflex.

Abdominal reflexes: the patient lies supine, with the abdomen relaxed. With a sharp object, the skin of the patient's abdomen is scraped quickly and lightly in each quadrant along a line toward the umbilicus. The umbilicus moves toward the stimulus.
Plantar response: the sole of the patient's foot is scratched firmly with a blunt instrument such as a key. The stimulus is begun at the heel and smoothly carried forward along the lateral border of the sole to the base of the toes and then medially to the base of the great toe. A normal response is curling of the toes. The Babinski sign is the extension of the great toe and fanning of the other toes.

Coordination

The ability to coordinate the movements of multiple muscle groups can be observed during ordinary activity, such as shaking hands, talking, dressing, and writing. Specific tests allow the assessment of coordination in localized areas. All these tests may be done with the patient sitting or supine, and each should be done individually for all four extremities.

Finger-to-nose testing: the patient is asked to touch alternately his or her own nose and the examiner's finger with the tip of his or her own index finger. The examiner's finger should be far enough away so that the patient must extend the arm fully. This test is performed with the patient's eyes open and then closed.
Heel-to-shin testing: the patient places the heel carefully on the opposite knee and slides it slowly along the edge of the tibia to the ankle and back up to the knee again.
Rapid alternating testing: the patient pats each hand or foot as rapidly and regularly as possible against a firm surface. A more difficult variation requires alternately patting the front and back of the hand on the knee as rapidly and regularly as possible.

Gait and Station

Tests of gait and station involve all areas of the motor system. Various patterns of gait abnormality occur with different disorders. The test of gait and station is perhaps the single most useful motor system test and should be observed in all patients.

> *Gait*: the patient walks normally back and forth at a moderate rate and then walks on the heels and toes and tandem along a straight line, touching heel to toe; the patient then hops on each leg.
> *Station*: the patient is asked to stand with the feet together, first with the eyes open and then with the eyes closed. There should be little or no sway.

Abnormal Movements

Because many motor disorders are manifested as abnormal involuntary movements, the patient should be examined when he or she is undressed, both sitting and supine, and fully relaxed for such movements. Fasciculations in particular require careful observation of each area under good lighting.

Additional Reading

Burke RE. Spinal cord: ventral horn. In: Shepherd GM, editor. The synaptic organization of the brain. 4th ed. New York: Oxford University Press; 1998, pp. 77-120.

Doya K. Complementary roles of basal ganglia and cerebellum in learning and motor control. Curr Opin Neurobiol. 2000;10:732-739.

Holstege G. The somatic motor system. Prog Brain Res. 1996;107:9-26.

Jankowska E. Spinal interneuronal systems: identification, multifunctional character and reconfigurations in mammals. J Physiol. 2001;533(Pt 1):31-40.

Luppino G, Rizzolatti G. The organization of the frontal motor cortex. News Physiol Sci. 2000;15:219-224.

Sanes JN. Donoghue JP. Plasticity and primary motor cortex. Annu Rev Neurosci. 2000;23:393-415.

Voogd J, Glickstein M. The anatomy of the cerebellum. Trends Neurosci. 1998;21:370-375.

Wichmann T, DeLong MR. Functional neuroanatomy of the basal ganglia in Parkinson's disease. Adv Neurol. 2003;91:9-18.

Chapter 9

The Internal Regulation System

Objectives

1. Describe the general organization and functions of the internal regulation system.
2. List the main components of the central circuits of the internal regulation system at the supratentorial, posterior fossa, and spinal levels.
3. List the main functions of the insular cortex, anterior cingulate cortex, amygdala, hypothalamus, periaqueductal gray matter, parabrachial nucleus, nucleus of the solitary tract and reticular formation of the ventrolateral medulla, and medullary raphe nuclei.
4. Describe the location and functions of the cranial parasympathetic nuclei, intermediolateral cell column, sympathetic ganglia, and parasympathetic ganglia.
5. Differentiate sympathetic pathways from parasympathetic pathways by their localization, function, and pharmacology.
6. Name the effects of the sympathetic and parasympathetic systems on the pupil, salivary glands, heart, blood vessels, sweat glands, respiratory tract, gastrointestinal tract, bladder, and sexual organs. Name the neurotransmitter and receptors that mediate these effects.
7. List the primary manifestations of generalized autonomic failure.
8. List the sites at which lesions can produce abnormalities of the pupil, and describe the types of abnormalities seen with each lesion.
9. List the sites at which lesions can produce bladder disorders and the type of neurogenic disorder produced by a lesion at each site.

Introduction

The internal regulation system consists of neurons and pathways that control functions necessary for survival of the individual and the species. These neurons are located at supratentorial, posterior fossa, spinal, and peripheral levels. The internal regulation system controls visceral, endocrine, and motor functions that maintain the internal environment and allow bodily adaptation in response to challenges from the external environment. These functions include 1) maintenance of blood flow to tissues, 2) regulation of the composition of the blood to provide an adequate internal environment for cell function (*homeostasis*), 3) adaptive responses to external and internal challenges, including stress and emotional reactions, 4) regulation of immune function, 5) modulation of pain sensation, and 6) reproductive behavior.

The internal regulation system performs all these important functions through four components: 1) the *autonomic nervous system*, which controls the activity of the heart; the smooth muscle of the blood vessels, pupil, and visceral organs; and the exocrine glands; 2) the *endocrine system*, including circulating hormones from the pituitary gland and peripheral endocrine organs; 3) connections with the somatic motor system required for automatic functions such as breathing and swallowing and complex behaviors such as drinking, feeding, and sexual behavior; and 4) interconnections with the consciousness system, which regulates the sleep-wake cycle and attention to external stimuli. The primary focus of this chapter is on the autonomic output of the internal regulation system. Autonomic disorders may be prominent manifestations of several neurologic diseases and, in some cases, may be valuable in localizing lesions in the nervous system.

Overview

The internal regulation system consists of 1) areas of the central nervous system that receive and integrate information from the external and internal environments and mediate visceral reflexes or adaptive autonomic, endocrine, and motor responses (integrating-coordinating circuits); 2) visceral, pain, and other sensory afferents; humoral signals; and cortical inputs that provide information about the state of the body and environment; and 3) the autonomic (visceral motor), endocrine, and somatic motor outputs that mediate the influence of these circuits on peripheral effectors (Fig. 9.1).

The integrating-coordinating circuits are located at the supratentorial, posterior fossa, and spinal levels. They include the *insular cortex*, *anterior cingulate cortex*, *amygdala*, *hypothalamus*, *periaqueductal gray matter* of the midbrain, *parabrachial nucleus* of the pons, *nucleus of the solitary tract*, ventrolateral reticular formation (ventrolateral medulla), and *medullary raphe nuclei* (Fig. 9.2). All these areas are reciprocally connected. The main functions of these structures are summarized in Table 9.1.

These areas receive input from visceral receptors innervated either by neurons in the dorsal root ganglia that synapse in the dorsal horn (*spinal visceral afferents*) or neurons in the visceral ganglia of the *vagus nerve* (cranial nerve X) and *glossopharyngeal nerve* (cranial nerve IX) that synapse in the nucleus of the solitary tract (*cranial visceral afferents*). Neurons in the dorsal horn and nucleus of the solitary tract convey the sensory information from these afferents to all the areas of the internal

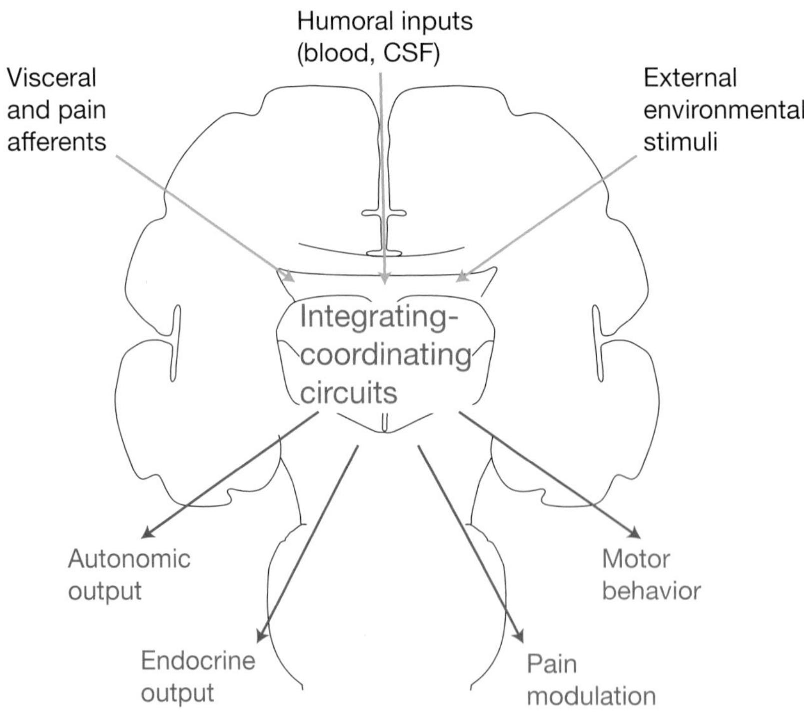

Fig. 9.1. Overview of the organization of the internal regulation system, including the inputs and outputs of its central integrating-coordinating circuits. CSF, cerebrospinal fluid. (Modified from Benarroch EE. Basic neurosciences with clinical applications. Philadelphia: Elsevier; 2006. Used with permission of Mayo Foundation for Medical Education and Research.)

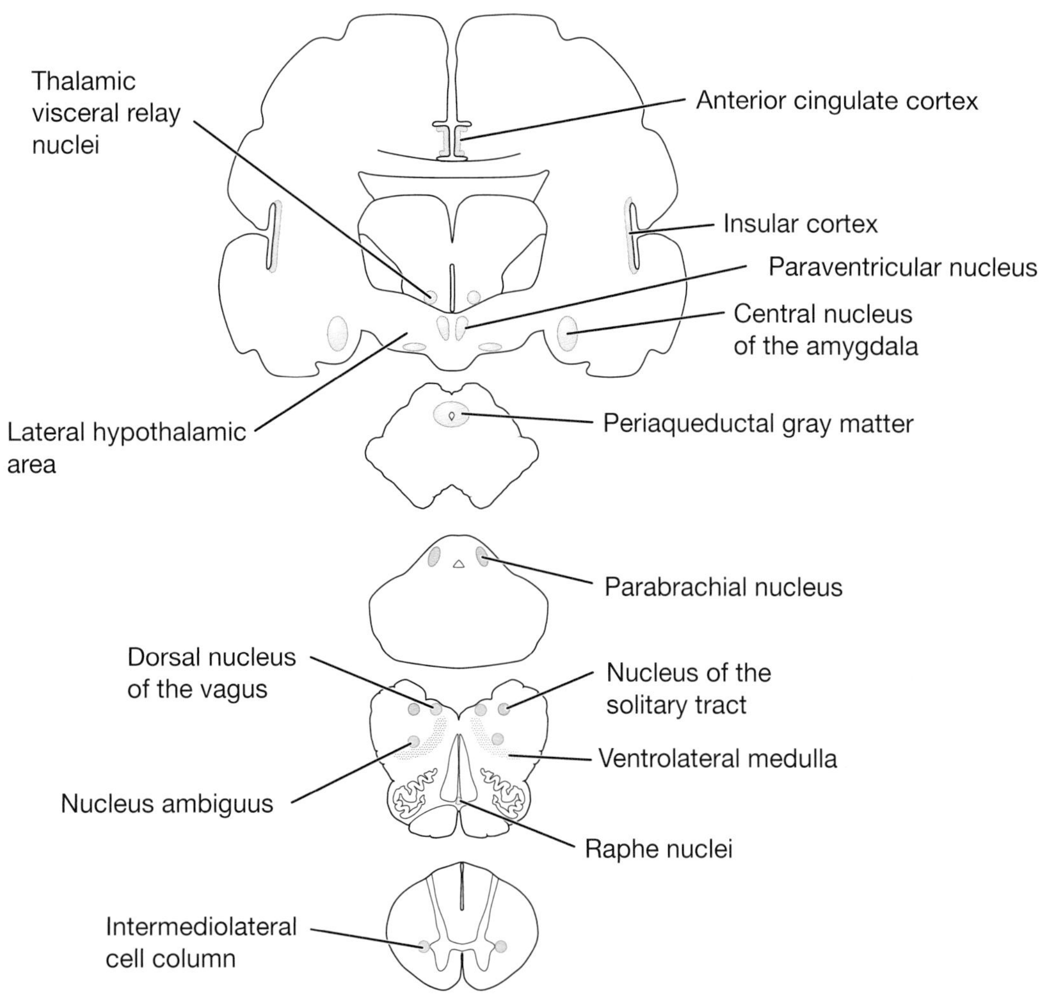

Fig. 9.2. Components of the internal regulation system. All these areas are reciprocally connected and contain various neurotransmitters. The main parasympathetic output is mediated by the dorsal nucleus of the vagus and the nucleus ambiguus, and the sympathetic output is mediated by the intermediolateral cell column. (Modified from Benarroch EE. Basic neurosciences with clinical applications. Philadelphia: Elsevier; 2006. Used with permission of Mayo Foundation for Medical Education and Research.)

regulation system. The central autonomic neurons also receive humoral information from the blood and cerebrospinal fluid and information about the external environment indirectly from sensory systems' relay stations in the cerebral cortex, amygdala, or hypothalamus.

The autonomic output of the internal regulation system is mediated by the *sympathetic* and the *parasympathetic* systems. This autonomic output consists of two neurons: 1) *preganglionic neurons* located in the brainstem or spinal cord and 2) neurons in the *autonomic ganglia*. Autonomic ganglion neurons called *postganglionic neurons* receive excitatory input from preganglionic neurons and send postganglionic axons to innervate peripheral visceral effectors (Fig. 9.3).

The preganglionic sympathetic neurons are located in the *intermediolateral cell column* of segments T1 to L3 of the spinal cord. These neurons innervate the paravertebral and prevertebral sympathetic ganglia. The preganglionic parasympathetic neurons are located in specific visceral efferent nuclei of the brainstem and in

Table 9.1. Functional Anatomy of the Central Components of the Internal Regulation System

Level	Area	Function
Supratentorial		
Telencephalon	Insular cortex	Visceral sensation
	Anterior cingulate cortex	Motivation and drive
	Amygdala	Emotion
Diencephalon	Hypothalamus	Circadian rhythms
		Sleep-wake cycle
		Thermoregulation
		Osmoregulation
		Response to stress
		Immune modulation
		Feeding and drinking
		Reproduction
Posterior fossa	Periaqueductal gray matter	Response to stress
		Pain control
	Parabrachial complex	Visceral sensory relay
		Respiration
		Micturition
	Nucleus of the solitary tract	First relay of visceral brainstem afferents
		Initiation of medullary reflexes
		Respiration
	Ventrolateral medulla	Vasomotor tone
		Respiration
		Afferent to hypothalamus
	Medullary raphe	Thermoregulation
	Dorsal nucleus of the vagus	Preganglionic parasympathetic input to gastrointestinal and respiratory tracts
	Nucleus ambiguus	Preganglionic parasympathetic input to heart
Spinal	Intermediolateral cell column (spinal levels T1-L3)	Preganglionic sympathetic input
	Sacral parasympathetic nucleus (levels S2-S4)	Preganglionic parasympathetic input to bladder, rectum, and sexual organs
	Dorsal horn	Relay of visceral, pain, and temperature sensations

spinal segments S2 to S4. A third division of the autonomic nervous system is the *enteric nervous system*, which is located in the walls of the gut. The neurotransmitter for all preganglionic neurons—both sympathetic and parasympathetic—is *acetylcholine*, which through *nicotinic* receptors excites the autonomic ganglion neurons. The primary neurotransmitter of sympathetic ganglion neurons is *norepinephrine*, which acts on *adrenergic* receptors to affect target organs. However, the sympathetic postganglionic neurons that innervate sweat glands have acetylcholine as a neurotransmitter. All parasympathetic postganglionic neurons have acetylcholine as the primary neurotransmitter. The effects of acetylcholine on effector organs are mediated through *muscarinic* receptors.

The sympathetic output, which is activated in a coordinated fashion, is critical for maintaining blood pressure during postural change and for thermoregulation and integrated responses to exercise, stress, and emotion. Sympathetic stimulation elicits pupillary dilatation, heart activation, vasoconstriction or vasodilatation of peripheral vessels, sweating, bronchodilatation, inhibition of gastrointestinal motility and secretion, relaxation of the bladder and rectum, and ejaculation. In contrast to the diffuse activation of the sympathetic system, activation of the parasympathetic system is more specific, usually affecting only one target organ. It elicits pupillary constriction, salivary gland and lacrimal gland secretion, heart inhibition, bronchoconstriction, increased gastrointestinal motility and secretion, evacuation of the bladder and rectum, and penile erection.

The endocrine output of the internal regulation system is mediated by circulating hormones, including those secreted by the pituitary gland under control of the hypothalamus and those secreted by peripheral endocrine organs under the influence of autonomic input. Somatic motor output controls the muscles of respiration,

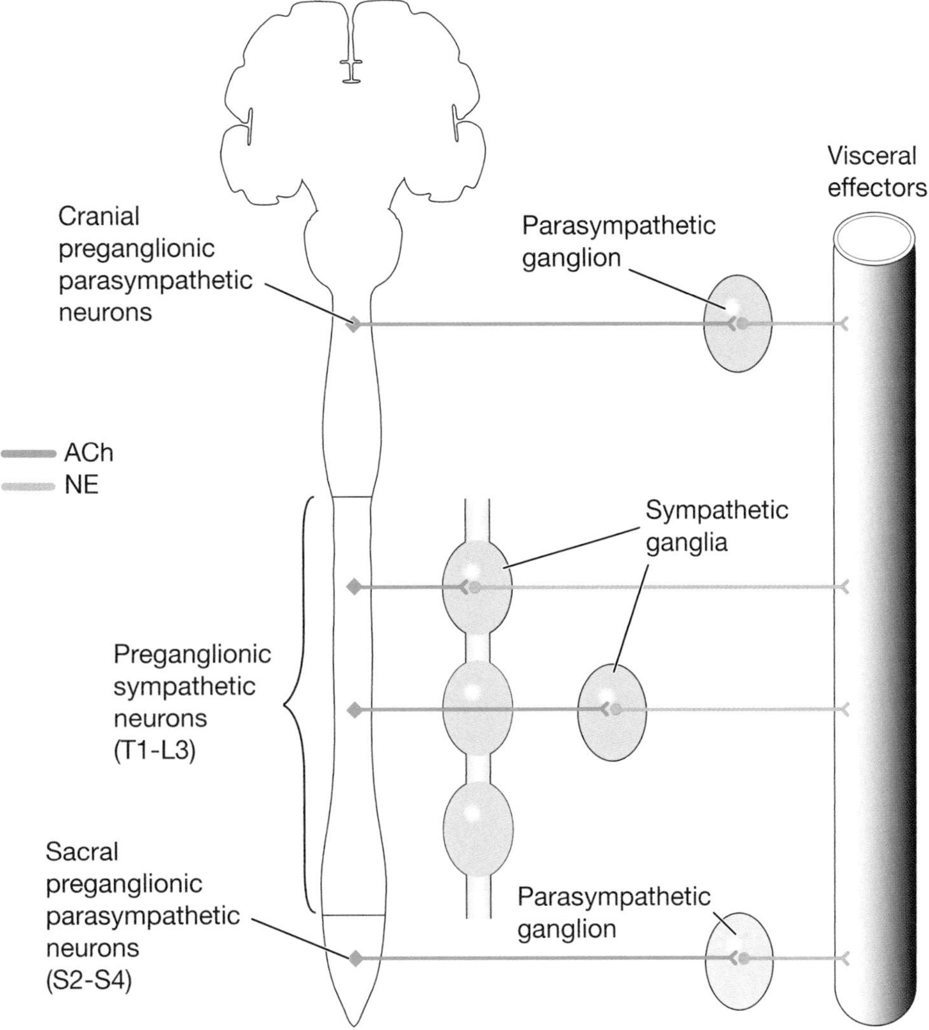

Fig. 9.3. General organization of the sympathetic and parasympathetic outputs of the internal regulation system. ACh, acetylcholine; NE, norepinephrine.

swallowing, and mastication and the external sphincters. The internal regulation system modulates pain by controlling the transmission of nociceptive information at the level of the dorsal horn.

The internal regulation system can be affected by diffuse or focal neurologic disorders. Diffuse disorders produce generalized autonomic failure by affecting both sympathetic and parasympathetic outflow. Important causes include central degenerative disorders, peripheral neuropathies involving autonomic axons, and drugs or toxins. Focal disorders usually affect the pupil, the bladder, or bowel function. Unilateral abnormality of the pupil indicates involvement of central or peripheral sympathetic or parasympathetic pupillomotor pathways on the same side. Impaired control of the bladder, rectum, or sexual organs commonly reflects a focal midline lesion at the spinal level.

- The internal regulation system controls responses critical for survival.
- The components of the internal regulation system are distributed throughout the neuraxis.
- The internal regulation system controls autonomic, endocrine, and motor outputs.
- Disorders of the internal regulation system may be manifested as autonomic failure or autonomic hyperactivity or impaired function of specific effector organs.

Anatomical and Functional Organization of the Internal Regulation System

Integrating-Coordinating Areas

The integrating-coordinating areas of the internal regulation systems are located in the supratentorial and posterior fossa levels. The supratentorial components of this system are the insular cortex, anterior cingulate cortex, amygdala, and hypothalamus (Fig. 9.4). All these areas are interconnected with one another, receive input from the nucleus of the solitary tract, parabrachial nucleus, and dorsal horn, either directly or through a relay in the thalamus, and project to the autonomic nuclei in the brainstem.

Telencephalic Components

The *insular cortex* is buried within the sylvian fissure and covered by the frontal and parietal opercula. The insula is the primary viscerosensory cortex. It receives visceral information from the dorsal horn, nucleus of the solitary tract, and parabrachial nucleus. The nucleus of the solitary tract and parabrachial nuclei also convey taste sensation, and the dorsal horn conveys pain and temperature sensation. All these inputs reach the insula through a relay in different portions of the ventromedial nucleus of the thalamus. Thus, the insula is the primary cortical representation of taste, visceral sensation, pain, and temperature sensation (Fig. 9.5).

The cingulate gyrus is located on the medial aspect of the hemisphere, just above the corpus callosum (Fig. 9.6). The *anterior cingulate* cortex is involved in behavioral drive and motivation triggered by emotionally significant stimuli. It receives pain and visceral sensory information from the thalamus and is connected with the amygdala, prefrontal cortex, basal ganglia, brainstem, and spinal cord. The anterior cingulate cortex initiates motor and autonomic responses associated with affective behavior, including responses to pain and emotional drive and motivation.

The *amygdala* is located in the anterior portion of the medial aspect of the temporal lobe, just anterior to the hippocampal formation (Fig. 9.4). Its main function is to provide emotional significance to sensory stimuli, ranging from pain to facial expression, and to initiate integrated responses to emotion, particularly fear.

The amygdala receives both elementary sensory input, such as pain or visceral sensation, directly from the brainstem or thalamus, and processed sensory information from the cerebral cortex. The amygdala provides emotional significance for these sensory stimuli and initiates conditioned responses, particularly conditioned fear. These responses are mediated by projections from the amygdala to the hypothalamus and autonomic and motor nuclei of the brainstem and spinal cord. Through these projections, the amygdala initiates coordinated autonomic, endocrine, and motor responses to emotionally relevant stimuli (Fig. 9.7).

- The insula is the primary cortical representation of visceral, pain, temperature, and taste sensations.

- The anterior cingulate gyrus is involved in high-level control of autonomic function during motivated motor responses to behaviorally relevant stimuli.
- The amygdala provides emotional significance to sensory stimuli and initiates an integrated autonomic, endocrine, and motor response to emotion, particularly conditioned fear.

Hypothalamus

The *hypothalamus* is the effector structure of the diencephalon (Fig. 9.8). It is essential for homeostasis, including thermoregulation, osmoregulation, control of food intake and reproduction, biologic rhythms (including the sleep-wake cycle), integrated responses to stress, and regulation of immune responses. All these functions are critical for survival and depend on the ability of different regions of the hypothalamus to receive and integrate visceral and other sensory input and humoral information and to initiate the appropriate autonomic, endocrine, and behavioral response to a challenge from the internal environment (e.g., hypoglycemia, hemorrhage, or dehydration) or external environment (e.g., changes in ambient temperature or exposure to danger).

Anatomically, the hypothalamus is subdivided into the preoptic, tuberal, and mammillary regions (Fig. 9.8 *A*). Functionally, it is subdivided into three longitudinally arranged zones: the periventricular, medial, and lateral zones (Fig. 9.8 *B*). These three zones contain several nuclei, each with different connections and functions, that are closely interconnected and interact, generating the appropriate autonomic, endocrine, and behavioral response (Fig. 9.9).

The periventricular zone contains nuclei involved in neuroendocrine control through projections to the posterior pituitary or medial eminence. The medial zone contains nuclei that are involved in thermoregulation, control of food intake, and reproduction. The lateral zone, through its connections with the cerebral cortex and brainstem, is

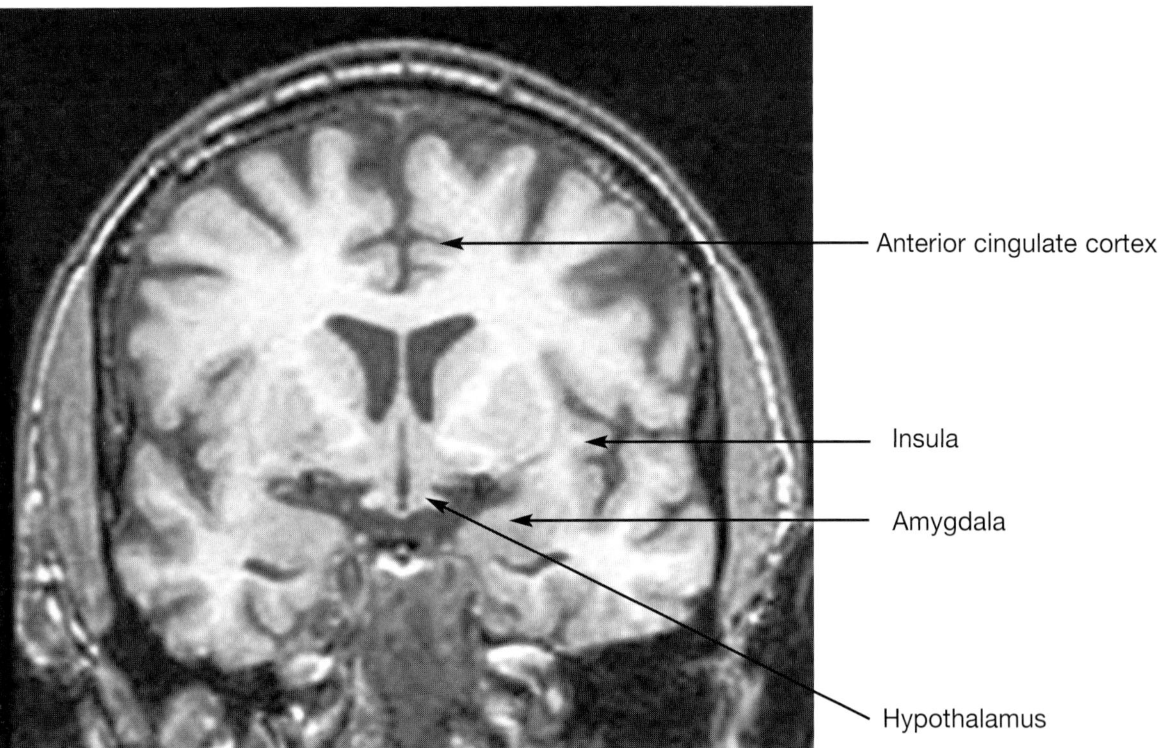

Fig. 9.4. Coronal magnetic resonance image showing the main components of the internal regulation system at the supratentorial level.

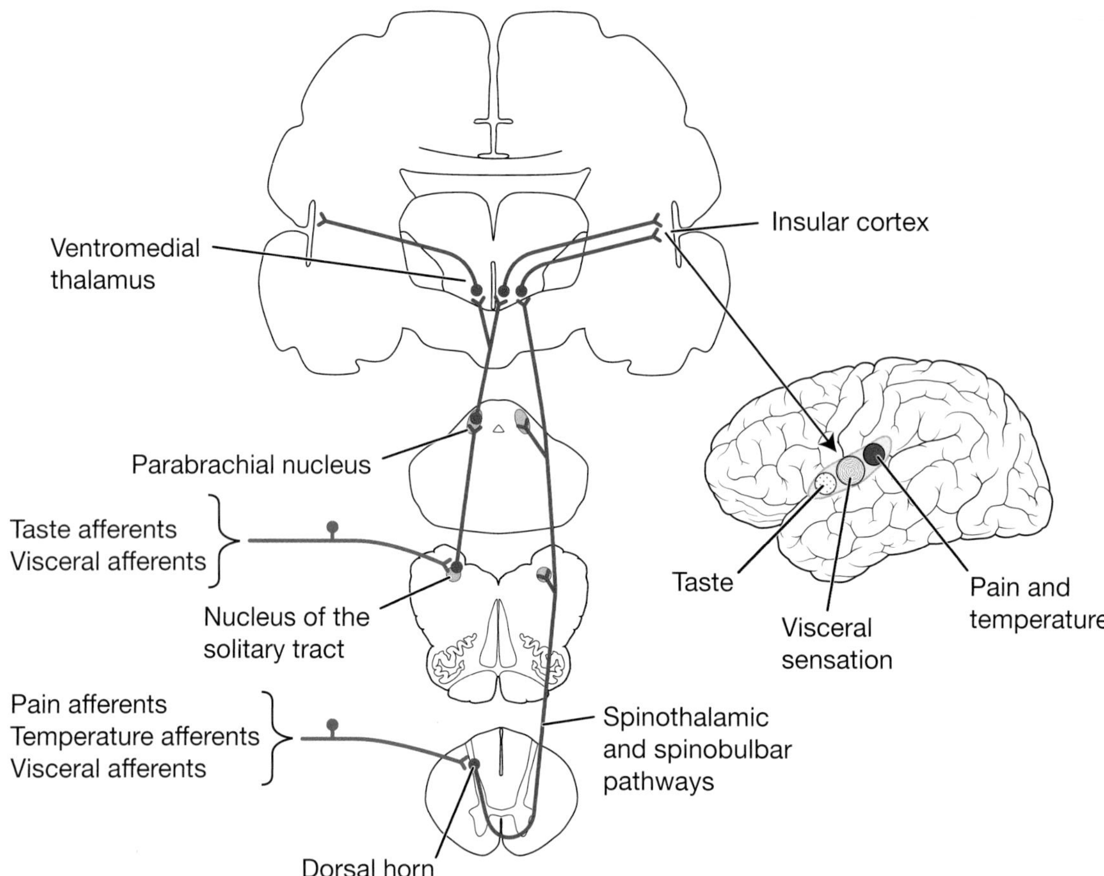

Fig. 9.5. Integration of visceral sensory, pain, and temperature information at the level of the insular cortex. The insular cortex is the primary viscerosensory cortex for taste, visceral, pain, and temperature sensations. Spinal visceral afferents, conveying visceral sensation, relay in the dorsal horn; brainstem visceral afferents, conveying taste and visceral sensation, relay in the nucleus of the solitary tract. Both the dorsal horn and nucleus of the solitary tract project to the parabrachial nucleus. All these areas convey taste, visceral, pain, and temperature sensations to the ventromedial region of the thalamus, which projects to the insular cortex. All these sensory modalities are represented topographically in the insula.

involved in control of the sleep-wake cycle; it also participates in control of food intake.

Although several hypothalamic nuclei project to autonomic nuclei in the brainstem and spinal cord, the two most prominent projections arise from the *paraventricular nucleus* and the *lateral hypothalamic area* (Fig. 9.10). These hypothalamic areas contain separate populations of neurons that project to different subsets of preganglionic neurons and generate distinct patterns of autonomic response according to the stimuli. The paraventricular nucleus is crucial for integrated autonomic and endocrine responses to stress.

- The hypothalamus is essential for thermoregulation, osmoregulation, control of food intake and reproduction, biologic rhythms (including the sleep-wake cycle), integrated responses to stress, and regulation of immune responses.
- The hypothalamus receives and integrates information from the viscera, blood, and external environment.
- The paraventricular nucleus and the lateral hypothalamic area provide most of the hypothalamic output to the autonomic nuclei in the brainstem and spinal cord.
- The endocrine output of the hypothalamus involves connections with the pituitary gland.

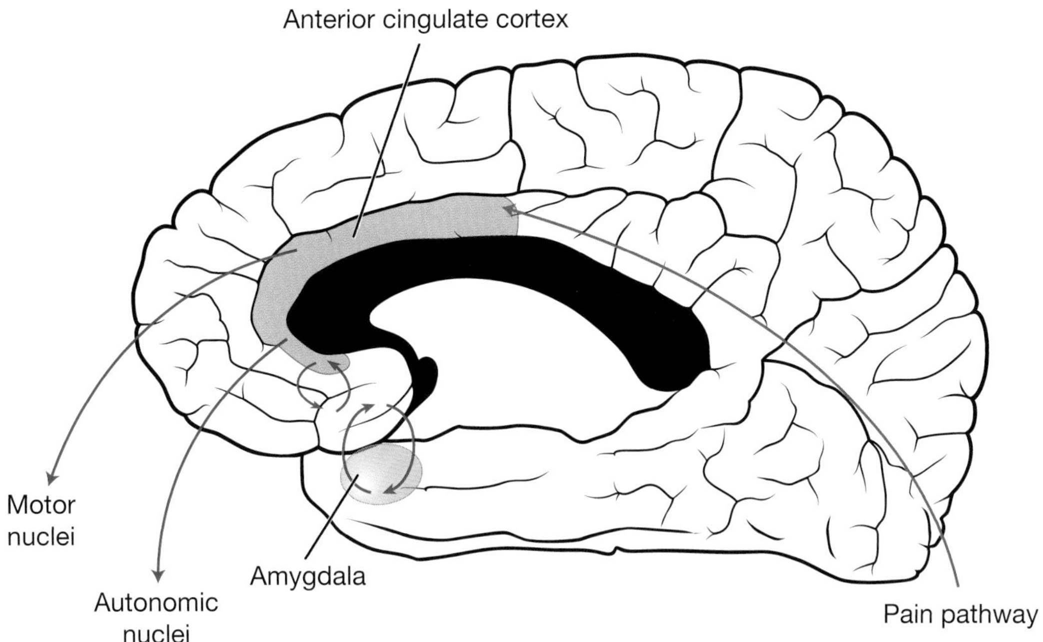

Fig. 9.6. The anterior cingulate cortex is involved in mechanisms of emotion, motivation, and behavioral drive through its reciprocal connections with the prefrontal cortex and amygdala. The amygdala has reciprocal connections with the orbitofrontal cortex. The anterior cingulate cortex receives input from pain pathways and is involved in affective components of pain sensation. It controls motor function through its output to the basal ganglia and motor nuclei of the brainstem and spinal cord. It also regulates autonomic function through its output to the hypothalamus and autonomic nuclei of the brainstem.

Brainstem Components

The brainstem components of the integrating-coordinating circuits of the internal regulation system include the periaqueductal gray matter, parabrachial nucleus, nucleus of the solitary tract, reticular formation of ventrolateral medulla, and medullary raphe nuclei (Fig. 9.2).

The periaqueductal gray matter surrounds the aqueduct of Sylvius. It contains different populations of neurons that project to different nuclei of the pons and medulla and coordinate different patterns of motor, autonomic, and pain-suppressing responses to stress. A lateral region initiates active ("fight-or-flight") responses, including sympathetic excitation, increased motor activity, and opioid-independent analgesia, that reflect an active response to stress. A medial region initiates passive ("avoidance" or "playing dead") responses, characterized by sympathetic inhibition, immobility, and opioid-dependent analgesia.

The *parabrachial nucleus* is located in the dorsolateral portion of the pons and is an important relay station for visceral sensation, taste, pain, and temperature sensation to rostral components of the internal regulation system. This information is relayed to the parabrachial nucleus from the nucleus of the solitary tract or the dorsal horn. The parabrachial nucleus then conveys this information to the thalamus (which projects to the insula and anterior cingulate cortex), hypothalamus, and amygdala. The parabrachial region also contains a group of neurons involved in control of respiration and another group that coordinates micturition, as described below in this chapter.

The *nucleus of the solitary tract* is the first relay station of the brainstem for visceral afferents in the facial, glossopharyngeal, and vagus nerves (Fig. 9.11). This nucleus has three important functions. First, it relays these inputs, both directly or through the parabrachial nucleus, to all the central autonomic areas, particularly the hypothalamus and amygdala. Second, it participates in several reflexes critical for control of blood pressure, heart rate,

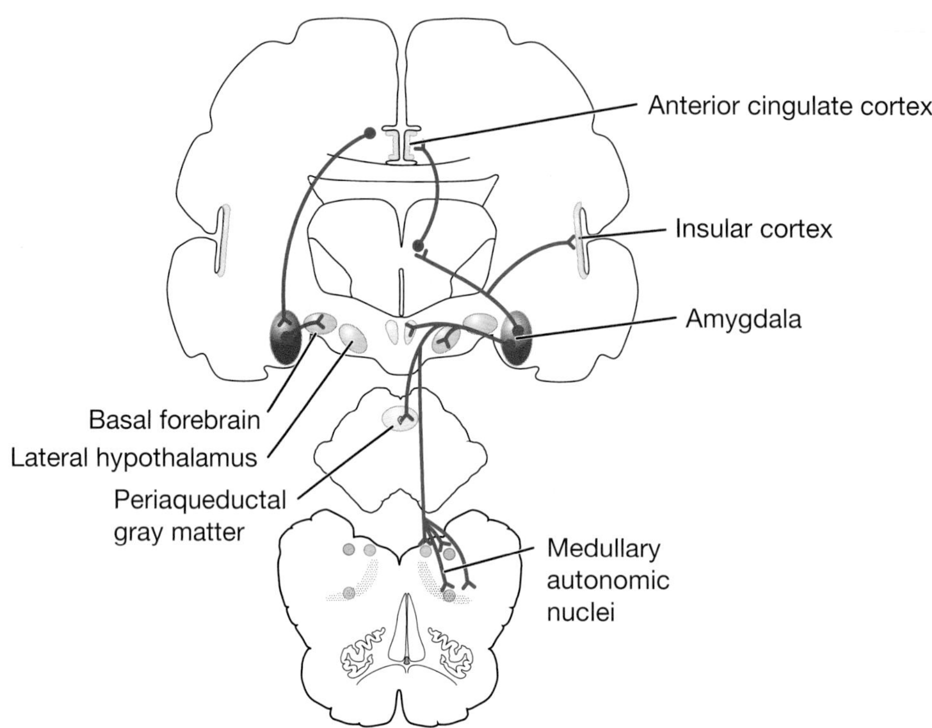

Fig. 9.7. Main connections of the amygdala. The amygdala receives sensory input from the thalamus and sensory association areas of the cerebral cortex and provides sensation with emotional significance through its interconnections with the basal forebrain and anterior cingulate cortex. Through its connections with the hypothalamus and brainstem, the amygdala coordinates autonomic, endocrine, and motor components of emotional responses.

and respiration. Third, it initiates complex patterns requiring the coordinated activity of medullary cranial nerve motor nuclei, for example, swallowing and vomiting.

Ventrolateral Medulla

The reticular formation of ventrolateral medulla contains several groups of neurons important for maintaining arterial blood pressure and respiratory rhythm (Fig. 9.12). It also contains catecholaminergic neurons that relay visceral input from the nucleus of the solitary tract to the hypothalamus. Rostral ventrolateral medulla contains neurons that provide continuous (tonic) excitation to preganglionic sympathetic neurons which control the heart and promote vasoconstriction of skeletal and visceral blood vessels. These neurons have a critical role in maintaining arterial blood pressure. Caudal ventrolateral medulla mediates the inhibitory control from the nucleus of the solitary tract to rostral ventrolateral medulla. It also contains noradrenergic neurons that project to the hypothalamus and control endocrine responses to hypotension and stress. The ventrolateral medulla contains a long column of neurons (extending from caudal pons to the rostral spinal cord) referred to as the ventral respiratory group. This consists of several regions critical for the control of respiration.

Medullary Raphe Nuclei

Neurons in the medullary raphe nuclei project to the intermediolateral cell column and synapse on preganglionic neurons that control skin vasomotor outputs important for thermoregulatory responses to cold. Through projections to the dorsal horn, medullary raphe nuclei modulate transmission of pain sensation, and through projections to the ventral horn, they modulate the activity of respiratory and other motor neurons. Some ventral medullary raphe neurons may have an important role in respiratory responses to hypercapnia.

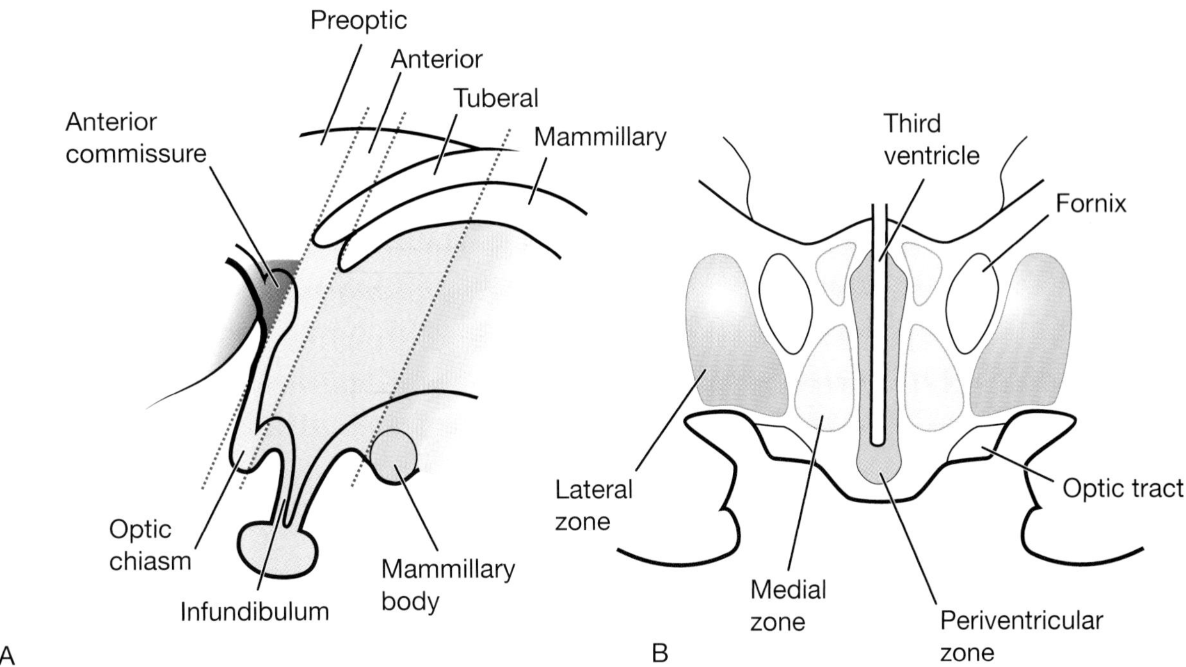

Fig. 9.8. General anatomical organization of the hypothalamus. *A*, The hypothalamus consists of four regions: preoptic, anterior, tuberal, and mammillary (posterior). *B*, Each of these main regions is subdivided into three zones: periventricular (surrounding the third ventricle), medial (in relation to the fornix), and lateral (in relation to the fornix).

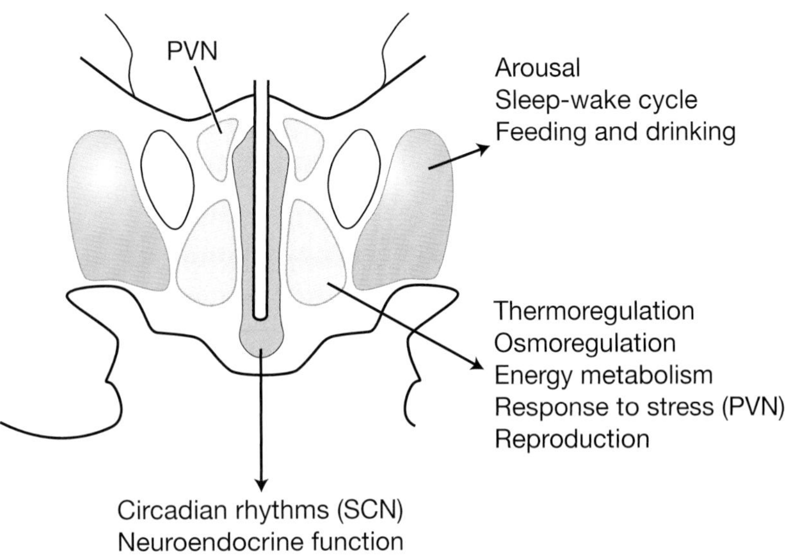

Fig. 9.9. Main functions of the periventricular, medial, and lateral zones of the hypothalamus. All these areas are intimately interconnected and act together to generate integrated responses. The paraventricular nucleus (PVN) and lateral hypothalamic zone provide the main output to autonomic nuclei in the brainstem and spinal cord. SCN, suprachiasmatic nucleus.

- The periaqueductal gray matter has a major role in the coordination of patterns of autonomic, motor, and antinociceptive responses to external stressors.
- The parabrachial nucleus is essential for relaying visceral, taste, pain, and temperature information from the brainstem to the thalamus, hypothalamus, and amygdala.
- The nucleus of the solitary tract is the first relay station for brainstem visceral afferents and mediates reflexes controlling cardiovascular function, respiration, vomiting, and swallowing.
- Different groups of neurons of the reticular formation of ventrolateral medulla are critical for maintenance of arterial blood pressure, respiratory rhythm, and cardiorespiratory interactions.
- The medullary raphe nuclei control the sympathetic response to cold and participate in respiratory chemosensitivity.

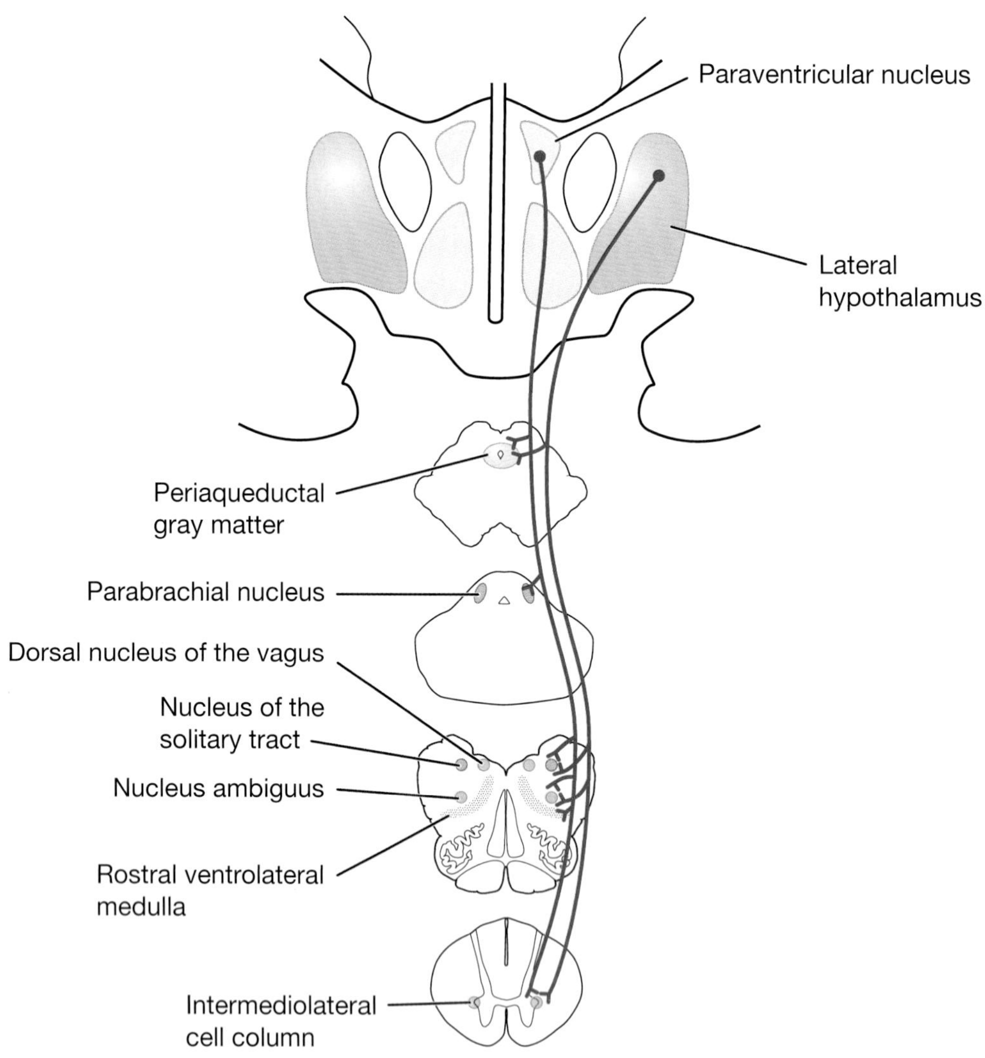

Fig. 9.10. The paraventricular nucleus and lateral hypothalamic area provide the main hypothalamic output to the autonomic nuclei in the brainstem and spinal cord. They control the activity of preganglionic neurons both directly and through projections to the rostral ventrolateral medulla and nucleus of the solitary tract.

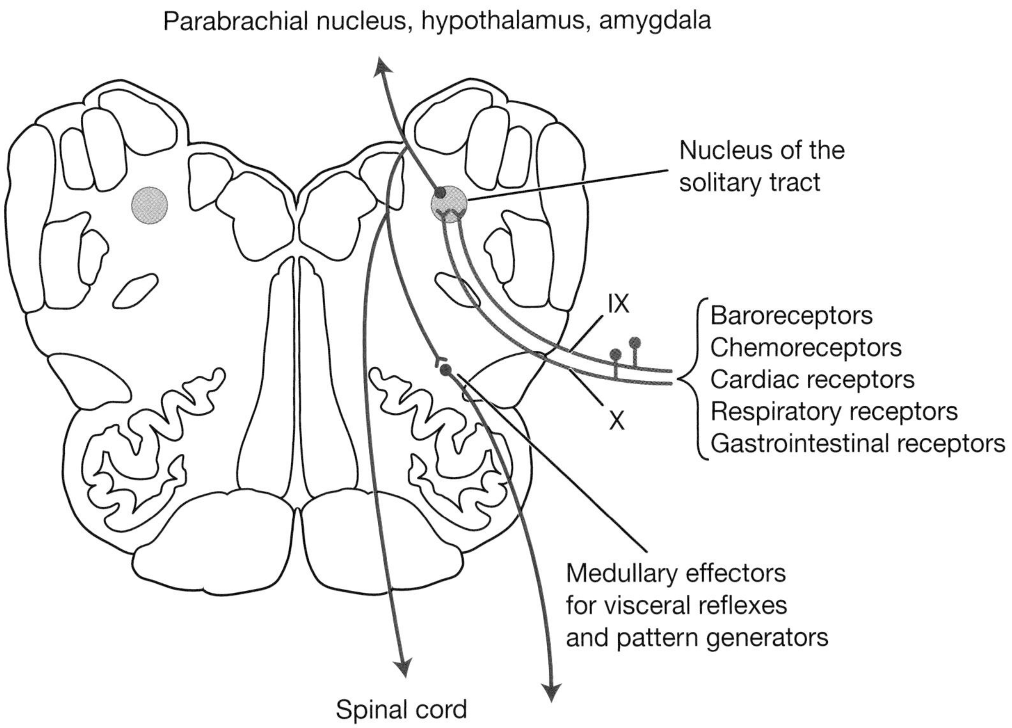

Parabrachial nucleus, hypothalamus, amygdala

Nucleus of the solitary tract

IX

X

Baroreceptors
Chemoreceptors
Cardiac receptors
Respiratory receptors
Gastrointestinal receptors

Medullary effectors for visceral reflexes and pattern generators

Spinal cord

Fig. 9.11. Main connections of the nucleus of the solitary tract. This nucleus is the first relay station for taste and general visceral afferents conveyed by cranial nerves. Its rostral portion, through the facial, glossopharyngeal (IX), and vagus (X) nerves, receives afferents from taste receptors. Its caudal portion, through the glossopharyngeal and predominantly vagus nerves, receives afferents from cardiovascular, respiratory, and gastrointestinal receptors. Different subgroups of neurons have ascending axons that project to the parabrachial nucleus, hypothalamus, and amygdala to generate adaptive and homeostatic responses; projections to pattern generator networks of the medullary reticular formation to coordinate the activity of cranial nerve nuclei involved in swallowing, vomiting, and other complex motor acts; and projections to the rostral ventrolateral medulla, nucleus ambiguus, and dorsal motor nucleus of the vagus to generate respiratory, cardiovascular, and gastrointestinal reflexes.

Input to the Internal Regulation System

Interoceptive Input: Visceral, Pain, and Temperature Sensations

Visceral, pain, and temperature sensations provide the internal regulation system with information about the state of the body, which is essential for the control of visceral function and emotional and adaptive responses. The pathways conveying pain and temperature sensations to the cerebral cortex (spinothalamic tract and trigeminothalamic tract) are described in Chapter 7. These pathways arise in the dorsal horn of the spinal cord and trigeminal nucleus and provide collateral pathways to several components of the internal regulation system. Through *spinobulbar pathways*, pain and temperature information from the dorsal horn (particularly lamina I) is relayed to the nucleus of the solitary tract, parabrachial nucleus, and periaqueductal gray matter. The dorsal horn and trigeminal nucleus also project directly to the hypothalamus and amygdala. All these structures also receive input from visceral receptors.

Visceral receptors are located in the muscular wall and the mucosal and serosal surfaces of internal organs, blood vessels, and the pleural and peritoneal cavities. Visceral receptors are activated by mechanical or chemical stimuli and are innervated by small myelinated and unmyelinated fibers. The density of innervation of the viscera is low compared with that of the skin and deep

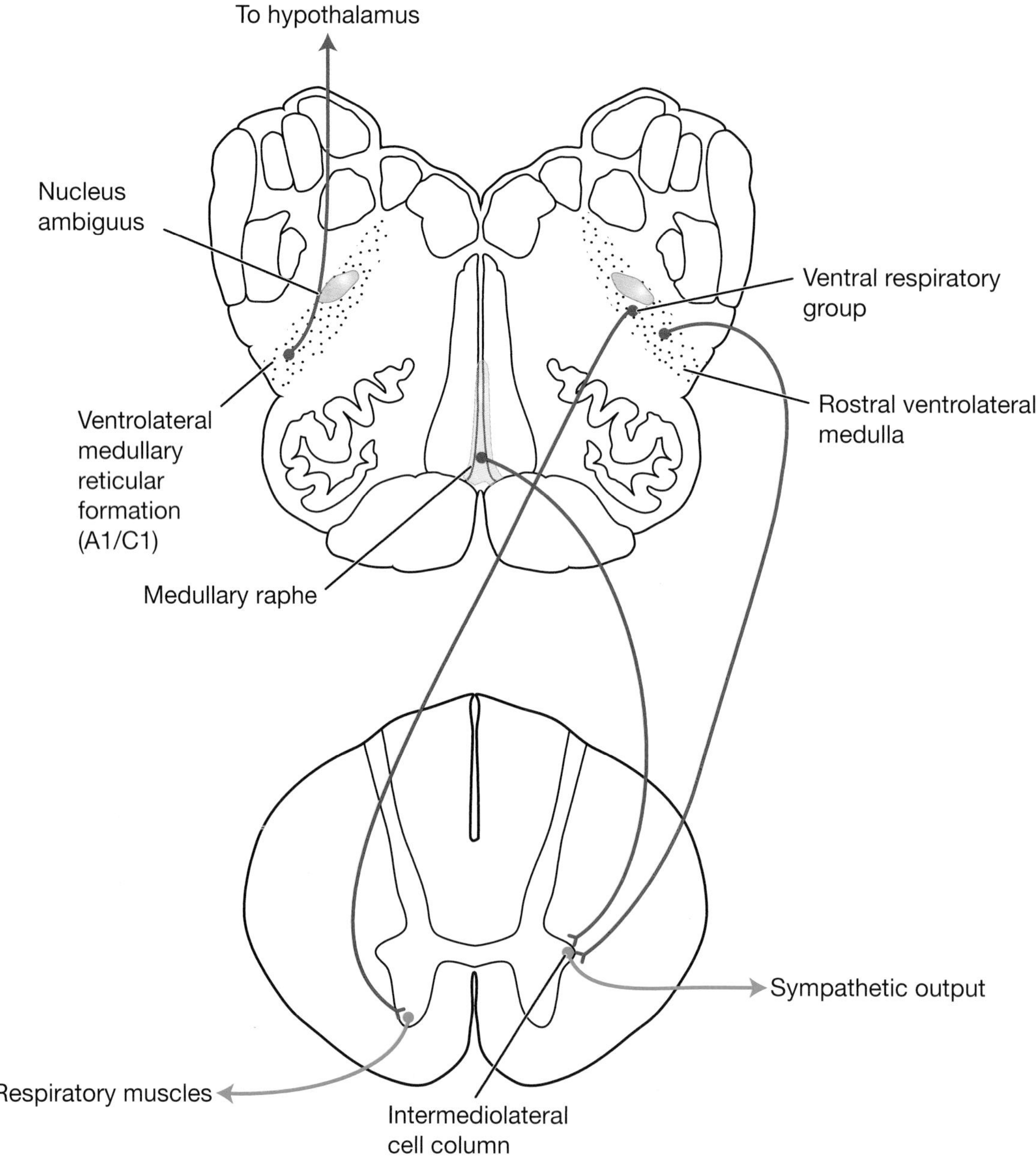

Fig. 9.12. Regions of the medulla involved in control of cardiovascular and respiratory functions. These regions receive input from the hypothalamus and nucleus of the solitary tract and mediate cardiovascular reflexes and coordinated homeostatic responses. The rostral ventrolateral medulla is critical for activation of preganglionic sympathetic neurons involved in maintaining blood pressure. The A1/C1 groups of catecholaminergic neurons in ventrolateral medulla convey visceral sensory and pain inputs to the hypothalamus. The medullary raphe projects to preganglionic neurons involved in thermoregulation and is important for respiratory responses to hypercarbia and hypoxia. Most vagal output to the heart arises from the nucleus ambiguus. The ventral respiratory group includes local neurons involved in generating the respiratory rhythm and neurons that project to the phrenic and other respiratory motor neurons. There are important interactions between the medullary cardiovascular and respiratory neurons.

somatic tissue. This partly explains the vague spatial resolution of visceral sensation.

General visceral afferent signals follow three main routes. Some remain in the peripheral organ and mediate local reflexes, some provide collateral input to autonomic ganglion cells and mediate ganglion reflexes, and some enter the central nervous system at the level of the spinal cord (spinal visceral afferents) or brainstem (brainstem visceral afferents).

> Unmyelinated visceral afferents contain several combinations of neuropeptides and, like nociceptive afferents, may release neuropeptides centrally (transmission of visceral sensory information) and locally (via axon reflexes), producing vascular and secretory changes at the level of the site of stimulation.

The cell bodies of spinal visceral afferents are small and located in dorsal root ganglia. The peripheral axons of these neurons pass through the paravertebral chain and enter sympathetic and sacral parasympathetic nerves to innervate visceral organs (Fig. 9.13). The central axons join the dorsal roots and enter the spinal cord. In the spinal cord, visceral afferents branch extensively, thus providing divergent input to many neurons in the dorsal horn and intermediate gray matter (Fig. 9.14). Many dorsal horn neurons, particularly in lamina I (superficial dorsal horn), receive input from both visceral and somatic afferents that convey pain and temperature sensation. These spinal neurons relay this sensory information to the brainstem, thalamus, amygdala, and hypothalamus. The spinothalamic pathways synapse in the ventromedial nucleus of the thalamus, which projects to the insular cortex, and in medial thalamic nuclei, which project to the anterior cingulate gyrus. The spinobulbar pathways terminate in the nucleus of the solitary tract, parabrachial nucleus, periaqueductal gray matter, and catecholaminergic neurons of ventrolateral medulla (A1/C1 groups). Although visceral sensation is transferred mainly along pathways in the ventrolateral quadrant of the spinal cord, some information is transferred by axons in the midline portion of the dorsal columns. This includes pain from midline structures of the pelvis and sensations related to micturition, defecation, and gastric distention.

Unlike somatic pain, visceral pain is generally vague and poorly localized. It usually is described as being abdominal, thoracic, or pelvic rather than being localized to a specific organ. It commonly activates autonomic and somatic reflexes. Because of the convergence of visceral and somatic afferents on dorsal horn neurons, visceral pain is often referred to as overlying or being near a somatic structure; this is called *referred pain* (Fig. 9.15).

Most visceral sensation is unconscious and serves to trigger visceral reflexes as well as integrated autonomic, endocrine, and other adaptive responses. Visceral afferents trigger viscerovisceral and viscerosomatic spinal reflexes through interneurons located in the intermediate gray matter of the thoracolumbar and sacral spinal cord (Fig. 9.14).

Brainstem visceral afferents are part of the vagus and glossopharyngeal nerves. The cell bodies of vagal afferents are in the *nodose ganglion*; they conduct sensory information from gastrointestinal, respiratory, cardiac, and aortic arch mechanoreceptors and chemoreceptors. The cell bodies of glossopharyngeal afferents are in the *petrosal ganglion*; they conduct sensory information from carotid sinus baroreceptors and carotid body chemoreceptors. All these vagal and glossopharyngeal afferents synapse in different regions of the caudal portion of the nucleus of the solitary tract. The rostral portion of the nucleus of the solitary tract receives information from taste receptors, carried primarily in the facial nerve (cranial nerve VII) (cell bodies in the *geniculate ganglion*); some taste fibers are also in the glossopharyngeal and vagus nerves.

The nucleus of the solitary tract conveys this information to the parabrachial nucleus, and both these nuclei send axons to a portion of the ventromedial nucleus of the thalamus that, in turn, projects to the insular cortex, the cortical area associated with conscious visceral sensation. In addition, both the nucleus of the solitary tract and the parabrachial nucleus project to the hypothalamus and amygdala to initiate complex adaptive and emotional responses to visceral input. Because both the nucleus of the solitary tract and parabrachial nucleus also receive spinobulbar input from the dorsal horn conveying pain and temperature sensation, they are sites for the integration of visceral and somatic bodily sensation.

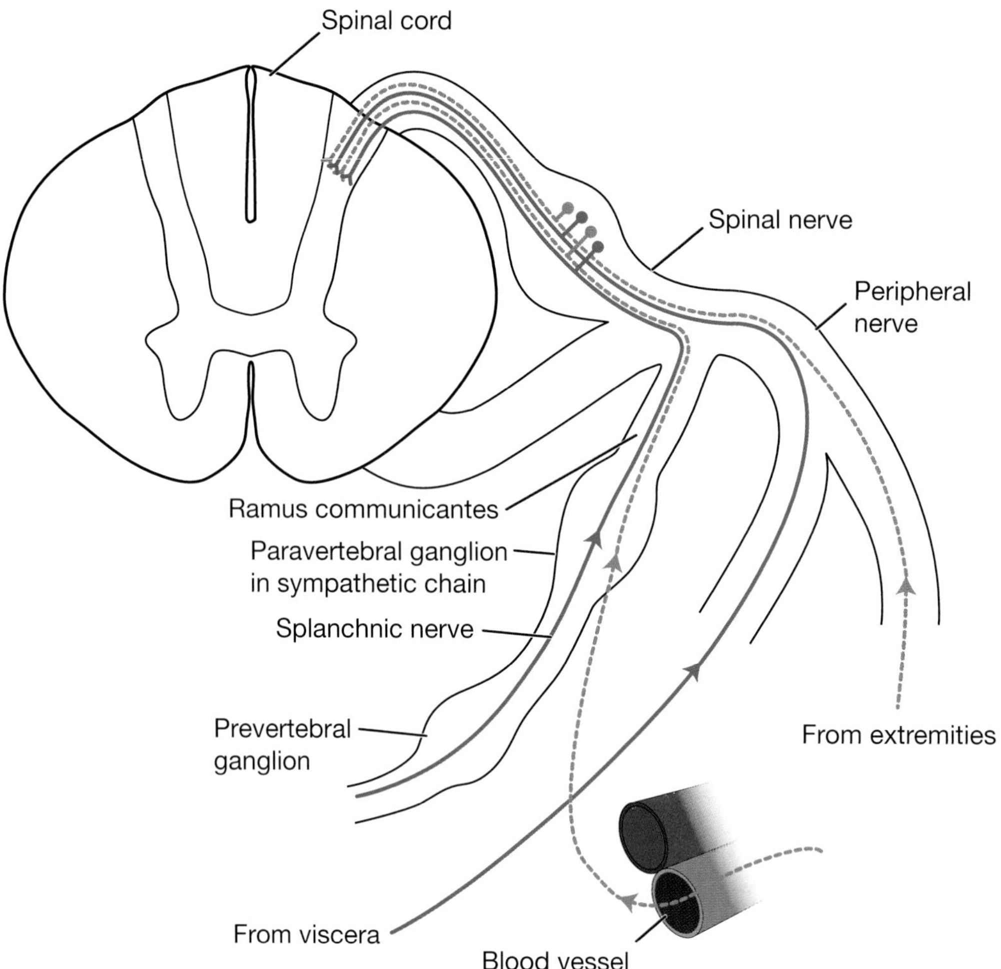

Fig. 9.13. Visceral afferents reach the spinal cord in several ways. All afferents are axons of small neurons in dorsal root ganglia. These afferents travel in peripheral nerves or through sympathetic paravertebral or prevertebral ganglia, whether coming from the extremities or viscera.

Vagal afferents sometimes mediate visceral pain, and they also may trigger central pain-controlling mechanisms through projections to the periaqueductal gray matter. Also, vagal afferents have a major role in conveying chemical information, such as levels of cytokines and gastrointestinal peptides, to the nucleus of the solitary tract and, thus, to all other components of the internal regulation system. This afferent information is important for the sensation of satiety after a meal and for generating febrile responses.

- Visceral afferents from taste, gastrointestinal, respiratory, and cardiovascular receptors project to different portions of the nucleus of the solitary tract.
- There is convergence of visceral, pain, and temperature sensations at the levels of the dorsal horn, nucleus of the solitary tract, and parabrachial nucleus.
- This integrated interoceptive information is relayed by the ventromedial thalamus to the insula. It also is relayed directly and by the parabrachial nucleus and A1/C1 neurons to the amygdala and hypothalamus.

Humoral Input

Changes in blood glucose, blood gases, electrolytes, temperature, osmolarity, and circulating steroid hormones exert a direct influence at all levels of the internal regulation

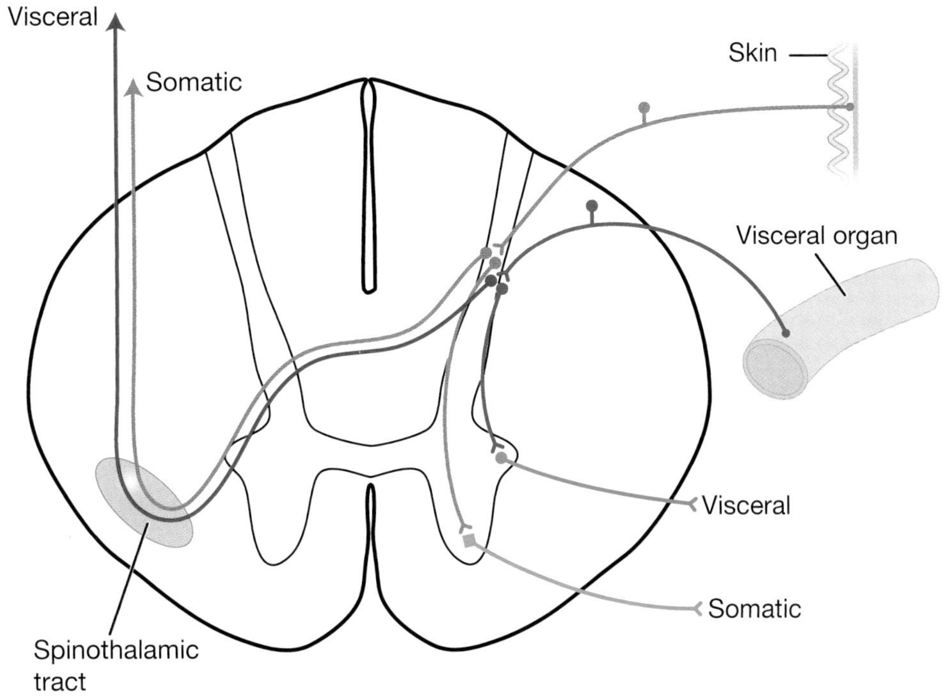

Fig. 9.14. Visceral afferents synapse with dorsal horn neurons and interneurons in the intermediate gray matter. Axons of dorsal horn neurons transmit information about visceral sensation, including visceral pain, in the spinothalamic tract. Many visceral afferents converge with somatic afferents on single dorsal horn neurons, providing the basis for referred pain. Local interneurons receiving visceral afferents project to preganglionic and somatic motor neurons to initiate segmental visceroviseral and viscerosomatic reflexes.

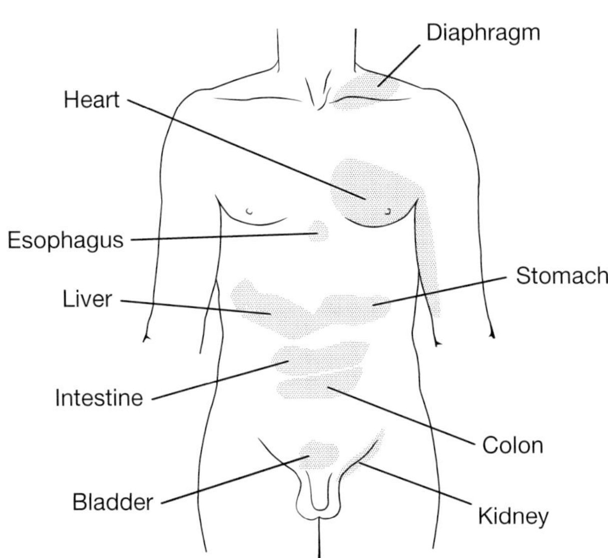

Fig. 9.15. Shading indicates dermatomal areas to which visceral pain is referred.

system. For example, the hypothalamus, medulla, and endocrine pancreas contain glucoreceptive neurons, and the skin, viscera, spinal cord, brainstem, and hypothalamus contain thermoreceptive neurons. Changes in pH and the partial pressure of carbon dioxide in the cerebrospinal fluid are detected by central chemosensitive areas of the ventral surface of the medulla.

Circulating peptides, monoamines, and other substances that do not readily cross the blood-brain barrier have a powerful influence on the internal regulation system by acting on receptors in the *circumventricular organs.* These organs are specialized structures in the walls of the ventricles that are characterized by fenestrated capillaries; thus, they lack a blood-brain barrier. Circumventricular organs detect chemical changes in the blood and cerebrospinal fluid and relay this information to the rest of the internal regulation system through connections to the hypothalamus, nucleus of the solitary tract, and ventrolateral medulla. Important examples include the *area postrema* in the walls of the fourth ventricle, the *subfornical organ* in the anterior wall of the third ventricle, and the *vascular organ of the lamina terminalis*, also in the anterior third ventricle immediately below the fornix.

> The area postrema is a chemoreceptor trigger zone for vomiting in response to toxic substances, including certain chemotherapy agents. The subfornical organ mediates the effects of circulating angiotensin II and natriuretic peptides on blood pressure, thirst, and sodium balance. The vascular organ of the lamina terminalis is the target for circulating cytokines that trigger the febrile response.

- The circumventricular organs lack a blood-brain barrier, thus permitting circulating peptides, monoamines, and other substances to influence the internal regulation system.

Inputs from the Amygdala and Orbitofrontal Cortex

Visual, auditory, somatosensory, and olfactory stimuli in addition to visceral, pain, and temperature sensations may reach the internal regulation system indirectly, primarily through connections of the amygdala and orbitofrontal cortex. The amygdala receives these sensory inputs from both the thalamus and cortical sensory association areas and assigns them emotional significance. The orbitofrontal cortex receives olfactory input directly (without thalamic relay) and taste, visual, and somatosensory input indirectly through the insula and anterior portions of the temporal lobe. Orbitofrontal cortex contains neurons that associate different types of stimuli, for example, the sight and taste of food, to determine the motivational value of the stimulus.

- The amygdala and orbitofrontal cortex provide information about the emotional and motivational value of sensory input to the internal regulation system.

Circadian Control: Suprachiasmatic Nucleus

The *suprachiasmatic nucleus*, located just above the optic chiasm, is the circadian pacemaker. It regulates several biologic rhythms, including the sleep-wake cycle, body temperature, and hormonal secretion (e.g., cyclic release of melatonin from the pineal gland). The endogenous rhythmic activity of the neurons of the suprachiasmatic nucleus is entrained by light during the day-night cycle. Light stimulates the ganglion cells of the retina, and axons of ganglion cells form the retinohypothalamic tract, which stimulates the suprachiasmatic nucleus.

> The suprachiasmatic nucleus inhibits the paraventricular nucleus of the hypothalamus. Through the sympathetic system, the paraventricular nucleus activates melatonin secretion of the pineal gland. Thus, melatonin secretion is maximal during darkness (at night).

- The suprachiasmatic nucleus is the circadian pacemaker and receives visual input that entrains autonomic and other biologic rhythms to the day-night cycle.

Output of the Internal Regulation System

The internal regulation system controls functions critical for adaptation and survival by four main groups of output: 1) autonomic, which controls the visceral organs; 2) endocrine, which exerts multiple effects by way of the bloodstream; 3) motor, which mediates automatic functions such as respiration; and 4) pain modulatory output. All these outputs are activated in a coordinated fashion.

Autonomic Output

The autonomic nervous system consists of three subdivisions: sympathetic, parasympathetic, and enteric nervous system. The sympathetic and parasympathetic outputs, referred to as *general visceral efferents*, differ from the somatic motor system in several important ways (Table 9.2). The output of both the sympathetic and parasympathetic systems consists of a two-neuron pathway: a preganglionic neuron and an autonomic ganglion neuron (see below) (Fig. 9.3).

Endocrine Output

The endocrine system elicits potent long-latency and prolonged responses that complement the fast, short-lasting effects of the autonomic system. The endocrine output originates from two main sources: 1) the hypothalamic-pituitary axis and 2) the peripheral endocrine organs. Some neurons of the hypothalamus produce peptides or dopamine that are released into the circulation. This process is known as *neurosecretion*. The hypothalamus has two neurosecretory systems. The *magnicellular system* consists of large neurons (hence, its name) in the paraventricular nucleus and supraoptic nucleus that synthesize either arginine vasopressin (AVP, antidiuretic hormone) or oxytocin and whose axons end in the posterior pituitary (*neurohypophysis*), where these neuropeptides are stored and released into the general circulation. The *parvicellular system* consists of neurons in the preoptic, paraventricular, and infundibular nuclei of the hypothalamus that secrete regulatory hormones into blood vessels of the median eminence and influence hormonal secretion by endocrine cells of the anterior pituitary (*adenohypophysis*). The hormones secreted by these hypothalamic-pituitary systems have multiple effects throughout the body. These neurosecretory systems are discussed in Chapter 16.

Autonomic output affects the function of peripheral endocrine organs. For example, sympathetic activation elicits the release of epinephrine from the adrenal medulla and renin from the juxtaglomerular apparatus of the kidney. Vagal output activates endocrine glands in the gastrointestinal tract and pancreas. The secretory effects of the vagus are both direct and indirect through the release of gastrointestinal peptides.

- Hormones secreted by the hypothalamic-pituitary axis or by peripheral endocrine organs produce potent and long-lasting effects that are coordinated with and potentiate the effects of the autonomic output.

Motor Output

The internal regulation system has important connections with the motor system at all levels of the neuraxis. At the supratentorial level, connections of the lateral hypothalamus and amygdala with the ventral striatum are important for complex motor behavior. At the posterior and spinal levels, brainstem and spinal motor neurons that innervate muscles involved in respiration, swallowing, and other automatic motor functions are important effectors of the internal regulation system. The activity of these motor neurons is controlled by *central pattern generators*. The internal regulation system controls the sacral motor neurons that innervate the external sphincters.

Networks of interneurons in the reticular formation of the lower pons and medulla coordinate the activity of spinal and cranial motor neurons that innervate the

Table 9.2. Comparison Between the General Visceral Efferent System and the General Somatic Efferent System

	Visceral	**Somatic**
Activity	Tonic, slow, diffuse	Phasic, fast, local
Output	Two neurons (preganglionic and postganglionic)	One neuron (alpha motor neuron)
Efferent axon	Small myelinated	Large myelinated
Effector neurotransmitter (receptor)	Acetylcholine (muscarinic) Norepinephrine (adrenergic)	Acetylcholine (nicotinic)
Effectors		
Type	Heart, smooth muscle, glands	Striated muscle
Spontaneous activity	Yes	No
Effect of denervation	Supersensitivity	Paralysis, atrophy

respiratory muscles. Important effector motor neurons are the *phrenic motor neurons* that are located at cervical levels C2 to C4 and innervate the diaphragm and *nucleus ambiguus motor neurons* that innervate the muscles of the larynx.

> The neurons of the respiratory central pattern generator network that control these motor neurons exhibit rhythmic activity due to intrinsic "pacemaker" activity or network interactions mediated by excitatory and inhibitory neurotransmitters (or both). This network includes neurons in the parabrachial nucleus of the pons (pontine respiratory group), the nucleus of the solitary tract (dorsal respiratory group), and the ventrolateral medulla (ventral respiratory group). These neurons, particularly those of the ventral respiratory group, project to the phrenic motor neurons that innervate the diaphragm and to the motor neurons that innervate the intercostal and abdominal muscles. A subgroup of local neurons of the ventral respiratory group, called the preBötzinger complex, is critical for generating the respiratory rhythm. Through these pathways, the medullary respiratory network controls the inspiratory and expiratory phases of the respiratory cycle.

Swallowing, vomiting, coughing, and sneezing are complex motor acts that, once initiated, cannot be interrupted voluntarily. They depend on the coordinated activation of respiratory, pharyngeal, and laryngeal motor neurons as well as vagal preganglionic neurons. The central pattern generator for these complex motor acts consists of a network of interneurons in the lateral reticular formation of the medulla.

- Respiration is controlled by a neuronal network of neurons located in the pons, nucleus of the solitary tract, and ventrolateral medullary reticular formation.
- Swallowing, vomiting, and other complex motor acts involve a medullary network that coordinates activity of branchiomotor and respiratory motor neurons and vagal preganglionic neurons.

The sphincter motor neurons of *Onuf nucleus*, located at spinal levels S2 and S3, innervate the external sphincter and pelvic floor muscles. Their activity is coordinated, in an antagonistic manner, with that of the sacral preganglionic neurons that innervate the ganglia of the bladder and bowel. Unlike other motor neurons, the motor neurons of Onuf nucleus receive input not only from the classic motor pathways but also from the pontine micturition center, hypothalamus, and ventral respiratory group.

- The Onuf nucleus, located at spinal levels S2 and S3, innervates the external sphincter muscle.

Pain Modulatory Output

Many components of the internal regulation system are part of a network involved in modulation of the sensation of pain. This network includes the hypothalamus, periaqueductal gray matter, noradrenergic neurons in the dorsolateral pons, and neurons in the rostral ventromedial medulla, including serotonergic neurons of the *nucleus raphe magnus*. Different portions of the periaqueductal gray matter initiate different autonomic and pain-suppressing responses through projections to the noradrenergic and serotonergic groups that project to the dorsal horn of the spinal cord and decrease the relay of nociceptive input. In some conditions, descending projections from the ventromedial medulla may increase the responsiveness to pain. All these areas of the internal regulation system contain receptors for opioids and are the target of action of morphine and related drugs.

Autonomic Output of the Internal Regulation System

General Organization

Preganglionic Neurons

The preganglionic sympathetic or parasympathetic neurons occupy the general visceral efferent column of the brainstem and spinal cord. Like skeletal motor neurons, the preganglionic neurons are derived from the basal plate, use acetylcholine as their neurotransmitter, and elicit fast excitation of autonomic ganglion neurons through *nicotinic receptors.* The preganglionic axons are small myelinated fibers that exit the brainstem or spinal level to innervate the autonomic ganglia.

Autonomic Ganglia

The autonomic ganglia are derived from the neural crest and contain neurons that have norepinephrine or acetylcholine as their primary neurotransmitter. The unmyelinated axons (postganglionic fibers) of autonomic ganglion neurons travel in peripheral nerves or perivascular plexuses to innervate the target organ. Postganglionic axons contain varicosities that generally do not form direct synaptic contacts with the target organs. The complex networks of neurons and axons that innervate the heart, respiratory system, and gastrointestinal tract are called *visceral plexuses.* They consist of preganglionic parasympathetic efferents, postganglionic sympathetic efferents, primary visceral afferents, and clusters of peripheral sympathetic or parasympathetic ganglion cells.

- Preganglionic neurons use acetylcholine as the neurotransmitter and produce fast excitation of autonomic ganglion neurons through nicotinic receptors.
- Autonomic ganglion neurons are derived from the neural crest, have unmyelinated axons, and have acetylcholine or norepinephrine as the neurotransmitter.

Effects on Target Organs

Norepinephrine and acetylcholine act on different subtypes of G protein-coupled receptors to modulate the activity of the target organs, including the heart, smooth muscle of the pupil and viscera, and glandular epithelia. Unlike skeletal muscle, which requires fast excitatory input from motor neurons for excitation and contraction, many visceral effectors are automatically active.

> Cardiac and visceral smooth muscles, for example, exhibit the properties of automatism, adaptation, and intramural conduction. Automatism is the ability to sustain rhythmic contractions in the absence of innervation and is due to spontaneous depolarizations that tend to spread to other cells. Adaptation is the ability of smooth muscle to modify its rhythmicity and contractility in response to mechanical stimuli, such as stretch or distention of an organ. Intramural conduction involves transmission of electrical input between syncytial fibers through gap junctions (as in the heart and blood vessels) or through local intramural connections (as in the gut).

There is a fundamental difference in the response of skeletal muscles and visceral organs to loss of innervation. As described in Chapter 8, the loss of motor axons results in atrophy and development of spontaneous activity (fibrillations) in the denervated skeletal muscle. In contrast, in response of loss of innervation by postganglionic axons, the responsiveness of the visceral target organ to the neurotransmitter or agonist that stimulates its receptors increases. This phenomenon is called *denervation supersensitivity.* It reflects the increased number of G protein-coupled receptors in the membrane. Normally, a tonic continuous release of neurotransmitter from postganglionic terminals regulates the number of postsynaptic receptors in the target organs. Denervation supersensitivity is important for localization of lesions in the autonomic system because its presence indicates a postganglionic lesion that deprives the target organ of the tonic release of neurotransmitter.

- Denervation supersensitivity indicates a postganglionic lesion.

There are important differences in the anatomical organization, neurochemistry, and functions of the sympathetic and parasympathetic systems (Table 9.3).

Sympathetic Output

Preganglionic Neurons

Preganglionic sympathetic neurons are located in the intermediolateral cell column of spinal segments T1 to L3. They are organized into different preganglionic sympathetic functional units that control specific targets. They include muscle vasomotor, splanchnic vasomotor, skin vasoconstrictor, skin vasodilator, cardiomotor, sudomotor, and visceromotor preganglionic neurons (Fig. 9.16).

The activity of preganglionic sympathetic neurons depends on descending input from several sources, particularly the rostral ventrolateral medulla, medullary raphe, paraventricular nucleus, and lateral hypothalamus. These inputs project differentially to the various functional units of preganglionic sympathetic neurons. The supraspinal inputs have three main functions: 1) to provide tonic excitation of preganglionic sympathetic neurons, 2) to mediate the effects of descending influences and brainstem reflexes on sympathetic activity, and 3) to allow a functionally selective pattern of sympathetic output according to the stimulus and required response. Descending sympathetic pathways occupy a narrow band in the lateral column of the spinal cord.

- Preganglionic sympathetic neurons are located in the intermediolateral cell column of spinal levels T1-L3.
- Preganglionic sympathetic neurons form functionally distinct subunits that receive different supraspinal input and mediate different patterns of sympathetic responses.

Although preganglionic sympathetic neurons have a segmental organization, the distribution of the preganglionic fibers does not follow the dermatomal pattern of somatic nerves. Thus, preganglionic neurons in spinal segments T1 and T2 provide the input to the ganglia that innervate the target tissues of the head and neck;

Table 9.3. Main Anatomical and Functional Differences Between the Sympathetic and Parasympathetic Systems

System	Sympathetic	Parasympathetic
Preganglionic neuron	Intermediolateral cell column (spinal level T1-L3)	Cranial nerve nuclei Sacral spinal cord (S2-S4)
Ganglia	Paravertebral Prevertebral	Near end organ
Preganglionic neurotransmitter	Acetylcholine	Acetylcholine
Effect on ganglion neurons	Fast excitation via nicotinic receptors	Fast excitation via nicotinic receptors
Ganglion neuron neurotransmitter	Norepinephrine (acetylcholine for sweat gland)	Acetylcholine
Receptor in target organ	α- and β-Adrenergic (muscarinic in sweat glands)	Muscarinic
Main targets	Blood vessels and sweat glands of limbs and trunk Pupil All visceral organs	Pupil All visceral organs
Activity	Coordinated pattern of activation of multiple effectors	Isolated activation of individual effector
Main functions	Maintenance of arterial blood pressure Thermoregulation Responses to exercise and stress Pupil dilatation	Nutrient digestion and absorption Micturition Defecation Penile erection Pupil constriction

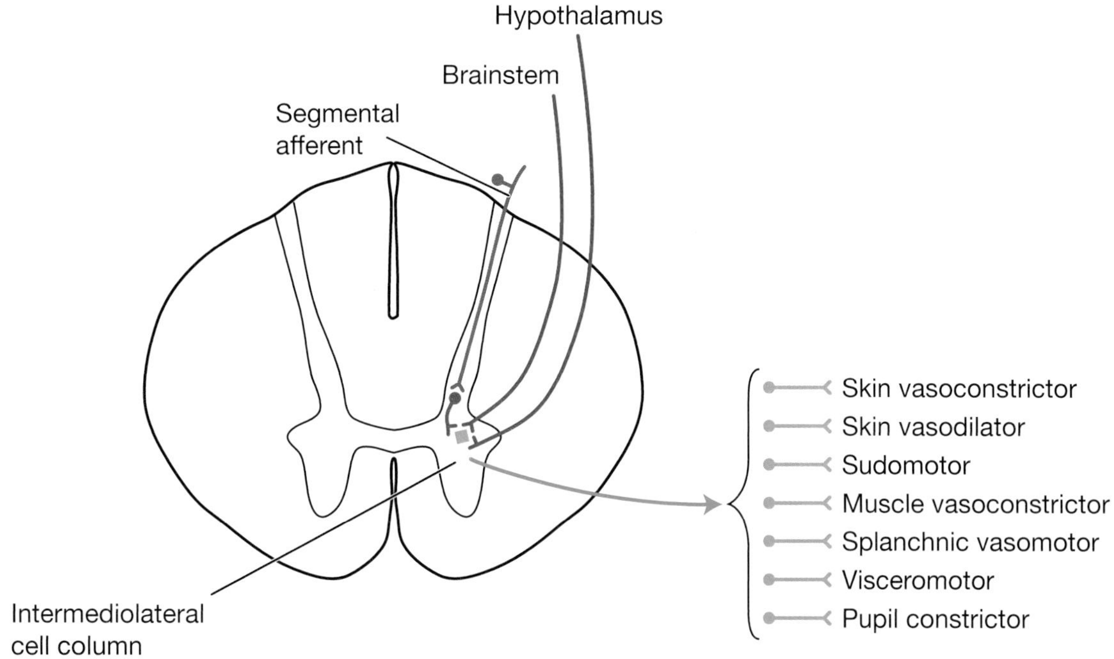

Fig. 9.16. Preganglionic sympathetic neurons are subdivided into units that control specific effectors and are recruited in a coordinated pattern by input from the hypothalamus and brainstem. Loss of this descending influence, as in spinal cord injury, results in massive sympathoexcitation in response to segmental input (e.g., from a distended bladder) called autonomic dysreflexia, which leads to severe hypertension.

T3 to T6, the upper extremities and thoracic viscera; T7 to T11, the abdominal viscera; and T12 to L3, the lower extremities and pelvic and perineal organs (Fig. 9.17, Table 9.4).

The preganglionic sympathetic axons exit through the ventral roots and join the *white rami communicantes* of the corresponding spinal nerve to reach the paravertebral sympathetic chain (Fig. 9.18).

At this level, preganglionic fibers 1) synapse on a postganglionic neuron in the *paravertebral ganglion* at the same level, 2) branch and go rostrally and caudally in the sympathetic chain to synapse on a large number of neurons in many paravertebral ganglia, 3) pass through the paravertebral chain without synapsing and form the *splanchnic nerves* that innervate *prevertebral ganglia*, or 4) pass through the chain as splanchnic nerves to innervate the *adrenal medulla*. The adrenal medulla is a homologue of a sympathetic ganglion, and its cells release epinephrine into the bloodstream.

Sympathetic Ganglia

The paravertebral (or sympathetic trunk) ganglia and prevertebral (or autonomic plexus) ganglia have several anatomical and functional differences. The paravertebral ganglia act primarily as a relay station for preganglionic input and provide long postganglionic axons to all sympathetically innervated tissues and organs except those in the abdomen, pelvis, and perineum (Fig. 9.17).

These fibers follow three main courses: perivascular, spinal, and visceral. Perivascular fibers course along arterial trunks and branches. For example, axons from the superior cervical ganglion (spinal segments T1 and T2) innervate the pupil, blood vessels and sweat glands of the face, salivary glands, cerebral blood vessels, and the pineal gland. Postganglionic axons from the superior cervical ganglion follow the course of branches of the internal and external carotid arteries. In contrast,

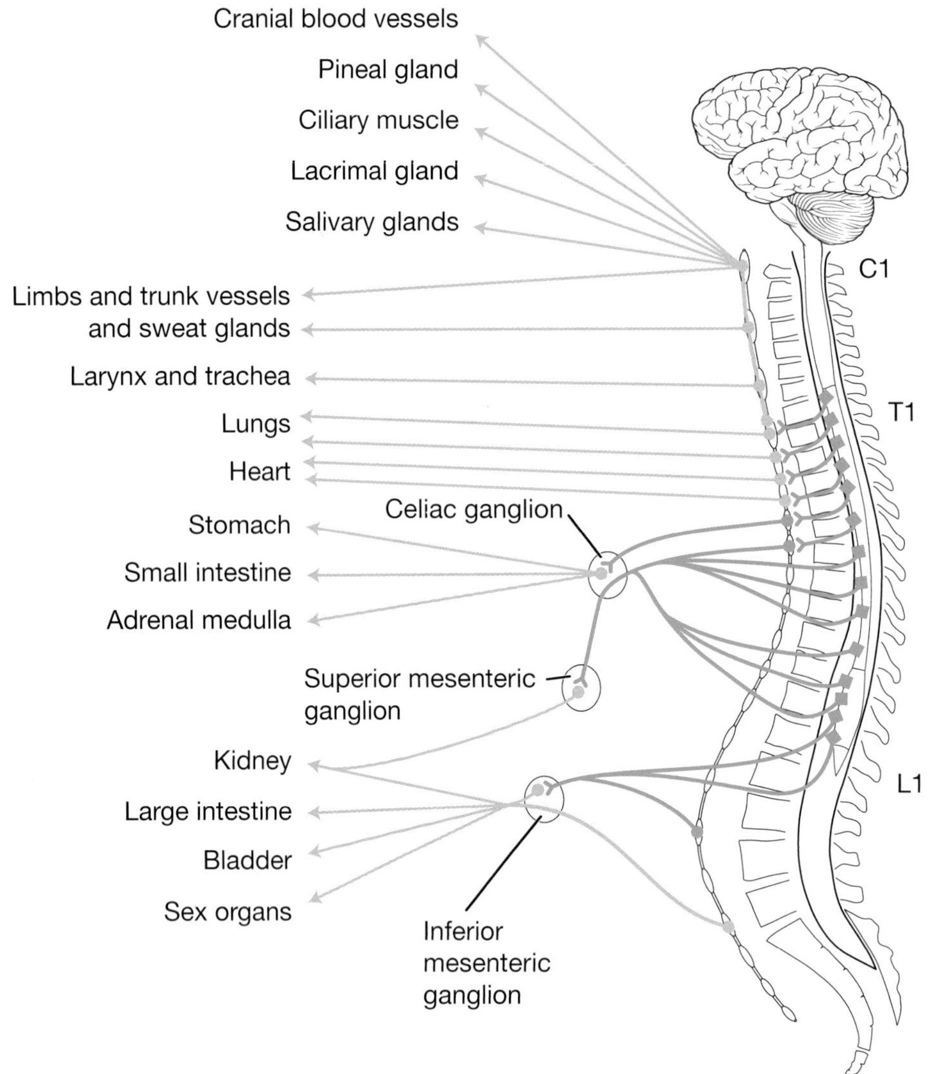

Fig. 9.17. General organization of the sympathetic outflow. The sympathetic system, via prevertebral ganglia, is the only innervation of muscle and skin blood vessels, sweat glands, and piloerector muscles in the limbs and trunk.

postganglionic axons innervating the blood vessels and sweat glands of the limbs and trunk join the peripheral nerves by way of the gray rami communicantes and follow the distribution of the corresponding somatic nerve. For example, axons from the stellate ganglion innervate the upper extremity through branches of the brachial plexus. Visceral fibers from the lower cervical and upper thoracic ganglia innervate the heart via the cardiac plexus to produce cardiac stimulation or reach the tracheobronchial tree via the pulmonary plexus to produce bronchodilatation.

The prevertebral ganglia are anterior to the abdominal aorta, close to the origin of the celiac and mesenteric arteries, and innervate all abdominal, pelvic, and perineal organs. Their preganglionic input travels in the splanchnic nerves (Fig. 9.17).

Table 9.4. Functional Organization of the Sympathetic Outflow

Spinal segment	Ganglion	Pathway	Organ	Effect
Paravertebral ganglion				
T1	Superior cervical	Perivascular (internal carotid)	Pupil	Dilatation (mydriasis)
T2	Superior cervical	Perivascular (external carotid)	Facial sweat glands	Sweating Vasoconstriction
T2 to T6	Stellate	Gray rami (brachial plexus)	Upper extremity	Vasoconstriction in skin Piloerection Sweating Vasodilatation in muscle
T9 to L1	Lumbosacral	Gray rami (lumbrosacral plexus) Perivascular	Lower extremity	
T2 to T8	Upper thoracic	Cardiac plexus Pulmonary plexus	Heart Tracheobronchial tree	Stimulation Bronchodilatation
Prevertebral ganglion				
T6 to T10	Celiac	Celiac plexus	Gastrointestinal tract	Inhibition of peristalsis and secretion
T11 to L1	Superior mesenteric	Celiac plexus	Gastrointestinal tract	
T12 to L1	Celiac	Celiac plexus	Kidney	Vasoconstriction Renin secretion
T10 to L1	Celiac	Celiac plexus	Adrenal gland	Epinephrine secretion
T12 to L3	Inferior mesenteric, hypogastric	Hypogastric plexus	Rectum Bladder Sex organs	Retention of feces Retention of urine Ejaculation

Preganglionic input from spinal segments T5 to L2 are carried in the splanchnic nerves to the celiac and superior mesenteric ganglia, which contribute postganglionic fibers to the celiac plexus that innervates all abdominal viscera except the descending colon. Preganglionic axons from spinal segments L1 to L3 travel in the lumbar splanchnic nerves, which synapse in the inferior mesenteric ganglion. This ganglion provides axons to the hypogastric plexus, which innervates the descending colon and pelvic and perineal organs (rectum, bladder, and genitalia).

Unlike the paravertebral ganglia, which serve primarily as a relay station, the prevertebral ganglia are a site of integration of input from preganglionic neurons with input from afferents with cell bodies in the dorsal root ganglia and sensory neurons of the enteric nervous system in the wall of the gut. Thus, the prevertebral ganglia can participate in peripheral reflexes that regulate the motility and secretion of the gut.

- Paravertebral ganglia innervate all target organs except those in the abdomen, pelvis, and perineum.
- The superior cervical ganglion innervates the pupil,

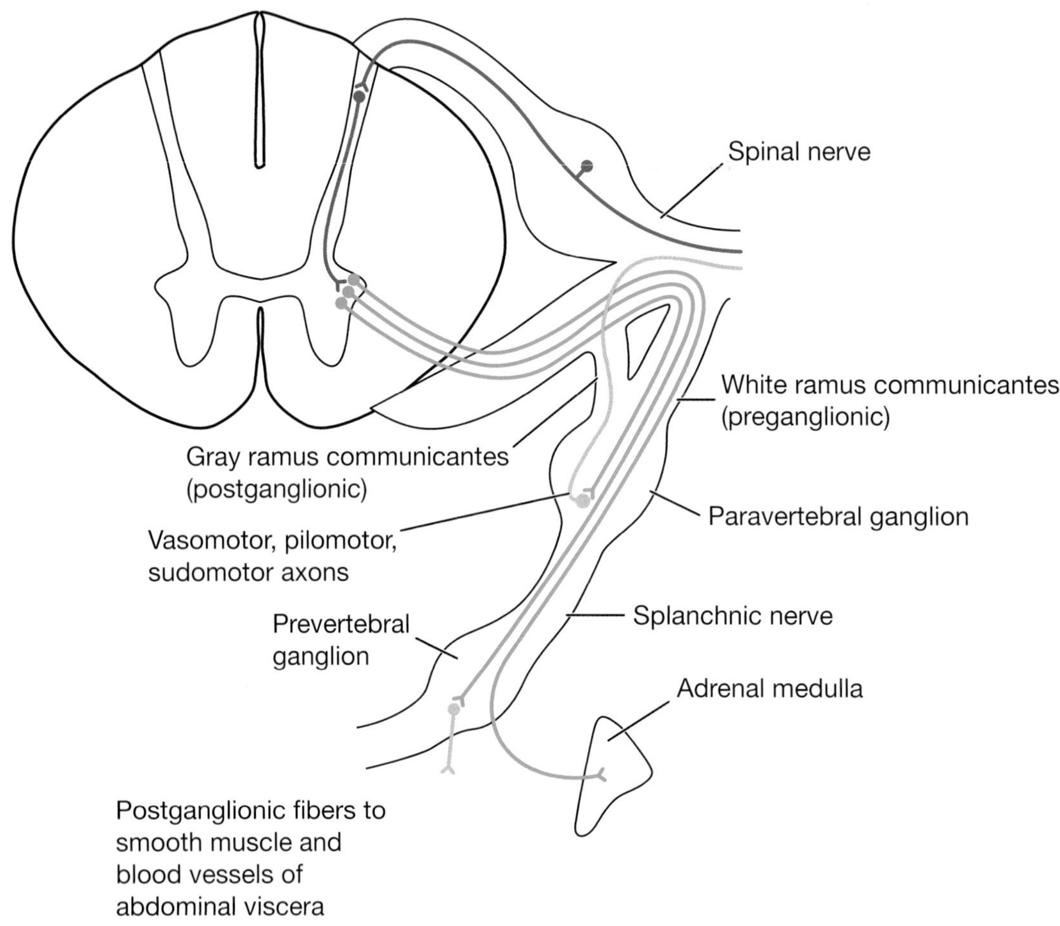

Fig. 9.18. Organization of the paravertebral and prevertebral sympathetic outflow.

blood vessels and sweat glands of the face, cerebral blood vessels, and the pineal gland.

- Axons from paravertebral ganglia join peripheral nerves to innervate the blood vessels and sweat glands of the limbs and trunk.
- Prevertebral ganglia receive input from splanchnic nerves and innervate the viscera and blood vessels of the abdomen and pelvis.

Sympathetic Neurotransmission

The primary neurotransmitter of sympathetic ganglion neurons is norepinephrine. The only exception is the sympathetic neurons that innervate the sweat glands; these neurons have acetylcholine as a neurotransmitter. The adrenal medulla secretes epinephrine into the general circulation. The synthesis, reuptake, and metabolism of norepinephrine are described in Chapter 6. The effects of norepinephrine and epinephrine are mediated by different subtypes of α (alpha)- and β (beta)-adrenergic receptors. α_1-Receptors mediate the sympathetically induced contraction of smooth muscle in blood vessels, pupillodilator muscles, vas deferens, and visceral sphincters. α_2-Receptors act mainly as inhibitory presynaptic autoreceptors, but they may also elicit smooth muscle contraction. β_1-Receptors mediate the sympathetic stimulation of cardiac automatism, conduction, excitability, and contractility. β_2-Receptors mediate the relaxation of the smooth muscle of the blood vessels, bronchi, gut, and bladder.

In addition to norepinephrine, postganglionic fibers innervating the vascular and visceral smooth muscle also release ATP and neuropeptide Y. ATP elicits rapid excitation of smooth muscle. Neuropeptide Y is a potent direct vasoconstrictor and modulates noradrenergic transmission by inhibiting the presynaptic release and potentiating the postsynaptic effects of norepinephrine.

- Norepinephrine acts on α_1-receptors and elicits vasoconstriction, pupillodilatation, and contraction of the internal anal and rectal sphincters and vas deferens.
- Norepinephrine stimulates the heart through β_1-receptors and relaxes vascular and visceral smooth muscle by acting on β_2-receptors.
- The sympathetic stimulation of sweat glands is mediated by acetylcholine acting on muscarinic receptors.

Functional Significance of the Sympathetic System

The sympathetic system initiates coordinated responses that are necessary for maintenance of blood pressure, thermoregulation, and integrated cardiovascular and metabolic responses to exercise, stress, and emotion. Sympathetically elicited vasoconstriction of skeletal muscle and splanchnic arteries and veins is critical for maintenance of arterial blood pressure on assuming the standing posture by preventing pooling of blood in the lower parts of the body. The output of the sympathetic system to the heart is important in increasing heart rate and cardiac output during exercise or other forms of stress. Under these conditions, the sympathetic system increases, through β-receptors, glycogenolysis and lipolysis, thus providing nutrients to the exercising muscle. Sympathetic output to the skin is important in thermoregulation. In response to cold, sympathetic activity elicits skin vasoconstriction and piloerection through α_1-receptors. In response to heat, the sympathetic system increases sweat production and skin vasodilatation. The activation of sweat glands is mediated by acetylcholine acting on muscarinic receptors. The mechanism of sympathetically mediated vasodilatation is still incompletely understood, but it involves inhibition of vasoconstrictor neurons and local release of the potent vasodilator nitric oxide (NO). In humans, skin sympathetic activity is activated by cold and emotional stimuli.

Through its action on β_2-receptors, the sympathetic system also elicits bronchodilation and inhibits motility of the gut and bladder. Through α_1-receptors, it elicits dilatation of the pupil (mydriasis), contraction of the smooth muscle of the internal sphincters of the bladder and rectum, and contraction of the vas deferens. Thus, through the combined effects of β_2- and α_1-receptors, the sympathetic system favors storage and prevents evacuation of the bladder and bowel.

- Sympathetically induced vasoconstriction of skeletal muscle and splanchnic vessels is critical for maintenance of arterial blood pressure upon standing.
- The sympathetic system elicits coordinated responses to exercise and stress.
- Sympathetic cholinergic stimulation of the sweat glands is critical for response to heat, and adrenergic vasoconstriction of the skin is critical for response to cold.

Parasympathetic Output

General Organization

The parasympathetic outputs arise from preganglionic neurons in the general visceral efferent column of the brainstem, the *cranial parasympathetic* output, and in the sacral spinal cord, the *sacral parasympathetic* output (Fig. 9.19, Table 9.5). Like the sympathetic preganglionic neurons, preganglionic parasympathetic neurons have acetylcholine as their neurotransmitter and activate the parasympathetic ganglia through nicotinic receptors. In the parasympathetic system, the myelinated preganglionic axons travel a long distance before reaching the effector target ganglia, which are typically located close to the target organs. This allows local parasympathetic control of specific visceral functions, unlike the generation of patterns of activity in different organs as with the sympathetic system.

Functions of the Cranial Parasympathetic Outflow

The brainstem preganglionic parasympathetic neurons are located in general visceral efferent nuclei; the preganglionic axons travel in cranial nerves III (oculomotor nerve), VII (facial nerve), IX (glossopharyngeal nerve), and X (vagus nerve). Cranial nerves III, VII, and IX provide parasympathetic input to structures of the face and head. These structures receive their sympathetic input from the superior cervical ganglia. The origin, trajectory, and functions of cranial nerves III, VII, IX, and X are discussed in Chapter 15. The *Edinger-Westphal nucleus* is part of the oculomotor complex in the midbrain. Its preganglionic axons occupy the peripheral portion of the oculomotor nerve and synapse on neurons of the *ciliary ganglion* in the orbit. These neurons innervate the pupillary constrictor muscle, producing *miosis*, and the ciliary muscle, producing accommodation of the lens.

Preganglionic axons from the *superior salivatory nucleus*, located in the pons, travel in the facial nerve to innervate the *sphenopalatine ganglion*, which provides input to the lacrimal gland (eliciting lacrimation) and the cranial and cerebral blood vessels (eliciting vasodilatation), and to the *submaxillary* and *submandibular* ganglia that stimulate the corresponding salivary glands. Preganglionic axons from the *inferior salivatory nucleus*, located in the medulla, travel in the glossopharyngeal nerve and synapse in the otic ganglion, which activates the parotid gland.

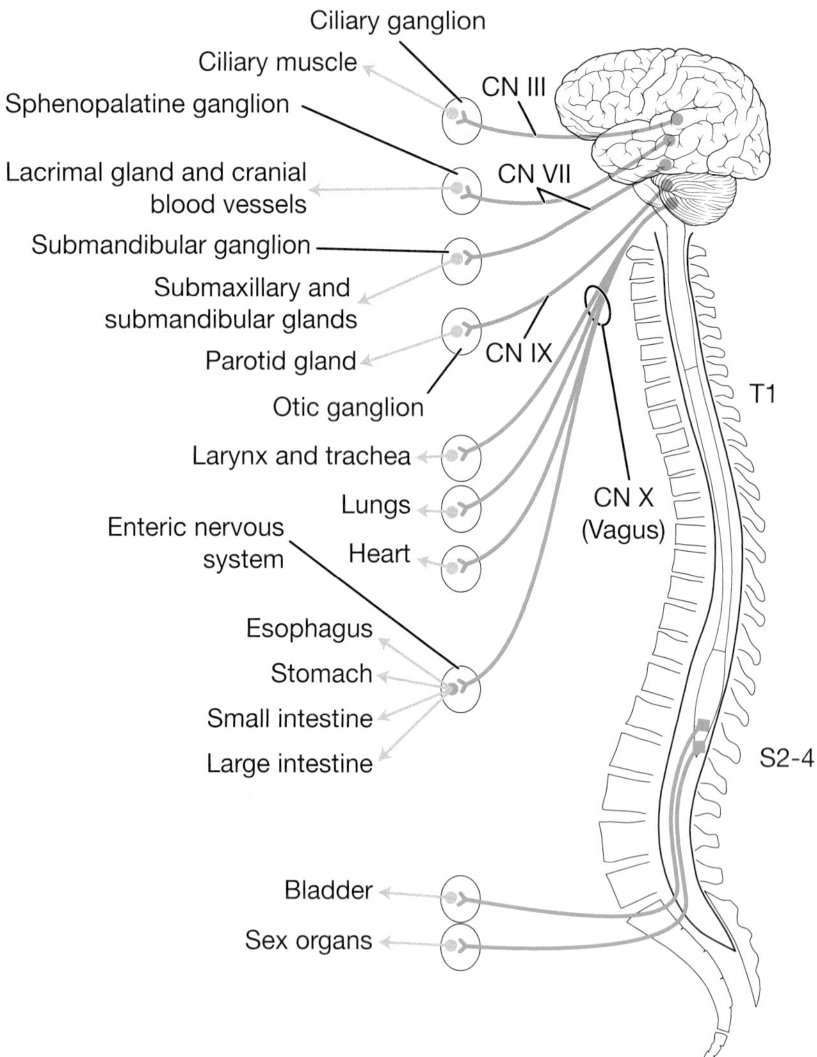

Fig. 9.19. General organization of the parasympathetic outflow.

Table 9.5. Functional Organization of the Parasympathetic Outflow

	Nucleus	Nerve	Ganglion	Effect
Cranial division				
Midbrain	Edinger-Westphal	CN III	Ciliary	Pupilloconstriction Accomodation
Pons	Superior salivatory	CN VII	Sphenopalatine Submandibular	Lacrimation Salivation (submaxillary and sublingual glands)
Medulla	Inferior salivatory Dorsal nucleus of the vagus	CN IX CN X	Otic Near end organs	Salivation (parotid gland) Bronchoconstriction Bronchosecretory Gastrointestinal peristalsis and secretion
	Ambiguus	CN X	Near end organs	Decreases heart rate and conduction
Sacral division				
Segments S2 to S4	Intermediolateral cell column	Pelvic Splanchnic	Near end organs	Emptying of bladder and rectum Erection

CN, cranial nerve.

- The Edinger-Westphal nucleus, through its axons in the oculomotor nerve, activates ciliary ganglion neurons that elicit pupillary constriction and accomodation of the lens.
- The superior salivatory nucleus, through its axons in the facial nerve, elicits lacrimation, cerebral vasodilatation, and salivation.
- The inferior salivatory nucleus, through its axons in the glossopharyngeal nerve, triggers salivation.

The most widespread preganglionic parasympathetic output from the brainstem is through the *vagus nerve*, arising in the medulla. It innervates the heart, the respiratory tract, and all the gastrointestinal tract down to the level of the descending colon. Most vagal preganglionic neurons are located in the *dorsal nucleus of the vagus*. A subpopulation of neurons in the *nucleus ambiguus* provides most of the preganglionic innervation to the heart (Fig. 9.20). As discussed in Chapter 15, most of the neurons in this nucleus innervate the striate muscles of the pharynx, larynx, and esophagus.

The vagus nerve innervates the parasympathetic ganglia located in or near the target organs. Its main effects are cardioinhibitory, visceromotor, and secretomotor. The parasympathetic innervation of the heart inhibits the automatism of the sinoatrial node and conduction in the atrioventricular node, producing bradycardia. Vagal input to the sinoatrial node provides beat-to-beat control of the heart rate. Vagal output also elicits constriction of the bronchial smooth muscle and stimulates bronchial gland secretion. In the gastrointestinal tract, the vagus nerve has complex effects. It innervates neuronal plexuses of the enteric nervous system and stimulates esophageal motility, gastric relaxation (to receive a meal) and evacuation, coordinated peristalsis along the gut, and secretion of electrolytes and digestive enzymes from the stomach, intestine, pancreas, and liver.

Despite the importance of the preganglionic parasympathetic component of the vagus nerve, most axons in this nerve are afferents from visceral organs, including the heart, large blood vessels, lungs, and abdominal organs. These afferents, with cell bodies in the *nodose ganglion*, synapse in the nucleus of the solitary tract (Fig. 9.20).

- The vagus nerve exerts a cardioinhibitory effect, elicits bradycardia and bronchial constriction and secretion, and facilitates gastrointestinal motility and secretion.

Sacral Parasympathetic Outflow

The sacral preganglionic output arises from neurons in the *sacral preganglionic nucleus*, located in the lateral gray matter of spinal segments S2 to S4 (Fig. 9.21). Their axons pass through the ventral roots to the *pelvic splanchnic nerves*, which join the inferior hypogastric plexus to innervate the colon, bladder, and sexual organs. Parasympathetic fibers to the bladder elicit contraction of the bladder detrusor muscle, and those to the rectum elicit contraction of the circular smooth muscle. The sacral preganglionic neurons are involved in reciprocal inhibitory interactions, through interneurons, with somatic motor neurons of Onuf nucleus that innervate the external urethral and rectal sphincters and pelvic floor muscles through the pudendal nerve. The sacral parasympathetic output also elicits vasodilatation of the cavernous tissue of the penis required for penile erection. This is coordinated with sympathetically mediated ejaculation.

- The sacral parasympathetic system is critical for defecation, micturition, and erection.
- There is coordinated reciprocal inhibitory interaction between sacral preganglionic neurons, which facilitate contraction of the bladder and rectum, and motor neurons in Onuf nucleus, which elicit contraction of the external sphincters.

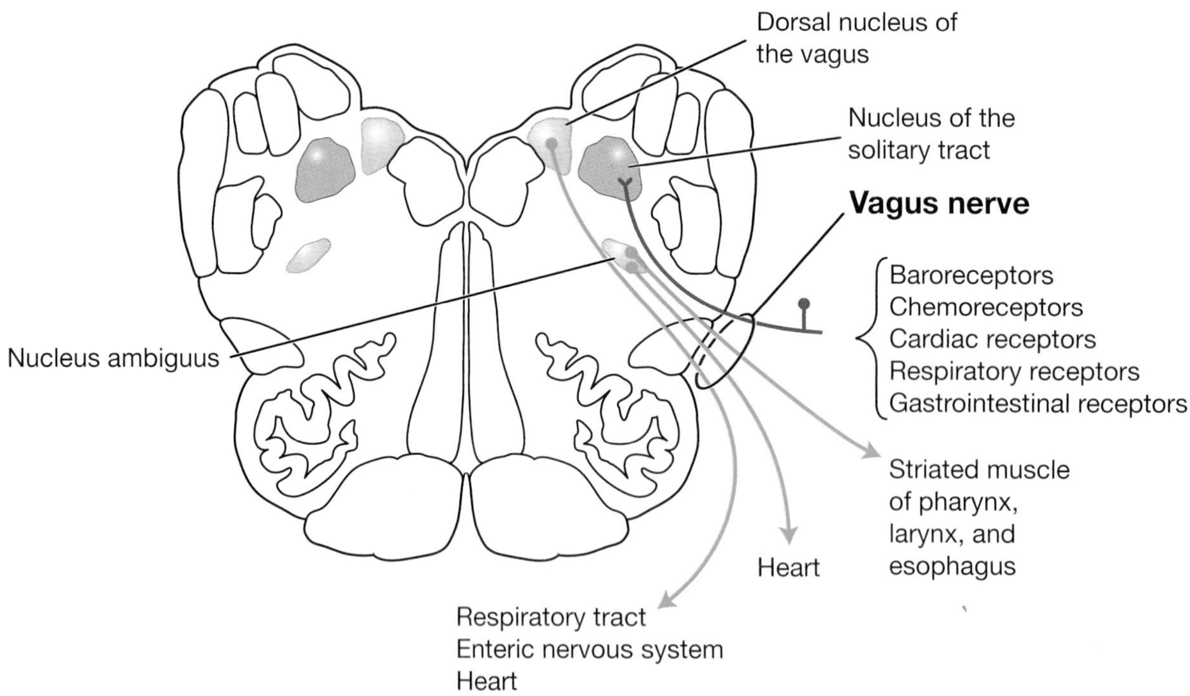

Fig. 9.20. Components of the vagus nerve. Most fibers of the vagus nerve are afferents that terminate in the nucleus of the solitary tract. The dorsal nucleus of the vagus contains preganglionic neurons whose axons enter the vagus nerve and project to the respiratory and gastrointestinal tracts. The nucleus ambiguus contains preganglionic neurons innervating the heart and branchiomotor neurons innervating muscles of the larynx and pharynx.

Parasympathetic Neurotransmission

The primary postganglionic parasympathetic neurotransmitter is acetylcholine, which acts on different subtypes of *muscarinic receptors*.

> The different effects of acetylcholine in various target organs are mediated by various subtypes of muscarinic receptors. Cardiac inhibition is mediated by M_2 receptors, whereas activation of visceral smooth muscle and exocrine glands is mediated by M_1 and M_3 receptors. Acetylcholine is hydrolyzed rapidly by acetylcholinesterase. Drugs that inhibit this enzyme indirectly potentiate the parasympathetic effects on target organs and the sympathetic effects on sweat glands. These effects are also elicited by drugs that directly activate muscarinic receptors. In contrast, drugs such as atropine, which block muscarinic receptors, elicit the opposite effects.

Some parasympathetic effects are mediated by other chemical transmitters such as vasoactive intestinal polypeptide and NO, which coexist with acetylcholine in some postganglionic parasympathetic sympathetic neurons. For example, NO is important in mediating the relaxation of the cavernous tissue required for penile erection.

- Acetylcholine, acting on muscarinic receptors, is the primary neurotransmitter of the parasympathetic postganglionic neurons.
- Parasympathetically triggered smooth muscle relaxation may be mediated by NO.

Interactions Between the Sympathetic and Parasympathetic Systems

Most visceral organs have a dual sympathetic and parasympathetic control. However, peripheral blood vessels, pilomotor muscles, and sweat glands receive only sympathetic innervation. Parasympathetic control predominates in the salivary glands, sinoatrial node, and gastrointestinal tract. The interactions between the sympathetic and parasympathetic systems may be antagonistic, as in the case of the pupil or sinoatrial node, or functionally complementary, as in the case of parasympathetically mediated erection and sympathetically

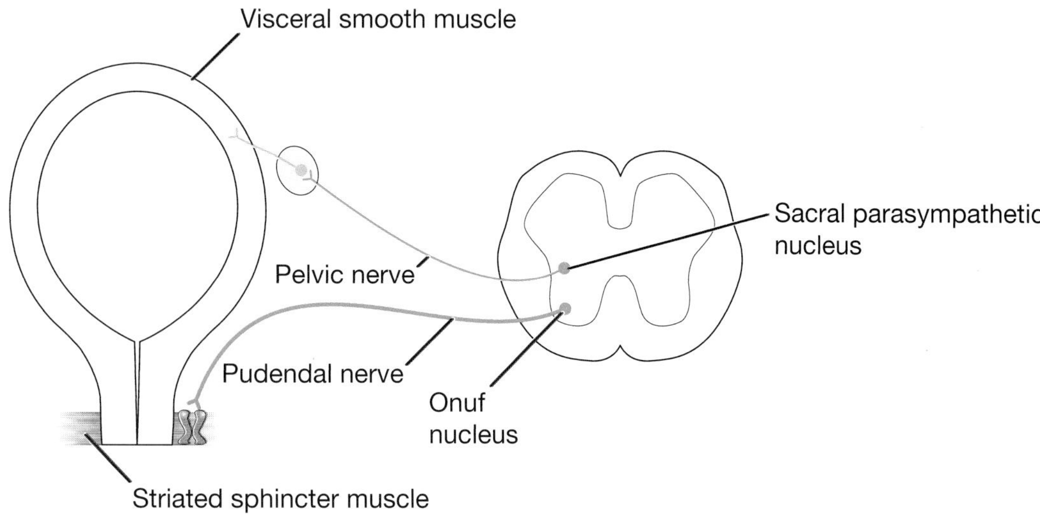

Fig. 9.21. Organization of the sacral parasympathetic outflow. Preganglionic neurons in the sacral parasympathetic nucleus (S2–S4) innervate ganglion neurons controlling the bladder, rectum, and sexual organs. They activate bladder and rectal evacuation and penile erection. Sacral parasympathetic neurons are involved in inhibitory interactions, through interneurons, with somatic motor neurons in Onuf nucleus, which innervate the striated muscles of the external sphincters and pelvic floor.

mediated ejaculation. The interactions between the sympathetic and parasympathetic systems may occur at the level of the neuroeffector junction or target organ. The effects of the sympathetic system and the neurochemical mechanisms are summarized in Figure 9.22 and Table 9.6.

Clinical Correlations

Diseases involving the internal regulation system may produce 1) generalized autonomic failure, 2) isolated disorders affecting a particular autonomic effector, 3) level-specific syndromes, and 4) syndromes of autonomic hyperactivity. The clinical manifestations of sympathetic or parasympathetic failure or hyperactivity are summarized in Table 9.7.

Generalized Autonomic Failure

Diffuse disorders involving preganglionic neurons, postganglionic neurons, or both, produce generalized autonomic failure affecting the outflow of both the sympathetic and the parasympathetic systems. The most important clinical manifestations of sympathetic failure are a decrease in arterial pressure upon standing, called *orthostatic hypotension*, and inability to sweat, called *anhidrosis*. Patients with orthostatic hypotension complain of lightheadedness, blurred vision, other symptoms of cerebral hypoperfusion, or neck and shoulder pain shortly after assumming an upright posture and have to sit down to avoid fainting. These symptoms are worse in the morning, after meals, or after exposure to heat. Anhidrosis produces intolerance to heat and the sensation

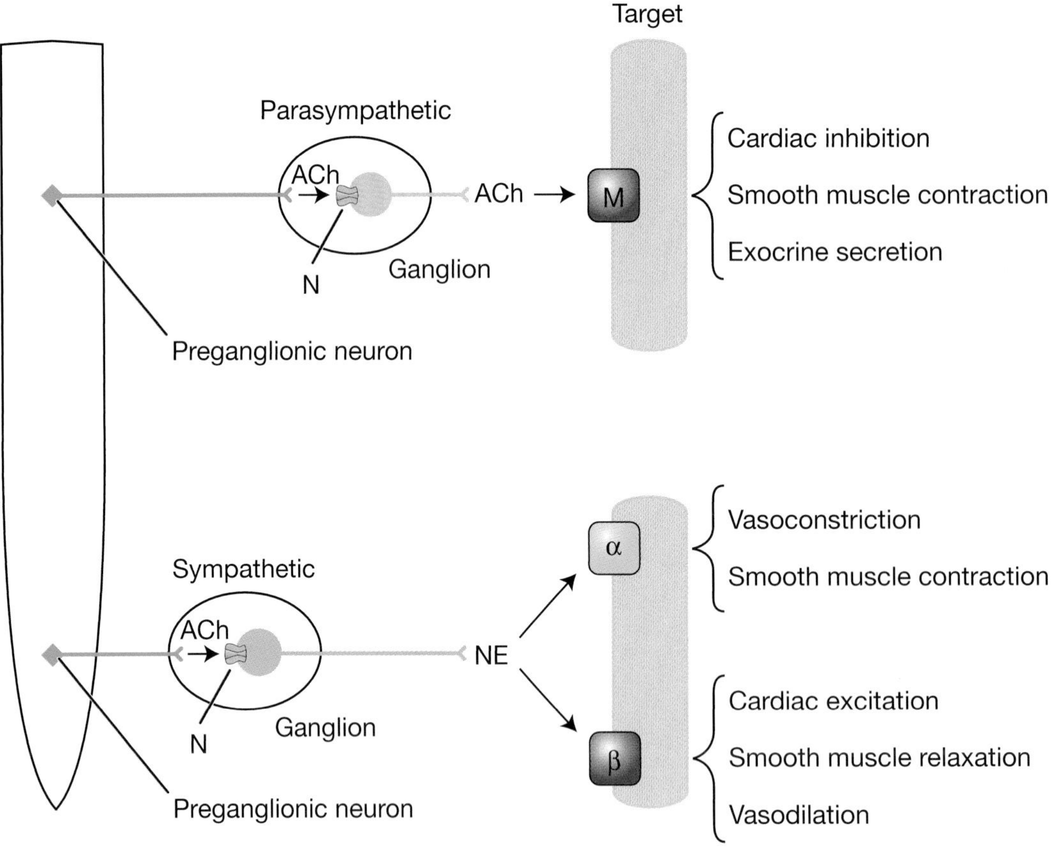

Fig. 9.22. Overview of the primary autonomic neurotransmitters and their receptors and effects on the target organ. α, α-receptor; ACh, acetylcholine; β, β-receptor; M, muscarinic receptor; N, nicotinic receptor; NE, norepinephrine. Acetylcholine is the neurotransmitter of sympathetic fibers innervating sweat glands.

Table 9.6. Peripheral Autonomic Effects

	Sympathetic		Parasympathetic
	α-Receptor	β-Receptor	Muscarinic receptor
Heart			
Heart rate		Increases	Decreases
Atrioventricular conduction		Increases	Decreases
Contractility		Increases	Antagonizes
Smooth muscle			
Pupil	Dilatation		Constriction
Lens			Accommodation
Bronchial		Dilatation	Constriction
Gastrointestinal			
Motility		Decreases	Increases
Sphincter			Decreases[a]
Bladder			
Detrusor		Relaxation	Contraction
Sphincter	Constriction		Relaxation[a]
Sex organs	Ejaculation		Erection[a]
Blood vessels			
Arteries	Constriction (skin, gut, kidney)	Dilatation (muscle, heart)	Dilatation[a] (gut, genital)
Veins	Constriction		
Pilomotor	Contraction		
Glands			
Salivary/lacrimal	Inhibits		Stimulates
Bronchial	Inhibits		Stimulates
Gastrointestinal	Inhibits		Stimulates
Sweat	Stimulates[b]		
Metabolism		Glycogenolysis Lipolysis Renin secretion	Insulin secretion

[a]Mediated by nitric oxide or vasoactive intestinal polypeptide or both.
[b]Postganglionic sympathetic fibers that innervate sweat glands are cholinergic axons, and they act on muscarinic receptors.

of flushing. The most important consequences of parasympathetic failure are impaired gastric emptying (producing early satiety, nausea, or vomiting), constipation, urinary retention, and erectile dysfunction.

- The main manifestations of generalized autonomic failure are orthostatic hypotension, anhidrosis, constipation, urinary retention, and erectile dysfunction.

The most common causes of generalized autonomic failure are degenerative, such as *multiple system atrophy* (a disorder also producing parkinsonism or ataxia or both); peripheral neuropathies that affect sympathetic

Table 9.7. Manifestations of Autonomic Failure and Autonomic Hyperactivity

Division and effector	Failure	Hyperactivity
Sympathetic		
Pupil	Horner syndrome	Mydriasis
Heart	Bradycardia	Tachycardia
Blood vessels	Orthostatic hypotension[a]	Hypertension
Sweat glands	Anhidrosis[a]	Hyperhidrosis
Gastrointestinal	Diarrhea	--
Bladder	--	--
Sexual	Impaired ejaculation	--
Parasympathetic		
Pupil	Mydriasis	Miosis
Heart	Tachycardia	Bradycardia
Lacrimal gland	Dry eyes (xerophthalmia)	Tearing
Salivary gland	Dry mouth (xerostomia)	Sialorrhea
Gastrointestinal	Impaired gastric emptying	
	Constipation[a]	Diarrhea
Bladder	Urinary retention[a]	Urinary urgency
Sexual	Erectile failure[a]	--

[a]The most prominent manifestations of generalized autonomic failure.

and parasympathetic outputs, most commonly due to *diabetes mellitus*; and effects of drugs or toxins that block adrenergic or muscarinic receptors.

Effects of Drugs or Toxins in the Autonomic Nervous System
Many drugs and toxins, including several medications, may affect sympathetic or parasympathetic neurotransmission and produce manifestations of sympathetic or parasympathetic failure or hyperactivity.

1. Drugs That Affect Adrenergic Transmission
Sympathetic effects, except on sweat glands, are mediated by norepinephrine acting on α- or β-adrenergic receptors. Norepinephrine is stored in synaptic vesicles. After release, its synaptic effects are terminated by presynaptic reuptake by a norepinephrine transporter. After reuptake, norepinephrine is either incorporated again into a synaptic vesicle or metabolized by monoamine oxidase. Many drugs or toxins may affect each of these processes and increase the level of norepinephrine in the synaptic space. Therefore, intoxication with any of these drugs may result in exaggerated activation of sympathetic noradrenergic effectors, which is manifested primarily by mydriasis, tachycardia, and hypertension (as well as anxiety, tremor, or even seizures due to central effects).

For example, stimulating drugs such as cocaine and amphetamine inhibit the presynaptic reuptake of norepinephrine. Amphetamine also competes with norepinephrine for vesicular storage, causing release of norepinephrine. Some drugs used for treatment of depression also inhibit norepinephrine reuptake. Monoamine oxidase inhibitors, also used to treat depression, impair norepinephrine metabolism.

Many therapeutic drugs act by stimulating or blocking α- or β-adrenergic receptors. For example, drugs that

Clinical Problem 9.1.

A 52-year-old man was referred for evaluation because of blackouts. The spells began a year before admission and were becoming more frequent. They occurred only when he arose from a supine or sitting position to a standing posture and were most severe in the morning. This change in position precipitated a giddy feeling in his head and dimness of vision and often was followed by complete loss of consciousness. No convulsive movements were observed, and shortly after hitting the floor, he regained consciousness, only to pass out again if he got up too quickly. In addition to this primary symptom, the patient complained that during the last 3 years, he became gradually unable to obtain a penile erection and had constipation. He felt very uncomfortable in hot weather and did not perspire as he had before. He feels that he cannot empty his bladder completely. On examination, his blood pressure was 130/70 mm Hg when he was supine, decreased to 110/50 mm Hg when he sat, and fell to 70/30 mm Hg when he stood; at this time, he began to complain of faintness. His pulse rate was 82 to 90 beats per minute during the entire episode. The skin was warm and dry and remained so after many minutes in a hot examining room. Results of the rest of the physical examination were normal.

a. What is the name of the syndrome?
b. What are possible causes?
c. Which of the patient's symptoms reflects a disorder of sympathetic outflow and which of parasympathetic outflow?
d. How can the affected system be evaluated clinically and by laboratory testing?

After the patient applied a nasal spray containing pseudoephedrine (a drug that stimulates α_1-receptors), he had a severe increase in arterial pressure.

e. How can this abnormal reaction be interpreted in the setting of this disorder?
f. How does it help to localize the lesion?

stimulate α_1-adrenergic receptors are used for the treatment of hypotension and those that stimulate β_2-adrenergic receptors are used to produce bronchodilation during asthma attacks. In contrast, drugs that block α- or β-adrenergic receptors are used for the treatment of hypertension. Therefore, for any patient who has manifestations of sympathetic failure, the use of these medications should be considered a possible cause.

2. Drugs that Affect Cholinergic Transmission

Several drugs and toxins affect the release or degradation of acetylcholine. By affecting synaptic levels of acetylcholine, these drugs alter the level of activation not only of visceral muscarinic receptors but also of nicotinic receptors in the skeletal muscle or sympathetic ganglia.

For example, botulinum toxin reduces the release of acetylcholine and thus impairs not only its muscarinic actions on visceral organs but also its nicotinic effects on the skeletal muscle, causing severe muscle weakness. In contrast, acetylcholinesterase inhibitors, such as those used for treatment of myasthenia gravis or as a warfare chemical weapon, increase synaptic levels of acetylcholine, leading to increased activation of both muscarinic and nicotinic receptors.

Several drugs or toxins stimulate or block muscarinic receptors. The effects of drugs that stimulate muscarinic receptors mimic the effect of acetylcholinesterase inhibitors on visceral effectors. They include miosis, increased lacrimation, salivation, bronchial secretion, sweating, bradycardia, bronchoconstriction, diarrhea, and urinary urgency. In contrast, drugs that block muscarinic receptors mimic the effects of toxins that block acetylcholine release. Manifestations of cholinergic muscarinic failure include mydriasis, tachycardia, dry mouth, dry eyes, anhidrosis, constipation, and urinary retention.

Control of Specific Effectors

There are several examples of integration of activity within the internal regulation system at the supratentorial, posterior fossa, spinal, and peripheral levels. Some

Clinical Problem 9.2.

An elderly retired oil tycoon was brought to the emergency department complaining of severe cramping abdominal pain, vomiting, diarrhea, and shortness of breath. He was able to relate that he became ill about half an hour after ingesting a hearty meal served to him by his young bride of only a month. The meal consisted of steak smothered in mushrooms, mashed potatoes, and home-canned green beans. His spouse had complained of not feeling well before dinner and had not eaten at all. Physical examination showed marked tearing. The pupils were pinpoint in size. The patient was salivating profusely. Pulse rate was 50 beats per minute. Examination of the chest disclosed diffuse rales in inspiration and wheezing in expiration. Markedly active bowel sounds were heard on auscultation of the abdomen, and the examination was frequently interrupted by the patient's urgent need for a bedpan.

a. What is the mechanism of these symptoms?
b. What are the type and location of the disorder?
c. If these symptoms occurred in a soldier engaged in warfare, what cause would you suspect?
d. What type of drug would you use to treat these symptoms?

examples of these are discussed below because of their clinical significance in neurology.

Control of the Pupil

The diameter of the pupil is controlled by the balanced activity of two sets of muscles. The pupilloconstrictor muscle is a circular band of muscle fibers innervated by the parasympathetic system. The pupillodilator muscle is a radial band of muscle fibers innervated by the sympathetic system. Pupillary constriction is called *miosis*, and pupillary dilatation is *mydriasis*. The size of the pupil is a function of the relative activity of parasympathetic and sympathetic influences (Fig. 9.23).

Parasympathetic Pathway and Reflexes

The parasympathetic pathway for pupillary constriction is a two-neuron system. Preganglionic axons from the Edinger-Westphal nucleus of the midbrain travel in the oculomotor nerve and synapse in the ciliary ganglion in the orbit. Postganglionic neurons innervate the pupil constrictor and ciliary muscle through the short ciliary nerves. By acting on muscarinic cholinergic receptors, this pathway elicits miosis and increased curvature of the lens.

The pathway for pupillary constriction is activated by stimulation with either light (light reflex) or near vision (accommodation). The pathway for the *light reflex* is discussed in Chapter 16. Briefly, it involves afferents in the optic pathway, a synapse in the pretectal area of the midbrain, excitatory input from this area to the Edinger-Westphal nucleus, and efferent axons to the constrictor muscle by way of the oculomotor nerve and ciliary ganglion (Fig. 9.24). Decussation of the pathway at the level of the pretectal and Edinger-Westphal nuclei allows stimulation of either eye to produce both an ipsilateral, or *direct*, response and a contralateral, or *consensual*, response. The *accommodation reflex* is activated by inputs from the visual cortex to a subnucleus of the oculomotor complex that coordinates the response to near vision. This includes convergence of the eyes, miosis, and increased curvature of the lens.

Clinical Problem 9.3.

A 72-year-old man with a history of depression, insomnia, diabetes mellitus, and hypertension is treated with a drug to improve his mood and sleep disorder. Within 24 hours after taking the medication, he became confused and agitated. Physical examination showed mydriasis, tachycardia, dry mouth, anhidrosis, and urinary retention.

a. What is the most likely cause of these symptoms?
b. How can you distinguish them from those produced by anxiety?
c. How do you explain the patient's confusional state?

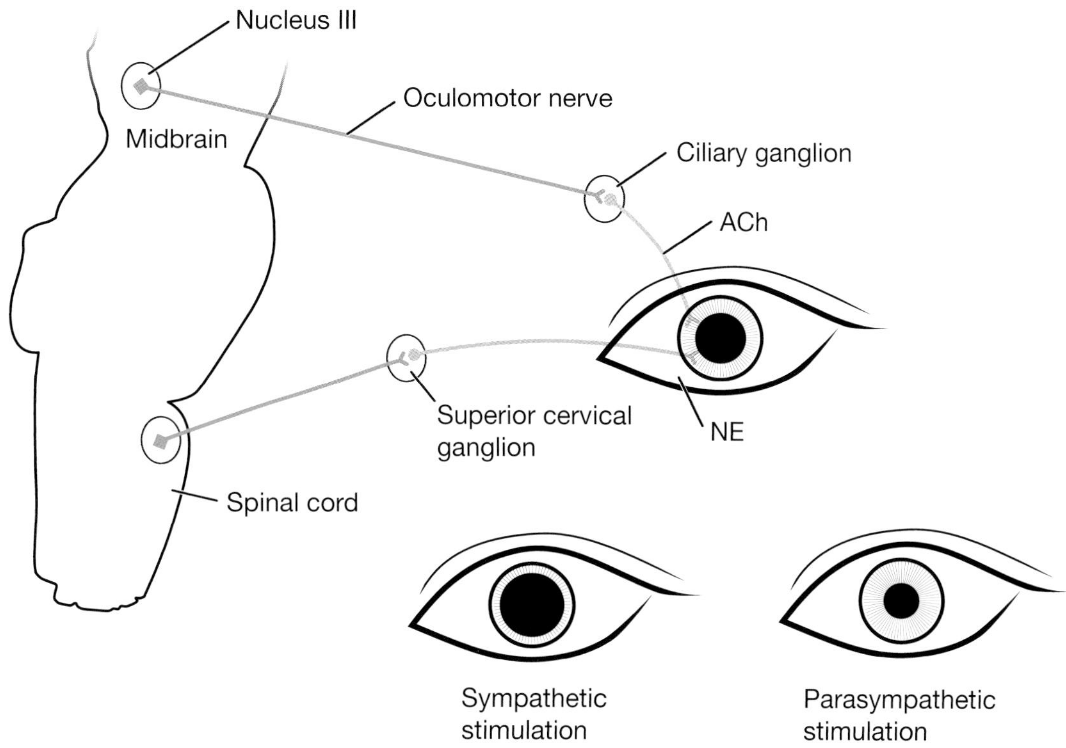

Fig. 9.23. Origin, pathways, and effects of autonomic neurotransmission on pupil size. ACh, acetylcholine; NE, norepinephrine.

Reflexes eliciting parasympathetically mediated miosis have localizing value. For example, lesions of the optic nerve (afferent pathway) of one eye impair both the direct (ipsilateral) and consensual (contralateral) light reflex, whereas lesions affecting the oculomotor nerve (efferent pathway) to one eye abolish the direct (ipsilateral) but not the consensual (contralateral) pupillary constrictor response on exposure of the affected eye to light. Lesions affecting the ciliary ganglion produce a large pupil (because of unopposed sympathetic influence) that does not respond to light. In the presence of this postganglionic lesion, the administration of a dilute solution of muscarinic agonist (such as pilocarpine) elicits a potent pupillary constriction at a dose that is ineffective in affecting a normal eye.

Sympathetic Pathway and Reflexes

The sympathetic pathway for pupillary dilatation is a three-neuron system (Fig. 9.25). The first neuron is located in the hypothalamus. Its axon descends in the dorsolateral portion of the brainstem to innervate the second neuron, which is a preganglionic sympathetic neuron in the intermediolateral cell column at spinal levels T1 and T2, referred to as the *ciliospinal center*. Preganglionic axons enter the sympathetic chain and ascend in the sympathetic trunk to synapse on the third (or postganglionic) neuron, which is in the superior cervical ganglion. Postganglionic fibers follow the course of the internal carotid artery and ophthalmic artery and then join the long ciliary nerves to innervate the dilator muscle. They produce mydriasis through α_1-adrenergic mechanisms.

The pathway for pupillary dilatation is activated by stress, including pain. The *ciliospinal reflex* consists of pupillary dilatation evoked by noxious cutaneous stimulation, such as pinching the face or trunk.

Clinical Correlations

A *unilateral large pupil* commonly results from hypoactivity of the ipsilateral parasympathetic outflow (Table 9.8).

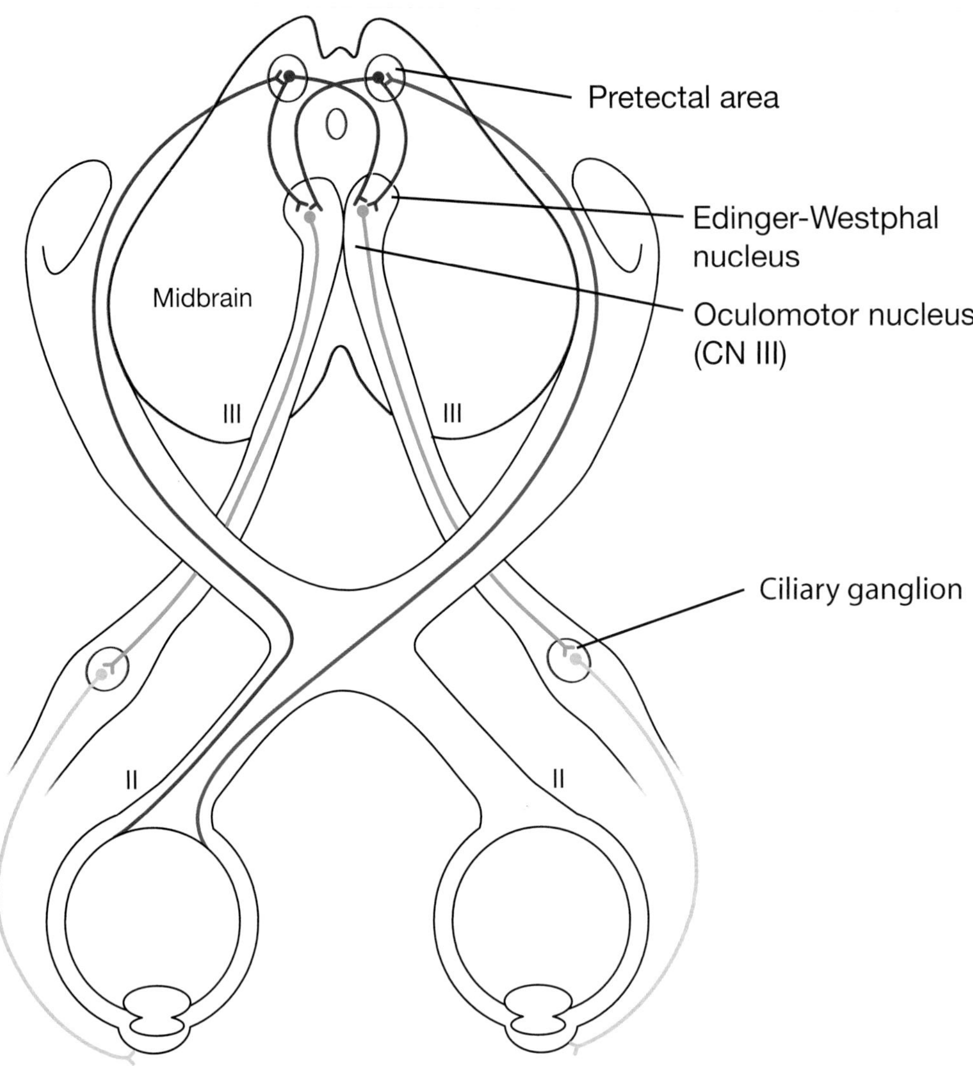

Fig. 9.24. Pathway of the light reflex involves afferents in the optic pathway (II), a synapse in the pretectal area of the midbrain, excitatory projection from this area to the Edinger-Westphal nucleus, efferent axons in the oculomotor nerve (III) to the ciliary ganglion, and postganglionic fibers to the constrictor muscle of the pupil. Decussation of the pathway at the level of the pretectal nuclei allows stimulation of either eye to produce both an ipsilateral, or direct, response and a contralateral, or consensual, response. (Modified from Adams AC. Neurology in primary care. Philadelphia: F. A. Davis Company; 2000. Used with permission of Mayo Foundation for Medical Education and Research.)

The lesion may occur at the level of the preganglionic neuron (oculomotor nerve), postganglionic neuron (ciliary ganglion), or muscarinic receptor (pharmacologic blockade) on the same side. Because of the superficial location of the pupilloconstrictor pathway on the oculomotor nerve, this pathway is commonly affected by compressive lesions, such as an aneurysm or uncal herniation. Stimulation of the affected eye fails to produce pupillary constriction in that eye, but because of the preservation of the optic nerve afferent and crossing of the light reflex pathway, pupillary constriction is preserved on the contralateral side. Lesions affecting the ciliary ganglion produce denervation supersensitivity of the pupillary constrictor muscle. In this situation, the topical application

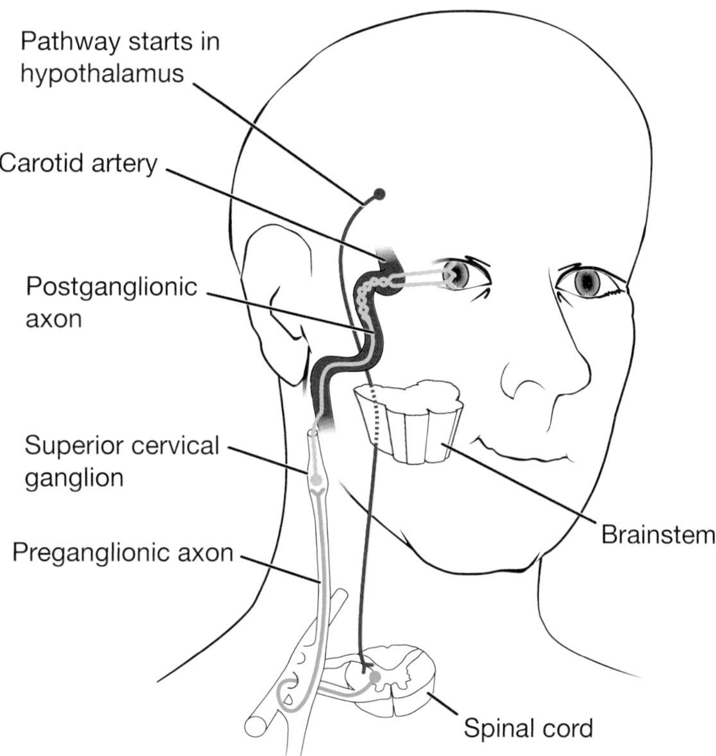

Fig. 9.25. The sympathetic pathway for pupillary dilatation is a three-neuron system. The first neuron is located in the hypothalamus; its axon decends through the dorsolateral portion of the brainstem to innervate the second neuron, which is a preganglionic sympathetic neuron in the intermediolateral cell column at spinal levels T1 and T2. Preganglionic axons enter the sympathetic chain and ascend in the sympathetic trunk to synapse on the third neuron, which is in the superior cervical ganglion. Postganglionic fibers follow the course of the internal carotid and ophthalmic arteries to innervate the dilator muscle. (Modified from Adams AC. Neurology in primary care. Philadelphia: F. A. Davis Company; 2000. Used with permission of Mayo Foundation for Medical Education and Research.)

Table 9.8. Large Dilated Pupil

	Preganglionic	Postganglionic	Pharmacologic blockade
Cause	Lesion of oculomotor nerve	Lesion of ciliary ganglion	Muscarinic blockade
Direct light reflex	No	No	No
Consensual reflex	No	No	No
Contralateral eye reflexes	Yes	Yes	Yes
Response to muscarinic agonists (pilocarpine)			
Low dose	No	Yes	No
High dose	Yes	Yes	No

of a dilute solution of pilocarpine (a drug that stimulates muscarinic receptors) produces a powerful pupillary constrictor response, but it is ineffective when applied to the normally innervated eye. This helps to differentiate a peripheral lesion from a central lesion affecting the pupilloconstrictor pathway. In contrast, the lack of a pupillary constrictor response to topical application of high doses of pilocarpine suggests blockade of muscarinic receptors.

- A unilateral, dilated, unreactive pupil indicates that a lesion is affecting the ipsilateral oculomotor nerve or ciliary ganglion.
- With oculomotor nerve lesions, a dilated and unreactive pupil is associated with ptosis and ocular motor paralysis.
- Ciliary ganglion lesions produce an exaggerated response to the topical application of pilocarpine (denervation supersensitivity).

A *unilateral small pupil* is commonly due to impaired activity of the ipsilateral sympathetic outflow. Miosis is commonly associated with ptosis (lid droop due to sympathetic denervation of the tarsal muscle) and facial anhidrosis. This combination is known as *Horner syndrome* (Table 9.9). Oculosympathetic paralysis can be caused by 1) central lesions that interrupt the hypothalamospinal pupillodilator pathway, 2) lesions that affect the preganglionic neuron (second neuron) of the pathway, and 3) lesions that affect the superior cervical ganglion (third neuron) or its projections to the eye. An important example of a lesion that interrupts the connection between the hypothalamus and preganglionic neuron is a focal lesion in the lateral part of the brainstem or upper cervical cord. Preganglionic axons can be affected by lesions that compress the sympathetic chain, for example, a tumor in the apex of the lung. The postganglionic fibers from the superior cervical ganglion can be compressed by a carotid dissection or a mass lesion in the cavernous sinus.

The localization of the lesion depends on associated neurologic findings and neuroimaging studies. The distinction between preganglionic and postganglionic lesions that cause Horner syndrome can also be made by pharmacologic testing of the pupil (Table 9.9). Application of a drug that stimulates the release of norepinephrine from the sympathetic terminals (e.g., dextroamphetamine) causes dilatation of the affected pupil in patients with preganglionic lesions (and with postganglionic axons intact) but not in patients with postganglionic lesions. Topical application of a dilute solution of a drug that stimulates α_1-receptors in the pupillary dilator muscle causes an exaggerated dilator response in the affected pupil in patients with postganglionic lesions (reflecting denervation hypersensitivity) but fail to elicit a response in the normal pupil.

Table 9.9. Horner Syndrome

Feature	Central or preganglionic	Postganglionic
Facial sweating	Abnormal	Normal (except above eyebrow)
Response to drugs releasing norepinephrine (methamphetamine)	Yes	No
Response to direct α-agonist (e.g., norepinephrine)	Normal	Exaggerated (denervation supersensitivity)
Localization of lesion	Hypothalamus Dorsolateral medulla Spinal cord	Superior cervical ganglion Cavernous sinus

Clinical Problem 9.4.

A 37-year-old man who had had a thyroid carcinoma completely resected had a 2-month history of progressive left shoulder pain and weakness of the hand. Neurologic examination showed drooping of the left eyelid, left pupil smaller than the right (both reacted normally to light), and dry skin on the left side of his face. There were weakness and atrophy of the thenar and hypothenar muscles and a left Babinski sign.

a. What is the location of the lesion?
b. What is the type of lesion?
c. What structures are most likely involved?
d. Does the lesion involve sympathetic or parasympathetic fibers?
e. List the structures where these pathways could be damaged to produce a similar syndrome.
f. What do you expect to be the effect on the affected pupil of topical application of a drug that causes the release of norepinephrine from nerve terminals in this patient?

In another patient with a similar syndrome, this drug has no effect.

g. What does this indicate?
h. What would you expect to occur with the topical application of a dilute α_1-adrenergic agonist in this patient?

- A unilateral small pupil associated with mild ptosis (Horner syndrome) indicates a lesion affecting the ipsilateral sympathetic pathway at the level of the hypothalamus, dorsolateral brainstem, cervical cord at or above T1, sympathetic chain or superior cervical ganglion (commonly, a neoplasm), or internal carotid artery (arterial dissection or cavernous sinus lesion).
- In a patient with Horner syndrome, the lack of a pupillary dilatation response to a topically applied drug that causes the release of norepinephrine and an exaggerated response to a drug that activates α_1-adrenergic receptors (denervation supersensitivity) indicates a postganglionic lesion (distal to the superior cervical ganglion).

Control of the Bladder

The control of the bladder is integrated at peripheral, spinal, posterior fossa, and supratentorial levels.

Peripheral Innervation

The bladder is controlled by input from sacral parasympathetic, lumbar sympathetic, and sacral somatic axons (Fig. 9.26). The sacral parasympathetic fibers are from preganglionic neurons at spinal cord segments S2 to S4. The axons of these neurons join the pelvic nerve and innervate ganglia located close to the bladder wall. Sacral parasympathetic fibers, acting on cholinergic muscarinic receptors, stimulate the contraction of the bladder detrusor muscle, promoting emptying of the bladder (*micturition*).

The lumbar sympathetic fibers, from spinal cord segments T11 to L3, are part of the hypogastric nerves. These fibers produce both relaxation of the detrusor muscle (via β-adrenergic receptors) and contraction of the bladder neck (via α_1-adrenergic receptors). These actions favor the storage of urine. The sacral somatic motor axons are from motor neurons in Onuf nucleus (spinal cord segments S2 and S3), which project through the pudendal nerves to innervate the external urethral sphincter and pelvic floor. These axons, through cholinergic nicotinic receptors, stimulate the contraction of the external sphincter (Table 9.10).

Storage and Micturition Reflexes

The storage of urine and micturition are two opposite functional states of the bladder. At low levels of bladder filling, low-frequency firing of bladder afferents initiates reflexes that promote urine storage. When bladder filling reaches a threshold volume (approximately 300 mL), high-frequency firing of bladder afferents triggers the *micturition reflex*.

During storage, the sacral parasympathetic neurons are inhibited and the lumbar sympathetic neurons and sacral motor neurons are activated, which leads to relaxation of the bladder detrusor muscle and contraction of the

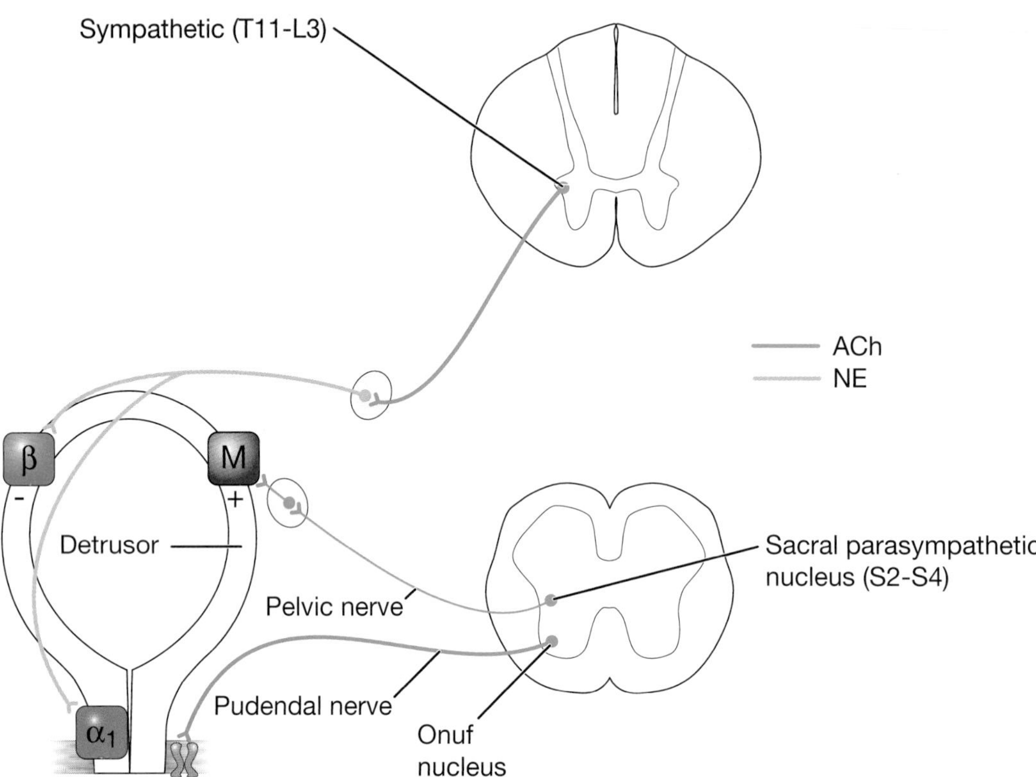

Fig. 9.26. Peripheral innervation of the bladder. ACh, acetylcholine; α_1, α-adrenergic receptor; β, β-adrenergic receptor; M, muscarinic receptor; NE, norepinephrine.

bladder neck and external sphincter muscles. In contrast, during micturition, the parasympathetic neurons are activated, which stimulates contraction of the bladder detrusor muscles. The sympathetic neurons and somatic motor neurons are inhibited; thus, the bladder neck and external sphincter muscles are relaxed. These coordinated patterns of response depend on reflexes initiated by afferents from the bladder that signal bladder distention.

The normal micturition reflex, which involves a supraspinal pathway, is coordinated by the *pontine micturition center* located in dorsal pons (Fig. 9.27). This center is activated, through the periaqueductal gray matter, by high-frequency bladder afferent discharges. Through projections to the sacral spinal cord, the pontine micturition center promotes the coordinated activation of the sacral parasympathetic neurons innervating the bladder detrusor muscle and inhibition of the motor neurons in Onuf nucleus innervating the external sphincter muscle. The pontine micturition center sends excitatory projections to the sacral parasympathetic nucleus and inhibits, through synapses on local interneurons, Onuf nucleus. This produces the coordinated contraction of the bladder detrusor muscle and relaxation of the external sphincter muscle, allowing complete emptying of the bladder.

Although the sacral spinal cord contains the neuronal circuitry for generating reflex contractions of the bladder detrusor and external sphincter muscles in response to afferent input from the bladder, this segmental reflex is poorly coordinated because the bladder detrusor and external sphincter muscles may contract at the same time. Normally, this sacral micturition reflex is inhibited by the pontine micturition center.

- Normally, the micturition reflex involves a supraspinal pathway and is coordinated by the pontine micturition center in dorsal pons.

Table 9.10. Innervation of the Bladder

Division	Spinal level	Nerve	Neurotransmitter	Receptor	Mechanism	Effect
Parasympathetic	S2 to S4	Pelvic	Acetylcholine	Muscarinic	Contraction of detrusor	Bladder emptying
					Relaxation of sphincter	Bladder emptying
Sympathetic	T11 to L3	Hypogastric	Norepinephrine	β-Adrenergic	Relaxation of detrusor	Retention of urine
				α-Adrenergic	Contraction of bladder neck	Retention of urine
Somatic	S2 to S4	Pudendal	Acetylcholine	Nicotinic	Contraction of external sphincter	Retention of urine

Voluntary Control of Micturition

Under normal conditions, the activity of the pontine micturition center, and thus the micturition reflex, may be transiently inhibited by input from the medial frontal lobe, possibly through a relay in the medial hypothalamus and periaqueductal gray matter. This frontal lobe input is the basis for voluntary control of micturition.

Control of Sexual Organs

The hypothalamus, receiving input from the cerebral cortex and circulating sex hormones (estrogens and testosterone), has a critical role in the regulation of sexual and reproductive behavior. The autonomic output is essential for penile erection and ejaculation in men and for control of the engorgement of the clitoris and vaginal lubrication in women. Sacral parasympathetic output is necessary for reflex penile erection; these effects are mediated primarily by NO. Lumbar sympathetic output, mediated by α_1-adrenergic receptors, is necessary for contraction of the vas deferens, which is required for ejaculation, and may also contribute to emotionally triggered erection in patients with spinal cord injury. However, excessive sympathetic input elicits vasoconstriction of erectile tissue, preventing penile erection.

- The sacral parasympathetic output, mediated by NO, is critical for penile erection.

Clinical Correlations

Disturbances at different levels of the system for bladder control result in the development of a *neurogenic bladder* (Fig. 9.28). The three major manifestations of neurogenic bladder are urinary incontinence, urgency, and urinary retention. The management of these disorders requires a careful history and examination, determination of residual volume, and urodynamic studies (Table 9.11).

Lesions that affect the inhibitory connections between the medial aspect of the frontal lobes and the pontine micturition center produce an *uninhibited bladder*. These patients complain of urinary urgency and incontinence, which is socially embarrassing. However, because the connections between the pontine micturition center and spinal cord are intact, the reflex arc is preserved, bladder size is normal, and there is no urinary retention. The anal reflex, which indicates the integrity of the sacral spinal cord and cauda equina, is also preserved. An uninhibited bladder is common in the elderly but is also a manifestation of dementia, hydrocephalus, and Parkinson disease.

A *spastic bladder* occurs with lesions that interrupt the connections between the pontine micturition center and the sacral spinal cord. The symptoms include urinary frequency and incontinence. In this disorder, the sacral micturition reflex is preserved, but because of the lack of pontine control, the contractions of the bladder detrusor and external sphincter muscles are not coordinated. This *detrusor-sphincter dyssynergia* increases the intravesical pressure during micturition (because the action of the bladder detrusor muscle is opposed by that of the external sphincter muscle). This leads to hypertrophy of the bladder wall and reduction of bladder volume and compliance. Eventually, urinary retention occurs, and this together with increased intravesical pressure predisposes to hydronephrosis, urinary tract infection, and renal failure. Spastic bladder occurs with midline or bilateral lesions of the cervical or thoracic spinal cord, for example, traumatic injury or multiple sclerosis. Neurologic examination of these patients commonly documents upper motor neuron and sensory findings. However, the anal reflex is intact because the sacral spinal cord is preserved.

A *flaccid bladder* occurs with midline or bilateral lesions of the segmental reflex arc at the level of the spinal

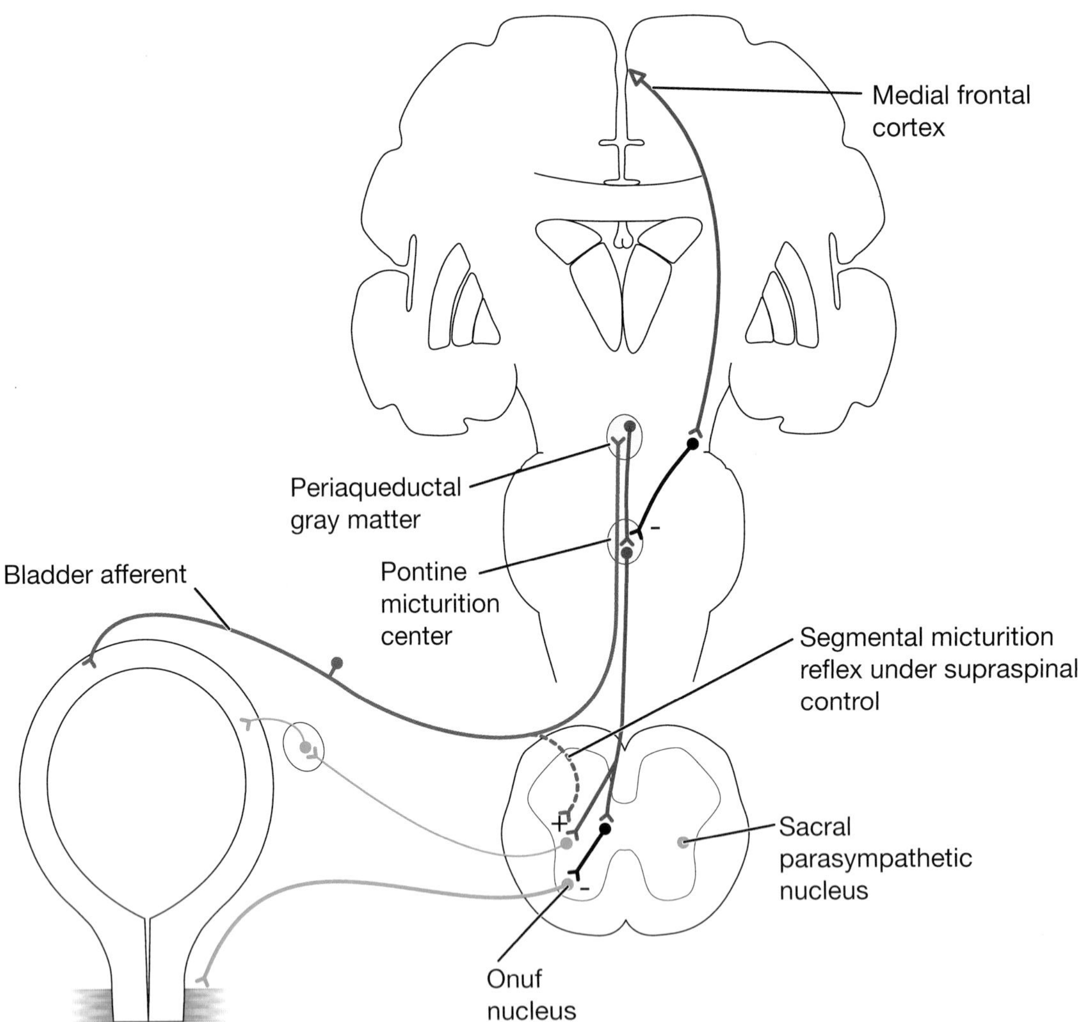

Fig. 9.27. The normal micturition reflex involves a supraspinal pathway. The reflex is coordinated by the pontine micturition center. This region, activated by input from the bladder, contains neurons that stimulate sacral preganglionic neurons and inhibit a lateral pontine region that activates neurons in Onuf nucleus. Thus, activation of the pontine micturition center leads to the coordinated contraction of the bladder detrusor muscle and relaxation of the external urethral sphincter muscle required for normal micturition. The excitability of the pontine micturition center is controlled by inhibitory input from the medial frontal lobe, which is the basis for voluntary control of micturition.

cord or its afferents or efferents in the cauda equina. With the lack of the micturition reflex, the bladder becomes distended with urine and hypotonic. Because of concomitant weakness of the external sphincter muscle, the bladder empties partially (*overflow incontinence*) but only infrequently. The patient has urinary retention, typically with a postvoid residual volume larger than 100 mL. Involvement of the caudal equina and sacral cord is manifested by perianal anesthesia and the absence of the anal reflex.

- Uninhibited bladder occurs with lesions of the medial frontal lobe.
- Spastic bladder occurs with cervical or thoracic spinal cord lesions and is manifested as detrusor-sphincter dyssynergia.
- Flaccid bladder usually occurs with midline lesions of the conus medullaris or cauda equina and is characterized by urinary retention from onset, overflow incontinence, and absence of the anal reflex.

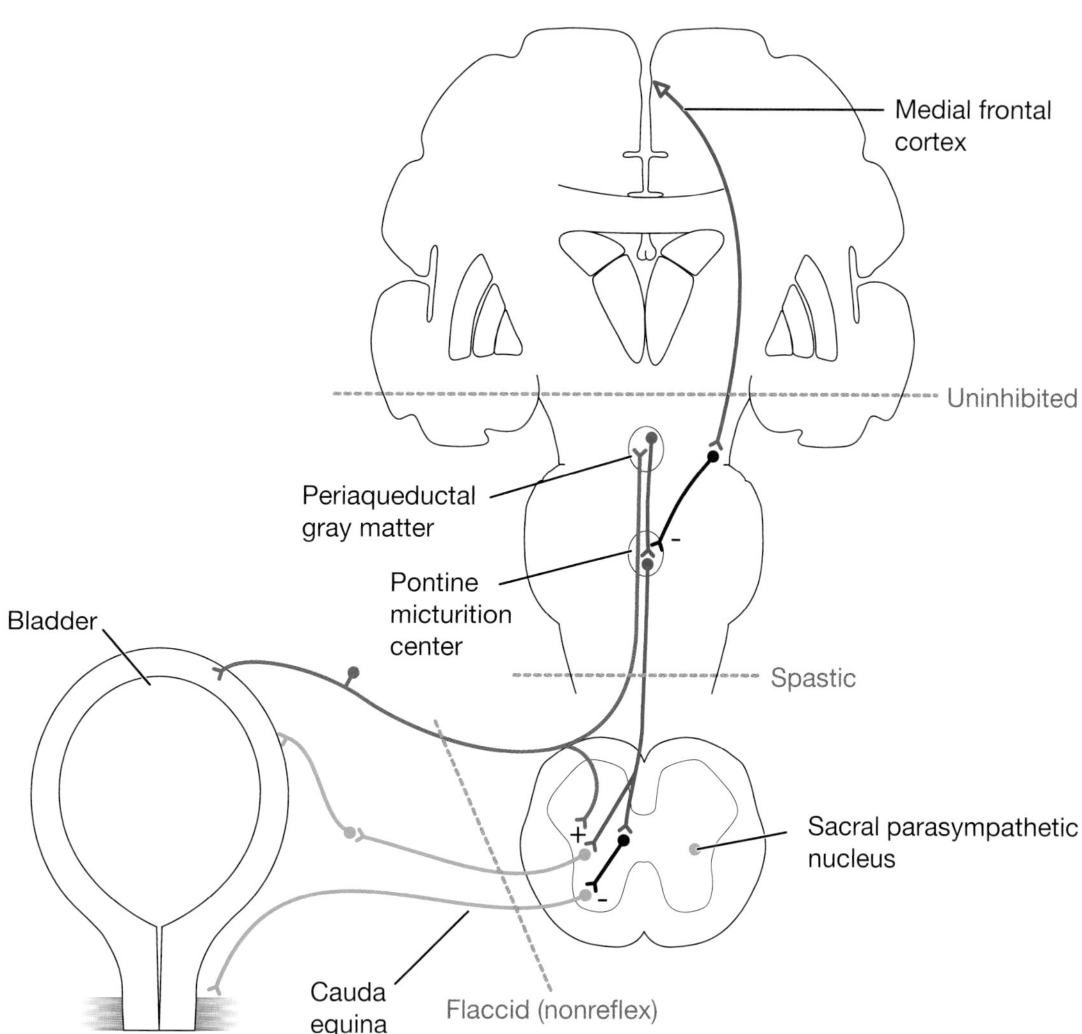

Fig. 9.28. Sites of lesions producing neurogenic bladder. Lesions affecting the frontal lobes or basal ganglia produce an uninhibited bladder. Lesions between the pontine micturition center and the sacral cord (in general, cervical and thoracic cord lesions) produce a spastic bladder. Lesions of the conus medullaris or cauda equina produce a flaccid bladder.

Table 9.11. Neurogenic Bladder

Feature	Uninhibited	Spastic	Flaccid
Incontinence	Yes	Yes	Yes
Retention	No	No or late (detrusor-sphincter dyssynergia)	Yes
Perianal sensation	Yes	Yes or decreased	No
Anal and bulbocavernous reflexes	Yes	Yes	No
Bladder volume	Normal	Decreased	Increased
Intravesical pressure	Normal	Increased	Decreased
Localization of lesion	Medial frontal lobes	Lower brainstem or spinal cord above level of conus medullaris	Conus medullaris or cauda equina
Example	Hydrocephalus Meningioma	Trauma Multiple sclerosis	Neoplasm Extruded disk Diabetes mellitus Motor radiculopathy

Cardiovascular Reflexes

The medulla is the site of reflex mechanisms critical for controlling circulation and respiration. These medullary reflexes are triggered by different types of receptors, including baroreceptors in the carotid sinus or aortic arch that respond to changes in arterial pressure; cardiac receptors in the atria, ventricles, or coronary arteries; chemoreceptors in the carotid bodies; and receptors in the airways. The axons from these receptors are in branches of the vagus or glossopharyngeal nerve that terminate in different portions of the nucleus of the solitary tract. Neurons in this nucleus control the sympathetic outflow to the heart and blood vessels by direct and indirect projections to rostral ventrolateral medulla and activate vagal output to the heart by connections with the dorsal vagal nucleus and nucleus ambiguus. The nucleus of the solitary tract also initiates respiratory reflexes through connections with the ventral respiratory group.

Clinical Problem 9.5.

A 51-year-old tree trimmer gradually experienced difficulty with urination during a 6- to 9-month period. He felt less urge to urinate, had difficulty in starting urination, and voided only small amounts. Recently, incontinence and a urinary tract infection have developed. On neurologic examination, he has decreased anal sensation and absence of anal and bulbocavernous reflexes. His bladder is distended, but he is unable to empty it.

a. What is the location of the lesion?
b. What is the type of lesion?
c. What type of bladder disturbance is this?
d. What abnormalities of sexual function might be expected?

Baroreceptor Reflex

The most clinically relevant medullary reflex for neurologic diagnosis is the baroreceptor reflex, or *baroreflex* (Fig. 9.29). This reflex is a critical buffering mechanism that prevents fluctuations of arterial pressure by providing rapid adjustment of the total peripheral resistance and cardiac output in response to postural change, emotion, and other stimuli. Through this reflex, an increase in arterial pressure produces compensatory vasodilatation (decreasing total peripheral resistance) and bradycardia (reducing cardiac output). In contrast, a decrease in arterial pressure, for example, when blood pools in the abdominal and lower limb vessels with standing, produces a sympathetically mediated vasoconstriction (increasing total peripheral resistance) and tachycardia. A baroreflex-triggered increase in sympathetic vasoconstrictor output to skeletal muscle and visceral vessels, mediated by α_1-adrenergic receptors, prevents blood from pooling in these regions and thus is essential to prevent a decrease in blood pressure when assuming an erect posture. Failure

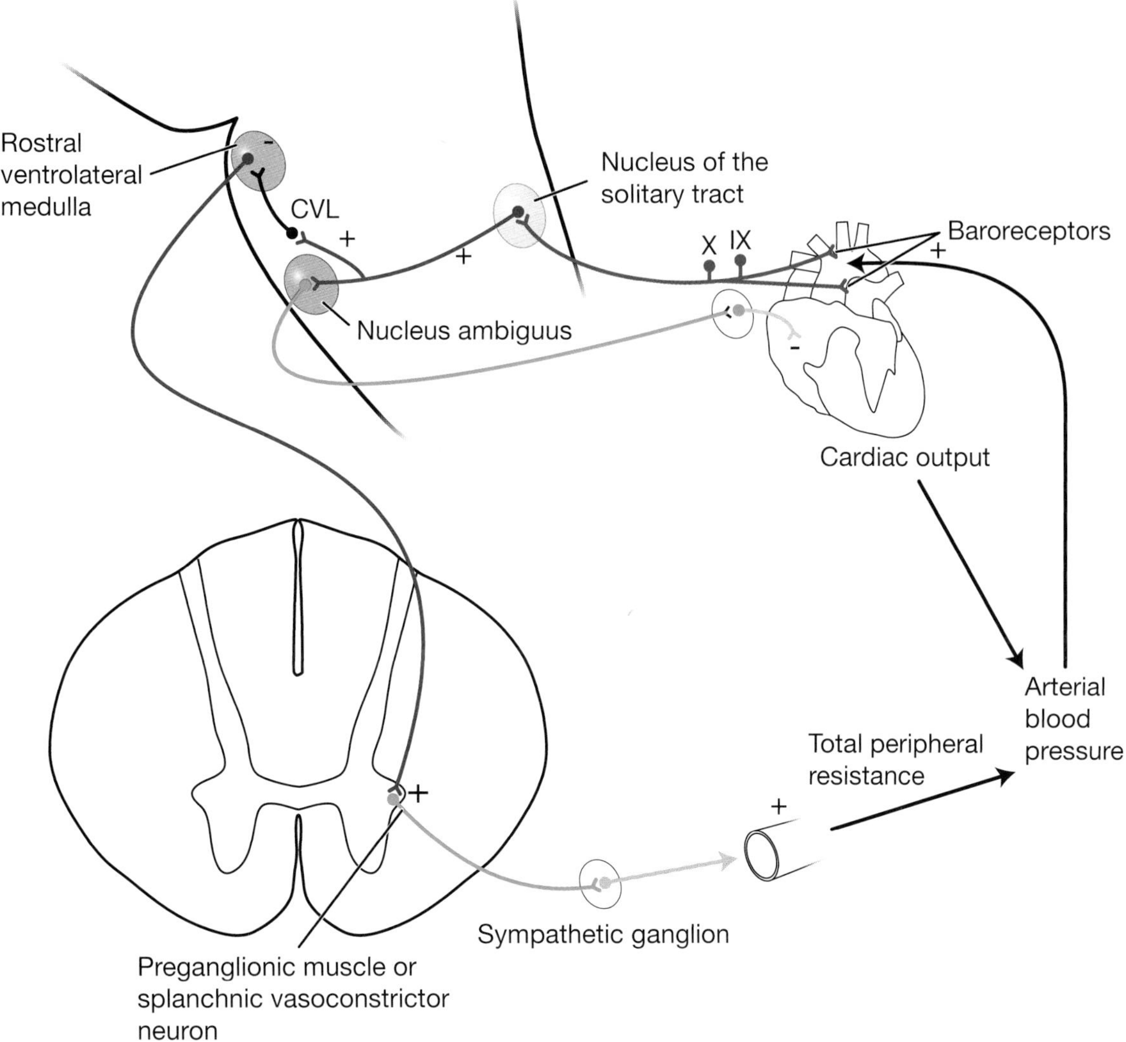

Fig. 9.29. The baroreceptor reflex is a critical buffering mechanism that prevents fluctuations of arterial blood pressure, thus rapidly adjusting total peripheral resistance and cardiac output. The carotid sinus and aortic baroreceptors provide excitatory input to the nucleus of the solitary tract through the glossopharyngeal (IX) and vagus (X) nerves, respectively. This baroreceptor input increases in response to an increase in arterial blood pressure, thus activating neurons in the nucleus of the solitary tract. These neurons send excitatory axons directly to the nucleus ambiguus (resulting in vagal-mediated bradycardia) and indirectly send inhibitory input via caudal ventrolateral medulla (CVL) to rostral ventrolateral medulla (resulting in inhibition of sympathetic vasomotor activity, which leads to vasodilatation). The result is a decrease in arterial blood pressure. In contrast, in response to a decrease in arterial blood pressure, as with standing, baroreceptor activity decreases, leading to sympathetically mediated vasoconstriction and tachycardia.

of baroreflex-mediated vasoconstriction produces orthostatic hypotension. Failure of baroreflex buffering leads to fluctuating hypertension.

> The carotid sinus and aortic baroreceptors are tonically active and provide excitatory input to the nucleus of the solitary tract through the glossopharyngeal and vagus nerves, respectively. Baroreceptor discharge increases in response to an increase in pulsatile arterial pressure, thus activating the nucleus of the solitary tract. This nucleus, in turn, sends excitatory fibers to the nucleus ambiguus, producing vagally mediated bradycardia, and indirect inhibitory fibers to the rostral ventrolateral medulla, resulting in inhibition of sympathetic vasomotor activity leading to vasodilatation. In contrast, in response to a decrease in arterial pressure, as when standing, baroreceptor activity decreases, producing sympathetically mediated vasoconstriction and tachycardia.

- Medullary reflexes are critical for cardiovascular and respiratory control.
- The arterial baroreflex is essential for preventing fluctuations of arterial blood pressure.
- Baroreflex-triggered sympathetic vasoconstriction of leg skeletal muscles and visceral blood vessels is important in preventing orthostatic hypotension.

Cardiorespiratory Interactions

Vasomotor, cardiovagal, and respiratory medullary neurons form an integrated cardiorespiratory network that is coordinated by local interneurons. For example, the activity of the cardiovagal neurons in the nucleus ambiguus is inhibited during inspiration (leading to tachycardia) and increases during expiration (leading to bradycardia). This respiratory modulation of the heart rate is known as *respiratory sinus arrhythmia*. It is an important indicator of the integrity of the vagal innervation of the heart.

All medullary reflexes are modulated by descending projections from the hypothalamus and amygdala, which may inhibit or facilitate these reflexes during complex adaptive responses such as exercise and emotion. For example, the baroreflex is inhibited during stress, affording a concomitant increase in arterial pressure and heart rate.

Clinical Correlations

The transient, reversible loss of consciousness due to global cerebral or brainstem hypoperfusion of rapid onset and followed by rapid, spontaneous, and complete recovery is called *syncope*. It can be classified into several categories. Syncope due to insufficient pumping action of the heart, as with severe arrhythmia or structural cardiac disease, is *cardiogenic syncope*. Syncope due to the inability to activate the sympathetic vasomotor output to leg muscles and viscera is *neurogenic orthostatic hypotension*. It is a prominent manifestation of autonomic failure and an important cause of syncope, and it should be differentiated from the effects of drugs or hypovolemia. A rapid decrease in arterial blood pressure and bradycardia due to a sudden loss of sympathetic vasomotor activity and activation of cardiovagal outputs cause *neurally mediated*, *reflex*, or *vasovagal syncope*. Triggers include prolonged standing (particularly in a hot environment), emotion, pain, and activation of depressor reflexes by, for example, micturition or coughing. Reflex syncope requires the functional integrity of the autonomic output to the cardiovascular system. The *postural tachycardia syndrome* consists of presyncopal symptoms associated with a marked increase in heart rate (more than 30 beats per minute from baseline or more than 120 beats per minute) and occurs upon standing. It reflects postural intolerance that can occur with venous pooling, hypovolemia, deconditioning, or neuropathies affecting the sympathetic innervation of the legs.

Supraspinal pathways that control the functions of the preganglionic sympathetic and sacral parasympathetic neurons descend ipsilaterally in the lateral columns of the spinal cord. Because of the bilateral innervation of blood vessels, only bilateral or midline lesions affecting the descending autonomic pathways impair cardiovascular control (this is similar to the bladder, as discussed above). Disorders of the spinal cord interrupt the supraspinal pathways that control the preganglionic neurons and cause abnormalities in both the tonic background excitation and coordination of the activity of preganglionic neurons. In the acute phase of spinal cord injury, lesions of the descending vasomotor pathways above spinal cord level T5 produce orthostatic hypotension and abolish skin vasomotor responses below the level of the lesion, leading to impaired responses to cold and hot environments. In patients with chronic bilateral or midline lesions above T5, stimulation of the skin, muscle, or viscera innervated by segments below the lesion may cause massive reflex activation of all sympathetic outputs. The result is severe hypertension and other effects, including headache, facial flushing, and bradycardia. This is called *autonomic dysreflexia.*

Thermoregulation

Role of the Hypothalamus

Changes in body temperature are detected by thermoreceptors in the skin, viscera, spinal cord, and brainstem, but the most important thermoregulatory center is the hypothalamus. The preoptic region (anterior to the optic chiasm) contains *warm-sensitive neurons* that increase in activity in response to an increase in core (blood) temperature above a given set point. These neurons initiate responses that lead to heat loss, including sweating and skin vasodilatation, and they inhibit *cold-sensitive neurons.* A decrease in the core temperature disinhibits the cold-sensitive neurons, thus triggering mechanisms for heat production and conservation, including skin vasoconstriction and shivering.

Role of the Sympathetic System

The two most important mechanisms of thermoregulation are sweating (for heat loss) and skin vasoconstriction (for heat conservation). They are mediated by the sympathetic innervation of the skin. The descending pathways that control preganglionic sudomotor and skin vasomotor neurons have not been well defined, but they involve connections within the hypothalamus and brainstem. The sympathetic ganglion neurons that innervate the sweat glands have acetylcholine as a neurotransmitter and activate sweating by stimulating muscarinic receptors. The skin vasomotor sympathetic ganglion neurons have norepinephrine as a neurotransmitter and elicit vasoconstriction through α_1-adrenergic receptors. Sympathetic skin vasodilatation may be mediated by NO.

Gastrointestinal Motility

Motility within the gastrointestinal tract depends on the interaction of local networks of neurons in the wall of the gut called the *enteric nervous system.* This system is controlled by the vagus and sympathetic ganglia.

Enteric Nervous System

The enteric nervous system consists of a large number of neurons in the submucosal plexus and myenteric plexus in the wall of the gut. These plexuses include afferent (sensory) neurons that are stimulated by intestinal distention, excitatory and inhibitory interneurons, and motor neurons. Most of the neurons contain acetylcholine, but different functional subtypes also use neuropeptides, ATP, or NO as neurotransmitters. The neurons of the enteric nervous system form integrative local circuits and reflexes that control motility, secretion, and blood flow throughout the gut. The activity of the enteric nervous system is independent of extrinsic innervation but is modulated by vagal and sympathetic input.

> Distention, mechanical distortion of the mucosa, or change in intraluminal chemistry (e.g., the presence of bile salts) elicits a reflex that leads to propulsion of the bolus along the gut. This peristaltic reflex consists of contraction of the circular smooth muscle that is oral to the bolus in the lumen (ascending excitatory reflex) and relaxation of the circular smooth muscle that is anal to the bolus (descending inhibitory reflex).

Vagal and Sympathetic Influences

Neurons in the dorsal vagal nucleus participate in vagovagal reflexes triggered by input to the nucleus of the solitary tract from gastrointestinal tract mechanoreceptors and chemoreceptors. Stimulation of the vagus nerve causes relaxation of smooth muscle in the proximal stomach during swallowing (receptive relaxation) and stimulates motility in the distal stomach and gastric emptying. The sympathetic preganglionic neurons that innervate the gastrointestinal tract have a relatively small input from the brain. The *sympathetic prevertebral reflex* is a feedback mechanism that regulates motor activity in the gut. Enteric afferents activated by gut distention activate prevertebral ganglion neurons that inhibit gut motility.

- The enteric nervous system consists of a large number of sensory and motor neurons and interneurons that control peristalsis and secretion throughout the length of the gut.

Responses to Emotion and Stress

A critical function of the internal regulation system is the integration of responses to emotion and stress. This consists of a highly interconnected functional unit that includes the anterior cingulate gyrus, ventromedial prefrontal cortex, amygdala, hypothalamus, and periaqueductal gray matter (Fig. 9.30). Physical or psychologic stressors activate sympathoadrenal and adrenocortical responses that promote adaptation and survival short term.

Amygdala and the Conditioned Fear Response

The amygdala provides sensory information with affective value and initiates adaptive visceral, endocrine, and motor responses associated with emotion, particularly fear.

> A conditioned fear response occurs when the subject is exposed to a stimulus, such as a sight, sound, or memory, that previously had been associated with a negative experience, for example, pain. This response is mediated by autonomic, endocrine, and motor outputs and is coordinated by the amygdala through its extensive connections with the hypothalamus, periaqueductal gray matter, and autonomic and motor nuclei of the medulla and spinal cord.

Defense Reaction

Acute, transient challenges that trigger successful, active adaptations produce a short-term response called the *defense reaction*. This consists of sympathetic and adrenomedullary activation and results in an increase in heart rate, cardiac output, and arterial pressure; redistribution of blood flow to the limbs; inhibition of the baroreflex; inhibition of pain; and active "fight" or "flight" responses. This reaction resembles the response to physical exercise and involves the lateral hypothalamus and periaqueductal gray matter. It is mediated by sympathoexcitatory neurons in rostral ventrolateral medulla.

> Depending on the stimulus and the subject's perception of the challenge and ability to cope with it, different regions of the periaqueductal gray matter may initiate the active fight-or-flight response (sympathoexcitation and increased motor activity) or a passive avoidance ("playing dead" response) characterized by hypotension, bradycardia, and immobility.

Stress Response

When the magnitude of the stressor reaches a certain threshold, both the sympathoadrenal and adrenocortical systems are activated by reciprocal interactions among the central nucleus of the amygdala, the paraventricular nucleus, and noradrenergic neurons of the locus ceruleus.

> The paraventricular nucleus of the hypothalamus generates coordinated endocrine and autonomic responses to internal and external stressors, including the secretion of antidiuretic hormone and activation of the sympathetic, adrenomedullary, and adrenocortical systems. The different neuronal groups in the paraventricular nucleus respond to visceral, limbic, and humoral signals such as pain, fear, and circulating cytokines. They are involved in responses to hypoglycemia and regulation of the immune response.

Normally, the responses to stress are short-lasting and adaptive, allowing energy mobilization and repair mechanisms. However, when these responses are abnormally intense or when the subject is exposed repeatedly to the stressor or is unable to turn off the responses, the excessive sympathoadrenal and adrenocortical activation may lead to such diseases as hypertension, diabetes mellitus, obesity, and depression.

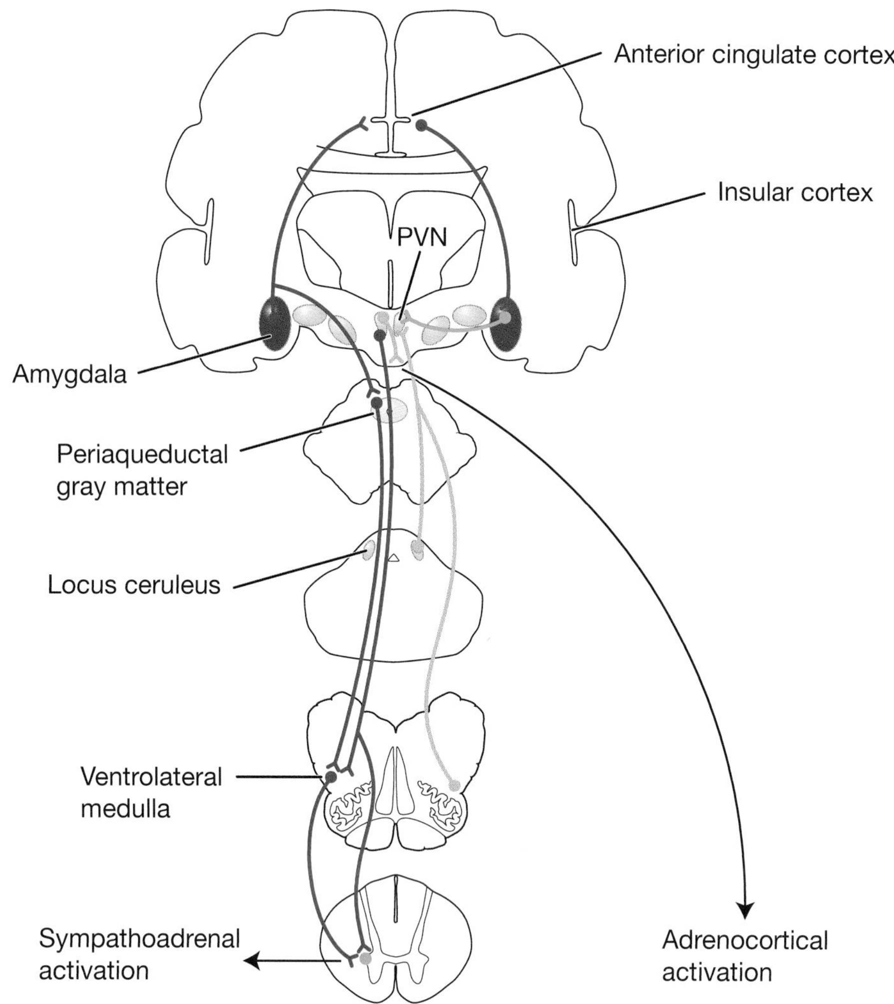

Fig. 9.30. The internal regulation system integrates and coordinates responses to emotion and stress. This involves a highly interconnected functional unit containing the anterior cingulate gyrus, amygdala, paraventricular nucleus (PVN) periaqueductal gray matter, rostral ventrolateral medulla, and medullary raphe nuclei. These structures are involved in the patterned activation of the sympathoadrenal, adrenocortical, and pain modulatory systems. (Modified from Benarroch EE. Basic neurosciences with clinical applications. Philadelphia: Elsevier; 2006. Used with permission of Mayo Foundation for Medical Education and Research.)

- The anterior cingulate gyrus, amygdala, hypothalamus, and periaqueductal gray matter form an interconnected network involved in responses to emotion and stress.
- The responses to stress depend on the nature of the stressor and the individual's perception of the ability to cope with it.

Clinical Evaluation of the Internal Regulation System

History and Examination

The clinical evaluation should include appropriate inquiry into a history of autonomic symptoms and examination of autonomic function. The size and symmetry of the pupils and their reactions to light should be noted carefully. Normal pupils are equal in size (2 to 4 mm in diameter) and react briskly to light in either eye. Pulse and blood pressure in the supine and standing positions can reflect alterations in neural input and must be part of each examination. A pronounced decrease in arterial blood pressure when the patient is standing (orthostatic hypotension), particularly when not associated with a compensatory increase in heart rate, indicates dysfunction of the afferent, central, or efferent component of the baroreceptor reflex. Lack of heart rate variability with deep respiration indicates failure of the vagal control of the heart. Skin temperature and sweating are controlled by sympathetic fibers. A search should be made for any localized absence of sweating, asymmetrical skin temperature or color, and absence of normal oral and conjunctival moisture.

The clinical evaluation of neurogenic bladder includes 1) assessing the ability of the patient to voluntarily control the initiation or interruption of micturition and bladder sensation and 2) examining reflexes integrated at the level of the conus medullaris and mediated by sensory and motor roots in the cauda equina. The *bulbocavernous* and *anal reflexes* are somatic reflexes integrated at spinal cord levels S2 to S4, and their loss indicates a lesion of the conus medullaris and cauda equina. Loss of perianal sensation is also consistent with a caudal equina lesion. Quantitation of residual volume, either by palpation and percussion of the bladder for evidence of abnormal bladder distention or by the postvoid residual after catheterization, is important in the evaluation of neurogenic bladder.

Laboratory Evaluation

There are several laboratory tests for autonomic function (Table 9.12). Cardiovascular reflex tests include beat-to-beat measurements of the arterial blood pressure and heart rate responses during standing or *head-up tilt* and during the *Valsalva maneuver* (a forced expiration against resistance) and assessment of the *heart rate responses to deep breathing*. For example, a decrease in systolic arterial blood pressure of more than 20 mm Hg or of diastolic arterial blood pressure of more than 10 mm Hg during standing or head-up tilt is an indication of the impairment of sympathetic vasoconstriction. Reduced heart rate responses to deep breathing indicate impaired vagal control of the heart. The Valsalva maneuver is a complex test of both reflex sympathetic and cardiovagal functions.

The sympathetic innervation of the skin is tested by determining the patient's ability to sweat. The *thermoregulatory sweat test* determines the ability to sweat throughout the body in response to an increase in central core temperature of 1°C. The *quantitative sudomotor axon reflex test* assesses the ability of peripheral sudomotor axons, which are stimulated antidromically with the iontophoretic administration of acetylcholine, to release acetylcholine and activate sweat glands.

The clinical evaluation of a neurogenic bladder is complemented by *urodynamic evaluation*, including cystometrography, measurement of bladder pressure and urinary flow, and electromyography of the external sphincter muscle. Evaluation of impotence includes measuring the levels of prolactin and testosterone and performing the *penile tumescence test* during sleep. Motor function of

Table 9.12. Autonomic Function Tests

Autonomic function	Laboratory test
Sympathetic sudomotor	Thermoregulatory sweat test
	Sudomotor axon reflex test
Sympathetic vasoconstrictor	Blood pressure responses to standing or head-up tilt
	Blood pressure response to Valsalva maneuver
Vagal cardiac	Heart rate response to deep breathing
Vagal gastrointestinal	Gastrointestinal motility studies
Bladder function	Urodynamic study
Erectile function	Nocturnal penile tumescence test

the gut is tested by measuring the magnitude, frequency, rhythm, and distribution of peristaltic waves with pressure transducers.

Pharmacologic testing with adrenergic and cholinergic agonists is useful for detecting a lack of response or denervation supersensitivity of effector organs. These tests often are used to assess pupillary control, sweating, and cardiovascular function. The presence of denervation supersensitivity indicates a postganglionic (peripheral) lesion.

- Denervation supersensitivity is a manifestation of postganglionic, as opposed to preganglionic, autonomic failure.

Unlike generalized autonomic failure, which reflects a diffuse central or peripheral lesion effect of drugs or toxins, focal disorders at the supratentorial, posterior fossa, spinal, or peripheral level may affect specific visceral effectors. In particular, abnormalities of the pupil or bladder function have an important localizing value in neurology. Other disorders produce level-specific syndromes that also have localizing value.

Additional Reading

Benarroch EE. The central autonomic network: functional organization, dysfunction, and perspective. Mayo Clin Proc. 1993;68:988-1001.

Grundy D. Neuroanatomy of visceral nociception: vagal and splanchnic afferent. Gut. 2002;51 Suppl 1:i2-i5.

Jänig W, Häbler H.-J. Organization of the autonomic nervous system: structure and function. In: Appenzeller O, editor. Handbook of clinical neurology: the autonomic nervous system. Part 1: normal functions. Amsterdam: Elsevier; 1999. pp. 1-52.

Kunze WA, Furness JB. The enteric nervous system and regulation of intestinal motility. Annu Rev Physiol. 1999;61:117-142.

Lundberg JM. Pharmacology of contransmission in the autonomic nervous system: integrative aspects on amines, neuropeptides, adenosine triphosphate, amino acids and nitric oxide. Pharmacol Rev. 1996;48:113-178.

Saper CB. The central autonomic nervous system: conscious visceral perception and autonomic pattern generation. Annu Rev Neurosci. 2002;25:433-469.

Shields RW Jr. Functional anatomy of the autonomic nervous system. J Clin Neurophysiol. 1993;10:2-13.

Chapter 10

The Consciousness System

Objectives

1. Describe the anatomy of the consciousness system, with special reference to the reticular formation, the cholinergic and monoaminergic cell groups, the thalamic nuclei, the ascending projection system, and the cerebral cortex.
2. List the major connections (input and output) of the reticular formation.
3. Describe the projection pathways of the consciousness system to the cerebral cortex.
4. Describe and differentiate the electrical activity of single neurons and neuronal aggregates.
5. Describe the neurophysiologic basis of the normal electroencephalogram (EEG) and the fundamental waking and sleep patterns.
6. List the functions of the consciousness system.
7. Describe the characteristics of the different sleep states and their anatomical substrate.
8. Define and list the characteristics of each of the following: narcolepsy, rapid eye movement (REM) sleep behavior disorder, confusional state (delirium), coma, concussion, seizure, and syncope.
9. State the anatomical locations of lesions that produce the loss of consciousness, and give examples of specific disease processes that affect each area.
10. Describe how the EEG is useful in evaluating patients who have disorders of consciousness.

Introduction

The major afferent pathways that provide the central nervous system with direct access to information about the external environment are described in Chapter 7. In parallel with these pathways at the posterior fossa and supratentorial levels is another ascending system, the consciousness system. This system extends from the medulla to the cerebral cortex. The consciousness system is a diffuse system that regulates the state of arousal, attention, and the sleep-wake states and modulates cortical reactivity to stimuli. The pathways of the consciousness system arise from the brainstem, hypothalamus, and basal forebrain and modulate activity of the cerebral cortex through projections to the thalamus or directly to the cerebral cortex. In this chapter, the anatomy and physiology of the consciousness system, its role in the regulation of wakefulness and sleep, and pathologic states of altered consciousness, which are a reflection of deranged activity within the system, are described.

Overview

Consciousness is defined as the state of awareness of self and the environment. This state is determined by two main functions: *arousal* (level of consciousness) and *awareness* (content of consciousness). The consciousness system is a diffuse yet organized neuronal system located in the brainstem, diencephalon, and cerebral hemispheres.

Structures in the system are 1) nuclei of the brainstem reticular formation, hypothalamus, and basal forebrain; 2) thalamic nuclei; 3) ascending projections from the brainstem, hypothalamus, and basal forebrain to the thalamus and cerebral cortex; and 4) widespread areas of the cerebral cortex (Fig. 10.1). Control of the behavioral states of arousal, wakefulness, and sleep and attention to the environment is related to specific changes in the activity of neurons in the brainstem and basal forebrain that produce functional changes in thalamic and cortical circuits. Proper functioning of the consciousness system, and hence the regulation of alertness, awareness, and attention, is predicated on continuous interaction among the cerebral cortex, thalamus, basal forebrain, hypothalamus, and brainstem reticular formation.

The *arousal* component of consciousness is achieved through the action of the ascending projections of the reticular activating system and basal forebrain on the thalamus and cerebral cortex. A normal cyclic physiologic alteration of consciousness is *sleep*, which is readily reversed by appropriate stimuli. Sleep has been divided into two stages, rapid eye movement (REM) sleep and nonrapid eye movement (NREM) sleep, which are controlled by the hypothalamus, thalamus, and brainstem reticular formation. The normal processing of information for conscious awareness (i.e., the content of consciousness) requires *attention*, which is determined by the interaction of different areas of the cerebral cortex under the coordinating and modulatory influences of the thalamus, cholinergic and monoaminergic cell groups of the basal forebrain and the brainstem reticular formation.

Pathologic processes that destroy or depress the function of the brainstem reticular formation, hypothalamus, basal forebrain, or thalamus, their ascending projection pathways, or both cerebral hemispheres produce alterations in consciousness. The evaluation of a patient who has a disorder of consciousness requires analysis of associated neurologic signs to determine whether the responsible lesion is 1) located at the supratentorial level, 2) located at the posterior fossa level, or 3) diffusely distributed at both levels.

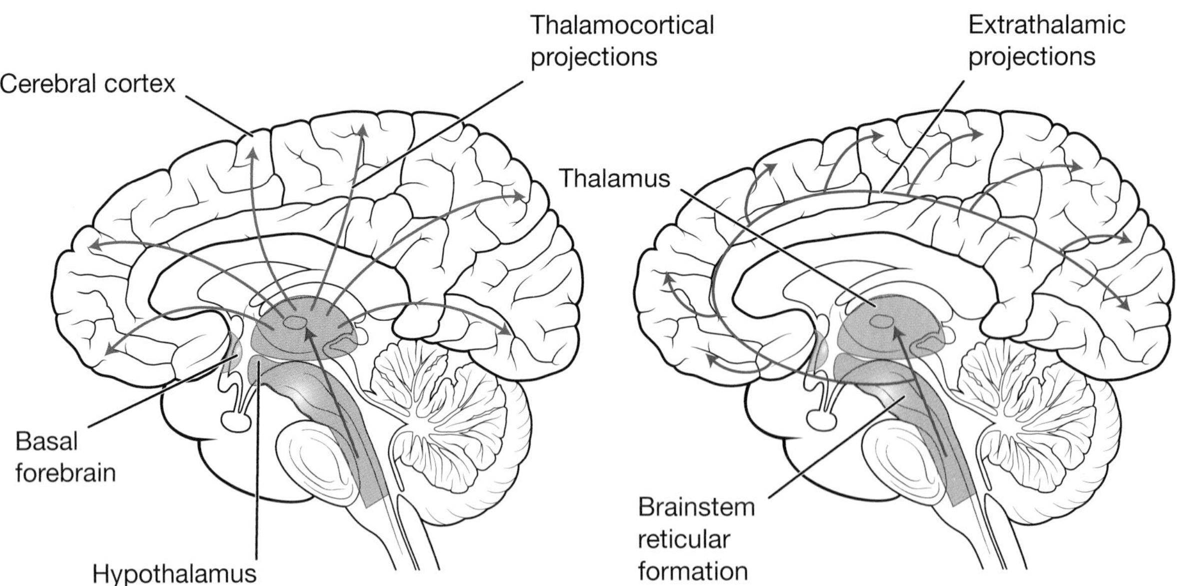

Fig. 10.1. Lateral view of the brain showing the components of the consciousness system. Note that neurons of the brainstem reticular formation may control activity of the cerebral cortex both through a relay in the thalamus and by direct projections to the cerebral cortex (extrathalamic pathways). The cholinergic and monoaminergic systems project directly to the cerebral cortex.

Anatomy of the Consciousness System

Structures of the consciousness system include nuclei of the brainstem reticular formation, hypothalamus, basal forebrain, and thalamus; the ascending projection pathways; and widespread areas of the cerebral cortex (Fig. 10.1).

Reticular Formation

The reticular formation is a complex aggregate of neurons whose cell bodies form clusters in the tegmental portion of the brainstem, the basal forebrain, and the thalamus. The neurons are characterized by long, radiating dendrites that have few branches and axons that have numerous collaterals and project for long distances along the neuraxis. The diffuse arrangement of these multipolar neurons and their many interconnections allow a single reticular neuron to receive afferents from many sources and to make synaptic contact with numerous neurons. This arrangement gives rise to the term *reticular* ("forming a network"). With phylogenic advancement, this centrally located network has become surrounded by structures that serve specific functions in the motor and sensory systems.

- The reticular formation consists of a network of neurons and ascending and descending pathways in the brainstem.

Anatomical Subdivisions

The reticular formation has been subdivided functionally into a *midline region* (the *raphe*), a *medial region* containing large neurons that project to the spinal cord and to ocular motor nuclei, and a *lateral region* that receives axon collaterals from many ascending sensory pathways. The rostral portions of the reticular formation at the level of the upper pons and midbrain contain neurochemically defined groups of neurons that project to the cerebral cortex either directly or by relay in the thalamus and are a key component of the consciousness system. The caudal portion of the reticular formation in the lower pons and medulla sends projections to the spinal cord and is involved in the control of motor function, respiration, and blood pressure. Neurons of the reticular formation also coordinate the function of cranial nerve nuclei. For example, neurons in the medial portion of the reticular formation of the pons (called the paramedian pontine reticular formation) activate fast horizontal eye movements, and neurons in the lateral portion of the reticular formation of the medulla coordinate complex motor patterns such as respiration, swallowing, and vomiting (Fig. 10.2).

Afferent and Efferent Connections

Afferent pathways to the reticular formation consist of 1) collateral branches from the primary ascending tracts of the sensory system (spinothalamic and spinoreticular pathways); 2) fibers from widespread areas of the cerebral cortex (corticoreticular fibers) as well as collaterals from the corticospinal and corticobulbar tracts of the motor system; 3) fibers from other structures, including the cerebellum, basal ganglia, hypothalamus, cranial nerve nuclei, and the colliculi; and 4) visceral afferents from the spinal cord and cranial nerves (Fig. 10.3).

- The afferent pathways to the reticular formation consist of collateral branches from ascending sensory pathways, corticoreticular fibers, other structures of the central nervous system (e.g., cerebellum and basal ganglia), and visceral afferents.

The efferent pathways from the reticular formation project rostrally to the forebrain, caudally to the spinal cord, and within the brainstem. The ascending projections to the thalamus and cerebral cortex are the anatomical substrate of the consciousness system. Projections of the reticular formation to spinal and ocular motor neurons are critical for the control of posture, locomotion, and eye movements. Projections to areas of the internal regulation system are critical for control of endocrine and autonomic function (Fig. 10.4). By means of these numerous connections and pathways, the reticular formation can integrate information from various levels of the neuraxis and thereby regulate and modify the activity of the nervous system.

- The efferent pathways of the reticular formation consist of projections to the forebrain, the spinal cord, and to motor and internal regulation systems.

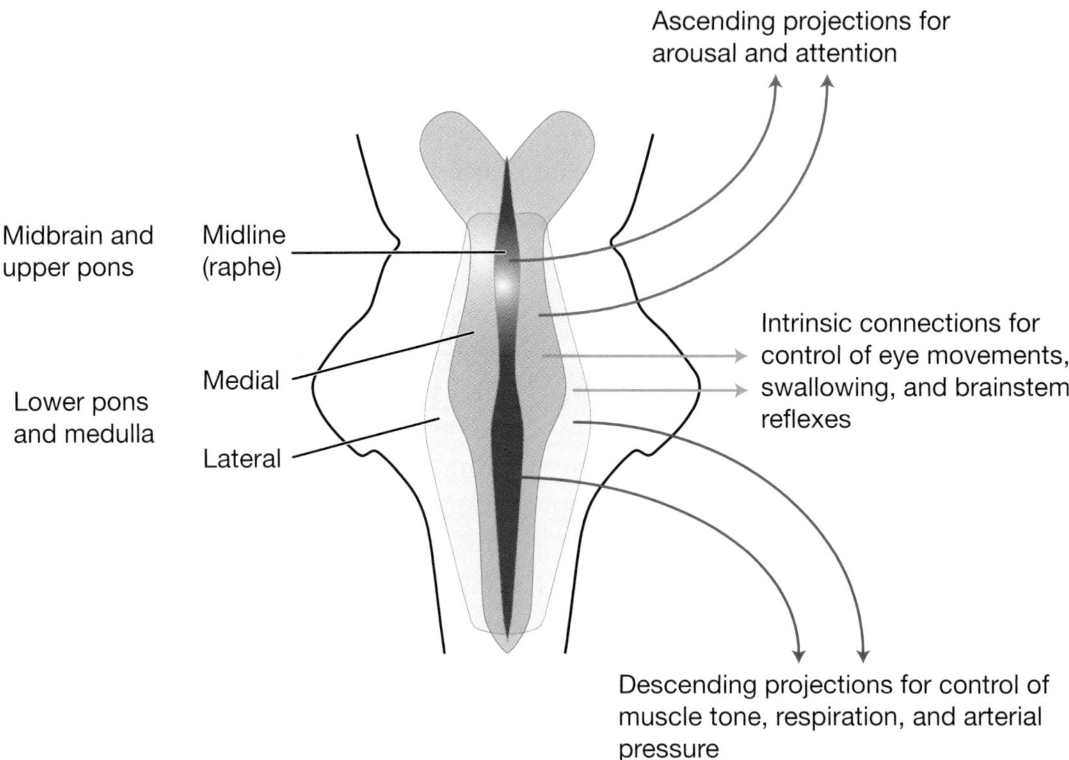

Fig. 10.2. General organization of the brainstem reticular formation.

The reticular formation extends functionally to include the areas of the posterior hypothalamus and basal forebrain. The concept of the reticular formation as a diffuse interconnected system that receives numerous converging inputs and gives rise to multiple divergent outputs has to be refined because of evidence that it includes distinct neurochemically and functionally defined nuclei, each with specific neuronal connections.

Cholinergic and Monoaminergic Systems

Several neurochemically defined nuclei are involved with the control of the different behavioral states of wakefulness and sleep and attention to environmental stimuli. They can be subdivided into two main groups: *cholinergic groups* and *monoaminergic groups* (Table 10.1). The cholinergic and monoaminergic cell groups project to the cerebral cortex through the *medial forebrain bundle*. This is a large tract that extends from the midbrain tegmentum through the lateral hypothalamus into the septum, preoptic area, and hypothalamus, and some of the axons in the bundle reach the cingulate gyrus. The medial forebrain bundle represents the most rostral extent of the reticular system and contains ascending and descending fibers that interconnect the brainstem and telencephalon.

Cholinergic Groups

The cholinergic nuclear groups of neurons synthesizing acetylcholine are located in the *basal forebrain* and in the dorsal tegmentum of the upper pons and midbrain, called the *mesopontine tegmentum* (Fig. 10.5). The cholinergic structures of the basal forebrain, including the *nucleus basalis of Meynert* and the *medial septum*, send diffuse projections to the cerebral cortex. These projections are critical for the regulation of attention, processing of sensory information, and learning and memory.

The cholinergic neurons of the mesopontine tegmentum project to the thalamus, forebrain, and brainstem. These mesopontine neurons are important in the mechanisms of arousal and the regulation of different stages of

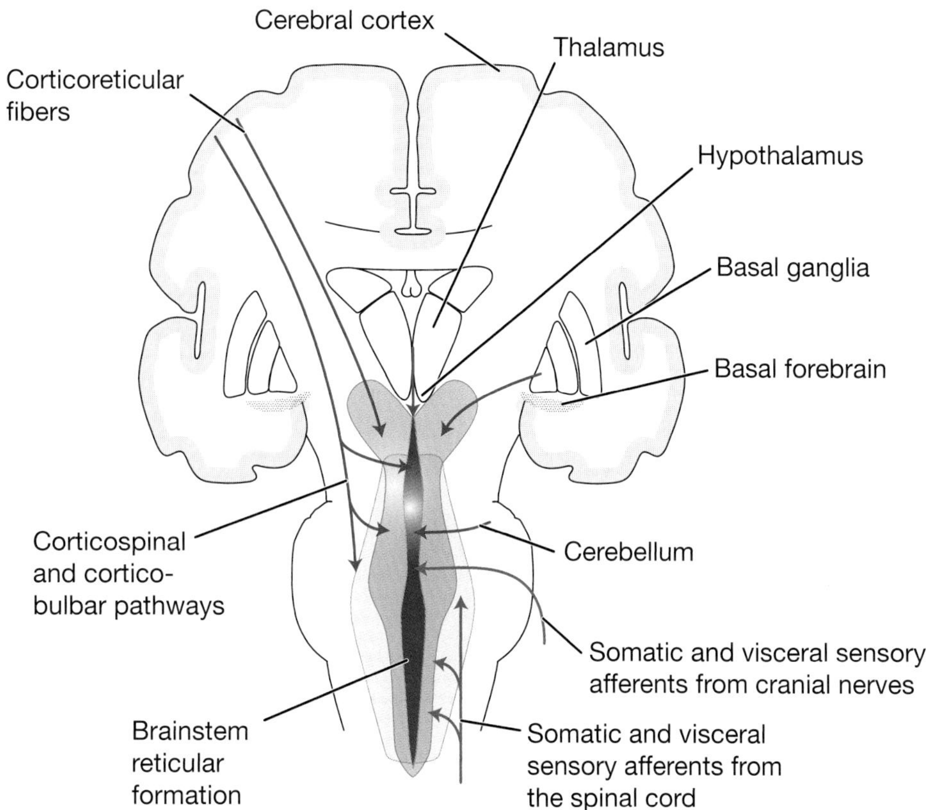

Fig. 10.3. Input to the brainstem reticular formation.

sleep. Thus, the cholinergic groups of the basal forebrain and upper brainstem, through their connections with each other, the thalamus, and the cerebral cortex, are involved in essentially all functions of the consciousness system.

Monoaminergic Groups

The monoaminergic groups important in regulating behavioral states and state-dependent cortical activity include neurons that synthesize dopamine, norepinephrine, serotonin, or histamine. The dopamine-synthesizing cells are located in the *substantia nigra pars compacta* and *ventral tegmental area* of the midbrain (Fig. 10.6 *A*). These cells project to the basal ganglia and frontal lobe. This dopaminergic system is activated by external rewards and exposure to novel stimuli and is important in controlling motivated motor behavior. The norepinephrine-synthesizing cells are located in the *locus ceruleus*, which is in the lateral part of the upper pons (Fig. 10.6 *B*). The locus ceruleus sends diffuse projections to areas that mediate responses to sensory stimuli and control motor behavior, including the cerebral cortex, thalamus, hypothalamus, basal forebrain, cerebellum, and spinal cord. The activity of neurons in the locus ceruleus increases in response to new and challenging stimuli; thus, this nucleus has an important role in the mechanisms of arousal and attention.

Both dopamine and norepinephrine are catecholamines. The metabolism of catecholamines produces neuromelanin; consequently, dopaminergic and noradrenergic neurons are pigmented neurons. These nuclei can be identified macroscopically by their black (in the case of the substantia nigra, hence its name) or bluish (in the case of locus ceruleus, hence its name) appearance in fresh specimens.

The serotonin-synthesizing neurons are located in the *raphe nuclei*, which occupy the midline of the

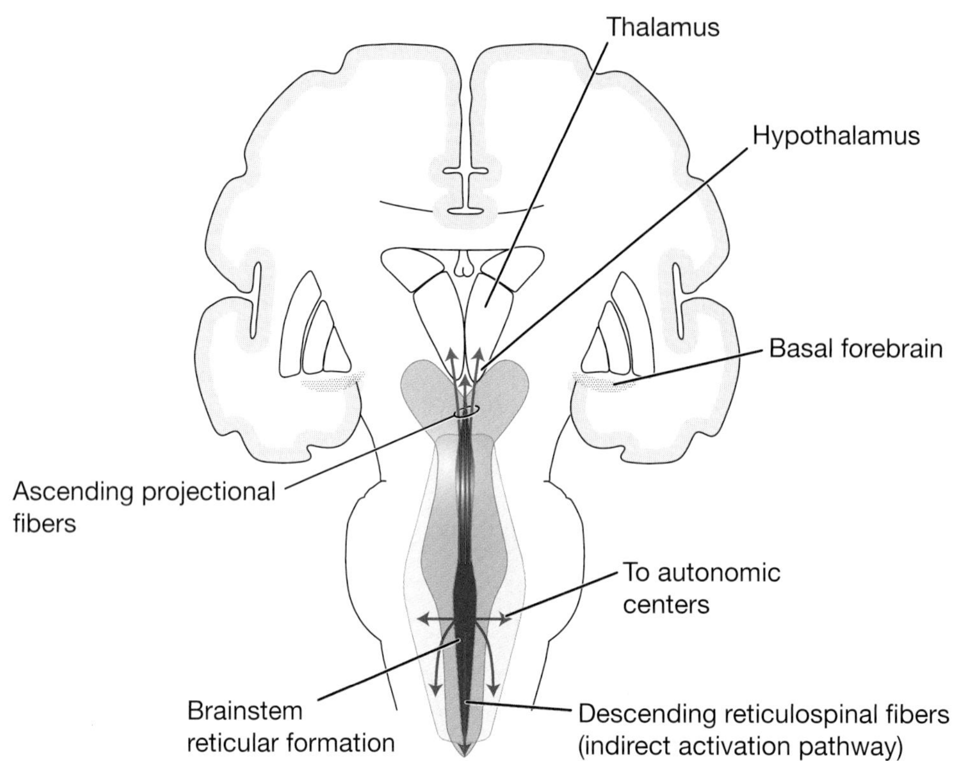

Fig. 10.4. Output pathways of the brainstem reticular formation.

Table 10.1. General Features of the Cholinergic and Monoaminergic Cell Groups of the Consciousness System

Location of nuclear group	Neurotransmitter	Main function
Basal forebrain	Acetylcholine	Attention Memory
Tegmentum of rostral pons and midbrain	Acetylcholine	Arousal REM sleep
Ventral tegmental area of the midbrain	Dopamine	Motivated motor behavior in response to reward
Locus ceruleus	Norepinephrine	Attention to novel and potentially challenging stimuli REM sleep inhibition
Raphe nuclei	Serotonin	Regulation of mood and affect REM sleep inhibition
Tuberomammillary nucleus of the hypothalamus	Histamine	Wakefulness

REM, rapid eye movement.

brainstem (Fig. 10.7 *A*). They include a rostral group and a caudal group. The rostral raphe nuclei, in upper pons and midbrain, give rise to ascending projections to the cerebral cortex, thalamus, hypothalamus, and basal forebrain. The caudal raphe nuclei, located in lower pons and medulla, project to other areas of the brainstem and spinal cord. The histamine-synthesizing neurons are located in the *tuberomammillary nucleus* in the posterior lateral hypothalamus (Fig. 10.7 *B*). These neurons have a critical role in the maintenance of wakefulness. Another important group of neurons in the posterior lateral hypothalamus synthesizes the neuropeptide *hypocretin* (also called *orexin*). These neurons send excitatory projections to all the cholinergic and monoaminergic groups and are important in regulating the transition between wakefulness and sleep. Thus, the tegmentum of the upper pons and midbrain contains three essential components of the

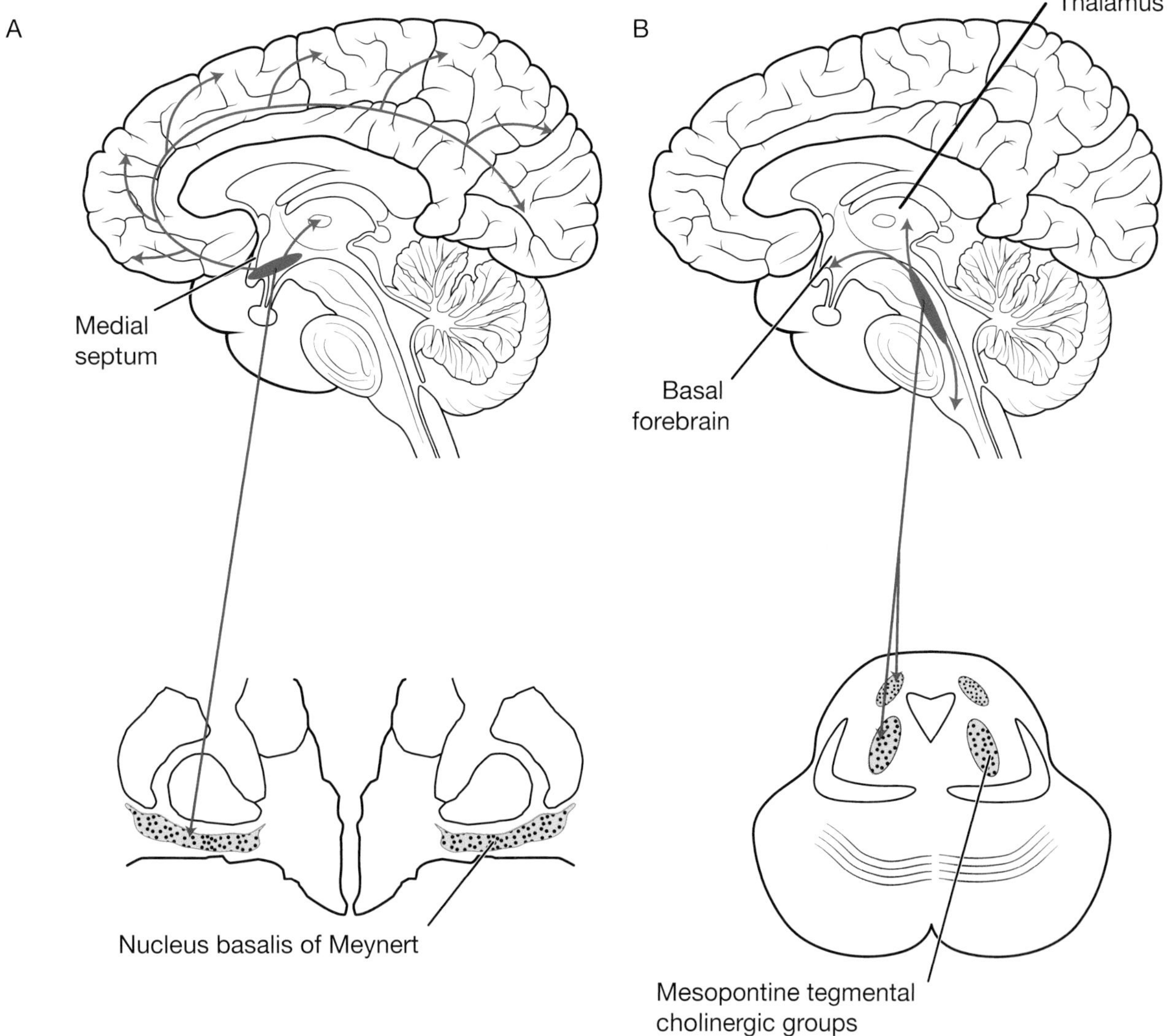

Fig. 10.5. Cholinergic groups of the consciousness system. *A*, The basal forebrain group, including the nucleus basalis of Meynert and medial septum, project to the cerebral cortex. *B*, The mesopontine cholinergic group, including the laterodorsal and pedunculopontine tegmental nuclei, project to the thalamus, basal forebrain, and brainstem.

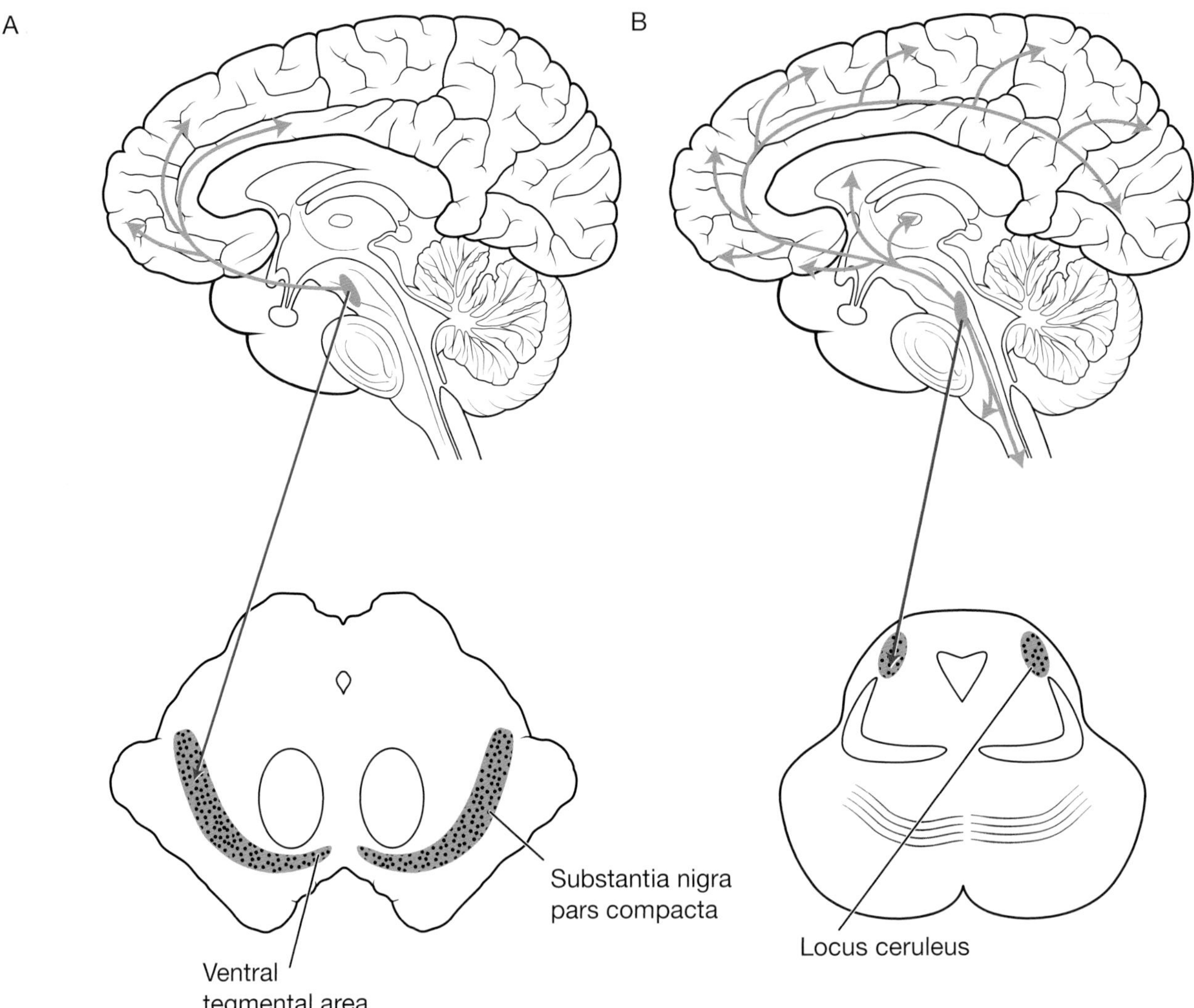

Fig. 10.6. Catecholaminergic groups of the consciousness system. *A*, The dopamine-synthesizing neurons are located in the substantia nigra pars compacta, which projects to the striatum, and the ventral tegmental area, which projects to the frontal cortex and limbic system. *B*, The norepinephrine-synthesizing neurons of the locus ceruleus project extensively to the cerebral cortex, thalamus, basal ganglia, brainstem, and spinal cord. Both cell groups contain neuromelanin, which makes them identifiable in fresh specimens.

consciousness system (the cholinergic, noradrenergic, and serotonergic systems) (Fig. 10.8). The posterior hypothalamus contains the histaminergic and hypocretin systems important for arousal.

- The cholinergic neurons are located in the brainstem and basal forebrain.
- The monoaminergic nuclear groups are located in the brainstem and hypothalamus.

Thalamus

The thalamus is the gateway to the cerebral cortex and subserves three important roles: 1) it acts as a relay station (relaying information to and from the cerebral cortex), 2) it filters and modulates the flow of information to the cerebral cortex from other areas, and 3) it coordinates the activity in widespread areas of the cerebral cortex. The thalamus is subdivided into two main components. The larger component is the *dorsal thalamus*,

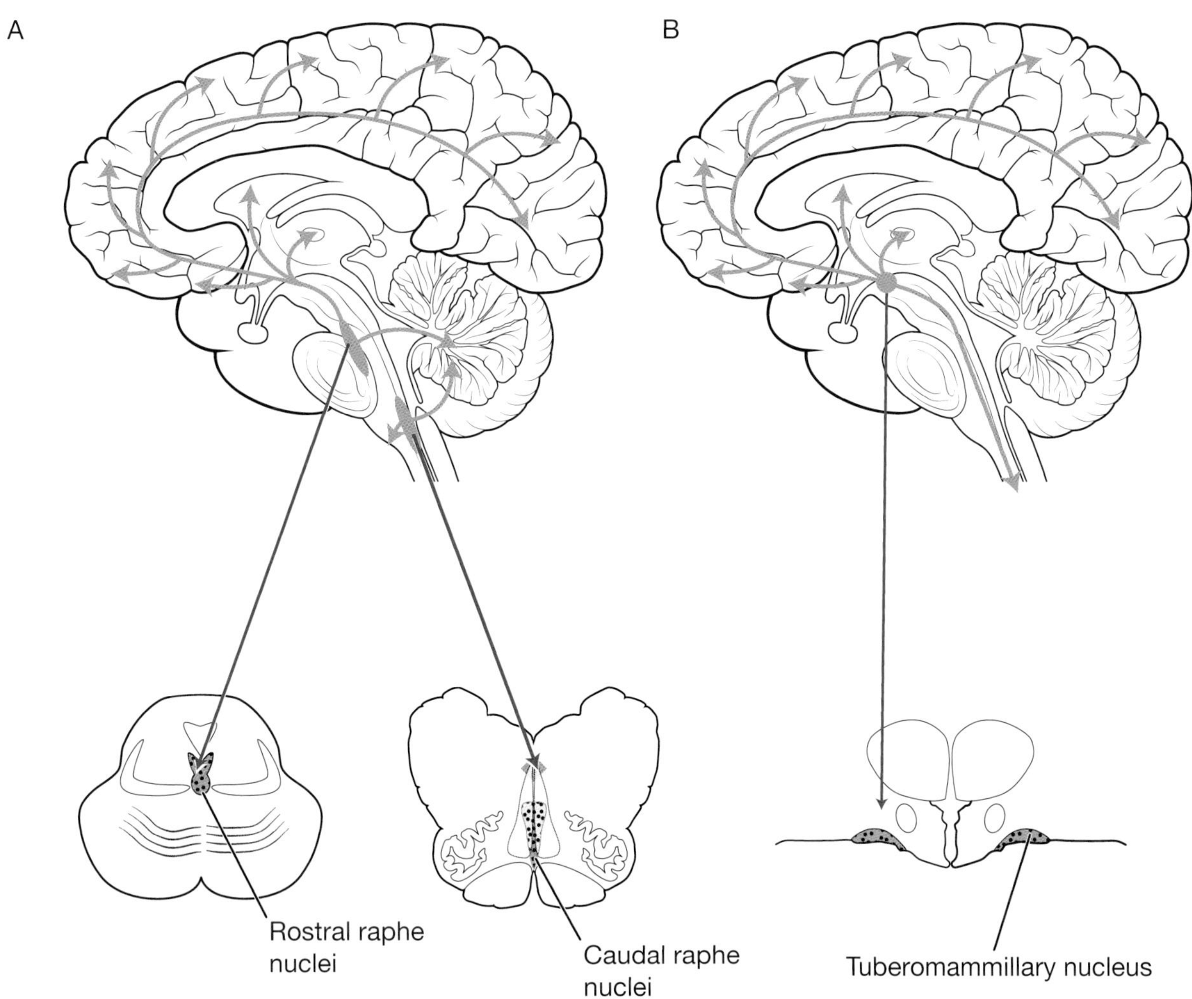

Fig. 10.7. Serotonergic and histaminergic groups of the consciousness sytem. *A*, The serotonin-synthesizing neurons are located in the raphe nuclei. The rostral raphe nuclei, located in the upper pons and midbrain, project to the cerebral cortex, thalamus, and hypothalamus and are an important component of the consciousness system. The caudal raphe nuclei, located in the caudal pons and medulla, project to the cerebellum and spinal cord and are important in controlling motor, respiratory, and autonomic functions. *B*, The histamine-synthesizing neurons of the tuberomammillary nucleus project heavily to the hypothalamus and cerebral cortex and are critical for wakefulness.

or thalamus proper, which contains the relay nuclei for sensory, motor, and association pathways and has reciprocal connections with the cerebral cortex. The smaller component is the *reticular nucleus* of the thalamus, which projects to other thalamic nuclei but not to the cerebral cortex (Fig. 10.9).

Dorsal Thalamus

The nuclei of dorsal thalamus are subdivided into three groups on the basis of their connections and functions (Fig. 10.10). The *specific thalamic relay* nuclei receive input from each sensory pathway (lemniscal, spinothalamic, visual, auditory), basal ganglia, or cerebellum; project to sensory or motor areas of the cerebral cortex; and have reciprocal connections with these cortical areas (Fig. 10.10 *A*). The relay nuclei are located in the ventral, lateral, and anterior portions of the thalamus and are described in the chapters on the sensory system and motor system and in Chapter 16 A. The *association nuclei* have reciprocal connections with association areas of the cerebral cortex, including the prefrontal cortex and posterior parietal cortex, and form part of the circuits that integrate sensory and motor information for such functions as visuospatial attention and voluntary motor control. The two most important association nuclei are the *pulvinar*, which interacts with the posterior parietal cortex, and the *mediodorsal nucleus*, which interacts with the prefrontal cortex (Fig. 10.10 *B*). The third group, erroneously referred to as "nonspecific" thalamic nuclei include the *intralaminar* nuclei and *midline* nuclei (Fig. 10.11). These nuclei are an important component of the consciousness system. They receive input from the spinothalamic tract, reticular formation, basal forebrain, basal ganglia, and limbic system and send axons to widespread areas of the cerebral cortex as well as the basal ganglia and hypothalamus (Fig. 10.10 *C*).

The intralaminar nuclei are located in the internal medullary lamina, a band of myelinated fibers that separates the anterior, medial, and lateral groups of relay and association nuclei. They are an important component of the basal ganglia circuits and project diffusely throughout the cerebral cortex. The midline nuclei are particularly interconnected with the components of the internal regulation system.

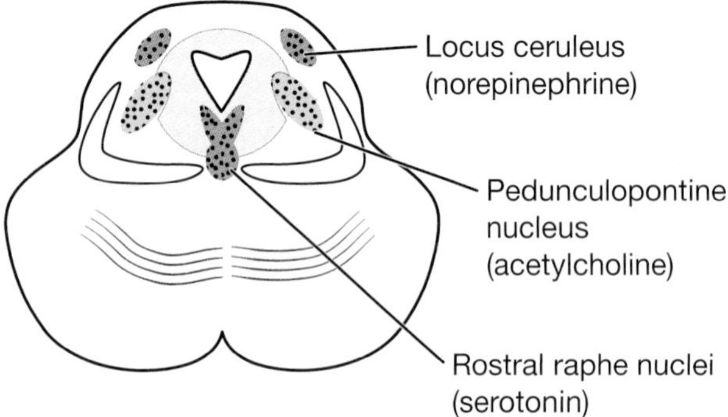

Fig. 10.8. Location of the cholinergic and monoaminergic nuclei in the rostral pontine tegmentum.

All the nuclei of the thalamus proper contain excitatory projection neurons that have L-glutamate as their neurotransmitter. These neurons project to the cerebral cortex and receive input from the cortical areas to which they project (reciprocal connections) (Fig. 10.9). These *corticothalamocortical loops* are important in coordinating activity initiated in different parts of the cerebral cortex involved in a specific task. The temporal synchronization of activity in separate cortical areas is critical for processing sensory information. Each thalamic relay nucleus also contains inhibitory local circuit neurons.

Reticular Nucleus of the Thalamus

The reticular nucleus of the thalamus is a key element of the consciousness system. This nucleus contains a network of highly interconnected neurons that synthesize γ-aminobutyric acid (GABA). The reticular nucleus GABAergic neurons, unlike the neurons of dorsal thalamus, do not project to the cerebral cortex but to the other thalamic nuclei (Fig. 10.9). The reticular nucleus receives excitatory input from the cerebral cortex and sends inhibitory input to all thalamic nuclei. The highly interconnected neurons of the reticular thalamic nucleus participate in reciprocal corticothalamocortical loops that are important for synchronized rhythmic activity of thalamocortical neurons during certain stages of sleep, as discussed below.

- The thalamus acts as a gateway to the cerebral cortex and serves as a relay station, filters information going to the cerebral cortex, and coordinates the activity of the cerebral cortex.

Ascending Pathways

The activating influences of the thalamus, hypothalamus, basal forebrain, and brainstem reticular formation are transmitted to the cerebral cortex by two main types of projection pathways: thalamocortical pathways and extrathalamic pathways (Table 10.2). The thalamic pathways involve the thalamic relay and intralaminar nuclei that project to the cerebral cortex. These thalamocortical inputs are phasic, excitatory, mediated by L-glutamate, and depend on the arrival of input from afferent pathways. The cholinergic and monoaminergic neurons of the basal forebrain, hypothalamus, and brainstem project to both the thalamus and the cerebral cortex (Fig. 10.1). Projections to the relay nuclei and reticular nucleus of the thalamus regulate the pattern of activity of thalamic neurons. This is critical for the gating function of the thalamus for controlling cortical arousal. Direct cholinergic and monoaminergic projections to the cerebral cortex modulate cortical excitability and response to thalamic input (extrathalamic cortical modulation). Unlike the phasic stimulus-specific activity of the direct thalamocortical projections, the modulatory effect

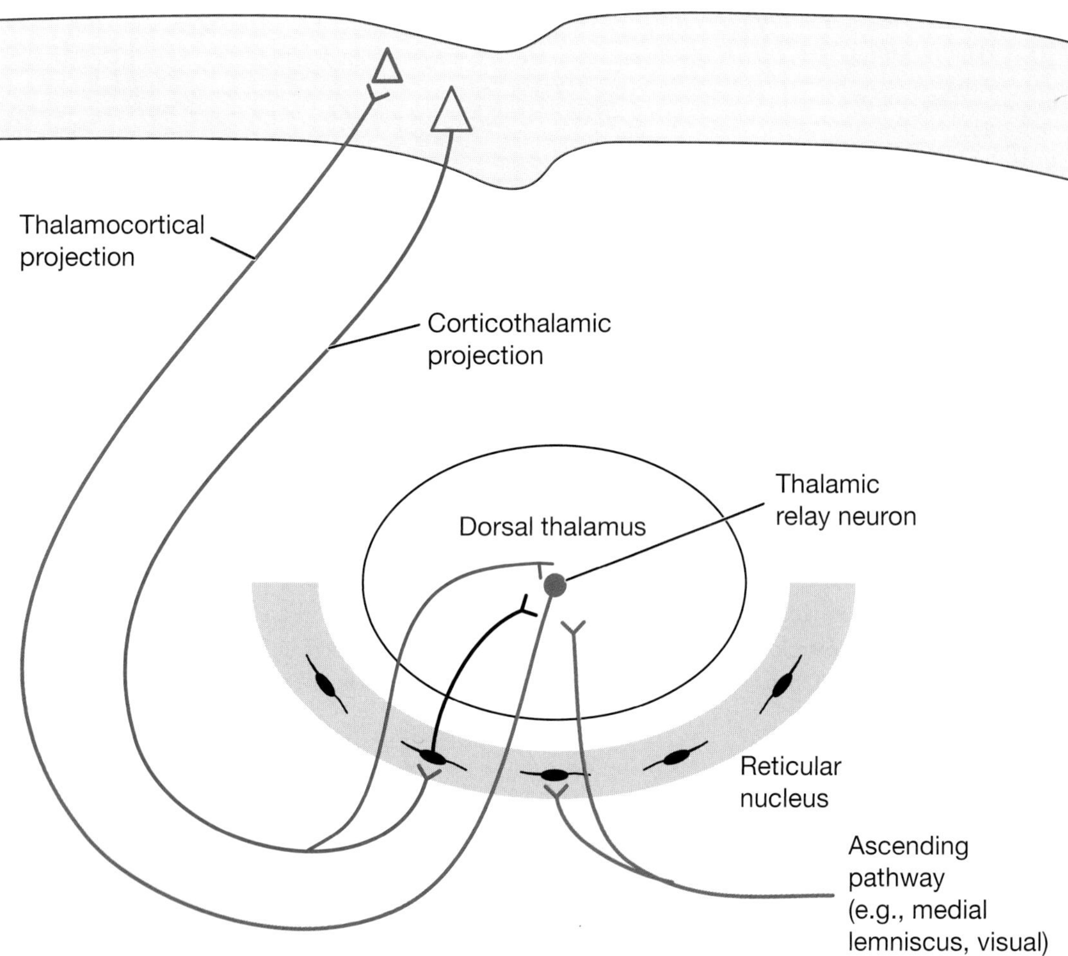

Fig. 10.9. General organization of the thalamus. The thalamus is subdivided into two main components: the dorsal thalamus, which contains the relay nuclei for sensory, motor, and association pathways, and the reticular nucleus of the thalamus. The relay neurons in the dorsal thalamus are excitatory and have L-glutamate as a neurotransmitter. They project to the cerebral cortex and receive reciprocal excitatory input from the cortical areas to which they project. The reticular nucleus contains a network of highly interconnected GABAergic neurons that do not project to the cerebral cortex but to the other thalamic nuclei. The reticular nucleus receives excitatory input from the cerebral cortex and sends inhibitory input to all thalamic nuclei. Reciprocal corticothalamocortical loops are critical for synchronization of activity in widespread areas of the cerebral cortex, during both wakefulness and sleep.

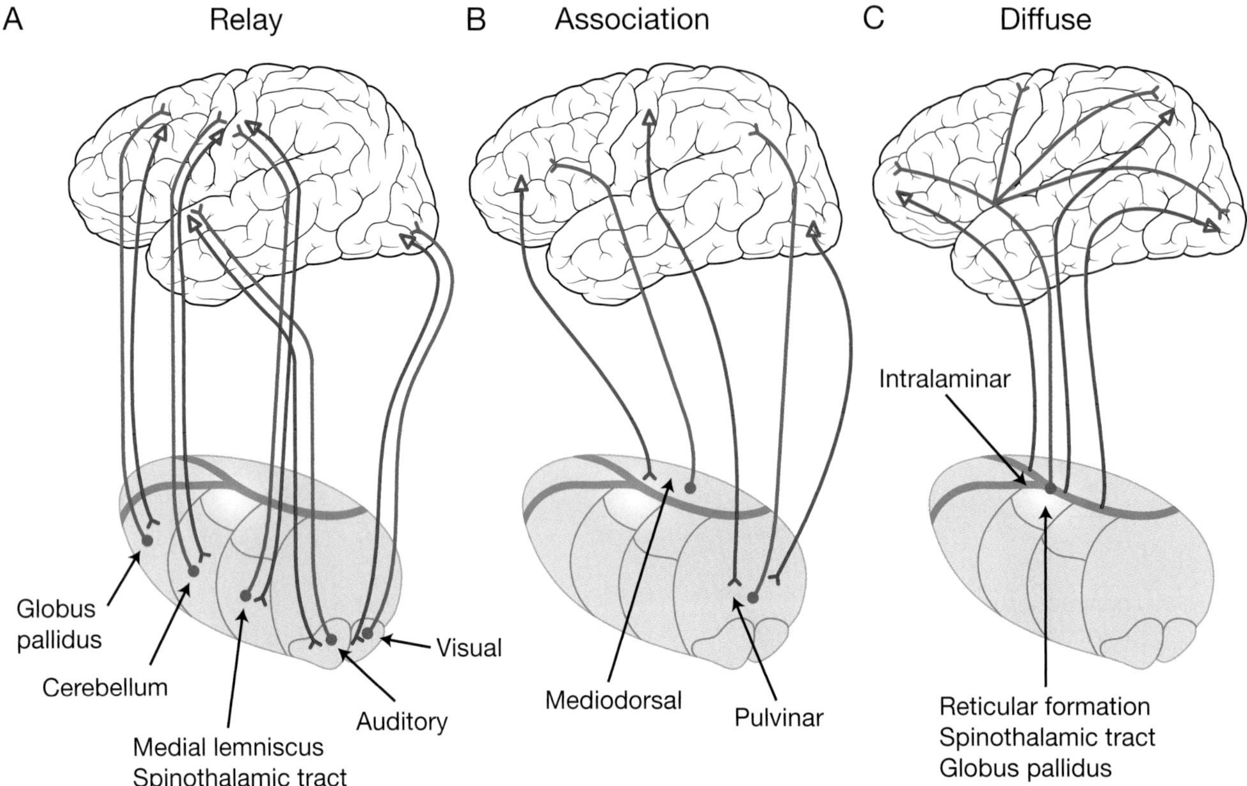

Fig. 10.10. The nuclei of the dorsal thalamus are subdivided into three groups on the basis of their connections and functions. *A*, The specific thalamic relay nuclei receive input from a specific sensory pathway (medial lemniscus, spinothalamic, visual, or auditory), basal ganglia, or cerebellum and project to sensory or motor areas of the cerebral cortex. These relay nuclei are located in the ventral, lateral, and anterior portions of the thalamus. *B*, The association nuclei, including the mediodorsal nucleus and pulvinar, have reciprocal connections with association areas of the cerebral cortex, including the prefrontal cortex and posterior parietal cortex, respectively. *C*, The third group is the so-called nonspecific thalamic nuclei, such as the intralaminar nuclei, whose axons project to widespread areas of the cerebral cortex, basal ganglia, and hypothalamus.

of cholinergic and monoaminergic inputs to the thalamus and cerebral cortex is continuous (tonic) and depends on the behavioral state of the person (e.g., arousal, sleep, or emotion). Because of the simultaneous effect on the thalamus and cerebral cortex, the state-dependent changes in activity of cholinergic and monoaminergic neurons cause profound and global changes in cortical activity.

In addition to the thalamic and cortical projections, the cholinergic and monoaminergic nuclei are intimately interconnected with each other. For example, the cholinergic neurons of the basal forebrain receive input from neurons in the mesopontine tegmentum and noradrenergic neurons in the locus ceruleus. Thus, through projections to the basal forebrain, monoaminergic neurons may indirectly affect cholinergic input to the cerebral cortex.

- **The activating influences of the reticular formation occur by way of the thalamocortical and extrathalamic pathways.**

Cerebral Cortex

Although many specific functions, such as somatic sensation and vision, are relayed and integrated in specific areas of the cerebral cortex, no single cortical area is responsible for the maintenance of consciousness. Indeed, because of the widespread interconnections between the nonspecific thalamic nuclei and the cerebral cortex, all areas of the cortex appear to participate in consciousness and, thus, are considered part of the consciousness system.

Cell Types in the Cerebral Cortex

The cerebral cortex consists of two types of neurons: *pyramidal neurons* and *local interneurons*. Pyramidal neurons are excitatory cells that have glutamate as their neurotransmitter; they project to other cortical areas and to all subcortical structures. Local interneurons have GABA as their neurotransmitter. They are reciprocally connected with pyramidal neurons and form interconnected networks through gap junctions. The pyramidal and local neurons in the cerebral cortex are organized into *functional columns* (Fig. 10.12).

Columnar Organization

Cortical columns are the elementary functional units of the cerebral cortex. Each column extends vertically through cellular layers II to VI and contains pyramidal neurons that are heavily interconnected vertically. The neurons within a column have similar properties, receive the same input from a thalamic relay nucleus, and respond to the same specific types of information. The

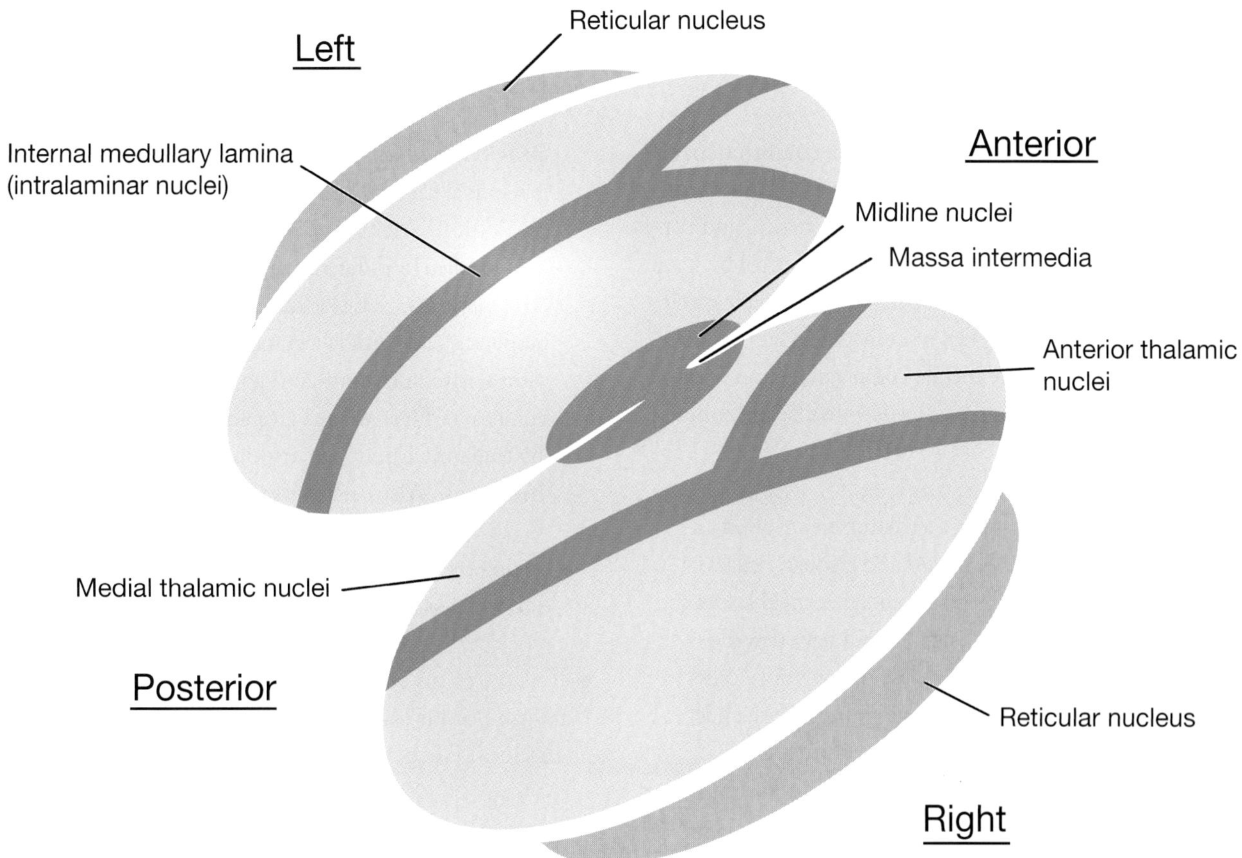

Fig. 10.11. Thalamic nuclei involved in the consciousness system. The intralaminar, midline, and reticular nuclei of the thalamus receive input from the reticular formation and cerebral cortex. The intralaminar and midline nuclei project diffusely to the cerebral cortex, exerting a facilitatory effect on cortical neuronal excitability. The thalamic reticular nucleus does not project to the cerebral cortex but controls the activity of other thalamic nuclei.

Table 10.2. Features of Thalamic and Extrathalamic Pathways to the Cerebral Cortex

Feature	Thalamocortical pathways	Extrathalamic pathways
Origin	Thalamic relay nuclei	Cholinergic and monoaminergic neurons of brainstem, hypothalamus, and basal forebrain
Projection pathway	Thalamic radiations	Medial forebrain bundle
Target	Specific primary and association areas of the cerebral cortex	All primary and association areas of the cerebral cortex Thalamus
Activity	Phasic	Tonic
Effect on cortical neurons	Excitatory	Modulatory
Function	Relays information to the cerebral cortex Filters information to the cerebral cortex Coordinates activity in the cerebral cortex	Modulates excitability of cortical neurons Modulates activity of the thalamus
Dependent on	Specific afferent information	Behavioral state Sleep-wake cycle

properties of cortical neurons within a column depend on the spatial and temporal integration of inputs from various excitatory inputs from thalamocortical and corticocortical connections and inhibitory control by local GABAergic interneurons. The input from each specific thalamic relay nucleus ends in individual columns; however, the input from the intralaminar nuclei and cholinergic and monoaminergic systems spreads horizontally across columns.

Pyramidal neurons within a column are involved in mechanisms of feed-forward and feedback excitation. Pyramidal cells in superficial cortical layers project to other cortical regions and have descending axon collaterals that synapse on pyramidal cells in the deep layers. Pyramidal neurons in deeper cortical layers project to subcortical structures and have ascending collaterals that synapse on pyramidal cells in more superficial layers. All pyramidal neurons within a column receive excitatory input from the thalamus, but this constitutes only 10% of the excitatory input to the column. Most excitatory input is from corticocortical connections from functionally related columns. These interactions provide the basis for abnormal recruitment of pyramidal neurons and the spread of seizure activity. Cortical excitation within and between columns is controlled by different types of local GABAergic interneurons. These interneurons limit the responses of pyramidal neurons to recurrent excitation within a column and participate in lateral inhibition. Thus, when a given column is activated by thalamic input, all surrounding columns are inhibited. Also, networks of interconnected GABAergic interneurons are critical for synchronizing the activity in widespread areas of the cortex, which is important for many cognitive tasks.

- The cerebral cortex is organized into functional columns consisting of excitatory pyramidal neurons and local GABAergic interneurons.

Physiology of the Consciousness System

Neurophysiology of Single Cells

As described in Chapter 5, neurons generate two types of potentials: synaptic potentials and action potentials

(Fig. 10.13). Neurons also have intrinsic membrane properties that are determined by the presence and distribution of different types of ion channels. Because of these intrinsic properties, neurons exhibit spontaneous oscillations of the membrane potential that determine whether, when, and how a neuron responds to a synaptic input. These oscillations allow the neuron 1) to respond only when the synaptic stimuli arrive at a particular time, 2) to serve as pacemakers, or 3) to initiate rhythmic patterns of activity transmitted to other areas of the nervous system.

Synaptic Potential

Synaptic potentials are local potentials generated in the dendrite or soma of a postsynaptic neuron as a result of a neurotransmitter interacting with receptors in the neuron's cell membrane. Synaptic potentials are localized,

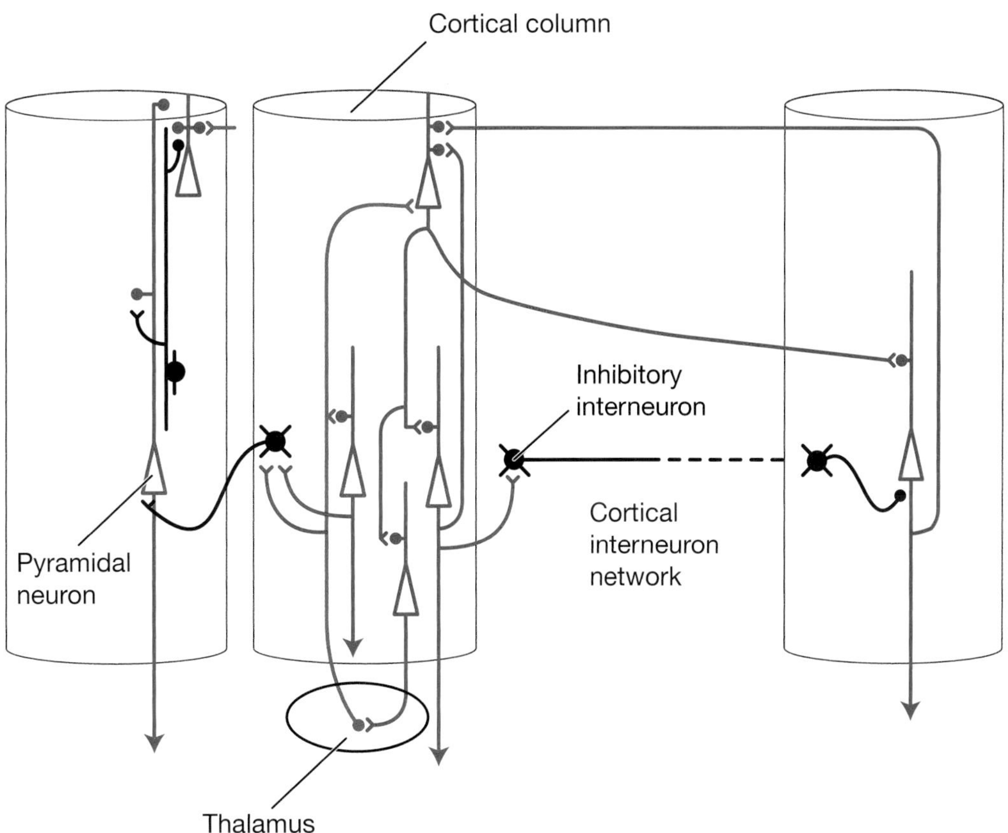

Fig. 10.12. Organization of the cerebral cortex. The cerebral cortex consists of two types of neurons, pyramidal neurons and local interneurons. The pyramidal neurons are excitatory and use glutamate as a neurotransmitter. They project to other cortical areas and all subcortical structures. The local interneurons use GABA as a neurotransmitter, are reciprocally connected with pyramidal neurons, and form interconnected networks through gap junctions. The pyramidal neurons and local interneurons are organized into functional columns. All the neurons in a given column have similar properties, which are determined by the spatial and temporal integration of inputs from several sources, including excitatory thalamocortical and corticocortical connections and local inhibitory interactions. Each column receives excitatory input from the thalamus and from pyramidal neurons in other columns. Within each column, there are excitatory interactions between pyramidal neurons, which are regulated by local GABAergic inhibition via interneurons. These interneurons also participate in lateral inhibition. Networks of interconnected GABAergic interneurons are important in synchronizing the activity in widespread areas of the cerebral cortex, which is critical for many cognitive tasks.

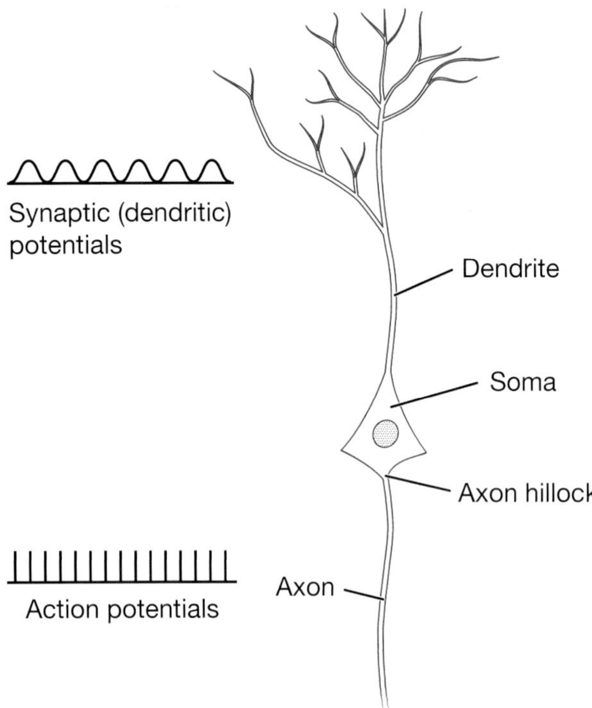

Fig. 10.13. Cortical neuron and synaptic potentials generated in a dendrite and action potentials generated in an axon.

nonpropagated, graded fluctuations of the postsynaptic membrane potential. They are excitatory (excitatory postsynaptic potentials [EPSPs]) when the neurotransmitter causes depolarization of the cell membrane and inhibitory (inhibitory postsynaptic potentials [IPSPs]) when the neurotransmitter causes hyperpolarization of the cell membrane. The duration of these potentials is usually 15 to 20 milliseconds. Because they do not have a refractory period, they can undergo both spatial and temporal summation (see Chapter 5), which determines the probability of a neuron reaching the threshold for generating an action potential.

> Fast EPSPs and IPSPs involve opening of ion channel receptors by excitatory (glutamate) or inhibitory (GABA) neurotransmitters, respectively. The ascending cholinergic and monoaminergic systems have a modulatory effect on the excitability of central nervous system neurons. With few exceptions, acetylcholine and monoamines do not elicit fast EPSPs or IPSPs in the central nervous system, but exert a major influence on the ability of the neuron to respond to excitatory and inhibitory inputs (see Chapter 6).

- Synaptic potentials are local, graded fluctuations of the postsynaptic membrane potential.
- The ascending cholinergic and monoaminergic systems control the excitability of neurons in the central nervous system.

Action Potential

An action potential usually arises in the initial segment (near the axon hillock) and propagates along the axon (Fig. 10.13). It occurs only when the neuronal membrane is depolarized beyond a critical (threshold) level. It is an all-or-none phenomenon propagated down the axon and followed by a temporary refractory period (Fig. 10.13). The duration of the action potential is brief (usually less than 1 millisecond).

- Action potentials are an all-or-none phenomenon and are propagated down the axon and, in some cases, dendrites.

Intrinsic Electrophysiologic Behavior of Neurons

The heterogeneous repertoire and distribution of ion channels in different types of neurons results in a wide variety of patterns of neuronal activity in the brain. For example, neurons may generate typical fast action potentials, slow action potentials, or long-duration potentials that allow repetitive firing in response to a single stimulus. There are relatively silent neurons that have generally steady resting potentials and require strong stimuli for activation. Others are pacing neurons that fire repetitively at a constant frequency. A typical example is a brainstem monoaminergic neuron, which discharges spontaneously at a low frequency. Bursting neurons generate regular bursts of action potentials that are separated by hyperpolarization of the membrane. This generates spontaneous rhythmic burst firing, which is a pattern seen in the cerebral cortex and thalamus. Thalamic neurons that project to the cerebral cortex have two basic modes of generating action potentials: *tonic* (single spike activity) and *rhythmic burst* activity. The pattern of activity of these neurons changes during the sleep-wake cycle according to the presence or absence of cholinergic input, and this has an important role in gating the transmission of sensory information to the cerebral cortex (Table 10.3).

> Whether a thalamocortical neuron fires in a tonic or rhythmic burst pattern depends on the value of the membrane potential at the time that the neuron is activated. The single spike mode occurs when the membrane potential is relatively depolarized from the excitatory influence of the cholinergic system. This allows precise transmission of sensory information to the cerebral cortex and is typical of the states of activation of the cerebral cortex, such as wakefulness, characterized by fast cortical electrical activity. In contrast, rhythmic burst firing occurs when the thalamic cell is relatively hyperpolarized because of the withdrawal of cholinergic activation. In this case, thalamocortical transmission does not reflect sensory input to thalamus because thalamic neurons discharge rhythmically at a frequency that depends on their intrinsic properties, independently of the frequency of the input. This pattern of activity is typical of states of inactivation of the cerebral cortex, such as during deep sleep, characterized by slow rhythmic electrical activity.

- Some neurons have electrophysiologic properties that determine their responsiveness to synaptic inputs.
- The pattern of activity of thalamocortical neurons gates the access of information to the cerebral cortex.

Neurophysiology of Neuronal Aggregates

Neurons in the central nervous system do not function in isolation but as part of neuronal aggregates. In particular, neurons of the cerebral cortex have rich synaptic interconnections within and between columns, and the electrical activity of the aggregate reflects the summated effect of all the dendritic potentials and action potentials occurring within that aggregate or cortical column. This activity is recorded as complex waveforms rather than as simple spikes of single cells. The cerebral cortex generates these electrical waves in response to local activity within each functional column and the combined activity of several columns in response to input from the specific and nonspecific thalamic nuclei and the extensive corticocortical connections. Because the intralaminar thalamic nuclei have widespread connections with the cerebral cortex, they can exert a strong synchronizing influence on cortical activity.

- Neurons have synaptic interconnections and function as neuronal aggregates (columns).

Table 10.3. Functional States of the Thalamocortical Circuits and Cerebral Cortex

Feature	Active state	Inactive state
Ascending input from cholinergic mesopontine neurons	Present	Reduced
Pattern of activity in thalamic relay nuclei	Single spikes	Rhythmic burst firing
Relay of sensory input to the cerebral cortex	Present	Impaired
Electroencephalogram	Low-voltage, fast activity	High-voltage, rhythmic slow activity
Examples	Wakefulness REM sleep	Non-REM sleep General anesthesia Absence seizure Coma

REM, rapid eye movement.

The Electroencephalogram

Electrical activity of the cerebral cortex can be detected with the *electroencephalograph* (EEG), which records cortical activity from electrodes placed on the scalp (Fig. 10.14). This brain wave activity consists of continuous rhythmic or arrhythmic oscillating waveforms that arise from the dendrites of pyramidal cells and vary in frequency, amplitude, polarity, and shape.

> These electrical potentials are usually in the range of 20 to 50 μV and reflect the summation of synaptic potentials of many dendrites lying near the surface of the cerebral cortex. The fluctuation of the EEG is due to varied excitatory and inhibitory synaptic potentials impinging on the dendritic membranes.

The cortical activity recorded in the EEG is the result of the activity of cortical ensembles modulated by synaptic input from other cortical regions and from the basal forebrain, thalamus, and brainstem. Thalamic influences determine the intrinsic resting frequencies of the brain waves, because structures in the thalamus serve as the "pacemakers" in producing widespread synchronization and rhythmicity of cortical activity over the cerebral hemispheres. Cholinergic and monoaminergic inputs modulate the excitability and pattern of activity of thalamic and cortical neurons.

Electrical activity recorded by the EEG from the cerebral cortex is classified into four main types, according to the frequency or number of waveforms per second (hertz) (Fig. 10.15).

1. *Beta activity* is low-amplitude fast activity occurring at a frequency of more than 13 Hz. This type of activity is usually seen over the anterior head regions.
2. *Alpha activity* is rhythmic activity at a frequency of 8 to 13 Hz. This rhythm occurs in the posterior head regions and is the predominant background activity during the relaxed waking state when the eyes are closed. With eye opening or with attention, the rhythmic alpha background is attenuated and replaced by a low-voltage pattern.

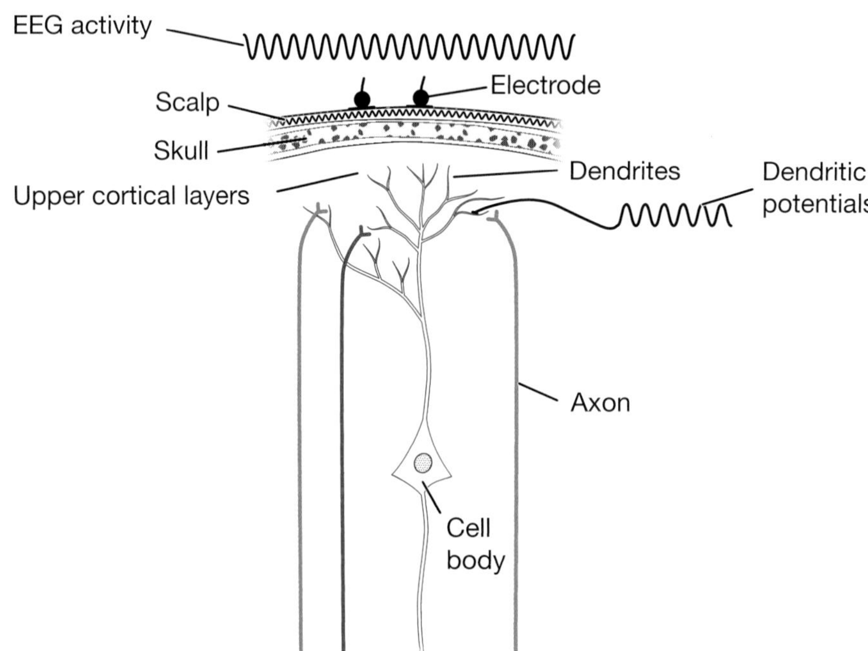

Fig. 10.14. The EEG is a recording of the dendritic potentials in the upper cortical layers as they appear at the scalp.

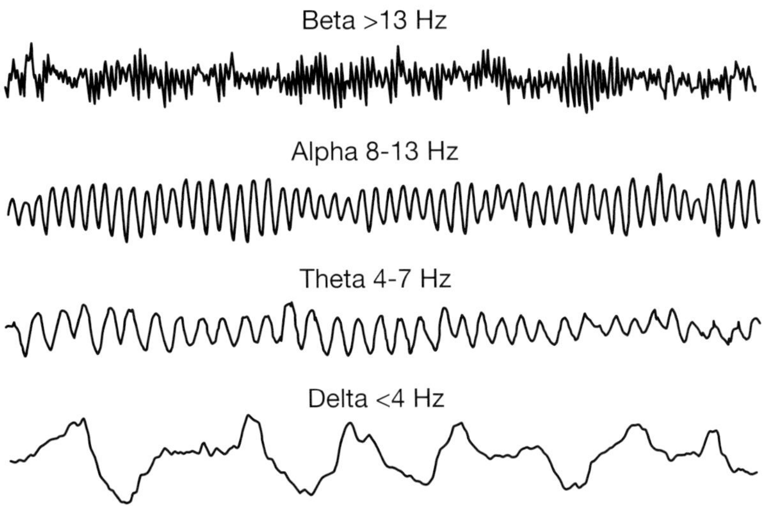

Fig. 10.15. Four basic EEG frequencies.

3. *Theta activity* ranges from 4 to 7 Hz and may be normal when present in a child or in an adult in a drowsy state, but in a fully awake adult, it is abnormal.
4. *Delta activity* is the slowest waveform, with a frequency less than 4 Hz. This activity is normal when present in an infant or a sleeping adult but is abnormal under any other circumstances.

■ The electroencephalogram is a record of the electrical activity of the cerebral cortex.

Functions of the Consciousness System

Consciousness is defined as *awareness of environment and self.* It implies a condition in which the person is capable of perceiving stimuli from the environment and, if the motor system is intact, responding appropriately to the stimuli. The consciousness system has two principal functions: 1) maintenance of the *waking state* (*arousal*, or level of consciousness) and 2) content of experience (*awareness*). In addition, the consciousness system regulates the sleep-wake cycle and is critical for attention.

■ Consciousness consists of wakefulness (arousal, or level of consciousness) and awareness (content of consciousness).

Maintenance of the Waking State (Arousal)

Arousal and wakefulness depend on 1) the integrity of the brainstem reticular formation, hypothalamus, basal forebrain, and thalamus; 2) their cortical projections; and 3) the cerebral cortex as a whole. The electrophysiologic correlates of wakefulness are the alpha rhythm (8 to 13 Hz), which is recorded in the posterior head regions and characterizes a waking state with the eyes closed, and a beta rhythm, which occurs in the anterior head regions at frequencies higher than 13 Hz and is associated with mental activity. The low-voltage, fast pattern of the waking state reflects activity synchronized across widespread areas of the brain at a *gamma frequency* (greater than 30 Hz) that correlates with information processing during cognitive tasks. With progressive decrease in the level of cortical arousal, the EEG shows progressive slowing and increased rhythmicity, manifested as a delta rhythm during deep sleep. This reflects the rhythmic burst activity of thalamic neurons that becomes synchronized throughout the cerebral cortex through corticothalamocortical interactions.

Direct electrical stimulation of the reticular formation in a sleeping animal produces a state of behavioral arousal, indicated by opening of the eyes, turning of the head, and movement of the limbs.

Associated with this is a change in the EEG from a low-frequency synchronous sleep pattern to the low-voltage, fast pattern of the waking state.

The reticular formation receives sensory input from collaterals of every major sensory pathway. This keeps the reticular activating system in an excited state and, in turn, activates the cerebral cortex to maintain wakefulness. The importance of sensory influences in maintaining a wakeful state is illustrated by the progressive decrease in the degree of wakefulness that occurs with loss or reduction in sensory input. If the consciousness system is intact, stimulation of the reticular activating system produces an arousal response; however, if a portion of the consciousness system is destroyed, particularly the rostral part of the brainstem and thalamus, a permanent sleep state ensues.

The pattern of EEG activity during wakefulness and sleep reflects the level of activity of cholinergic and monoaminergic neurons of the basal forebrain, hypothalamus, and brainstem. During wakefulness, the tonic activity of cholinergic and monoaminergic neurons maintains a state of excitability in the thalamocortical circuits and facilitates sensory processing. A progressive decrease in the activity of these neurons results in progressive synchronization and slowing of thalamic activity and decreased excitability of cortical neurons.

Cholinergic and monoaminergic inputs have a dual effect on thalamocortical circuits: 1) at the level of the thalamus, they inhibit rhythmic burst activity and facilitate sensory transmission, and 2) at the level of the cerebral cortex, they increase excitability and responsiveness of cortical neurons to thalamic and cortical inputs.

- Maintenance of the wake state (arousal) depends on the tonic activity of brainstem cholinergic and monoaminergic neurons and their thalamocortical targets.

Attention and Awareness

A second function of the consciousness system is conscious awareness, that is, the content of consciousness. This is determined by the integrated activity of the cerebral cortex, including the primary sensory areas and association areas involved in high-level cognitive processing. These association areas include the prefrontal cortex and posterior parietal cortex, areas that have a critical role in *attention*. Attention is a cognitive function that allows the selection of only those sensory stimuli that are meaningful for controlling action, according to the goals and motivations of the subject. Attention selectively enhances the response to a specific stimulus and filters unwanted information. For example, when reading a book, a person is absorbed by the words on the page and is not aware of body contact with the chair or outside noises. The consciousness system selectively sends alerting signals to the cerebral cortical area that receives visual input and suppresses sensory input in auditory or somatic pathways. Thus, the consciousness system acts in an adaptive manner to prevent the cerebral cortex from being overwhelmed and to permit selective attention to specific external and internal stimuli. Attention is a mechanism by which only one of a large number of stimuli reaches conscious awareness. This may depend on the stimulus itself (its intensity, salience, or novelty) or on the influence that the prefrontal cortex exerts on the responsiveness of cortical sensory areas to input. Cholinergic and monoaminergic inputs are critical for selective attention and awareness.

Cholinergic neurons in the nucleus basalis of Meynert receive excitatory input from the prefrontal cortex and project to the primary and associative sensory areas. These cortical areas contribute to the selection and processing of behaviorally significant sensory stimuli. The dopaminergic system, which arises from neurons in the ventral tegmental area and projects to the prefrontal cortex, is activated by reward and is important in motivated behavior. Noradrenergic neurons of the locus ceruleus project to the basal forebrain and sensory cortex and mediate stress-induced increase in attention. The cholinergic and monoaminergic systems also affect the selection of specific sensory stimuli by modulating the relay of sensory information in the thalamus.

- Selective attention allows selection of a specific sensory stimulus while preventing distracting stimuli from reaching awareness.
- Attention depends on a network that includes the prefrontal and parietal cortices, cholinergic and monoaminergic neurons, and thalamus.

Sleep-Wake Cycle

Consciousness may be altered by several conditions. However, a normal physiologic alteration is that associated with sleep, which is defined as a cyclic, temporary, and physiologic loss of consciousness that is readily, promptly, and completely reversed by appropriate stimuli.

Sleep is an active phenomenon. Hypnogenic areas of the brain and neurochemical substances actively promote sleep and inhibit the arousal system. The structures involved in the regulation of the wake-sleep cycle include several areas of the hypothalamus, the basal forebrain, the cholinergic and monoaminergic groups of the brainstem, and the reticular nucleus of the thalamus (Fig. 10.16).

- Sleep is a cyclic, temporary, physiologic loss of consciousness that is reversible.

Two distinctive patterns of sleep are seen in normal persons: *rapid eye movement* (REM) *sleep* and *non–rapid eye movement* (non-REM or NREM) *sleep* (Table 10.4). These states are reflected by typical patterns in the EEG (Fig. 10.17).

Phenomenology

Non-REM Sleep

Non-REM sleep is sleep during which no rapid eye movements occur. There is widespread decrease in brain activity. Vital signs and autonomic activity are more

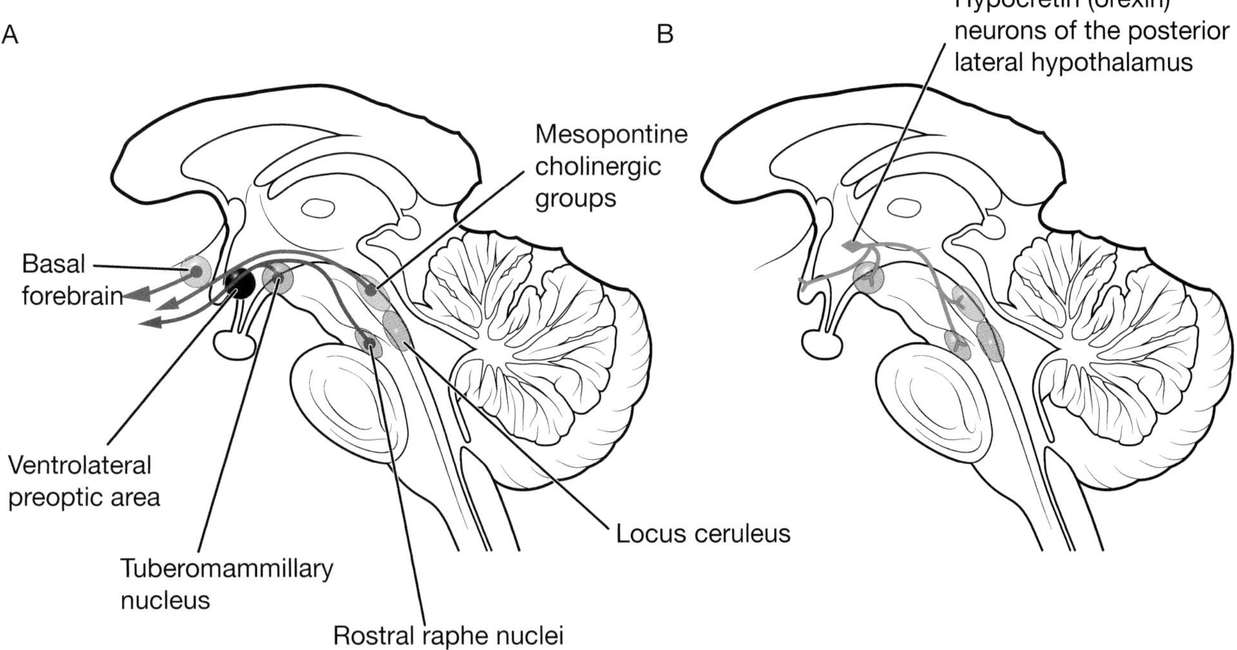

Fig. 10.16. Areas of the brain related to sleep. *A*, The ventrolateral preoptic area is necessary for onset of sleep. It inhibits the arousal-inducing cholinergic neurons of the basal forebrain and mesopontine tegmentum, histamine neurons of the tuberomammillary nucleus, norepinephrine neurons of the locus ceruleus, and serotonin neurons of the rostral raphe. *B*, The hypocretin (orexin) neurons of the posterior lateral hypothalamus prevent abrupt transitions between wakefulness and sleep through excitatory projections to the cholinergic and monoaminergic cell groups. The cholinergic neurons in the mesopontine tegmentum, via reciprocal interactions with the raphe nuclei and locus ceruleus, are critical for the transition between non-rapid eye movement and rapid eye movement sleep.

Table 10.4. Characteristics of the Two Major Patterns of Sleep (Non-REM and REM)

Feature	Non-REM sleep	REM sleep
Electroencephalogram	Spindles, V waves, K-complexes, delta waves	Low-voltage pattern
Eye movements	Slow (during drowsiness)	Rapid
Muscle tone	Some tone in postural muscle groups	Muscle atonia except in diaphragm, sphincter, and eye muscles
Muscle twitches	No	Yes
Vital signs	Stable	Fluctuating
Penile erection	Rare	Common
Dreams	Rare	Common
Percentage of sleep in adults	75-80	20-25
Percentage of sleep in infants	50	50

REM, rapid eye movement.

stable. During non-REM sleep, the EEG shows different patterns, depending on the depth of sleep (Fig. 10.17). During drowsiness, the EEG has a low-amplitude background with an attenuation of rhythmic activity. During light-to-medium levels of sleep, specific EEG waveforms (sleep spindles, V waves, and K complexes) are present. The sinusoidal waveforms ranging from 10 to 14 Hz and usually present over the frontal head regions are called *sleep spindles*. High-amplitude, sharply contoured waveforms occurring over the frontal and parietal regions are *V waves* (vertex waves). High-amplitude diphasic V waves, called *K complexes*, often signify a partial arousal response in the EEG. During deep levels of sleep, widespread high-amplitude slow waves are present. Deep stages of non-REM sleep are characterized by the presence of delta waves (1 to 4 Hz).

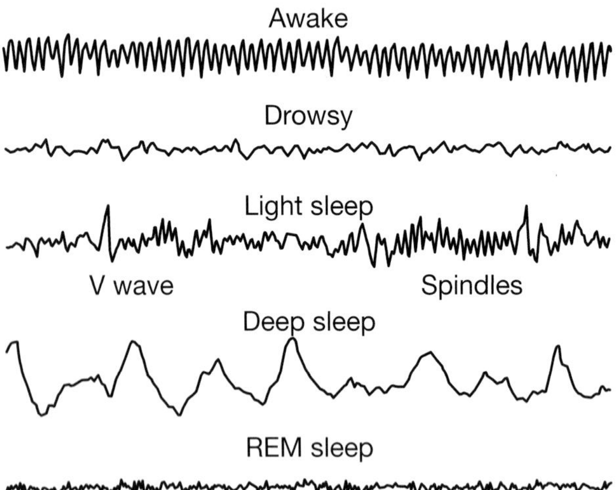

Fig. 10.17. EEG patterns of wakefulness and different levels of sleep. The awake EEG is recorded from occipital areas with the eyes closed. With the eyes open, the EEG resembles the rapid eye movement (REM) sleep pattern.

REM Sleep

Features of REM sleep include rapid conjugate eye movements; fluctuations in blood pressure, heart rate, and respiration; poikilothermia; a decrease in muscle tone; muscle twitches; and penile erection. This is also the stage of sleep during which dreams occur. An EEG recorded during REM sleep shows a low-amplitude fast pattern resembling that of a person in an alert state with the eyes open (Fig. 10.17). Because of the above characteristics, REM sleep is also known as *paradoxical*, *active*, or *dream sleep*.

During a night's sleep in adults, non-REM sleep occurs first and generally lasts for 60 to 90 minutes. It is then interrupted by a REM period, which may last from several minutes to half an hour and is followed by another non-REM period. A total night's sleep usually consists of four to six cycles of alternating non-REM and REM sleep. Non-REM sleep is the predominant type of sleep in adults and accounts for 75% to 80% of the nocturnal sleep pattern, whereas REM sleep accounts for only 20% to 25%. In newborn infants, however, 50% of sleep is REM sleep.

- The two main types of sleep states are REM sleep and non-REM sleep.

Physiology

The three behavioral states of wakefulness, non-REM sleep, and REM sleep are regulated by complex interactions among the hypothalamus, brainstem, thalamus, and cerebral cortex (Fig. 10.16). During the sleep-wake cycle, fluctuations in the activity of hypothalamic and brainstem cholinergic and monoaminergic neurons are responsible for the transition between these three behavioral states (Fig. 10.18).

Wakefulness

During wakefulness, both mesopontine cholinergic neurons and monoaminergic neurons (locus ceruleus, raphe nuclei, and tuberomammillary nucleus) are active (Table 10.5). In particular, the activity of the histamine neurons in the tuberomammillary nucleus is critical for maintenance of wakefulness (this explains why over-the-counter "cold pills" containing antihistamines cause drowsiness).

> Cholinergic and monoaminergic activity maintain an active state in the thalamocortical circuits that is characterized by tonic activity in thalamic relay neurons and low-amplitude fast cortical oscillations in the EEG. During this stage, neurons in the cerebral cortex are receptive to peripheral sensory input and there is temporal synchronization of firing of separate groups of neurons in different areas of the cerebral cortex engaged in a particular task.

Non-REM Sleep

The sleep-wake cycle is only one of several circadian rhythms that occur approximately every 24 hours. Many other biologic systems, such as hormonal secretion, have a circadian pattern. Circadian rhythms are controlled by a biologic clock located in the *suprachiasmatic nucleus*, located just above the optic chiasm in the anterior hypothalamus. Neuronal activity in this nucleus is synchronized with the diurnal light-dark cycle through input from the retina. Among other rhythms, the suprachiasmatic nucleus controls the cyclic secretion of *melatonin* from the *pineal gland*.

The transition between wakefulness and sleep results from a combination of circadian factors triggered by

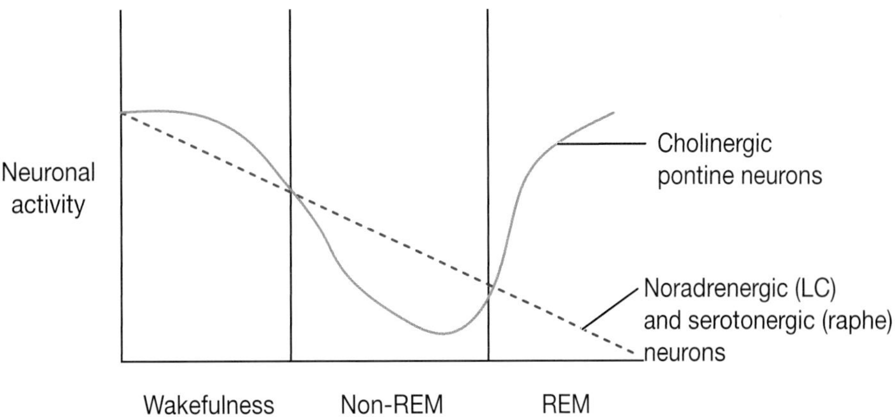

Fig. 10.18. Changes in neurochemical activity during wake-sleep states. LC, locus ceruleus; REM, rapid eye movement (sleep).

Table 10.5. Activity Within the Consciousness System During the Sleep-Wake Cycle

Feature	Wakefulness	Non-REM sleep	REM sleep
Hypothalamic influence	Posterior lateral hypothalamus	Ventrolateral preoptic area	Ventrolateral preoptic area
Cholinergic input	Active	Reduced	Active
Monoaminergic input	Active	Reduced	Absent
Electroencephalogram	Alpha rhythm (8-10 Hz) with eyes closed; low-voltage, fast activity with eyes open	Sleep spindles K-complex High-voltage, slow rhythm (delta rhythm)	Low-voltage, fast activity
Attention	Present	Absent	Absent
Content of consciousness	Outside and stored information	Not accessible	Stored information (dreams)

REM, rapid eye movement.

signals from the suprachiasmatic nucleus and homeostatic factors determined by the duration of previous wakefulness. The suprachiasmatic nucleus is activated by light and inhibits the secretion of melatonin by the pineal gland. Therefore, melatonin secretion increases during darkness, corresponding to the night period in humans. Sleep deprivation leads to progressive accumulation of adenosine in the basal forebrain. This inhibitory neurotransmitter inhibits the activity of basal forebrain neurons involved in wakefulness and, thus, induces sleep. The stimulating effects of caffeine may partly reflect blockade of adenosine receptors in the brain.

The major sleep-promoting region is the *ventrolateral preoptic area* of the hypothalamus (Fig. 10.16). This area receives input from the suprachiasmatic nucleus and basal forebrain and contains GABAergic neurons that project to and inhibit the activity of hypothalamic and brainstem monoaminergic and cholinergic neurons involved in arousal. Sleep induction may constitute a thermoregulatory mechanism leading to heat loss. Heat-sensitive neurons in the preoptic region of the hypothalamus are connected with sleep-promoting neurons in the ventrolateral preoptic area.

The abrupt transition between wakefulness and sleep is prevented by a group of neurons in the posterior lateral hypothalamus that synthesize *hypocretin,* also called *orexin* (Fig. 10.16). These neurons have widespread projections that activate the cholinergic and monoaminergic neurons, thus preventing sudden transition from wakefulness to sleep (particularly REM sleep). The inhibitory action of the ventrolateral preoptic area eventually causes a progressive decrease in activity of both the cholinergic and monoaminergic neurons during non-REM sleep (Fig. 10.18). The interruption of the tonic influence of these neurons on the thalamus is manifested by increased oscillatory activity within thalamocortical circuits, reflected by the appearance of sleep spindles and then by delta waves in the EEG. Functional neuroimaging studies indicate that during non-REM sleep, there is a global decrease in cerebral energy metabolism and blood flow compared with those of the waking state.

REM Sleep

The appearance of REM sleep is marked by increased activity of cholinergic neurons in dorsal pons and maximally suppressed activity of monoaminergic neurons (Fig. 10.18). These pontine cholinergic neurons are called *REM-on cells.* They provide excitatory input to the thalamus and brainstem and have reciprocal excitatory interactions with glutamatergic neurons in rostral pons. The activating effects of cholinergic and glutamatergic neurons on the thalamus lead to cortical activation. This is reflected in the EEG as a low-amplitude fast activity similar to that seen during the wake state. Functional neuroimaging studies indicate that during REM sleep metabolic activity increases in the pons, midbrain, thalamus, hypothalamus, amygdala, basal ganglia, and particularly anterior cingulate cortex, but activity remains depressed in dorsolateral prefrontal cortex. The activity of cortical circuits, particularly those involved in memory and emotion, is dominated by internal stimuli (e.g., from stimuli stored as memories), and these provide the content of dreams during REM sleep.

The pontine REM-on neurons project to the pontine paramedian reticular formation, which activates ocular motor neurons responsible to rapid eye movements. They also project to the reticular formation of the medulla that is the origin of reticulospinal inhibitory pathways that use glycine and reduce the excitability of spinal reflexes, producing muscle atonia.

The noradrenergic neurons of the locus ceruleus and the serotonergic neurons of the raphe nuclei are called *REM-off neurons* because their activity is suppressed during REM sleep. These neurons inhibit the REM-on neurons; thus, withdrawal of this inhibition may contribute to the triggering of REM sleep.

- The cycle of wakefulness, non-REM sleep, and REM sleep is regulated by specific neurochemical systems of the brainstem, hypothalamus, and thalamus.
- During wakefulness, the cholinergic system is responsible for thalamocortical activation, and the monoaminergic systems are responsible for the processing of external inputs.
- Induction of non-REM sleep involves the inhibition of cholinergic and monoaminergic neurons by the ventrolateral preoptic area.
- The hypocretin (orexin) hypothalamic neurons prevent abrupt transitions between wakefulness and sleep.
- During REM sleep, pontine cholinergic (REM-on) neurons are active and monoaminergic (REM-off) neurons are silent.
- Activity of cholinergic REM-on neurons also triggers cortical activation, rapid eye movements, and muscle atonia.

Clinical Correlations

Sleep Disorders

A disorder of sleep control mechanisms characterized by excessive sleepiness is called *narcolepsy*. The patient falls asleep spontaneously and precipitously at any time during the day. These episodes are most frequent during monotonous situations. In addition, the patient may have cataplexy, sleep paralysis, hypnagogic hallucinations, and disturbed nocturnal sleep. An abrupt loss of muscle tone that may cause the patient to fall suddenly to the ground is called *cataplexy*. It is precipitated by emotional events such as laughter, fright, and excitement. During the transition between wakefulness and sleep, *sleep paralysis* occurs. This is a temporary state involving the inability to move. False visual or auditory perceptions, called *hypnagogic hallucinations*, occur just before the patient falls asleep and often in conjunction with sleep paralysis. Narcolepsy is the manifestation of the intrusion of REM sleep phenomena during wakefulness. It is associated with the loss of hypocretin neurons in the posterior lateral hypothalamus.

- Narcolepsy is characterized by excessive sleepiness, cataplexy, sleep paralysis, hypnagogic hallucinations, and disturbed nocturnal sleep.

The condition in which the patient stops breathing when asleep is *sleep apnea*. This may be due to upper airway obstruction or depression of central respiratory mechanisms. After a period of apnea, which may last up to a minute, a patient with obstructive sleep apnea arouses from sleep with noisy gasping respirations. When the patient goes back to sleep, the cycle is repeated. As a result, the patient has fragmented sleep and is excessively drowsy when awake.

The inappropriate enactment of dreams and intermittent motor activity during REM sleep is referred to as *REM sleep behavior disorder*. In this disorder, the motor atonia that usually occurs during REM sleep is lost; consequently, patients can perform various movements such as jumping or falling out of bed, hitting objects or bed partners, and vocalizing. These patients can injure themselves or bed partners. Some patients with REM sleep behavior disorder have or develop a neurodegenerative disorder characterized by α-synuclein inclusion bodies in neurons or glial cells. This includes Parkinson disease, Lewy body dementia, and multiple system atrophy.

The disorder consisting of periodic or repetitive stereotyped flexion-extension movements of the limbs, usually the legs, that occur during sleep and cause intermittent arousal or awakening is *periodic limb movement*. Other types of sleep disorders are *sleep walking* (*somnambulism*) and *sleep terrors*. They occur predominantly during arousal from deep levels of non-REM sleep. Prolonged sleep deprivation can cause decreased vigilance and attention span, poor performance of tasks, increased irritability, diplopia, unsteadiness, slurring of speech, and, occasionally, hallucinations.

■ Sleep disorders include narcolepsy, sleep apnea syndrome, REM sleep behavior disorder, periodic limb movement disorder, sleep walking, and sleep terrors.

Clinical Problem 10.1.

A 33-year-old man is evaluated for excessive sleepiness over the past 8 years. He falls asleep uncontrollably during conferences at work. He also describes episodes in which he drops an object held in his hand after he laughs.

a. What is the name of this disorder?
b. What are other features of this disorder?
c. What physiologic abnormality causes this disorder?
d. What is the pathologic substrate of this disorder?

Disorders of Consciousness

As described above in this chapter, consciousness is a function of the combined activity of the reticular activating system, thalamus, and cerebral cortex. Major damage to or depression of the brainstem or bilateral hemispheric dysfunction (or both) produces a pathologic alteration in consciousness. Lesions that alter consciousness are located at the supratentorial or posterior fossa level. Clinical and experimental evidence indicates that the functional integrity of the rostral pontine and mesencephalic reticular formation, thalamus, and cerebral cortex bilaterally is critical for the maintenance of consciousness. The three basic mechanisms that affect the consciousness system are 1) lesions of the brainstem reticular activating system or posterior hypothalamus bilaterally, 2) bilateral interruption of the ascending projections at the level of the thalamus, and 3) diffuse or bilateral hemispheric cortical lesions. These lesions may affect awareness, arousal, wake-sleep states, or vital functions, depending on the level of involvement (Fig. 10.19). Focal or unilateral lesions of the cerebral hemispheres do not cause loss of consciousness as long as the projections of the consciousness system to at least one cerebral hemisphere are intact. However, if there is bilateral destruction of the cerebral hemispheres or if a unilateral hemispheric lesion produces a mass effect resulting in the interruption of the reticular activating pathways at the level of the diencephalon, there is no longer a substratum for consciousness, and unconsciousness ensues.

Disorders of consciousness may be transient or prolonged and may vary from mildly increased sleepiness to deep coma. Transient causes include concussion, seizures, syncope, and metabolic encephalopathy. They reflect reversible functional impairment of the neurons of the consciousness system. Prolonged or irreversible states include coma, persistent vegetative state, and minimal conscious state. They reflect severe and irreversible damage of some or all components of the consciousness system.

■ Loss of consciousness can occur with lesions of the brainstem reticular activating system or posterior hypothalamus bilaterally, interruption of the ascending projections at the level of the thalamus, or diffuse or bilateral cortical lesions.

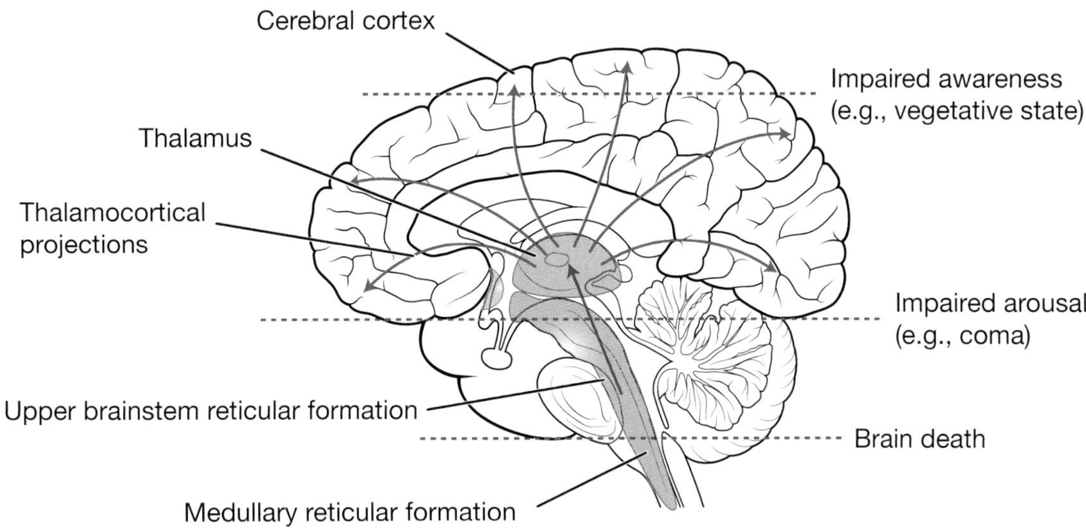

Fig. 10.19. Clinical consequences of impairment at different levels of the consciousness system.

Coma and Related Disorders of Arousal

Coma is a state of extended unconsciousness in which the patient is unarousable and shows little or no spontaneous movement and little or no alerting response to painful or noxious stimuli. Often, the muscle-stretch reflexes, the plantar responses, and the pupillary light reflexes are depressed or absent. Vital signs are usually altered, particularly with lesions affecting the brainstem; the patient has a slow and variable pulse rate and a periodic respiratory pattern.

Less severe degrees of impaired arousal are referred to as somnolence, obtundation, and stupor. In *somnolence*, the patient is easily aroused and shows appropriate verbal and motor responses to sensory stimuli. When the stimulus stops, the patient drifts back to sleep. In *obtundation*, the alertness of the patient is mildly to moderately decreased. When left undisturbed, the patient falls asleep; when aroused, he or she shows a slowed or reduced response to all forms of stimuli. In *stupor*, the patient often shows a moderate amount of spontaneous movement and can be aroused to respond purposefully to afferent stimuli. If sufficiently aroused, the patient can give a brief response to questions or simple commands.

The definitions of somnolence, obtundation, and stupor lack precision, and the degree of impaired consciousness can be assessed more objectively with measurements of eye opening, verbal responses, and motor responses elicited by stimuli of different intensity. One such measurement is the *Glasgow Coma Scale*, discussed below.

In contrast to the pathologic alterations described above, *sleep* is a normal physiologic state, but one that also can be associated with pathologic involvement of the consciousness system. A sleeping person, compared with one in coma, is fully aroused by appropriate stimuli. During sleep, the eyes are closed, the muscles are relaxed, and cardiac output, pulse rate, blood pressure, and respiration are decreased.

- There are various degrees of altered arousal: coma, stupor, obtundation, and somnolence.

Coma may result from structural or metabolic disorders. Direct damage or depression of the consciousness system in the posterior fossa or diencephalon may occur from infarction, hemorrhage, neoplasm, trauma, metabolic disturbances, or anesthetic agents and drugs. Unilateral lesions of the cerebral hemispheres do not usually cause coma if the consciousness system is intact. However, a unilateral lesion that causes a pressure effect or swelling of the brain can involve the cerebral hemispheres or brainstem (or both) bilaterally and impair consciousness. Thus, indirect involvement of the consciousness system also can result in coma. This involvement is usually from mass lesions that are extrinsic to the consciousness system and compress or distort the diencephalon and brainstem. Common examples are mass lesions of the posterior fossa (e.g., a cerebellar neoplasm) or expanding unilateral cerebral masses that cause herniation of the brain contents and secondary compression of diencephalic or midbrain structures (see Chapter 15).

Coma can also result from bilateral processes that diffusely affect the cerebral hemispheres, such as encephalitis, meningitis, subarachnoid hemorrhage, metabolic disturbances (e.g., hypoglycemia), hypoxia, some degenerative diseases, and certain drugs.

- Coma can be produced by the following: 1) focal lesions of the posterior fossa that involve the brainstem; 2) focal supratentorial lesions, if they are large enough to involve directly or indirectly the deep midline diencephalic structures necessary for the maintenance of consciousness; and 3) diffuse lesions, generally of an anoxic, toxic-metabolic, or inflammatory nature, capable of causing widespread depression of neural activity.

Clinical Problem 10.2.

A 74-year-old woman with a history of hypertension had sudden onset of a severe right-sided headache, followed by weakness of the left side of her face and body and somnolence. When hospitalized 1 hour later, she had severe weakness on the left side of the body and face and decreased sensation on the left side of the body and face. During the next few hours, she became progressively less responsive and finally comatose.

a. Before the time the patient entered the hospital, what would be the most appropriate anatomicopathologic diagnosis?
b. What is the nature of the lesion?
c. What is the mechanism of her becoming comatose?
d. What changes would be expected in the EEG?

Generally, comatose patients who survive the initial brain insult begin to awaken and recover gradually within 2 to 4 weeks. This recovery may not progress further than a vegetative state or minimally conscious state. Patients in *vegetative state* are awake but unaware of themselves or the environment. Persistent vegetative state has been defined as that remaining 1 month after brain damage. Vegetative state may be regarded as permanent 3 months after nontraumatic brain injury and 12 months after traumatic brain injury.

The so-called minimally conscious state refers to patients who are not in vegetative state but are not able to communicate consistently. These patients show clear but limited evidence of awareness of themselves or their environment by following simple commands, yes/no responses (regardless of accuracy), intelligible speech, and purposeful behavior.

The disorders of consciousness should be differentiated from the *locked-in syndrome*. These patients cannot communicate or move in response to stimuli because they are quadriplegic and anarthric. However, they are fully alert and aware and may communicate by blinking or moving the eyes vertically. This syndrome results from bilateral disruption of the corticospinal and corticobulbar pathways, most commonly at the level of the pons, or as a consequence of a severe peripheral nerve disorder such as Guillain-Barré syndrome. The differences between coma, vegetative state, minimally conscious state, and locked-in syndrome are summarized in Table 10.6.

Confusional State (Delirium)

A transient state, distinct from dementia, is *confusion* (also called quiet delirium) in which cognitive function progressively declines in the presence of normal alertness. A characteristic feature of delirium is impaired attention. As a consequence, the patient has difficulty maintaining a coherent sequence of thought, is distractible, has slow responses to verbal stimuli, is less able to recognize and understand what is occurring in the environment, and is disoriented to place and time.

Delirium is an agitated state of confusion associated

Table 10.6. Comparison of the Clinical Features of Coma, Vegetative State, Minimally Conscious State, and Locked-in Syndrome

Feature	Coma	Vegetative state	Minimally conscious state	Locked-in syndrome
Arousal	Absent	Present	Present	Present
Sleep-wake cycle	Absent	Present	Present	Present
Awareness	Absent	Absent	Partial	Full
Motor function	Reflex and postural responses	Postures or withdrawal to noxious stimuli	Response to noxious stimuli, reaching for objects Inconsistent command following	Paralysis of face, bulbar, and limb muscles
Visual function	None	Startle Brief visual fixation	Sustained visual fixation or pursuit	Preserved
Communication	None	None	Contingent vocalization or inconsistent but intelligible verbalization	By means of vertical eye movements or blinking
Emotion	None	None or reflexive crying or smiling	Contingent crying or smiling	Preserved

with *illusions* (false interpretations or misrepresentations of real sensory images), *hallucinations* (false sensory perceptions for which there is no external basis), and *delusions* (false beliefs or misconceptions that cannot be corrected by reason). Patients with confusional state and delirium may have alterations in the sleep-wake cycle. They may be vigilant (hyperalert) or have different degrees of reduced level of arousal. Typical features of confusional state and delirium are acute onset and a fluctuating course.

Common causes of confusion and delirium include primary neurologic disorders (head injury, vascular, inflammatory, or neoplastic), metabolic or nutritional disorders (hypoglycemia, hypoxia, or thiamine deficiency), and drugs (especially anticholinergics) or withdrawal (especially alcohol). These causes may selectively affect components of the consciousness system involved in attention, including the cholinergic and noradrenergic neurons in the brainstem reticular activating system and the basal forebrain, association nuclei of the thalamus, prefrontal cortex, and posterior parietal cortex. Occasionally, focal lesions affecting these structures may also produce confusion and delirium.

Confusion or delirium may occur in a previously healthy person, but in most cases, there is some vulnerability because of old age, preexisting cognitive dysfunction (e.g., dementia), or chronic illness.

Transient Causes of Loss of Consciousness

The consciousness system may be impaired only transiently. A transient disturbance of consciousness may result from 1) metabolic encephalopathy, 2) concussion, 3) generalized seizure, or 4) syncope.

Several systemic disorders produce *metabolic encephalopathy*, which diffusely affects the consciousness system and causes a transient alteration in consciousness, often without localizing signs, or, if more severe, a confusional state. Hypoxemia, hypoglycemia, hyponatremia, and drug overdose are common causes of metabolic encephalopathy.

A brief loss of consciousness that usually occurs after a sudden blow to the head is called *concussion*. Although the patient is unconscious, he or she often can be aroused by vigorous stimuli. After the return of consciousness, some confusion and *amnesia* (loss of memory) persist for a variable period, but there usually are no permanent neurologic sequelae.

Clinical Problem 10.3.

A 56-year-old man with diabetes mellitus became confused and then unresponsive over a period of several hours. He had given himself his usual injection of insulin on awakening in the morning. Because of an upset stomach, he failed to eat anything during the day. When brought to the emergency department, he was comatose but did not have localizing neurologic signs.

a. What is the anatomicopathologic diagnosis?
b. What portions of the consciousness system are involved?
c. What is the precise etiologic diagnosis?
d. What changes might be found in the EEG?

Mechanisms postulated to cause transient loss of consciousness include a sudden increase in intracranial pressure, cerebral ischemia, or sudden depolarization or hyperpolarization (or both) affecting of brainstem, diencephalic, or cortical neurons by mechanical distortion of their axons. Although no gross neuropathologic change is usually apparent, diffuse axonal injury and individual neuronal alterations have been found on microscopic examination, particularly in the brainstem reticular formation.

- Concussion is a brief loss of consciousness usually caused by a blow to the head; it may be followed by confusion and amnesia.

A *seizure* (convulsion) is a transient episode of supratentorial origin in which there is an abrupt and temporary alteration in cerebral function. Seizures may consist of abnormal movements (such as tonic or clonic movements), an abnormal sensation (such as paresthesia or visual hallucination), or a disturbance in behavior or consciousness. They are caused by a spontaneous, excessive discharge of cortical neurons, which may be the result of an increase in neuronal excitability, excessive excitatory synaptic input impinging on neurons, or a decrease in normal inhibitory mechanisms.

Seizures can be either focal or generalized. A *focal seizure*, also called *partial seizure*, involves only a localized area of the cerebral cortex. Partial seizures have been subdivided into simple partial seizures, in which there is no loss of consciousness, and complex partial seizures, in which there is some alteration of consciousness. A *generalized seizure* involves widespread and bilateral areas of both hemispheres simultaneously. Because it may spread to the thalamus and reticular activating system, it may be associated with loss of consciousness. Seizures can occur from generalized processes or focal lesions affecting the brain, including inflammatory, vascular, neoplastic, degenerative, toxic-metabolic, and traumatic disorders.

- Seizures result from excessive discharge of cortical neurons and may be focal or generalized.

Fainting, or *syncope*, is a transient loss of consciousness due to a decrease in cerebral blood flow and ischemia of the entire brain. It is the result of decreased cardiac output, slowing of the heart rate, or pooling of blood in the periphery. The loss of consciousness is usually brief (a matter of seconds to minutes) and is preceded by lightheadedness, weakness, giddiness, sweating, and dimming of vision. During this time, the patient is pale and sweaty, the pulse is weak, and blood pressure is reduced. Syncope accompanied by brief generalized tonic, clonic, or tonic-clonic movements is called *convulsive syncope*.

- Syncope is a transient loss of consciousness due to a decrease in cerebral blood flow and ischemia of the entire brain.

Clinical Problem 10.4.

A 38-year-old woman had a 3-year history of generalized tonic-clonic seizures. On the day of admission to the hospital, she was found unresponsive on the floor of her living room. When brought to the emergency department, she was stuporous, with continuous bilateral convulsive movements of the face and upper and lower extremities. These subsided, and within 24 hours, the results of a neurologic examination were normal.

a. What is the anatomicopathologic diagnosis?
b. What changes might be seen in the EEG during the seizure?
c. List six types of conditions that cause generalized seizures.
d. If focal seizures were also present in this patient, would that influence your choice about the possible cause of her seizures?

Role of the EEG in the Evaluation of Disorders of Consciousness

The EEG is helpful in studying normal physiologic activity; however, its greatest usefulness is in detecting abnormalities of cerebral functioning and, thus, is a useful adjunct to neurologic diagnosis. The EEG of a normal subject who is awake but with eyes closed shows alpha activity in the posterior head regions (Fig. 10.20). The EEG reflects the intrinsic cortical activity as modified by subcortical structures (the thalamus and ascending projections of the reticular activating system). Therefore, an EEG abnormality is the result of a disturbance of 1) cortical neuronal activity, 2) subcortical structures that regulate cortical neuronal activity, and 3) thalamocortical projection pathways.

The two main types of EEG abnormalities are 1) slow-wave abnormalities and 2) epileptiform abnormalities; both can be either focal or generalized (Table 10.7). A focal EEG abnormality indicates a localized disturbance of cerebral function, whereas a generalized EEG abnormality indicates a bilateral and diffuse disturbance of cerebral function or a disturbance that is projected to the surface from subcortical structures. Thus, the EEG helps to distinguish between a focal and a generalized disturbance of cerebral function and helps to determine the level of the brain involved.

In coma due to diffuse cerebral disease, the EEG shows widespread, generalized slowing (Fig. 10.21), with the degree of slowing often paralleling the degree of coma. When there is dysfunction of subcortical structures, the EEG shows different types of abnormalities depending on the level of the neuraxis involved. With diencephalic or midbrain involvement, the EEG shows intermittent, rhythmic slow waves that occur bilaterally and synchronously over both hemispheres. If the pons or lower brainstem is involved, the EEG may contain alpha activity and resemble an abnormal waking record, but unlike the normal alpha rhythm in an alert person, this activity does not show normal reactivity to light, noise, or noxious stimuli. In addition, there may be cyclic sleep patterns consisting of sleep spindles, V waves, and delta waves. With focal cerebral lesions, the EEG shows focal slowing (Fig. 10.22). If the primary cerebral lesion is large enough to distort or to cause a pressure effect on diencephalic or mesencephalic structures, the EEG may show intermittent, widespread, rhythmic slow-wave abnormalities in addition to the focal slow-wave abnormality.

If the patient has a seizure disorder, the EEG shows epileptiform abnormalities consisting of *sharp waves*, *spikes*, or *spike and slow-wave* discharges that may occur in a focal or generalized manner (Fig. 10.23). During an actual seizure, these occur in a sustained, repetitive, and rhythmic fashion (Fig. 10.24).

- The EEG is useful in evaluating patients who have alteration of consciousness and helps determine whether the underlying condition or lesion is focal or generalized.

Brain Death

Brain death occurs when neural damage is irreversible, and although cardiac activity may be present, there no longer is evidence of cerebral function. The patient is unresponsive and shows no spontaneous movement or behavioral response to external stimuli. The absence of

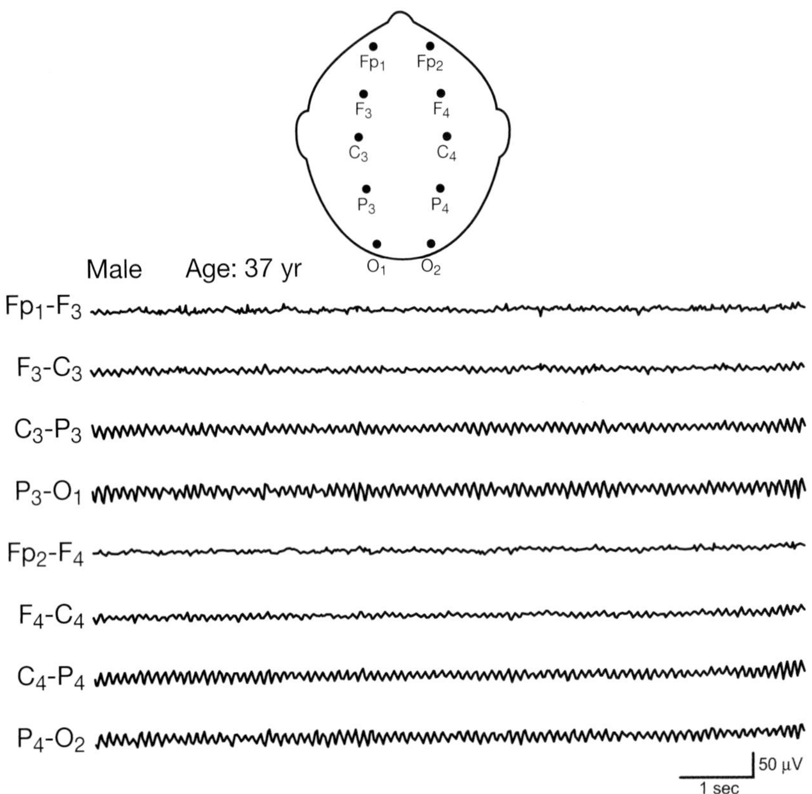

Fig. 10.20. Normal EEG pattern during the wakeful state, showing presence of alpha activity in the posterior head region. (In each EEG illustration, electrical activity is a bipolar recording of the potential difference between electrodes, indicated by letters and numbers to the left of each line. The location of each electrode is shown on the diagram of the head.)

Table 10.7. Electroencephalographic (EEG) Changes in Various Disease Processes

	EEG changes	
Disease process	**Focal**	**Generalized**
Infarct	Slow	
Tumor	Slow	
Focal seizure	Spikes, sharp waves	
Hypoxia		Slow
Hypoglycemia		Slow
Generalized seizure		Spikes, sharp waves
Brain death		No activity

brainstem function is manifested by the loss of respiratory activity and all brainstem reflexes. The absence of cerebral function can be confirmed by blood flow studies that show cessation of blood flow in the brain or by EEG, which shows a flat pattern with no sign of electrocerebral activity. Because brain function is markedly depressed by hypothermia, certain anesthetic agents, and other drugs that also can produce a flat EEG, these causes have to be excluded before concluding that irreversible brain death is present.

- Brain death occurs with the loss of cerebral and brainstem function and no detectable cerebral activity on the EEG.
- Reversible causes of coma and a flat EEG can result from anesthesia, certain drugs, and hypothermia.

Neurologic Examination of the Consciousness System

Examination of a patient who has altered consciousness is a challenge to physicians. The situation is often emergent, and the patient is frequently uncooperative. Furthermore, an assessment of the functions of the consciousness system alone seldom provides sufficient information for anatomicopathologic diagnosis, and one must rely on other associated clues from the history and results of a physical examination to determine the location and cause of the lesion responsible.

Assessment of the Consciousness System

Involvement of the consciousness system is evaluated by noting the patient's ability to perceive and attend to the external environment. The degree of coma is determined by the patient's response to stimuli such as touch, pinprick, calling the patient's name, a hand clap, or some other form of loud noise. If the patient is unresponsive to milder forms of stimulation, then noxious or painful stimuli such as pinching or deep pressure in sensitive areas are used. The patient's response is observed to define the presence of delirium, confusion, somnolence, stupor, or coma (as described above), any of which would suggest some involvement of the consciousness system.

The Glasgow Coma Scale allows a quantitative recording of the patient's responses, which is helpful for patient follow-up.

This scale analyzes three markers of consciousness: eye opening (E), motor responses (M), and verbal responses (V) and provides a score according to the intensity of the stimulus required to obtain the response and the type of response. According to this scale, coma is arbitrarily defined as failure to open eyes in response to verbal commands (E2),

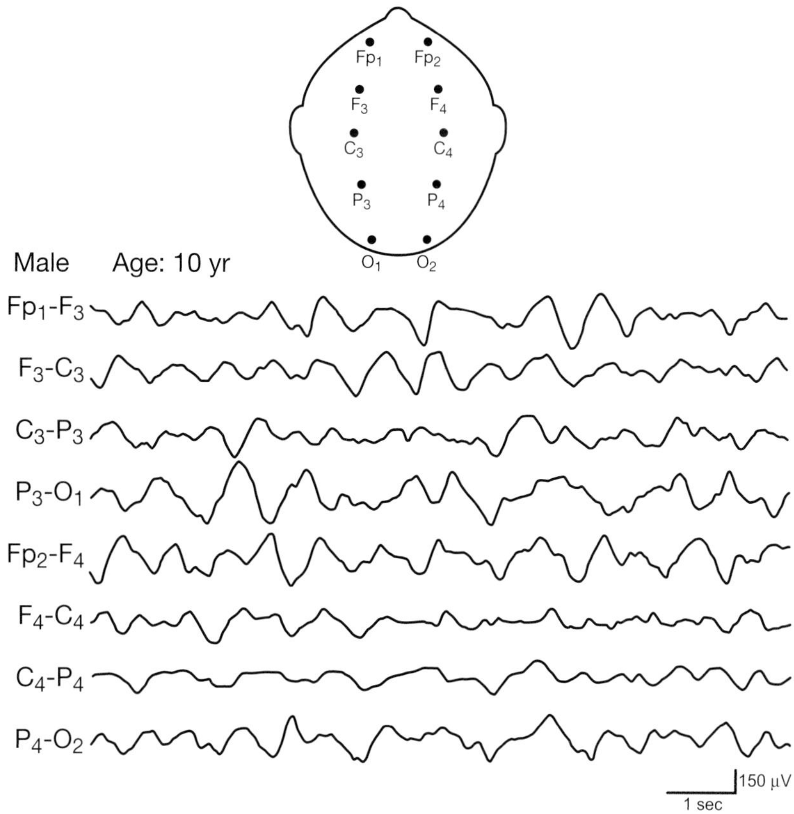

Fig. 10.21. EEG of a comatose patient with encephalitis, showing widespread delta slowing.

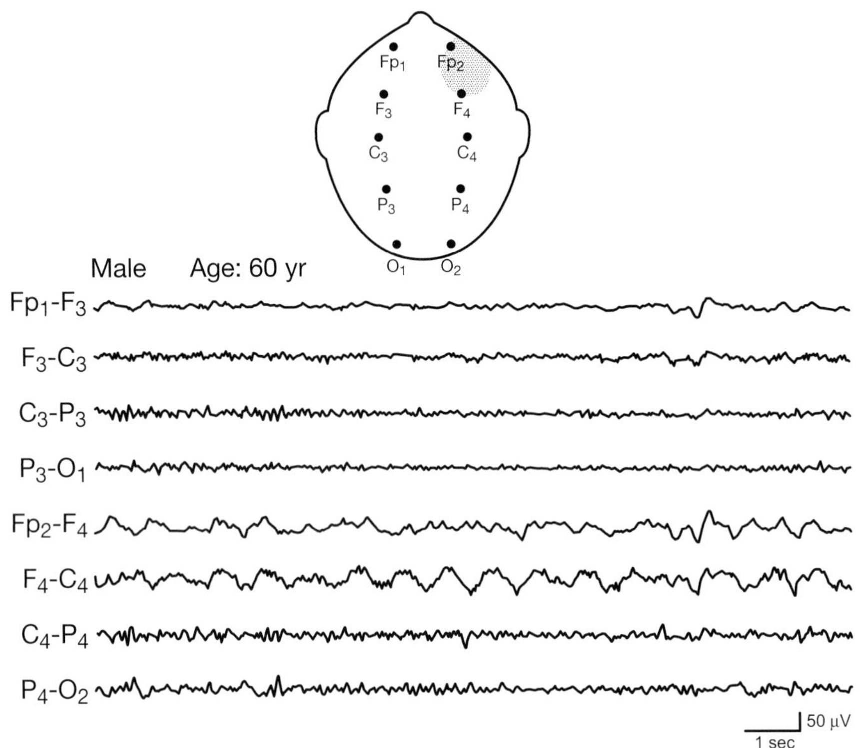

Fig. 10.22. EEG showing focal delta slowing over the right frontal area (stippled) due to right frontal tumor.

perform no better than weak flexor motor responses to stimuli (M4), and utter only unrecognizable words in response to pain (V2).

Anatomicopathologic Diagnosis

Lesions affecting the consciousness system are located at the supratentorial level or posterior fossa level (or both); therefore, one must seek clues that suggest involvement at these levels by noting the vital signs (pulse, blood pressure, respiration, temperature) and examining motor, sensory, and cranial nerve functions. Precise anatomical localization is seldom necessary, but some attempt should be made to apply the general principles of anatomical diagnosis described in Chapter 3 and the brainstem reflexes described in Chapter 15 to decide if the lesion responsible is located at the supratentorial level or the posterior fossa level or if it is diffusely distributed at both levels.

This seemingly crude localization is extremely useful in the clinical setting, and when combined with information about the temporal evolution of the illness, it is used (as described in Chapter 4) to establish a cause (vascular, inflammatory, toxic-metabolic, traumatic, neoplastic, or degenerative).

Judicious selection of appropriate ancillary studies such as blood tests, including determination of glucose and electrolyte levels, arterial blood gases, toxicologic screen, computed tomography or magnetic resonance imaging of the head, cerebrospinal fluid examination, and EEG, is often required to establish a precise anatomicopathologic diagnosis. For all patients, however, basic management includes an assessment of the airway (A), breathing (B), and cardiovascular (C) function. This ABC approach, together with the administration of glucose and thiamine, should be performed in all patients, regardless of the suspected cause of loss of consciousness. For patients with focal deficits, a mass lesion should be suspected and an imaging study, usually computed tomography of the head in the emergency department, should be performed as soon as possible after the airway is protected. For patients with fever, blood cultures and empiric antibiotic therapy should be started as

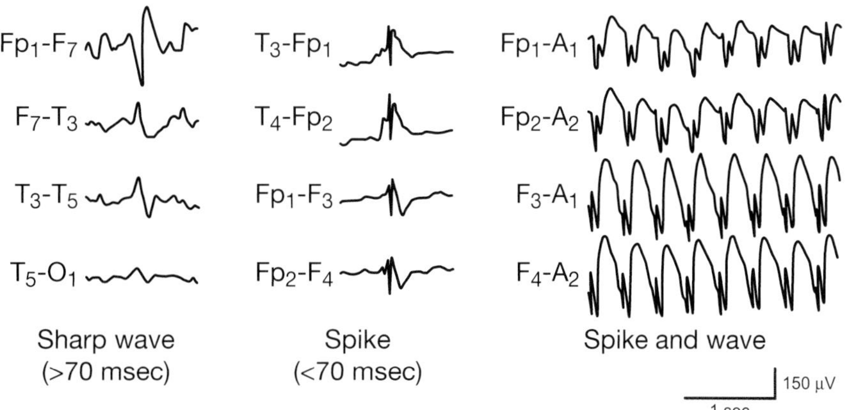

Fig. 10.23. Three types of epileptiform discharges. The sharp-wave discharge (*left*) was recorded from the left temporal region. The spike (*center*) and spike and (slow) wave discharges (*right*) were recorded from widespread areas of cerebral cortex.

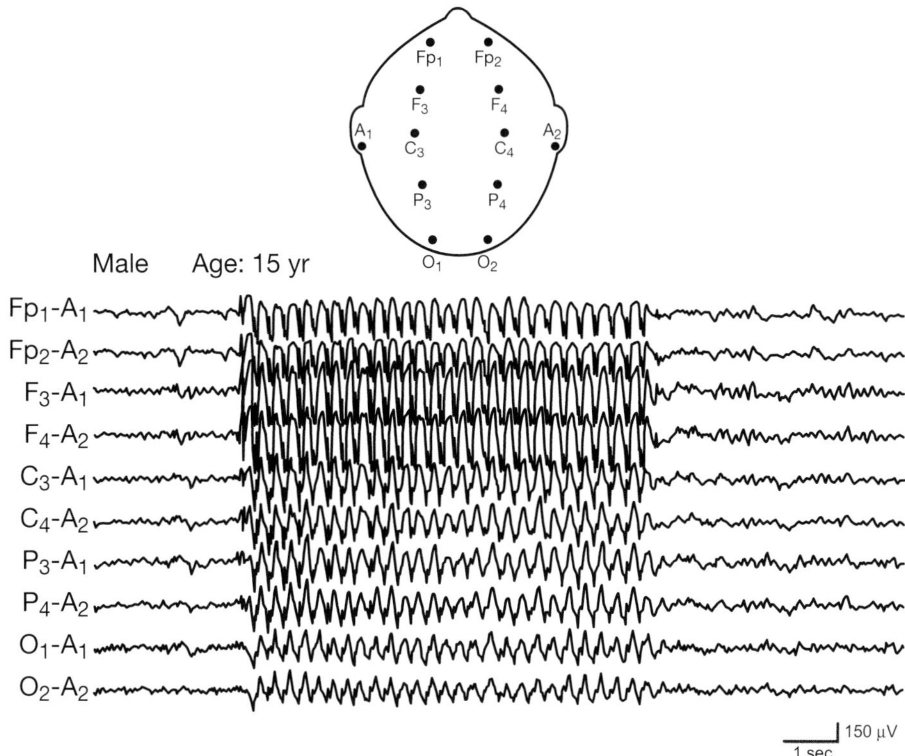

Fig. 10.24. Generalized 3-Hz spike and wave discharge with an absence seizure, during which the patient was unresponsive.

soon as possible, followed by a cerebrospinal fluid examination. The CSF analysis should be done only after computed tomography has excluded a mass lesion.

- The neurologic assessment of patients who have altered consciousness includes determining reactivity to stimuli, the degree of altered consciousness, and whether the process involves the supratentorial or posterior fossa level or is diffuse.

Additional Reading

Fisch BJ. Fisch & Spehlmann's EEG primer: basic principles of digital and analog EEG. 3rd ed. Amsterdam: Elsevier; 1999. Chapter 11, pp 185-198; Chapter 12, pp 199-210; Chapter 16, pp 245-260.

Laureys S, Owen AM, Schiff ND. Brain function in coma, vegetative state, and related disorders. Lancet Neurol. 2004;3:537-546.

Pace-Schott EF, Hobson JA. The neurobiology of sleep: genetics, cellular physiology and subcortical networks. Nat Rev Neurosci. 2002;3:591-605.

Schenck CH, Mahowald MW. REM sleep behavior disorder: clinical, developmental, and neuroscience perspectives 16 years after its formal identification in SLEEP. Sleep. 2002;25:120-138.

Silber MH, Krahn LE, Morgenthaler TI. Sleep medicine in clinical practice. London: Taylor & Francis; 2004. Chapter 1, pp 3-24; Chapter 7, pp 91-116; Chapter 16, pp 321-346.

Steriade M. Arousal: revisiting the reticular activating system. Science. 1996;272:225-226.

Wijdicks EF. Determining brain death in adults. Neurology. 1995;45:1003-1011.

Wijdicks EFM. Coma and other states of altered awareness. In: Neurologic complications of critical illness. 2nd ed. Oxford: Oxford University Press; 2002. pp 3-27.

Zeman A. Consciousness. Brain. 2001;124:1263-1289.

Chapter 11

Cerebrospinal Fluid: Ventricular System

Objectives

1. Define or identify the following: dura mater, arachnoid, pia mater, epidural space, subdural space, subarachnoid space, dural sinuses, falx cerebri, tentorium cerebelli, blood-brain barrier, choroid plexuses, lateral ventricles, foramen of Monro, third ventricle, aqueduct of Sylvius, fourth ventricle, and foramina of Luschka and Magendie.
2. Describe and trace the formation, circulation, and absorption of cerebrospinal fluid (CSF).
3. Define communicating hydrocephalus and noncommunicating hydrocephalus. Give an example of each type, describe its location, and state the anatomicopathologic consequences of a lesion in that location.
4. Discuss the relation between the contents of the cranial cavity and intracranial pressure, and give examples of general pathologic states that may result in increased intracranial pressure.
5. Interpret the significance of abnormalities in CSF color, cellular composition, serologic findings, total protein level, gamma globulin concentration, glucose level, and culture, and list the CSF findings in meningitis, encephalitis, subarachnoid hemorrhage, and traumatic puncture.
6. Describe or list the features of the syndrome of meningeal irritation.
7. Describe or list the features that indicate increased intracranial pressure.
8. Describe the neuroanatomical basis for the following neurodiagnostic studies: myelography, computed tomography, magnetic resonance imaging, and radioisotope cisternography.

Introduction

The meninges, ventricular system, subarachnoid space, and cerebrospinal fluid (CSF) constitute a functionally unique system that has an important role in maintaining a stable environment within which the central nervous system can function. The membranes that constitute the meninges serve as supportive and protective structures for neural tissue. The CSF itself provides a cushioning effect during rapid movement of the head and mechanical buoyancy to the brain. In addition to providing a pathway for the removal of brain metabolites, it functions as a chemical reservoir that protects the local environment of the brain from changes that may occur in the blood, thus ensuring the brain's continued undisturbed performance. The CSF system occurs at the supratentorial, posterior fossa, and spinal levels. Because of this extensive anatomical distribution and function, pathologic alterations of the CSF system can occur in many neurologic disorders.

Overview

Structures included in the CSF system are the meninges and meningeal spaces formed between the meningeal linings and the brain, the ventricular system, and the CSF itself. The *meninges* consist of three mesodermally derived membranes: the dura mater (outermost), arachnoid, and the thin pia mater (innermost), which adheres closely to the external surface of the central nervous system. The epidural space is external to the dura mater, between it and bone. The subdural space is between the dura mater and the arachnoid, and the subarachnoid space is between the arachnoid and the pia mater. The subarachnoid space contains CSF. CSF also fills the cavities in the brain: the two lateral ventricles, the third ventricle, the aqueduct of Sylvius, and the fourth ventricle.

The composition of CSF is similar but not identical to that of plasma. CSF is formed by a combination of processes that include passive diffusion, facilitated diffusion, and active transport. It is produced primarily, but not exclusively, by the choroid plexus of the ventricular system. The CSF circulates through the ventricular system into the subarachnoid space and over the surface of the brain and spinal cord. Most of the CSF passes through the arachnoid villi into the venous sinuses.

Because of the close relation between the CSF system and neural tissue, pathologic processes that primarily alter the function of the CSF system may secondarily alter nervous system function. Furthermore, because the central nervous system is bathed and surrounded by CSF, disease processes that primarily affect the nervous system may be reflected by changes in the anatomy and physiology of the CSF system. Therefore, an examination of the composition of the CSF and the structure of this system is an important and useful neurodiagnostic tool.

Anatomy of the CSF System

Dura Mater and Its Major Folds

The *dura mater* is a tough, fibrous membrane. In the cranial cavity, it consists of two almost inseparable layers. The outer (periosteal) layer of the dura mater corresponds to the periosteum of the cranial bones. Therefore, the epidural space between the dura mater and bone normally is not present. It is a potential space that becomes of pathologic importance if the dura mater is separated from bone by blood (epidural hematoma) or by pus (epidural abscess). The inner (meningeal) layer of the dura mater remains attached to the outer layer except where they are separated to form venous channels, the *dural venous sinuses*.

The *falx cerebri* is a sickle-shaped reflection of meningeal dura that extends into the interhemispheric fissure to separate the two cerebral hemispheres. It extends from the base of the anterior fossa to the internal occipital protuberance. Its upper margin contains the *superior sagittal sinus*, and its lower free edge, which arches over the corpus callosum, contains the *inferior sagittal sinus* (Fig. 11.1).

At the level of the internal occipital protuberance, the dura mater forming the falx cerebri extends laterally to form a winglike structure, the *tentorium cerebelli*. The outer border of the tentorium cerebelli is attached to the occipital bone and along the upper edges of the petrous bones. Thus, it separates the ventral surface of the cerebral hemispheres from the dorsal surface of the cerebellum and divides the cranial cavity into the supratentorial compartment (anterior and middle cranial fossae and their contents) and the infratentorial, or posterior fossa, compartment (Fig. 11.1). The cerebellar hemispheres are partially separated by a downward extension of dura mater, the *falx cerebelli*. The wings of the tentorium cerebelli converge and attach to the posterior clinoid processes of the sella turcica. The free border of the tentorium cerebelli thus forms an opening, the tentorial notch, that surrounds the midbrain at the transition between the posterior fossa and the middle fossa.

The two layers of the dura mater remain tightly attached as they pass through the foramen magnum into the spinal canal. At the level of the second or third cervical vertebra, the meningeal dura separates widely from the inner periosteum of bone and forms a narrow sac that extends to the level of the second sacral vertebra. The spinal epidural space thus formed between the dura mater and the periosteum contains fat and vascular structures (principally veins). The conus medullaris, the lower end of the spinal cord (Fig. 11.2), terminates at the level of the second lumbar vertebra. A thin remnant of central nervous system tissue, the *filum terminale*, extends caudally from the conus medullaris to the termination of the dural sac at the second sacral level. The filum terminale is composed of glial cells, ependyma, and astrocytes covered

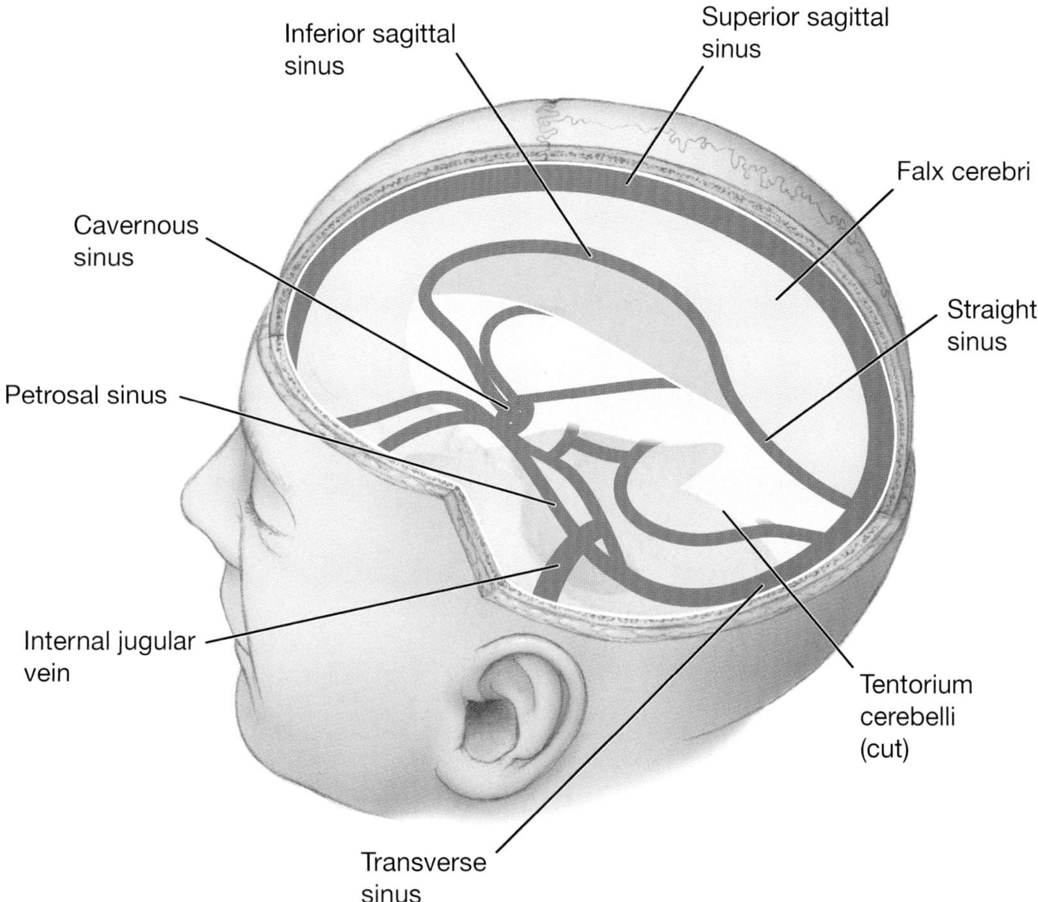

Fig. 11.1. The dura mater and its major sinuses. Dorsolateral view showing the falx cerebri (located at the midline in the interhemispheric fissure), the tentorium cerebelli (separating the supratentorial compartment from the infratentorial, or posterior fossa, compartment), and the dural lining of the base of the skull. The dural venous sinuses are shown in blue.

by pia mater. The dura mater is pierced by the roots of the spinal and cranial nerves along the length of the brainstem and spinal cord.

- The dura mater is attached to cranial bones.
- The epidural space is a potential space between the dura mater and bone.
- The falx cerebri separates the two hemispheres.
- The tentorium cerebelli separates the cerebral hemispheres and the cerebellum.
- The conus medullaris, the lower end of the spinal cord, terminates at the second lumbar vertebra.

Leptomeninges (Arachnoid and Pia Mater)

Embryologically, the leptomeninges (the arachnoid and pia mater) begin as a single membrane that becomes separated by numerous confluent subarachnoid spaces containing CSF. However, the arachnoid remains attached to the pia mater by numerous weblike trabeculae (Fig. 11.3). Although the pia mater adheres tightly to the surfaces of the brain and spinal cord, the arachnoid is closely applied to the inner surface of the meningeal dura mater throughout the neuraxis. The potential space between the dura mater and the arachnoid is termed the *subdural space*. It normally

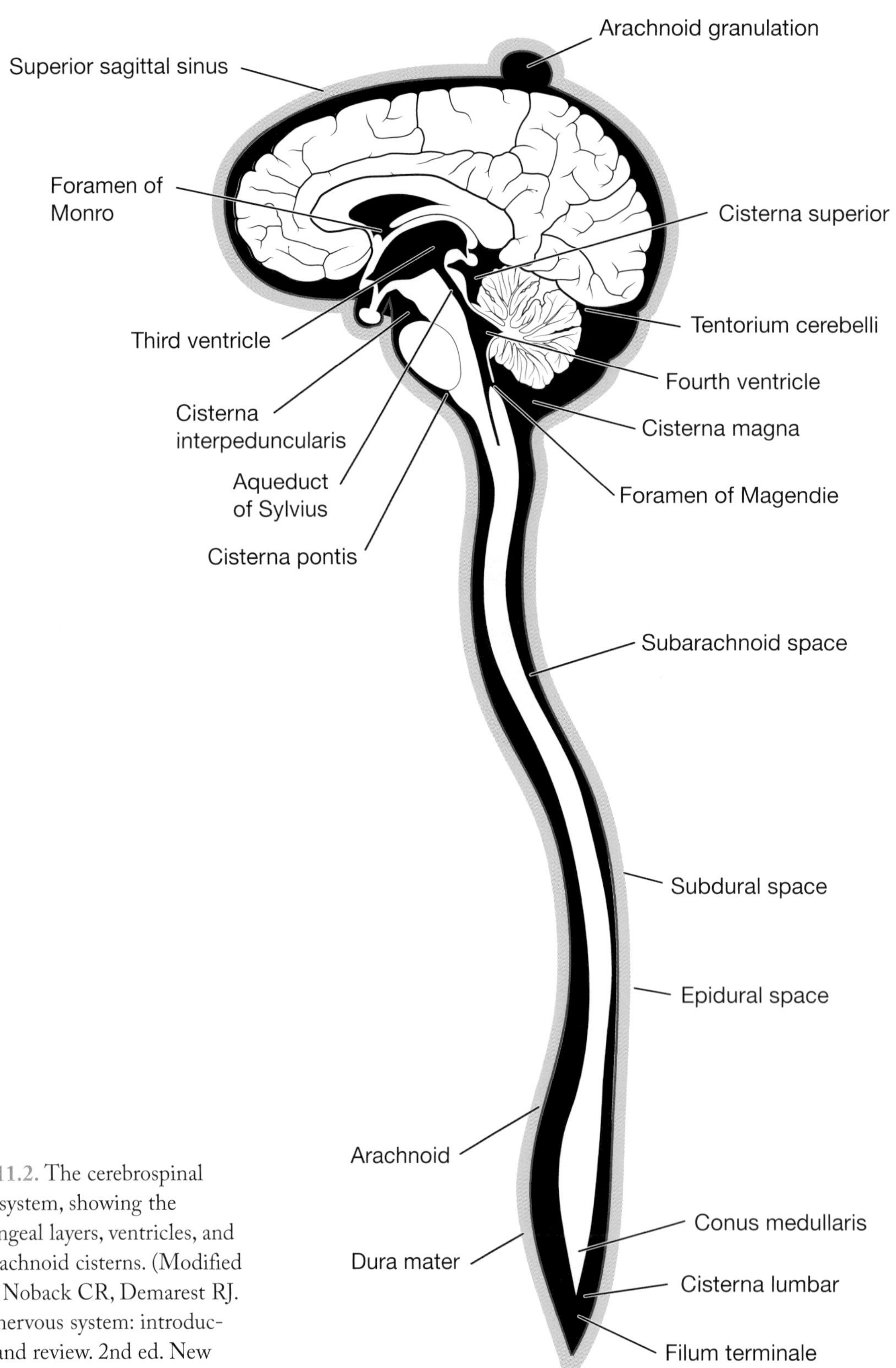

Fig. 11.2. The cerebrospinal fluid system, showing the meningeal layers, ventricles, and subarachnoid cisterns. (Modified from Noback CR, Demarest RJ. The nervous system: introduction and review. 2nd ed. New York: McGraw-Hill; 1977. Used with permission.)

contains a thin layer of fluid. In pathologic states, blood may accumulate in this space and produce a *subdural hematoma*.

- The arachnoid layer is applied to the dura mater.
- The pia mater adheres to the brain and spinal cord.
- The potential space between the dura mater and arachnoid is the subdural space.

As a result of the relation of the arachnoid with the dura mater and of the pia mater with neural tissue, the *subarachnoid space* varies greatly in size and shape, particularly over the surfaces of the brain and in the lumbar region of the spinal canal (Fig. 11.2).

In the cranial cavity, enlargements of the subarachnoid space are called cisterns, which usually are named for their anatomical location (e.g., the interpeduncular cistern is located between the cerebral peduncles). The large subarachnoid cistern below the cerebellum is the cisterna magna. In the spinal canal, where the spinal cord ends at the level of the second lumbar vertebra and the arachnoid remains closely applied to the dura mater to the level of the second sacral vertebra, a large lumbar subarachnoid space is formed that contains a reservoir of CSF, the filum terminale, and the nerve roots of the cauda equina as they pass to their intervertebral foramina.

The major arterial channels of the brain are located in the subarachnoid space. Bleeding from these vessels results in subarachnoid hemorrhage.

- The space between the arachnoid and pia mater (and brain) is the subarachnoid space.
- Major arterial channels are located in the subarachnoid space.

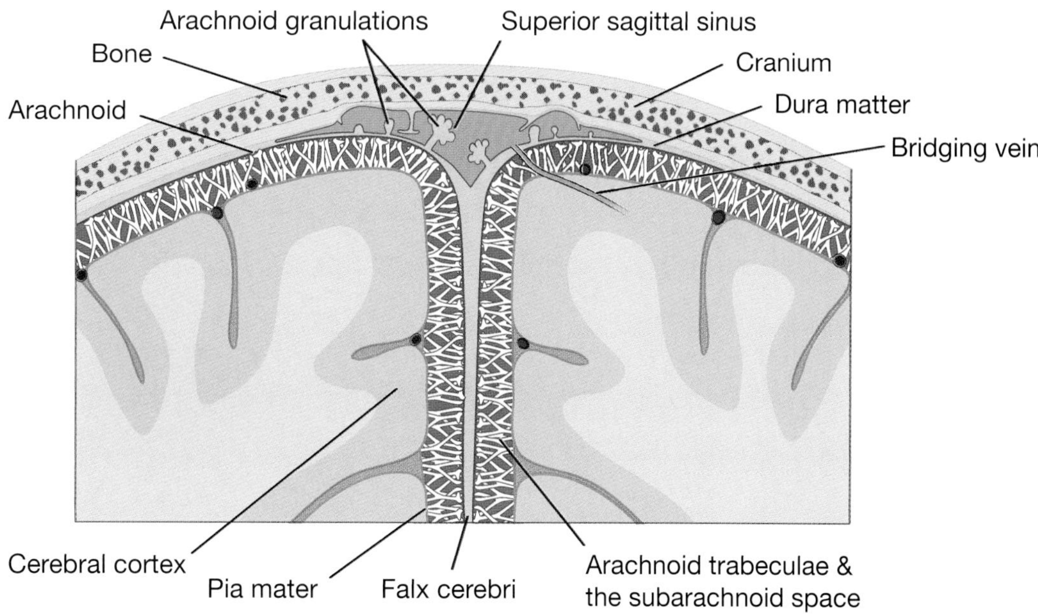

Fig. 11.3. Meninges and meningeal spaces. Diagrammatic coronal section through the paramedian region of the cerebral hemispheres. Note the bridging vein that extends from the cerebral cortex to the superior sagittal sinus. Tearing of this type of vein where it joins the dural sinus is a common cause of subdural bleeding.

On gross inspection, the pia mater cannot be seen except at intervals in the spinal canal, where it extends laterally to attach to the dura mater as the denticulate ligaments (Fig. 11.4). Throughout the rest of its distribution, the pia mater closely invests the central nervous system, with its few cell layers being separated from the outermost neural tissue, the astrocytic glia limitans, by a thin layer of collagen.

In the arachnoid trabeculae, the cells of the pia mater and arachnoid are contiguous and are called pia-arachnoid (Fig. 11.5). As arterioles dip into the parenchyma of the brain, they are invested with a sheath of pia-arachnoid that disappears at the capillary level, leaving only the endothelium of the blood vessel and its basement membrane in direct contact with the astrocytic glia limitans (Fig. 11.5). These structures, particularly the tight junctions between endothelial cells, form the blood-brain barrier.

The descriptive term *blood-brain barrier* was first used many years ago when it was observed that certain dyes injected intravenously would stain all body organs except the brain; yet, the same dyes injected into the CSF would stain brain tissue. Consequently, it was postulated that a barrier to the passage of dye was located between the blood and the brain. The tight junctions of the unfenestrated endothelial cells are of major importance in maintaining the integrity of the blood-brain barrier. These junctions are not, however, the only blood-brain barrier but merely part of a system of barriers (some anatomical, others physiologic) that produce differences in the chemical composition of the brain, CSF, and blood.

The invaginations of the arachnoid into the dural venous sinuses are called the *arachnoid villi* (or granulations) (Fig. 11.2). Fluid circulating through these villi passes into the venous blood and systemic circulation. In this way, the CSF ventricular system provides a pathway for the removal of products of cerebral metabolism.

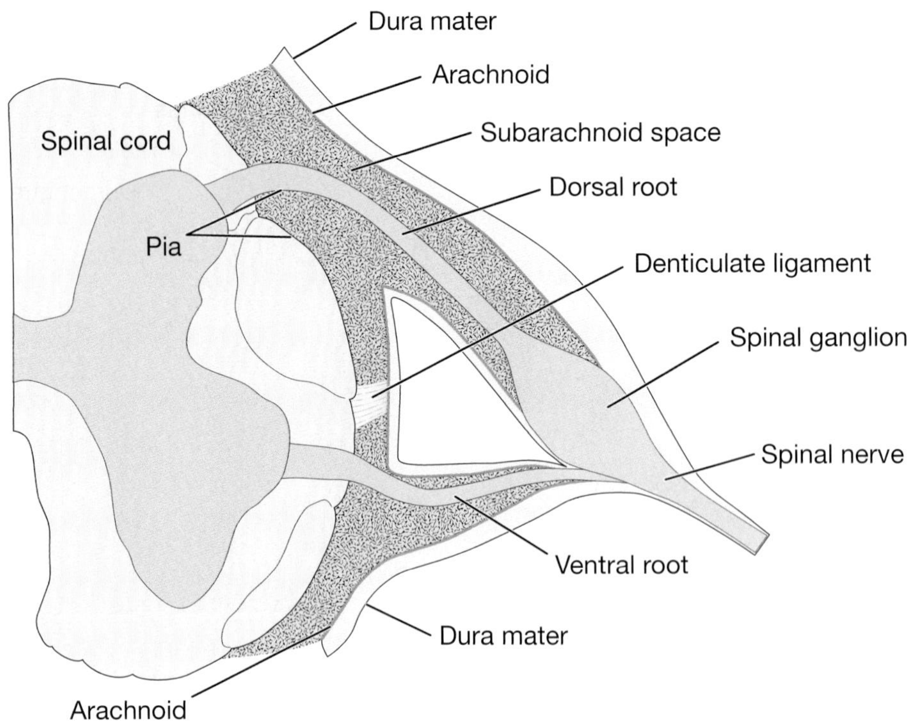

Fig. 11.4. Meningeal relationships at the spinal level. Note that as the spinal nerve leaves the spinal canal it is invested by dura mater. The denticulate ligaments attach the spinal cord to the dura mater laterally.

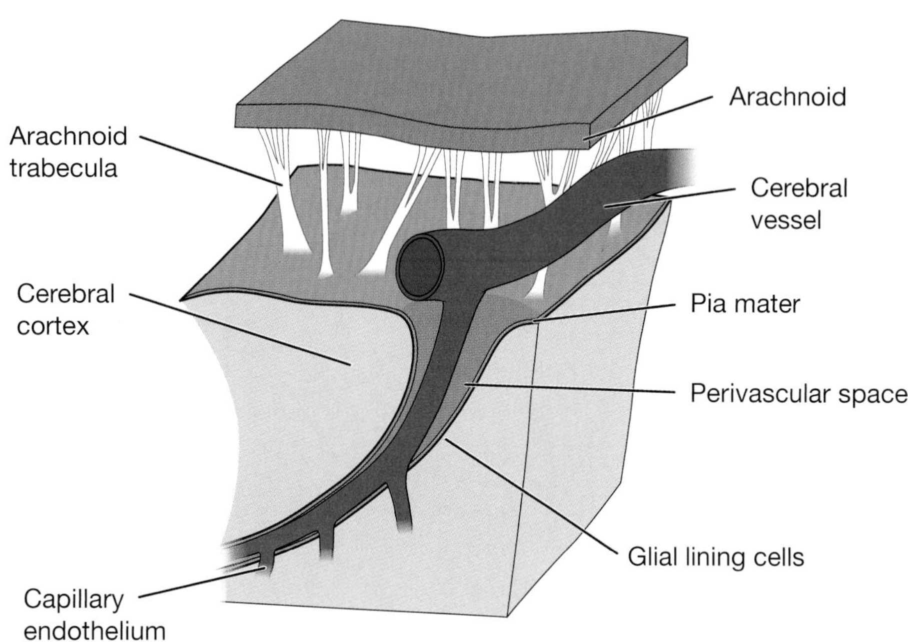

Fig. 11.5. Detailed relations of the meninges and structures in the subarachnoid space. An arteriole carries pia mater into the cerebral cortex.

- The CSF ventricular system provides a pathway for the removal of products of cerebral metabolism.
- The blood-brain barrier is a system of barriers between the blood vessels and brain.

Ventricular System of the Brain

The ventricular system (Fig. 11.6) is lined with ciliated cuboidal epithelium (derived from ectoderm) called the *ependyma.*

> Tanycytes are specialized ependymal cells that lack cilia and are located in the lining of the floor of the third ventricle. They may be involved in the release of hypophysiotropic hormones from the hypothalamus into the portal circulation.

The lateral, third, and fourth ventricles contain choroid plexuses. They are multitufted vascular organs that arise embryologically when ependyma, leptomeninges, and blood vessels fold into the ventricles. These structures, rich in enzymes found in other secretory organs, are the main (but not only) source for the production of CSF.

> Pinocytosis is the movement of substances across the cell membrane in the form of tiny vesicles formed by pinching off a section of the surface membrane. The process of pinocytotic transport has been identified in the choroid plexus.

Each cerebral hemisphere contains a *lateral ventricle* (Fig. 11.7), and each lateral ventricle is divided into an anterior horn located in the frontal lobe, body and atrium (or trigone) in the parietal lobe, posterior horn in the occipital lobe, and inferior horn in the temporal lobe. The lateral ventricles communicate with each other and the *third ventricle* of the diencephalon through the *interventricular foramina of Monro.* The *aqueduct of Sylvius* traverses the mesencephalon and leads from the third ventricle to the *fourth ventricle*, located dorsal to the pons and medulla. The communication between the ventricular system and the

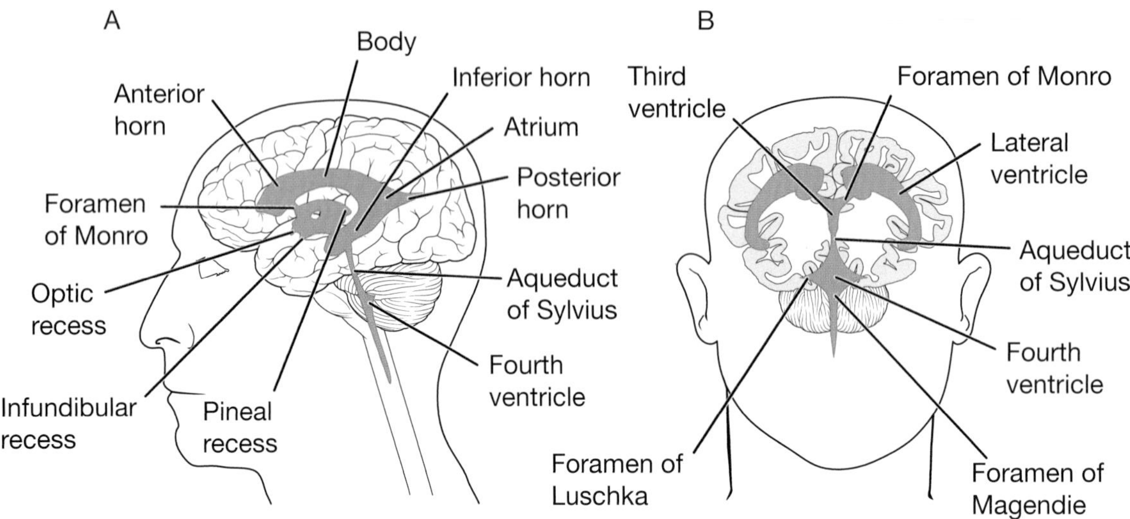

Fig. 11.6. Ventricular system. *A*, Lateral view. *B*, Anterior view. The pons has been removed from *B* to show the anatomy of the fourth ventricle.

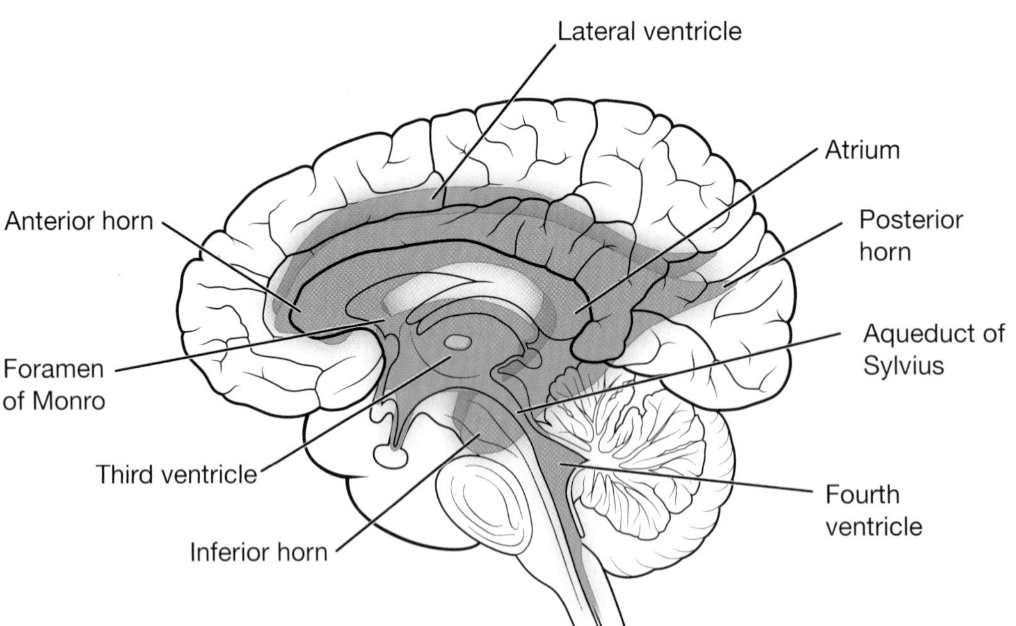

Fig. 11.7. Sagittal image of a brain showing the ventricular system and related structures.

subarachnoid space occurs in the fourth ventricle through two foramina of Luschka and the foramen of Magendie.

A small and discontinuous central canal extends for a short distance caudally from the fourth ventricle. This canal is usually obliterated at the spinal level, and in normal adults, only a few ependymal cells remain as remnants of the once prominent central canal of the embryo.

- Choroid plexuses occur in the lateral, third, and fourth ventricles and are the main source of CSF.
- CSF circulates from the fourth ventricle into the subarachnoid space.

The Cerebrospinal Fluid

Formation and Circulation of CSF

The rate of CSF formation remains relatively constant at approximately 0.35 mL per minute (500 mL/day). Because the total volume of CSF in the adult is 90 to 150 mL, the processes of CSF formation and resorption must remain in delicate balance to prevent any alteration in the structure and function of the brain.

The production of CSF is an active process, mediated partly by the enzyme carbonic anhydrase. CSF production is relatively independent of hydrostatic forces; however, a decrease in choroid plexus perfusion pressure to 50 mm Hg causes a decrease in CSF production. In contrast, the rate of CSF absorption is proportional to the hydrostatic pressure, with greater absorption occurring in the presence of increasing CSF pressure.

Nerve terminals have been identified on plexus arterioles and on the cells of the secretory epithelium. Thus, alterations in CSF production may occur in response to both intrinsic and extrinsic neurotransmitter systems, including norepinephrine and vasopressin.

Most of the CSF is actively secreted into the ventricular system by the choroid plexuses; however, these are not the only source of CSF. Some is derived directly from the interstitial fluid of the brain and crosses the ependyma to enter the ventricles. Additional exchange may take place between the neural tissue and the subarachnoid space across the pia mater.

Circulation of the CSF is pulsatile and promoted by the beating of the cilia of the ependymal cells and pulsatile changes in the volume of intracranial blood that occurs with cardiac systole and respiratory movements. The to-and-fro movement of CSF results in a directional flow that is from the lateral, third, and fourth ventricles into the subarachnoid space, where CSF then circulates in two major directions. The more important pathway is rostrally through the tentorial notch and dorsally toward the intracranial venous system, where CSF exits through the arachnoid villi projecting into the dural venous sinuses, particularly the superior sagittal sinus. Although the exact mechanism of transfer of CSF to venous blood through the arachnoid villi is incompletely understood, transcellular transport in giant vacuoles seems most likely.

The villi act as one-way valves, preventing blood from entering the CSF. A hydrostatic pressure of 70 mm H_2O or more forces the CSF into the sinuses. The second pathway, a quantitatively less important and slower route taken by the CSF after its exit from the ventricular system, is downward through the foramen magnum into the spinal subarachnoid space, where it is partially resorbed through the leptomeninges.

CSF Pressure

The craniovertebral cavity and its dural lining form a closed space. Any increase in the volume of one of the three compartments (blood, CSF, brain) in the cavity can occur only in conjunction with an equal reduction in the volume of the others or with a consequent increase in pressure. Normally, however, the contents of the three compartments are relatively constant, producing a CSF pressure of 50 to 200 mm H_2O when recorded in the lumbar subarachnoid sac, with the patient in a lateral recumbent position.

- The CSF pressure obtained during a lumbar puncture should be less than 200 mm H_2O.

Minor oscillations occur in CSF pressure recorded in this manner in response to respiration and arterial pulsation, as various amounts of blood enter and leave the craniovertebral cavity. Certain additional maneuvers cause wider oscillations in CSF pressure. Compression of the jugular veins, for example, impedes the outflow of blood from the brain, expands the venous vascular bed, and causes a rapid increase in intracranial pressure. Because the lumbar subarachnoid sac is directly continuous with the intracranial subarachnoid space, an increase in pressure is transmitted throughout the ventricular system and subarachnoid space (as long as there is no obstruction to the flow of CSF). The spinal epidural venous plexuses normally contribute to CSF pressure by continuous tamponade of the spinal dural sac. Increased intrathoracic or intra-abdominal pressure (coughing, sneezing, straining at stool, or abdominal compression) can increase CSF pressure.

In certain pathologic conditions, the increase in the volume of some of the components of the cranial cavity cannot be compensated for by readjustments in the volume of the other constituents. In this situation, intracranial pressure increases to abnormal levels. In addition, plateau waves, a pathologic increase in intracranial pressure, are occasionally noted. These acute increases in pressure may be as high as 600 to 1,300 mm H_2O and may last for 5 to 20 minutes. The cause of these pressure increases, which are accompanied by a reduction in cerebral blood flow, is not known.

Monitoring of CSF pressure has been used in various clinical situations (most notably in cases of head trauma) to help guide the management of patients with known or suspected increased intracranial pressure. The symptoms and consequences of increased intracranial pressure are discussed below in the chapter.

The Blood-Brain–CSF Barrier System

The central nervous system contains two basic fluid compartments: extracellular (CSF and interstitial fluid) and intracellular (primarily fluid within the cytoplasm of neurons and glial cells). The chemical compositions of these two fluid compartments are dissimilar, and the composition of each fluid differs significantly from that of blood. The chemical composition of the central nervous system fluid compartments is maintained within relatively narrow limits despite large fluctuations in the composition of extracellular fluid elsewhere in the body. Therefore, factors other than simple diffusion must be responsible for the passage of chemicals from one compartment to another.

Historically, reference has been made to a blood-brain barrier, implying an anatomical structure that would explain the variable distribution of substances in each compartment. Although not the sole explanation for the blood-brain barrier, anatomical considerations do have an important role. Morphologically, the choroidal epithelium, arachnoid, and capillary endothelial cells have tight junctions that obliterate the intercellular clefts that are normally between cells. This anatomical feature impedes the diffusion of larger molecules. Some areas of the brain, however, are excluded from this blood-brain barrier system (perhaps as a means of allowing neuronal receptors to sample plasma directly). In these regions, the capillary endothelium contains fenestrations that allow proteins and small molecules to pass from the blood to adjacent tissue. These regions are called circumventricular organs. They include the area postrema in the walls of the fourth ventricle (chemicals acting at this level may produce vomiting), the subfornical organ and neighboring structures in the anterior wall of the third ventricle (chemicals acting here regulate thirst, water balance, and body temperature), the median eminence of the hypothalamus, the neurohypophysis, and the pineal gland. These areas have fenestrated capillaries rather than tight junctions, abundant capillary loops, and large perivascular spaces. Because of their unique structure and connections (neural and humoral sampling), circumventricular organs are important for homeostasis.

There are also other physicochemical factors, such as lipid solubility, protein binding, and state of ionization, that alter the passage of substances from one fluid compartment to another. In addition, certain substances are transported across membranes by carrier-mediated, facilitated diffusion systems, and others are transported by energy-requiring active transport systems. Thus, the blood-brain barrier is a wide variety of barrier systems, some anatomical and physicochemical, that act together to maintain homeostasis.

With the breakdown of the blood-brain barrier in various pathologic conditions, several changes occur that are reflected as alterations in the composition of the CSF. Four major mechanisms are believed to be involved in the increased vascular permeability noted in disease states: 1) interendothelial passage across tight junctions, 2) transendothelial flow, 3) vesicular transport, and 4) neovascularization.

Characteristics of CSF

Another function of the CSF is to provide a pathway for the removal of the products of cerebral metabolism. In this regard, the CSF has been referred to as a large metabolic sink, a reservoir for brain metabolites to drain into and then to enter the systemic circulation. Thus, the composition of the CSF reflects the processes described above as well as the metabolic activity of the central nervous system.

Appearance

The CSF normally is clear and colorless; turbidity or discoloration is always abnormal. Turbidity most commonly is due to an increased number of red or white blood cells. The most important cause of discoloration of the CSF is bleeding in the subarachnoid space. With subarachnoid hemorrhage (usually from trauma or rupture of an intracranial vessel), the fluid is initially pink to red, depending on the severity of the bleeding. For 2 to 10 hours after such an event, the red blood cells undergo lysis, and the liberated hemoglobin is broken down to form bilirubin, which imparts a yellow color (xanthochromia) to the CSF. A yellow discoloration also may be due to a markedly increased level of CSF protein or to an increase in the level of plasma bilirubin.

Cellular Elements

Normal CSF contains no more than five lymphocytes per microliter. A cell count of 6 to 10 cells is very suspicious, and a count greater than 10 is definitely abnormal and suggests the presence of disease in the central nervous system or meninges. The presence of polymorphonuclear leukocytes always indicates disease.

Microbiologic Features

CSF is normally sterile. Therefore, results of microbiologic studies (Gram stain, cultures) should be negative.

Protein

The normal total CSF protein concentration is no greater than 45 mg per deciliter. The capillary endothelial membrane is highly effective in limiting the concentration of protein in the CSF, and an increase in the CSF protein concentration is a frequent (but nonspecific) pathologic finding, suggestive of disease involving the central nervous system or meninges.

The amount of protein normally present in the CSF is much less than that in plasma, although the relative proportions of the protein fractions are similar. Most of the CSF protein is probably derived from the plasma. One protein of clinical significance is the gamma globulin fraction. Normally, gamma globulin is synthesized outside the central nervous system. The normal concentration of gamma globulin in lumbar fluid is less than 13% of the total CSF protein concentration. In conditions such as multiple sclerosis, neurosyphilis, and some other subacute or chronic infections of the central nervous system, the gamma globulin level increases in association with a normal or slightly increased total protein level. (For this observation to be valid, there must be no change in the level of serum gamma globulin.) Such an increase in the concentration of gamma globulin in the CSF suggests an abnormal formation of gamma globulin by chronic inflammatory cells within the nervous system, with diffusion of the protein from the brain into CSF.

Measurement of immunoglobulin G (IgG), which accounts for almost all the gamma globulin in normal CSF and in most disease states, is a more sensitive indicator of central nervous system inflammation and immunoglobulin production than is total gamma globulin in disorders such as multiple sclerosis.

> Qualitative changes in the IgG fraction can be identified with agar gel electrophoresis of concentrated CSF. In normal CSF and in most noninflammatory neurologic diseases, the IgG fraction forms a diffuse, homogeneous zone of migration. Normal CSF IgG is less than 8.4 mg per deciliter. In multiple sclerosis and some other subacute and chronic inflammatory diseases, two or more discrete subfractions, which represent specific antibody populations called oligoclonal bands, are identified within the IgG migration zone. Another protein fraction derived from the central nervous system, myelin basic protein, can be identified with radioimmunoassay. It is not present in normal CSF and is an indicator of active demyelination.

Glucose

The glucose level in the CSF is normally about 60% to 70% of that in plasma. Therefore, the normal CSF range is between 45 and 80 mg per decileter for patients with plasma glucose levels of 80 to 120 mg per deciliter. Values less than 35 to 40 mg per deciliter are abnormal.

Glucose enters the CSF from plasma by facilitated diffusion through a specific transport system. Similar mechanisms are responsible for its removal. Glucose is also metabolized by arachnoidal, ependymal, neuronal, and glial cells, or it may leave the CSF with water (bulk flow).

Changes in CSF glucose levels reflect similar changes in the blood, but a variable time is required before the CSF glucose equilibrates with serum glucose. Thus, the CSF level does not reach a maximum for about 2 hours after rapid intravenous injections of hypertonic glucose, and there is a similar delay in the CSF glucose level decreasing after insulin-induced hypoglycemia. Therefore, if it is diagnostically important to measure the CSF glucose level, the CSF and plasma levels should be measured simultaneously, with the patient in a fasting state.

An increase in CSF glucose level is of little diagnostic importance and likely reflects an increase in the plasma glucose level. However, a low CSF glucose level (in association with a normal plasma concentration) is very important. The CSF glucose level is characteristically low in acute bacterial and chronic fungal infections of the central nervous system. (It is frequently normal in viral infections.) Low CSF glucose values are thought to be due primarily to a breakdown of facilitated diffusion of glucose, which effectively slows the rate of entry of glucose into the central nervous system.

- CSF is a clear, colorless fluid with fewer than 5 lymphocytes per microliter, a protein concentration less than 45 mg/deciliter, and a glucose level that is 60% to 70% of that of plasma.

Clinical Correlations I: Disorders of the CSF System

Syndrome of Increased Intracranial Pressure

An uncompensated increase in the volume of any of the constituents of the cranial vault increases intracranial pressure. It can occur from an increase in the total volume of brain tissue (as with diffuse cerebral edema), a focal increase in brain volume (as with intracerebral hemorrhage, neoplasm, or other mass lesion), an increase in CSF volume without an associated loss of brain tissue (as in hydrocephalus), or diffuse vasodilatation or venous obstruction (from any of several causes). Although many clinical symptoms may be associated with increased intracranial pressure, none is individually diagnostic of this condition; yet, together these symptoms form a characteristic clinical pattern consisting of the following:

1. *Headache* is believed to be due to traction on pain-sensitive structures within the cranium. Factors that tend to increase this traction, such as coughing, straining, or position change, often precipitate or aggravate the headache.
2. *Nausea and vomiting* are associated with the vagal motor centers, which are located in the floor of the fourth ventricle and affect motility of the gastrointestinal tract. Increased ventricular pressure transmitted to these vagal motor centers may account for nausea and vomiting.

3. *Increased blood pressure* is related to intracranial pressure; as intracranial pressure increases, arterial blood pressure also must increase if blood flow is to continue in the brain. This response is mediated by neurons in ventrolateral medulla.
4. *Bradycardia* is presumed to be due to pressure on a vagal control mechanism similar to that proposed for nausea and vomiting.
5. *Papilledema* is characterized by elevation and blurring of the optic disc margin, as viewed with an ophthalmoscope (Fig. 11.8). The subarachnoid space of the brain extends along the course of the optic nerve (Fig. 11.9). Thus, increased pressure within the skull and subarachnoid space can be transmitted to the optic nerve, impairing axonal transport. This causes edema of the nerve head.
6. *Alterations in consciousness* occur if the pressure increase is large. As further pathologic change develops, consciousness may be lost because of diffuse hypoperfusion and secondary brainstem compression (see Chapter 10).
7. *Changes in the skull* occur in children and adults. In children, in whom the bones of the cranial vault have not yet fused permanently, chronic increases in pressure may be partially compensated for by a modest separation of the bones along the suture lines. In infants, in whom a soft spot (fontanelle) has not yet ossified, the membranous fontanelle at the vertex of the head may become tense and bulge outward. In adults, in whom bony fusion is complete and the skull is incapable of further expansion, demineralization of bone, especially around the sella turcica, is occasionally seen.

The clinical syndrome of increased intracranial pressure may occur in isolation, but more commonly it is superimposed on the signs and symptoms of the underlying lesion. If this syndrome occurs with signs of a focal lesion, whether acute, subacute, or chronic in evolution, the most likely diagnosis is a mass lesion.

- Increased intracranial pressure is associated with headache, nausea and vomiting, increased blood pressure, bradycardia, papilledema, and alteration in consciousness.

Intracranial Hypotension

Intracranial hypotension due to leakage of CSF is a common complication following lumbar puncture. It also can occur spontaneously. It usually is manifested by postural

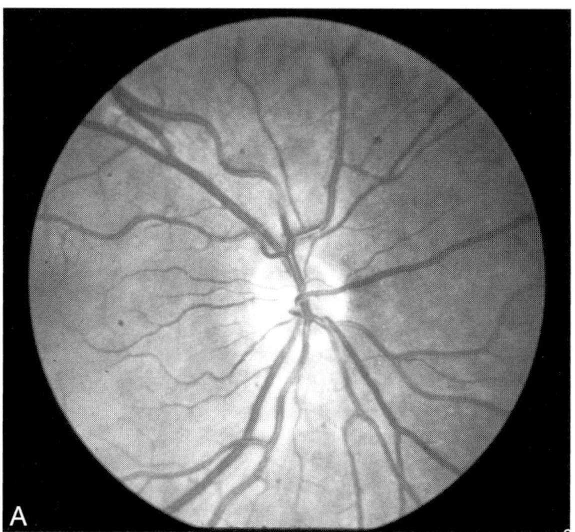

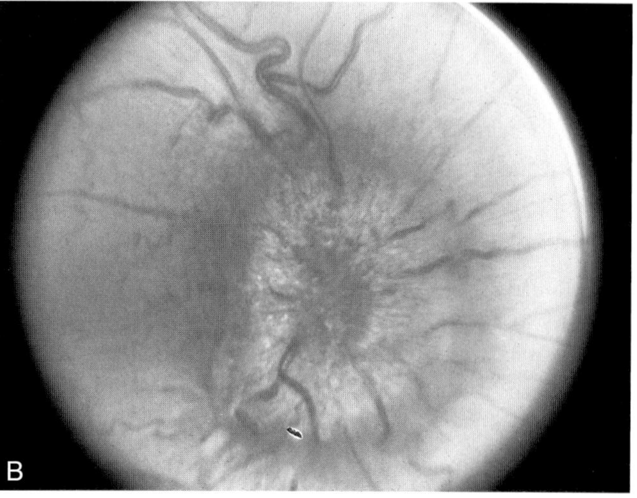

Fig. 11.8. Optic fundus and optic nerve head. *A*, Normal optic disc. *B*, Papilledema. The disc margins are elevated and blurred; venous congestion and hemorrhages are seen surrounding the disc.

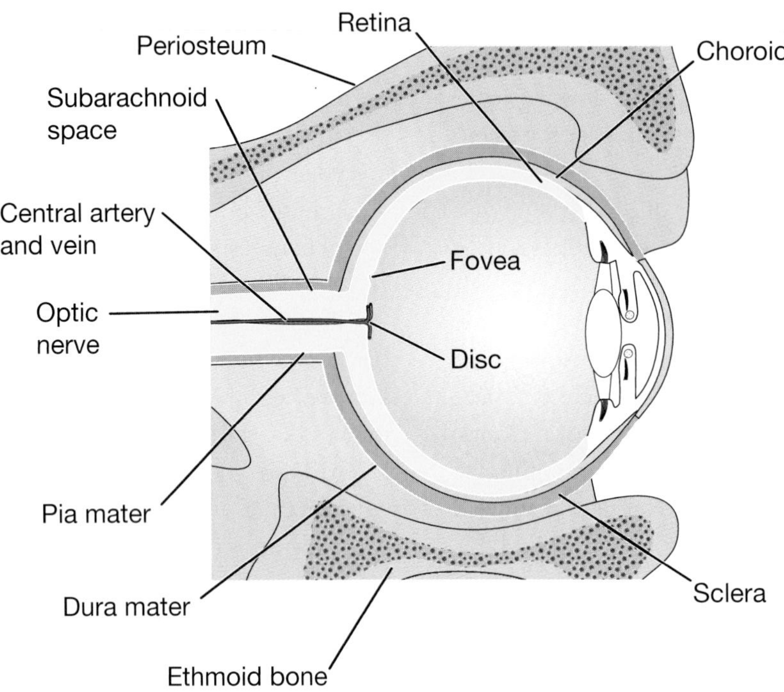

Fig. 11.9. Relation of the meninges and meningeal spaces to the optic nerve. Increased intracranial pressure may cause edema of the optic nerve head.

headache, which occurs or is made worse by assuming an upright position.

Hydrocephalus

In certain pathologic conditions, the pathway for CSF circulation is blocked and absorption is impaired. The rate of CSF formation by the choroid plexus remains relatively constant, and because the amount of CSF increases, there is a corresponding increase in ventricular pressure. Also, the ventricular system proximal to the blockage progressively dilates (hydrocephalus) (Fig. 11.10). Signs and symptoms of increased intracranial pressure also may develop. Studies have shown that the obstruction is most commonly either 1) within the ventricular system itself, that is, proximal to the outlets of the fourth ventricle, for example, aqueductal stenosis (obstructive hydrocephalus), or 2) outside the ventricular system where inadequate circulation over the convexities of the brain prevents adequate resorption, for example, after meningitis or subarachnoid hemorrhage (communicating hydrocephalus) (Fig. 11.11).

- Hydrocephalus is dilation of the ventricles and is caused most often by obstruction of CSF flow in the ventricles or out of the ventricles.
- Communicating hydrocephalus occurs when there is inadequate reabsorption of CSF.

The term hydrocephalus also describes the situation that occurs in brain atrophy. Coincident with the reduction in volume of brain tissue, the ventricles and subarachnoid space enlarge, with an increase in the amount of CSF. The total volume of the intracranial contents is unchanged, however, and there is no increase in intracranial pressure. This type of process is referred to as hydrocephalus ex vacuo.

Cerebral Edema

Brain swelling, or edema, is an increase in brain volume due to an increase in the water content of the brain. It is a nonspecific condition that can be associated with a wide variety of cerebral disorders, including hypoxia,

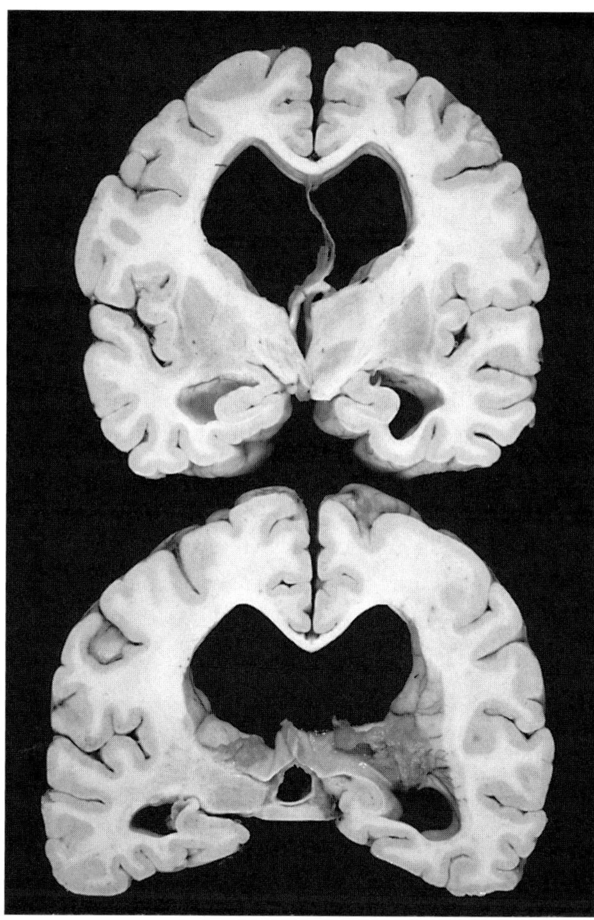

Fig. 11.10. Coronal sections of the cerebral hemispheres showing hydrocephalus. Note marked dilatation of the lateral ventricles, with thinning of the cerebral walls at the expense of the white matter. In the lower (more posterior) section, the thin septum pellucidum has been artificially torn.

Clinical Problem 11.1.

A 10-month-old infant has an enlarging head and a delay in reaching developmental milestones. The neurologic examination confirms developmental delay and also shows a tense, bulging, enlarged anterior fontanelle; opthalmoscopic examination shows normal fundi. The head circumference is 50 cm. The opening CSF pressure is 200 mm H_2O on lumbar puncture. On the basis of these findings, answer the following questions:

a. How do we know the head is abnormally large?
b. What are the possible causes of a large head?
c. What tests might be useful in obtaining information about the infant's ventricular system?
d. Does the lesion found in this patient produce a communicating or noncommunicating type of hydrocephalus?
e. What changes would you expect to find in the configuration of the ventricular system in a computed tomographic scan or magnetic resonance image of
   i. this patient
   ii. a patient with chronic obstruction of the foramina of Luschka and Magendie
   iii. a patient with inflammatory obliteration of the intracranial arachnoid villi
   iv. a patient with an acute subarachnoid hemorrhage

meningitis, neoplasm, abscess, and infarction. Three major types of brain edema have been described:

1. *Vasogenic edema* results from an increase in permeability of brain capillary endothelial cells and produces an increase in extracellular fluid volume.
2. *Cytotoxic edema* is an increase in the intracellular fluid volume of the brain. This form of edema is presumably caused by failure of the ATP-dependent Na^+ pump mechanism, with the result that Na^+ efflux is altered and water enters the cell, maintaining osmotic equilibrium.
3. *Interstitial edema* is a periventricular transudate found in cases of communicating hydrocephalus, with increased CSF pressure and passive movement of CSF from the ventricles into the surrounding periventricular regions.

Although vasogenic edema is seen most often surrounding focal brain lesions and cytotoxic edema is

Clinical Problem 11.2

A 38-year-old man with the same pathologic condition as the infant in Clinical Problem 11.1 has normal head size, papilledema, and an opening CSF pressure of 500 mm H_2O on lumbar puncture. How can you explain the differences in these two cases?

seen in association with hypoxia, either type may be relatively well localized or diffuse and widespread. Both types produce an increase in intracranial volume and pressure, causing symptoms of increased intracranial pressure that may be superimposed on the underlying pathologic process (Fig. 11.12).

Intracranial pressure can be monitored clinically with a transducer surgically placed through the skull. The constant assessment of pressure-related changes provides a physiologic basis for therapeutic intervention.

- Cerebral edema is an increase in brain volume due to an increase in the water content of the brain.

Syndrome of Acute Meningeal Irritation

Several noxious agents produce meningeal irritation, but regardless of the cause, the clinical manifestations are similar and consist of the following:

1. Headache is usually prominent and severe and due to vasodilatation or chemical irritation or inflammation (or both) of the major pain-sensitive structures.
2. Stiff neck is caused by irritation of the meninges in the posterior fossa and upper cervical spinal canal, which stimulates spinal nerve roots and results in reflex spasm and contraction of the posterior neck muscles. This increased resistance to neck flexion is termed nuchal rigidity.
3. Alteration in consciousness results from a pathologic process that is widespread and severe, causing diffuse depression of cortical function and change in the level of consciousness.

The common causes of the syndrome of acute meningeal irritation are bacterial meningitis, viral

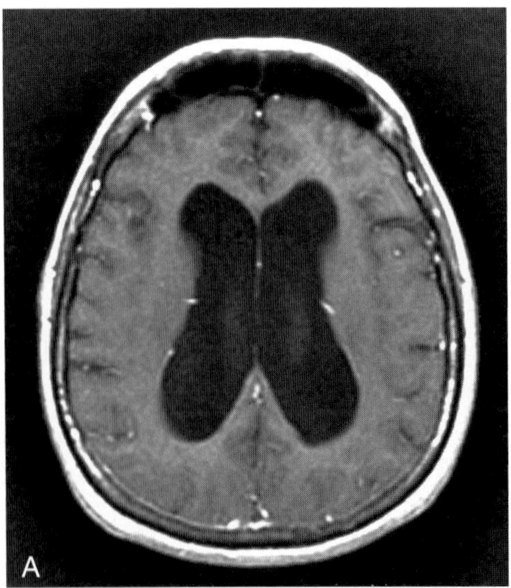

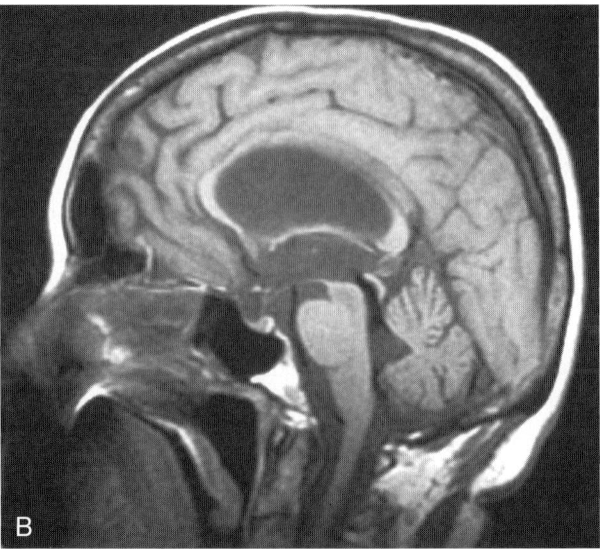

Fig. 11.11. Communicating hydrocephalus as shown by magnetic resonance imaging. *A*, Axial view. *B*, Sagittal view.

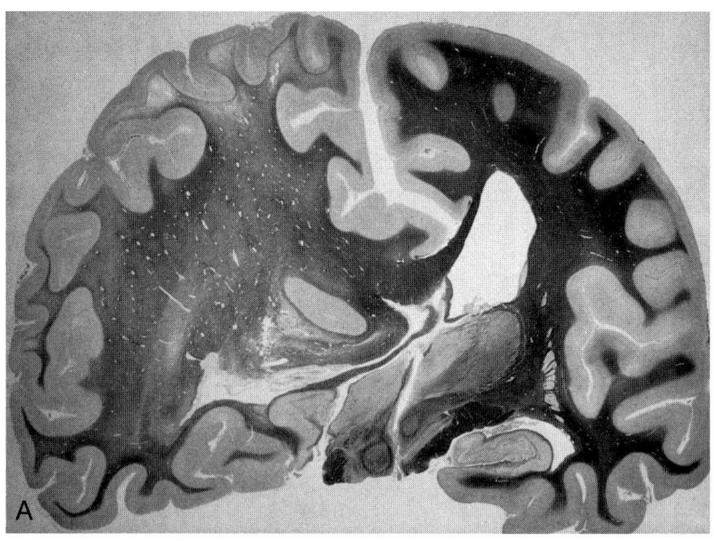

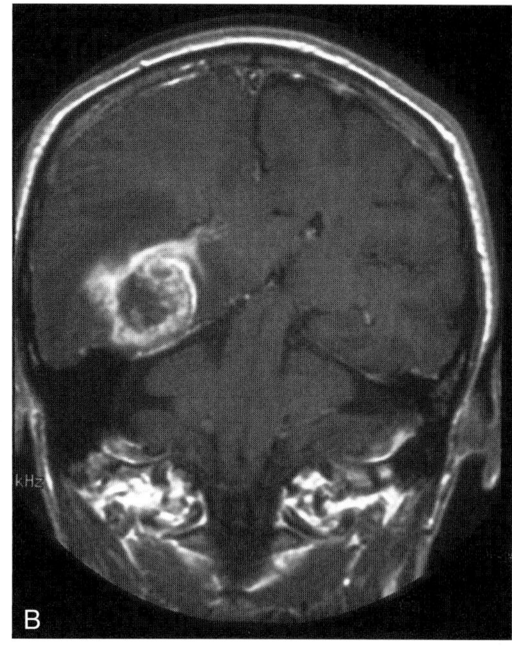

Fig. 11.12. *A*, Cerebral edema (associated with neighboring meningioma, not shown). Note pallor and swelling of the white matter of the left cerebral hemisphere, with marked shift of the midline structures from left to right. (Luxol-fast blue stain; ×1.) *B*, Magnetic resonance image of the brain showing vasogenic edema surrounding a malignant glioma in the right temporal lobe. The increased permeability of the blood-brain barrier is demonstrated by leakage of the contrast material gadolinium (shown as white). Note the mass effect, with distortion and shift of the midbrain to the opposite side.

encephalitis, and subarachnoid hemorrhage. Each of these superimposes its own characteristic signature on the general pattern of meningeal irritation.

- The signs of meningeal irritation are headache, stiff neck, and alteration in consciousness.

Bacterial Meningitis

An inflammation of the CSF system can be caused by bacterial invasion and can be accompanied by a characteristic leukocytic exudate in the pia mater and arachnoid as well as in structures adjacent to the leptomeninges (Fig. 11.13). Bacteria may be found in the CSF and within neutrophils. The type of leukocytic exudate reflects the nature of the invading organism. Most commonly, acute infections are caused by meningococcus, *Haemophilus influenzae*, and pneumococcus organisms and accompanied by a polymorphonuclear exudate. More indolent infections, such as those caused by *Myobacterium tuberculosis* or fungi, are associated with a predominance of lymphocytes. Immunosuppressed patients, for example, those with acquired immunodeficiency syndrome or those who take drugs to prevent rejection of a transplanted organ, commonly have meningitis due to opportunistic organisms such as fungi or parasites. In these patients, the cellular response may be poor. The pathologic reaction is distributed widely throughout the leptomeninges, but it may be most extensive in the basal subarachnoid cisterns. The clinical-anatomical-temporal profile of this disorder is that of diffuse, subacute, and progressive involvement of the nervous system, with the superimposed features of fever and systemic reaction and the syndrome of meningeal irritation, and with or without evidence of increased intracranial pressure. After treatment or subsidence of the infection, reactive changes may occur within the CSF system, impairing CSF absorption and producing hydrocephalus.

Viral Encephalitis

Viral infections usually induce remarkably few gross pathologic changes in the brain. Vascular dilatation, congestion, and edema are not uncommon, and occasional petechial hemorrhages may be seen in the cerebral cortex. The histopathologic features are necrosis of nerve cells and neuronophagia, perivascular cuffing by lymphocytes and mononuclear leukocytes, and meningeal infiltration by similar cells. The clinical-anatomical-temporal profile of this disorder is virtually identical to that noted for bacterial meningitis (diffuse, subacute, and progressive); however, because of the difference in the inflammatory response, the findings on examination of the CSF may be different (Table 11.1).

Subarachnoid Hemorrhage

The acute rupture of an intracranial vessel may produce little pathologic change in the brain itself. As red blood cells intermix with CSF, the signs and symptoms of meningeal irritation are to be expected. Most commonly, subarachnoid hemorrhage is a result of trauma, rupture of an intracranial aneurysm, or leakage from an arteriovenous malformation. Although the bleeding is often from a single, well-localized source, blood rapidly mixes with CSF and is distributed throughout the neuraxis (Fig. 11.14). A diffuse, acute, and sometimes progressive disorder results. Only rarely does an aneurysm produce focal signs.

Examination of the CSF by lumbar puncture is the usual means of initially differentiating the disorders that produce the syndrome of meningeal irritation (Table 11.1).

Intracranial Epidural Hematoma

An epidural hemorrhage lies between the dura mater and the inner table of the skull and usually occurs from a skull fracture or traumatic laceration of the *middle meningeal artery*. Blood dissects the dura mater from the bone, forming a localized, rapidly expanding intracranial mass. Typically, the patient receives an injury to the head of sufficient force to produce a period of unconsciousness. Thereafter, depending on the rate of bleeding, the patient becomes increasingly drowsy and lapses into stupor and finally into deep coma. The cerebral hemisphere is pushed

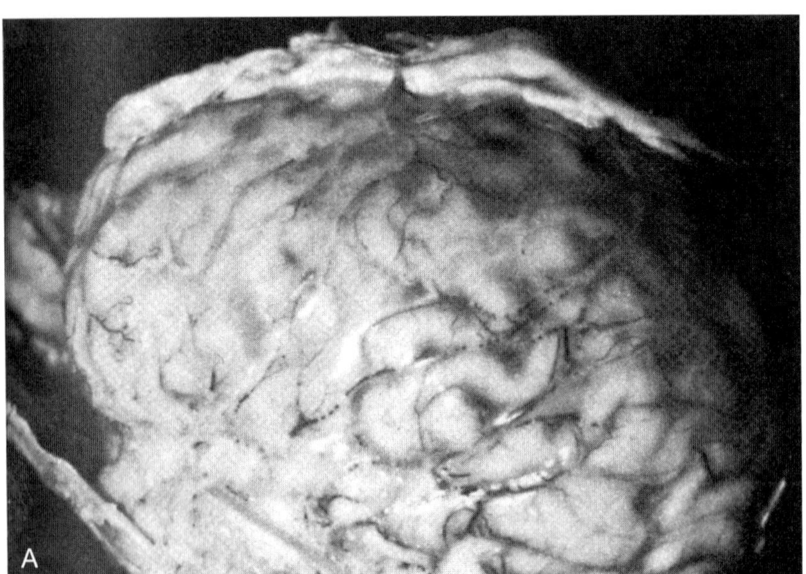

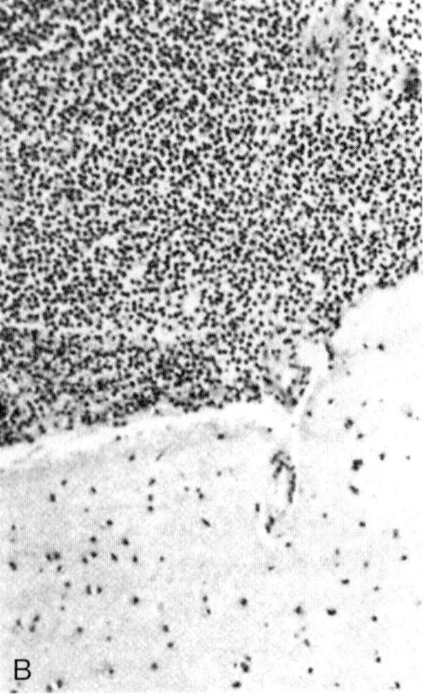

Fig. 11.13. Acute purulent bacterial meningitis. *A*, Brain in situ viewed from the left side showing marked clouding of the subarachnoid space. *B*, Section of cerebral cortex, with the adjacent subarachnoid space filled with acute inflammatory cells. (H&E; ×250.)

Table 11.1. CSF Findings in Syndromes Involving Meningeal Irritation

CSF	Normal	Subarachnoid hemorrhage	Bacterial meningitis	Viral encephalitis
Appearance	Clear	Bloody	Cloudy	Clear to slightly cloudy
Cell count	<5 lymphocytes	Red blood cells present White blood cells in proportion to red blood cells in the peripheral blood cell count	Usually >1,000 white blood cells, mostly polymorphonuclear leukocytes	Usually 25-500 white blood cells, mostly lymphocytes
Protein	<45 mg/dL	Normal to slightly increased	Usually increased >100 mg/dL	Minimally increased, usually <100 mg/dL

CSF, cerebrospinal fluid.

medially by the enlarging mass and compresses the midbrain against the unyielding free edge of the tentorium cerebelli. The patient will die unless emergency measures are taken to evacuate the blood clot.

The clinical-anatomical-temporal profile of this lesion is that of an acute, focal, and progressive lesion, with evidence of increased intracranial pressure. The patient often has a history of trauma.

Intracranial Subdural Hematoma

Subdural hematomas are most common in infants and adults of middle age and older, particularly adults who are likely to have head injury (e.g., alcoholics). The injury that produces the hematoma may be severe or so mild that it is forgotten.

At the time of injury, a cortical vein usually tears at the point where it attaches to the superior sagittal sinus. As a result, a small amount of bleeding occurs in the subdural space. Often, the initial bleeding is not enough to cause noticeable symptoms. Fibroblasts and capillaries proliferate and surround the blood with a fibrous membrane derived from the dura mater. The hematoma enlarges from recurrent bleeding of the neomembrane or from increased osmotic activity of disintegrating red blood cells. With further increase in size, the intracranial volume increases, compressing the underlying brain (Fig. 11.15). The typical clinical-anatomical-temporal profile of this not uncommon and potential treatable disorder is that of a chronic, focal, progressive lesion with symptoms of increased intracranial pressure.

- A subarachnoid hemorrhage occurs with an acute rupture of a blood vessel in the subarachnoid space.
- An intracranial epidural hemorrhage is usually caused by rupture of the middle meningeal artery.
- A subdural hematoma is caused by rupture of a cortical vein and usually is a result of trauma.

Clinical Correlations II: Diagnostic Studies Using the CSF System

The anatomy, physiology, and known pathologic changes that may occur within the CSF system are the basis for many neurodiagnostic tests.

Lumbar Puncture

Although lumbar puncture is a procedure with little risk or discomfort to the patient, examination of the CSF by puncture of the lumbar subarachnoid sac is not a routine diagnostic test. Lumbar puncture is indicated only when it is necessary to obtain specific information about

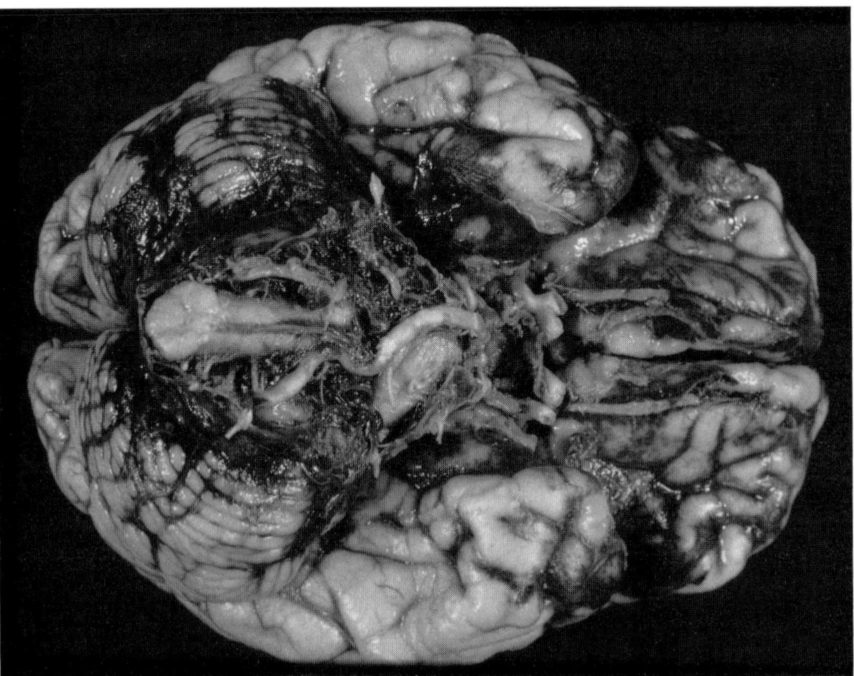

Fig. 11.14. Base of the brain after acute subarachnoid hemorrhage from a ruptured aneurysm. Note that blood occurs throughout the subarachnoid space but is concentrated in major cisterns.

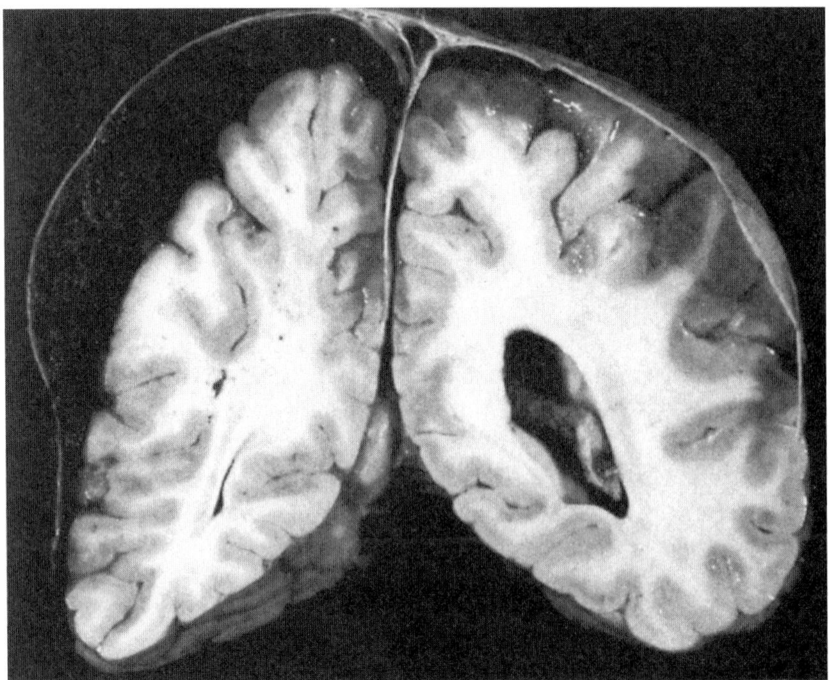

Fig. 11.15. Left subdural hematoma. Note the accumulation of blood between the dura mater and arachnoid, with compression of the left cerebral hemisphere.

the cellular or chemical constituents of the CSF. The procedure usually is contraindicated if there is known or suspected increased intracranial pressure, because in certain instances (especially those of localized mass lesions) sudden alteration in CSF pressure dynamics can lead to herniation of the brain contents through the foramen magnum and clinical decompensation or death. Usually when increased intracranial pressure is suspected, a brain imaging study (such as computed tomography or magnetic resonance imaging) is performed to help define the nature of the intracranial pathologic process before a decision is made about whether lumbar puncture is needed.

The examination is performed in one of the three lower lumbar interspaces (Fig. 11.16). Puncture above the L2-3 interspace (the region of the conus medullaris) is inadvisable. In infants or children in whom the spinal cord may be situated at a lower level, the puncture should be performed in the L4-5 or L5-S1 interspace.

With the patient in a lateral recumbent position, a simple manometer is used to measure CSF pressure (normally less than 200 mm H_2O). To ensure that the needle is placed properly in the subarachnoid sac, the pressure response to gentle coughing, straining, or abdominal compression should be observed. Normally, a prompt increase in pressure of at least 40 mm H_2O results from the increase in central venous pressure that accompanies these maneuvers.

After the initial pressure is measured, the appearance of the fluid is noted, and 5 to 15 mL of CSF is removed for cell count, protein analysis, measurement of glucose level, and microbiologic and other studies. A serologic test for syphilis is generally performed on all CSF specimens because that disease, characterized partly by a chronic inflammatory reaction in the central nervous system, may mimic many other disorders.

Even with the most experienced examiners, one of the veins in the spinal epidural space is nicked occasionally by the lumbar puncture needle, producing a "traumatic tap." Bloody fluid is obtained, and this must be differentiated from a true subarachnoid hemorrhage. In a traumatic tap, fluid collected in successive test tubes usually shows a decreasing amount of red blood cells, but in cases of hemorrhagic disease, the blood staining of the fluid is uniform. Furthermore, in a hemorrhagic disorder, several hours often elapse between the onset of symptoms and the performance of a lumbar puncture, and xanthochromic staining of the supernatant fluid is seen in a centrifuged specimen; this staining is not noted in the case of a traumatic puncture.

- Lumbar puncture is used to obtain information about the cellular and chemical components of the CSF.

Neuroimaging Studies

Myelography

Myelography consists of the introduction of a radiopaque substance, usually by lumbar puncture, into the subarachnoid space. Myelography can be used to study the spinal canal (Fig. 11.17 *A*) and posterior fossa (Fig. 11.17 *B*) and is often combined with computed tomography for better definition of abnormality at the spinal level.

Computed Tomographic Imaging

Computed tomography is another method for studying the anatomy of the intracranial space in patients. This

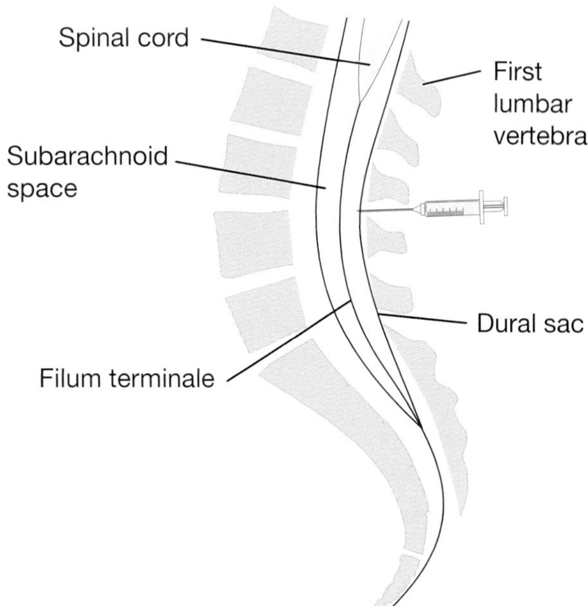

Fig. 11.16. Site of lumbar puncture. Note that in a normal adult, the caudal border of the spinal cord lies at the L1-L2 vertebral level.

Clinical Problem 11.3.

You are called to the emergency department to evaluate a semicomatose elderly woman who responds to painful stimuli with movement of all four extremities. She was brought to the hospital by police ambulance after being found in her apartment by neighbors who had not seen her for 3 days. On physical examination, blood pressure is 120/80 mm Hg, pulse 120 per minute, respiration 124 per minute, and temperature 39.5°C rectally. There is marked resistance to flexion but not to lateral rotation of the neck. Results of the rest of the examination are normal. Opening CSF pressure on lumbar puncture is 270 mm H_2O. Examination of the CSF shows the following:

1) Appearance before centrifugation:
   tube #1—2+ pink, 2+ turbid
   tube #3—slightly pink, 2+ turbid
2) Appearance after centrifugation: all tubes clear and colorless
3) Cell counts:
   tube #1—300 white blood cells (90% polymorphonuclear leukocytes) and 2,800 red blood cells
   tube #3—320 white blood cells (90% polymorphonuclear leukocytes) and 700 red blood cells
4) Protein:
   tube #1—180 mg/dL
   tube #3—176 mg/dL
5) Glucose: 10 mg/dL in all tubes

On the basis of these findings, answer the following questions:

a. What is the location of the lesion (level? lateralization?)? Is this a mass lesion? What is the cause?
b. How do you explain the differences in appearance and cellular count of the CSF between tubes #1 and #3?
c. What would you expect to find on Gram staining of the CSF? On culture of the CSF?
d. How would you explain the CSF glucose result?
e. What structures did the lumbar puncture needle penetrate before it reached the subarachnoid space?

technique, which is rapid, painless, and almost free of risk, permits visualization of the ventricular system, subarachnoid space, and parenchymal structures at the spinal, posterior fossa, and supratentorial levels (Fig. 11.18).

All computed tomographic imaging techniques are based on four general principles. First, they all focus on a physical characteristic of small volumes of tissue (voxels) within a "slice" of the body in a particular plane. Second, they have an array of detectors that allow that characteristic to be measured in each voxel from many different directions. Third, they use a computer to mathematically process the data collected in the detectors in such a way that it localizes each voxel within the slice and assigns it a relative value. Fourth, they use a display module to create a map of the location and relative value of the characteristic in each voxel addressed. This produces a picture in which each voxel is represented by a dot (pixel) of relative intensity on a black-white (or sometimes color) scale. The shade is proportional to the magnitude or intensity of the tissue characteristic measured. The resolution of anatomical and pathologic detail of the resulting picture depends on the matrix (number of pixels per unit area) and the range of differences in the characteristic under study that can be measured. In x-ray computed tomographic scanning, the tissue characteristic measured is electron density as manifested by the attenuation of an x-ray beam. In positron emission tomographic scanning, it is the ability of tissue to take up molecules containing positron-emitting isotopes. In magnetic resonance imaging, it is the density and physical state of mobile hydrogen nuclei (protons) in the tissue.

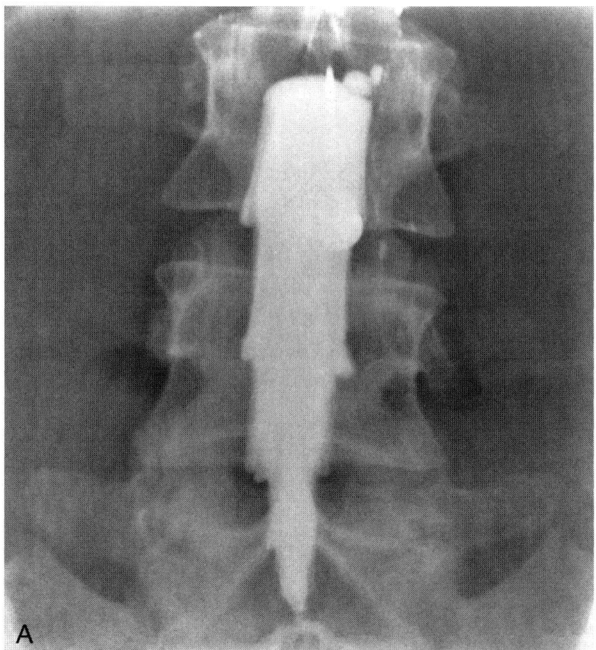

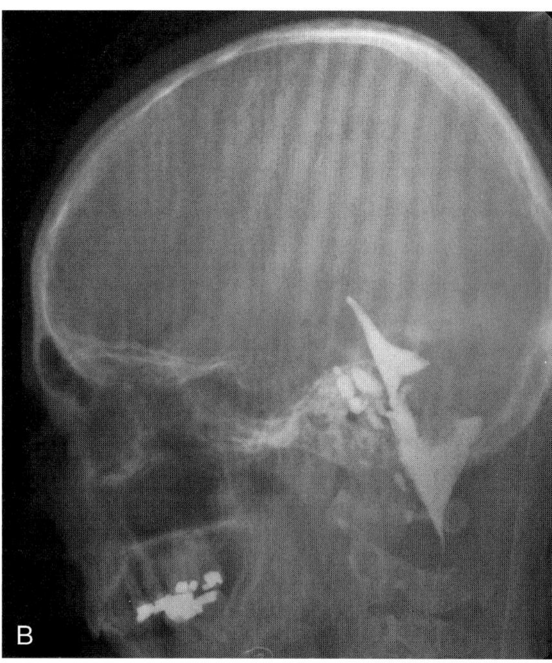

Fig. 11.17. Myelograms. *A*, Anteroposterior view showing filling of the lumbar subarachnoid space. *B*, By tilting the patient downard, contrast medium can be used to visualize the entire spinal canal and structures contained in the posterior fossa (lateral view).

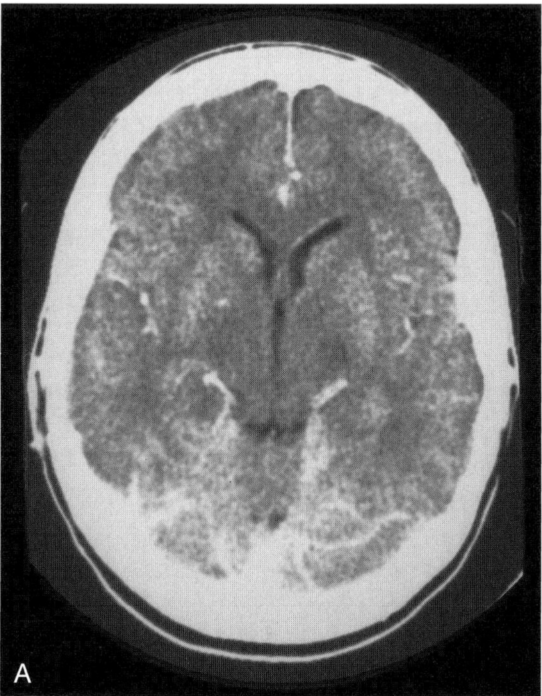

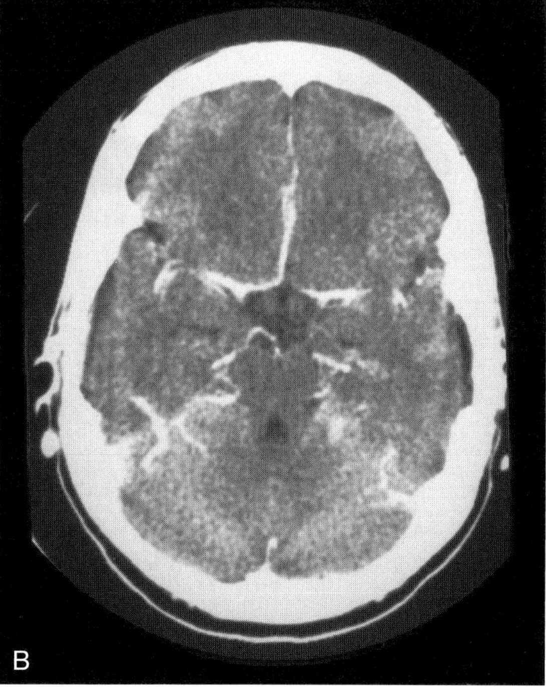

Fig. 11.18. Computed tomograms (axial sections). *A*, Level of the caudate nucleus and thalamus. *B*, The base of the brain at the level of the midbrain.

X-Ray Computed Tomography

Computed tomographic techniques using x-rays to generate the scan were the first to be developed for clinical use. Thin beams of x-rays are passed through the patient's head, and the amount of energy transmitted (not absorbed by structures in its path) is measured with an x-ray detector on the opposite side of the head. This is repeated thousands of times (within a few seconds) from every point around the circumference of the head. The absorption data are processed by a computer, which reconstructs a horizontal section of the head about 1 cm thick. The entire cranial contents can be demonstrated by generating a series of adjacent sections. The ventricular system and any distortions and displacements can be identified. Most hemorrhages, infarcts, and tumors in the substance of the brain can be detected because their density (x-ray absorption) differs from that of normal brain. Intravenously administered contrast media (iodine-containing compounds) aid in visualizing lesions that are vascular or in which the blood-brain barrier is disturbed.

Magnetic Resonance Imaging

Magnetic resonance imaging is the most recently developed technique for imaging the internal structures of the body, including the central nervous system and spinal cord.

- The anatomy of the CSF system can be visualized with myelography, computed tomography, or magnetic resonance imaging.

The physics of magnetic resonance imaging are complicated and beyond the scope of this book. Briefly, hydrogen nuclei (protons) in tissue, mostly as part of water molecules, normally are aligned randomly. When the body is placed in a strong magnetic field, the protons, which behave as tiny magnets because of their spin, align longitudinally in the direction of the flux lines of the field. When a pulse of energy in the form of radio-frequency waves is delivered to the tissue, the aligned protons absorb energy and tilt away from the longitudinal toward the transverse axis of the magnetic field. When the radio-frequency pulse is turned off, the protons begin to realign in the axis of the main magnetic field. It is during this process that they emit radio-frequency energy that is picked up by the detectors. Protons spin at a frequency directly proportional to the local magnetic field. The frequency of this spin is the frequency picked up by the detectors. The different frequencies seen by the detector array allow the voxels to be localized in space.

Signals are only sent from the tissue during the return, or relaxation phase, from transverse magnetization back to longitudinal magnetization. Loss of transverse magnetization occurs from reorientation of protons in the main magnetic field and from magnetic interactions of spinning protons in the tissue, causing them to become out of phase with one another. These two phenomena occur at exponential rates that have time constants referred to as T1 and T2, respectively. In addition to local tissue factors, the intensity of the signal in each voxel is determined by the sequence of radio-frequency pulses, the interval between the pulses, the interval between excitation and detection, and the number of times the sequence is repeated. These factors are under operator control and can be manipulated to emphasize signals generated by either T1 or T2 relaxation phenomena. The resulting images are referred to as being T1- or T2-weighted. They display somewhat different tissue characteristics and, thus, different signal intensities in the same tissue. The T1-weighted images are better for defining normal anatomy. The T2-weighted images are more sensitive for most pathologic conditions, including those producing edema (e.g., infarcts and tumors) or loss of myelin (e.g., multiple sclerosis). Magnetic resonance imaging is especially useful in visualizing posterior fossa structures, the craniocervical junction, and the spinal cord. A contrast material such as gadolinium can be used to enhance lesions associated with increased permeability of the blood-brain barrier.

From a practical clinical standpoint, the major advantage of magnetic resonance imaging over computed tomography is the greater sensitivity of the technique and

Clinical Problem 11.4

A 37-year-old man is evaluated because of a 6-month history of progressive weakness in his legs and loss of pain and thermal sensation to the level of his nipples. On the basis of your findings on physical examination, answer the following questions:

a. What is the location of this lesion (level? localization?)? Is this a mass lesion? What is the cause?
b. What radiologic studies might help you locate the lesion(s) accurately?

greater anatomical detail of the images (Fig. 11.19). Other advantages are listed in Table 11.2. Currently, the drawbacks to the use of magnetic resonance imaging are the need for greater patient cooperation because of the time required to generate images (which are degraded by any motion), the inability to scan patients who have pacemakers or other electronic or metallic implants that could be affected by a magnetic field, and the cost.

Nuclear Medicine Techniques

Radioisotope brain scanning is based on the detection of focal areas of increased permeability of the blood-brain barrier (e.g., tumor or abscess) shown by leakage and accumulation of a normally nondiffusible molecule labeled with a radioisotope. After the labeled molecule is injected into the lumbar subarachnoid space, the circulation of CSF is observed. Localization of the labeled molecule within the ventricles and its failure to circulate over the brain surface after 48 hours are suggestive of a blockage in the extraventricular CSF pathways. A similar procedure can be used to evaluate a CSF leak in patients who have intracranial hypotension. For example, after a skull fracture, CSF may leak through the cribriform plate and produce CSF rhinorrhea. The site of the leak can be identified by detecting where the isotope accumulates.

Neurologic Examination of the CSF System

As part of the neurologic examination of patients who have suspected disease of the CSF system, it is necessary to search specifically for signs of increased intracranial pressure and meningeal irritation. In addition, assessment of this system occasionally requires lumbar puncture.

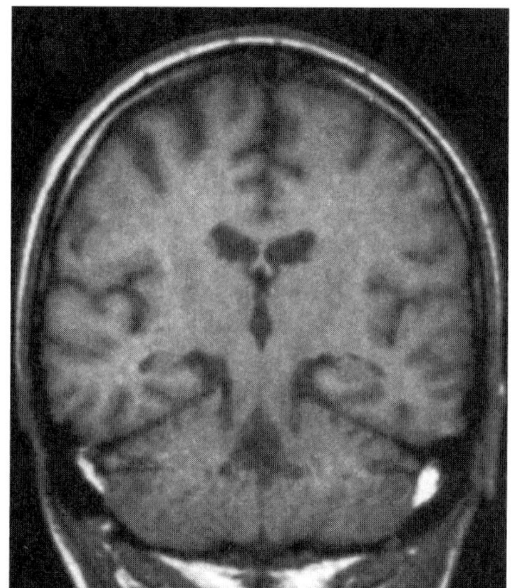

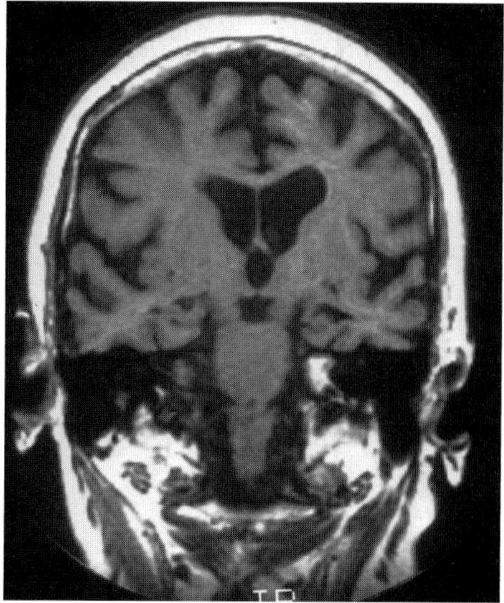

Fig. 11.19. Magnetic resonance images—coronal sections of the brain. *A*, Normal brain. *B*, Brain with atrophy and enlarged ventricles.

Table 11.2. Advantages of Magnetic Resonance Imaging Compared With X-Ray Computed Tomography

No exposure to ionizing radiation
No interference by surrounding bone
Superior resolution of soft tissue
Images can be produced in virtually any plane
Able to image flowing blood
Physiologic imaging

An increase in intracranial pressure is suspected on the basis of the clinical-anatomical-temporal profile of the illness and the constellation of signs and symptoms outlined above. Many patients with increased intracranial pressure have papilledema, and ophthalmoscopic visualization of the optic nerve head in search of papilledema should be performed carefully on all such patients. One must be cautious; although the presence of edema of the nerve head should always raise the possibility of an increase in intracranial pressure, it may be associated with other conditions.

The presence of meningeal irritation is best determined by examining for *nuchal rigidity*. When there is meningeal irritation, the side-to-side movement of the neck causes little discomfort, and frequently the first 10 to 15 degrees of neck flexion meet with little resistance, but with additional flexion, resistance and discomfort increase rapidly. To reduce the effects of traction on the lumbosacral roots when the neck is flexed, a patient with meningeal irritation may automatically flex the hips and knees. (This type of abnormal response seen with meningeal irritation is referred to as the Brudzinski sign.) An additional and related test can be performed with the patient recumbent and the legs flexed at the hips and knees. In this position, the lumbosacral nerve roots are relatively slack, and maneuvers designed to stretch these nerve roots (such as extension of the knee) normally produce no discomfort. In the presence of meningeal irritation, pain and increased resistance (Kernig sign) occur. The presence of Kernig sign without nuchal rigidity (and especially if it is unilateral) is indicative of an irritative process involving the lumbosacral nerve roots rather than diffuse meningeal irritation.

- Neurologic examination of patients with suspected disease of the CSF system should look for signs of increased intracranial pressure and meningeal irritation.

Additional Reading

Fishman RA. Cerebrospinal fluid in diseases of the nervous system. 2nd ed. Philadelphia, PA: W. B. Saunders; 1992.

Junck L, Albers JW, Drury I. Laboratory evaluation. In: Gilman S, editor. Clinical examination of the nervous system. New York: McGraw-Hill; 2000. pp. 269-303.

Rekate HL. Recent advances in the understanding and treatment of hydrocephalus. Semin Pediatr Neurol. 1997;4:167-178.

Rosenberg GA. Brain edema and disorders of cerebrospinal fluid circulation. In: Bradley WG, Daroff RB, Fenichel GM, Jankovic J, editors. Neurology in clinical practice. 4th ed., Vol. 2. Philadelphia, PA: Butterworth Heinemann; 2004. pp. 1745-1762.

Wiebers DO, Dale AJD, Kokmen E, Swanson JW, editors. Mayo Clinic examinations in neurology. 7th ed. St. Louis, MO: Mosby; 1998. (Chapter 14, pp. 331-356; Chapter 16, pp. 469-475.)

Zunt JR, Marra CM. Cerebrospinal fluid testing for the diagnosis of central nervous system infection. Neurol Clin. 1999;17:675-689.

Chapter 12

The Vascular System

Objectives

1. Identify on a diagram the following major vessels, and list the symptoms that might develop in a patient with a lesion of the affected artery:
   a. Vertebral artery
   b. Posterior communicating artery
   c. Common and internal carotid arteries
   d. Anterior cerebral artery
   e. Middle cerebral artery
   f. Basilar artery
   g. Posterior cerebral artery
2. Describe the methods of formation and the role of adenosine triphosphate in brain metabolism.
3. Describe the mechanisms of cell damage that occur with ischemia.
4. Define autoregulation, and discuss the factors that can alter cerebral blood flow.
5. Define ischemia, infarction, intracerebral hemorrhage, epidural hemorrhage, subdural hemorrhage, and subarachnoid hemorrhage.
6. Describe what tests can assess the brain and vasculature for ischemic stroke and hemorrhage.
7. Given a patient protocol:
   a. Recognize when the problem suggests cerebrovascular disease, and list those aspects of the protocol that led to this conclusion.
   b. Localize the area of abnormality to a specific area of the neuraxis, and identify whether that area of abnormality occurs within the distribution of the internal carotid, vertebrobasilar, or spinal arterial systems.
   c. Decide if the basic pathologic mechanism is hemorrhage or infarction, and state the reasons for your choice.

Introduction

The blood vessels to an organ provide it with a relatively constant supply of oxygen and other nutrients and a means for removal of metabolic waste. Failure to meet these vital requirements results in disease in that organ. Because of the unique structure and organization of the nervous system, localized abnormalities in its blood supply may produce devastating alterations in neural function. In this chapter, the normal anatomy and physiology of the vascular supply to neural tissue and the clinical manifestations of pathologic processes affecting this system are described.

Of all neurologic diseases likely to be encountered, cerebrovascular disease (stroke) is among the more common. Cerebrovascular disease represents a major cause of disability and death throughout the world. In the United States, stroke ranks third, after cancer and heart disease, as a cause of death. The amount of money spent annually on diagnosis, treatment, and rehabilitation is extremely large. Because many stroke victims survive the acute phase of illness and live for years thereafter in a disabled condition, the social and economic impact of stroke is immeasurable.

Vascular disease involving cerebral vessels is no different from vascular disease involving other organ systems. The processes of atherosclerosis and thromboembolism differ little whether they involve the cerebral, peripheral, or coronary circulation. However, understanding the clinical problems in patients with cerebrovascular disease depends on more detailed knowledge of the anatomy and physiologic principles unique to the nervous system.

In other longitudinal systems described in accompanying chapters, the manifestations of disease are a direct result of damage to neural tissue within that system. The vascular system, however, is a supporting system, and diseases of the vascular system are manifested as secondary alterations in function in other neural systems. The vascular cause of disease is identified by the characteristic temporal profile of sudden onset and rapid evolution of symptoms involving other systems.

Overview

Arterial Supply

To sustain aerobic metabolism, the brain is supplied by two major arterial systems: the carotid arterial system and the vertebrobasilar arterial system. A series of anastomotic channels, including the circle of Willis located at the base of the brain, connect these two systems.

The *carotid arterial system*, commonly referred to as the *anterior circulation*, supplies much of the cerebral hemispheres. Lesions involving the carotid arterial system may alter function in the distribution of any or all of its three clinically important branches: ophthalmic artery (supplies the retina and choroid), anterior cerebral artery (supplies the medial cerebral hemisphere), and middle cerebral artery (supplies the lateral cerebral hemisphere, basal ganglia, and internal capsule). Therefore, various combinations of hemiparesis, hemisensory deficit, monocular visual loss, homonymous hemianopia, and aphasia are suggestive of a lesion in this system.

The *vertebrobasilar arterial system* (two vertebral arteries and the basilar artery) is often designated as the *posterior circulation* because it supplies the posterior fossa, occipital lobes, and portions of the posterior and inferior temporal lobes. Lesions of the vertebrobasilar system may alter function in the distribution of its branches to the brainstem, cerebellum, occipital lobes, and portions of the temporal lobe. The various combinations of diplopia, dysarthria, dysphagia, and disequilibrium associated with hemiparesis, hemisensory deficit, or homonymous hemianopia are suggestive of a lesion in the vertebrobasilar system.

The blood supply to the spinal cord is through the anterior spinal artery and paired posterior spinal arteries (branches of the vertebral arteries and descending aorta). The vascular supply to the peripheral nerves is usually from nutrient vessels of accompanying major arteries.

Cerebral Blood Flow and Pathophysiology

Cerebral blood flow is normally maintained at a relatively constant rate of approximately 20 to 70 mL/100 g brain tissue per minute. A process called *autoregulation* helps maintain perfusion pressure despite fluctuations in blood pressure and cerebrovascular resistance. A decrease in blood flow below a critical threshold level results in ischemia and infarction.

Occlusive-Ischemic Vascular Disease

When a portion of neural tissue is deprived of its blood supply, *ischemia* develops. If the normal protective mechanisms are insufficient to compensate for this deprivation, death of tissue, or *infarction*, results. The process of metabolic failure leading to cell death involves the cessation of blood flow, loss of energy, and neuronal depolarization. The resultant release of glutamate, entry of calcium ions into the cell, generation of oxygen free radicals and nitric oxide, and the activation of proteases and lipases all contribute to cell breakdown and infarction.

Disease of a blood vessel may result in local thrombus formation, which may progress to occlusion-thrombosis of the vessel, or a portion of the thrombus (embolus) may break loose and lodge in a distal portion of the circulation. Both processes may result in localized areas of neural tissue being deprived of blood, and both may produce a focal destructive lesion (infarct). The clinical symptoms reflect tissue damage in the regions of ischemia and infarction. Atherosclerosis is the most important disease process responsible for thromboembolic disease;

however, it is not the only disease process responsible for it. Ischemia may occur without occlusive disease if there is hemodynamic failure of the circulatory system, as might be seen with cardiac disease or profound hypotension. This type of ischemia also may result in infarction, but the defect, anoxic encephalopathy, is usually distributed diffusely throughout the brain.

Hemorrhagic Vascular Disease

A diseased blood vessel may rupture and leak, producing hemorrhage. Depending on the site of accumulation of the blood, focal or diffuse neurologic symptoms may result. Types of hemorrhage may include epidural, subdural, subarachnoid, and intraparenchymal or intracerebral hemorrhage.

Blood that extravasates throughout the subarachnoid space is a *subarachnoid hemorrhage* and results in diffuse neurologic signs. Subarachnoid hemorrhage is commonly the result of trauma, rupture of an intracranial aneurysm, or bleeding from an arteriovenous malformation.

Blood within the epidural space is an *epidural hemorrhage*. It is usually due to trauma. The onset is generally acute, with focal signs contralateral to the lesion because of significant mass effect.

Blood that accumulates between the dura mater and arachnoid is a *subdural hemorrhage*. The subdural space is a potential space. The cerebral veins in the subarachnoid space travel through the subdural space to drain into the dural venous sinuses. Subdural hemorrhage generally results from traction on these bridging veins. The venous blood leak is slower than an arterial blood leak, and these patients often present with a subacute focal neurologic deficit contralateral to the side of the lesion.

Blood that accumulates within the substance of the brain is an *intracerebral hemorrhage*. It produces signs of a focal, mass lesion. Intracerebral hemorrhage is commonly the result of hypertensive arteriolar disease or bleeding from an arteriovenous malformation.

Clinical Correlation

The clinical pattern seen with disease in the cerebrovascular system is distinctive. The cardinal identifying feature is its *acute* onset. The symptoms of vascular disease may be *focal* or *diffusely distributed*. The symptoms produced reflect the location and mechanism of the pathologic process. The parenchymal lesions, which are the result of either occlusive-ischemic or hemorrhagic disease processes, may be of a *mass* or *nonmass* type (Table 12.1).

Several radiographic techniques can evaluate the cerebral vasculature. *Cerebral angiography* is an examination of the cerebral blood vessels by injection of a radiopaque substance into the arterial system. This study is considered the gold standard test for blood vessel lesions, but it is an invasive test with some risk of complication. Often, before conventional angiography is considered, noninvasive angiography is performed with *magnetic resonance angiography*, *magnetic resonance venography*, or *computed tomographic angiography*. Another noninvasive study of blood vessels that uses ultrasound technology is *ultrasonography*, but the sensitivity and specificity of this technique for intracranial vessels are not as good as the sensitivity and specificity of magnetic resonance angiography or computed tomographic angiography.

Table 12.1. Correlation of Vascular and Parenchymal Disease

	Resultant parenchymal lesion	
Type of vascular disease	**Focal**	**Diffuse**
Occlusive-ischemic	Infarct (nonmass)	Anoxic encephalopathy
Hemorrhagic	Intracerebral hemorrhage (mass)	Subarachnoid hemorrhage

Anatomy of the Vascular System

Blood Supply to the Brain

All the arteries that supply the supratentorial and posterior fossa levels arise from the aortic arch (Fig. 12.1). The *innominate (brachiocephalic) artery* divides into the right common carotid and right subclavian arteries. The left *common carotid artery* arises directly from the apex of the aortic arch. The right and left common carotid arteries ascend in the neck lateral to the trachea. Slightly below the angle of the jaw, the common carotid artery bifurcates into the internal and external carotid arteries.

The *internal carotid artery* on each side enters the skull, without branching, through the carotid canal in the petrous portion of the temporal bone. The petrous segment of the internal carotid artery enters the cranium through the foramen lacerum. After entering the cranium, each internal carotid artery forms an S-shaped curve, the carotid siphon, and lies within the cavernous sinus. As the artery leaves the cavernous sinus, it pierces the cranial dura mater and arachnoid to enter the subarachnoid space at the base of the brain. Just distal to the cavernous segment within the subarachnoid space, the internal carotid artery gives rise to the *ophthalmic artery*,

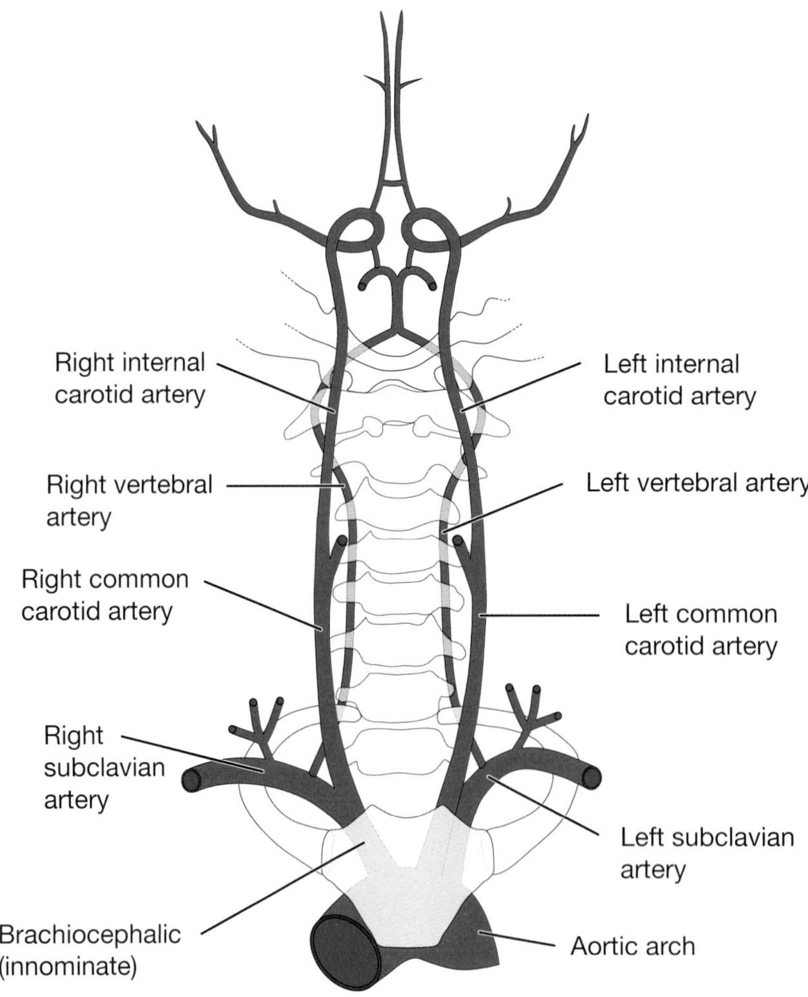

Fig. 12.1. Major arteries supplying the supratentorial and posterior fossa levels.

which makes an important anastomotic communication with branches of the external carotid artery. The ophthalmic artery supplies the retina and choroid of the eye. The internal carotid artery also gives rise to the *posterior communicating* and *anterior choroidal arteries* (Fig. 12.2). The posterior communicating artery connects the internal carotid artery with the posterior cerebral artery. The anterior choroidal artery supplies the ipsilateral internal capsule and a portion of the basal ganglia. At the carotid terminus, each internal carotid artery divides into the anterior cerebral artery and middle cerebral artery.

The *vertebral arteries* are the first branches of the right and left *subclavian arteries*. Each artery ascends through foramina in the transverse processes of the upper six cervical vertebrae, curves behind the articular process of the atlas, pierces the dura mater, and enters the subarachnoid

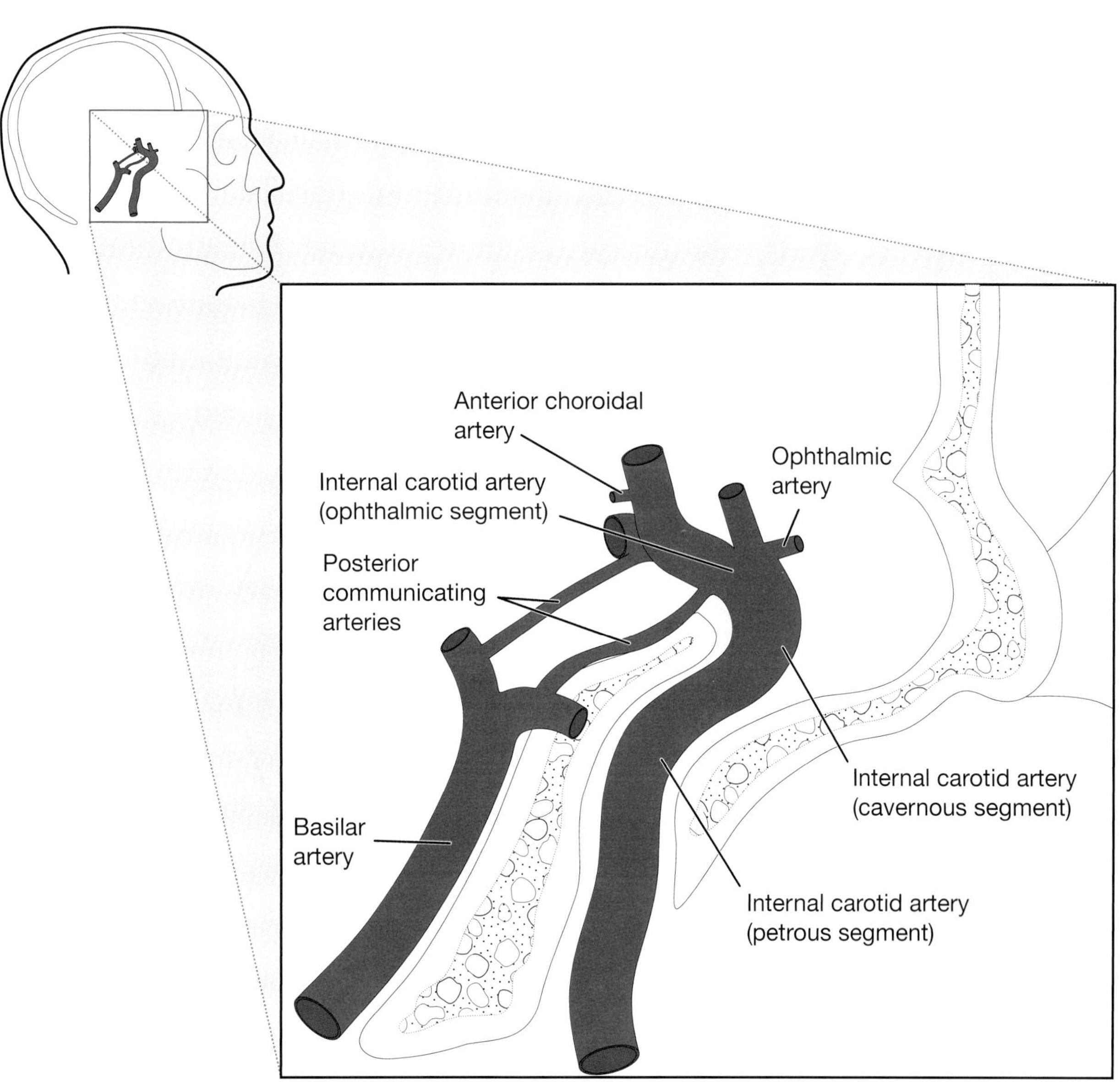

Fig. 12.2. The internal carotid artery.

space at the level of the upper cervical spinal cord. The vertebral arteries enter the cranial cavity through the foramen magnum. The vertebral arteries are subject to normal anatomical variations. For example, the left vertebral artery may arise directly from the arch of the aorta. Also, the two vertebral arteries are often of unequal caliber, one being dominant. The major branches from the vertebral artery include the *anterior spinal artery*, *posterior spinal artery*, and *posterior inferior cerebellar artery*.

The vertebral arteries enter the cranium and ascend on the ventrolateral surface of the medulla oblongata. At the lower border of the pons, they unite to form the *basilar artery*. The major branches of the basilar artery include the *anterior inferior cerebellar artery*, *superior cerebellar artery*, and numerous *median* and *paramedian perforators*. At the level of the midbrain, the basilar artery divides into the right and left *posterior cerebral arteries* (Fig. 12.3).

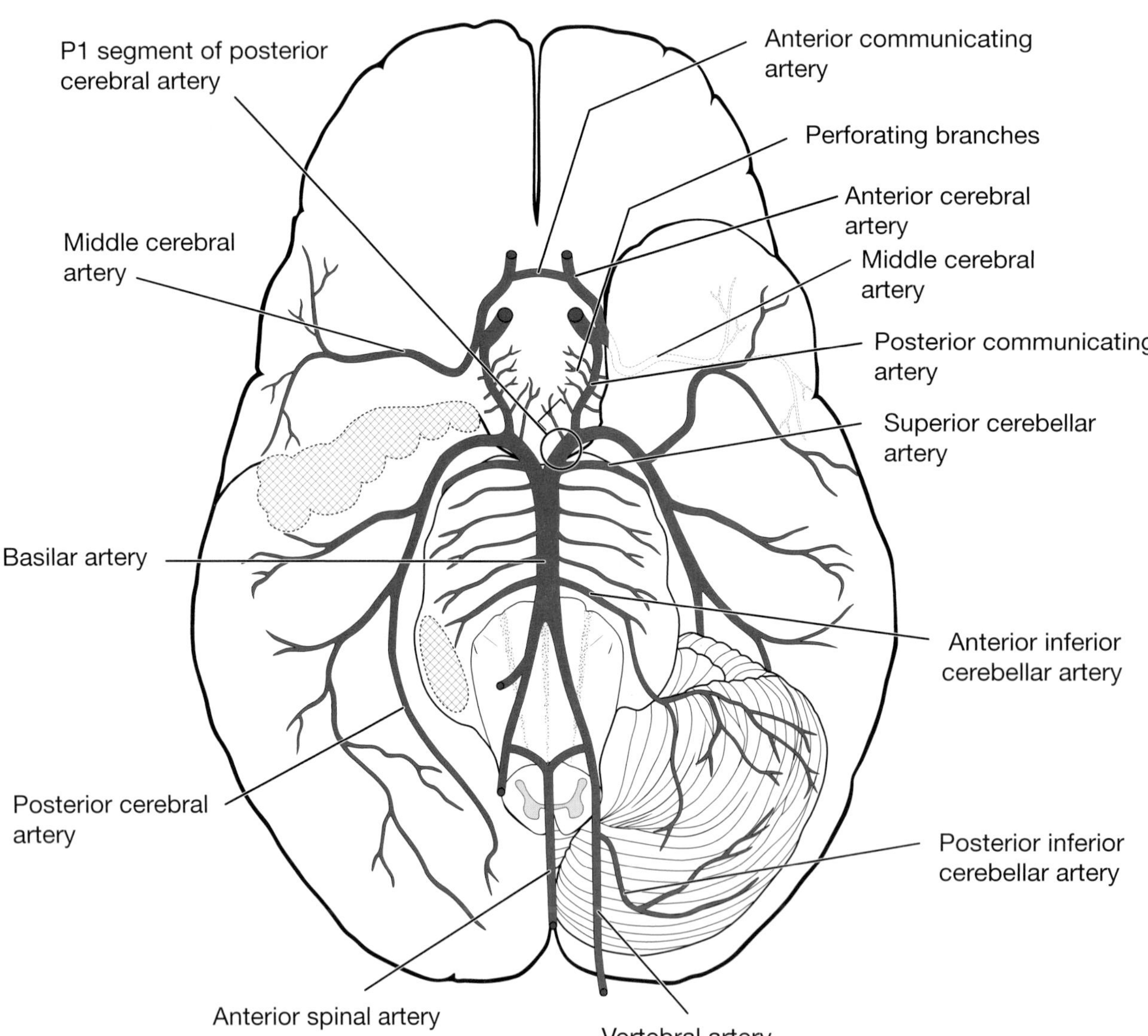

Fig. 12.3. Major arteries on the basal aspect of the brain.

Circle of Willis

At the base of the brain, surrounding the optic chiasm and pituitary stalk, anastomotic connections occur between the internal carotid and vertebrobasilar arterial systems. This ringlike series of vessels is called the *circle of Willis* (Fig. 12.4). It consists of the anterior communicating artery, which unites the two anterior cerebral arteries, and the posterior communicating arteries, which join the internal carotid arteries with the posterior cerebral arteries. The circle of Willis is subject to frequent anatomical variation, and a normal circle is seen in only approximately 30% of the population. Common variations in the circle

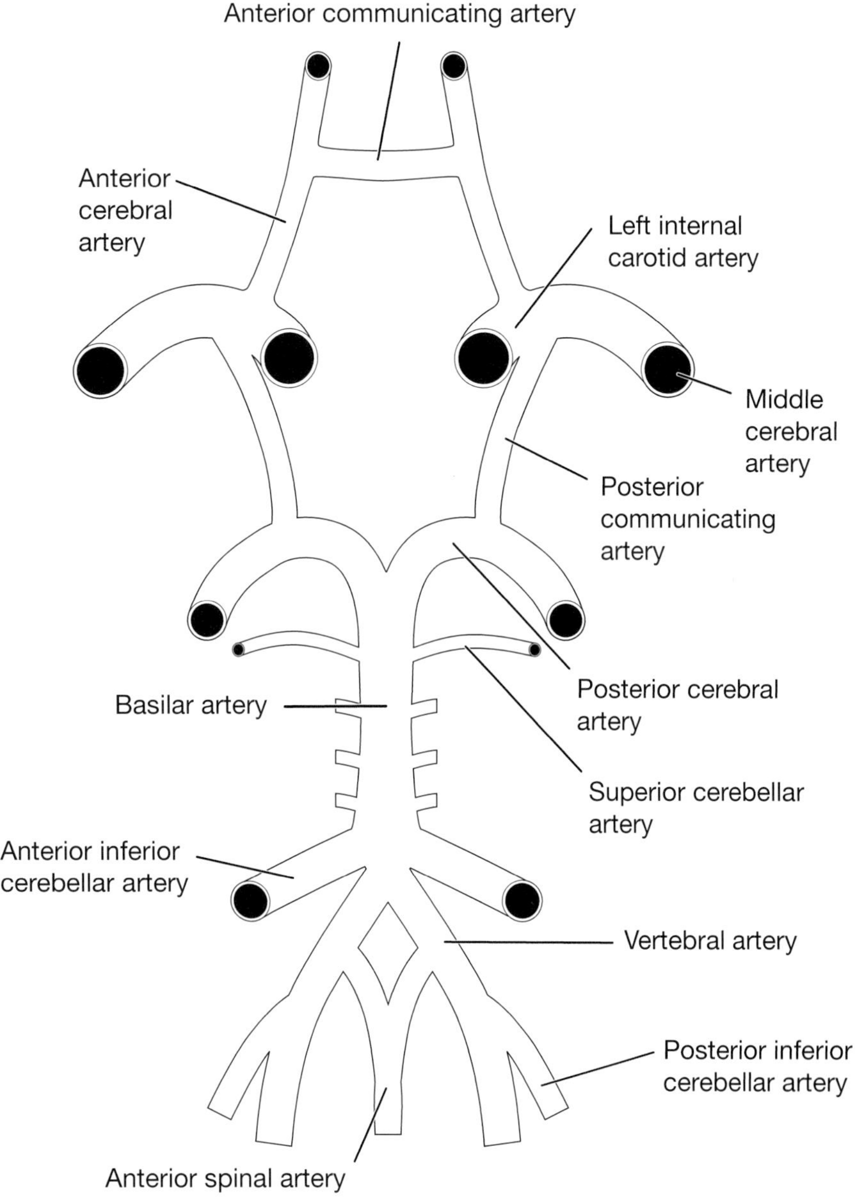

Fig. 12.4. The major intracranial arteries and the circle of Willis (anterior cerebral, anterior communicating, posterior communicating, and posterior cerebral arteries).

include posterior cerebral arteries that arise from the internal carotid artery via an enlarged posterior communicating artery, the absence of one or both posterior communicating arteries, and the presence of multiple small anterior communicating arteries.

Blood Supply to the Outer Tube and Inner Tube of the Neuraxis

The basic concept of neural organization being an outer tube and an inner tube is reflected in the vascular supply to the brain. The cerebral cortex (outer tube), involved in high-order processing in the sensory and motor systems, receives its blood supply from the large anastomotic circumferential arteries, or cortical arteries, that are easily seen in the subarachnoid space. These vessels are responsive to chemical and metabolic regulation and are susceptible to the pathophysiologic processes of atherosclerosis and thromboembolism, often resulting in large areas of infarction. In contrast, the blood supply to the deep structures (inner tube), including the diffuse internal regulation and consciousness systems, is from penetrating or perforating vessels and end arterioles. These vessels are less responsive to chemical and metabolic regulation and are susceptible to the pathologic changes accompanying blood pressure change, which predispose to small (lacunar) infarction and intracranial hemorrhage.

Blood Supply to the Cerebral Hemispheres

The supratentorial level is provided with blood from the *anterior*, *middle*, and *posterior cerebral arteries* (Fig. 12.5). The *anterior cerebral artery* (Fig. 12.6) supplies the medial surface of the cerebral hemisphere and the superior border of the frontal and parietal lobes. The *middle cerebral artery* (Fig. 12.7) supplies most of the lateral surface of the cerebral hemisphere, including the lateral portions of the frontal lobe, the superior and lateral portions of the temporal lobe, and the deep structures of the frontal and parietal lobes. The *posterior cerebral artery* supplies the entire occipital lobe and the inferior and medial portions of the temporal lobe (Fig. 12.3). The deeper structures of the cerebral hemispheres are supplied by penetrating branches of the larger arteries.

Of notable importance are the perforating *lenticulostriate arteries* (Fig. 12.7), which supply the basal ganglia and internal capsule, and the perforating branches of the posterior cerebral artery, which supply the thalamus (Fig. 12.8).

Anastomoses and Collateral Circulation

Extensive communications exist between the arterial systems that supply the brain. Because of the potential for additional circulation through these alternate channels, occlusion of one or more intracranial or extracranial vessels may occur occasionally, with few or no neurologic signs and symptoms.

The major anastomoses are 1) the circle of Willis, 2) corticomeningeal (leptomeningeal) communications between the three major cerebral vessels on the surface of the hemispheres at the junctions between the areas supplied by these vessels, and 3) communications between extracranial and intracranial arteries.

The most important extracranial to intracranial anastomoses occur in the regions of the face and orbit, where the ophthalmic artery, a branch of the internal carotid artery, communicates with the superficial temporal and facial branches of the external carotid artery. Occasionally, anastomoses between the external carotid and vertebral arteries occur in the neck.

Blood Supply to the Posterior Fossa

The structures contained in the posterior fossa (midbrain, pons, medulla, and cerebellum) are supplied by branches of the vertebral and basilar arteries (Fig. 12.3). Although these vessels have numerous branches, the pattern of blood supply from the branches is relatively constant (Fig. 12.9). At each level of the brainstem, short median and paramedian perforating branches supply a zone on either side of the midline. The paramedian area of the caudal medulla is supplied by the anterior spinal artery, which arises from the union of branches from each vertebral artery. The paramedian area at higher levels is supplied by penetrating branches of the basilar artery. An intermediate zone is supplied by short circumferential branches of the vertebrobasilar system. The lateral areas of the brainstem and the cerebellum are supplied by three pairs of long circumferential arteries. The *posterior inferior cerebellar artery* arises from the vertebral artery and supplies the lateral medulla and posterior inferior aspect of the cerebellum.

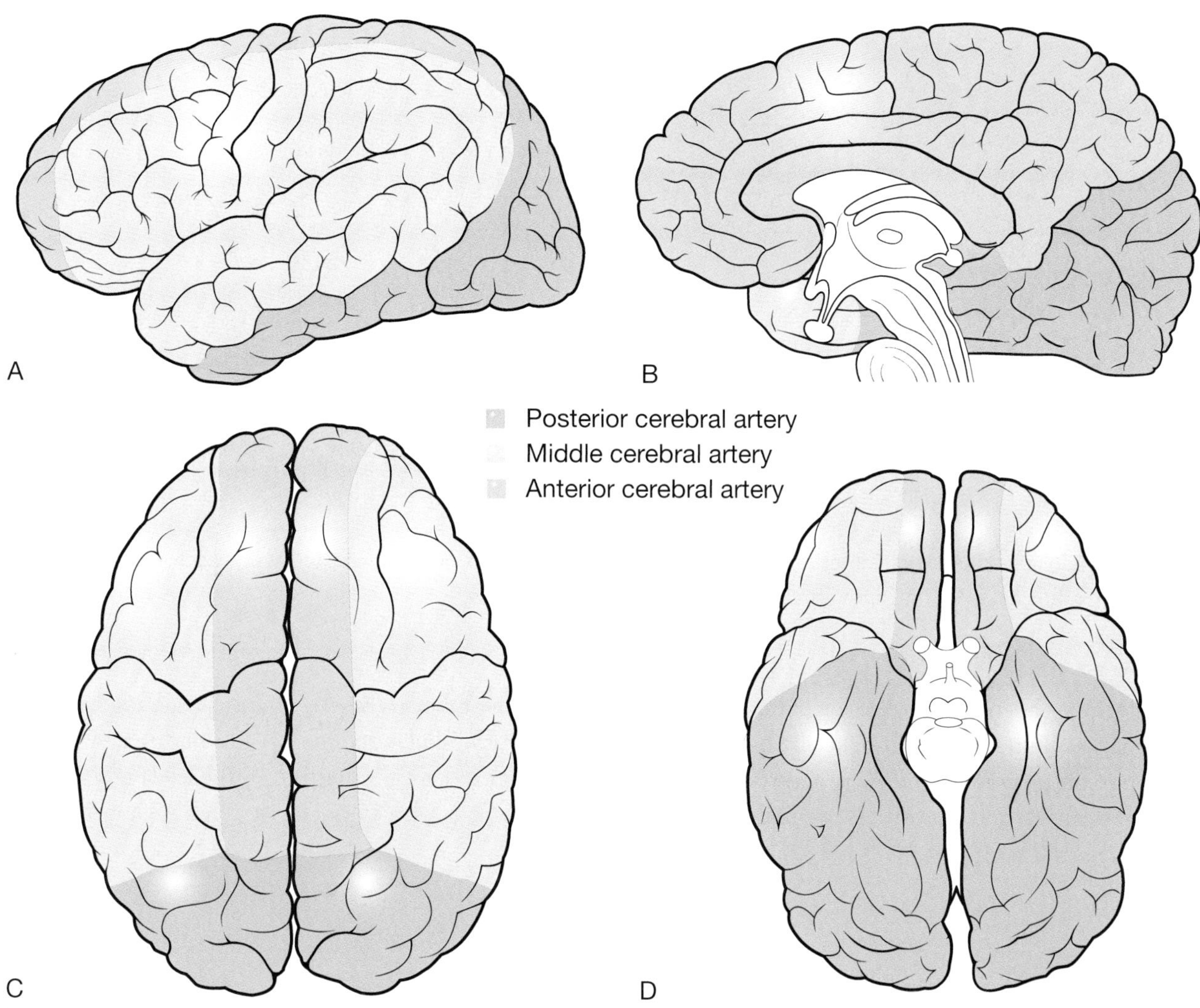

Fig. 12.5. Distribution of the anterior, middle, and posterior cerebral arteries. *A*, Lateral, *B*, medial, *C*, superior, and *D*, inferior views.

The *anterior inferior cerebellar artery* is a branch of the basilar artery and supplies the lateral aspect of the pons and the anterior inferior aspect of the cerebellum. The *superior cerebellar artery* is a branch of the basilar artery and supplies the lateral midbrain and superior surface of the cerebellum.

Functional Anatomy of the Cerebral Vasculature

Clinically, the distribution of a presumed arterial lesion can be inferred by relating the observed signs and symptoms to the anatomy of the cerebral vessels. Although precise localization to a specific blood vessel is sometimes desirable, it is essential to be able to determine whether a lesion lies in the distribution of either the carotid (anterior circulation) or vertebrobasilar (posterior circulation) arterial systems (Table 12.2). Lesions may be due to involvement of the entire carotid or vertebrobasilar system or their distal branches.

Lesions involving the internal carotid artery may alter function in the distribution of any or all of its three

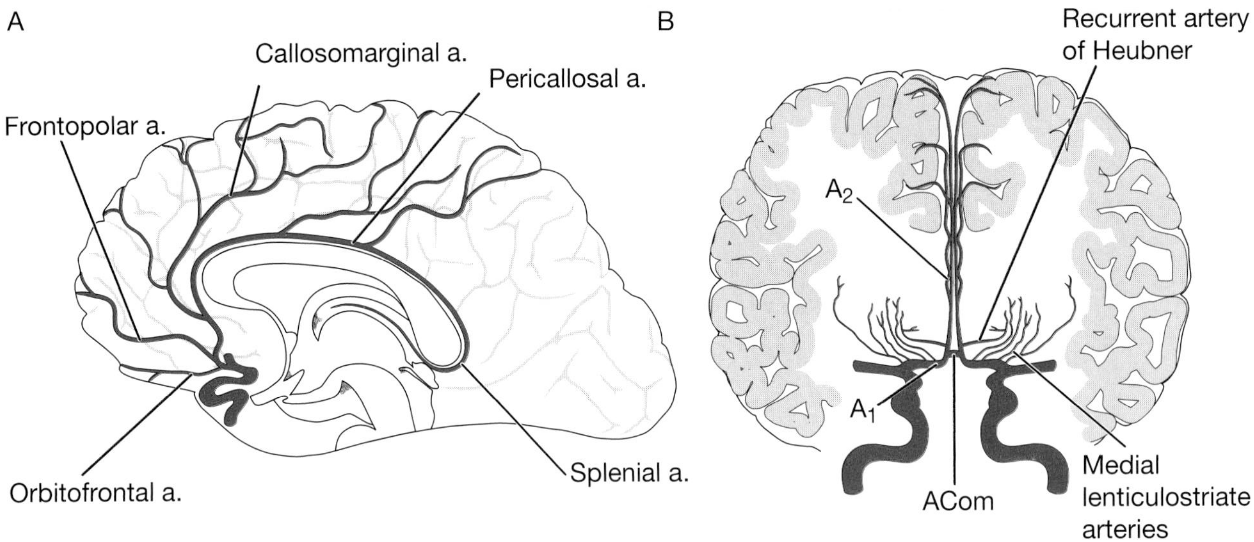

Fig. 12.6. Major branches of the anterior cerebral artery. *A*, Lateral and *B*, coronal views. A_1 and A_2, Segments of the anterior cerebral artery; ACom, anterior communicating artery.

clinically important branches. A lesion of the *ophthalmic artery* may result in ipsilateral monocular loss of vision. A lesion of the *anterior cerebral artery* may result in contralateral weakness and sensory loss primarily in the leg. A lesion of the *middle cerebral artery* may result in contralateral weakness and sensory loss maximal in the face and arm and, to a less degree, in the leg (Fig. 12.10). If the optic pathways are involved, a contralateral

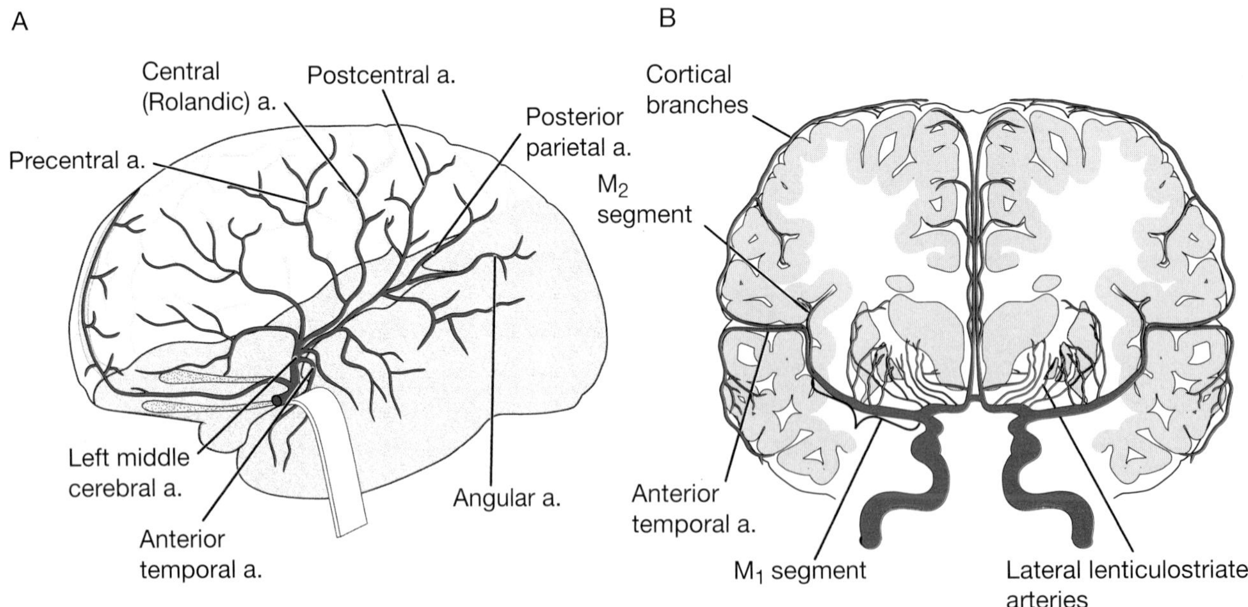

Fig. 12.7. Major branches of the middle cerebral artery. *A*, Lateral, and *B*, coronal views. M_1 and M_2, segments of middle cerebral artery.

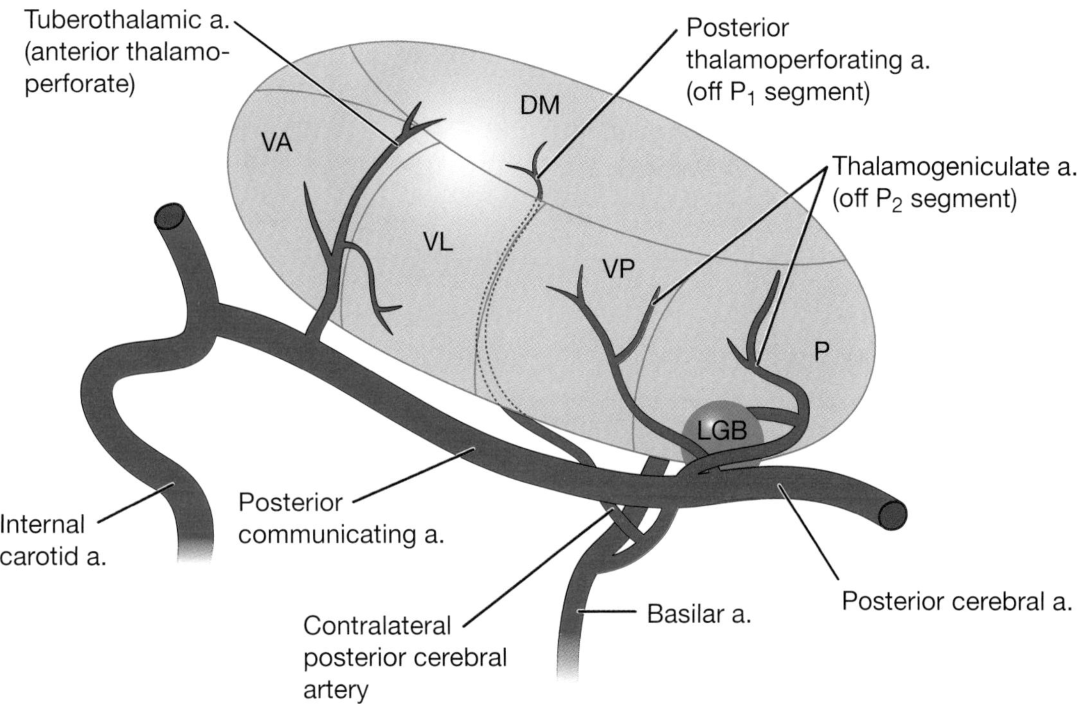

Fig. 12.8. Blood supply to the thalamus. Thalamic nuclei: *DM*, dorsomedial; *LGB*, lateral geniculate body; *P*, pulvinar; P_1 and P_2, segments of the posterior cerebral artery; *VA*, *VL*, *VP*, ventral anterior, lateral, and posterior, respectively.

homonymous hemianopia may be produced. With dominant hemisphere lesions, the speech areas may be involved, which will result in aphasia. Nondominant hemisphere lesions may result in hemineglect of space. Therefore, the various combinations of hemiparesis, hemisensory deficit, monocular loss of vision, homonymous hemianopia, and aphasia are suggestive of a lesion in the carotid arterial system.

Lesions involving vertebral and basilar arteries may alter function in the distribution of any or all of their clinically important branches. A lesion affecting branches that supply the brainstem may result in loss of brainstem function, cranial nerve abnormalities (with or without hemiparesis), and hemisensory deficits. A lesion affecting branches that supply blood to the cerebellum may result in ataxia and disequilibrium. A lesion of branches of the posterior cerebral artery, which supply the occipital lobe, may produce unilateral or bilateral hemianopia. Therefore, the various combinations of diplopia, dysarthria, dysphagia, and disequilibrium associated with hemiparesis, hemisensory deficit, and homonymous hemianopia are suggestive of a lesion in the vertebrobasilar arterial system.

Clinical Problem 12.1.

A 50-year-old man experienced sudden onset of vertigo. Neurologic examination showed dysarthria, difficulty with swallowing, left Horner syndrome, left palatal weakness, and loss of pain sensibility over the left face and right limbs and trunk. He had coarse ataxia and incoordination of his left arm.

a. What is the location of the lesion?
b. List the tract or nucleus responsible for each of the symptoms or signs in this patient.
c. What is the vascular supply of this region?

Clinical Problem 12.2.

A 78-year-old man acutely develops upper motor neuron weakness in the right arm and face and difficulty expressing himself. One week earlier, he had a single transient episode of left monocular blindness.

a. What tracts or areas of the brain are affected?
b. What is the vascular supply to this region of the brain?
c. What is the significance of the episode 1 week earlier? Is episode 1 in the same or a different vascular territory?

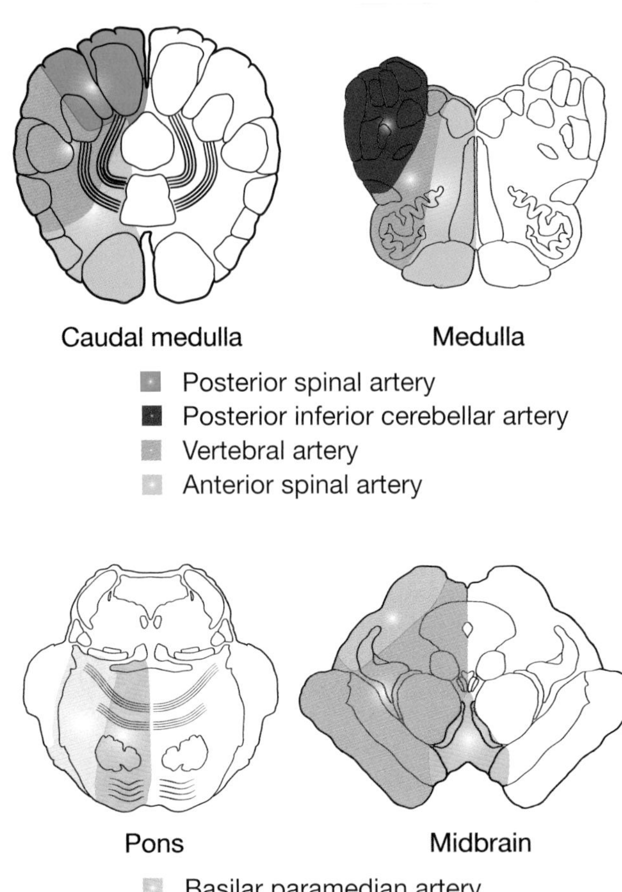

Fig. 12.9. Blood supply to the medulla, pons, and midbrain.

Blood Supply to the Spinal Cord

The spinal cord is supplied with arterial blood by one anterior and two posterolateral vessels that run along the length of the cord and by an irregular plexus of segmentally arranged vessels that encircle the cord and interconnect the major vessels. The *anterior spinal artery* is a single vessel in the ventral median fissure. It arises from a pair of small branches of the vertebral arteries that fuse along the caudal medulla and descend along the cervical spinal cord (Fig. 12.3). A series of six to eight ventral *radicular arteries* that arise from the intercostal, lumbar, and sacral arteries connect with the anterior spinal artery at various levels along the length of the spinal cord (Fig. 12.11). The largest of these radicular arteries is located in the low thoracic or upper lumbar region. Because of this uneven blood supply, the spinal cord is most vulnerable to ischemia at the midthoracic and upper lumbar levels, as indicated by the stippled areas in Figure 12.11. Sulcal branches of the anterior spinal artery pass alternatively to the right and left at each segment to supply blood to the interior of the spinal cord (Fig. 12.12).

The *posterior spinal arteries* are paired structures that run along the posterolateral aspect of the cord near the dorsal roots. They receive contributions from the posterior radicular arteries and supply the dorsal funiculus and dorsal horns (Fig. 12.12).

Vascular disease is less common in the spinal cord than in the brain. When ischemic disease occurs, however, it is most often confined to the distribution of the anterior spinal artery, where it produces loss of motor function and loss of pain and temperature sensation below the level of the lesion; the functions associated with the dorsal columns are spared.

Blood Supply to Peripheral Structures

All neural structures must receive adequate arterial blood supply to sustain life and maintain their integrity. Axons traveling to the periphery are gathered into bundles or

Table 12.2. Neurologic Signs Associated With Lesions of the Carotid and Vertebrobasilar Arterial Systems

Carotid system	Vertebrobasilar system
Hemiparesis (contralateral body and face)	Hemiparesis (ipsilateral face and contralateral body)
Hemisensory loss (contralateral body and face)	Hemisensory loss (ipsilateral face and contralateral body)
Homonymous hemianopia	Diplopia (double vision)
Monocular loss of vision	Dysphagia (swallowing difficulty)
Aphasia	Dysarthria
	Dysequilibrium and/or incoordination

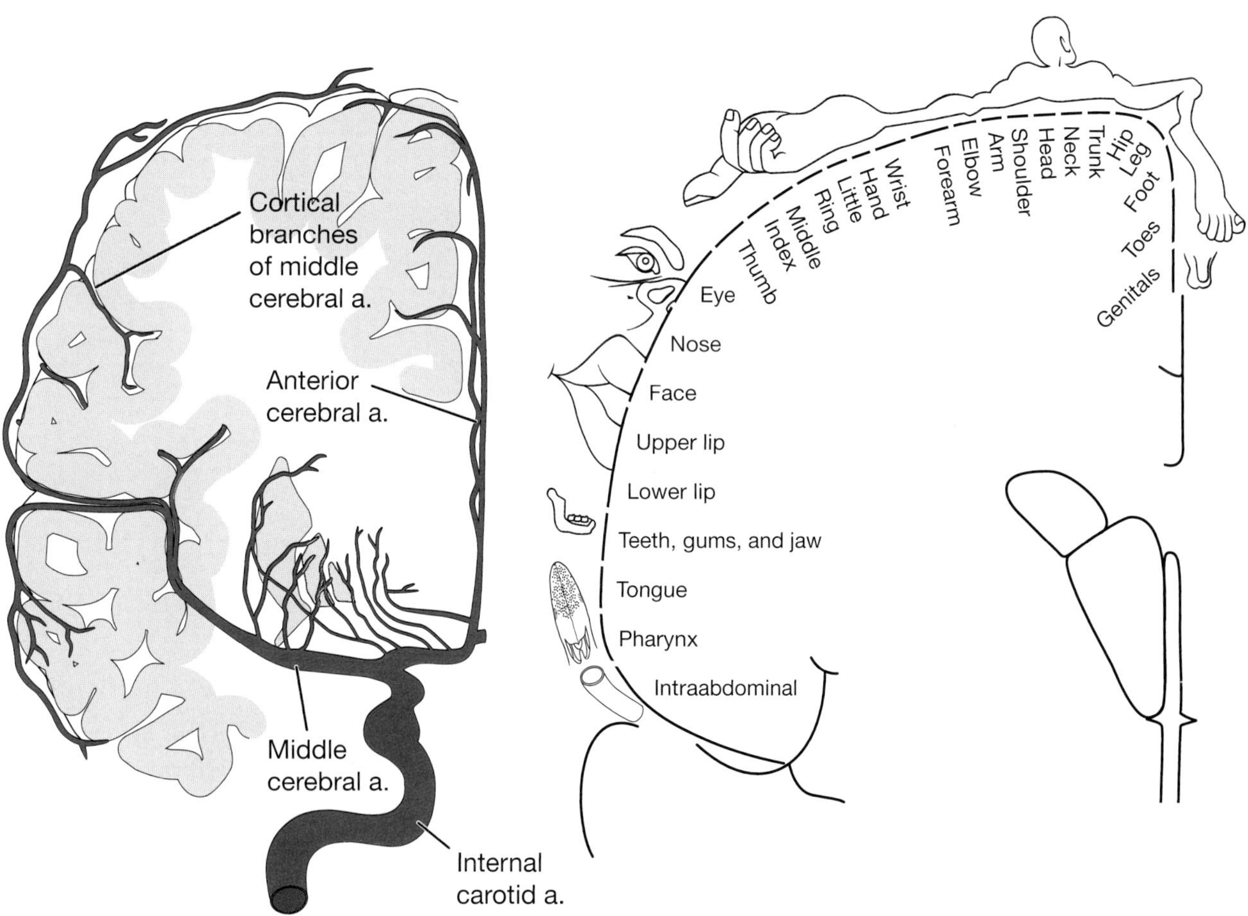

Fig. 12.10. The middle cerebral artery supplies the lateral surface of the cerebral hemisphere, including the representations of the face and arm of the homunculus. The anterior cerebral artery supplies the medial surface, including the representation of the leg of the homunculus.

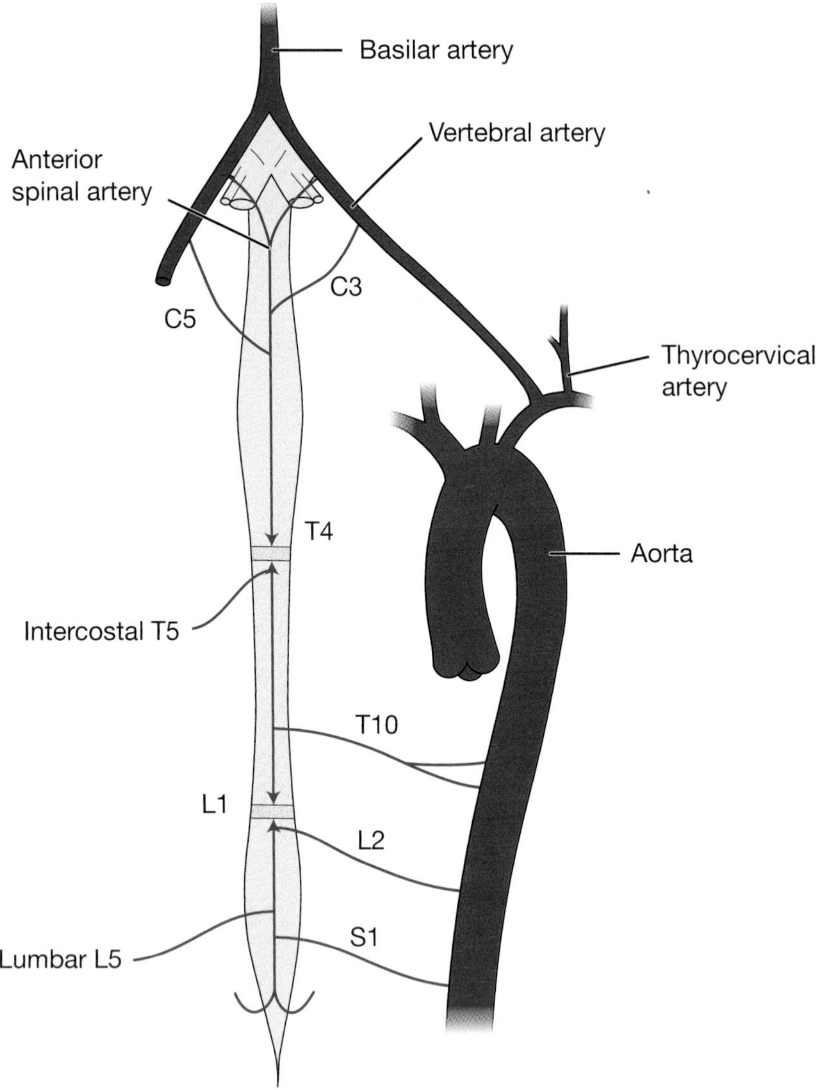

Fig. 12.11. Anterior spinal artery. Radicular arteries vary in location but are shown here at spinal cord levels C3, C5, T5, T10, L2, L5, and S1. Stippled areas, zones of marginal blood supply at T4 and L1.

fascicles that have a connective tissue covering. Within this covering, along the entire course of the nerve, is a rich and highly anastomotic plexus of small arterioles derived from the branches of the major extremity vessels (Fig. 12.13). This dense anastomosis renders the peripheral nerve relatively immune to ischemic vascular disease. Such abnormality, when noted in peripheral neural structures, is usually associated with either direct compression of the nerve or with multiple segmental vascular lesions from small-vessel arterial disease.

Venous Drainage of the Central Nervous System

The venous drainage of the brain is divided into superficial and deep systems. The cerebral cortex and outer half of the white matter drain into the superficial system of veins located over the convexity of the brain in the subarachnoid space. The superficial veins of the superior half of the brain drain into the superior sagittal sinus, and those from the inferior half drain into the transverse sinuses. The deep white matter and deep nuclei of the brain drain into the deep venous system, which includes the *great cerebral vein*

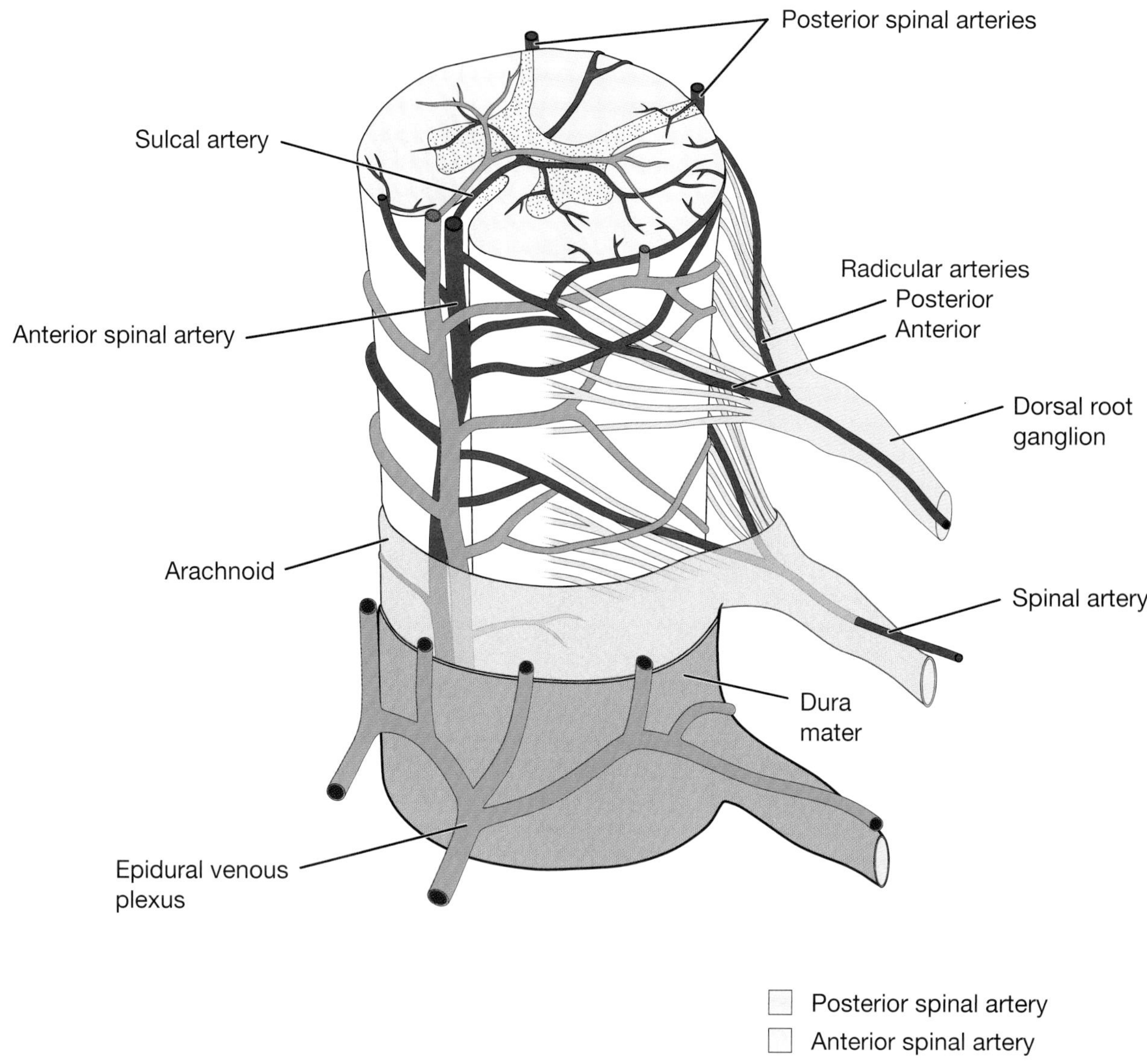

Fig. 12.12. Vascular supply of the spinal cord.

of Galen, *inferior sagittal sinus*, and *straight sinus*. From these venous channels, blood empties into the *transverse sinuses*, *sigmoid sinuses*, and ultimately the *jugular veins* (Fig. 12.14). Veins on the inferior surfaces of the cerebral hemisphere end directly or indirectly in the *cavernous sinus*, an important dural structure located on either side of the pituitary fossa and containing the carotid artery; cranial nerves III, IV, and VI; and branches of cranial nerve V (V1 and V2). The spinal cord is drained by an anastomotic venous plexus surrounding the dural sac. Veins drain outward along both the dorsal and ventral roots into this plexus, which has numerous connections with the veins of the thoracic, abdominal, and pelvic cavities.

- The main branches from the internal carotid artery before it branches into the middle and anterior cerebral arteries are the ophthalmic, posterior communicating, and anterior choroidal arteries.

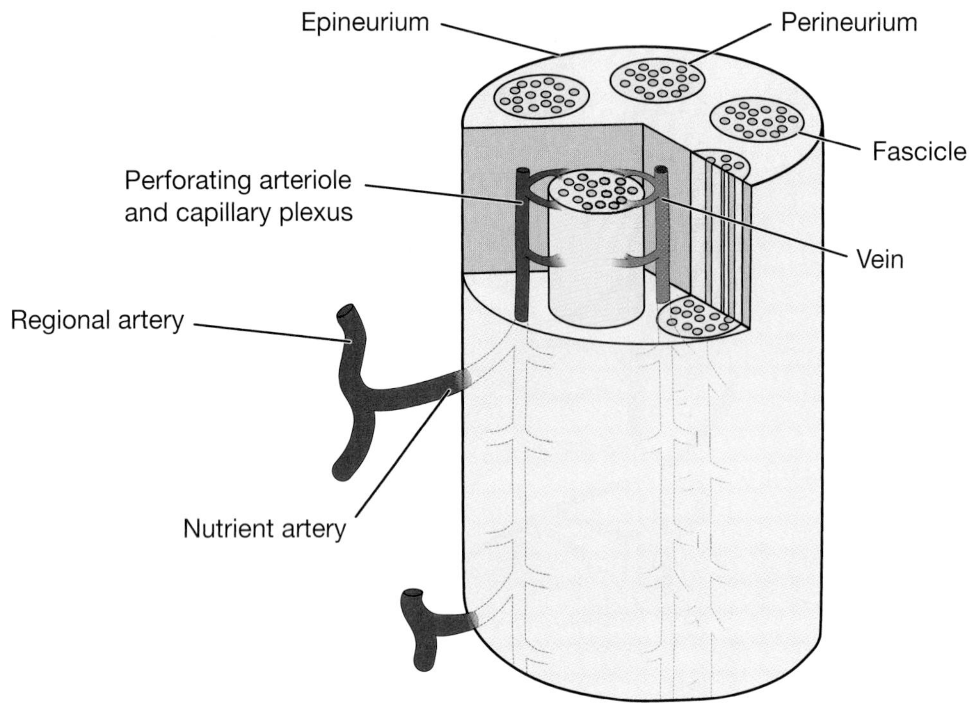

Fig. 12.13. Blood supply of a peripheral nerve. Multiple anastomotic channels are derived from regional arteries.

- The middle cerebral artery supplies the lateral cerebral hemisphere, internal capsule, and basal ganglia.
- The anterior cerebral artery supplies the medial cerebral hemisphere.
- The two vertebral arteries join to form the basilar artery. The vertebrobasilar arterial system supplies the posterior fossa.
- The posterior cerebral artery arises from the basilar artery and supplies a portion of the midbrain as well as the inferior temporal and occipital lobes.
- Sources of collateral circulation to the brain include 1) the circle of Willis, 2) extracranial arteries, and 3) intracranial arteries.
- The blood supply to the spinal cord is from the anterior and posterior spinal arteries, with segmental contributions from radicular arteries.
- Cerebral veins drain into dural venous sinuses. Important sinuses to remember include the superior sagittal sinus, inferior sagittal sinus, transverse sinus, sigmoid sinus, and cavernous sinus.

Physiology of the Vascular System

Cerebral Blood Flow

Adequate blood flow and oxygenation must be maintained for normal neural function. Normal blood flow through the brain is approximately 750 mL/min, or about 20 to 70 mL/100 g brain tissue per minute. Although the brain constitutes only 2% of the body weight, it receives 15% of the cardiac output and uses 20% of the oxygen consumed in the basal state. The total oxygen consumption of the brain is approximately 50 mL/min, or 3.7 mL/100 g brain tissue per minute. Any decrease in the amount of available oxygen provided to the brain reduces neural activity. Under normal conditions, the total oxygen consumption and blood flow to the brain are nearly constant. Cortical gray matter, with its greater metabolic demand, has about six times the blood flow of white matter. Local changes in blood flow may occur with changing demands of varying neural activity.

In any hemodynamic system, blood flow is directly proportional to the perfusion pressure and inversely proportional to the total resistance of the system. For the brain, this can be expressed by the following equation:

$$\text{Cerebral blood flow} = \frac{\text{Mean arterial pressure} - \text{Central venous pressure}}{\text{Cerebrovascular resistance}}$$

Several factors can modify cerebral blood flow by altering different elements in this equation. These have been divided arbitrarily into two groups: extracerebral factors and intracerebral factors (Table 12.3).

Extracerebral Factors

Factors outside the cranial cavity that modify or regulate cerebral blood flow are related primarily to the cardiovascular system and include systemic blood pressure, efficiency of cardiac function, and blood viscosity. The principal force in maintaining the cerebral circulation is the pressure difference between the arteries and veins. Because cerebral venous pressure normally is low (approximately 5 mm Hg), arterial blood pressure is the more important factor in maintaining cerebral blood flow. Variations in systemic arterial blood pressure do not, however, ordinarily produce changes in cerebral blood flow in a healthy person if the intrinsic regulatory mechanisms are intact, unless the mean arterial pressure decreases to less than 50 to 70 mm Hg. Systemic arterial blood pressure depends on the efficiency of cardiac function (cardiac output) and peripheral vasomotor tone or resistance. These factors are governed principally by autonomic control from the vasomotor center in the medulla. Alterations in cardiac rhythm and myocardial function or the presence of cardiac disease may cause a change in cardiac output that may secondarily influence cerebral blood flow. Baroreceptors in the carotid sinus and aortic arch participate in reflexes that mediate cardiovascular tone and help maintain a constant blood pressure. Advancing age, atherosclerosis, and certain drugs may alter these reflex mechanisms, and a simple physiologic act such as assuming an upright posture may result in severe orthostatic hypotension and a pronounced decrease in cerebral blood flow (causing fainting or syncope). Also, the viscosity of the blood may alter cerebral blood flow; severe anemia may increase flow as much as 30%, and polycythemia may decrease it by more than 50%.

Intracerebral Factors

The state of the cerebral vasculature also can influence cerebral blood flow. Widespread intracranial arterial disease increases cerebrovascular resistance and can decrease cerebral blood flow, whereas pathologic processes associated with rapid shunting of blood from arteries to veins (as in arteriovenous malformation) may produce both an increase in total cerebral blood flow and a local decrease in tissue perfusion.

Any increase in intracranial pressure is transmitted directly to the low-pressure venous system and increases cerebral venous pressure, thus decreasing cerebral blood flow. In pathologic states frequently accompanied by increased intracranial pressure (see Chapter 11), this decrease in blood flow may further accentuate the signs and symptoms produced by the primary lesion.

Regulation of Cerebral Blood Flow

Several factors can modify cerebral blood flow: metabolic regulation, autoregulation, chemical factors, and neurogenic control (Fig. 12.15).

Metabolic Regulation

Normally, cerebral blood flow is coupled directly to neuronal metabolic activity, with a linear increase or decrease in cerebral blood flow resulting from a corresponding change in brain metabolic activity.

> This coupling of blood flow occurs with a short latency of 1 to 2 seconds and is a strictly regional effect, producing little alteration in overall total blood flow despite measurable local change. Local metabolic coupling can be demonstrated during sleep and various sensorimotor tasks and in pathologic conditions such as coma and seizure. The mechanism of metabolic coupling involves vasodilator metabolites such as adenosine, potassium and hydrogen ions, prostaglandins, oxygen free radicals, and nitric oxide.

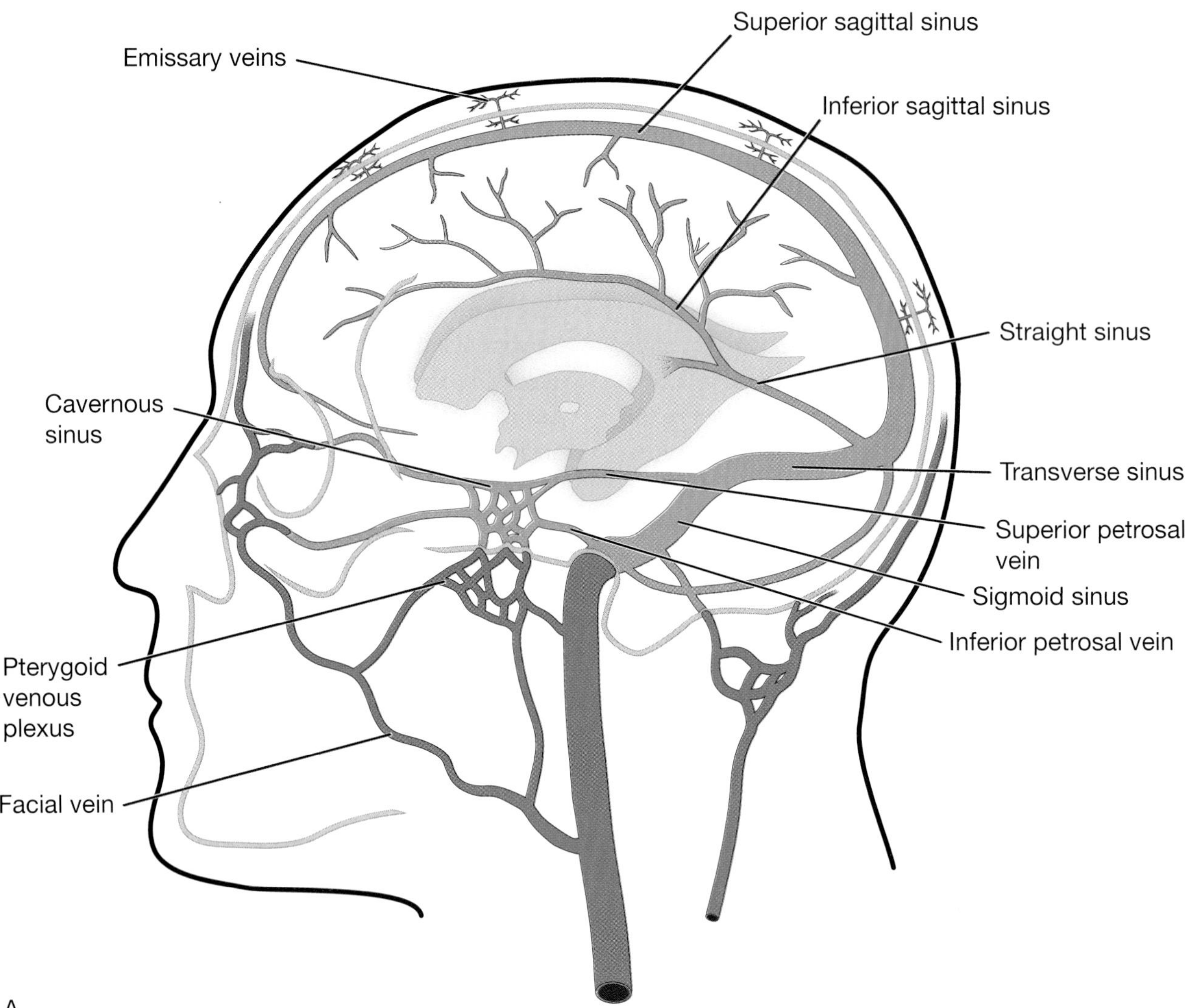

Fig. 12.14. Venous drainage of the brain. *A*, Sagittal view of major dural venous sinuses. *B*, Superior view of deep cerebral veins.

Autoregulation

The normal brain is able to regulate its own blood supply, *autoregulation*, in response to changes in arterial blood pressure and metabolic demand. Autoregulation is defined as the ability of an organ (e.g., the brain) to maintain blood flow constant for all but the widest extremes in perfusion pressure. Autoregulation of cerebral blood flow occurs when the mean arterial blood pressure is between 60 and 150 mm Hg; when it is less than 60 mm Hg, blood flow decreases, and when it is more than 150 mm Hg, blood flow increases.

Autoregulation is achieved with myogenic, neurogenic, and chemical-metabolic mechanisms. Autoregulation occurs in both large and small arterioles. Cerebral vessels, like other hollow organs that contain smooth muscle, can change diameter in response to intraluminal pressure. This effect, called the *Bayliss effect*, results in vasoconstriction with increased intraluminal pressure and vasodilatation with decreased intraluminal pressure. Therefore, autoregulation is primarily a pressure-controlled myogenic mechanism that operates independently but synergistically with other neurogenic and chemical-metabolic factors.

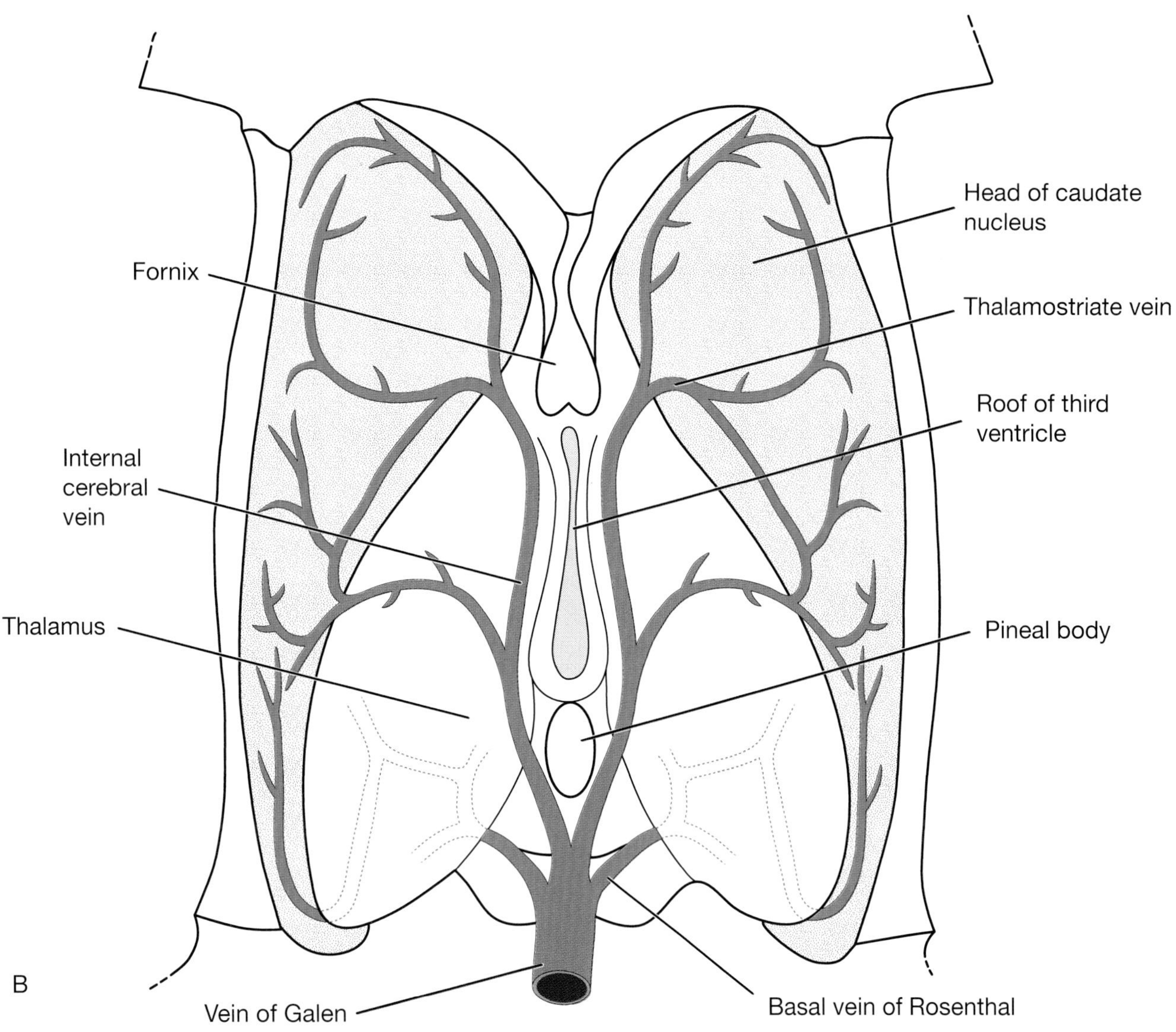

Autoregulation is a major homeostatic and protective mechanism. In normal persons, it prevents alterations in cerebral blood flow despite variations in systemic blood pressure or regional increases in metabolic demand on the brain. With a regional increase in metabolism, there is a corresponding increase in carbon dioxide, which produces local vasodilatation and increased blood flow, thus accommodating the increased metabolic demand. In certain disease states associated with vascular occlusion, an area of regional ischemia develops because of the reduction in available blood supply; intraluminal pressure decreases, oxygen is no longer available, carbon dioxide tension increases, lactate is produced, and the tissue becomes acidotic. All these factors produce vasodilatation of nearby vessels and may provide increased blood flow to an area of ischemia. In certain situations, this is sufficient to increase regional cerebral blood flow and prevent infarction; in other situations, it may decrease the size of the resultant infarct. In a region of cerebral infarction, these protective mechanisms have reduced cerebrovascular resistance to a very low value. Because there is little acute change in the

Table 12.3. Factors Regulating Cerebral Blood Flow

Factor	Cerebral blood flow	
	Increased	Decreased
Extracerebral		
Systemic blood pressure		Mean arterial pressure <50-70 mm Hg
Cardiovascular function		Arrhythmia; orthostatic hypotension; loss of carotid sinus and aortic arch reflexes
Blood viscosity	Anemia	Polycythemia
Intracerebral		
State of vasculature	Arteriovenous malformation	Atherosclerosis
Intracranial cerebrospinal fluid pressure		Increased intracranial pressure
Cerebral autoregulatory mechanisms	Result in vasodilation	Result in vasoconstriction
Myogenic factors	↓ Intraluminal pressure	↑ Intraluminal pressure
Neurogenic factors	Parasympathetic stimulation	Sympathetic stimulation
Biochemical-metabolic factors	↑ Carbon dioxide ↓ Oxygen ↓ pH (acidosis) ↑ Lactic acid	↓ Carbon dioxide ↑ Oxygen ↑ pH (alkalosis)

central venous pressure, the major determinant of blood flow in the region of ischemic tissue is the mean arterial blood pressure. Therefore, the proper maintenance of systemic blood pressure may be of prime importance in the treatment of ischemic infarcts, and any pronounced decrease in systemic pressure or the presence of cerebral edema (which will secondarily increase venous pressure) may further alter cellular function.

Chemical Factors

Chemical factors exert a strong influence on cerebral blood flow. Carbon dioxide, an end product of cerebral metabolism, diffuses rapidly across the blood-brain barrier. It is the most potent physiologic and pharmacologic agent that influences cerebral blood flow. Cerebral blood vessels react rapidly to any change in local carbon dioxide tension ($Paco_2$). Any increase in $Paco_2$ produces vasodilatation and increases cerebral blood flow, and a decrease in $Paco_2$ has the opposite effect. The cerebral circulation reacts to oxygen in the reverse manner: a decrease in local oxygen tension (Pao_2) produces vasodilatation and increases cerebral blood flow, and an increase in Pao_2 produces vasoconstriction and decreases cerebral blood flow. The exact mechanism by which carbon dioxide and oxygen exert their effects on cerebral blood vessels is not known. They may act directly on the smooth muscle of the vessel wall or indirectly through neurogenic chemoreceptors or they may alter the pH of the brain. A decrease in brain

Clinical Problem 12.3.

Hyperventilation is sometimes used to reduce increased intracranial pressure acutely. Why would this type of therapy potentially be harmful if used for a prolonged time?

pH (acidosis) from any cause produces vasodilatation and increases cerebral blood flow, whereas an increase in brain pH (alkalosis) is associated with vasoconstriction and decreased cerebral blood flow. Lactic acid, which is produced by the shift to anaerobic metabolism in regions of ischemia, is a potent vasodilator.

Neurogenic Control

Although extracranial and intracranial arteries are richly innervated, neurogenic factors do not seem to have as great a role in the regulation of cerebral blood flow as chemical and metabolic factors. Neurogenic control can be considered to consist of extrinsic, intrinsic, and local components in the brain (Table 12.4).

Extrinsic neurogenic control is provided by postganglionic fibers from the superior cervical sympathetic ganglion. These axons innervate the carotid and vertebral arteries and their major intracranial branches. Norepinephrine released from these sympathetic fibers produces vasoconstriction. This neurogenic control protects capillaries against hyperperfusion when blood pressure is increased. Parasympathetic fibers in the facial and superficial petrosal nerves innervate large- and small-diameter cerebral blood vessels. These fibers have acetylcholine as a neurotransmitter. Fibers from the facial nerve are a source of nitric oxide, a potent vasodilator substance. Fibers from the

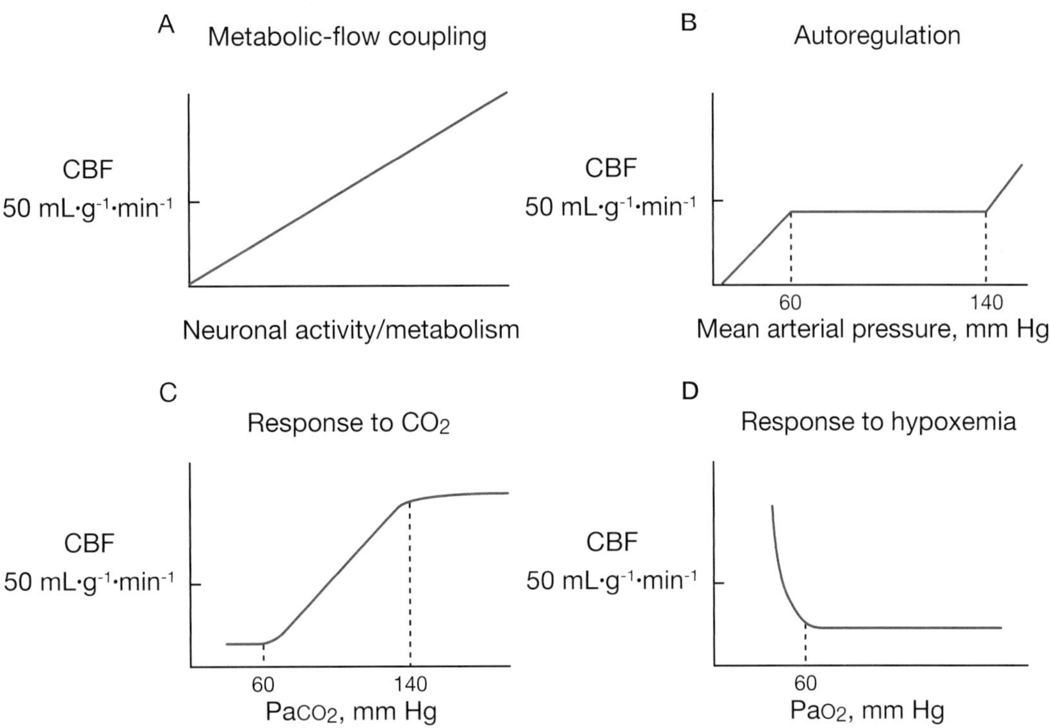

Fig. 12.15. Factors that regulate cerebral blood flow (CBF). *A*, Linear relation between focal neuronal metabolism and blood flow. This coupling involves local factors affected by neuronal activity and consumption of adenosine triphosphate by the sodium-potassium pump, particularly at the level of synapses (gray matter). These local factors include extracellular acidosis, potassium, adenosine, and nitric oxide. *B*, Cerebral autoregulation maintains CBF constant despite changes in mean arterial blood pressure between approximately 60 and 140 mm Hg; it depends on myogenic mechanisms. *C*, Carbon dioxide (CO_2) is a potent vasodilator even at physiologic $Paco_2$, whereas hypoxemia, *D*, produces vasodilatation only when it is severe.

Table 12.4. The Effect of Neurogenic Factors on Arteries

Type	Source	Neurotransmitter	Effect
Extrinsic	Sympathetic (superior cervical ganglion)	Norepinephrine	Constrict
		Neuropeptide Y	Constrict
	Parasympathetic (facial and superficial petrosal nerves)	Acetylcholine	Dilate
		VIP	Dilate
		Nitric oxide	Dilate
	Trigeminal nerve	Substance P	Dilate
		CGRP	Dilate
Intrinsic	Locus ceruleus	Norepinephrine	Dilate (microcirculation)
	Raphe nuclei	Serotonin	Constrict
Local	Interneurons	Neuropeptide Y	Constrict
		VIP	Dilate
		Nitric oxide	Dilate

CGRP, calcitonin gene-related peptide; VIP, vasoactive intestinal polypeptide.

trigeminal ganglion that use substance P and calcitonin gene-related peptide also innervate cerebral vessels and produce vasodilatation and increased permeability.

Intrinsic neurogenic control of the cerebral circulation is provided by pathways originating in the brainstem and by interneurons in the cerebral cortex. The major brainstem pathways are from the locus ceruleus, whose neurons use norepinephrine to produce microcirculatory vasodilatation, and the raphe nuclei, whose neurons use serotonin, a vasoconstrictor substance. Some cortical interneurons contain neuropeptide Y (a vasoconstrictor) or vasoactive intestinal polypeptide (a vasodilator) and, thus, could contribute to local regulation of blood flow.

Cerebral Metabolism

High metabolic activity and high oxygen consumption characterize cerebral metabolism. A constant supply of energy is necessary for the support of neuronal and neurologic functions. These vital energy-dependent processes include the establishment of membrane potentials, maintenance of transmembrane ionic gradients, membrane transport, and the synthesis of cellular constituents such as proteins, nucleic acids, lipids, and neurotransmitters. The energy needed is supplied in the form of high-energy phosphate bonds from adenosine triphosphate (ATP), which is synthesized in the brain, as in other organ systems, through the glycolytic pathway, the Krebs (citric acid) cycle, and the respiratory (electron-transport) chain (Table 12.5).

Under aerobic conditions, glucose is effectively metabolized through the glycolytic pathway, citric acid cycle, and respiratory chain to yield 38 moles of ATP per mole of glucose. Under anaerobic conditions, the Krebs (citric acid) cycle and respiratory chain cannot be activated because of lack of oxygen; therefore, the pyruvate derived from glycolysis is metabolized to lactate and yields only 2 moles of ATP per mole of glucose. Another source of high-energy phosphate bonds is creatine phosphate. This compound, which is even more abundant than ATP in the brain, is used to regenerate ATP from adenosine diphosphate and is thus important for maintaining the level of tissue ATP. Although glycogen is present and the brain is

Table 12.5. Glucose Metabolism

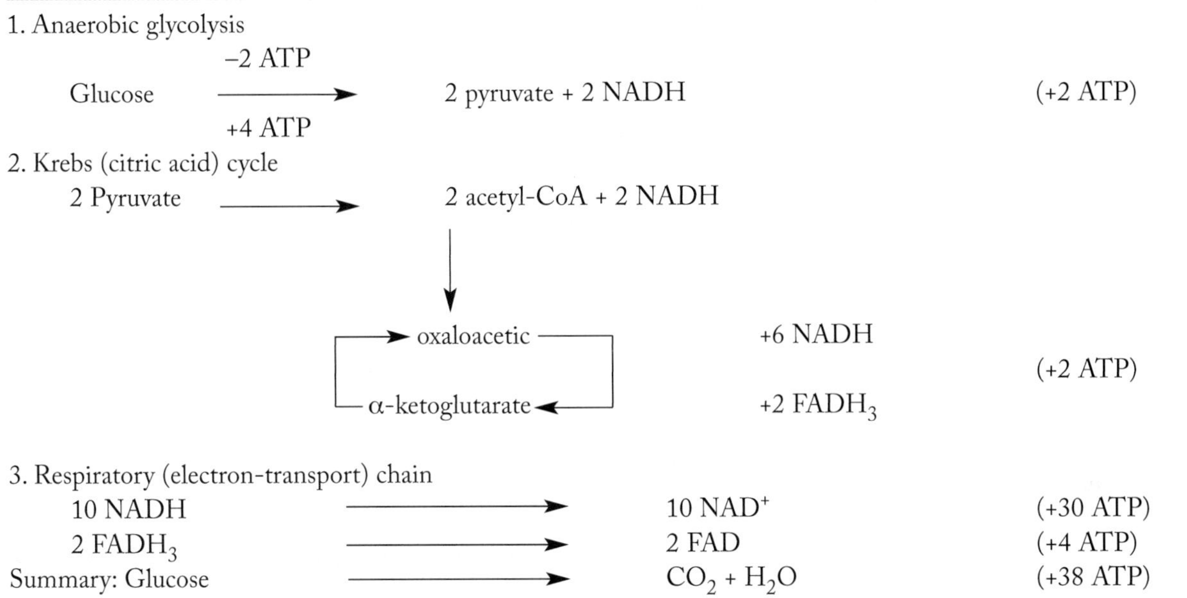

1. Anaerobic glycolysis			
Glucose	−2 ATP → +4 ATP	2 pyruvate + 2 NADH	(+2 ATP)
2. Krebs (citric acid) cycle			
2 Pyruvate	→	2 acetyl-CoA + 2 NADH	
	↓ oxaloacetic ⇄ α-ketoglutarate	+6 NADH +2 $FADH_3$	(+2 ATP)
3. Respiratory (electron-transport) chain			
10 NADH	→	10 NAD^+	(+30 ATP)
2 $FADH_3$	→	2 FAD	(+4 ATP)
Summary: Glucose	→	CO_2 + H_2O	(+38 ATP)

ATP, adenosine triphosphate; CO_2, carbon dioxide; FAD, flavin adenine dinucleotide; $FADH_3$, reduced form of flavin adenine trinucleotide; NADH, reduced nicotinamide adenine dinucleotide.

capable of its rapid synthesis and breakdown, the role of glycogen in brain metabolism is not completely understood. Glucose is the basic substrate for brain metabolism. The astrocytes store glycogen and are the source of lactate, which can be used by neurons to produce glucose.

Pathophysiology

Reversible alteration in cell function from the lack of oxygen results in ischemia, and irreversible alteration results in infarction. After vessel occlusion and deprivation of blood flow to the brain, a series of events unfold, the *ischemic cascade* that lead ultimately to neuronal dysfunction and death (Fig. 12.16).

Cerebral blood flow and cerebral oxygen and glucose consumption decrease in the center of the ischemic area. These functions are less impaired at the periphery of the ischemic area (the "ischemic penumbra") where there are accompanying metabolic and electrophysiologic changes but where blood flow is sufficient to prevent irreversible cell damage (Fig. 12.16).

Local autoregulatory mechanisms are impaired, and local responsivity of vessels to chemical and metabolic changes and to alterations in perfusion pressure is lost.

Anaerobic glycolysis is initiated as the vital substrates, oxygen and glucose, are decreased and brain glycogen content diminishes. Tissue lactate increases but pH decreases, and a zone of hyperemia and increased perfusion develops in the periphery of the ischemic zone.

Substrate depletion leads to failure of mitochondrial function and inefficient ATP generation, with leakage of potassium (K^+) from cells and the intracellular accumulation of sodium (Na^+), chloride (Cl^-), and calcium (Ca^{2+}) ions, and free fatty acids. The net effect is neuronal depolarization, loss of the transmembrane potential, and increase in tissue water. This also impairs ATP-dependent neurotransmitter reuptake.

Energy loss also results in increased release of excitatory neurotransmitters such as glutamate. The neurotoxic effect of this large accumulation of glutamate in the extracellular space is exerted through activation of *N*-methyl-D-aspartate (NMDA) and α-amino-3-hydroxy-5-methyl-4-isoxazole propionic acid (AMPA) receptors, causing increased permeability to Na^+, cellular swelling

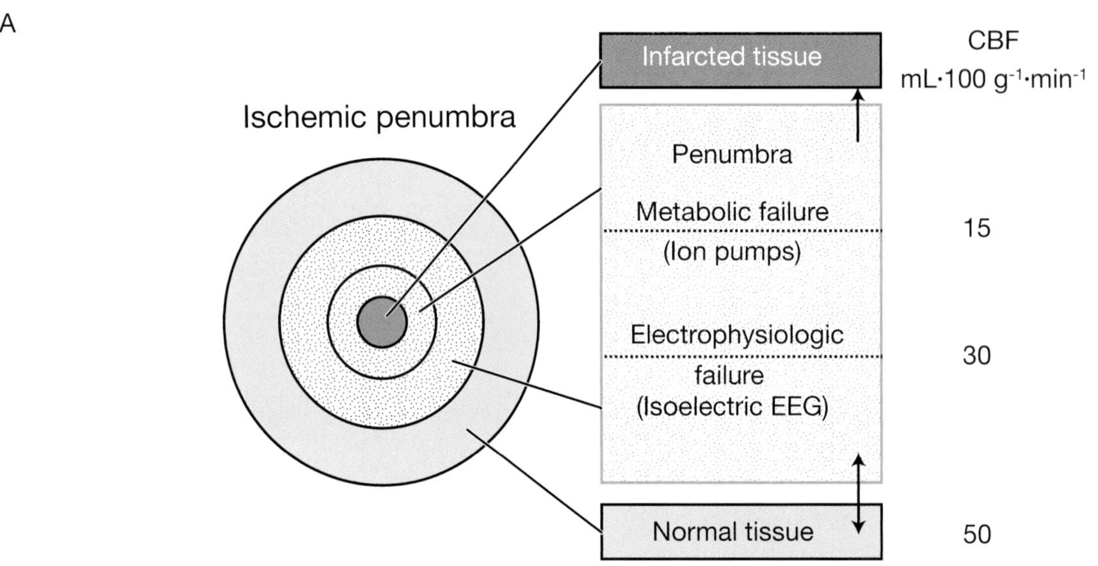

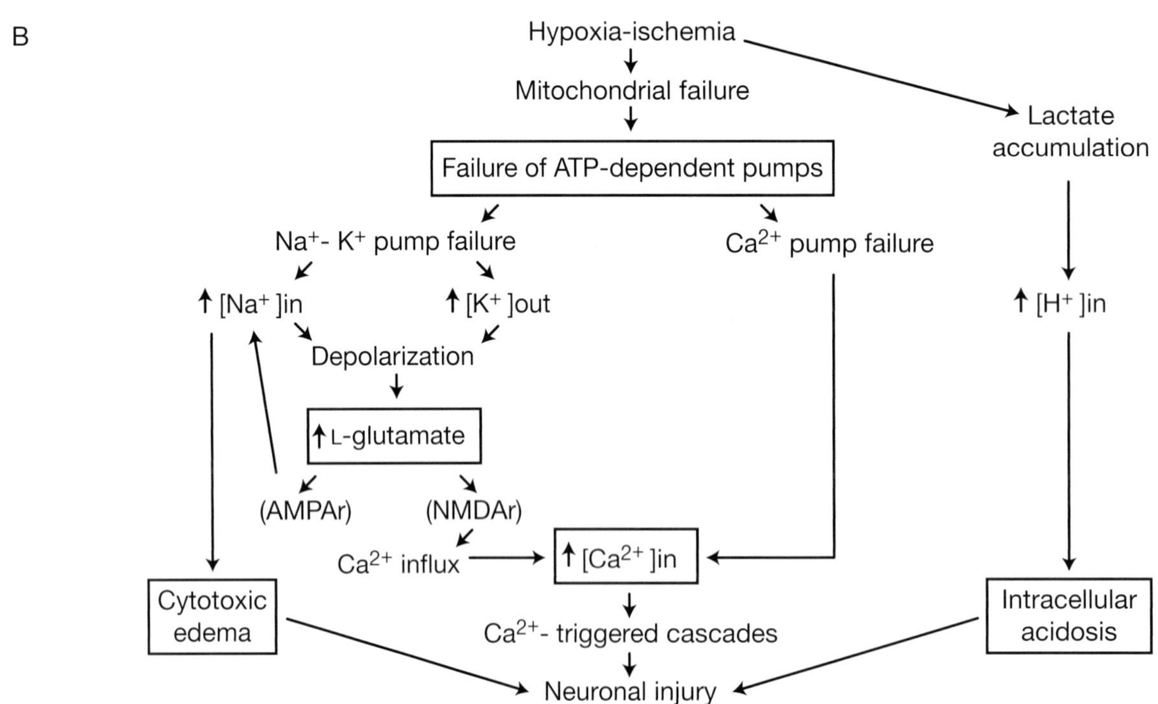

and lysis, and massive entry of Ca^{2+} into the postsynaptic neuron. Additional calcium-induced release of excitatory neurotransmitters during the ischemic process heightens neuronal necrosis.

The increase in intracellular Ca^{2+} activates phospholipases, proteases, and endonucleases and generates oxygen free radicals and nitric oxide. This leads to membrane, mitochondrial DNA, and microtubular damage and, eventually, cell destruction (Fig. 12.16 *B*).

If the period of ischemia is short and the supply of high-energy phosphate bonds can be reestablished, neuronal function can resume. The local accumulation of adenosine, K^+, and hydrogen, which occurs in response to the production of lactic acid, produces local vasodilatation in an attempt to restore an adequate blood supply. However, if the cell continues to be deprived of nourishment, catabolic and morphologic changes occur. Initially, the cell begins to swell (acute cell change); if its metabolic needs are not met, the cell becomes irreversibly damaged. This is referred to as *infarction*, the morphologic correlate of which is ischemic cell change (see Chapter 4). If the area of infarction is large, other cellular elements and the blood-brain barrier are affected. In the region of maximal change, cell death and destruction occur. With the catabolic changes and breakdown of the blood-brain barrier, the water content of the tissue increases. The associated brain edema may further impair the function of cells in the regions surrounding the infarction. After scavenger cells enter the area and the cellular debris is removed, a cystic cavity remains.

In conditions of partial ischemia, the decrease in high-energy phosphate bonds is less precipitous, and the irreversible damage occurs only after a more prolonged period of ischemia. Thus, in cerebral hypoxia, the metabolic changes are similar to those of anoxia but to a lesser extent because there is an abudant supply of glucose. However, if the hypoxia is prolonged, the accumulation of lactate from accelerated glycolysis becomes significant, and ischemia and infarction may result.

In hypoglycemia, the brain is supplied with adequate oxygen but lacks glucose as a substrate. Hypoglycemia produces a different metabolic pattern from that of cerebral ischemia. In hypoglycemia, the brain can maintain high-energy phosphate bonds through the use of creatine phosphate and other substances. Function is temporarily altered; however, if the glucose deficiency is not present for a prolonged period, catabolic changes do not develop and recovery can occur with reversal of the hypoglycemic state.

- Normal blood flow to the brain depends on the mean arterial pressure, central venous pressure, and cerebrovascular resistance.
- Cerebral blood flow can be influenced by neuronal metabolic activity, autoregulation, chemical factors (pH, carbon dioxide, oxygen), and neurogenic factors.
- Cerebral autoregulation is the process whereby cerebral blood flow is maintained despite a change in mean arterial blood pressure. In humans, this occurs

Fig. 12.16. *A*, The ischemic penumbra. Decreased cerebral blood flow (CBF) produces a gradient of severity of deprivation of oxygen and glucose in brain tissue. Between the area of infarction and normal tissue is an area of jeopardized brain tissue called the ischemic penumbra. Neurons in this region have potentially reversible electrophysiologic failure due to energy deprivation but have not experienced the cascade leading to neuronal death. The ischemic penumbra is the target of neuroprotective treatment in ischemic stroke. *B*, Cascade of events leading to ischemic neuronal injury. The initial mechanism is mitochondrial failure, adenosine triphosphate (ATP) depletion, and pump failure. This leads to neuronal depolarization due to increase of extracellular potassium (K^+), decrease in uptake of L-glutamate, and increase in intracellular sodium (Na^+) and calcium (Ca^{2+}). Calcium-triggered cascades, including phospholipases, proteases, and nucleases together with intracellular acidosis (from accumulation of lactate), lead to production of oxygen free radicals, disruption of the cytoskeleton, and neuronal death. AMPAr, α-amino-3-hydroxy-5-methyl-4-isoxazole propionic acid receptor; EEG, electroencephalogram; NMDAr, *N*-methyl-D-aspartate receptor.

between a mean arterial blood pressure of 60 and 150 mm Hg.

- With prolonged lack of oxygen, an irreversible alteration of cells occurs, setting in motion a series of events, called the ischemic cascade, that lead to infarction.

Pathology of the Vascular System

The symptoms and signs produced by vascular disease reflect altered neuronal function in focal or diffuse areas of the nervous system. The location and nature of the underlying neural-parenchymal lesion are related directly to the abnormalities found in the blood vessels or circulatory system. Therefore, this discussion of the pathology of the vascular system considers the major derangements involving blood vessels and the neural-parenchymal lesions produced by these vascular abnormalities.

Vascular Pathology

Normal Arterial Histology

The normal arterial wall contains three distinct layers (Fig. 12.17): 1) the *intima* is a layer of connective tissue lined by endothelium on the luminal surface and is separated from the media by the internal elastic lamina; 2) the *media* is a layer of diagonally oriented smooth muscle cells surrounded by collagen and mucopolysaccharides; and 3) the *adventitia* is the outermost layer and contains fibroblasts and smooth muscle cells intermixed with bundles of collagen and mucopolysaccharides. An external elastic lamina generally is not found in intracerebral arteries.

Intracranial Arterial Aneurysms

An abnormal, localized dilatation of the arterial lumen is called an *aneurysm*. The most commonly encountered type is a round or oval-shaped, berrylike structure that arises at the bifurcation of cerebral vessels (Fig. 12.18). The majority of cerebral aneurysms are located in the anterior half of the circle of Willis, with the most frequent sites being the internal carotid-posterior communicating artery junction, the anterior cerebral-anterior communicating artery junction, and the middle cerebral artery bifurcation. A ballooning of the intima is associated with a defect in the media and internal elastic lamina, perhaps from a developmental anomaly. These lesions vary in size from 1 mm to more than 10 mm. They occasionally produce symptoms by exerting pressure on adjacent structures but more often they are diagnosed after rupturing and bleeding into the subarachnoid space or brain. Occasionally, aneurysms are due to destruction of the arterial wall by atherosclerosis (atherosclerotic aneurysm) or to infected emboli arising from the heart (septic or mycotic aneurysm).

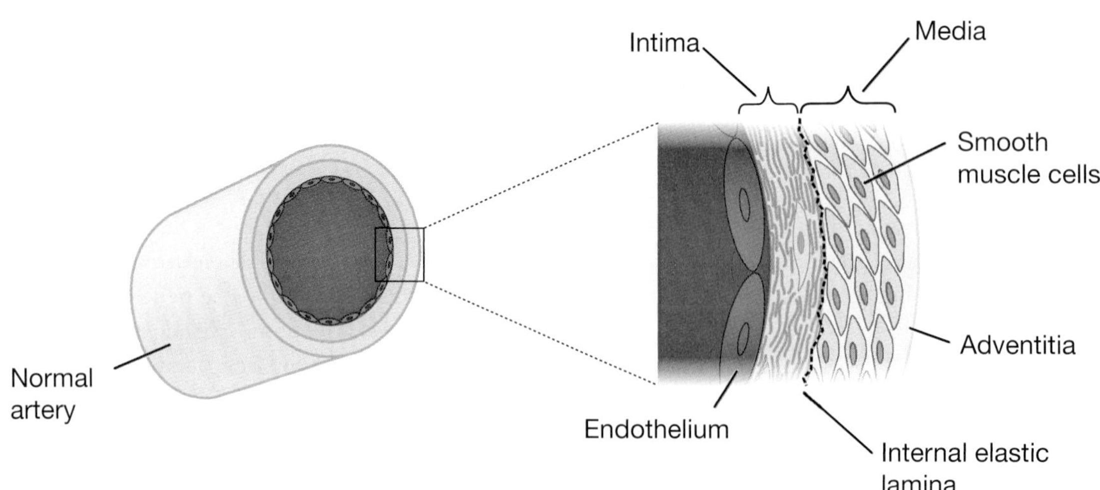

Fig. 12.17. Cross section of a normal arterial wall showing the intima, internal elastic lamina, media, and adventitia.

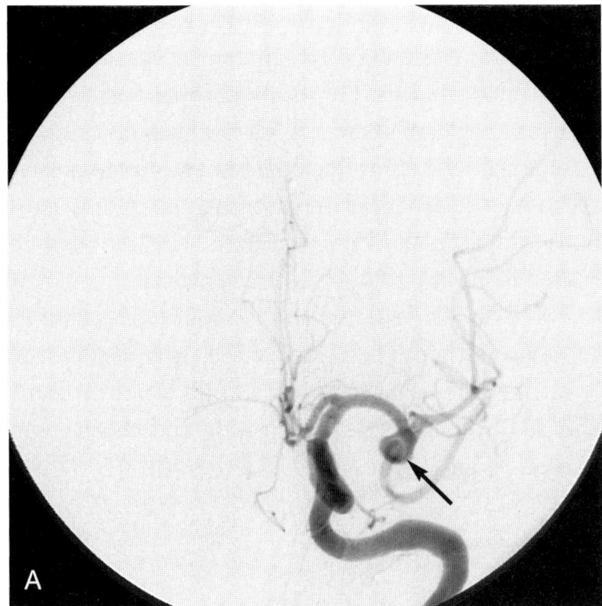

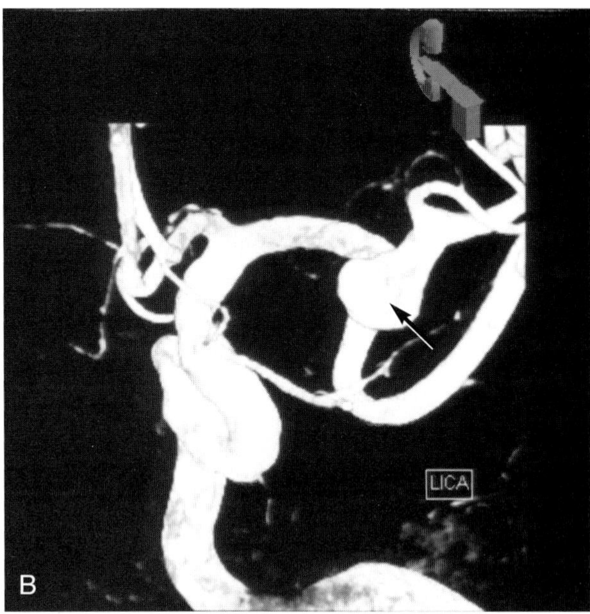

Fig. 12.18. Cerebral aneurysm. *A*, Conventional angiogram, anteroposterior view, showing a 7-mm left middle cerebral artery bifurcation aneurysm (*arrow*) after a left internal carotid artery injection. *B*, The same aneurysm (*arrow*) seen after three-dimensional rotational angiography.

Arteriovenous Malformations

Developmental abnormalities often encountered in young adults are *arteriovenous malformations*. They result from defective communication between arteries, capillaries, and veins, with dilatation of one or more of the vascular elements, and form a variable-sized meshwork of tortuous blood vessels. The walls of these abnormal vessels may be thin (and predisposed to rupture) or they may be hypertrophic. Rapid shunting of blood generally occurs and may produce a chronic ischemic state in the neighboring brain. Depending on the location and structure of the malformation, associated seizures and focal neurologic deficit, infarction, or bleeding into the subarachnoid space or brain may occur.

Atherosclerosis

One of the most important pathologic lesions responsible for cerebral infarction is *atherosclerosis*. The basic lesion is the atherosclerotic plaque. Atherosclerotic plaque formation requires several sequential steps that are set into motion by certain triggers: hypertension, diabetes mellitus, obesity, chronic inflammation or infection, and oxidized lipoproteins. Initially, the trigger results in the activation of endothelial cells and the expression of white blood cell adhesion proteins. Certain adhesion molecules allow the migration of white blood cells into the intima, and these monocytes transform into macrophages. These macrophages have certain receptors that allow them to engulf specific lipoproteins, and they become "foam" cells. Foam cells, in turn, secrete mediators that allow the continued accumulation of other monocytes and promote smooth muscle cell proliferation in the vessel and change the extracellular matrix, degrading the collagen protective structure. It is possible that early atherogenic lesions may regress; however, with further arterial injury, the process is repeated and the plaque becomes altered by increased lipid content, intramural hemorrhage, and calcification. The artery may show progressive narrowing of the lumen to the point of occlusion or the integrity of the endothelium may become vulnerable because of the proliferation of metalloproteinases that degrade the stability of the plaque. If the plaque becomes unstable and ruptures, the subendothelium is exposed and platelets can adhere and aggregate, resulting in thrombus formation (Fig. 12.19).

An additional danger is the development of local intra-arterial thrombosis, with subsequent embolization to distal vessels. Furthermore, sudden hemodynamic failure with decreased cerebral blood flow can also result in ischemia.

The basic processes of platelet aggregation and release can be inhibited by certain drugs. Platelet-vessel wall interaction is influenced by the selective oxygenation of arachidonic acid in both the platelet and vascular endothelium. In the platelet, thromboxane synthase converts prostaglandin H_2 to thromboxane A_2, which is a potent aggregator of platelets as well as a constrictor of arterial conductance vessels. However, vascular endothelium metabolizes prostaglandin H_2 to prostacyclin, a compound that antagonizes platelet aggregation and dilates blood vessels. These observations suggest that pharmacologic agents which selectively inhibit thromboxane synthase or facilitate the biosynthesis of prostacyclin may be beneficial in preventing the thromboembolic complications of atherosclerosis. Medications such as acetylsalicylic acid (aspirin) are beneficial.

The vascular endothelium is a source of vasoactive substances. Endothelium-derived relaxing factors such as nitric oxide produce vasodilatation. Endothelium-derived constricting factors such as the endothelin group of peptides are potent vasoconstrictors.

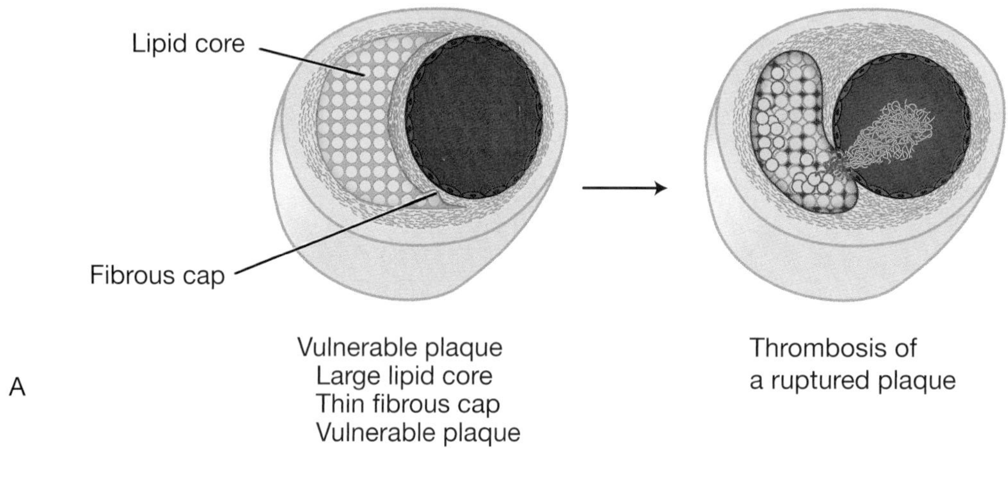

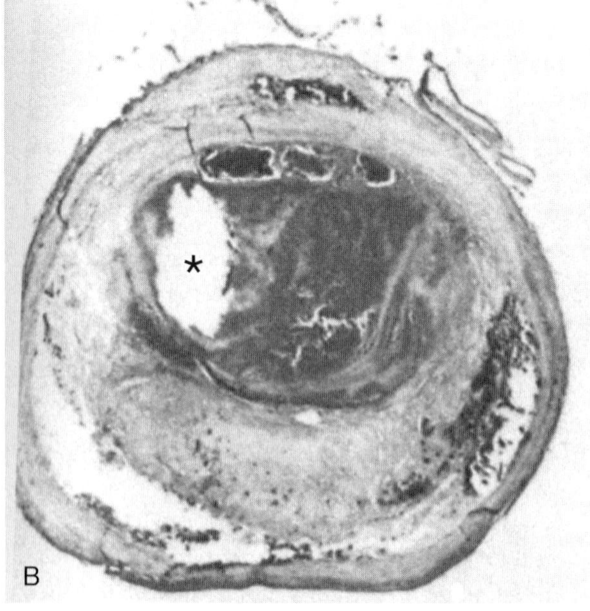

Fig. 12.19. An atherosclerotic plaque. *A*, A large lipid core and thin fibrous cap make the atherosclerotic plaque more vulnerable to rupture and thrombosis. *B*, Cross section of an atherosclerotic plaque in the carotid artery showing arterial wall necrosis with mural thrombosis and stenosis of the lumen (*). (H&E; ×3.5.)

Atherosclerosis tends chiefly to affect large-caliber blood vessels; in the cerebral circulation, both intracranial and extracranial arteries may be involved (Fig. 12.20). Although minimal patchy involvement of the carotid and vertebral arteries is seen, significant stenosis or occlusion commonly occurs at selected sites. The extracranial portion of the carotid arteries tends to develop atherosclerotic plaques at the carotid bifurcations and in the proximal portions of the internal carotid arteries, whereas the vertebral arteries are especially likely to develop lesions at the site of origin from the subclavian arteries. Atherosclerosis of the intracranial arteries is usually limited to the larger arteries related to the circle of Willis and is found most frequently in the internal carotid, proximal middle cerebral, vertebral, and basilar arteries. The smaller distal branches of the major cerebral arteries are seldom involved by gross atheromatous plaques.

Fibrinoid Necrosis

The segmental, nonatherosclerotic arteriopathy that involves primarily smaller intraparenchymal blood vessels is *fibrinoid necrosis* (also called lipohyalinosis and arteriolar sclerosis). It is found almost exclusively in the brains of patients with hypertension. The lesion is characterized by a fibrinoid material and lipid-laden macrophages in the subintimal layer of cerebral vessels (Fig. 12.21). It has

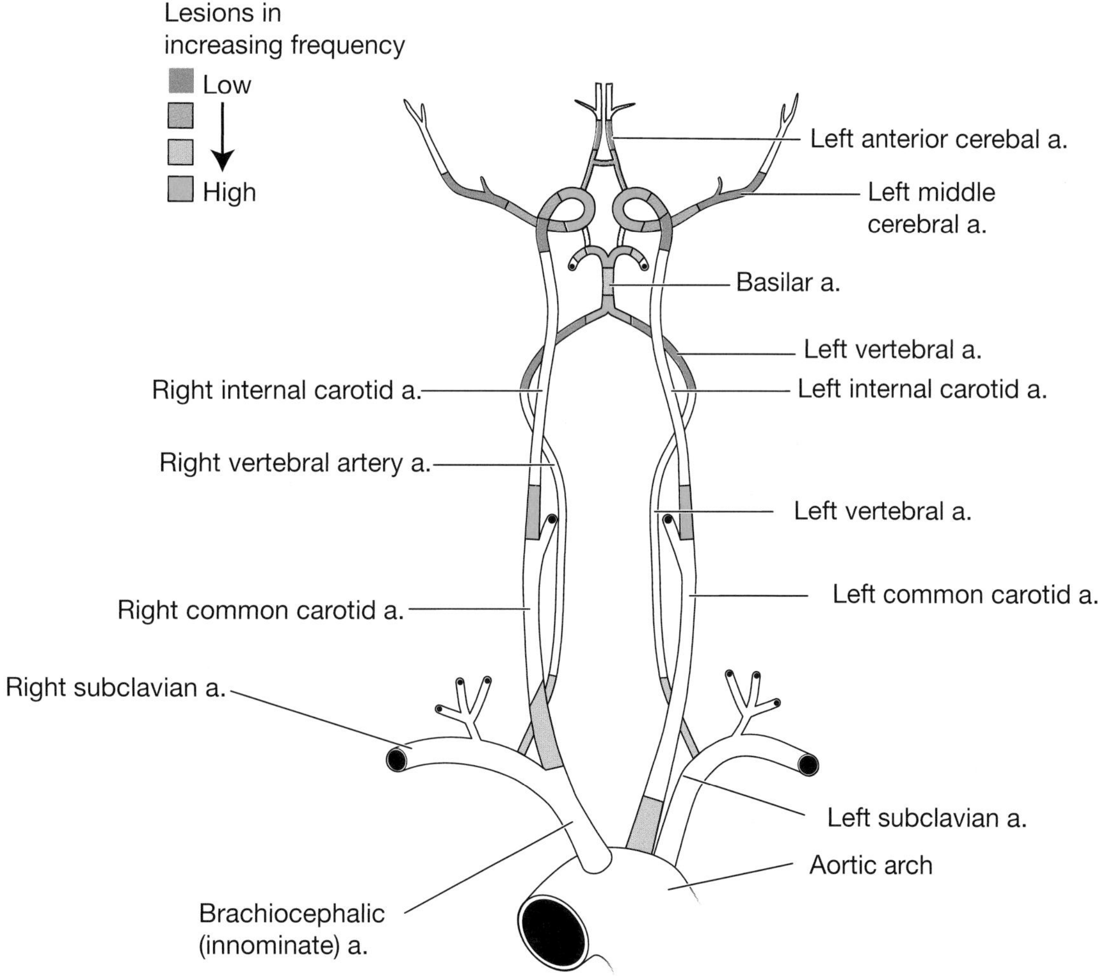

Fig. 12.20. Location and severity of atherosclerotic lesions in major extracranial and intracranial vessels.

been postulated that a sustained increase in blood pressure causes further arterial disorganization. Some of these lesions show progressive luminal obliteration and eventually result in small areas of infarction called lacunae, but others produce progressive weakening of the vessel wall and microaneurysm formation and eventually rupture, producing an intracerebral hemorrhage.

Other Types of Blood Vessel Lesions

Other pathologic processes that may result in disease of the intracranial arteries and veins can produce local thrombosis and, thus, infarction or hemorrhage. Common examples include inflammatory involvement of cerebral blood vessels (*vasculitis*), noninflammatory vasculopathies, and dissection (intimal tear).

Neural-Parenchymal Pathology

The neural-parenchymal lesions produced by the vascular lesions discussed above are of two major types: hemorrhage and infarction (Fig. 12.22). Lesions of both types are common at the supratentorial and posterior fossa levels but less frequent at the spinal level. Symptomatic vascular disease involving the peripheral level is distinctly rare and generally occurs with lesions involving smaller arteries and arterioles that secondarily alter the blood supply to peripheral nerves.

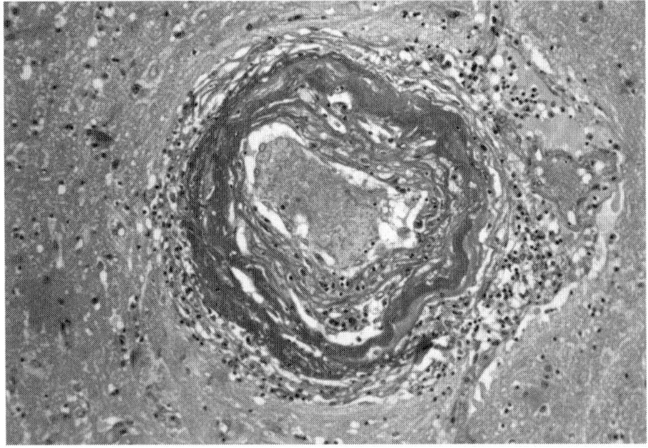

Fig. 12.21. Hypertensive fibrinoid necrosis. Note irregular degeneration and dilatation of the vessel wall associated with infiltration by fibrinoid material and lymphocytes. (H&E; ×100.)

Hemorrhagic Lesions

Pathologic examination shows that nontraumatic intracranial hemorrhagic disease may be defined by its anatomical location. Blood within the subarachnoid space is referred to as *subarachnoid hemorrhage*, and blood within the parenchyma of the brain is referred to as *intracerebral hemorrhage* (Fig. 12.23). Hemorrhage in either of these locations may be produced by various pathophysiologic mechanisms, the most common being 1) rupture of an intracranial aneurysm, usually producing subarachnoid hemorrhage (occasionally with an associated intracerebral hemorrhage); 2) rupture of an intraparenchymal vessel, usually producing a variably sized, blood-filled mass lesion (intracerebral hemorrhage), which often has some extension of bleeding into the ventricles; and 3) bleeding from an arteriovenous malformation, commonly producing either a subarachnoid hemorrhage or an intracerebral hemorrhage, alone or in combination.

Traumatic intracranial hemorrhagic disease may also be defined by its anatomical location. Trauma may result in epidural, subdural, subarachnoid, or intraparenchymal blood. An *epidural hemorrhage* is generally the result of blunt trauma in which a meningeal artery is ruptured. Epidural hemorrhage thus presents as an acute focal mass. A *subdural hemorrhage* generally results from the rupture of the veins traversing the subdural space en route to the venous sinuses. This also causes a focal deficit with mass effect, but it may be more subacute in onset.

Infarction

With prolonged tissue ischemia, permanent pathologic change occurs in neuronal function and structure. In the presence of diffuse oxygen deprivation, wide areas of the cerebral cortex (which is more sensitive to metabolic alteration than other cerebral structures) show evidence of necrosis and cell loss, *anoxic encephalopathy*. More commonly, the area of infarction is localized to the distribution of a diseased blood vessel (Fig. 12.24). In that region, softening and necrosis with ischemic cell change (see Chapter 4) are observed. The size of the infarct varies; smaller lesions (0.5 to 10 mm) are often referred to as lacunar infarctions and are common in the brains of patients with hypertension (Fig. 12.25). Occasionally, especially with large infarctions, the original nonmass

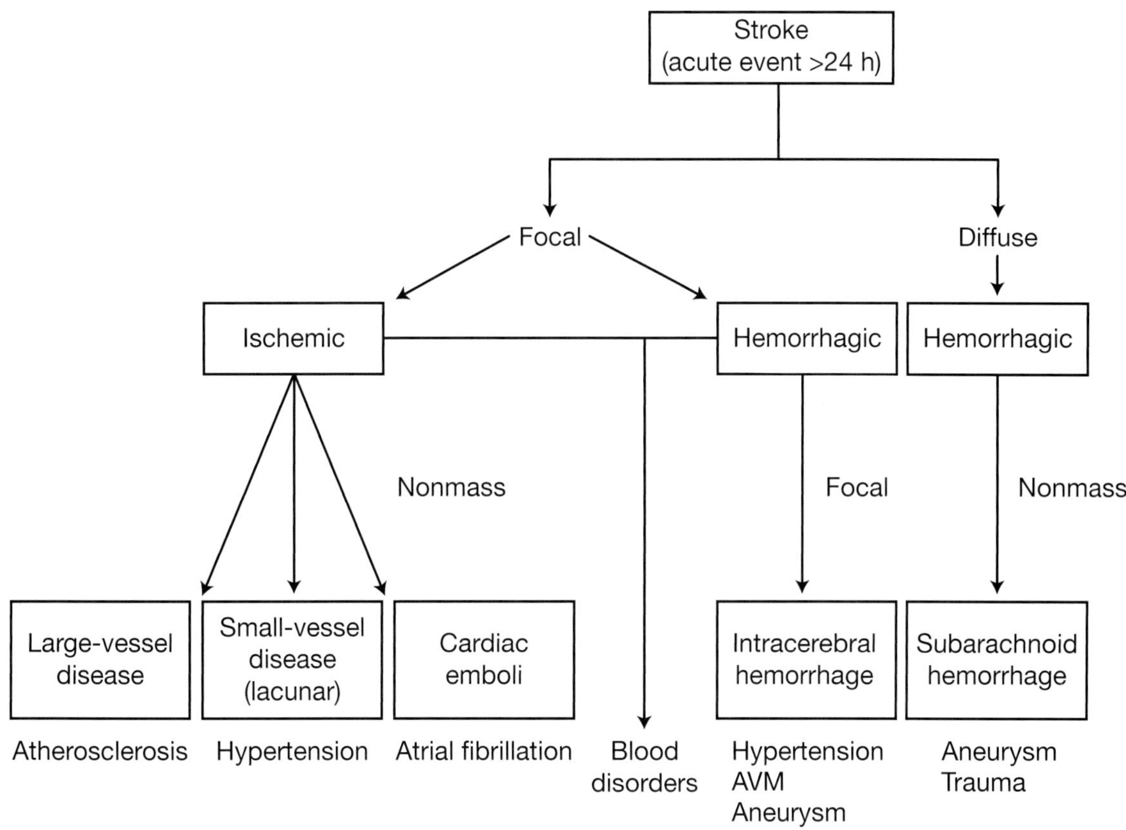

Fig. 12.22. Stroke, typically an acute event, can be divided into two main groups. Ischemic stroke produces focal nonmass lesions (infarction). Common causes are large-vessel disease due to atherosclerosis, small-vessel disease due to hypertension, and cardiac emboli due to atrial fibrillation. Intraparenchymal hemorrhage is a focal mass lesion. It may occur as a consequence of hypertension, vascular malformations, or a coagulation disorder. Subarachnoid hemorrhage is a diffuse nonmass lesion. The most common cause is rupture of a saccular aneurysm. Rupture of an arteriovenous malformation (AVM) can produce either an intraparenchymal or a subarachnoid hemorrhage and can be manifested by seizures or headache.

lesion may become edematous and assume the characteristics of a mass lesion. With time, the necrotic tissue in an infarcted area is removed by phagocytes and replaced by a cavity that contains cystic fluid and is surrounded by an area of glial tissue.

- Pathologic changes that may occur in the cerebral blood vessels which may result in cerebral infarction include atherosclerosis, fibrinoid necrosis, inflammation (vasculitis), and thromboembolism (artery-to-artery or cardiac).
- Cerebral infarction may be focal and due to focal arterial occlusion or thrombus or it may be diffuse, as with cardiac arrest and anoxic brain injury.
- Pathologic changes of the cerebral vasculature that may result in hemorrhagic stroke include aneurysm, arteriovenous malformation, and trauma.
- The location of the hemorrhage (epidural, subdural, subarachnoid, or parenchymal) may provide clues to the cause of bleeding.

Clinical Correlations

Ischemic Stroke and Transient Ischemic Attacks

The term *ischemic stroke* refers to sudden focal neurologic deficit that occurs in a vascular territory and lasts more than 24 hours. In comparison, a *transient ischemic attack*

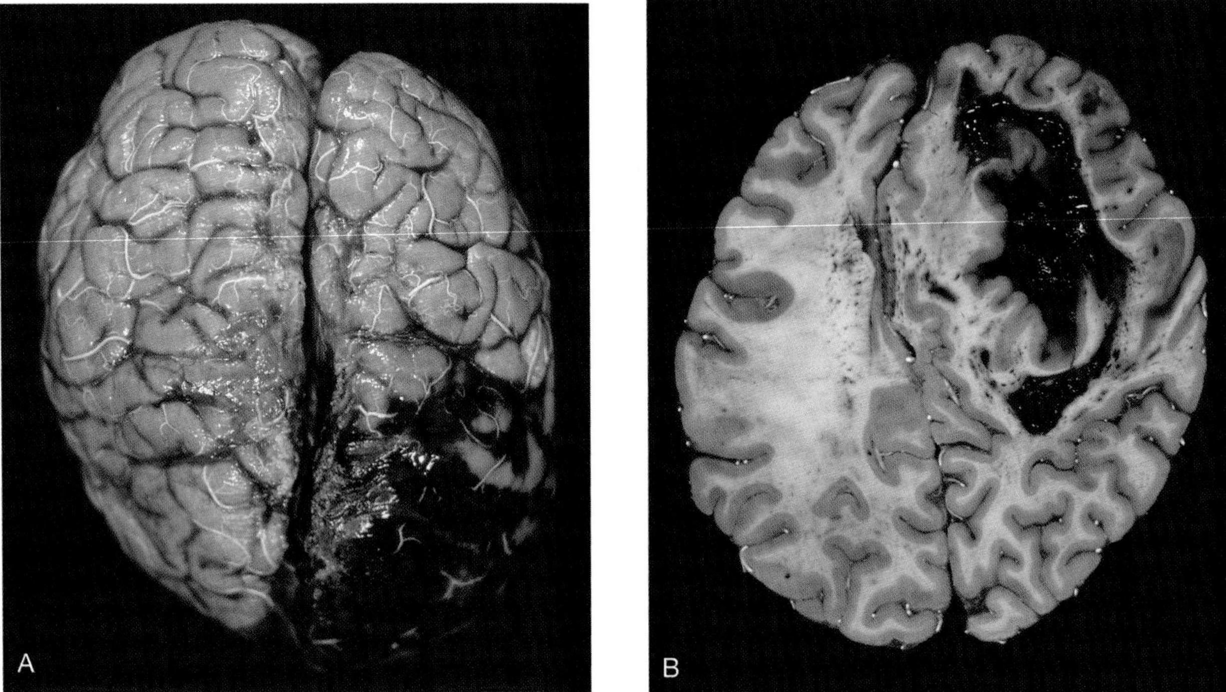

Fig. 12.23. Pathology specimens showing, *A*, subarachnoid hemorrhage and, *B*, intraparenchymal hemorrhage.

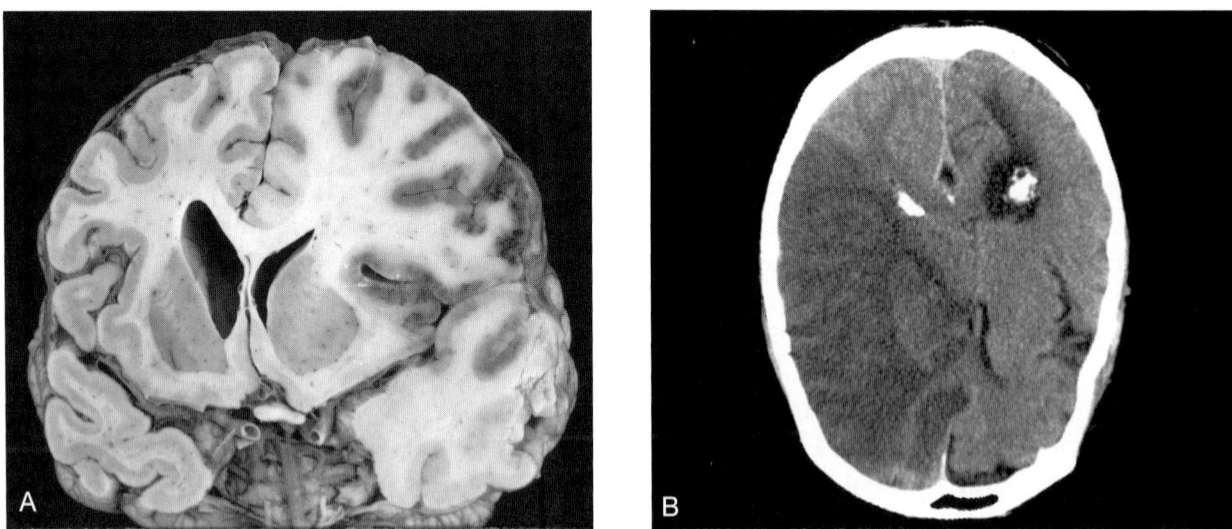

Fig. 12.24. *A*, Pathology specimen showing an acute infarction in the distribution of the middle cerebral artery. Note swelling and cortical discoloration and petechial hemorrhages in the infarcted territory, with marked shift of midline structures. *B*, Computed tomogram of the brain of a similar patient showing hypodensity in the distributions of the left middle cerebral and anterior cerebral arteries, with mass effect and midline shift.

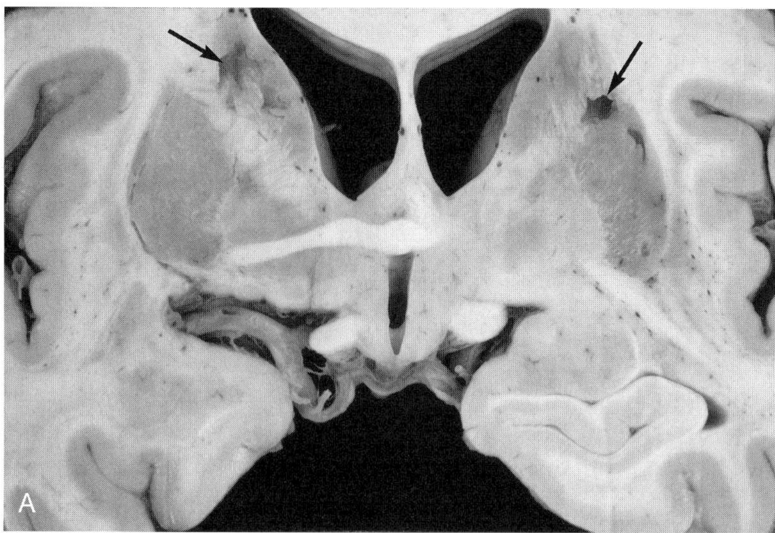

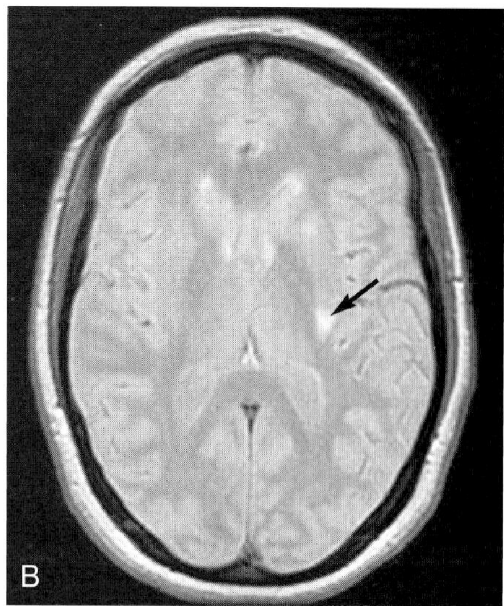

Fig. 12.25. *A*, Pathology specimen showing lacunar infarcts (*arrows*) in the basal ganglia bilaterally. *B*, Magnetic resonance image (T2 weighted) of a lacunar infarction (*arrow*) in the left posterior limb of the internal capsule.

is a spell of focal neurologic dysfunction that clears within 24 hours without permanent neurologic dysfunction. Most transient ischemic attacks commonly last 5 to 30 minutes. Transient ischemic attacks and strokes can occur in either the carotid or vertebrobasilar arterial system. These may also be the result of thrombosis, artery-to-artery emboli, or cardiac emboli. Lesions in the region of the carotid bifurcation are a common source of transient ischemic attack. A related episode is *amaurosis fugax* (fleeting blindness), which consists of transient monocular blindness that often arises from temporary alteration of the retinal blood supply (ophthalmic artery) caused by ipsilateral carotid artery disease. These events must be recognized because between 20% and 35% of patients who experience them subsequently have permanent cerebral infarction.

The goal of intervention in ischemic stroke is to prevent further damage to the brain from lack of blood flow and to preserve the ischemic penumbra from infarcting. Thrombolytics, mechanical disruption of clot, and antiplatelet agents are used for acute treatment of ischemic stroke.

The secondary goal of treatment is the prevention of recurrent stroke or transient ischemic attack. Antiplatelet agents and, in some cases, anticoagulants have a role in preventing clot formation. Because atherosclerosis is a major cause of stroke, treatment of associated risk factors is important. These risk factors include hyperlipidemia, hypertension, tobacco use, diabetes mellitus, obesity, and metabolic syndrome. In addition to atherosclerosis and lipohyalinosis, important causes of stroke to recognize are cardiac disorders such as atrial fibrillation.

Hypertension

Sustained elevation in systemic blood pressure increases the risk of subsequent stroke (ischemic and hemorrhagic) by at least four times when compared with normotension. Hypertension of even modest degree affects the cerebral vasculature by two distinct mechanisms. 1) Acceleration of atherosclerosis—patients of any age with hypertension have a greater amount of atherosclerotic disease than those without hypertension and are at higher risk for the forms of atherothrombotic disease described above. 2) Initiation of pathologic change in small arterioles (fibrinoid necrosis)—this type of arterial degeneration is found almost exclusively in patients with hypertension and seems to be the vascular lesion that predisposes to both lacunar infarction and intracerebral hemorrhage.

Certain Forms of Cardiac Disease

Valvular heart disease of various types, endocarditis, and various cardiac arrhythmias (primarily atrial fibrillation) are associated with intracardiac thrombus formation. Because a large proportion of the cardiac output supplies the cerebrum, the nervous system remains a major target organ for all forms of cardiac emboli.

Generalized Cerebral Ischemia-Syncope

Under normal circumstances, cerebral blood flow remains relatively constant in spite of minor fluctuations in blood pressure. When systemic blood pressure decreases to extremely low levels and the cerebral autoregulatory mechanisms are no longer effective, a state of generalized cerebral ischemia develops. An example of this is the momentary giddiness and light-headedness occasionally experienced when a person abruptly assumes an upright posture. If cerebral perfusion remains inadequate, *syncope* results and consciousness is lost. States of decreased cardiac output, hypotension from many causes, vagal hyperactivity, and impairment of sympathetic vasomotor reflex activity are common causes of syncope, which should not be confused with a transient ischemic attack, as defined above. Transient ischemic attack is a focal ischemic event, but syncope is a generalized ischemic event that results from very different pathogenetic mechanisms and has a different prognosis. With severe focal intracranial vascular disease, syncope may infrequently be associated with focal neurologic signs and symptoms.

Subarachnoid Hemorrhage

With subarachnoid hemorrhage, the person generally presents with a sudden, severe headache oftentimes described as the "worst headache of my life." Subarachnoid hemorrhage can be associated with nausea, vomiting, and reduced level of consciousness. Sometimes, there are also focal neurologic deficits. Diagnosis can be made with computed tomography of the brain, but occasionally lumbar puncture is required if the computed tomographic findings are negative and clinical suspicion is high. The cerebrospinal fluid may have an increased number of red blood cells and evidence of xanthochromia (a yellow tinge to the cerebrospinal fluid from breakdown of red blood cells). Treatment is aimed at discerning the cause of the subarachnoid bleeding, which usually requires imaging and angiography. Typical nontraumatic causes include rupture of an aneurysm or arteriovenous malformation, both of which require surgical repair.

Radiographic Anatomy

Vascular Imaging Techniques

The cerebral blood vessels cannot be examined directly until autopsy. Noninvasive and invasive tests are used to examine the arteries of patients. The choice of test depends on the clinical scenario and the risk of the procedure to the patient. These procedures allow structural abnormalities of vessels, alterations in the position of vessels, and alterations in flow patterns to be identified.

In *cerebral arteriography*, or conventional angiography, an extracranial artery is cannulated and a radiopaque material is injected to achieve high-resolution images of the cerebrovascular anatomy. As the contrast medium circulates through the cerebral vessels, serial radiographs are obtained in both the lateral and anteroposterior projections. The contrast medium outlines the interior of the blood vessels, and the arterial, capillary, and venous phases of the circulation can be assessed. This procedure carries a very small risk of ischemic stroke because of the potential of the catheter dislodging atherosclerotic plaque. Also, the contrast sometimes can adversely affect the kidneys.

Normal vascular anatomy as seen in a conventional cerebral angiogram is shown in Figure 12.26. Deviations from the normal vascular pattern may indicate disease and should be correlated with the clinical history and examination findings.

Both *magnetic resonance angiography* and computed tomographic angiography alleviate the potential risks of an arterial puncture and may be a useful alternative to conventional angiography in many patients. Similarly, magnetic resonance imaging and computed tomography can be used to view the venous system (Fig. 12.27). Ultrasound technology also allows visualization of the common, external, and internal carotid arteries in the neck. Degrees of stenosis are inferred by changes in velocity

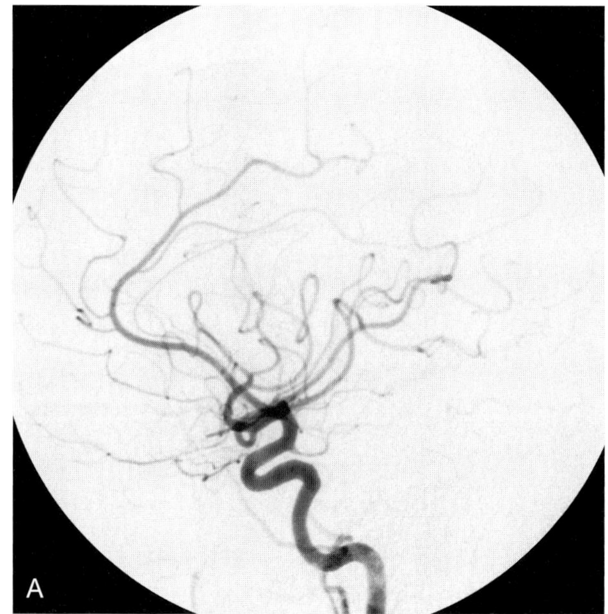

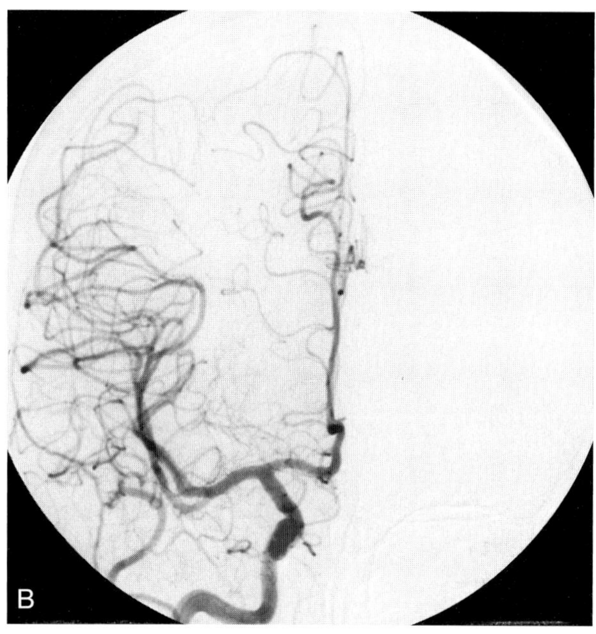

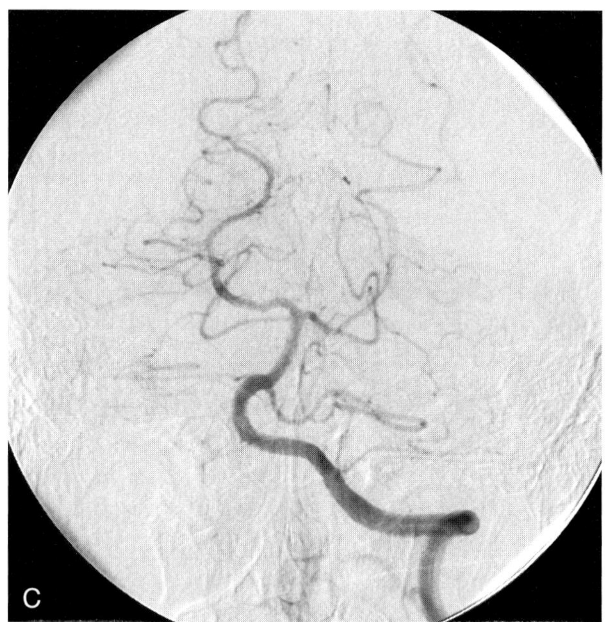

Fig. 12.26. Conventional angiography of the brain showing the intracranial segment of the right internal carotid artery in, *A*, lateral and, *B*, anteroposterior views. *C*, Anteroposterior view of the vertebrobasilar arterial system.

and the use of color flow technology. *Transcranial Doppler* ultrasonography can be used to noninvasively assess intracranial arteries, including the middle, anterior, and distal internal carotid arteries as well as the vertebral arteries and proximal basilar artery. Abnormalities evaluated with these imaging techniques include structural abnormalities of the vessels, alterations in the position of vessels, and alterations in flow patterns.

Structural Abnormalities of Vessels

Stenosis (narrowing) or occlusion (nonfilling) of a vessel may be seen. Vascular malformations and aneurysms are examples of this type of change. Conventional angiography may show collections of abnormal vessels within neoplasms, in particular, gliomas, meningiomas, and metastatic lesions. These collections may be responsible for the so-called tumor blush or stain seen as an area of increased dye concentration.

Alterations in the Position of Vessels

Mass lesions commonly cause vessels to be displaced. Such displacement may be local and delineate the mass or it may be distant and indirect. Examples of the latter include a shift in the position of the anterior cerebral artery with anteriorly placed lesions or a shift in the position of the internal cerebral vein with more posteriorly placed lesions.

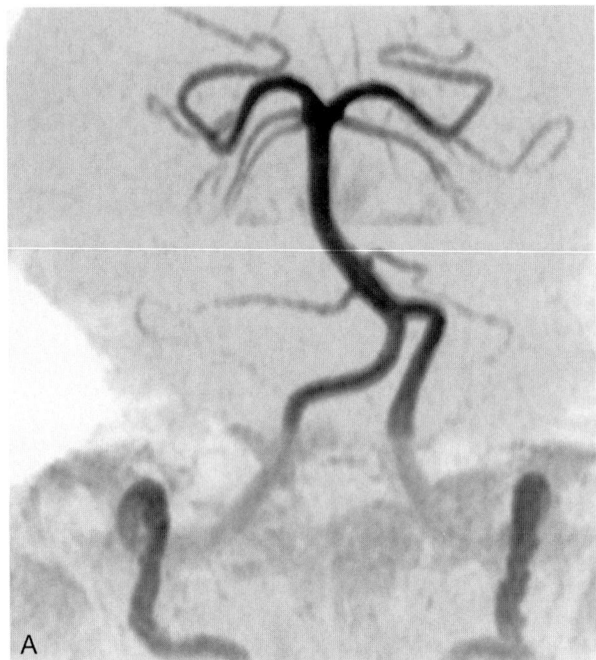

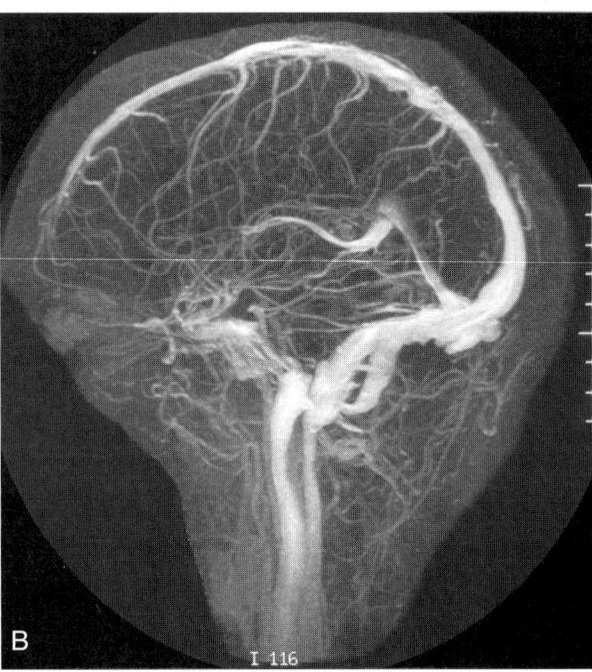

Fig. 12.27. *A*, Magnetic resonance angiogram showing the intracranial portion of the posterior circulation. *B*, Magnetic resonance venogram from a sagittal view.

Alterations in Flow Patterns

Changes in the circulatory pattern may be evident as an expression of abnormal vascular shunts, as with arteriovenous malformations and some tumors. Collateral flow patterns may be identified in instances of thrombosis of major arteries, for example, through the ophthalmic artery in cases of carotid artery occlusion; the diminution or absence of flow is found distal to the site of the vascular occlusion. A general slowing of the circulation may be noted when intracranial pressure is increased.

Brain Imaging Techniques

Both *magnetic resonance imaging* and *computed tomography* allow visualization of the brain parenchyma. These techniques are commonly used to visualize infarction and hemorrhage associated with disease of the vasculature.

Computed tomography is a radiographic technique capable of visualizing intracranial anatomy and abnormality. Often, it is used to evaluate a patient who presents with acute stroke. Areas of infarction (Fig. 12.28 *A*) often appear as regions of reduced attenuation, whereas regions of hemorrhage (Fig. 12.28 *B*) show increased attenuation. The vascular structures of the brain can be enhanced with the injection of intravenous contrast material, and this can be used to identify large vascular anomalies such as an arteriovenous malformation.

Magnetic resonance imaging is another imaging technique that can provide useful information about the status of the cerebral vasculature and brain parenchyma. This technique is more sensitive than computed tomography for detecting ischemic stroke, especially acutely. Also, magnetic resonance imaging provides more detailed information about both ischemic and hemorrhagic lesions. An example of an acute cerebral infarction is shown in Figure 12.29. A magnetic resonance image of a hemorrhage due to a vascular malformation is shown in Figure 12.30.

- Ischemic stroke is a sudden focal neurologic deficit in a vascular territory due to ischemia lasting more than 24 hours. A transient ischemic attack has a similar pathologic mechanism, but clinically lasts less than 24 hours.

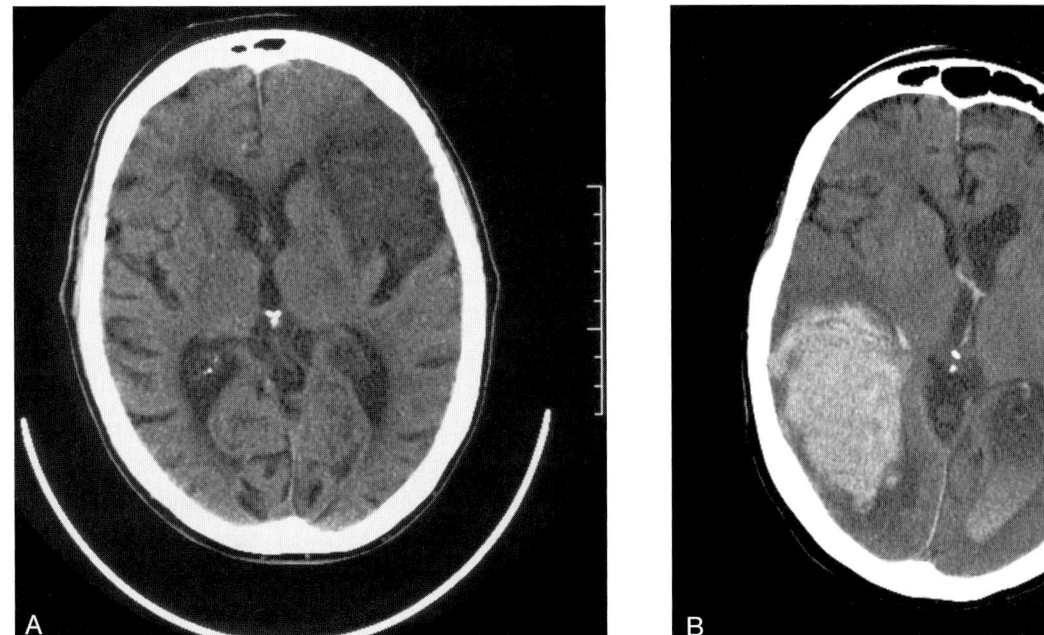

Fig. 12.28. Computed tomograms of the brain. *A*, In ischemic stroke, there is hypodensity of the brain parenchyma, in this case, in the distribution of the left middle cerebral artery. *B*, In a hemorrhagic stroke, there is increased attenuation, or hyperdensity, of the brain parenchyma.

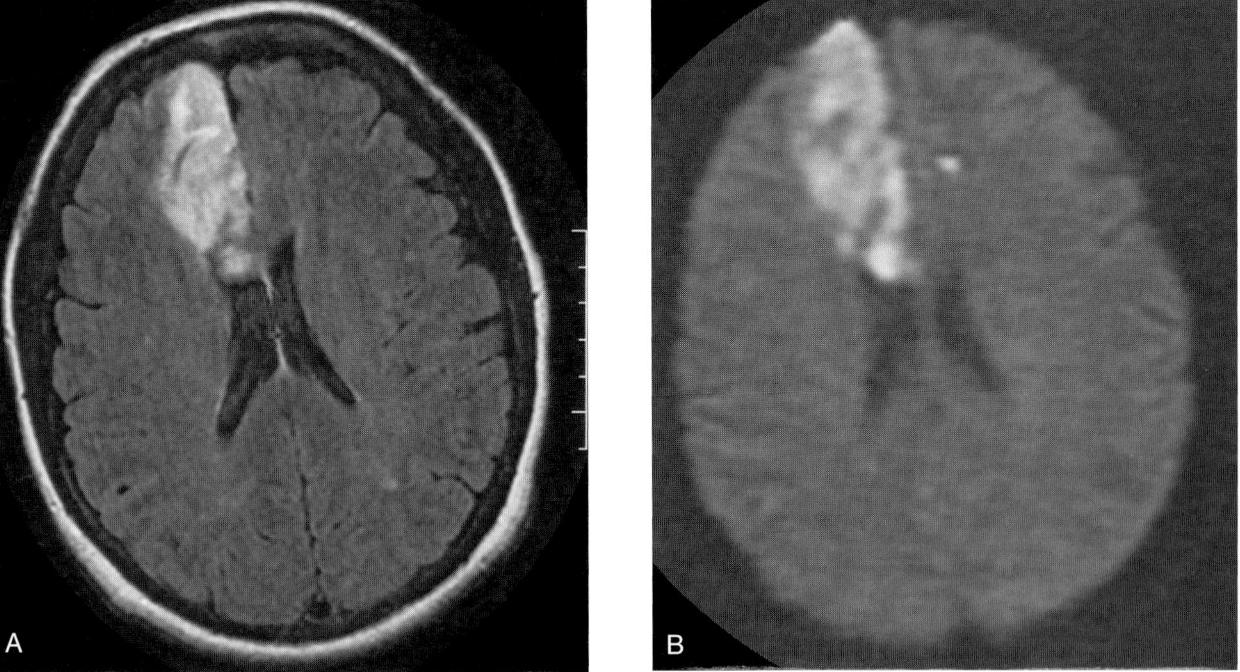

Fig. 12.29. Magnetic resonance image showing an acute cerebral infarction. *A*, The fluid attenuation inversion recovery (FLAIR) sequence shows an area of increased signal in the distribution of the right anterior cerebral artery. *B*, The accompanying diffusion-weighted image also shows increased signal in the same location. The diffusion-weighted image sequence indicates that the cerebral infarction occurred within the past 2 weeks.

- Amaurosis fugax is a type of transient ischemic attack resulting from temporary lack of blood flow in the ophthalmic artery.
- Acute treatments for ischemic stroke improve blood flow and reduce the damage from infarction. Also, treatments are available for secondarily preventing additional strokes.
- Hypertension, diabetes mellitus, tobacco use, hyperlipidemia, and atrial fibrillation are major risk factors for ischemic stroke or transient ischemic attack.
- Various invasive and noninvasive imaging techniques are available for the diagnosis of ischemic and hemorrhagic stroke. Computed tomography of the brain can readily distinguish between hemorrhage and ischemia. Magnetic resonance imaging provides more detail about both ischemic and hemorrhagic stroke. Angiography (conventional, magnetic resonance angiography, computed tomographic angiography) anatomically demonstrates the cerebral vasculature and can provide information about blood flow and collateral circulation.

Examination of the Vascular System

Because "vascular" refers to both an anatomical system and an etiologic category, its evaluation requires both historical data and information obtained from the physical examination. Patients with cerebrovascular disease may present with a wide range of symptoms of diverse cause. The evaluation of these patients should be designed to enable the clinician to determine 1) the nature of the presenting symptoms and signs; 2) the type, location, and extent of the pathologic process in the neural parenchyma; 3) the type, location, and extent of the pathologic process in the vasculature; and 4) the pathophysiologic mechanism responsible for the observed symptoms and signs. This evaluation

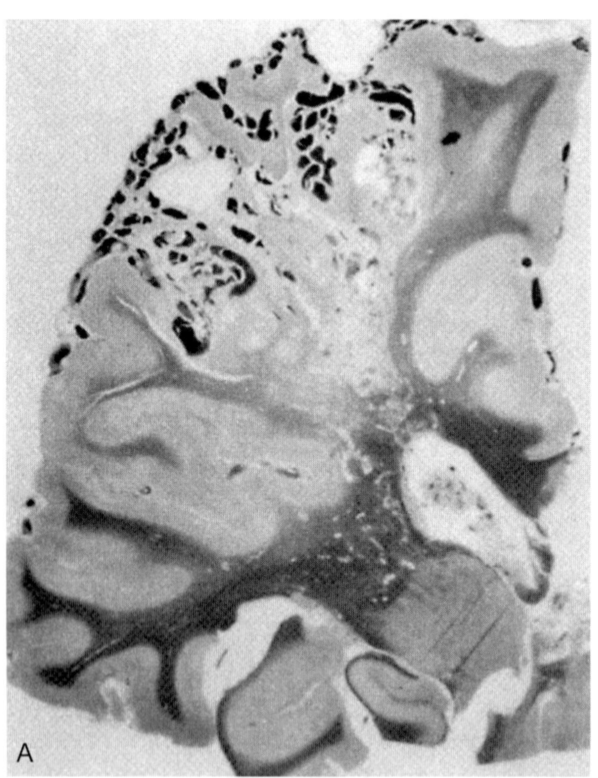

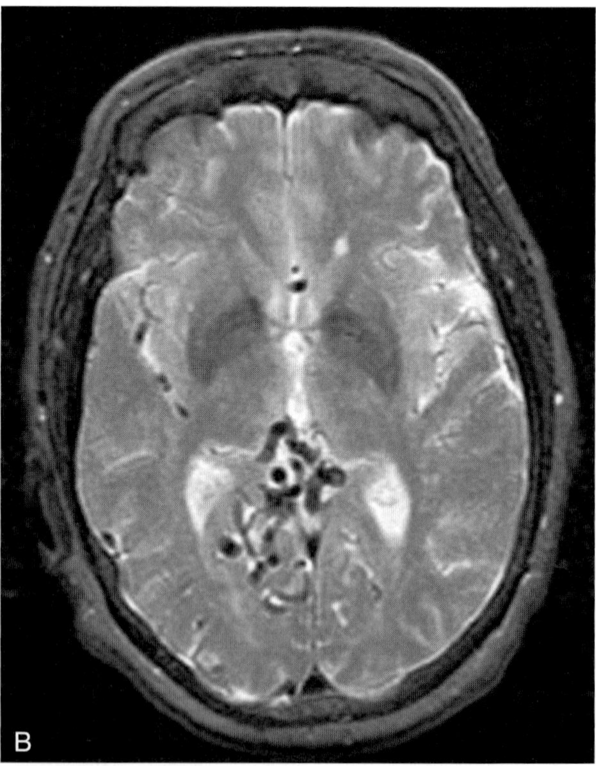

Fig. 12.30. *A*, Arteriovenous malformation of the left parietal lobe. Note the tangled mass of dilated vessels in a roughly wedge-shaped area pointing toward the ventricle, with degeneration of the cerebral tissue between vessels. (Celloidin section, Luxol fast blue stain; ×1.) *B*, A T2-weighted magnetic resonance image of the brain of a different patient shows several flow voids in the right posterior head region. This is suggestive of an arteriovenous malformation.

Clinical Problem 12.4.

A 62-year-old man had frequent, highly stereotyped episodes. He suddenly felt giddy and lightheaded, lost consciousness, and fell to the ground. A physician observed one of these spells and noted that during the episode the patient had no peripheral pulse and the blood pressure was too low to be detected. Both blood pressure and peripheral pulse returned to normal coincident with the patient's regaining consciousness.

a. What is the anatomicopathologic nature of the lesion?
b. What is the pathophysiologic mechanism responsible for the symptoms?
c. Define autoregulation.
d. Under normal physiologic conditions, which of the following could be expected to produce cerebral vasodilation: inhalation of oxygen, 20% decrease in arterial blood pressure, 20% increase in arterial blood pressure, inhalation of carbon dioxide?
e. How do these spells differ from a transient ischemic attack?

Clinical Problem 12.5.

A 38-year-old man suddenly experienced a severe headache that was associated with nausea, vomiting, and neck stiffness. When examined 2 hours later, he was somnolent but easily aroused. He had no focal neurologic findings but had marked nuchal rigidity. A computed tomographic scan from this patient is shown in Figure 12.31.

a. What is the anatomicopathologic nature of the lesion?
b. What is the pathophysiologic mechanism responsible for the symptoms?
c. What test might you order to determine the cause?

Clinical Problem 12.6.

A 16-year-old boy with endocarditis noted the sudden onset of complete loss of vision. Within minutes, this partially cleared, and he noted only a loss of vision in the left half of the visual field of each eye. His condition had improved slightly by the time he reached the hospital, but examination still showed a left homonymous hemianopia.

a. What is the anatomicopathologic nature of the lesion?
b. How could you determine if this were hemorrhagic or ischemic?
c. If it is ischemic, what is the vascular supply to this region of the brain?
d. List possible causes of an ischemic stroke or transient ischemic attack. What is the most likely cause in this patient?
e. If ischemic, is this a stroke or transient ischemic attack? When would you know?

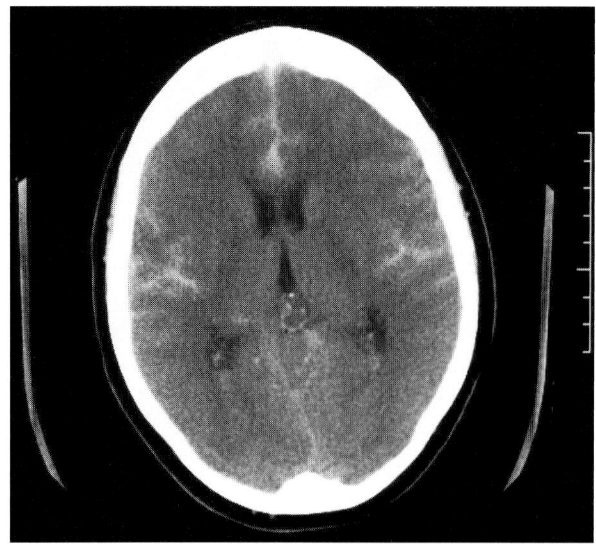

Fig. 12.31. Computed tomogram of the brain of a patient presenting with sudden, severe headache.

usually can be accomplished with reasonable accuracy through a detailed history and physical examination, aided by the judicious selection of ancillary diagnostic studies.

Historical Aspects

From the history, it is possible to determine if a problem is vascular and if the primary pathologic process is hemorrhage or infarction and to define the likely pathophysiologic mechanism responsible for the problem.

The judgment about whether a problem is vascular is made almost exclusively from the temporal profile, with the onset, evaluation, and course of the presenting symptoms. An acute onset with rapid evolution (minutes to hours) to maximal deficit implies a vascular cause. Without a history of a clearly defined acute onset, the diagnosis of nontraumatic cerebrovascular disease must remain uncertain.

Patients with symptoms of acute onset may be seen at any stage in the development of their symptoms. Some patients have symptoms that have resolved completely by the time they present for evaluation. They may describe the focal symptoms of transient ischemic attacks, but such events must be distinguished from other causes of transient neurologic deficits (Table 12.6).

Acute symptoms may progress, and the patient may display increasing deficit while being evaluated (a progressing stroke). With these patients, a careful historical inquiry must be made to uncover the possibility of an underlying neoplasm, other mass lesions (i.e., subdural hematoma), or superimposed metabolic or inflammatory encephalopathy (Table 12.7).

At the time of evaluation, the condition of some patients with symptoms of acute onset may have stabilized with residual deficit or may show some improvement. Most of these patients have a completed stroke. The historical inquiry must be directed at uncovering the pathophysiologic mechanism responsible for the deficit and must take into account other intracranial processes that could explain the symptoms.

The distinction between hemorrhage and infarction is of major clinical importance and readily made in most cases, but it may be difficult in some instances. The onset of symptoms in association with severe headache, although not invariably associated with hemorrhage, favors a hemorrhagic process. If the primary lesion is located at the supratentorial rather than posterior fossa level, then alteration in consciousness, stupor, or coma coincident with or shortly after the onset of symptoms favors the diagnosis of hemorrhagic disease.

When hemorrhage is suspected, the location of the hemorrhage can often be determined clinically. The early absence of focal neurologic symptoms favors a subarachnoid hemorrhage and, in the absence of trauma, suggests the possibility of a ruptured intracranial aneurysm. Focal neurologic symptoms suggest an intracerebral hemorrhage. In patients with suspected intracerebral hemorrhage, a history of significant, untreated hypertension makes the diagnosis more likely. In the absence of hypertension, one must consider the possibility of either a ruptured aneurysm with associated intracerebral hemorrhage or a parenchymal hemorrhage due to an arteriovenous malformation, which also can present as a subarachnoid

Table 12.6. Differential Diagnosis of Transient Focal Neurologic Deficit

Transient ischemic attack
Seizure
Migraine
Metabolic disturbances
Labyrinthine disease (vertigo)
Syncope
Myasthenia gravis

Table 12.7. Differential Diagnosis of a Fixed Focal Neurologic Deficit

Ischemic stroke
Intraparenchymal hemorrhage
Subdural hemorrhage
Epidural hemorrhage
Encephalitis
Neoplasm
Metabolic dysfunction

hemorrhage. A history of preexistent focal seizures, localized headache, or previous intracranial bleeding supports the diagnosis of an arteriovenous malformation.

When an ischemic process is suspected, it is necessary first to distinguish between carotid and vertebrobasilar arterial system disease. Although in most patients ischemic lesions are related to atherosclerosis, the patient's entire medical and neurologic history should be examined to determine whether the symptoms are a consequence of 1) intracranial pathologic processes involving large-caliber or small-caliber arteries and arterioles, 2) thromboembolic disease in the major extracranial vessels, 3) emboli arising from distant sources (most often, the heart), or 4) another systemic disorder.

The Neurovascular Examination

The physical evaluation of patients with suspected cerebrovascular disease must include an assessment of the neurovascular system in addition to a general physical examination and more detailed study of neurologic function. Cerebrovascular disease seldom occurs in isolation; the basic pathologic process often exerts its effect on multiple target organs, and therapeutic intervention can be planned only after the general well-being of the patient is considered. A careful cardiac, pulmonary, and peripheral vascular examination, including recording of pulse rate and rhythm and measurement of brachial blood pressure bilaterally and in the lying and standing positions, is essential. Also, the degree to which underlying disorders such as hypertension, diabetes mellitus, hyperlipidemia, and hematologic abnormalities may be contributing to the cerebrovascular symptoms must be determined. The neurovascular examination includes examining neck flexion for evidence of nuchal rigidity in patients with suspected hemorrhagic disease and three additional procedures designed to provide evidence of disease in the cerebrovascular system: auscultation of the head and neck, palpation of the cephalic vessels, and neuro-ophthalmologic examination.

Auscultation of the Head and Neck

The examiner should gently apply the stethoscope over the great vessels arising from the aortic arch, the carotid bifurcations, the orbits, and the skull and listen for evidence of bruits. A bruit is an abnormal pulsatile sound that indicates turbulent blood flow through a vessel. It is usually, but not always, associated with stenosis of that vessel. A bruit may be audible over an area of abnormal arteriovenous communication and at times may be heard over an anatomically normal vessel if flow is turbulent.

Palpation of the Cephalic Vessels

The carotid arteries in the neck and the superficial temporal arteries anterior to the ear should be palpated gently. Altered pulsation, especially if unilateral, usually indicates proximal obstructive vascular disease. Although palpation of the peripheral pulses is an important part of the assessment of the general vascular system, palpation of the carotid pulses is less reliable and has the potential danger of dislodging material from an atheromatous plaque. If pulsation of the carotid artery cannot be felt on gentle palpation, vigorous compression will add little diagnostic information.

Neuro-ophthalmologic Examination

The optic fundus should be examined in all patients because this provides valuable information about intracranial vascular disease. Atherosclerosis, hypertension, diabetes mellitus, and other systemic disorders produce recognizable retinal and vascular changes (Fig. 12.32). For

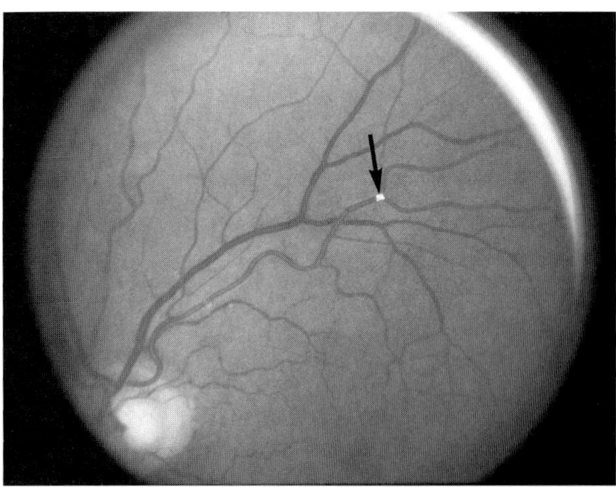

Fig. 12.32. Small cholesterol embolus (*arrow*) seen in a distal arteriole of the optic fundus of a patient with atherosclerosis of the proximal internal carotid artery.

example, *subhyaloid* (preretinal) *hemorrhages* may be observed in patients with subarachnoid hemorrhage. Evidence of retinal embolic events in the form of retinal infarcts and cholesterol (Fig. 12.32), platelet-fibrin, or calcific emboli may be seen in patients with carotid occlusive disease. These intra-arterial fragments are presumed to be from an ulcerated atheromatous lesion in the circulation proximal to the ophthalmic arteries, and their presence correlates well with demonstrable lesions in the ipsilateral internal carotid artery.

- Important aspects of the history of the present illness when considering cerebrovascular disease include the onset and course of the illness, specific symptoms, and risk factors for ischemic and hemorrhagic stroke.
- Important aspects of the physical examination in addition to a standard neurologic examination include assessment of blood pressure in both arms, pulse, auscultation of the head and neck for bruits, palpation of the cephalic vessels, and a neuro-ophthalmologic examination.

Additional Reading

Flemming KD, Brown RD Jr, Petty GW, Huston J III, Kallmes DF, Piepgras DG. Evaluation and management of transient ischemic attack and minor cerebral infarction. Mayo Clin Proc. 2004;79:1071-1086.

Powers WJ. Cerebral hemodynamics in ischemic cerebrovascular disease. Ann Neurol. 1991;29:231-240.

Rhoton AL Jr. The cerebellar arteries. Neurosurgery. 2000;47(3 Suppl):S29-S68.

Rhoton AL Jr. The supratentorial cranial space. Neurosurgery. 2002;51(4 Suppl):S1-S410.

PART III

Horizontal Levels

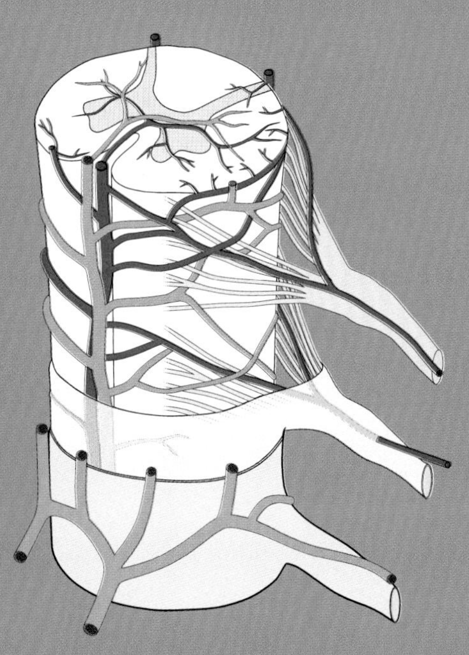

Chapter 13

The Peripheral Level

Objectives

1. Name the four major systems represented at the peripheral level, and describe the location, histologic features, and function of each.
2. Name the three major subdivisions of the peripheral level at which lesions occur, and describe their gross anatomical location, histologic features, and physiology.
3. List the neurologic deficits that would occur with damage in each of the subdivisions of the peripheral level, and explain their mechanism of occurrence.
4. Describe the mechanisms of neuromuscular transmission and muscle contraction.
5. Name the location, function, and deficit (motor, sensory, and reflex) resulting from a lesion of each of the following: spinal nerves C5, C6, C7, C8, L4, L5, and S1; brachial and lumbosacral plexuses; and radial, ulnar, median, sciatic, femoral, peroneal (fibular), and tibial nerves.
6. Describe the main clinical features that distinguish large-fiber neuropathies from small-fiber neuropathies.
7. Describe the major electromyographic characteristics of axonal neuropathy, demyelinating neuropathy, neuromuscular transmission defect, and myopathy.
8. Describe the major clinical, electrophysiologic, laboratory, and biopsy findings that distinguish a neuropathy, neuromuscular junction disorder, and myopathy.
9. Name examples of immunologic and genetic tests used to assess neuromuscular disorders.

Introduction

Precise anatomical localization is one of the major goals of neurologic diagnosis. The study of the major longitudinal systems and the manifestations of diseases within each system permit localization of a lesion in one or more systems. Chapters 13 through 16 present the patterns of disease at each of the four major levels. The combination of signs and symptoms resulting from damage to the systems at each major level often allows highly specific localization of the underlying disorder.

The peripheral level includes all neuromuscular structures outside the skull and spinal column. This includes spinal and peripheral nerves, nerve plexuses, sensory receptors, neuromuscular junctions, muscles, and the portions of cranial nerves outside the cranium. Diseases at the peripheral level are among the most common neurologic diseases and are encountered by physicians in all medical specialties. The anatomy, physiology, pathophysiology, and clinical disorders of these peripheral structures are considered in this chapter.

Overview

The peripheral level contains four of the longitudinal systems: the motor, sensory, internal regulation (autonomic component), and vascular systems. The peripheral axon of the lower motor neuron, the neuromuscular junction, and the muscle fibers of the motor unit are found at the peripheral level. The distal axon of the primary sensory neuron and the sensory receptors are peripheral. The distal axon of the autonomic preganglionic neuron, the entire postganglionic neuron, and the visceral afferent axons are peripheral. The cell bodies of motor neurons, second-order sensory neurons, and preganglionic autonomic neurons and the central processes of dorsal root ganglion cells are located in the spinal cord or brainstem, but some of their disorders have features similar to those of the peripheral level and are considered in this chapter.

Axons of the motor, sensory, and autonomic systems travel together in the periphery. Peripheral lesions typically produce combinations of symptoms and signs from all three of these neural systems. Diseases at the peripheral level may be focal (e.g., involving a single nerve) or diffuse (involving all spinal nerves). A focal lesion may be a mass or a nonmass lesion. Diffuse lesions often involve only one type of structure in the periphery, as in primary disease of muscle. However, disorders of the blood vessels of the peripheral vascular system can damage nerves or muscles. The temporal profile of peripheral diseases may be transient, acute, subacute, or chronic, corresponding to the major disease types, that is, vascular, traumatic, metabolic, inflammatory, neoplastic, or degenerative.

The peripheral nerves transmit information to and from the peripheral end organs, including sensory receptors, muscles, and autonomic receptors and effectors. Each of these has different clinical functions, and their diseases produce different clinical features.

Nerves

Peripheral nerves are the gross structures that carry motor, sensory, and autonomic (internal regulatory) axons to their end organs. (Some nerves contain only autonomic fibers, e.g., splanchnic nerves.) Cranial and spinal peripheral nerves transmit information between the central nervous system and the periphery (sensory organs, muscles, and viscera). Spinal nerves combine in the brachial plexus in the shoulder and the lumbosacral plexus in the pelvis to form a complex network of axons traveling peripherally and centrally from the spinal nerves to the peripheral nerves. Peripheral nerves provide the axonal innervation of the end organs.

Each type of nerve in the periphery consists of axons that have similar histologic, physiologic, and pathophysiologic features. Peripheral disorders of nerves may be axolemmal (involving the axon membrane) or axoplasmic (involving the entire axon) or may involve myelin, resulting in demyelination of the axon.

End Organs

The end organs include sensory receptors, muscle and autonomic receptors, and effectors. The somatic sensory receptors for the sensations of pain, touch, position, vibration, and muscle proprioception are considered in detail in the chapters on the sensory and motor systems and are not discussed in this chapter. The special sensory receptors of the cranial nerves are considered in Chapters 15 and 16.

Movement is produced by muscle. Within the muscles are neuromuscular junctions and muscle fibers and their contractile elements. Tendons, bones, and joints have an integral part in movement by converting the contraction of muscle into the movement of a limb. They are not considered further.

The autonomic receptors and effectors are a widespread and diverse group of visceral structures and are discussed in Chapter 9. Although diseases of these structures are common in general medical practice, they are not considered further because they are more properly studied with specific organ systems.

Peripheral Axons

The major peripheral structures are nerves and muscles. Nerves are a collection of nerve fibers called axons, which are bound together by connective tissue as they travel between the central nervous system and a peripheral end organ. They have similar microscopic features, physiologic characteristics, and pathophysiologic alterations with disease. The general features common to all types of nerves are considered first.

Histology

A nerve consists of thousands of axons that range in size from less than 1 μm to 20 μm in diameter. In each nerve trunk, individual fibers are surrounded by a connective tissue sheath, the *endoneurium*. Axons are bundled together into fascicles. Each fascicle is surrounded by *perineurium*. Groups of fascicles are bound together by an outer covering of connective tissue, the *epineurium* (Fig. 13.1). Each nerve has its own blood supply. Nutrient arteries enter a nerve at intervals along its length and form anastomotic channels within the connective tissue framework of the nerve. These anastomoses make nerves relatively resistant to vascular disease except in watershed zones where the anastamotic channels between nutrient arteries may not overlap sufficiently.

Axons can be differentiated histologically on the basis of diameter and the presence or absence of myelin. Unmyelinated axons have a small diameter and include autonomic fibers and sensory fibers transmitting pain and temperature information. Proprioceptive and somatic motor fibers have a large diameter (Table 13.1). However, the function of an individual axon cannot be specified on the basis of these characteristics because afferent (carrying information centrally) axons and efferent (carrying information peripherally) axons have a similar microscopic appearance.

Each myelinated nerve fiber has a series of Schwann cells arranged longitudinally along its length. Each Schwann cell forms the myelin cover of 0.5 to 1.0 mm of axon. The junctions between Schwann cells along a myelinated axon are seen as constrictions of the nerve fiber and are called the *nodes of Ranvier* (Fig. 13.1 and 13.2). These nodes divide myelinated axons into internodes, nodes, and paranodal regions. The voltage-gated sodium and potassium channels in the region of a node mediate the current flow of action potentials. Although the fibers in a nerve are adjacent to one another, the electrical activity in each axon is independent of the activity in the other axons. The action potentials are isolated from each other by the myelin sheath and endoneurium.

A single Schwann cell surrounds either a number of unmyelinated axons or one myelinated axon. During development, either many unmyelinated axons become enclosed by a Schwann cell or the cytoplasm of a Schwann cell wraps around one axon in concentric circles to form the myelin of a myelinated nerve fiber (Fig. 13.3). Interactions between the axon and Schwann cell are necessary for normal nerve function.

As the cytoplasm of a Schwann cell encircles an axon, its layers of plasma membrane fuse to form myelin (Fig. 13.4). Compact myelin, which is restricted to the internode, is a series of concentric layers of lipids and proteins that form major dense lines and interperiod lines. The

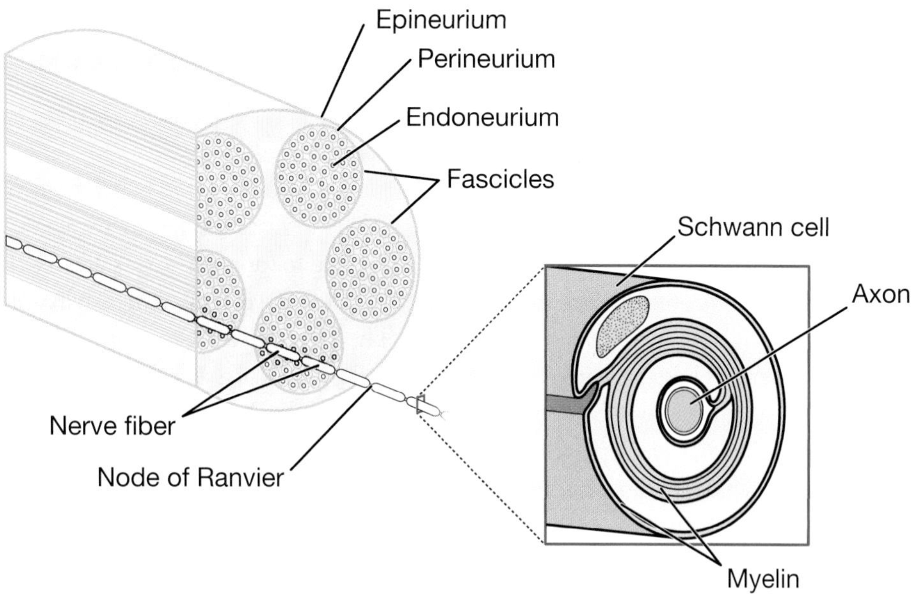

Fig. 13.1. Histologic features of a peripheral nerve. A nerve is subdivided into fascicles by the perineurium, with multiple motor and sensory nerve fibers intermingled in each fascicle.

Table 13.1. Nerve Fiber Types

Type	Diameter, μm	Conduction velocity, m/s	Function
Muscle nerve afferents			
Ia	12-20	70-120	Afferents from muscle spindle (primary endings—annulospiral)
Ib	12-20	70-120	Afferents from Golgi tendon organs
II	6-12	30-70	Afferents from muscle spindle (secondary endings—flower spray)
III	2-6	4-30	Pressure-pain afferents
IV	<2	0.5-2.0	Pain afferents
Cutaneous nerve afferents			
Aα	12-20	70-120	Joint receptor afferents
Aα	6-12	30-70	Paccinian corpuscle and touch receptor afferents
Aδ	2-6	4-30	Touch, temperature, and pain afferents
C	<2	0.5-2.0	Pain, temperature, and some mechanoreceptors
Visceral nerve afferents			
A	2-12	4-70	Internal regulation receptors
C	<2	0.2-2.0	
Efferents			
Alpha	12-20	70-120	Extrafusal skeletal muscle innervation from alpha motor neurons
Gamma	2-8	10-50	Intrafusal muscle spindle innervation from gamma motor neurons
B	<3	3-30	Preganglionic autonomic efferents
C	<1	0.5-2.0	Postganglionic autonomic efferents

lipids include cerebrosides, sulfatides, proteolipids, sphingomyelin, inositol phosphatides, phosphatidylserine, glycolipids, glycoproteins, and cholesterol.

Myelin contains specific proteins synthesized by myelin-forming Schwann cells (or by oligodendrocytes in the central nervous system). These proteins are adhesion molecules involved in the processes of wrapping and compaction of the myelin sheath. Myelin proteins in the peripheral nervous system include myelin *protein zero* and peripheral myelin *protein 22*. Another protein critical for myelination is the gap junction protein *connexin*, which is also synthesized by Schwann cells. Mutations of the genes encoding for myelin proteins produce several types of hereditary sensory and motor neuropathies.

Although myelin is relatively inert metabolically, its chemical constituents have a high rate of turnover and respond to various disease states. For instance, myelin may be lost (demyelination) in certain immunologic disorders. The loss of myelin along a peripheral nerve usually occurs in the region of a single Schwann cell, which extends from one node of Ranvier to another. This loss is called *segmental demyelination*. It alters the function of a nerve fiber.

Also, myelin may form abnormally or may accumulate myelin metabolites in abnormal quantities. This condition occurs in genetic disorders due to enzyme defects, such as metachromatic leukodystrophy, in which a deficit of arylsulfatase A results in the accumulation of metachromatic sulfatides in axons and the loss of function of these axons.

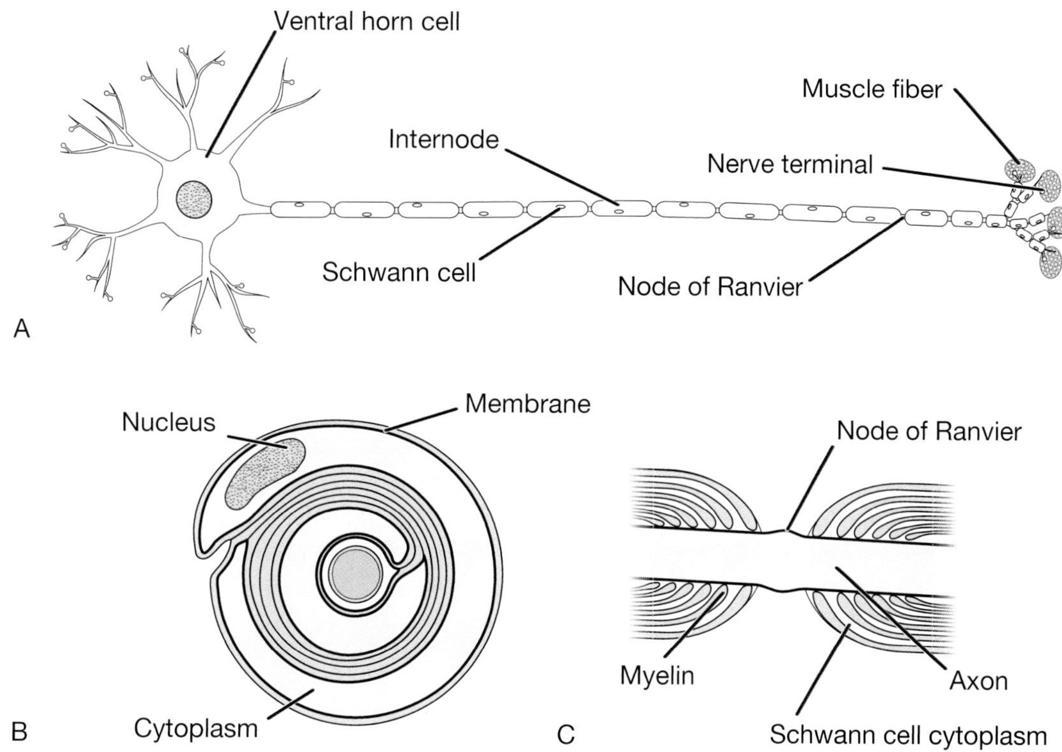

Fig. 13.2. Histologic features of a myelinated motor nerve fiber. *A*, Single myelinated axon extends from a ventral horn cell to nerve terminals on muscle fibers. *B*, Cross section through an internode of a nerve fiber, with layers of myelin formed by Schwann cell membrane wrapped around the axon. *C*, Longitudinal section of a node of Ranvier, with Schwann cell and myelin terminations abutting the axon. The region of the axon at the node (paranodal) has distinct ionic characteristics.

The axons of all nerve fibers consist of the axon membrane, or *axolemma*, and the axoplasm (the material within the axon). The axoplasm contains mitochondria, microtubules, microfilaments, and neurofilaments. The mitochondria generate the energy needed to establish the concentration gradients across the axolemma. The *microtubules* participate in the transport of proteins, enzymes, and other materials along the axon between the cell body and axon terminal. The function of *neurofilaments* and *microfilaments* is related to axonal transport and growth.

- The histologic features of a peripheral nerve are common to all types of nerves.
- Axons are surrounded by endoneurium and organized into fascicles by perineurium. The nerve is surrounded by epineurium.
- Axons and their function can be distinguished in part by their size and whether they have a myelin sheath.
- Axons are embedded in Schwann cells, which support axonal function.
- Myelin is formed by layers of Schwann cell cytoplasm wrapped around the axon.
- The axon contains mitochondria, neurofilaments, and microtubules needed for axonal transport.

Axonal Transport

The continuous and regulated flow of material from the cell body to the axons and synaptic terminals (and in the reverse direction) is critical for neuronal function and survival. Transport of substances along axons is not random but directed by the microtubules, which give polarity to the transport. Axonal transport includes

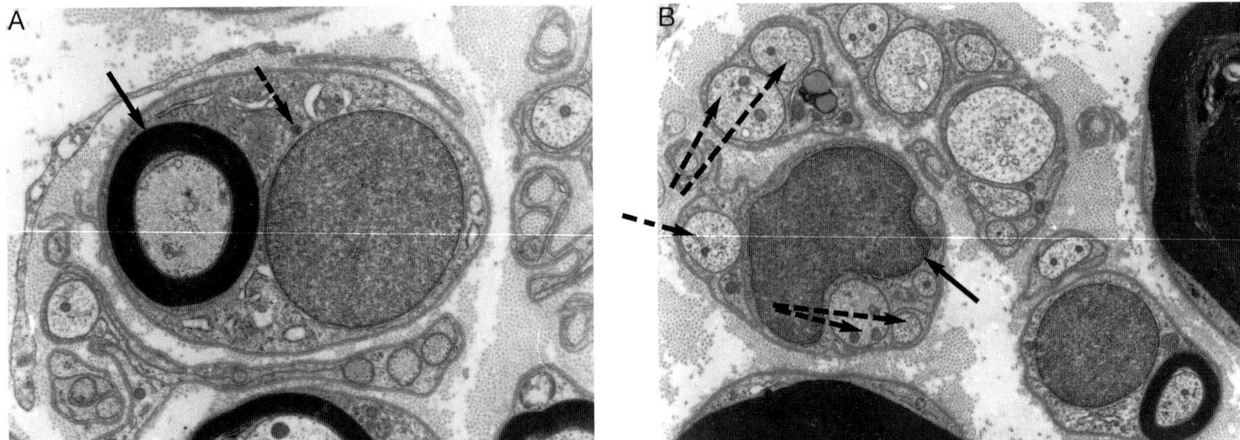

Fig. 13.3. Electron micrograph of a cross section of a peripheral nerve (×8500). *A*, Single, myelinated axon (*solid arrow*) is embedded in the cytoplasm of a Schwann cell (*dashed arrow*). Two other myelinated and several unmyelinated axons are visible below and to the right. *B*, Five unmyelinated axons (*dashed arrows*) are embedded in the cytoplasm of a Schwann cell (*solid arrow*). Other unmyelinated axons and two myelinated axons are visible below and to the right. (Courtesy of P. J. Dyck, MD, Peripheral Nerve Laboratory, Mayo Clinic College of Medicine, Rochester, MN.)

anterograde transport, the constant flow of material synthesized in the cell body and dendrites to the axon terminals, and *retrograde* transport, the transport of material from axon terminals to the cell body. Retrograde transport is a mechanism for the cell body to sample the environment around the synaptic terminals of its axon. Fast axonal anterograde transport occurs at a rate of 200 to 400 mm/day and is involved in the movement of proteins associated with membrane vesicles. These include glycosylated proteins that are delivered preferentially to synaptic terminals (e.g., synaptic vesicles, receptors, ion channels, neuropeptides, and enzymes for neurotransmitter biosynthesis). Slow anterograde axonal transport occurs at a rate of 0.1 to 4 mm/day and is involved in the movement of cytoskeletal proteins (e.g., tubulin, actin, and neurofilament proteins). Retrograde transport occurs at a rate of 100 to 200 mm/day and is an exaggerated manifestation of endocytosis. It is involved with the incorporation and recycling of lysosomes, pinocytotic vesicles, synaptic vesicle proteins, and neurotrophic factors. Retrograde transport is the mechanism by which some viruses (e.g., rabies and herpes simplex viruses) and toxins (e.g., tetanus and botulinum toxins) enter the nervous system.

Organic solvents (used in industry for cleaning, extraction, laboratory work, paint, and printing ink), pesticides, and some antineoplastic drugs can produce axonal neuropathy by disrupting the normal mechanisms of axonal transport and cytoskeletal assembly. Overexposure to these toxic chemicals produces a distal symmetrical sensorimotor axonal neuropathy that affects large-diameter sensory and motor axons in peripheral nerves and, in severe cases, long tracts in the spinal cord.

- Axonal transport is bidirectional, with fast and slow rates in both directions mediated by the microtubules.
- The anterograde transport of materials provides the axon terminals with the energy source and materials needed for synaptic transmission.
- Axonal transport is particularly susceptible to chemical agents.

Physiology

The resting potential and action potentials of single axons are described in detail in Chapter 5. This chapter focuses on the physiology of whole nerve trunks. The function of axons is to carry information in the form of electrical activity from one area to another. A measure of the ability of a

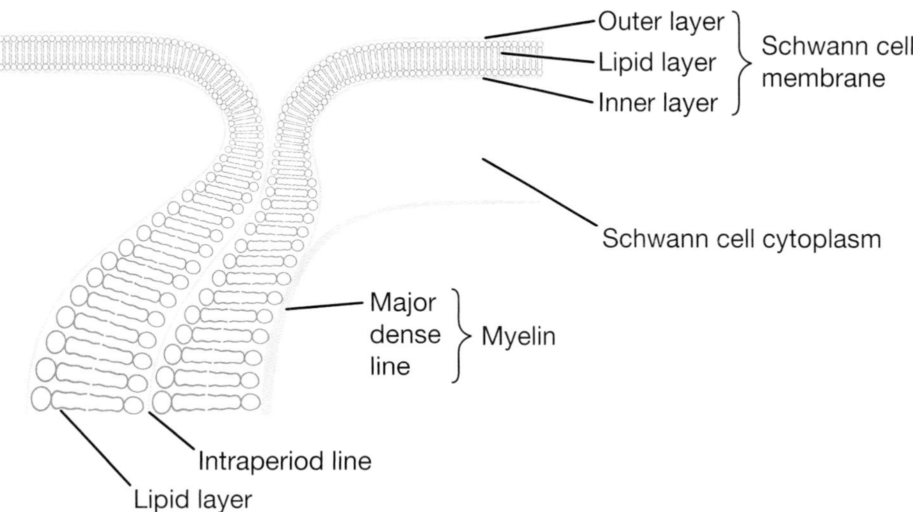

Fig. 13.4. Formation of myelin from layers of Schwann cell membrane. Major dense lines are formed from protein layers of membrane and are separated by the lipid layer, which contains cholesterol, cerebroside, sphingomyelin, and phospholipids.

nerve to perform this function is of major clinical value in the identification of disease involving a nerve.

The action potential of a single axon in a nerve can be recorded experimentally with an intracellular microelectrode, which records the action potential as a monophasic wave of depolarization. The electrical activity in a single nerve fiber can be monitored by placing electrodes in the extracellular fluid close to the nerve fiber. This method does not detect transmembrane potential changes; instead, it senses potential changes in the extracellular fluid that result from longitudinal current flow between the depolarized and nondepolarized regions of the axon. Experimentally, extracellular recording is improved (a bigger voltage change is measured) if the extracellular resistance is artificially increased by recording from the nerve exposed to air or immersed in oil.

Extracellular recording from single axons is difficult because of their small size; however, it is possible to record from groups of axons or from whole nerve trunks, if all the axons discharge synchronously. Such recordings are obtained experimentally and from patients by applying an electrical shock that activates many axons simultaneously. The potential recorded from a nerve activated in this way is the *compound nerve action potential*. The configuration of the signal obtained from an extracellular recording of the nerve impulse depends on the arrangement of the electrodes. A monophasic potential change is observed if only one of the electrodes is placed over the active nerve. A biphasic potential is recorded if both electrodes are placed over the active nerve (Fig. 13.5).

As in the stimulation of a single axon, the whole nerve trunk is activated by passing a current between the cathode (negative pole) and the anode (positive pole). The cathode depolarizes the underlying axons, and the anode hyperpolarizes them. Depolarization requires current flow inside the axons. Because large axons have lower internal resistance, the threshold for activation is lowest for the larger fibers. The *threshold stimulus* for a nerve trunk is that stimulus which just excites the large fibers (Fig. 13.6). Supramaximal stimuli activate all myelinated fibers, including the small fibers, and require greater current flow. Therefore, excitability depends on axon size.

The excitability of a nerve can be defined in terms of the two variables of a stimulus: voltage and duration. Plotting the strength of the current (or voltage)

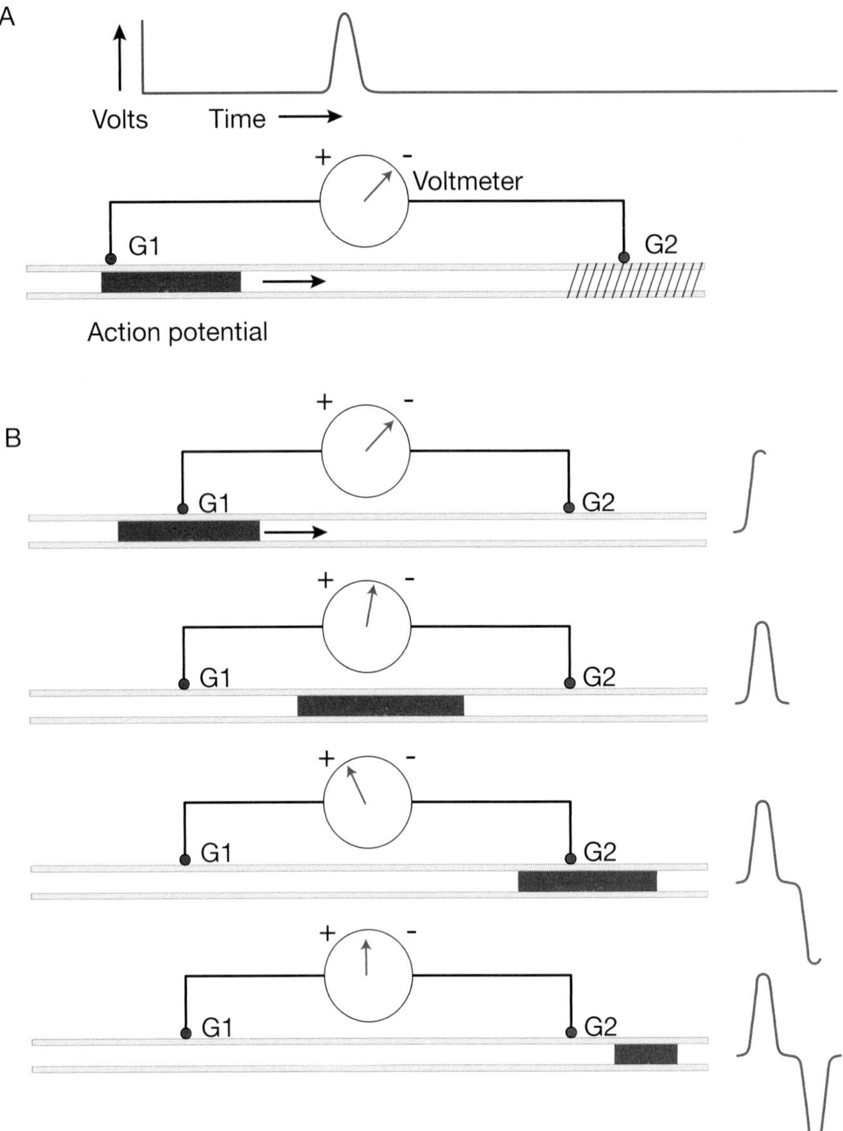

Fig. 13.5. Recording action potentials from a nerve trunk with electrodes G1 and G2. *A*, With G2 over damaged nerve (*hatched area*) and G1 over active nerve, a monophasic action potential is recorded as the depolarization passes under G1. *B*, If both electrodes are over active nerve fibers, potentials of opposite polarity are recorded as the depolarization passes under G1 and G2, a biphasic action potential. When G1 and G2 are close together, the two potentials fuse to form a smooth biphasic response.

against the duration of the stimulus needed to excite the nerve provides a strength-duration curve. This curve is often characterized in relation to two points. The rheobase is the minimal voltage needed to produce excitation with a long stimulus duration (usually 300 milliseconds), and chronaxie is the time required to excite a nerve by a stimulus with a voltage twice as large as the rheobase (Fig. 13.6). Changes in the chronaxie may be early markers of axonal disease.

The compound action potential recorded from a nerve trunk after supramaximal stimulation is the summation of action potentials from many axons. Its amplitude can be changed by varying the strength of the stimulus. A threshold stimulation evokes only a small potential, which is the result of activity in a few large fibers. As stimulus strength is increased, more fibers are excited, with each additionally activated fiber producing a small increment in the recorded voltage, and their activity is added to the compound action potential. When all the fibers are excited, the amplitude of the compound action potential is maximum; it will not increase in amplitude with further increase in stimulus strength (supramaximal). Thus, compound action potentials can be graded in amplitude, whereas action potentials in single axons are not graded but fire in an all-or-nothing fashion.

Because a nerve trunk contains axons of various diameter, a nerve has different conduction velocities and different thresholds for activation. The rate at which an axon conducts is a function of the amount of longitudinal current flow and is greater with larger axons. Conduction velocity is calculated by dividing the distance a potential travels by the time it takes to travel that distance. It is approximately five times the diameter of the axon in microns, for example, 5 to 100 meters/second for axons of 1 to 20 μm in diameter. If a nerve trunk is stimulated at a distance from the recording electrodes, the compound action potential exhibits several components (Fig. 13.7) because of the dispersion of potentials from fibers of different diameters. Impulses in the large, fast-conducting fibers reach the recording site first. Consequently, the components of the compound action potential distinguish activity in groups of fibers with diameters within a certain size range. The afferent fibers in cutaneous nerves (from receptors in joints and skin) are subdivided into groups named by letters (Aα, Aδ, and C). The afferent fibers in muscle nerves (from muscle receptors) are subdivided into groups designated by Roman numerals (I, II, III, IV). These are listed in Table 13.1.

Nerves that innervate muscle contain both sensory and motor fibers. The motor fibers arise from the alpha and gamma motor neurons and innervate extrafusal and intrafusal muscle fibers, respectively. The sensory fibers are group Ia and II fibers from muscle spindles and group Ib fibers from Golgi tendon organs. Cutaneous nerves innervate joints and skin and are commonly considered sensory nerves, although both they and muscle nerves

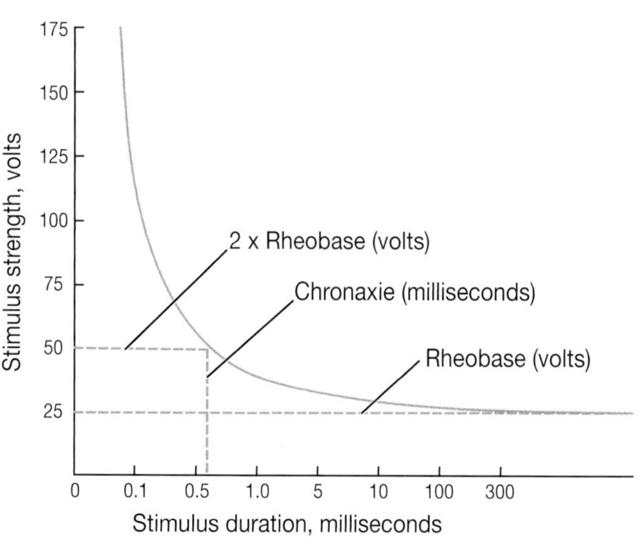

Fig. 13.6. Strength-duration curve. Threshold voltage for each duration is plotted. Rheobase is 25 V, and chronaxie is 0.6 millisecond.

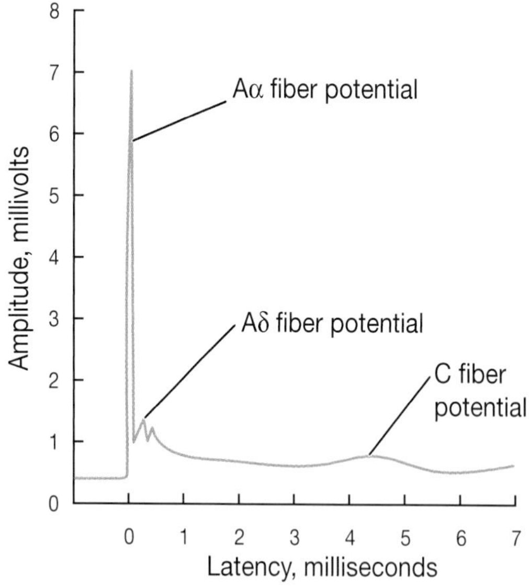

Fig. 13.7. Compound action potential recorded directly from a cutaneous nerve, showing peaks generated by different fiber types.

contain efferent and afferent fibers of the internal regulation system, the C or group IV fibers. The components of a mixed nerve are listed by size in Table 13.2.

In addition to transmitting action potentials, axons move proteins along their length. This process of axonal transport is important for making available the enzymes needed for the production of neurotransmitter in the nerve terminal, for maintaining the integrity of the distal parts of the axon, and for the release of *trophic factors* from the nerve terminal. Trophic factors released from nerve terminals are necessary for the normal function of the postsynaptic cell. These trophic factors are lost in some nerve diseases, causing physiologic and histologic abnormalities of the end organ.

- Action potentials in individual axons transmit information peripherally or centrally at rapid rates.
- Summation of the action potentials in all the axons in a nerve can be readily recorded as a compound nerve action potential.
- The range of axon size explains the differences in threshold for activation and different conduction velocities.
- Sensory axons are classified by size and function: cutaneous afferents into Aα, Aδ, and C fibers and muscle afferents into I, II, III, and IV fibers.
- Motor axons are classified as alpha, gamma, B, and C fibers.

Table 13.2. Fiber Types in a Mixed Nerve

Diameter, μm	Conduction velocity, m/s	Fiber type
12-20	70-120	Ia, Ib, Aα, alpha efferent
6-12	30-70	II, Aα, gamma efferent, visceral afferent
2-6	4-30	III, Aδ, gamma efferent, visceral afferent
<2	0.5-2.0	IV, B, C

Pathophysiology

A nerve may be altered in several ways by disease processes. These can be classified as diseases of the axolemma, the axoplasm, or the myelin sheath.

Axolemmal Disorders

The axon membrane may undergo physicochemical alterations that block conduction without destruction or histologic alteration of the axon. Such alterations may occur by electrical, pharmacologic, thermal, or mechanical means. The alterations are usually transient and reversible and include the familiar phenomenon of a leg "going to sleep."

Electrical conduction blocks do not occur clinically but can be produced by the application of steady depolarizing (cathodal block) or hyperpolarizing (anodal block) currents to a nerve fiber or nerve trunk. A depolarizing current may initially evoke an action potential and then block impulse transmission. An anodal block results from hyperpolarization of the axon membrane, which moves the membrane potential away from threshold.

A clinically useful method of producing conduction block is the application of a pharmacologic agent (local anesthetic) to a nerve. These agents include compounds such as procaine hydrochloride (Novocain), benzocaine, cocaine, and other esters of benzoic acid. Local anesthetics interfere with nerve conduction by preventing the membrane permeability changes that occur with depolarization (Table 13.3). The membrane is said to be "stabilized" by local anesthetics. Small, unmyelinated nerve fibers, such as those mediating pain, are more sensitive to local anesthetics than the larger myelinated fibers and are blocked at low concentrations of the drug that do not appreciably affect large fibers. Thus, pain sensation can be reduced without loss of proprioceptive sense or motor function.

A transient, reversible conduction block can be obtained by lowering the temperature of nerve fibers. This method of blocking nerve impulse transmission is achieved with the local application of ice or an ethyl chloride spray. It is used clinically to produce superficial anesthesia. Mechanical conduction blocks occur with distortion of a nerve and may be due to alteration

Table 13.3. Sequence of Events of Local Anesthetic Block

Displacement of calcium ions from nerve receptor site
↓
Binding of local anesthetic to receptor site
↓
Blockade of sodium channel
↓
Decrease in sodium conductance
↓
Decreased depolarization of nerve membrane
↓
Failure to achieve threshold potential level
↓
Lack of development of propagated action potential
↓
Conduction blockade

of the blood supply or to changes in the configuration of the membrane, with secondary changes in its ionic permeability.

Axoplasmic Disorders

Axons may be affected by acute or chronic disorders of the axoplasm. An acute lesion is one in which the axon is disrupted. This may occur with complete division of the nerve in a laceration or with a severe local crush, traction, or ischemia. In laceration, the connective tissue framework of the nerve is destroyed, but in the other lesions, it remains intact. In each instance, the continuity of the axons is lost; the axon distal to the lesion is deprived of axonal flow from the cell body and undergoes dissolution, a process called *wallerian degeneration*. Central chromatolysis and peripheral muscle atrophy accompany wallerian degeneration (Fig. 13.8). In most lesions other than laceration, not all axons are destroyed and some function may remain. The smaller fibers are more resistant to such injuries and are more likely to be spared. The terminals of motor axons remaining after axonal damage send out collateral sprouts to reinnervate denervated muscles in the region. Nearly complete recovery can occur in a mild or moderately severe neurogenic disorder if the remaining axons have normal function and axonal transport. After acute axonal disruption of all axons, recovery occurs only through the growth of new axons from the site of damage.

If a nerve is severed completely, reinnervation is poor because the axonal sprouts have no pathway to follow. Axonal sprouts may grow in the wrong direction and produce spirals or large bulbous tips. These sprouts, with their Schwann cells and connective tissue, may form a *neuroma*. A neuroma may not only prevent proper regrowth of the nerve but may also be painful.

The activity of Schwann cells in the distal nerve stump helps axons grow across a gap, as they divide, elongate, and migrate toward the proximal nerve stump. If axonal sprouts manage to reach this Schwann cell outgrowth, they may eventually reinnervate the denervated organs. However, the amount of functional recovery is always less than that after a crush injury. One reason for this is that most axonal sprouts do not find their way along the pathway originally followed by the parent fibers and reinnervate an inappropriate organ. A motor axon that establishes a connection with a sensory receptor will not function, and a motor axon that reinnervates a muscle different from the one it originally supplied cannot participate in the same reflex actions. The result of such aberrant reinnervation, called *synkinesis*, is the concomitant contraction of other muscles innervated by a nerve with attempts to activate a single muscle. The patient can no longer selectively activate a single muscle by itself. This commonly occurs after a facial nerve injury; a blink is associated with a twitch of the mouth. In injuries to long nerves, the end organs may atrophy before reinnervation can occur, thus preventing normal recovery.

The rate of nerve regeneration varies with the type of injury. Recovery is quicker with crush injuries than with nerve severance. The delay in recovery depends on axonal growth, reversal of atrophy of the end organ, reinnervation of the end organ, and remyelinization and maturation of the axon. In humans, the overall rate of functional recovery under optimal conditions is about 1 to 3 mm/day. The recovery rate in a limb may be quicker proximally than distally. Regeneration depends on the growth cone of the regenerating axon responding to extracellular signals.

Axoplasmic disorders may be chronic or slow in evolution and may present with findings different from those of acute lesions. When the process is complete, the axons degenerate just as they do in acute lesions; however, there are intermediate stages in which the axons first lose their integrity distally, a so-called dying back. This occurs first in the longest axons and results in loss of function in the most distal parts of the body. The axons also may atrophy or become narrowed in chronic disorders, referred to as *axonal atrophies* or *axonal dystrophies* (Fig. 13.8). In either situation, abnormalities develop in the axon before changes occur in the myelin. Therefore, unless major narrowing of an axon is present, the conduction of the axons is slowed very little. Chronic axonal disorders occur with many diseases, including genetic, toxic, metabolic, and deficiency states.

The narrow axons found in some axoplasmic disorders also occur with local compression of a nerve and in regenerating fibers. Moderate narrowing of an axon results in slowing of conduction velocity, but by itself, this usually causes little functional impairment. A nerve with slowed conduction velocity can still transmit impulses, but not at rates as high as normal. High-frequency impulses, such as those associated with rapid vibrations, output from muscle spindles, and motor activity in strong muscle contraction, are poorly transmitted so that vibratory sensation and reflexes are lost.

Myelin Disorders

Genetic, immunologic, and toxic disorders can produce primary damage to myelin. In these disorders, myelin is usually lost at some internodes but is normal at others. This scattered loss of myelin is *segmental demyelination* (Fig. 13.8). The loss of myelin results in slowing of conduction velocity, with mild impairment of vibratory sensation, loss of reflexes, some loss of proprioceptive sensation, and loss of strong muscle contractions. However, with moderate demyelination, the action potential is blocked, producing more severe deficits.

Immune-mediated demyelinating neuropathies occur with monoclonal antibodies to glycoproteins and to G_{M1} ganglioside. Genetic disorders can be associated with a lack of myelin (hypomyelination) or abnormal myelin and can cause functional disturbances similar to those of segmental demyelination.

In each of these disorders, the severity of damage and selective involvement of one or another fiber type may vary. In localized lesions, function is lost in the areas supplied by the nerve. In generalized nerve disease, the axons are affected randomly throughout the cross section of the nerve and randomly along the length of the nerve, so that the areas most likely to lose function are the distal regions supplied by the longest nerves. This produces a characteristic distribution of abnormalities in the distal portions of the extremities. This distal deficit also occurs in primary neuronal disease in which the neuron is unable to provide sufficient nutrients to the most distal portion of the nerve, with a resultant dying back of the distal portions of the long nerves.

Identification of the underlying genetic defect can lead to clinical genotyping as a predictive tool for drug choice. These are several areas of potential application, but routine application generally has not been performed. Azathioprine therapy for chronic inflammatory demyelinating polyradiculopathy (CIDP) is an example of a potential application of genotyping. Thiopurine methyltransferase (TPMT) is a key enzyme in the metabolism of the immunosuppressant drug azathioprine. This drug has been used in the treatment of CIDP and other neuromuscular diseases, including polymyositis and myasthenia gravis. Persons who have specific polymorphisms within the gene encoding for TPMT are more prone to develop liver and blood toxicity. An enzyme assay for TPMT activity has been used to identify those at risk. A recent report has suggested that genotyping is superior to TPMT enzyme assay, with improved risk assessment.

- Axolemmal disorders result in loss of function of individual axons by localized conduction block or loss of function over a longer segment of axon.
- Acute and chronic axoplasmic disorders have different abnormalities.
- Acute damage disrupts axons, causing wallerian

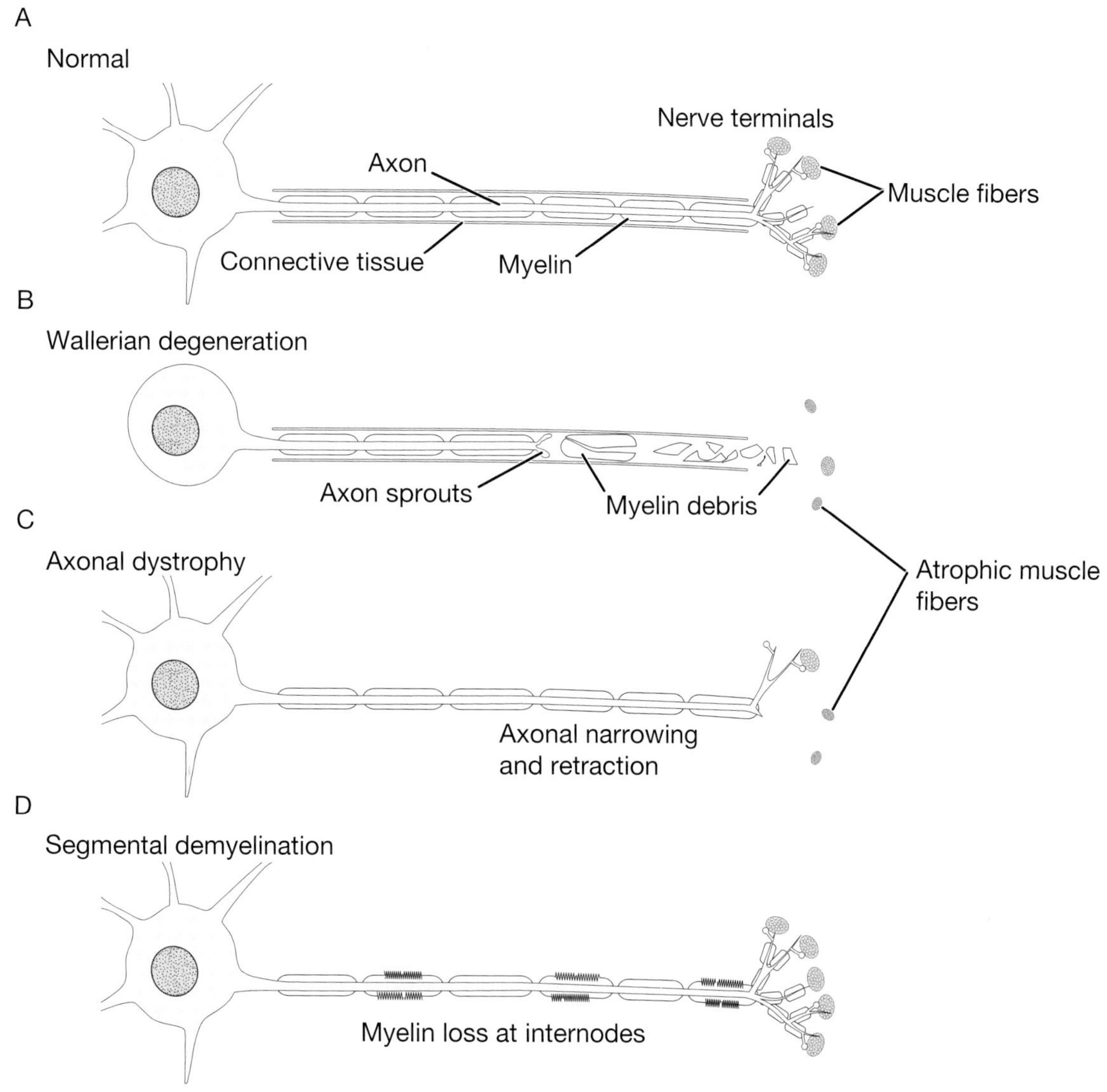

Fig. 13.8. Diagram of pathologic changes in peripheral nerve fibers. *A*, Normal axon. *B*, Wallerian degeneration occurs distal to local destruction of an axon and is associated with central chromatolysis of the cell body and muscle fiber atrophy. Regeneration occurs along the connective tissue path. *C*, Axonal dystrophy results in distal narrowing and dying back of nerve terminals because of either intrinsic axon or motor neuron disease. *D*, Segmental demyelination destroys myelin at scattered internodes along the axon without causing axonal damage.

degeneration distal to the site of damage.

- Chronic damage causes distal narrowing and atrophy, slow conduction, and eventually wallerian degeneration distally.
- Myelin disorders can also result in conduction block or slow conduction, particularly in acute segmental demyelination.

Pathophysiology Summary

Impairment of the ability of peripheral nerves to conduct action potentials normally, a change in threshold for activation, and loss of axonal transport result in five distinct clinical findings.

1. The inability to conduct an action potential is the result

of either transient metabolic changes or structural damage to the axon. If an axon is severed, the distal portion undergoes wallerian degeneration, but the distal part is able to conduct impulses for 3 to 5 days. The proximal part of the axon continues to function normally. Patients experience numbness and loss of sensation in proportion to the loss of sensory fibers, weakness with loss of motor fibers, and impairment of reflexes with loss of either sensory or motor fibers.

2. Axons may conduct impulses slowly or less rapidly with loss of myelin, axonal narrowing, or deformation of the axon. The latter may be seen in the area of compression or in regenerating fibers. Slow conduction produces mild clinical symptoms or signs except for the ability to transmit high-frequency information such as vibratory sensation, which is severely impaired, and the loss of reflexes.
3. The threshold for activation of the axon or the lower motor neurons may be so low that they discharge spontaneously. If this occurs, all the muscle fibers in the motor unit contract simultaneously. Such a single, spontaneous contraction of a motor unit, called a *fasciculation*, is visible as a small twitch under the skin. It is evidence of irritability of the motor unit. Similar irritability of large sensory fibers is perceived as paresthesia (tingling), and irritability of small fibers is perceived as pain, particularly with repetitive firing. Spontaneous firing occurs normally and in many peripheral disorders, especially ischemic or metabolic diseases.
4. With the loss of axonal transport and trophic factors from the axons, the denervated muscle becomes atrophic in proportion to the duration of denervation.
5. Also, because of membrane changes, the muscle fiber becomes hypersensitive to acetylcholine. Normally, most acetylcholine receptors are confined to the area immediately adjacent to the end plate. However, after denervation, the receptors spread along the surface and the entire muscle fiber responds to the drug. This is one form of denervation hypersensitivity (Table 13.4). Approximately 2 weeks after muscle fibers lose their innervation, they begin to discharge and twitch because of denervation hypersensitivity. This spontaneous, regular twitching of single muscle fibers is called *fibrillation*. Unlike fasciculations, fibrillations are not visible.

Nerves at the Peripheral Level

Peripheral axons are bundled together in nerves organized to serve different components of the body. Motor, sensory, and visceral axons leave the posterior fossa and spinal canal as cranial nerves and spinal nerves, respectively. The axons of spinal nerves form somatic and visceral plexuses from which the peripheral nerves emerge. After rearrangement they form the peripheral nerves proper. Each peripheral nerve has essentially the same histology, physiology, axonal transport, and pathophysiology described above for axons.

Spinal Nerves

Spinal nerves are formed by the dorsal sensory roots and ventral motor roots, which join in the neural foramina at the C1-C7, T1-T12, L1-L5, and sacral levels of the vertebral column. They include sympathetic fibers from the thoracic spinal cord to the paravertebral

Table 13.4. Examples of Denervation Hypersensitivity

Site	Clinical finding	Due to destruction of	Hypersensitivity to
Striated muscle	Fibrillation	Alpha efferents	Acetylcholine
Ventral horn cell	Spasticity, clonus, hyperreflexia	Descending pathway	Local sensory input
Pupil	Miosis	Postganglionic sympathetic	Epinephrine analogues
Pupil	Mydriasis	Postganglionic parasympathetic	Acetylcholine analogues

ganglia and parasympathetic fibers from the lumbosacral spinal cord and from the brainstem through the cranial nerves.

Clinical Correlations

Spinal nerves can undergo the physiologic and histologic alterations described above. Most commonly, these nerves are involved by bony spine disease, especially herniated discs. They can also be involved by tumor and inflammation. The damage involves both motor and sensory fibers. The diagnosis of disease of spinal nerves depends on recognizing the involvement of the paraspinal muscles and other muscles innervated by individual spinal nerves and the selective sensory loss in the dermatomes innervated by the spinal nerve. There is also specific loss of reflexes. When severe, spinal nerve injury produces autonomic disturbances such as loss of sweating, thinning of the skin, and trophic changes in the skin.

Plexus

A plexus is a complex recombination of axons as they rearrange themselves in passing from one area to another. The three major somatic plexuses are the brachial, lumbar, and sacral (lumbosacral) plexuses. The *brachial plexus* is derived from spinal nerves C5 through T1 and gives rise to the major nerves of the upper extremity. The axons of the spinal nerves are rearranged into trunks, divisions, and cords of the brachial plexus just beneath and behind the clavicle (Fig. 13.9 *A*).

The *lumbar plexus*, derived from L2 through L4 spinal nerves, and the *sacral plexus*, derived from L4 through S3 spinal nerves, give rise to the major nerves of the lower extremity. The femoral and obturator nerves arise from the lumbar plexus, and the sciatic nerve arises from the sacral plexus. The rearrangements of the axons in the lumbosacral plexus occur in the pelvis, posteriorly, deep to the psoas major muscle (Fig. 13.9 *B*).

Clinical Correlations

Each of these plexuses may undergo the same physiologic or histologic alterations described above for axons. They most commonly are involved by trauma, tumor, or hemorrhage. The diagnosis of disease in these regions depends on the presence of involvement of proximal

Clinical Problem 13.1.

For many years, a 43-year-old healthy farmer had occasional low back pain, which was treated successfully with chiropractic manipulation. One episode of "sciatica," with some ankle plantar flexion weakness, occurred 5 years ago. It was treated symptomatically, and the patient recovered without any residual effects. Three weeks ago, he awoke with moderate back pain that radiated into his left hip and leg. There was no improvement with chiropractic manipulation, and the pain in his leg steadily worsened until he began having tingling in the lateral calf and dorsum of the foot. The left Achilles reflex was reduced, but other reflexes were normal. He had mild weakness of foot dorsiflexion and hip abduction. There was mild hypalgesia over the lateral calf.

Nerve conduction studies were normal except for a low-amplitude peroneal motor response, with mild slowing of conduction. Electromyography showed a decreased number of motor unit potentials, with fibrillation potentials in the left L5 muscles, including the lumbar paraspinal muscle. The medial gastrocnemius and other S1 muscles showed a decreased number of motor units that were of long duration with no fibrillation potentials.

a. Describe how you would localize this disorder in the periphery.
b. Correlate the clinical findings with the anatomy.
c. What is the temporal profile, and how would you interpret it?
d. What diagnosis would you give the patient?
e. What is the significance of the fibrillation potentials?
f. Why was the conduction velocity only mildly slow?
g. What would a gastrocnemius biopsy show and why?

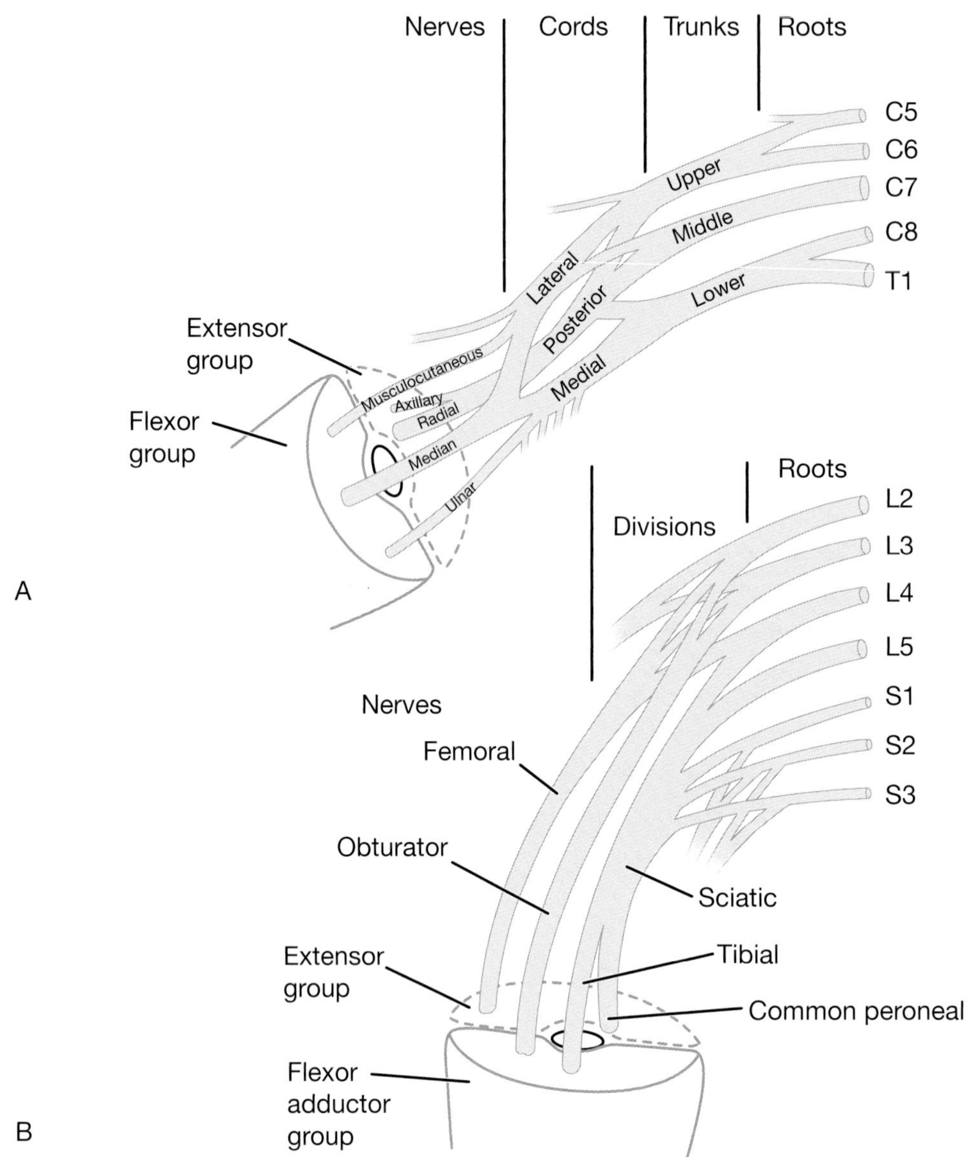

Fig. 13.9. Major components of nerve plexuses. *A*, Brachial plexus showing the origin of the three trunks, three cords, and peripheral nerves. *B*, Lumbosacral plexus divisions forming the nerves of the lower extremity.

muscles innervated by multiple roots, multiple dermatomal involvement, and sparing of the paraspinal muscles. The changes involve motor and sensory fibers and, when severe, cause autonomic disturbances such as loss of sweating, thinning of the skin, and trophic changes in the skin. Reflexes are also lost.

Several major plexuses are purely visceral and are part of the internal regulation system. Although these plexuses may be involved in localized disease processes, this is not common or of clinical significance.

- From the rearrangement of motor and sensory fibers of spinal nerves in the major plexuses, the peripheral nerves contain axons of more than one spinal nerve. Hence, muscles are innervated by multiple spinal nerves.

- The brachial plexus is made up of spinal nerves C5-T1.
- The lumbosacral plexus is made up of spinal nerves L2-S3.
- Autonomic axons also traverse the plexuses to reach peripheral nerves.
- Damage to one of the major nerve plexuses is characterized by widespread motor, sensory, and autonomic disturbances in an entire limb.

Individual Peripheral Nerves

Peripheral nerves are the major nerve trunks in the extremities and are derived from the plexuses. They have the histologic and physiologic features described in the previous section. Each nerve has a well-defined anatomical course in an extremity, supplies a specific area of skin, and innervates specific muscles (Fig. 13.10). The major peripheral nerves and their important areas of innervation are listed in Table 13.5. More detailed distributions are shown in Figure 13.11.

Clinical Correlations

The peripheral nerves may be involved individually at sites of common compression or diffusely in systemic, immune-mediated, or genetic disorders. The proximity of some nerves to bony structures makes them particularly vulnerable to lesions at those sites. The *median nerve* passes through a tunnel at the wrist (the carpal tunnel) where it is easily and often compressed, producing arm pain, sensory loss in the first three digits, and weakness of the thenar muscles. This is the carpal tunnel syndrome. The *ulnar nerve* is commonly compressed at the elbow, where it passes around the medial epicondyle in an exposed position (the "funny bone"). Lesions here produce sensory loss in the ring and fifth fingers, with flaccid weakness and atrophy of the intrinsic muscles of the hand. The *radial nerve* is particularly susceptible to injury where it curves around the humerus in the spiral groove in the mid-upper arm. Lesions at this site produce weakness of wrist and finger extension. The *peroneal (fibular) nerve* is in an exposed position over a bony prominence where it curves around the head of the fibula at the knee. Damage at this site produces footdrop, with inability to dorsiflex the foot, and sensory loss on the dorsum of the foot. Because of deep, protected locations, the sciatic, tibial, and femoral nerves have fewer injuries.

These and all other lesions of the peripheral nerves can be recognized by an analysis of the distribution of the motor, sensory, and reflex changes. The type of lesion may be any of those previously described with total, irreversible destruction due to wallerian degeneration or with mild, reversible changes due to membrane or myelin alterations.

Clinical Problem 13.2.

A 35-year-old farmer awoke with numbness and weakness in his feet. Five hours later, the numbness ascended to involve both lower extremities as well as the hands, and he noticed he was unable to climb stairs. Three hours later, he was unable to raise his arms, and his handgrip strength had decreased. The next day, he was unable to stand or walk and had difficulty lifting his head off the pillow.

Neurologic examination showed severe proximal and distal weakness in all limbs, areflexia, and loss of vibration and position sense in the fingers and toes. He also complained of shortness of breath. Nerve conduction studies showed marked slowing in conduction velocities, with evidence of conduction block. Needle electromyography did not show fibrillation potentials.

a. Describe how you would localize this disorder in the periphery.
b. Localize the disorder in that structure.
c. What is the temporal profile, and how would you interpret it?
d. Correlate each of the elements of the physical examination with the system involved.
e. What diagnosis would you give the patient?
f. What would a sural nerve biopsy be likely to show?
g. How could recovery occur?

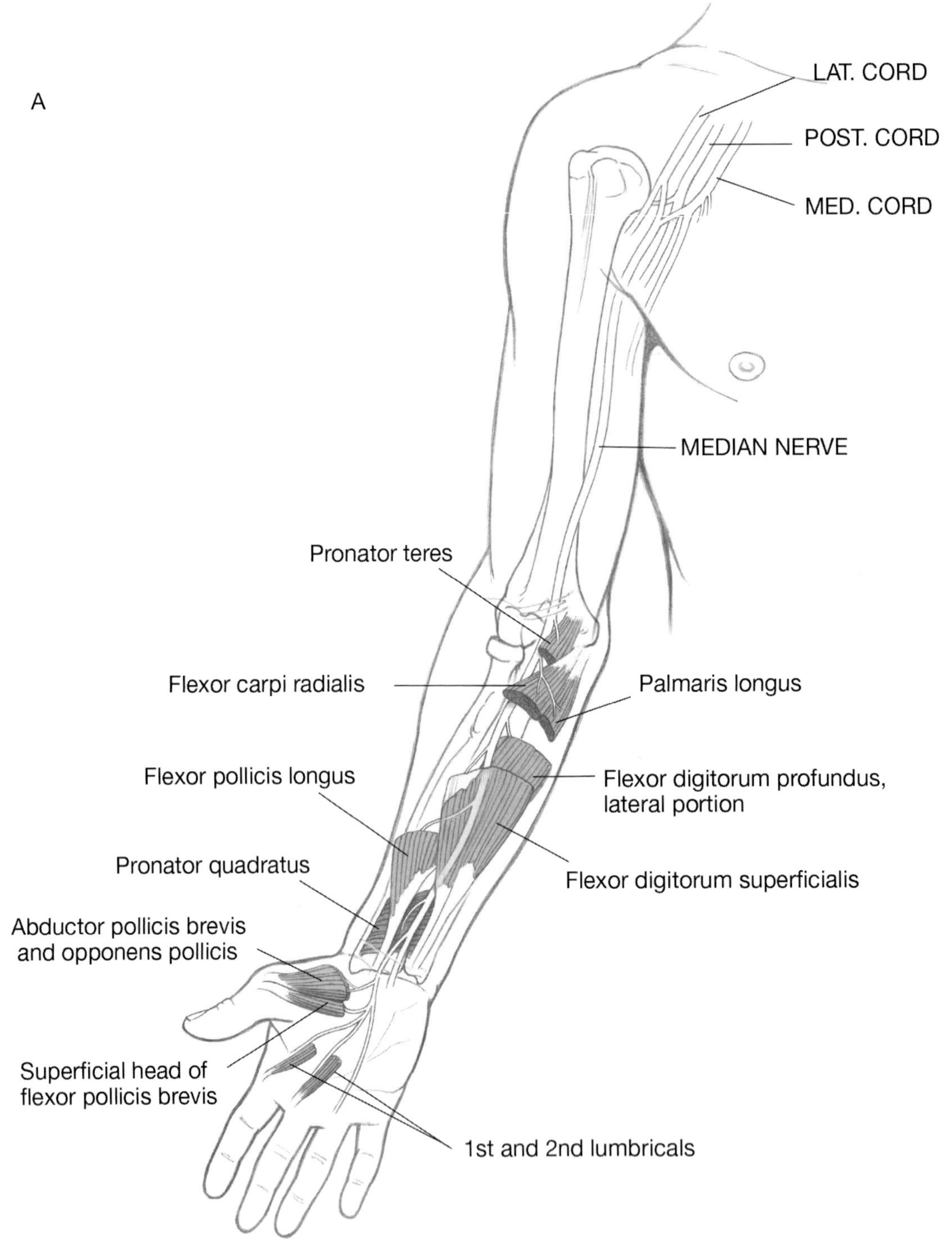

Fig. 13.10. Major nerves in the upper and lower extremities, showing their location and the muscles they innervate. *A-C*, Arm and hand. *D-I*, Hip, thigh, leg, lower leg, and foot. ANT, anterior; LAT, lateral; MED, medial; POST, posterior. (*A*, *B*, and *D-I* from Rosse C, Gaddum-Rosse P. Hollinshead's textbook of anatomy. 5th ed. Philadelphia: Lippincott-Raven; 1997. Used with permission. *C* from Hollingshead WH and Rosse C. Textbook of anatomy, 4th ed. Philadelphia: Harper & Row; 1985. Used with permission.)

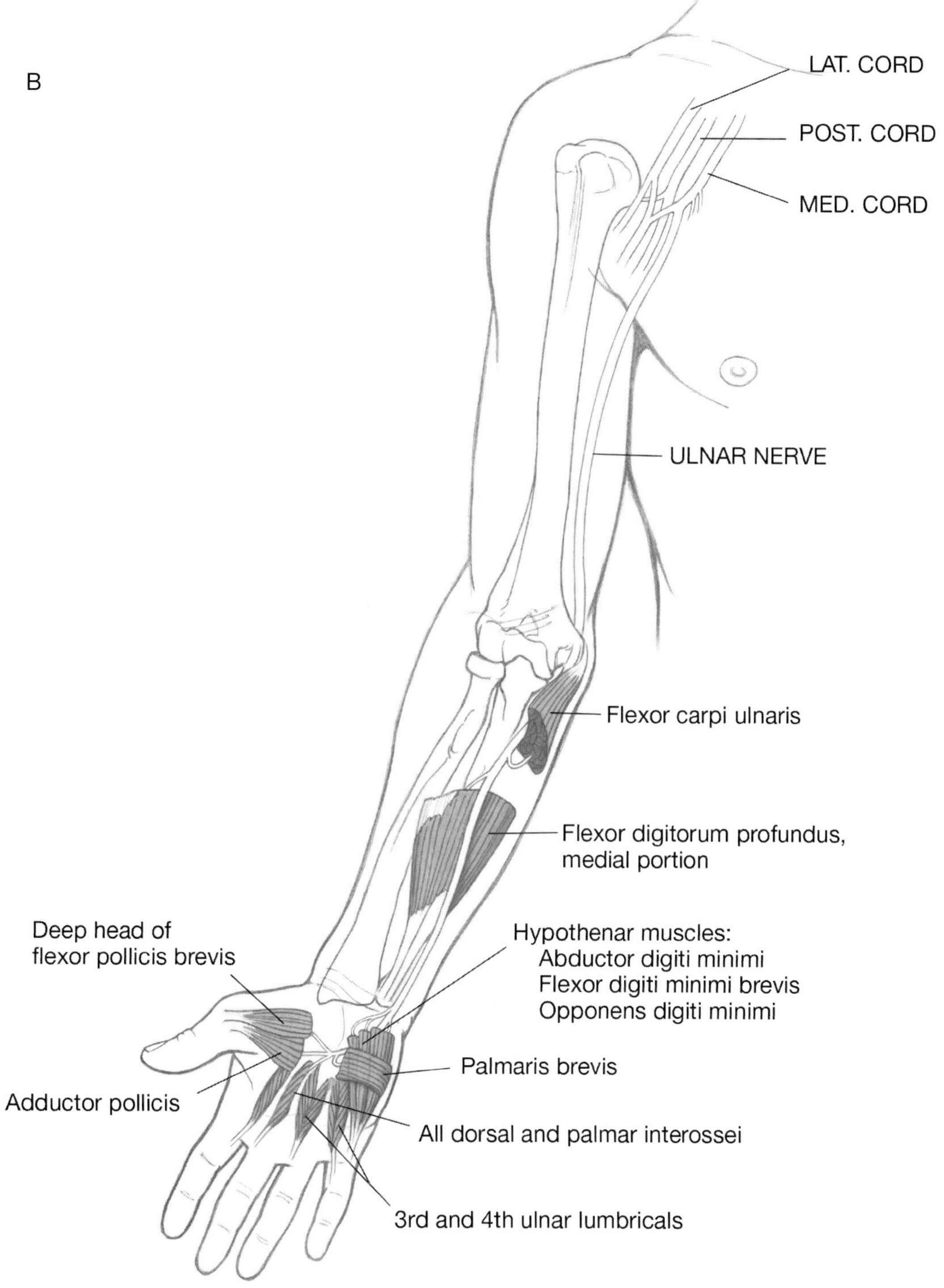
B
LAT. CORD
POST. CORD
MED. CORD
ULNAR NERVE
Flexor carpi ulnaris
Flexor digitorum profundus, medial portion
Deep head of flexor pollicis brevis
Hypothenar muscles:
Abductor digiti minimi
Flexor digiti minimi brevis
Opponens digiti minimi
Palmaris brevis
Adductor pollicis
All dorsal and palmar interossei
3rd and 4th ulnar lumbricals

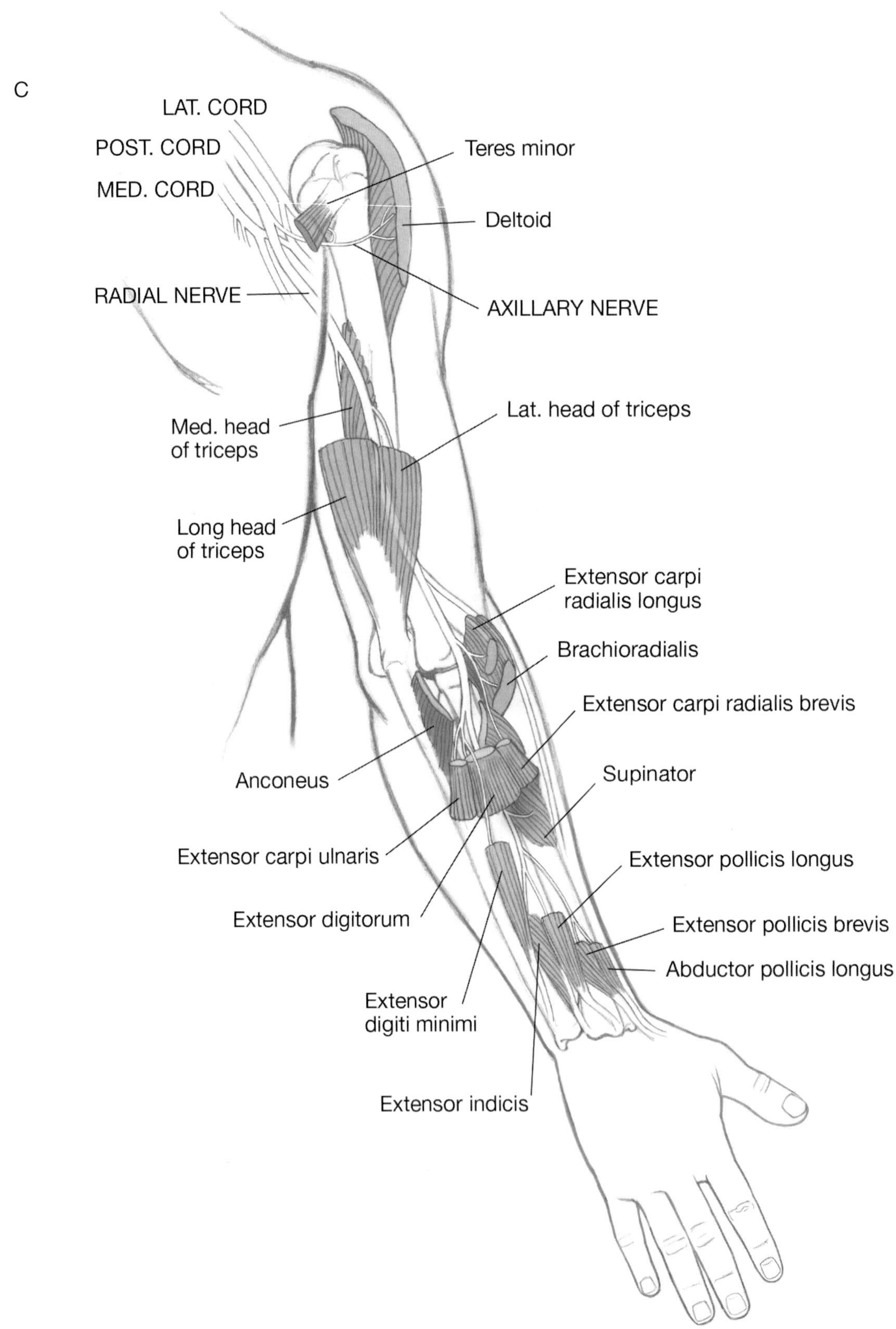
C
LAT. CORD
POST. CORD
MED. CORD
RADIAL NERVE
Teres minor
Deltoid
AXILLARY NERVE
Med. head of triceps
Lat. head of triceps
Long head of triceps
Extensor carpi radialis longus
Brachioradialis
Extensor carpi radialis brevis
Anconeus
Supinator
Extensor carpi ulnaris
Extensor pollicis longus
Extensor digitorum
Extensor pollicis brevis
Abductor pollicis longus
Extensor digiti minimi
Extensor indicis

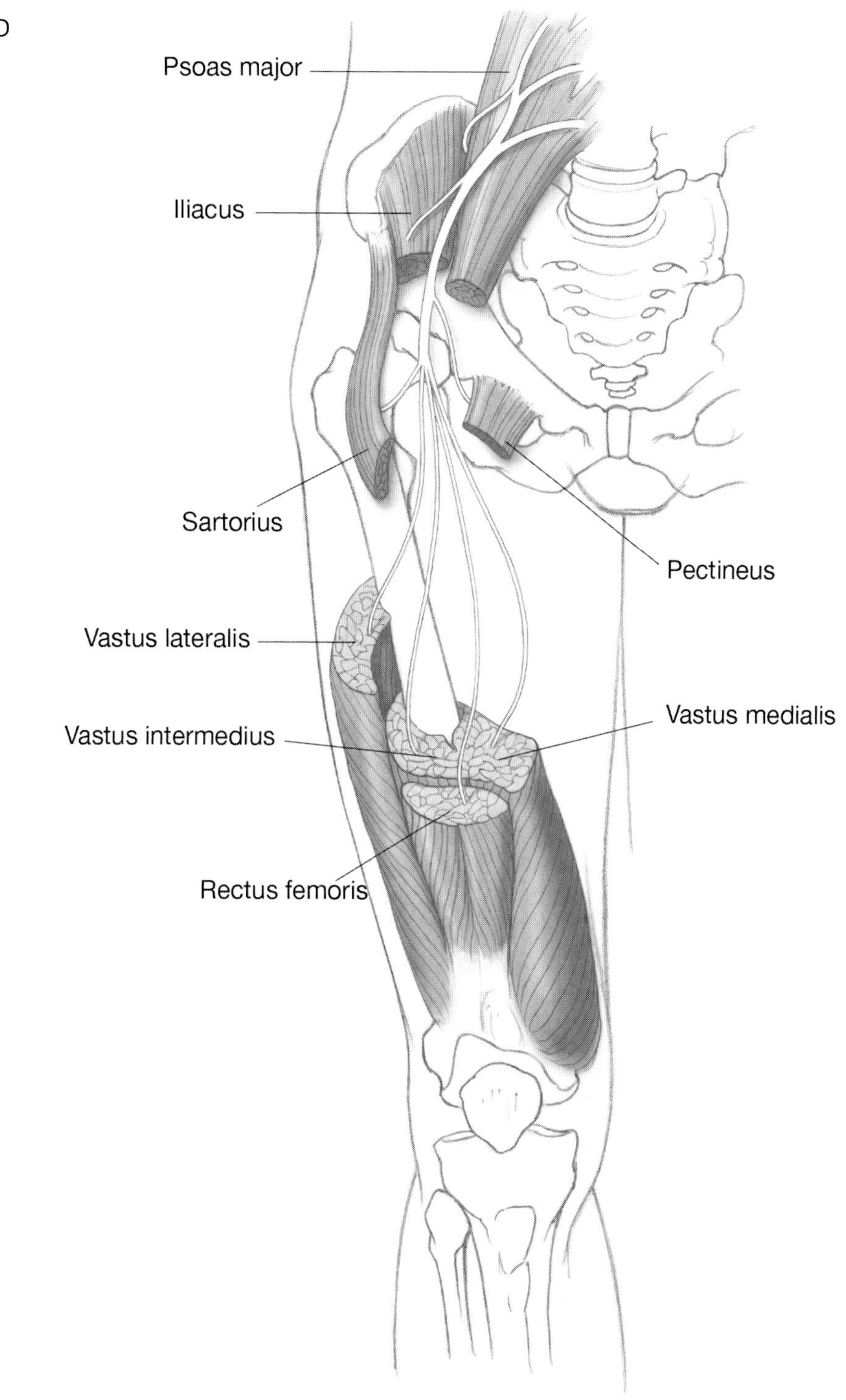
D
Psoas major
Iliacus
Sartorius
Pectineus
Vastus lateralis
Vastus medialis
Vastus intermedius
Rectus femoris

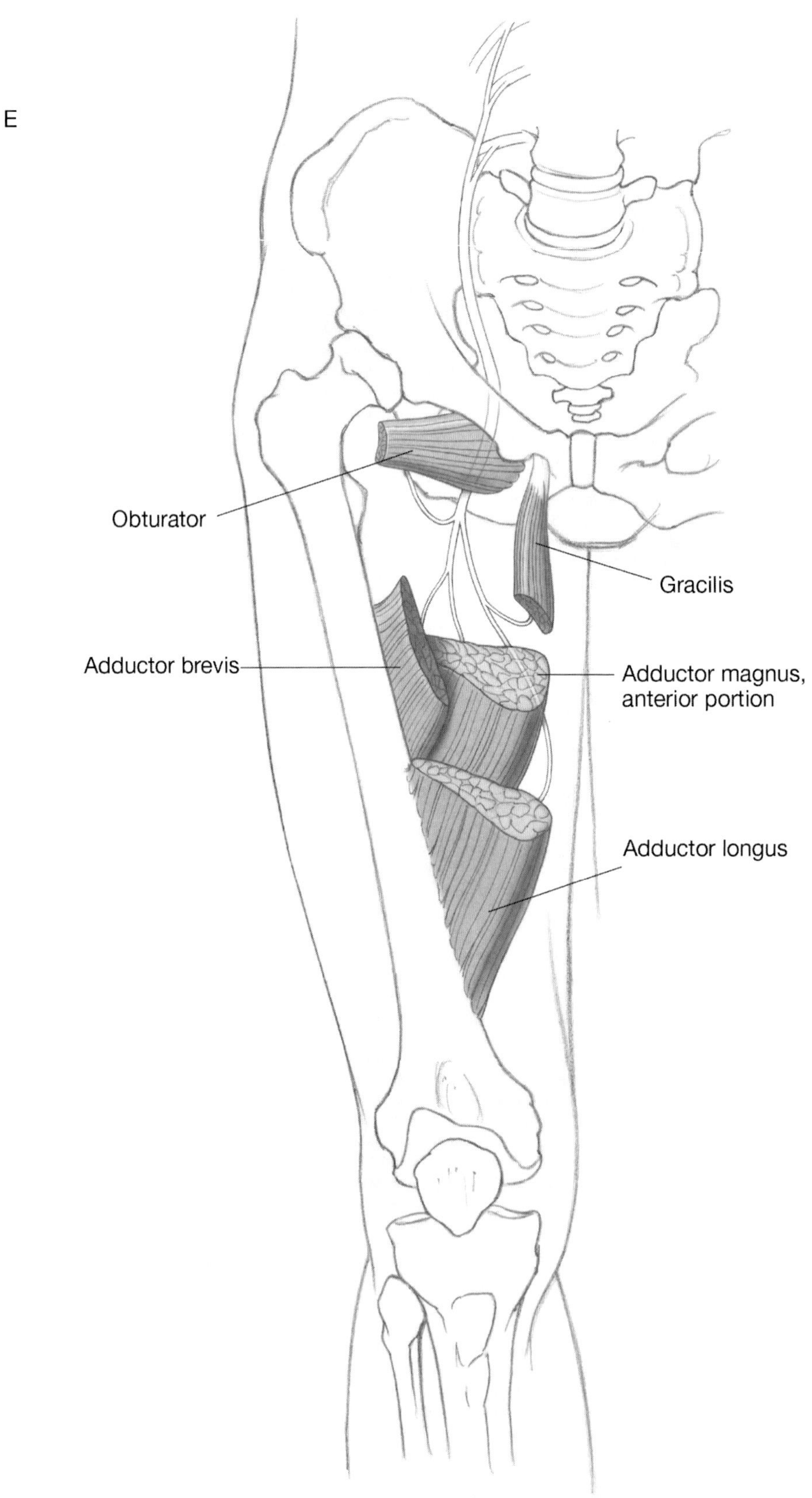
E
Obturator
Gracilis
Adductor brevis
Adductor magnus, anterior portion
Adductor longus

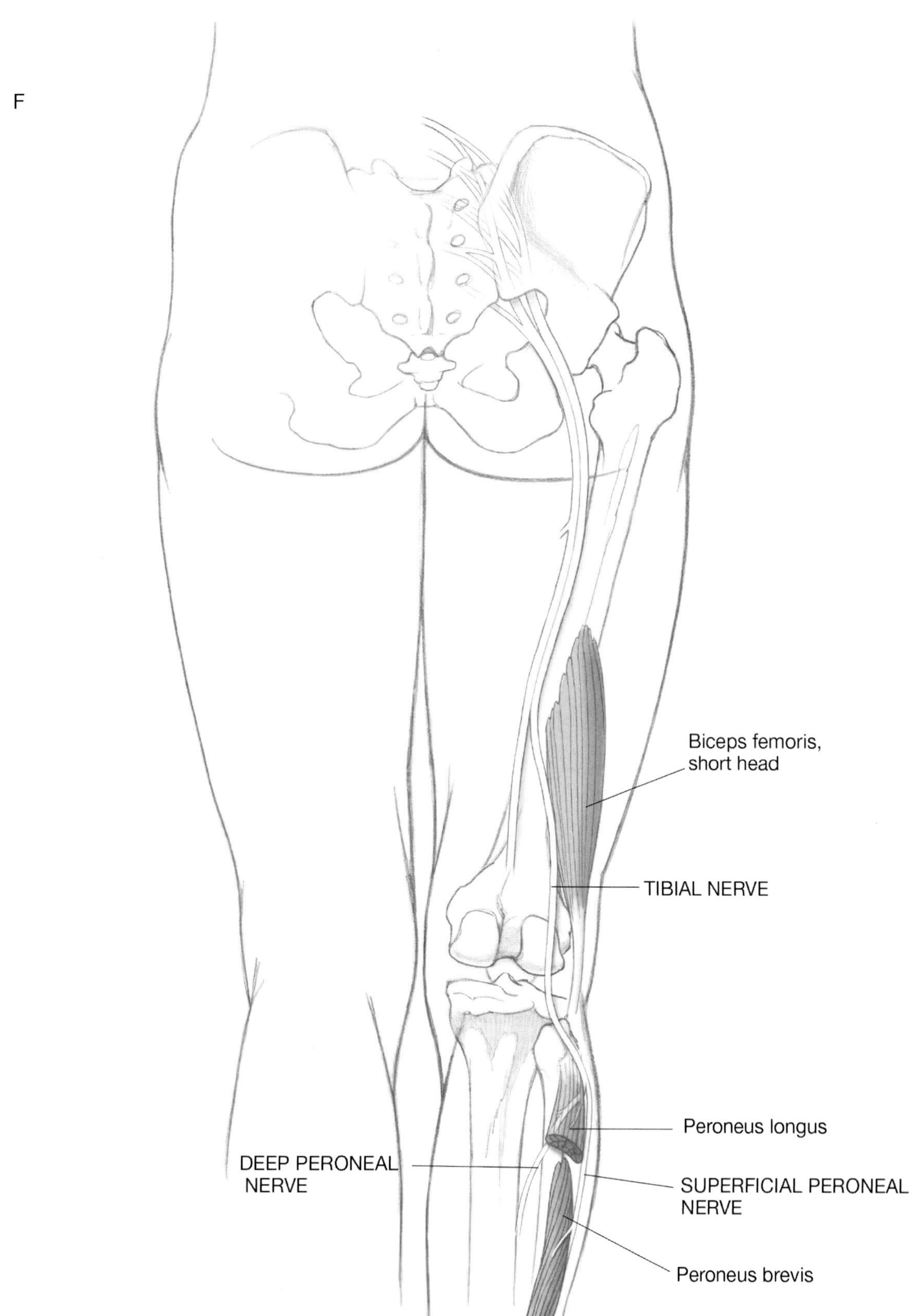
F
Biceps femoris, short head
TIBIAL NERVE
Peroneus longus
DEEP PERONEAL NERVE
SUPERFICIAL PERONEAL NERVE
Peroneus brevis

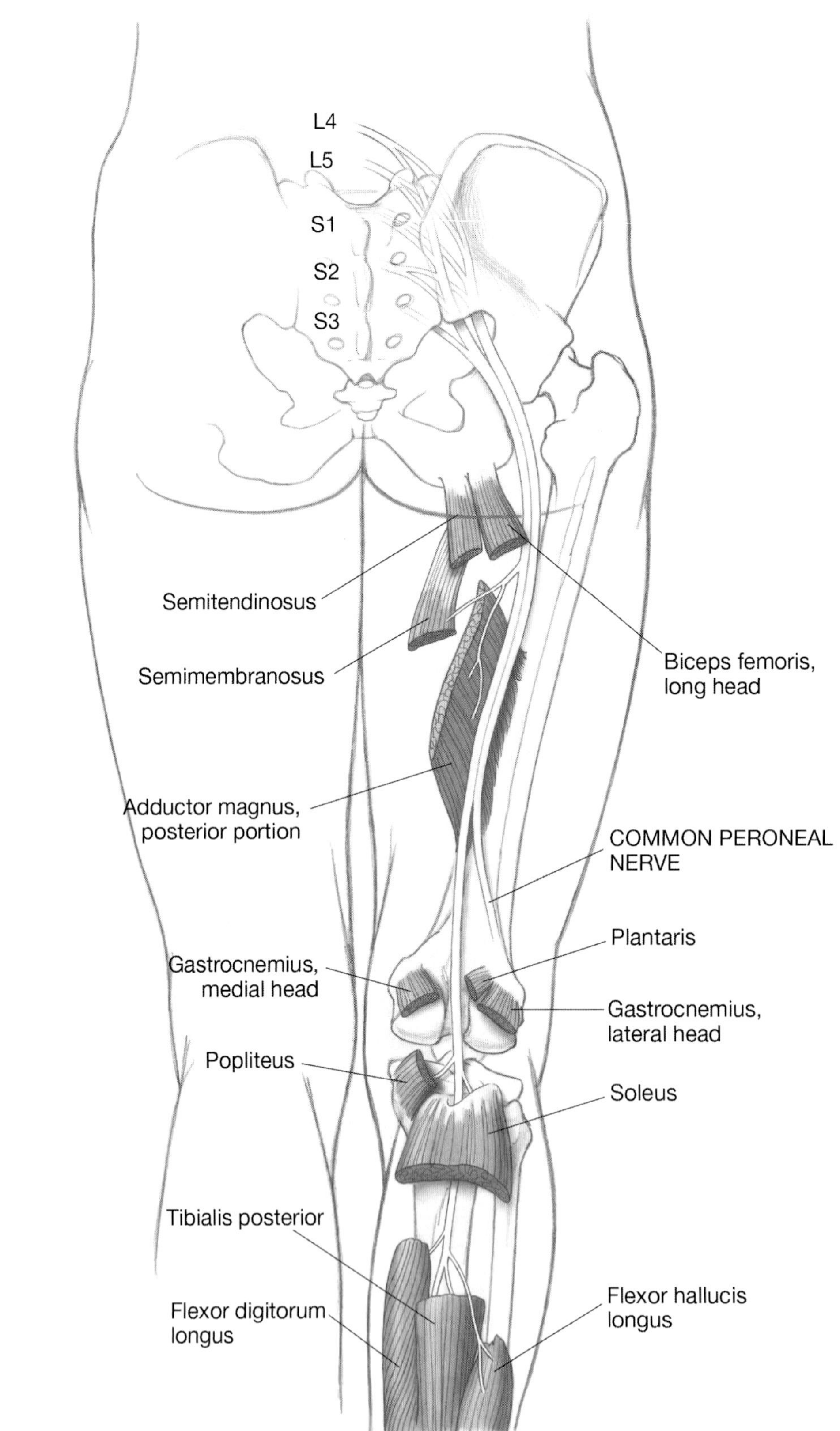
G
L4
L5
S1
S2
S3
Semitendinosus
Semimembranosus
Biceps femoris, long head
Adductor magnus, posterior portion
COMMON PERONEAL NERVE
Plantaris
Gastrocnemius, medial head
Gastrocnemius, lateral head
Popliteus
Soleus
Tibialis posterior
Flexor digitorum longus
Flexor hallucis longus

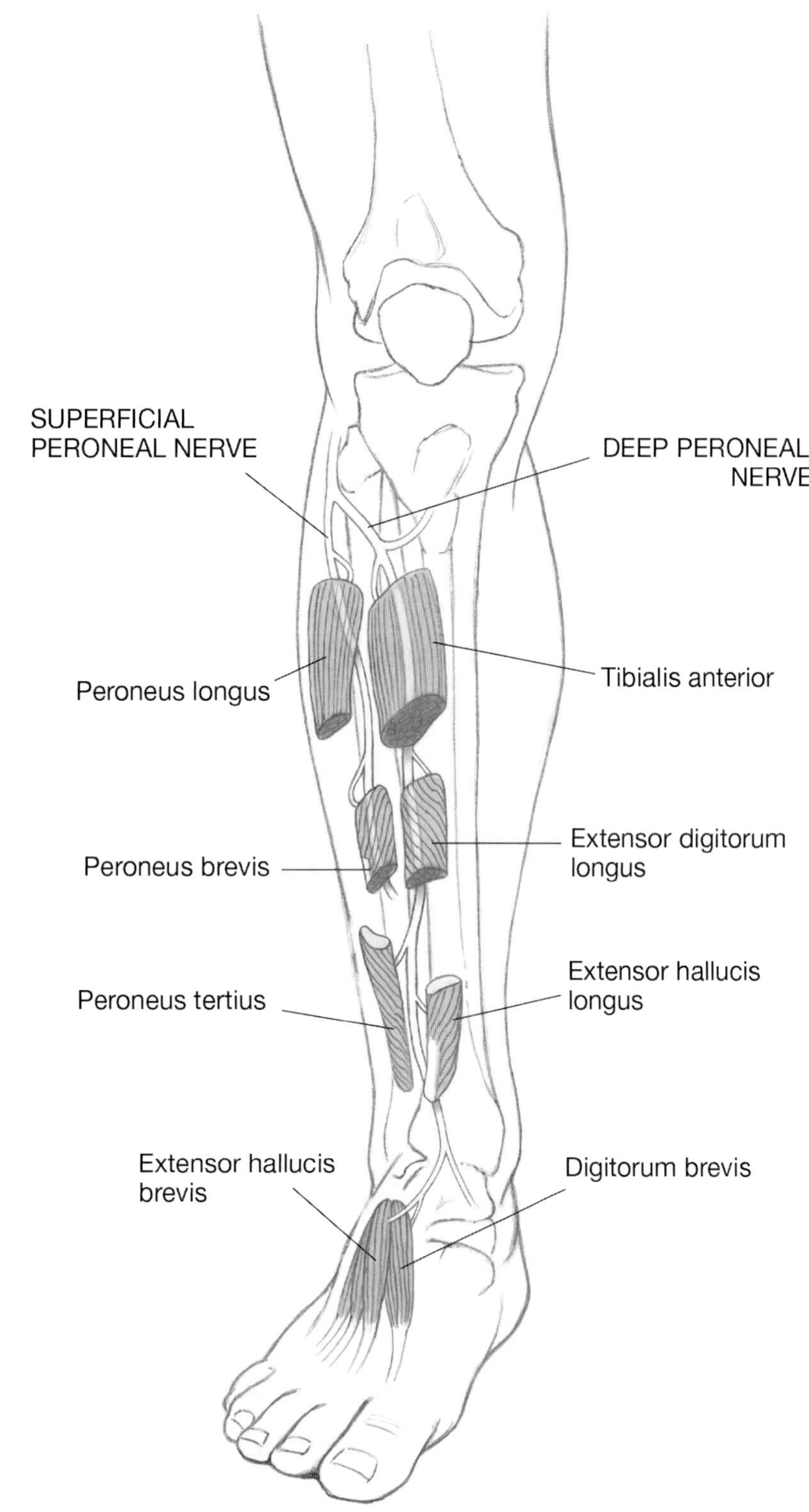
H
SUPERFICIAL
PERONEAL NERVE
DEEP PERONEAL
NERVE
Peroneus longus
Tibialis anterior
Peroneus brevis
Extensor digitorum
longus
Peroneus tertius
Extensor hallucis
longus
Extensor hallucis
brevis
Digitorum brevis

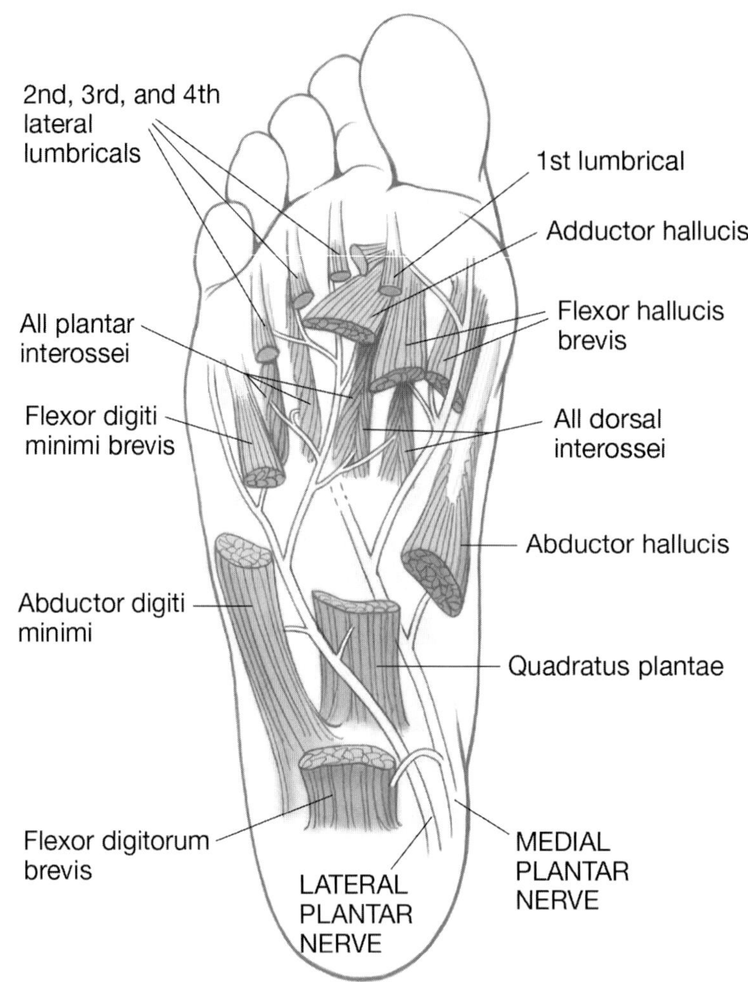

The use of nerve conduction studies to determine the location of slowing or block of conduction is particularly valuable in identifying the location and severity of lesions.

Peripheral nerves also may be involved in diffuse disease of the myelin or axons. In either instance, the clinical features are similar. There is distal loss of sensation in the upper and lower extremities (more prominent in the lower extremities), usually for all modalities. However, in some disorders, certain fiber types may be selectively involved, thus affecting certain sensory modalities. There may be paresthesia, dysesthesia, or hyperalgesia, usually in the same distribution. Reflexes are generally lost. Distal muscles are weak and flaccid and eventually atrophy. Atrophy of distal muscles produces deformities, for example, pes cavus and hammer toes (high arches with cocked-up toes) with the loss of intrinsic foot muscles.

- Individual peripheral nerves innervate defined skin segments (the dermatomes) and specific muscles. Thus, damage to peripheral nerves can be recognized by the distribution of the motor and sensory deficits.
- Weakness, atrophy, numbness, paresthesia, and loss of reflexes are typical signs of peripheral nerve damage.

Some neuropathies have a predilection for the large myelinated fibers involved in touch, proprioception, joint position sense, and reflexes. These large-fiber neuropathies

Table 13.5. Distributions of Major Peripheral Nerves

Nerve	General innervation
Median	Sensory: palmar surface of thumb and first three fingers Motor: finger and wrist flexion
Ulnar	Sensory: fourth and fifth fingers Motor: intrinsic hand muscles
Radial	Sensory: dorsum of the hand Motor: forearm, wrist, and hand extension
Femoral	Sensory: anterior aspect of thigh and medial part of leg Motor: hip flexion and knee extension
Sciatic	Sensory: posterior aspect of thigh and portion of leg below the knee Motor: knee flexion and all ankle and foot motion
Peroneal	Sensory: lateral aspect of leg and dorsum of foot Motor: foot and toe dorsiflexion
Tibial	Sensory: posterior part of leg and sole of foot Motor: foot and toe plantar flexion

may be manifested by paresthesia, sensory ataxia (Romberg sign), areflexia, and loss of tactile discrimination, joint position sense, and vibratory sensation. Important examples are neuropathies caused by vitamin B_{12} deficiency, immune or inflammatory demyelinating neuropathies, and paraneoplastic neuropathies. In other neuropathies, small myelinated or unmyelinated sensory and autonomic fibers are selectively affected. They are manifested by burning pain, lack of temperature and pain sensation, and autonomic manifestations that include orthostatic hypotension, impaired sweating, and gastrointestinal, sexual, or bladder dysfunction. Strength, reflexes, vibration and joint position sense, and the results of nerve conduction studies and needle electromyography (see below) may be normal. An important example is a form of diabetic neuropathy. Most neuropathies affect both motor and sensory fibers and large and small fibers and produce a combination of clinical features.

Although many peripheral nerve diseases affect both the axon and myelin, if the disease process primarily affects the axon, atrophy is more severe, with loss of innervation and prominent fibrillation in distal muscles. Disorders primarily producing damage to myelin are associated with less atrophy, are more readily reversible, and have little or no fibrillation.

The Neuromuscular Junction

The neuromuscular junction is the site at which the motor nerve terminal meets a muscle fiber and evokes contraction of the muscle. This contraction is accomplished through the production of an excitatory synaptic potential called an *end plate potential*. In a normal skeletal muscle fiber, the end plate potential always reaches threshold for the production of an action potential, which then propagates along the muscle fiber. The action potential, in turn, triggers a contraction.

Histology

Each neuromuscular junction consists of a presynaptic portion (the nerve terminal) and a postsynaptic portion (the muscle fiber). As an axon enters a muscle, it branches into many nerve terminals, each of which innervates one muscle fiber. As the terminal approaches the muscle fiber, the axon loses its myelin sheath and comes to lie in a depression in the muscle fiber. The nerve terminal is covered by a Schwann cell, except for the part of the

Clinical Problem 13.3.

A 47-year-old bank manager has had diabetes mellitus for 14 years. The diabetes is controlled with insulin. He complains of impotence of 6 months' duration. He has had 2 to 3 years of gradually progressive burning sensations and numbness, first in his feet and recently in his hands. He has occasional dizzy spells on arising.

On examination, his blood pressure is 115/75 mm Hg supine but decreases to 80/40 mm Hg, with no change in pulse, when he arises. He has mild weakness of his toe and foot dorsiflexors but no other weakness. Ankle reflexes are absent. Other reflexes are hypoactive. He has moderate loss of all modalities of sensation in a glove-and-stocking distribution. There is an absence of hair on his legs, and his skin is very dry. On nerve conduction studies, no sensory potentials could be obtained and motor responses were of low amplitude, with a mild slowing of conduction velocity. Electromyography showed fibrillation potentials in distal muscles bilaterally.

a. Describe how you would localize this disorder in the periphery.
b. Localize the disorder in that structure.
c. What is the temporal profile, and how would you interpret it?
d. Correlate each of the elements of the history and physical examination with the system involved.
e. What diagnosis would you give the patient?
f. What do the low-amplitude motor responses and fibrillation potentials mean for this patient?
g. What would electromyography and nerve conduction studies show if only the small, autonomic fibers were involved?

axolemma that is directly apposed to the sarcolemma of the muscle fiber and separated from it by an intervening synaptic cleft of 500 μm. The postsynaptic portion of the junction consists of complex folds of *sarcolemma* immediately beneath the nerve terminal (Fig. 13.12). This region can be demonstrated with histochemical techniques that stain acetylcholinesterase. The sarcolemma and its folds form the subneural apparatus.

The cytoplasm of the nerve terminal contains a concentration of mitochondria and many synaptic vesicles. Often, the synaptic vesicles seem to be clustered near a region of density of the presynaptic membrane. These specialized areas are located opposite the postsynaptic folds. Acetylcholine is bound to the vesicles in the nerve terminal.

There is a precise coordination between presynaptic and postsynaptic elements in the mature neuromuscular junction that ensures rapid synaptic transmission at the neuromuscular junction. Synaptic vesicles containing acetylcholine are clustered around the voltage-gated calcium channels in the *active zones*. The active zones are precisely apposed to the *postsynaptic* folds, which contain the densely clustered nicotinic acetylcholine receptors. During development, the growth cone of a motor neuron induces a local clustering of nicotinic receptors in the muscle membrane, precisely at the site of acetylcholine release.

This involves signals from the motor axon, including a protein called agrin. This protein, together with dystroglycans in the muscle basal membrane, interacts with a molecular complex related to the submembrane cytoskeleton, including a protein called dystrophin. This dystrophin-associated complex includes proteins that serve to anchor the nicotinic receptor at the level of the folds. Both survival of the motor neuron and stabilization of its synapses depend critically on the level of activity in the muscle.

Physiology

Small electrical potentials can be recorded from the region of the neuromuscular junction of skeletal muscle fibers, even in the absence of nerve impulses in the motor fibers. These potentials have all the electrical and pharmacologic properties of end plate potentials, except that they are small and occur randomly without the need

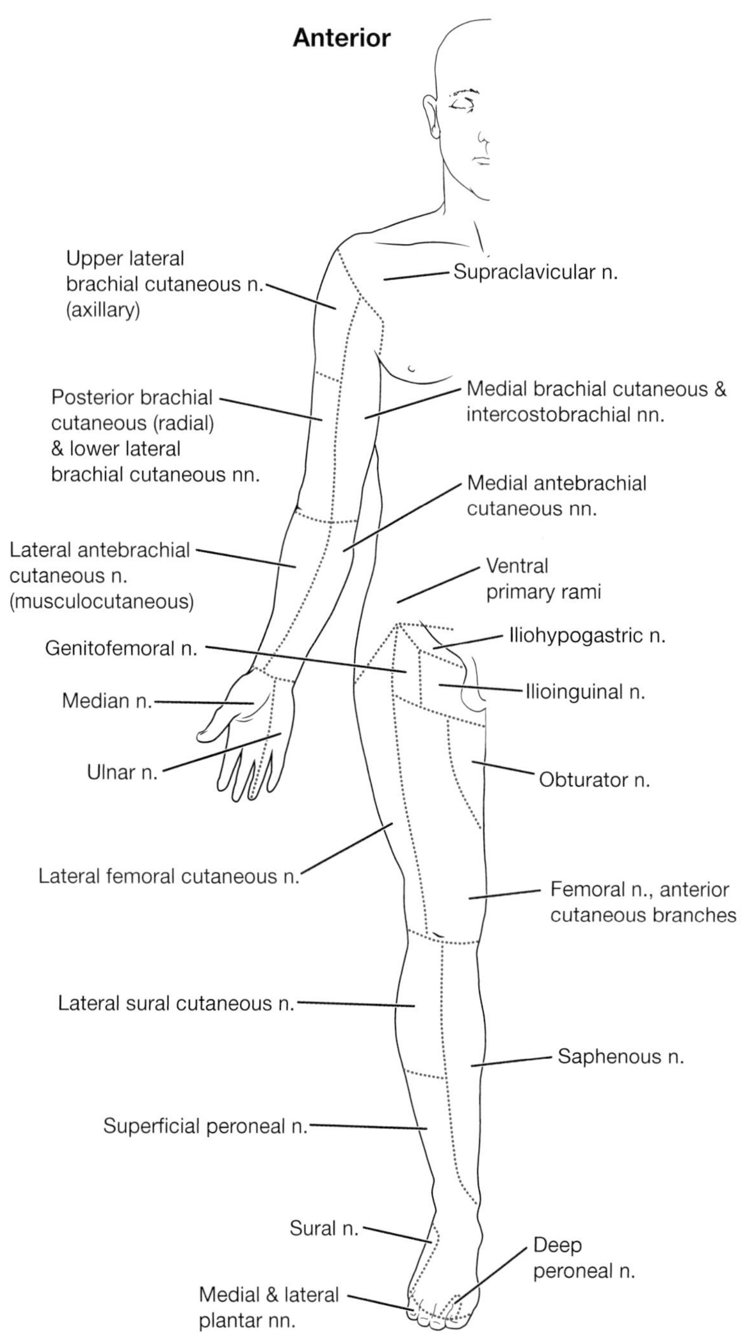

Fig. 13.11. Cutaneous distribution of peripheral nerves. n, nerve.

of nerve activity. These are called *miniature end plate potentials*.

Miniature end plate potentials are due to leakage of the neurotransmitter acetylcholine from the presynaptic terminals. The leakage occurs in quanta of transmitter; that is, miniature end plate potentials are produced by thousands of molecules of acetylcholine released together. The end plate potential, in contrast, is produced by the near-synchronous release of many quanta triggered by the nerve impulse. The

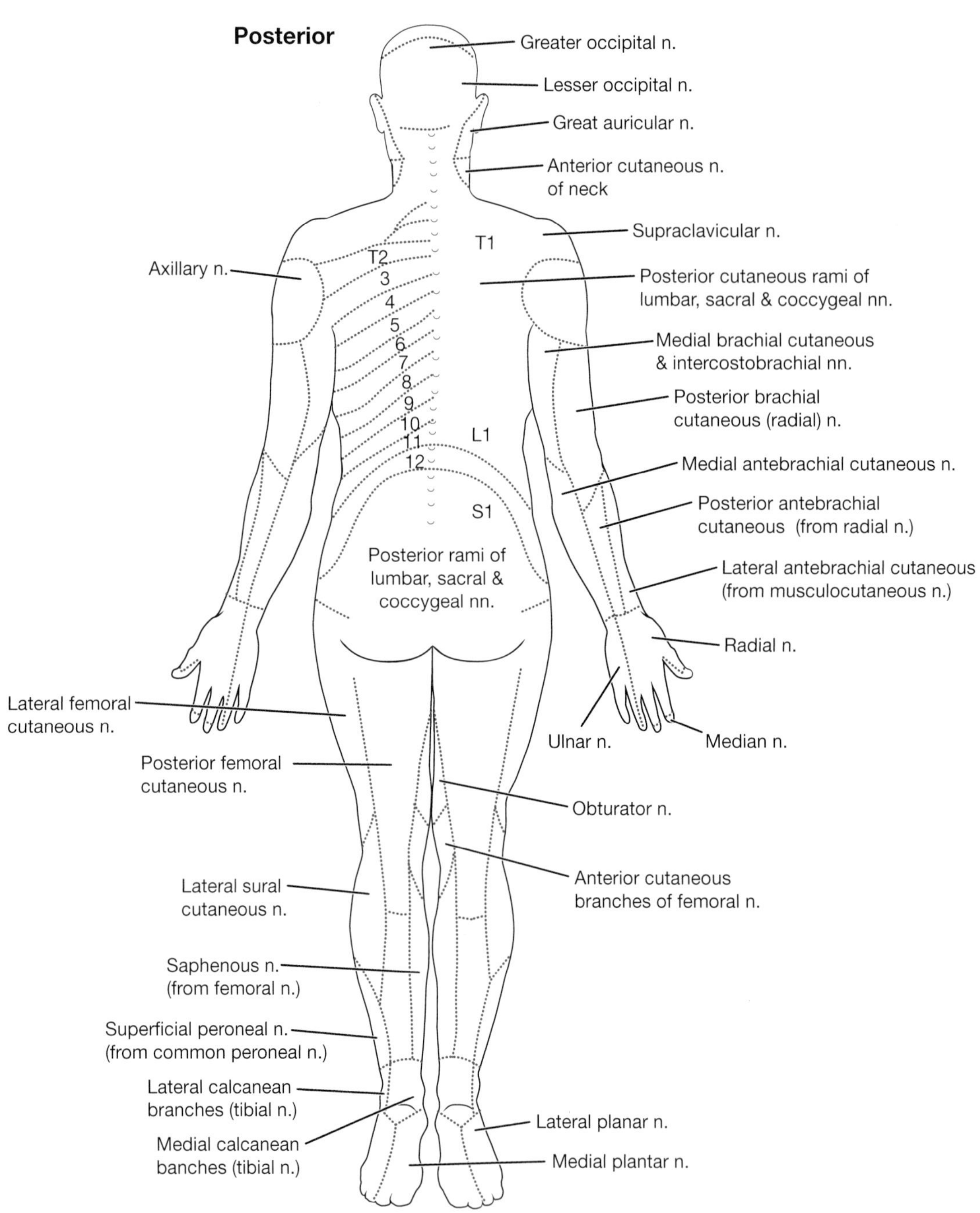

synaptic vesicles are the storage sites of quanta of acetylcholine.

When the resting potential of the motor axon terminal at the neuromuscular junction decreases, the frequency of miniature end plate potentials increases. However, the relationship is not a linear one. There is a tenfold increase in frequency for every 15 mV of depolarization. Depolarization of the motor axon terminal associated with an action potential triggers calcium influx through voltage-gated channels. The large increase in

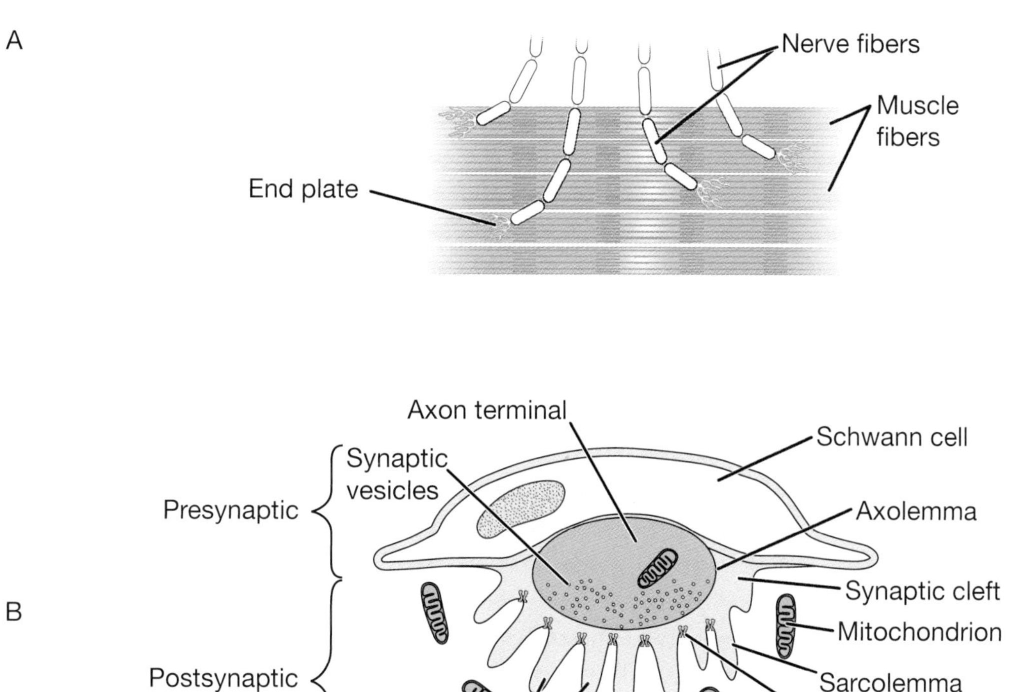

Fig. 13.12. Neuromuscular junction. *A*, End plate, where a single nerve terminal innervates a single muscle fiber. *B*, Cross section of an end plate. The axon terminal lies in a depression on the surface of a muscle fiber and is covered by a Schwann cell process. Postsynaptic folds of the sarcolemma contain acetylcholine receptors. Acetylcholine is stored in synaptic vesicles in the nerve terminal.

intracellular calcium causes the release of a burst of several hundred acetylcholine quanta, thus accounting for the end plate potential. The number of quanta (M) released by a presynaptic action potential can be calculated by dividing the average amplitude of the end plate potential (EPP) by the average amplitude of the miniature end plate potential (MEPP):

$$M = EPP/MEPP$$

Acetylcholine increases the permeability of the postsynaptic membrane to both sodium and potassium ions. Thus, the membrane potential is only partially depolarized; the synaptic currents do not flow long enough for the membrane to depolarize to zero. Therefore, the end plate potential is considerably smaller than the action potential; nevertheless, it is well above the threshold for generating a muscle fiber action potential. This is referred to as the *safety margin* of neuromuscular transmission. When the end plate potential reaches threshold, it triggers the action potential of the muscle. Acetylcholine is rapidly broken down by the enzyme acetylcholinesterase after binding with the postsynaptic membrane and producing the end plate potential.

Acetylcholine is synthesized by *choline acetyltransferase* from acetyl coenzyme A (CoA) and choline in the nerve terminal. It is stored in the vesicles and released by the action potential through calcium binding in the membrane. Acetylcholine diffuses across the synapse and binds with the cholinergic receptor until it is broken down by acetylcholinesterase. The events that occur at the neuromuscular junction are summarized in Figure 13.13.

Pharmacology

Many drugs affect neuromuscular transmission. For instance, curare, the poison once used by some South American Indians on the tips of their blowgun arrows, prevents acetylcholine from reacting with the receptor sites of the muscle membrane by competitively binding with the sites and causes paralysis. In contrast to the effect of acetylcholine, the reaction between the curare molecule and the acetylcholine receptor molecule does not change conductance in the membrane. Thus, curare blocks neuromuscular transmission.

Another substance that blocks neuromuscular transmission is botulinum toxin, the agent in food contaminated by *Clostridium botulinum* that causes botulism. By blocking the release of acetylcholine from motor nerve terminals, botulinum toxin causes a loss of end plate potentials and paralysis.

Neuromuscular transmission is enhanced by drugs that block the action of acetylcholinesterase. Without this enzyme, the acetylcholine released by nerve impulses has a greater and more prolonged action. However, the accumulation of too much acetylcholine may cause a depolarizing block of the muscle membrane. Excess acetylcholine may also desensitize acetylcholine receptor molecules and reduce the response to acetylcholine. This interaction occurs normally but is only transient because

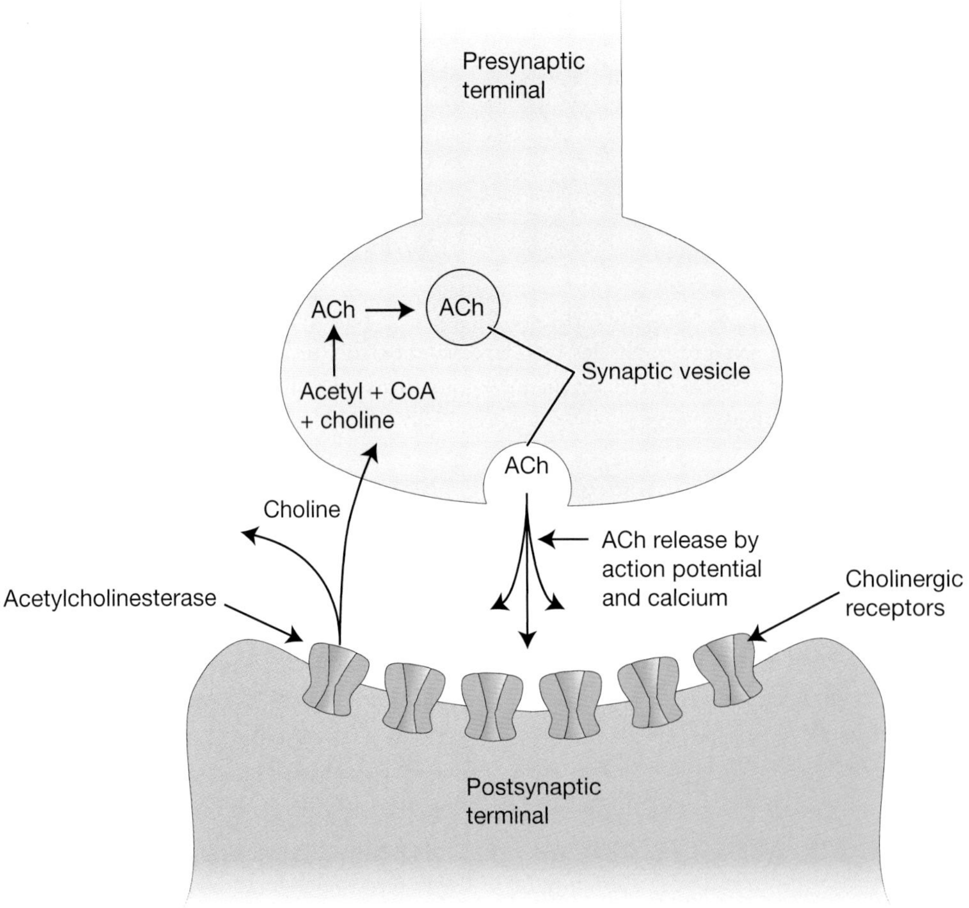

Fig. 13.13. Neurotransmitter action at the neuromuscular junction. Acetylcholine (ACh) is formed and stored in the presynaptic (nerve) terminal. It is released by depolarization of the nerve terminal in the presence of calcium and binds with receptors on the postsynaptic membrane. After producing an ionic conductance charge, it is hydrolyzed by acetylcholinesterase. CoA, coenzyme A.

the acetylcholine is removed by the esterase. An example of an anticholinesterase used clinically in the treatment of myasthenia gravis is physostigmine. Some insecticides and nerve gases are also anticholinesterases. Several drugs can mimic the action of acetylcholine at the neuromuscular junction. One of these is nicotine. In low doses, nicotine has an excitatory effect on skeletal muscle, but in high doses it blocks neuromuscular transmission.

Clinical Correlations

Disorders of neuromuscular transmission theoretically can involve several mechanisms, including the synthesis of acetylcholine, packaging of acetylcholine into vesicles, release of vesicles from the nerve terminal, diffusion of acetylcholine across the synaptic cleft, binding of acetylcholine with the receptor, response of the receptor to the transmitter, and breakdown of the acetylcholine by acetylcholinesterase. Two of these disorders, myasthenia gravis and Lambert-Eaton myasthenic syndrome, are well known clinically. Both are manifested as weakness without sensory loss. In *myasthenia gravis*, partial receptor blockade produces weakness that increases after exercise. In *Lambert-Eaton myasthenic syndrome*, the release of acetylcholine from the nerve terminal is impaired. This also produces weakness; however, it can be partially overcome by continued activity because, with continued activation, changes in the nerve terminal membrane facilitate acetylcholine release. Thus, patients with this syndrome show increasing strength with a brief period of exercise. In myasthenia gravis, both the end plate potentials and the miniature end plate potentials are small. In Lambert-Eaton myasthenic syndrome, which is often associated with carcinoma, the miniature end plate potentials are normal but the end plate potentials are small because fewer quanta are released. Several congenital myasthenic syndromes have been described that are due to defects in the packaging or release of acetylcholine, decreased acetylcholinesterase activity, or abnormal kinetics of the nicotinic acetylcholine receptor.

Muscle

All body movements are produced by muscle contraction. Through muscle activity, all behavior of the organism is effected. The function of muscle is to produce force and movement and to stabilize joints. Striated muscles act through their attachment to tendons and bones, but they depend foremost on their contractile elements. They vary in size and structure, from the tiny stapedius muscle in the middle ear to the large, powerful gastrocnemius muscle of the leg. Each performs specific functions, whether they be finely controlled, rapid, skilled movements or powerful, sudden contractions or slow, continuous, steady exertion of force. The size, shape (fusiform, unipennate, bipennate, and multipennate), and microscopic anatomy of muscles vary with their function. Muscles that produce sudden, strong, or phasic contractions consist predominantly of type II, white, fast-twitch muscle fibers that can function anaerobically; muscles that produce steady, continuous contractions consist primarily of type I, red, slow-twitch muscle fibers that depend on aerobic metabolism. The size of motor units, the innervation ratios, and the number of motor units vary among muscles and reflect the activity. The extraocular muscles, which perform rapid, quick, very finely controlled movements, have a large number of motor units, more than 1,000 per muscle. Each motor unit has a low innervation ratio, controlling only five to ten muscle fibers. In contrast, the gastrocnemius muscle is a much larger muscle but has approximately the same number of motor units. However, the innervation ratio is much higher, with each motor neuron controlling as many as 2,000 muscle fibers.

Muscles are classified as red or white on the basis of the staining properties of the fibers, which reflect underlying biochemical and histochemical differences, such as the content of glycogen, mitochondria, and particular enzymes. These can be used to identify different types of muscle fiber (Fig. 13.14). Type I fibers (red) contain large amounts of oxidative enzymes (lactic dehydrogenase, succinic dehydrogenase, and cytochrome oxidase). Type II fibers (white) contain little of these enzymes but relatively large amounts of phosphorylase and glycolytic enzymes such as adenosine triphosphatase (ATPase). All the muscle fibers of a motor unit are uniform; that is, all muscle fibers innervated by a single anterior horn cell have identical histochemical and physiologic properties. These properties are determined by the anterior horn cell. Reinnervation of muscle fibers by other anterior horn

Clinical Problem 13.4.

A 57-year-old man has been in good health except for a chronic "smoker's cough." During the past 6 months, he has noted gradually increasing difficulty in climbing steps. More recently, he has had trouble in arising from a chair. He has had some dryness of his mouth. Neurologic examination showed no abnormality other than weakness of proximal muscles and very hypoactive reflexes. The strength and reflexes appeared to improve somewhat with brief exercise.

The results of laboratory studies were unremarkable other than for changes in the electromyogram that suggested the presence of a defect of neuromuscular transmission. Chest radiography showed a mass in the right hilum of the lung. Electrophysiologic recordings were made from an intercostal muscle biopsy. The data obtained are shown in the Table.

	Patient	Normal
Average resting membrane potential, mV	75.6	74.7
Average miniature end plate potential amplitude, mV	0.3±0.3	0.3±0.4
Average end plate potential amplitude, mV	3.2±0.9	15±2.3
Average single fiber action potential, mV	97±3	98±3
Threshold, mV	60	60

a. Describe how you would localize this disorder in the periphery.
b. Localize the disorder in that structure.
c. What is the temporal profile, and how would you interpret it?
d. What diagnosis would you give the patient?
e. How might this disorder be treated?
f. What two factors determine the size of the end plate potential?
g. Which of these is abnormal in this patient?
h. What is the acetylcholine quantum content in this patient?

cells after denervation can change the type as well as the size of the muscle fiber. Some of the differences of type I and type II muscle fibers are listed in Table 13.6.

Histology

Each muscle consists of a large number of muscle fibers arranged in parallel with the longitudinal axis of the muscle. The fibers range from 2 to 15 cm in length and from 30 to 60 μm in diameter. Each is attached to the tendon of the muscle by connective tissue. Individual muscle fibers are multinucleated cells that contain myofibrils (the contractile elements) as well as mitochondria, nuclei, T tubules, and other cellular constituents. Each muscle fiber has a single end plate located approximately halfway along its length.

The myofibrils of a muscle are banded, giving muscle fibers a characteristic appearance. Each muscle fiber contains bundles of myofibrils arranged with their bands in register (Fig. 13.15). The bands are caused by the overlapping of the component fibrillar protein of the myofibrils. Each myofibril is approximately 1 μm in diameter and contains two types of filaments: thin filaments and

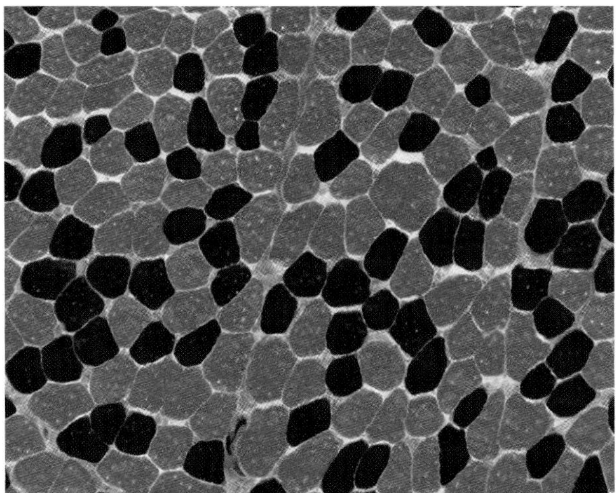

Fig. 13.14. Transverse section of muscle fibers treated with an adenosine triphosphatase stain showing the normal random checkerboard pattern of the two types of muscle fibers. Type I fibers are stained lightly; type II fibers are stained darkly. (ATPase stain; ×200.) (Courtesy of A. G. Engel, MD, Muscle Laboratory, Mayo Clinic College of Medicine, Rochester, MN.)

thick filaments. The thick filament contains myosin, a large protein material approximately 0.1 μm in diameter, with lateral projections of meromyosin. The thin filament is actin, which is 0.05 μm in diameter. The two proteins associated with actin are troponin and tropomyosin, and they can prevent the interaction of actin and myosin. The actin and myosin filaments have a hexagonal arrangement where they overlap (Fig. 13.16). The area of overlap is darker and called the A band. The area that includes only thin actin filaments is lighter and called the I band. The thin actin filaments are attached to a crystalline structure, which is also dark, called the Z disk. The region including only myosin filaments is the H zone. The myosin filaments are bound together at a dark area centrally called the M line, which is within the H band.

A muscle fiber can be divided longitudinally into areas called sarcomeres, which extend from one Z disk to the next. A sarcomere is approximately 2 μm long and consists (in order) of an I band, A band, H zone, A band, and I band between two Z disks.

Table 13.6. Characteristics of Motor Units

Tonic	Phasic
Motor neuron	Motor neuron
Small alpha motor neuron	Large alpha motor neuron
Small-diameter axon	Large-diameter axon
Low firing frequency	High firing frequency
Slow-twitch fibers	Fast-twitch fibers
Muscle fibers (red) (type I)	Muscle fibers (white) (type II)
Aerobic oxidative enzymes (lactic and succinic dehydrogenase, cytochrome oxidase)	Anaerobic glycolytic enzymes and phosphorylase
Small quantities of glycogen	Large quantities of glycogen
Rich in myoglobin	Poor in myoglobin
Lower threshold to stretch	Higher threshold to stretch
Longer contraction time	Shorter contraction time
More mitochondria	Fewer mitochondria
Lower muscle tension	Higher muscle tension
High oxygen consumption	Low oxygen consumption
Constant good blood flow	Rapidly insufficient blood flow
Low fatigability	Pronounced fatigability

Extending throughout the muscle fiber is sarcoplasmic reticulum, which forms a longitudinal, anastomotic network of irregular tubular spaces surrounding the myofibrils (Fig. 13.17). At specific locations along the length of the myofibrils, usually at the junction of the A and I bands, are transverse tubular structures, the T tubules, which are near the sarcoplasmic reticulum. T tubules are hollow and continuous with the surface membrane (sarcolemma); thus, they are open to the extracellular fluid. They run perpendicularly from the surface membrane into the muscle fiber, encircling the myofibrils.

Physiology

The contraction of a muscle fiber is initiated by an action potential. When the end plate potential reaches threshold, an action potential is initiated in the end plate region and propagates in both directions along the length of the muscle fiber.

Depolarization of the muscle membrane is initiated by the nicotinic receptor and involves activation of voltage-gated sodium channels. As the action potential sweeps down the muscle fiber, the current flow generated by the potential passes into the depth of the fiber through the T tubule system. The T tubule contains voltage-sensitive calcium channels and, when depolarized, triggers the release of calcium stored in the adjacent sarcoplasmic reticulum.

> The sarcoplasmic reticulum balances the process of calcium storage, release, and reuptake through calcium regulatory proteins, including three calcium-binding proteins in the lumen for calcium storage, calcium release channels, and sarcoplasmic reticulum calcium-ATPase pumps for calcium reuptake. Disorders of these mechanisms produce specific clinical syndromes such as malignant hyperthermia.

Depolarization results in the opening of calcium-release channels in the sarcoplasmic reticulum, referred to as the ryanodine receptors. Calcium binds to troponin C, leading to the detachment of tropomyosin from actin. Actin then attaches to the cross-bridges provided by the myosin heads protruding from the thick filaments, which contain an ATPase site. In the relaxed state when there is no interaction between actin and myosin, these cross-bridges bind adenosine diphosphate and phosphate.

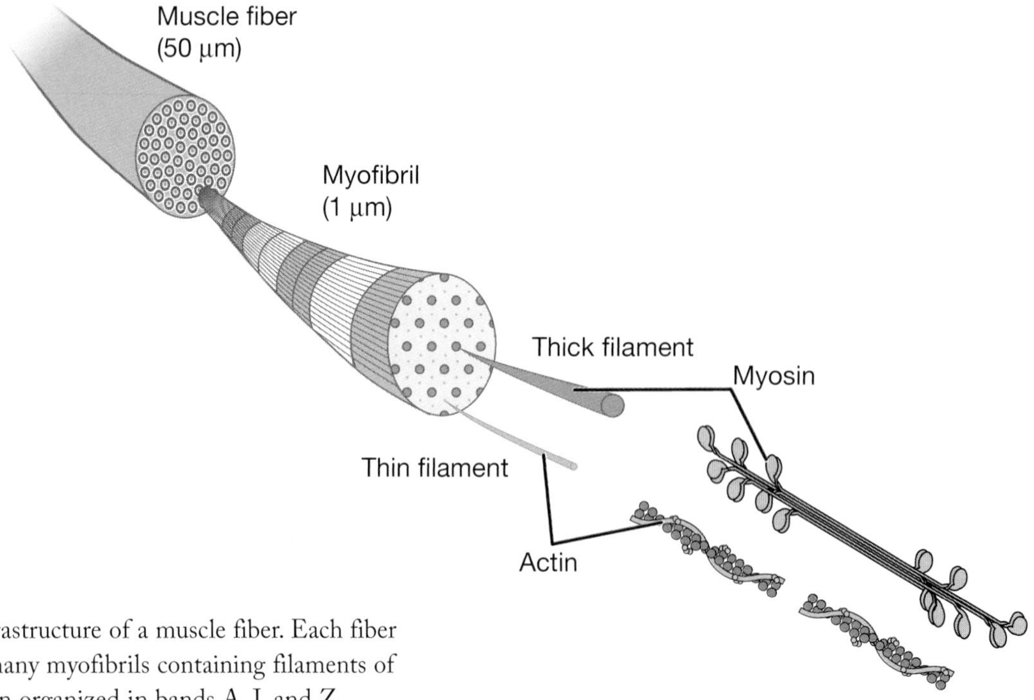

Fig. 13.15. Ultrastructure of a muscle fiber. Each fiber is made up of many myofibrils containing filaments of actin and myosin organized in bands A, I, and Z.

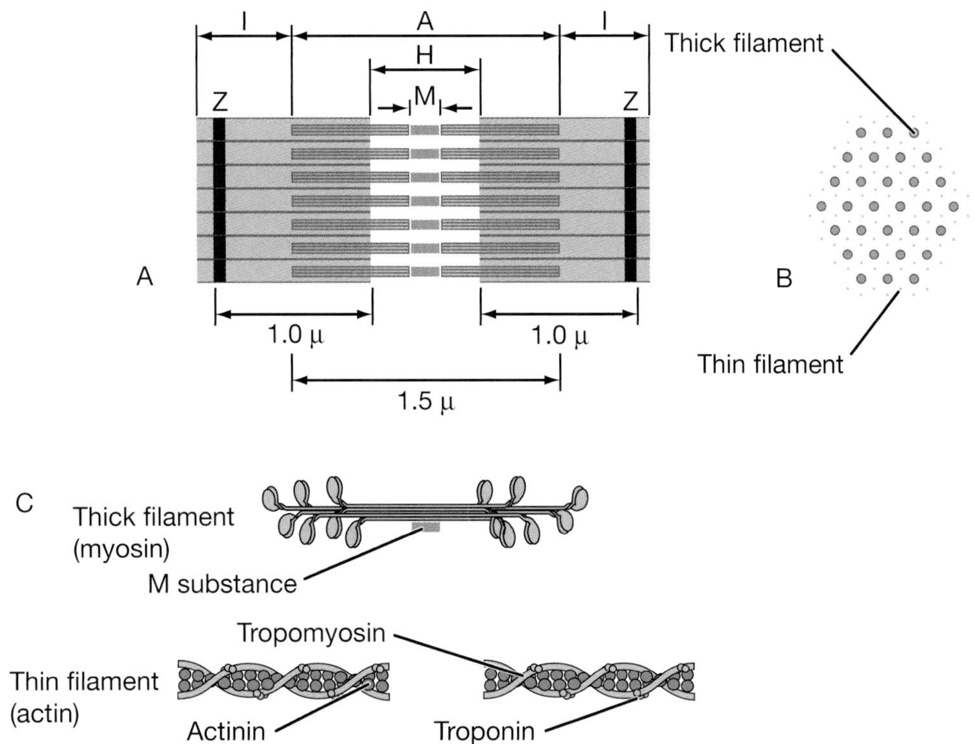

Fig. 13.16. Organization of protein filaments in a myofibril. *A*, Longitudinal section through one sarcomere (Z disk to Z disk) showing overlap of actin and myosin. *B*, Cross section through A band, where the thin actin filaments interdigitate with the thick myosin filaments in a hexagonal formation. *C*, Location of specific proteins in a sarcomere. (For definitions of A, H, I, M, and Z, see text.)

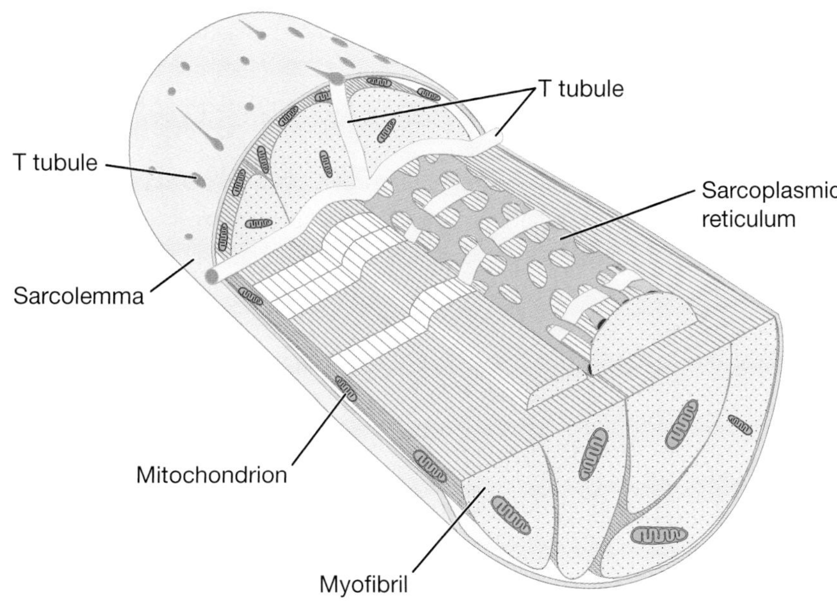

Fig. 13.17. Structure of a single muscle fiber cut longitudinally and in cross section. Individual myofibrils are surrounded and separated by sarcoplasmic reticulum. T tubules are continuous with the extracellular fluid and interdigitate with the sarcoplasmic reticulum.

When the inhibitory effect of tropomyosin is removed by calcium binding with troponin C, the myosin cross-bridges attach to actin and tilt toward the midsarcomere, driving the thin filament toward the midsarcomere, thus shortening the sarcomere. The length of the thick (myosin) filament and the thin (actin) filament does not change during muscle contraction. The interaction between actin and myosin is rapid and short lasting. In the presence of adenosine triphosphate (ATP), there is reuptake of calcium by the sarcoplasmic reticulum. This terminates the active state and produces relaxation.

The cross-bridges bind ATP and detach from actin, then they split ATP into adenosine diphosphate and phosphate and assume a relaxed position perpendicular to the shaft of the thick filament. If the ATP in muscle is depleted, the myosin cross-bridges remain attached to actin, and the muscle becomes rigid (as in rigor mortis). Mutations of the gene encoding for the calcium-release channel of the sarcoplasmic reticulum (the ryanodine receptor) lead to leakage of calcium from the sarcoplasmic reticulum on exposure to anesthetics such as halothane. This promotes severe and prolonged muscle contraction on recovery from anesthesia, a serious condition called malignant hyperthermia.

The generation of tension depends on the overlap of actin and myosin filaments. If a muscle is stretched too far, the overlap is minimal and affords little opportunity for interaction. Therefore, muscle has optimal lengths for contraction, as shown by a length-tension diagram (Fig. 13.18).

The rate at which tension develops varies with muscle fiber type. In a slow-twitch muscle in which the twitch lasts 100 milliseconds, repetitive stimulation at 10 per second produces a steady contraction. The same rate of activation in a fast-twitch fiber with a twitch time of 25 milliseconds produces a series of brief distinct twitches with each impulse. The sequence of events leading to muscle contraction is illustrated in Figure 13.19.

Clinical Correlations

Disease may damage muscle directly, as in myopathy, or indirectly by affecting nerves and causing neurogenic atrophy. In both instances, weakness and atrophy of the muscle result. However, myopathy and neurogenic atrophy are histologically and physiologically distinct. If a muscle loses its innervation because of disease of the lower motor neuron, the muscle fibers fibrillate and atrophy. In disorders with incomplete denervation, scattered muscle fibers atrophy. If the process is chronic, the viable axons in the muscle reinnervate the denervated fibers, resulting in motor units with a higher innervation ratio and large motor unit potentials. If the large units are lost, the atrophy subsequently appears in large groups of fibers to produce the typical histologic pattern of neurogenic atrophy (see below).

In many myopathies, entire muscle fibers degenerate randomly, affecting muscle fibers of many motor units, with a loss of fibers from all motor units. With this loss, a smaller force is generated when the motor units are activated. In addition to weakness, the loss of muscle fibers results in smaller motor unit potentials, a feature that can be recognized with needle electromyography. Although many primary muscle diseases, or myopathies, have specific histologic changes, some features are common to all myopathies: random variation in fiber size, internal migration of nuclei, increased connective tissue, and degenerative changes in the muscle fibers (see below).

Although these abnormalities may affect all muscles in the body, most primary muscle diseases affect proximal muscles more than distal muscles. Therefore, proximal muscle weakness is characteristic of myopathy. It is associated with normal sensation and normal reflexes as long as there is sufficient muscle to contract. The weakness is not associated with an alteration of tone.

Destruction of muscle fibers in their entirety or segmentally along their length is the most common way for disease processes to affect muscle. The major categories

Clinical Problem 13.5.
What deficit would a disorder of the interaction of T tubules, sarcoplasmic reticulum, and calcium due to prolonged treatment with high doses of prednisone be likely to cause?

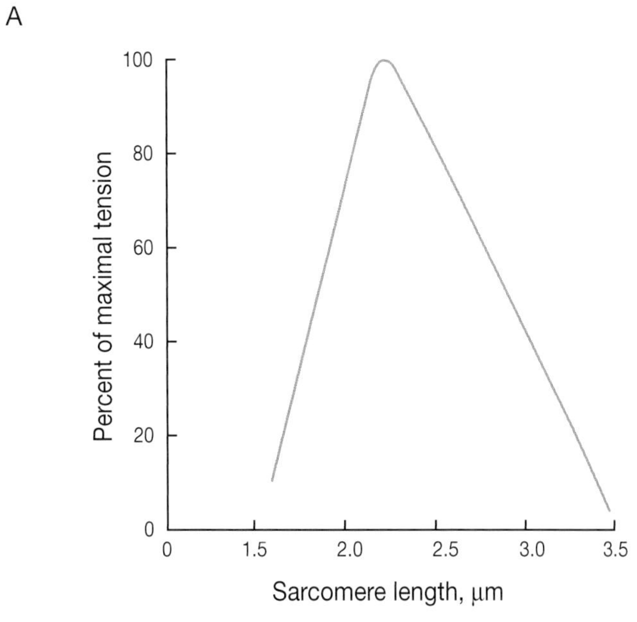

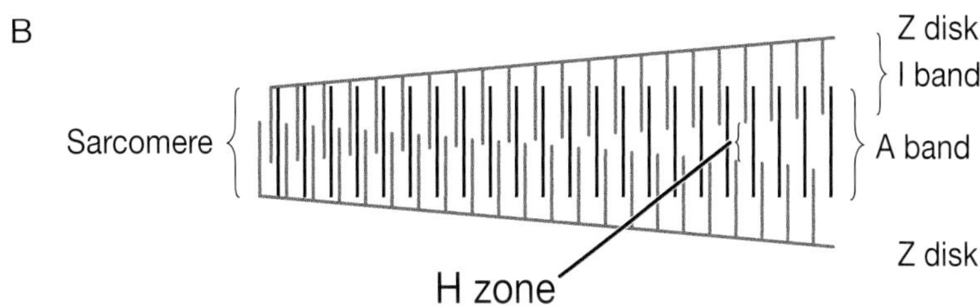

Fig. 13.18. Length-tension diagram of a muscle fiber in relation to its sarcomere length. *A*, Tension generated at different sarcomere lengths. *B*, Extent of overlap of actin and myosin filaments at different sarcomere lengths. (For definitions of A, H, I, and Z, see text.)

of myopathy are listed in Table 13.7. Three specific pathophysiologic alterations among these myopathies are worth mentioning specifically:

1. Disorder of the sarcolemma, due to an abnormality of the dystrophin-associated protein complex associated with the sarcolemma
2. Ion channelopathies
3. Disorder of the excitation-contraction coupling mechanism within the muscle fiber

Clinical Problem 13.6.

How could a patient in whom West Nile virus infection destroyed one-third of the anterior horn cells that innervate the biceps muscle recover with normal strength after 6 months?

Disorders of the Sarcolemma or Dystrophinopathies

In both Duchenne muscular dystrophy and Becker muscular dystrophy, the attachment of myofibrils to the sarcolemma is impaired, with abnormal transmission of force to the sarcolemma. There also are sarcolemmal defects and secondary muscle fiber necrosis. Other forms include limb-girdle muscular dystrophy with abnormal sarcoglycans and congenital muscular dystrophy with basal lamina defects.

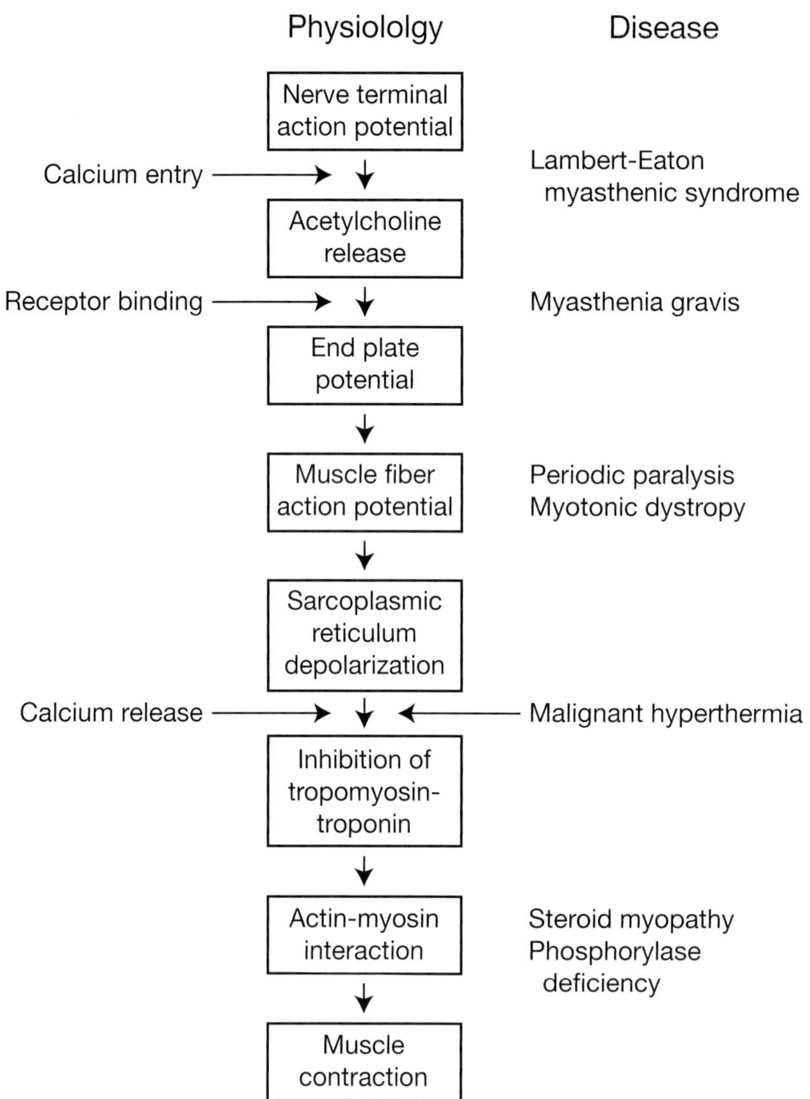

Fig. 13.19. Sequence of events leading to muscle contraction and pathophysiologic correlations.

Ion Channelopathies

Mutations encoding for subunits of the sodium, chloride, or calcium channel result in disorders of muscle excitability, referred to as muscle channelopathies. The two manifestations are 1) periodic paralysis due to transient inability to generate action potentials, and 2) myotonia, which consists of excessive muscle contraction, prolonged contraction, or the inability to stop contraction because of increased excitability of the muscle membrane. Sometimes both phenomena occur together. For example, mutations that impair inactivation of the sodium channel produce a transient increase in excitability, followed by the inability to generate new action potentials because of membrane depolarization. This may be triggered by an increase in extracellular potassium, as in hyperkalemic periodic paralysis. Mutations in the chloride channel result in increased excitability of the muscle membrane, as in congenital myotonia. Congenital myasthenic syndromes have a variety of causes.

Disorders of the Contractile Mechanism

In these disorders, muscle fibers generate normal electrical activity but do not generate enough energy to support normal muscle contraction and relaxation. Muscle depends on the metabolism of glycogen and glucose for a short-term energy supply. In genetic defects of glucose metabolism (e.g., muscle phosphorylase deficiency), sufficient energy cannot be produced. As muscle energy is depleted, the muscle cramps without electrical discharges. Other metabolic and toxic disorders interfere with the excitation-contraction coupling and produce weakness similar in distribution and character to that described in muscle fiber degeneration.

Clinical Findings in Peripheral Disorders

Peripheral Nerve Disease

Diseases involving the peripheral nerves have a combination of motor, sensory, and autonomic symptoms and signs. This includes flaccid weakness and atrophy and sensory loss involving all modalities of sensation in the same distribution as the motor findings. Deep tendon reflexes and superficial reflexes are absent in the distribution of the involved peripheral nerves. Damage to the sympathetic fibers in the peripheral nerves may alter sweating and skin temperature. Other internal regulation disturbances such as hypotension and impotence may also occur.

Diseases of the peripheral nerves are of two types: 1) symmetrical polyneuropathies, usually distal and due to a disturbance involving many nerves, and 2) localized mononeuropathies involving a single peripheral nerve, often from trauma, neoplasm, or compression. In mononeuropathy, or plexus disease, the weakness, pain, sensory deficit, and reflex loss are within the distribution of a specific peripheral nerve, for example, the sciatic, radial, median, or ulnar nerve.

Table 13.7. Classification of Myopathies

Congenital myopathies
Dystrophinopathies
Inflammatory myopathies
Ion channelopathies
Metabolic myopathies
Mitochondrial myopathies
Myopathies related to systemic disorders
Endocrinopathies
Toxins and drugs

Peripheral neuropathy with destruction of a segment of axon results in degeneration of the distal part of the axon in a process called axonal degeneration in diffuse disorders and called wallerian degeneration in focal lesions (see Chapter 4). Axonal degeneration occurs in generalized disorders of peripheral nerve, such as toxic neuropathies, diabetic neuropathies, and neuropathies due to nutritional deficiencies. In these disorders, the peripheral nerves show loss of axons, fragmentation of axis cylinders, and breakdown of myelin into fragments or myelin ovoids (Fig. 13.8).

Other peripheral neuropathies are characterized primarily by segmental demyelination. In Guillain-Barré syndrome (acute inflammatory demyelinating neuropathy), there are edema and swelling of the myelin and Schwann cell cytoplasm, with cellular infiltration and segmental loss of myelin. If severe, this may be associated with axonal destruction and wallerian degeneration. In genetic hypertrophic neuropathies such as Charcot-Marie-Tooth disease, nerve fibers are repeatedly demyelinated and remyelinated. Each episode leaves a layer of connective tissue, which forms concentric layers around the axon. These nerves become very large and firm, and the axons may finally be lost, leaving only the connective tissue stroma.

Peripheral neuropathy may be only one manifestation of a widespread genetic error of metabolism. In metachromatic leukodystrophy, there is a deficit of arylsulfatase, an enzyme that is active in the breakdown of myelin products. With the absence of this enzyme, abnormal sulfatides accumulate in peripheral nerves and produce the clinical pattern of peripheral neuropathy. The white matter of the central nervous system is also involved. Pathologically, metachromatically staining material accumulates along the axons in addition to the breakdown of myelin.

In Refsum disease, another genetically determined

disease, the metabolic defect results in an accumulation of phytanic acid, a fatty acid. The disease is characterized by a chronic sensorimotor polyneuropathy associated with hypertrophic changes and onion-bulb formation of peripheral nerves. The patient also has ichthyosis (dry, rough, scaly skin), retinitis pigmentosa, and deafness. In the past, this was considered an untreatable degenerative neurologic disorder; however, a diet low in phytanic acid has been shown to be helpful in treating this disease.

Neuromuscular Junction Disease

The major symptom of patients with defects of neuromuscular transmission is weakness, usually in proximal or cranial muscles. There is no atrophy, and muscle tone is normal. The major features that differentiate neuromuscular junction disease from muscle disease are fluctuation of weakness with exertion and the response to drugs acting at the neuromuscular junction, which do not occur in myopathies.

Myasthenia gravis, a disorder affecting the neuromuscular junction, is an autoimmune disease in which antibodies are formed against acetylcholine receptors in the postsynaptic membrane at the motor end plate. The decrease in the number of receptor sites at the motor end plate results in a decrease in the response of the muscle fiber to acetylcholine. Clinically, myasthenia gravis is characterized by fatigable weakness that is induced or increased by exercise and improved by rest or anticholinesterase agents.

Lambert-Eaton myasthenic syndrome is another immune-mediated disorder that affects neuromuscular junctions. In contrast to myasthenia gravis, it affects the presynaptic terminal and blocks the release of quanta of acetylcholine. This syndrome is usually a paraneoplastic disorder in which circulating antibodies secreted by small cell carcinoma of the lung bind with calcium channels in the nerve terminal to prevent the entry of calcium and the quantal release of acetylcholine. Lambert-Eaton myasthenic syndrome is similar to myasthenia gravis in that strength fluctuates with activity, but in contrast to myasthenia gravis, strength may improve with activity because more quanta of acetylcholine are released with continued activation. In this syndrome, the associated findings of muscle weakness and reduced reflexes are due to the neuromuscular junction effects; the dry mouth is due to involvement of parasympathetic junctions.

Muscle Disease

Patients with primary myopathy have weakness often accompanied by marked muscle atrophy. Voluntary movement is otherwise normal, with no involuntary movements or spasticity. The common types of myopathy, such as muscular dystrophy and polymyositis, involve proximal muscles. Reflexes are relatively preserved because the neural apparatus is intact. Fasciculations (twitching of the muscles), which indicate disease of the lower motor neuron, are not present. Patients with muscle disease show no evidence of damage to the longitudinal systems of the central nervous system. Cognitive function is not involved, and sensory symptoms or signs are not present.

Muscular dystrophy is a genetic disease that primarily affects muscle. One form (Duchenne) is due to a defect in dystrophin, the protein needed to maintain an intact sarcolemma. Muscular dystrophy has several forms, with different clinical patterns. The three major types are Duchenne, fascioscapulohumeral, and limb-girdle. Each has the histologic alterations typical of myopathy, with random, patchy degeneration of muscle fibers, central nuclei, and proliferation of connective tissue. Polymyositis, a connective tissue disease, is an immunologic disorder. Its pathologic changes are similar to those of dystrophy but with inflammatory cell infiltrates, particularly in and around blood vessels. These changes are more prominent in the peripheral areas of the muscle. Muscular dystrophies have the temporal profile characteristic of degenerative disorders; that is, they are diffuse, chronic, and progressive. However, polymyositis has the histologic features of an inflammatory disorder and often has a subacute temporal profile.

Laboratory Studies in the Identification of Peripheral Disease

In addition to the clinical features listed above, several laboratory tests are helpful in differentiating diseases involving peripheral structures. These include biochemical, electrophysiologic, and histologic studies.

Clinical Problem 13.7.

A 55-year-old woman developed symmetrical, proximal weakness with mild muscle soreness over 2 weeks. Examination showed normal reflexes, sensation, and mentation. All proximal muscles were moderately weak, distal muscles mildly so. There was no fatigue with exercise. The serum level of creatine kinase was increased.

a. Describe how you would localize this disorder in the periphery.
b. What is the temporal profile, and how would you interpret it?
c. What diagnosis would you give the patient?

Motor and sensory nerve conduction studies were normal, except for a borderline low-amplitude compound muscle action potential. Needle electromyography showed two abnormalities of the motor unit potentials: the potentials were small and they fired rapidly with minimal contraction. Fibrillation potentials were also noted.

d. What is the mechanism of weakness in this patient?
e. What are the two physiologic mechanisms used to increase force of contraction with weakness?
f. What mechanism explains the increased creatine kinase level and fibrillation potentials?
g. What pattern of histologic change would you expect in this patient?

Biochemical Tests

General Medical

Peripheral neuromuscular disorders are often found with, or secondary to, systemic disease processes. For example, the most common cause of peripheral neuropathy is diabetes mellitus. The cause can often be identified by testing for medical and toxic disorders. Kidney disease, porphyria, nutritional deficiencies, and toxic causes can often be recognized with biochemical tests.

Myopathies are particularly common with endocrine disease, connective tissue disease, and metabolic disorders that can be identified biochemically. Therefore, a general medical assessment is important in the evaluation of peripheral neuromuscular disease.

Muscle Enzymes

Muscle fibers contain several enzymes that are important in their metabolism, such as aldolase, serum glutamic-oxaloacetic transaminase, and lactic dehydrogenase. Muscle damage from any disease that causes the destruction or degeneration of muscle fibers releases these enzymes into the general circulation. Consequently, the levels of these enzymes are commonly increased in the blood of patients who have active primary muscle disease. However, these enzymes are also found in many other tissues, and their levels can be increased with other diseases, especially those that damage the heart or liver. Creatine kinase, which transfers a phosphate group from creatine phosphate to adenosine diphosphate to form creatine and adenosine triphosphate, occurs mainly in muscle and, thus, is a more specific indicator of muscle disease. Creatine kinase levels may be increased in the serum of patients with early or mild myopathy who have minimal clinical evidence of disease and in persons who are carriers of the abnormal gene in recessively inherited muscle disease.

Immunologic Tests

Circulating antibodies are becoming increasingly important in the diagnosis of nerve, neuromuscular junction, and muscle diseases. Many of these antibodies can now be identified with blood tests performed by commercial laboratories, as described below.

Peripheral Neuropathy

Previously, peripheral neuropathy was classified in many patients as idiopathic (cause unknown) after a full neurologic investigation excluded toxic disorders and those associated with medical disorders. A wide range of causes of immune-based peripheral neuropathies can be identified with blood tests for specific immunologic markers. For example, in some patients, paraneoplastic sensory neuropathy due to involvement of the dorsal root ganglion cell can be confirmed by the presence of antineuronal nuclear antibodies, and G_{M1} ganglioside antibodies are markers for multifocal motor neuropathies with conduction block.

Neuromuscular Junction Disease

Both prejunctional (with impairment of acetylcholine release) and postjunctional (due to abnormalities in the number or function of nicotinic receptors) disorders of neuromuscular transmission may result from immune, toxic, or congenital mechanisms. The diagnosis of immune-mediated disorders is supported by the presence of circulating autoantibodies against the ion channels involved in the disorder.

Myasthenia gravis, a postjunctional disorder, is characterized by the presence of acetylcholine receptor antibodies. Lambert-Eaton myasthenic syndrome, a prejunctional disorder, is associated with antibodies against voltage-gated calcium channels.

Muscle Disease

Several muscle diseases are likely immune mediated, but for most of them, the specific antibodies responsible have not been identified. The Jo-1 antigen involved in polymyositis is a major candidate.

Genetic

Important advances have been made in the detection of the genetic defects in each major group of neuromuscular disease, including the abnormal gene and, in some cases, the secondary abnormality. These advances have been most prominent in peripheral neuropathies.

Peripheral Nerve Disease

The genetic defects in the axonal and hypertrophic forms of Charcot-Marie-Tooth neuropathy are listed in Tables 13.8-13.10, along with examples of the many recently described genetic disorders of peripheral nerve. The genetic bases of motor neuron diseases have also been defined, such as X-linked spinobulbar muscular atrophy (Kennedy disease with CAG trinucleotide expansion in the androgen receptor gene on the X chromosome) and hereditary neuropathy with liability to pressure palsy with focal neuropathies (deletion of one of the two PMP-22 alleles).

Neuromuscular Junction Disease

The underlying mechanisms of the congenital defects of neuromuscular transmission are genetic in origin. More than 15 distinct loci for these defects have been defined that produce a wide variety of presynaptic and postsynaptic syndromes, including disorders of packaging of acetylcholine in the nerve terminal, formation of too few quanta of acetylcholine, acetylcholinesterase deficiency, slow- and fast-channel postsynaptic syndromes, and acetylcholine receptor deficiencies.

Muscle Disease

Deletions in the dystrophin gene are the hallmark of X-linked Duchenne muscular dystrophy. Expanded CTG trinucleotide repeats on chromosome band 19q13.3 are the basis of classic myotonic dystrophy type 1, and CCTG repeats on chromosome band 3q21.3 are the basis of proximal myotonic myopathy type 2.

Electrophysiologic Testing

Electrophysiologic testing is a major part of identifying and characterizing specific disease of nerve, muscle, and neuromuscular junction. Electromyography, with recording of spontaneous and voluntary activity from muscles, and nerve conduction studies, with stimulation of nerve and recording responses from nerve and muscle, are the major forms of electrophysiologic testing. Electrophysiologic assessment can confirm a clinical diagnosis, quantitatively define the severity, localize the damage to individual segments along the length of nerves, distinguish involvement of different components of nerve, muscle, or neuromuscular junction, recognize subclinical disorders, distinguish the residual effects of an old process from a new or progressing disorder, and, in some cases, define the underlying pathophysiologic mechanism.

> Specialized electrophysiologic techniques have been developed to answer specific clinical questions, for example, single fiber electromyography, fiber density, spike-triggered averaging, F and H wave latency, blink reflex latency measurement, motor unit number estimates, somatosensory

Table 13.8. Examples of Hereditary Demyelinating Neuropathies

Disease	Locus	Gene	Putative function	Clinical
Autosomal dominant				
Type 1				
HMSN 1A	17p11.2-12	*PMP22*	Myelin structure	Onion bulb formation[a]
HMSN 1C	16p13.1-12.3	*LITAF*	Possible neuronal apoptosis	Onion bulb formation[a]
Type 3				
HMSN 3A	17p11.2-12	*PMP22*	Myelin structure	Onion bulb formation[a]
Autosomal recessive				
Type 4				
HMSN 4A	8q13-21.1	*GDAP1*	Neuronal development	± Rare vocal cord paresis
HMSN 4D	8q24.3	*NDRG1*	Transcription regulation	± Deafness

HMSN, hereditary motor sensory neuropathy.
[a]Indicates repeated demyelination and remyelination.
Modified from Klein CJ, Dyck PJ. Genetic testing in inherited peripheral neuropathies. J Peripher Nerv Syst. 2005;10:77-84. Used with permission.

evoked potential and motor evoked potential latencies, jaw jerk latency, masseter inhibitory reflex, microneurography, and facial nerve lateral spread responses. A few of these are described below.

Nerve Conduction Studies

Often, it is not possible to be certain on the basis of clinical findings whether a patient has a peripheral disorder. To help identify the disease, the function of peripheral nerves can be evaluated with nerve conduction studies

Table 13.9. Examples of Hereditary Axonal Sensory Neuropathy (HMSN)

Disease	Locus	Gene	Putative function	Clinical
Autosomal dominant (HMSN 2 and CMT 2)				
A	1p35-36	*MFN2*	Mitochondiral fusion	Multiple different families
B	3q13-22	*RAB7*	Axonal transport	±Foot ulcers
E and 1F	8p21	*N-FL*	Neurofilament organization	±Hyperkeratosis
Autosomal recessive and X-linked (CMT 2)				
G and K	8q21	*GDAP1*	Neuronal development	±Vocal cord involvement
X1-linked	Xq13.1	*GJB1*	Myelin gap junctions	±CNS, hearing loss, thenar atrophy

CMT, Charcot-Marie-Tooth neuropathy; CNS, central nervous system.
Modified from Klein CJ, Dyck PJ. Genetic testing in inherited peripheral neuropathies. J Peripher Nerv Syst. 2005;10:77-84. Used with permission.

Table 13.10. Examples of Hereditary Multisystem Disorders With Neuropathy

Disease	Inheritance	Locus	Gene	Clinical	Possible treatment
Familial amyloidosis					
Transthyretin amyloidosis	AD	18q11	*Transthyretin*	Varied presentation	Liver transplant
Leukodystrophy					
Metachromatic leukodystrophy	AR	22q13	*Arylsulfatase*	Schwann cell metachromatic granules	Bone marrow transplant
Krabbe disease	AR	14q13	*GALC*	Inclusions in endoneurial macrophages	Bone marrow transplant
Peroxisomal					
Refsum disease	AR	10p	*PAHX*	Varied onion bulb formations	Low phytol—low phytanic acid diet
Fabry disease	XR	Xq22	*Alpha galactosidase*	Osmophilic granules	α-Glactosidase A
Lipoprotein deficiency					
Tangier disease	XR	9q22	*ABC1*	Myelin drops	----
Cerebrotendinous xanthomatosis	AR	2q33	*CYP27A1*	Schwann cell lipids	Chenodeoxycholic acid
Porphyrias					
Acute intermittent porphyria	AD	11q	*Porphobilinogen deaminase*	Axonal>demyelination	Avoidance of precipitant factors
Defective DNA					
Ataxia telangiectasia	AR	11q22	*ATM*	Sensory>motor	Early cancer screening
Mitochondrial defects					
Kearns-Sayre syndrome	Varied	Mt	Varied mutations	Demyelinating radiculopathy	? Superoxide scavengers

AD, autosomal dominant; AR, autosomal recessive; Mt, multiple; XR, X-linked recessive.
Modified from Klein CJ, Dyck PJ. Genetic testing in inherited peripheral neuropathies. J Peripher Nerv Syst. 2005;10:77-84. Used with permission.

that quantitatively measure the responses of nerves to stimulation. Normal findings on nerve conduction studies are of particular value in distinguishing between a central nervous system disorder and myopathies from peripheral nerve disease. Also, nerve conduction studies can localize disease in peripheral nerves, assess the severity of the disease, and characterize nerve disease.

The natural activity in peripheral nerve axons is independent of that in other axons and cannot be recorded readily; however, with the application of an electrical stimulus, all the large myelinated fibers can be discharged simultaneously and the resulting compound action potential can be recorded and measured. If an electrical stimulus (20-100 V for 0.1 millisecond) is applied to a mixed peripheral nerve, action potentials will be initiated that travel in both directions along the nerve. Action potentials traveling centrally are perceived by the patient as an electric shock in the distribution of the nerve stimulated. Action potentials traveling peripherally invade each terminal branch of the nerve, where they can be recorded either from cutaneous sensory branches or from muscles innervated by motor branches. Thus, either the motor or sensory components of the peripheral nerves can be studied selectively. The small, autonomic fibers cannot be readily stimulated and are not assessed with electrophysiologic methods.

The two types of potentials, the compound sensory nerve action potential and the compound muscle action potential, are measured on an oscilloscope. The smaller sensory nerve action potential amplitude is a function of the number of axons that can transmit activity from the point of stimulation to the recording site. The amplitude of a compound muscle action potential is a function of both the number of motor axons in the nerve and the number of muscle fibers that can be activated. The latency is a function of the rate at which the largest fibers in the nerve propagate action potentials along the axon. By measuring the distance traveled and dividing this value by the time, the conduction velocity can be determined (Fig. 13.20). Conduction velocity depends on the diameter of the axon and the extent of myelination of the axons.

No change in the sensory nerve action potential and compound muscle action potential occurs in normal axons or muscle fibers with repetitive stimulation at rates of up to 40 per second. In disorders of the neuromuscular junction and some nerve disorders, the axons cannot respond this rapidly.

Peripheral Nerve Diseases

The presence of peripheral nerve disease is reflected primarily in nerve conduction studies. In an axolemmal disorder, the action potential is blocked in the region of the abnormality. Stimulation distal to this point produces normal responses, but stimulation proximal to the abnormality produces either no response or only a response with reduced amplitude. Axoplasmic disorders with axonal narrowing result in slowing of conduction, whereas those with axonal degeneration result in decreased amplitude or absence of response to stimulation. In myelin disorders, slowing of conduction is more prominent, with progressive loss of amplitude on more proximal stimulation.

Localized lesions of a peripheral nerve produce a local block or a localized slowing of conduction in the region of the damage. The block results in a smaller evoked response with proximal rather than with distal stimulation (Fig. 13.21). In diffuse nerve disease, segmental demyelinating disorders have prominent slowing of conduction (Fig. 13.22) with dispersion of the compound muscle action potential, and axonal dystrophies have predominantly a loss of amplitude, especially distally.

Neuromuscular Junction Diseases

Disorders of neuromuscular transmission are characterized by progressive loss of amplitude of an evoked motor response with repetitive stimulation, especially at rates of 2 to 5 per second. The two major forms, myasthenia gravis and Lambert-Eaton myasthenic syndrome, can be distinguished by their response to exercise or rapid repetitive stimulation. Lambert-Eaton myasthenic syndrome shows an increment of the compound muscle action potentials, whereas myasthenia gravis shows a decrement.

Muscle Disease

In primary muscle disease, sensory nerve action potentials are normal. Compound muscle action potentials have normal conduction velocity; amplitude is reduced only if atrophy is pronounced.

Electromyography

Nerve conduction studies are usually performed in conjunction with electromyography because they use similar techniques and complement each other in arriving at diagnoses for both peripheral nerve and muscle diseases.

Muscle function can be evaluated by measuring the electrical activity with electromyography during a needle examination (Fig. 13.23). The spontaneous and voluntary electrical potentials in muscle are less than 50 μV recorded on the surface and need to be recorded with a small needle electrode inserted into the muscle and with amplification to both hear and see them. Electromyography provides information about the presence and type of disease involving muscle. Because nerve disorders produce

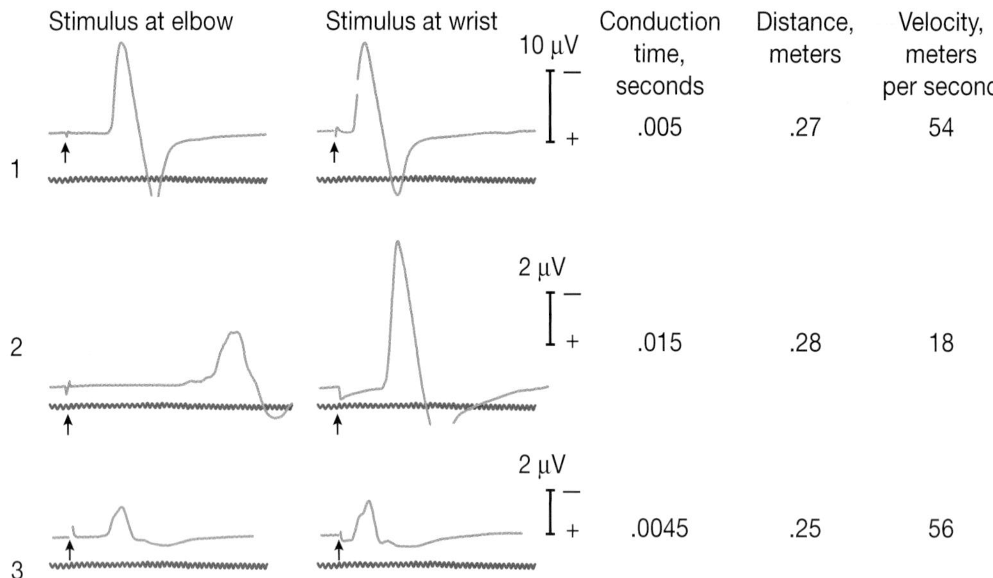

Fig. 13.20. Measurement of conduction velocity (distance traveled divided by time required). *1*, Normal. *2*, Neuropathy: conduction velocity is slowed along entire nerve, and amplitude is reduced with proximal stimulation because of dispersion of the response. *3*, Myopathy: conduction velocity is normal, but amplitude is reduced because of muscle atrophy. (From Department of Neurology, Mayo Clinic and Mayo Foundation, Clinical examinations in neurology. 6th ed. St. Louis: Mosby Year Book; 1991. Used with permission.)

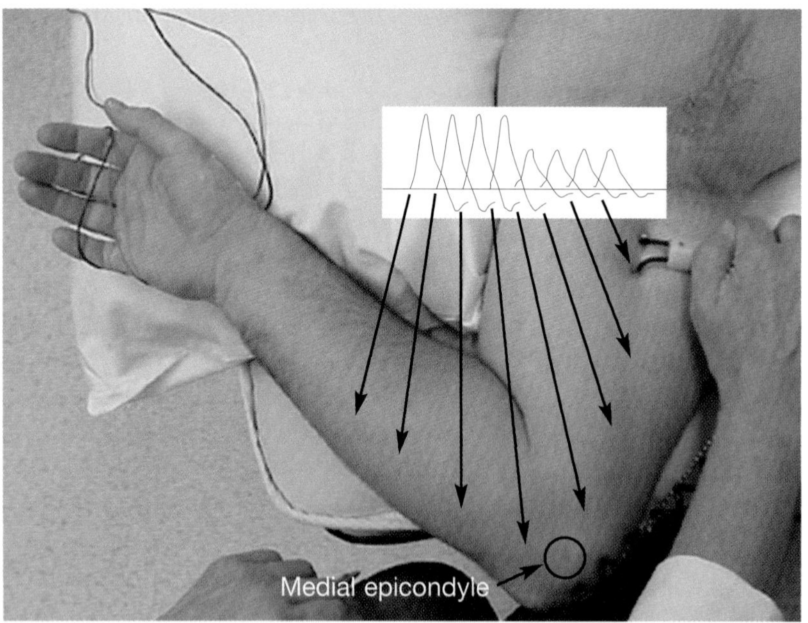

Fig. 13.21. Nerve conduction studies in a patient with ulnar neuropathy at the elbow. Stimulation is applied at 2-cm intervals along the nerve proximal and distal to the elbow (*arrows*). Note the localized partial block of conduction (decreased amplitude proximal to the elbow) at the medial epicondyle. Weakness is proportional to the reduction in the amplitude of the compound muscle action potential. This is usually due to acute local compression and can recover quickly.

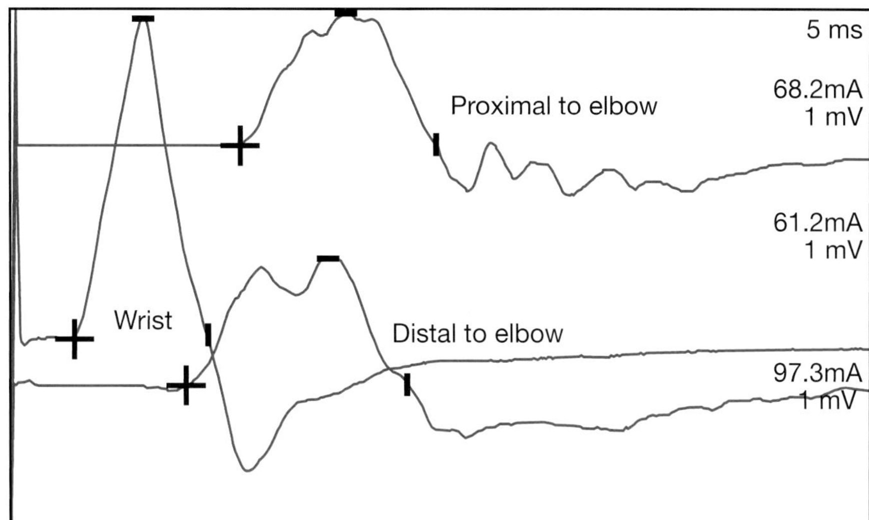

Fig. 13.22. Ulnar nerve conduction study in Guillain-Barré syndrome, or acute inflammatory demyelinating neuropathy. The compound muscle action potentials with nerve stimulation at the wrist, distal to the elbow, and proximal to the elbow show progressive dispersion because of differential slowing of conduction in the axons. Conduction velocity is markedly slowed for the fastest conducting fibers at 23 m/s.

secondary changes in muscle, electromyography is valuable not only in diagnosis of primary muscle disease but also in differentiating neurogenic disorders, diseases of neuromuscular transmission, and diseases of the central nervous system.

In electromyography, a needle electrode is inserted into a muscle and the electrical activity at rest and with voluntary activation is recorded on an oscilloscope and loudspeaker. The recorded potentials are characterized by their amplitude, duration, and firing patterns. Recordings are made in multiple muscles in three states: at rest, with needle movement, and with voluntary activity. With voluntary contraction of the muscle, the motor units fire repetitively, in an orderly fashion, with a frequency and number of motor unit potentials proportional to the effort exerted. Motor unit potentials are measured to determine their amplitude, duration, and firing rate. Myopathies can be differentiated on the basis of the characteristic motor unit potentials (Fig. 13.23). In a primary myopathy with random degeneration of muscle fibers, each motor unit has a reduced innervation ratio and the motor unit potentials are of short duration and low amplitude (Fig. 13.24). Because of the decrease in power of each motor unit, many more will fire for any given strength than in a normal muscle (rapid recruitment).

At rest, there is electrical silence in a normal muscle, except in the region of motor end plates where end plate potentials may be recorded (Fig. 13.25). If some muscle fibers are partially destroyed in a myopathy, the still viable portions may fire spontaneously (fibrillate) (Fig. 13.25). In sarcolemmal disorders, there is an overall reduction in activity, with small motor unit potentials. Myopathies, like the myotonic dystrophies with membrane irritability, have characteristic, spontaneous discharges called *myotonic discharges* (Fig. 13.25). In disorders of excitation-contraction coupling, no abnormality is recorded on electromyography.

In contrast to the changes in myopathy, a neurogenic disorder produces primarily a loss in the number of motor unit potentials and is seen as poor recruitment with increasing effort and a small number of units firing rapidly with stronger effort. In addition, if there has been chronic denervation with opportunity for reinnervation and a resultant increase in innervation ratio, the motor unit

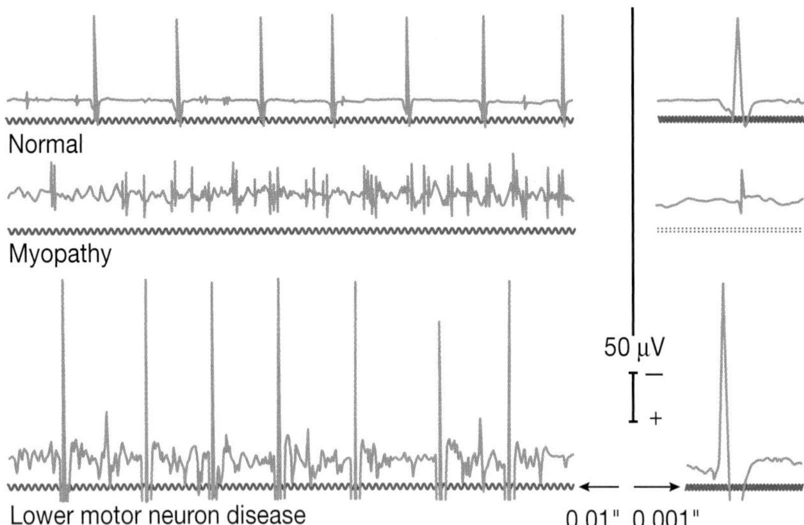

Fig. 13.23. Changes in voluntary motor unit potentials with disease during electromyography. Motor unit potentials during voluntary contraction in a normal person, small motor unit potentials in muscular dystrophy (myopathy), and large motor unit potentials in amyotrophic lateral sclerosis (lower motor neuron disease). Potentials on the left are displayed with a slow time base and those on the right, with a fast time base.

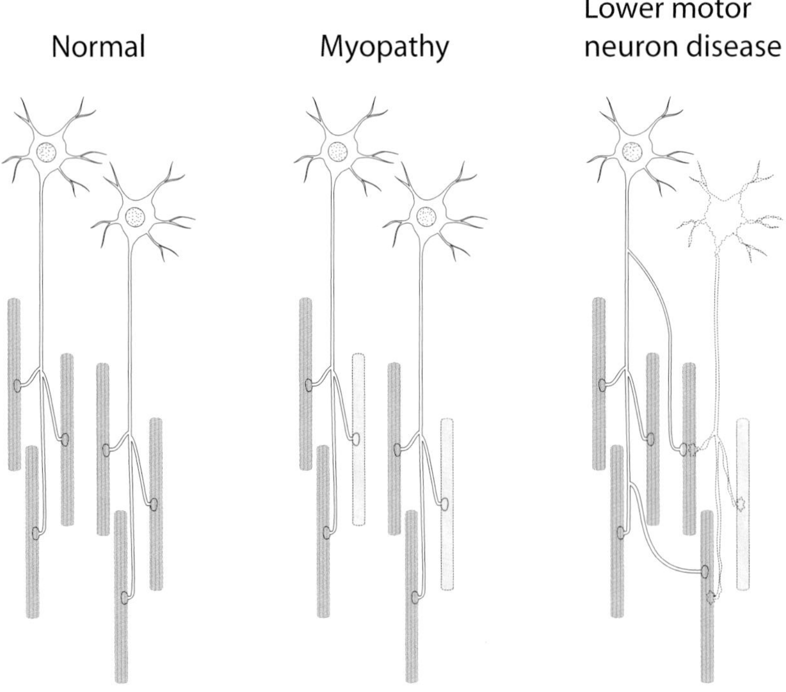

Fig. 13.24. Alteration in innervation patterns in peripheral disease. Myopathy shows random loss (green) of muscle fibers from all motor units. Neurogenic atrophy (lower motor neuron disease) shows loss of innervation of all fibers in a motor unit, with partial reinnervation by surviving axons.

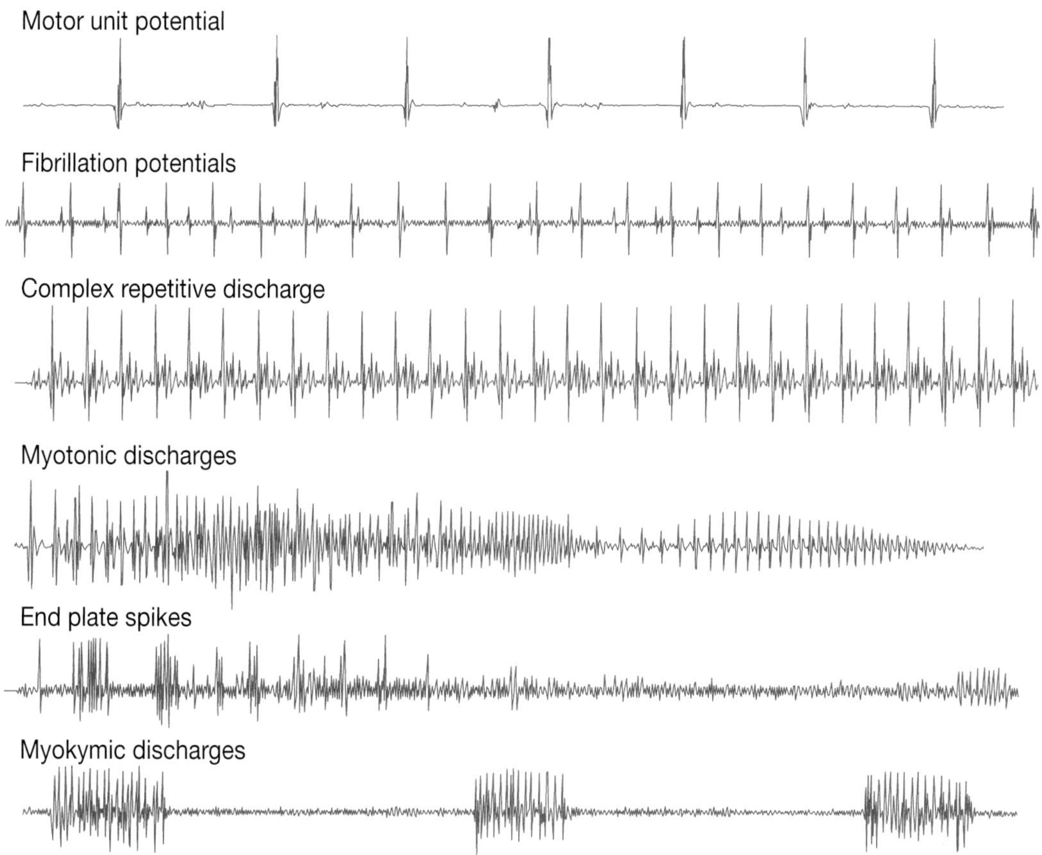

Fig. 13.25. Potentials recorded during clinical electromyography. A single, normal motor unit potential is shown in the top trace. Fibrillation potentials that occur with muscle fiber denervation are shown in the second trace. End plate spikes are normal discharges recorded in the end plate region. Complex repetitive discharges and myokymic discharges occur in different neurogenic disorders, and myotonic discharges occur with several muscle diseases.

potentials will show long duration and high amplitude (Fig. 13.23 and 13.25). Any muscle fibers that are denervated because of axonal degeneration fibrillate (Fig. 13.25). If a motor unit is irritable, single brief twitches (fasciculation) of the muscle fibers in a motor unit occur.

Diseases of neuromuscular transmission are characterized by variable conduction blocks in individual neuromuscular junctions with variations in the amplitude of the motor unit potentials during voluntary contraction. If a sufficient number are blocked, the motor unit potentials will be small as well as unstable.

In upper motor neuron disease, the motor units appear normal and recruit normally but fire slowly (poor activation).

By combining the findings from electromyography and nerve conduction studies, it is often possible to localize the disease in the periphery and, at times, to specific sites to characterize the general type of disorder and to assist in determining the severity or prognosis of the disorder.

Biopsy

Nerve Biopsy

In some peripheral nerve diseases, clinical, biochemical, genetic, and immunologic testing and electrophysiologic studies do not identify the nature of the abnormality. For these patients, a nerve biopsy specimen, usually of a fascicle of the sural nerve, is studied. Nerve biopsy specimens are best studied in three ways: by light microscopy of nerve bundles, teased fiber studies, and cross-sectional fiber counts. For ordinary light microscopy, a piece of nerve is fixed and stained with standard histologic stains and special stains for specific diseases. For instance, in leprosy, *Mycobacterium leprae* can be stained with acid-fast stains. In metachromatic leukodystrophy or amyloidosis, specific stains demonstrate the accumulation of abnormal materials.

If another portion of the nerve is fixed and stained for myelin, it can be teased or pulled apart into single fibers. These single fibers can be examined for the presence of segmental demyelination, paranodal loss of myelin, or other characteristic changes such as the presence of linear rows of myelin ovoids after axonal degeneration (Fig. 13.26). Also, the diameter and length of the internodes can be measured. Plots of the internodal length compared with the axon diameter can give quantitative estimates of the presence of myelin disorders.

Cross sections of a portion of the nerve can be studied with myelin stains, and the diameters of the fibers can be measured and plotted as density of fibers. The selective loss of certain fiber types can be determined quantitatively.

Muscle Biopsy

Although at times the clinical history or pattern of muscle impairment can permit the diagnosis of a myopathy, the clinical, biochemical, immunologic, and electrophysiologic findings often do not provide a specific diagnosis. In these situations, muscle biopsy can identify the presence of a myopathy (Fig. 13.27). Biopsy, like electromyography and nerve conduction studies, can differentiate muscle abnormalities due to neurogenic disorders (neurogenic atrophy) (Fig. 13.28) from those due to primary myopathy (Fig. 13.27). In the latter case, muscle biopsy can often provide an even more specific diagnosis (Fig. 13.29).

Muscle biopsy specimens are taken from a muscle that shows moderate (but not severe) weakness. In

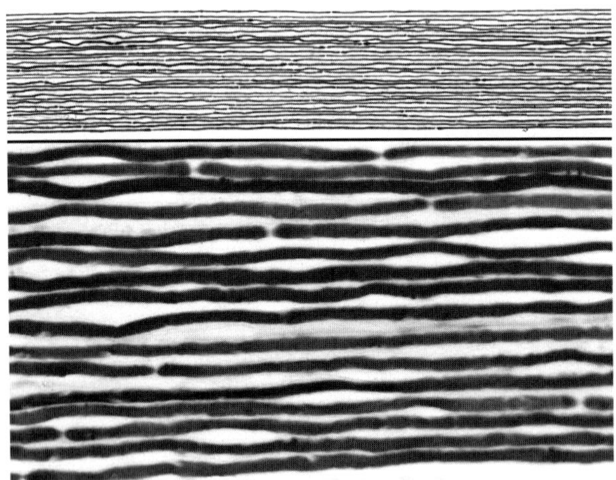

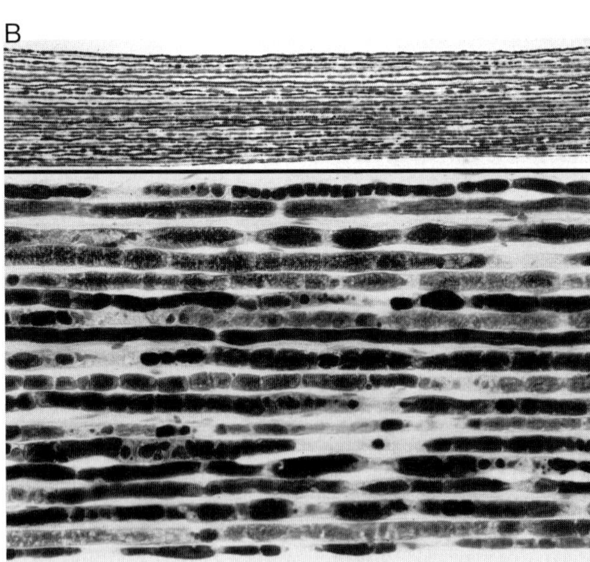

Fig. 13.26. *A*, Low- (*upper*) and intermediate- (*lower*) power light microscopic views of about one-quarter of the length of teased fibers laid side by side to illustrate that the method of teasing allows fibers to be visualized for long distances along their length. The teased fibers are from the sural nerve of a healthy subject. All fibers would be graded as normal. *B*, Low- (*upper*) and intermediate- (*lower*) power light microscopic views of teased fibers from the sural nerve of a patient with necrotizing vasculitis, showing severe axonal degeneration. (From Dyck PJ, Dyck PJB, Engelstad J. Pathologic alterations of nerves. In: Dyck PJ, Thomas PK, editors. Peripheral neuropathy. 4th ed. Philadelphia: Elsevier; 2005. Used with permission.)

severe weakness, so much muscle may be replaced by fat or connective tissue that a diagnosis cannot be made. The specimen is treated with standard stains such as hematoxylin and eosin or trichrome and histochemical stains that show different fiber types to identify inflammation, muscle fiber destruction, or specific structural changes in the fibers. Myositis of different types is the most common myopathy and shows inflammatory cells. Biopsy can differentiate forms of myositis. Specific stains can identify the glycogen in glycogen storage diseases or lipid in lipid storage disease. Fiber-type grouping provides evidence of neurogenic disease, and the presence of specific materials may allow the diagnosis of a specific myopathy.

Summary

Diagnosis of diseases at the peripheral level is based on the medical history, clinical findings, and laboratory tests. Peripheral lesions that affect the axon, neuromuscular junction, and muscle produce a lower motor neuron pattern of weakness that can be differentiated from disorders that involve the alpha motor neuron or ventral root (Fig. 13.30). Involvement of sensory and autonomic functions as well as motor function suggests peripheral neuropathy. Clinical and electrophysiologic features can identify a pathologic process such as demyelination, axonal loss, or both (Table 13.11). Fluctuating weakness (fatigability) is typical of a neuromuscular transmission defect. In prejunctional disorders with impaired release of acetylcholine (Lambert-Eaton myasthenic syndrome), there is hyporeflexia or areflexia and cholinergic autonomic impairment (dry mouth, impotence) and normal sensation with the fatigability. Fatigability with normal sensation and preservation of reflexes suggests myasthenia gravis. Proximal muscle weakness with or without atrophy in association with normal sensation and preservation of reflexes suggests muscle disease. The main clinical and pathophysiologic features that typically differentiate neuropathy from myopathy are summarized in Table 13.12 and Figure 13.31.

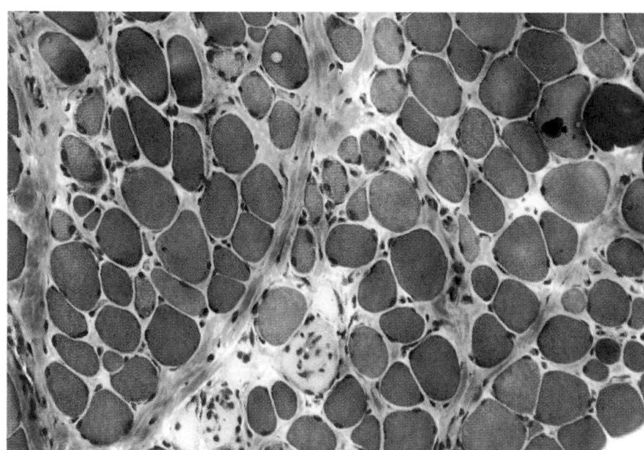

Fig. 13.27. Transverse section of muscle from a patient with Duchenne muscular dystrophy showing the general histologic features of myopathy. There is random variation in fiber diameter, with both large and small fibers. Some fibers have internal migration of nuclei, some are splitting or degenerating, and there is an increase in connective tissue. (Trichome stain; ×200.) (Courtesy of A. G. Engel, MD, Muscle Laboratory, Mayo Clinic College of Medicine, Rochester, MN.)

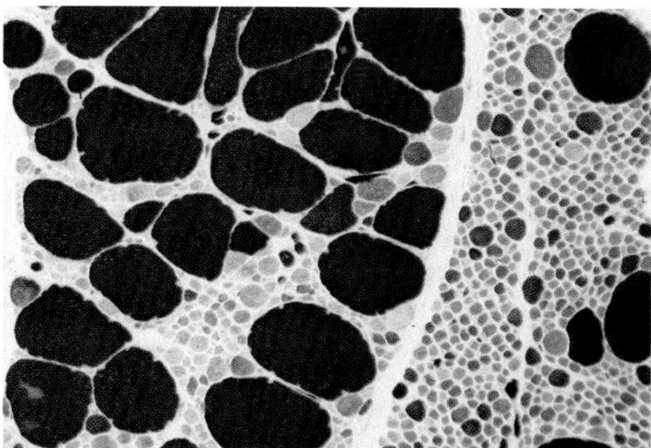

Fig. 13.28. Histologic changes in neurogenic atrophy in a transverse section of partially reinnervated muscle fibers. Type I fibers are stained lightly and type II fibers darkly. Note the loss of the normal checkerboard pattern; instead, there is grouping of similar fiber types and a mixture of hypertrophic fibers and atrophic fibers that have not been reinnervated. (ATPase stain; ×200.) (Courtesy of A. G. Engel, MD, Muscle Laboratory, Mayo Clinic College of Medicine, Rochester, MN.)

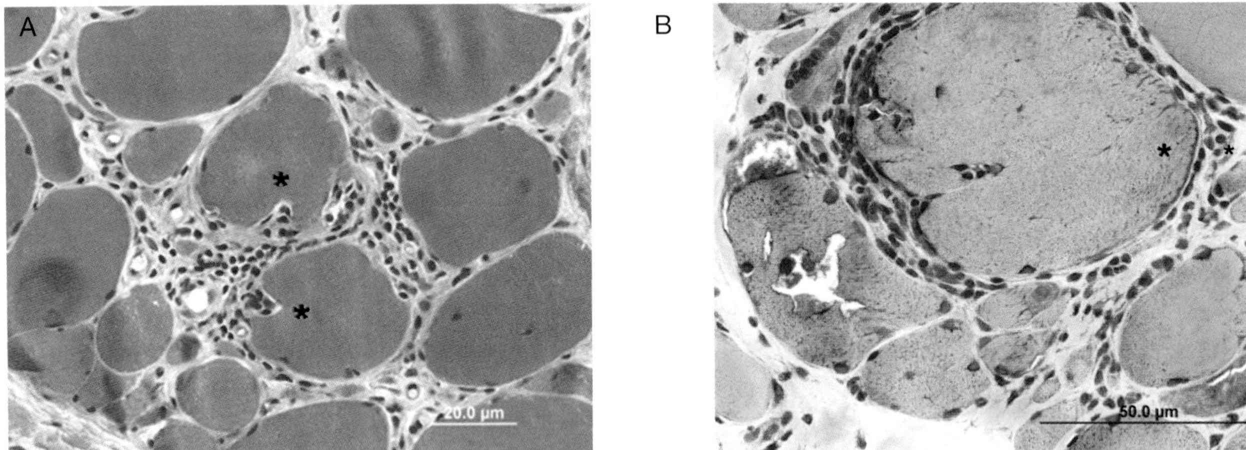

Fig. 13.29. Two forms of myositis. *A*, Polymyositis with inflammatory cells in the endomysium surrounding the muscle fibers and variation in fiber diameter (both large and small fibers). Some fibers have internal migration of nuclei, some are splitting or degenerating, and there is an increase in connective tissue. Two fibers in the center of the field are being invaded by inflammatory cells (*). (H&E; ×200.) *B*, Like polymyositis, inclusion body myositis has inflammatory cells in the endomysium, fibers invaded by inflammatory cells, internal migration of nuclei, fiber splitting, fiber degeneration, and an increase in connective tissue. Inclusion body myositis is differentiated by the subsarcolemmal granules (*). (Trichrome stain; ×200.) (Courtesy of A. G. Engel, MD, Muscle Laboratory, Mayo Clinic College of Medicine, Rochester, MN.)

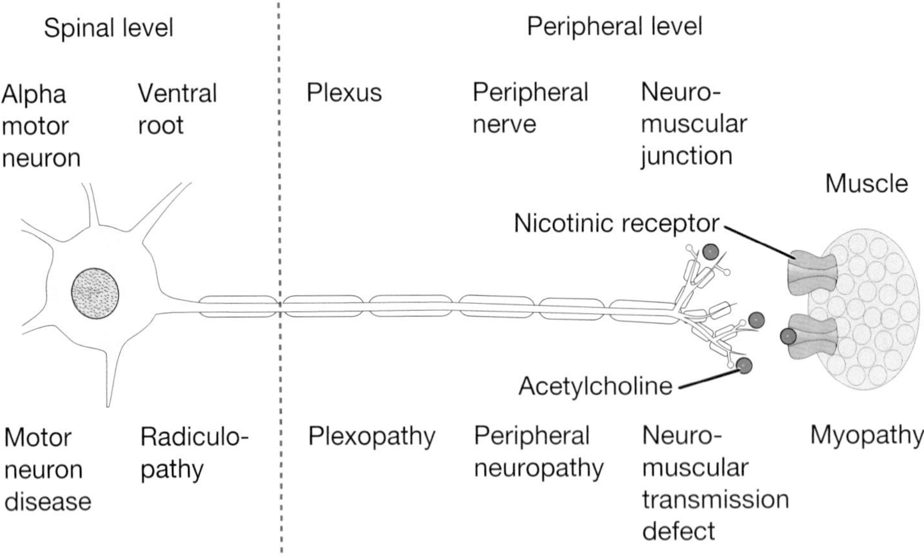

Fig. 13.30. Localization of lesions producing lower motor neuron syndromes at the central and peripheral levels. Disorders of the spinal nerve, plexus, and peripheral nerves may produce demyelination, axon loss, or both. They generally are associated with sensory and autonomic manifestations because of the involvement of several types of axons. Disorders of neuromuscular transmission may be prejunctional (due to impaired release of acetylcholine) or postjunctional (disorders involving the nicotinic acetylcholine receptor). Muscle disorders may produce muscle fiber loss or affect membrane excitability or force of muscle contraction.

Table 13.11. Differences Between Demyelinating and Axonal Neuropathies

Feature	Neuropathy type	
	Demyelinating	Axonal
Mechanism of weakness	Conduction block	Axonal loss
Atrophy	No or late (disuse)	Yes
Fasciculations	No	Yes
Mechanism of recovery	Remyelination	Axonal sprouting (reinnervation)
Nerve conduction velocities	Slow	Normal or slightly decreased
Motor action potential amplitudes	Normal or smaller distally than proximally, with temporal dispersion	Equally small distally and proximally
Fibrillation potentials	No	Yes
Recruitment	Poor	Poor
Motor unit potentials	Normal	Large, long duration, polyphasic

Table 13.12. Differences Between Neuropathy and Myopathy (Typical Cases)

Feature	Neuropathy	Myopathy
Distribution of weakness	Distal more than proximal	Proximal more than distal
Atrophy	Yes (mostly distal)	Yes (generally proximal)
Fasciculations	Yes	No
Reflexes	Decreased	Normal or decreased (late)
Sensory loss	Yes	No
Autonomic dysfunction	Sometimes	No
Creatine kinase	Normal	Increased levels (in most cases)
Electromyography		
Conduction velocity	Decreased	Normal
Sensory action potential amplitude	Decreased	Normal
Fibrillation potentials	Yes	Occasionally
Recruitment	Decreased	Increased
Motor unit panel	Long duration, large amplitude, polyphasic	Short duration, low amplitude, polyphasic
Muscle biopsy	Group atrophy	Variable muscle fiber size
	Fiber-type grouping	Inclusions

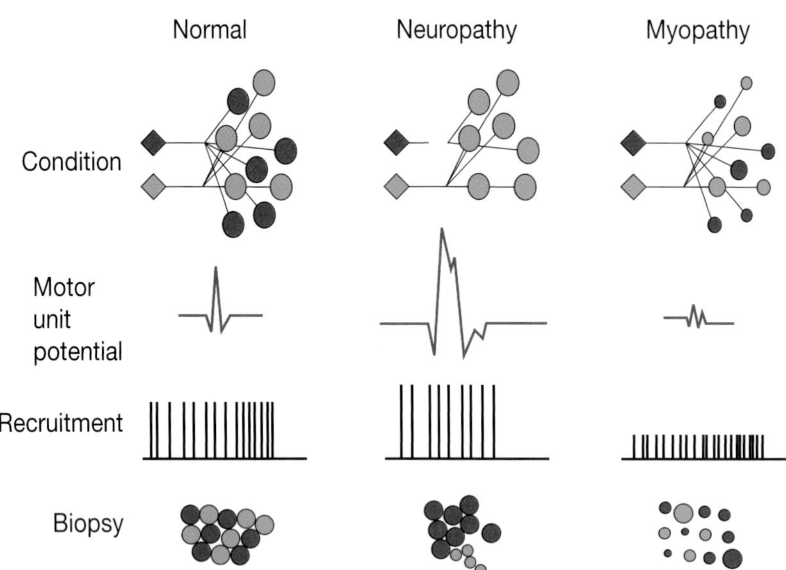

Fig. 13.31. Organization of the motor unit in normal conditions, neuropathy, and myopathy. In neuropathy, there is loss of motor units and axonal sprouting, with reinnervation of the muscle fibers by surviving axons. This is characterized by reduced motor unit recruitment during increased effort; long duration, large-amplitude polyphasic motor unit potentials; and group atrophy, with fiber-type grouping seen in a muscle biopsy specimen. In myopathy, there is a loss of muscle fibers in the motor units, but the total number of motor units is preserved. This is characterized by increased motor unit recruitment with increased effort, short duration, small-amplitude polyphasic motor unit potentials, and variable size and intermingling of normal and atrophic muscle fibers seen in muscle biopsy specimen.

Additional Reading

Daube JR, editor. Clinical neurophysiology. 2nd ed. Oxford: Oxford University Press; 2002.

Dyck PJ, Thomas PK, editors. Peripheral neuropathy. 4th ed. Philadelphia, PA: Elsevier; 2005.

Engel AG, Franzini-Armstrong C, editors. Myology: basic and clinical. 3rd ed. New York: McGraw-Hill; 2004.

Kimura J. Peripheral nerve diseases. Philadelphia, PA: Elsevier; 2006.

Stalberg E. Clinical neurophysiology of disorders of muscle and neuromuscular junction, including fatigue. Philadelphia, PA: Elsevier; 2003.

Chapter 14

The Spinal Level

Objectives

1. Name and identify the longitudinal systems and the transverse segments at the spinal level.
2. Describe the components of the dorsal roots and ventral roots of the spinal nerves.
3. Describe the relation between the spinal cord segments or spinal nerves and the corresponding vertebral level.
4. Describe the blood supply of the spinal cord, and name the segments most vulnerable to ischemia.
5. Describe the morphology of the spinal cord in a transverse section, and identify the different spinal cord levels on this basis.
6. Describe the types of projection neurons and interneurons that form the different laminae of Rexed in the gray matter.
7. Describe the origin and functions of the dorsal columns, dorsal spinocerebellar tract, spinothalamic tract, spinoreticular tract, and propriospinal system.
8. Describe the wind-up phenomenon and the consequences of central sensitization of dorsal horn neurons.
9. Describe the pathway and function of the muscle stretch reflex and the effects of fusimotor inputs and Ia inhibitory interneurons.
10. Describe the functions of the Golgi tendon organ and polysynaptic proprioceptive and nociceptive reflexes.
11. Describe the functions of spinal cord interneurons.
12. Describe functions of the corticospinal, rubrospinal, lateral vestibulospinal, and reticulospinal systems.
13. Describe reciprocal inhibition, recurrent inhibition, presynaptic inhibition, and spinal shock.
14. Describe and give examples of the stretch reflex and flexion reflex.
15. List the spinal nerves and cord segments that mediate the biceps, triceps, knee, and ankle reflexes.
16. List the symptoms and signs associated with lesions of the spinal cord at levels C3, C6, T6, L5, and S2.
17. List the features that differentiate an extramedullary lesion from an intramedullary lesion.
18. List the major clinicopathologic features of multiple sclerosis and pernicious anemia.

Introduction

The spinal level includes the vertebral column and its contents. The spinal canal within the vertebral column is the passage formed by the vertebrae. It extends from the foramen magnum of the skull through the sacrum of the spinal column and contains the spinal cord, nerve roots, spinal nerves, meninges, and the vascular supply of the spinal cord. Five of the major systems are represented in the spinal canal: the sensory, motor, internal regulation, vascular, and cerebrospinal fluid systems. The vascular and cerebrospinal fluid structures are the support systems of the spinal cord. Diseases of the spinal canal involve one or more of these systems and produce patterns of disease distinctive to this level. The anatomical and physiologic characteristics of the spinal cord and spinal nerves that permit the identification and localization of diseases in the spinal canal are presented in this chapter.

Overview

The spinal cord and nerve roots have a segmental organization. The segments along the length of the spinal cord are named to correspond to the vertebrae related to the spinal nerve roots. Nerve roots may be located above or below the corresponding vertebra, according to the longitudinal level of the spinal cord:

1. Cervical: the cephalad portion of the spinal cord from which eight pairs of ventral and seven pairs of dorsal roots arise to form the cervical spinal nerves.
2. Thoracic: the middle portion of the spinal cord from which 12 pairs of nerve roots arise to form the thoracic spinal nerves.
3. Lumbar: the upper caudal portion of the spinal cord from which five lumbar nerve roots arise to form the lumbar spinal nerves.
4. Sacral: the caudal end of the cord from which five pairs of sacral nerve roots arise. The conus medullaris is the termination of the spinal cord from which sacral nerve roots arise.

As seen in cross section, the spinal canal is divided into major structures from the center to the periphery: central canal, gray matter, white matter, blood vessels, nerve roots and spinal nerves, meninges, and subarachnoid and epidural spaces.

As in other areas of the nervous system, two distinct patterns of abnormality occur with disease of the nervous system: segmental and longitudinal. Damage to segmental structures, including the dorsal roots, dorsal horn, ventral horn, or ventral roots, produces signs localized to one segment of the body. The dorsal roots entering at a given spinal cord segment contain the central processes of dorsal root ganglion neurons and thus convey all types of sensory information from the corresponding dermatome and myotome. Therefore, segmental lesions that affect the dorsal roots cause the loss of all sensory modalities in the corresponding segment of the body. Segmental lesions that affect the alpha motor neurons in the ventral horn deprive the effector muscle of its excitatory and trophic innervation, leading to flaccid paralysis, atrophy, and fasciculation of that muscle. Segmental lesions also lead to loss of the corresponding segmental muscle stretch reflex. Segmental damage of preganglionic autonomic neurons may result in loss of activity of the corresponding effector ganglion neurons and, thus, their target. In summary, segmental signs of lesions at the spinal level include the following:

1. Loss of all sensory modalities in the corresponding segment of the body (dermatome), reflecting loss of dorsal root axons or dorsal horn neurons.
2. Flaccid weakness, atrophy, and fasciculations because of damage of the alpha motor neurons in the ventral horn or their axons traveling in the ventral root and innervating specific myotomes.
3. Absence of segmental muscle stretch reflexes because of impairment of the afferent or efferent (or both) limb of the reflex arc.
4. In some cases, segmental loss of function of specific visceral effectors, reflecting damage of preganglionic neurons of the intermediate gray matter.

These segmental findings allow lesions to be localized along the length of the spinal cord.

These segmental signs are recognized as originating at the spinal level, as opposed to the peripheral level, by the associated involvement of ascending or descending tracts in the spinal white matter, which produces intersegmental signs. The most important white matter pathways are the dorsal column, spinothalamic, and corticospinal paths. Damage to any of these systems produces intersegmental deficits in that system for all functions below the level of the lesion. Damage to the dorsal columns impairs discriminative touch, vibration, and proprioceptive information from the same side of the body. Damage to the spinothalamic tract, located in the anterolateral quadrant of the spinal cord, impairs pain, temperature, and visceral sensations from the contralateral side of the body. Involvement of the corticospinal tract, which descends in the dorsolateral quadrant of the spinal cord, and reticulospinal pathways, which descend in the anterior and anterolateral quadrants, produces ipsilateral weakness, hyperreflexia, spasticity, and the Babinski sign. The varied combination of deficits resulting from damage to these pathways, alone or in combination, produces specific syndromes that allow the lesion to be localized across the transverse plane of the spinal cord.

Spinal Cord Anatomy

External Morphology

Spinal Nerve Roots and Spinal Nerves

The spinal cord in the adult extends from the foramen magnum to the lower border of the first lumbar vertebra (L1). The spinal cord is roughly cylindrical, with a slight anteroposterior flattening. Two areas along its length are wider than other areas. These are the cervical and lumbar enlargements, from which arises the innervation of the upper and lower extremities. The caudal end of the spinal cord tapers to form the *conus medullaris* (Fig. 14.1).

Nerve fibers enter the spinal cord and exit from it by the *spinal nerve roots* (Fig. 14.2 and 14.3). They are subdivided into *dorsal* (or posterior) *roots* containing sensory (afferent) axons, and *ventral* (or anterior) *roots* containing motor (efferent) axons. The *dorsal root ganglia* contain the cell bodies of the nerve fibers in the dorsal root and are seen as an enlargement of the dorsal root.

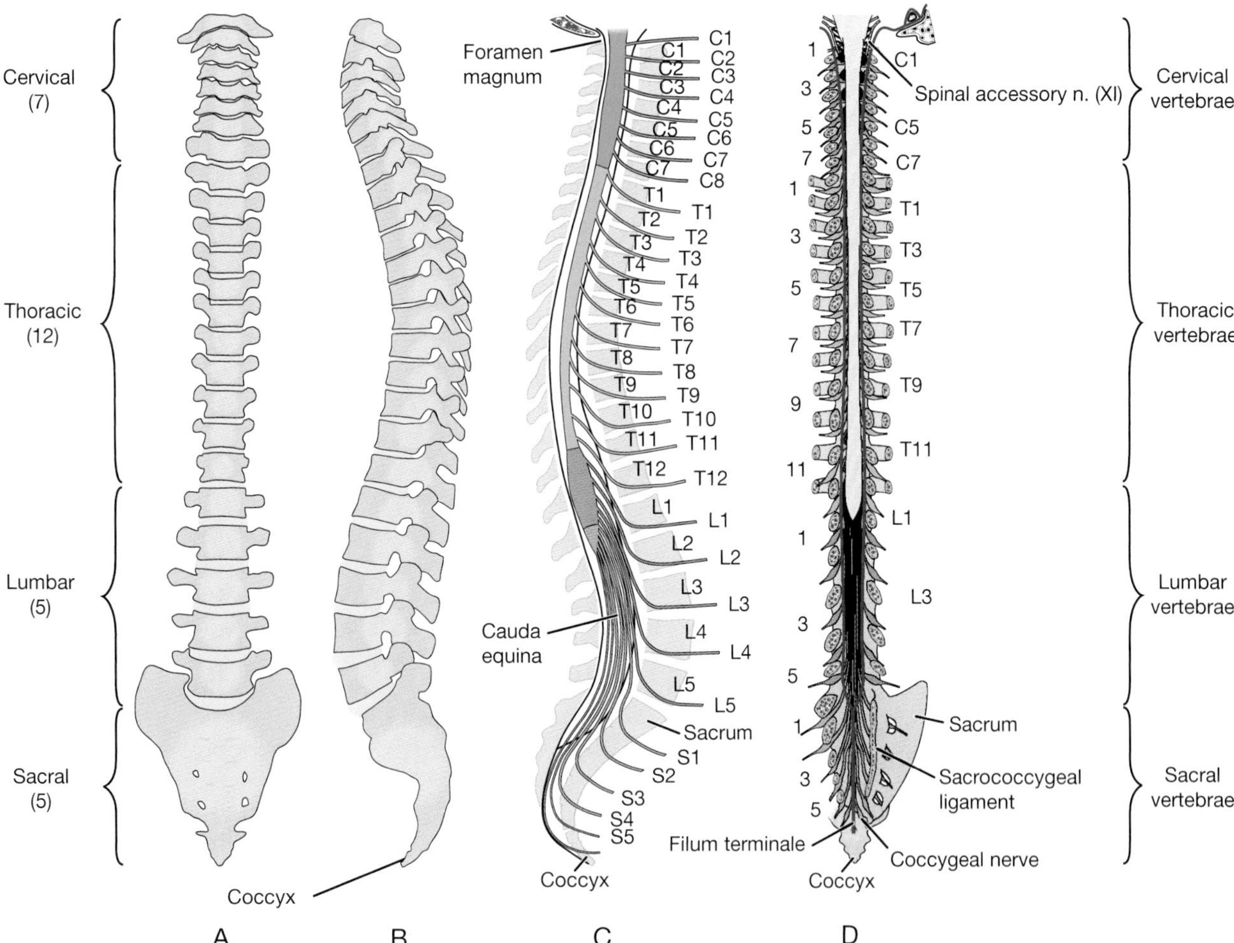

Fig. 14.1. The relation between the spinal column and cord. *A*, Ventral view of the spine. *B*, Left lateral view of the spine. *C*, Right lateral view of the spinal cord and roots in the spine. *D*, Dorsal view of the spinal cord.

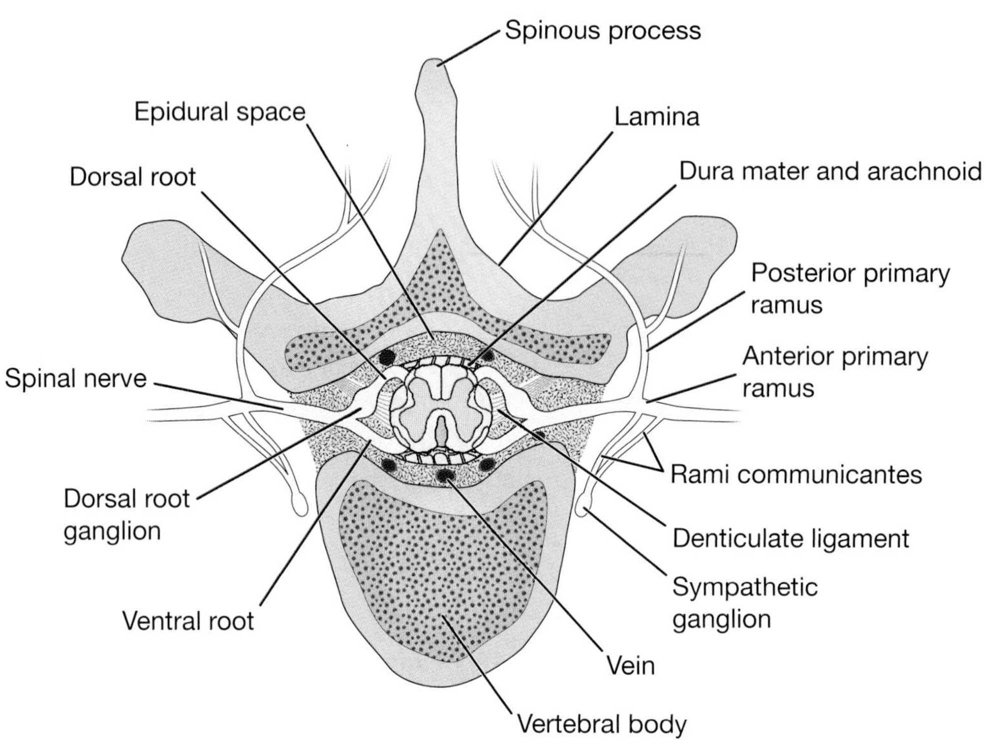

Fig. 14.2. Cross section of the spinal canal showing the spinal cord, its meningeal coverings, and the formation and exit of the spinal nerves.

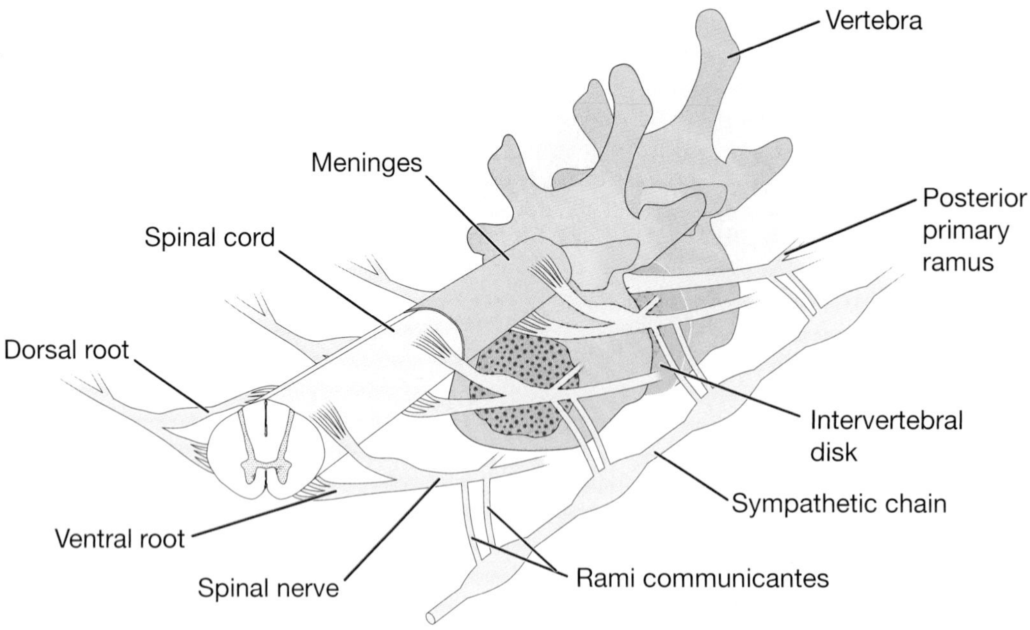

Fig. 14.3. Formation of a spinal nerve as it leaves the spinal canal through the intervertebral foramen.

The surface of the spinal cord has several longitudinal furrows. The ventral (anterior) surface is indented by the deep ventral median fissure. The dorsal (posterior) surface contains a shallow dorsal median sulcus. The dorsal spinal roots enter each side of the spinal cord along the dorsolateral sulcus. Dorsal intermediate sulci extend from the rostral cervical to the midthoracic spinal cord, between the dorsal root entry zone and the midline.

The dorsal and ventral roots join laterally at the *intervertebral foramen* to form a *spinal nerve* (Fig. 14.2). The foramen is the bony canal formed by two adjacent vertebrae. Thirty-one pairs of spinal nerves are formed and divide the cord into 8 cervical, 12 thoracic, 5 lumbar, and 5 sacral segments and 1 coccygeal segment. Each spinal segment except the first and last has a dorsal and ventral root. Spinal roots emerge on each side of a spinal segment and become ensheathed by dura mater as they unite to form a spinal nerve. In the intervertebral foramen, the dura mater merges with the perineurium of peripheral nerves.

The dorsal and ventral roots are contained entirely within the spinal canal, are bathed in cerebrospinal fluid, and are anchored in the intervertebral foramina at the point where their dural sleeves terminate. Spinal nerves are very short nerves in which the motor, sensory, and autonomic components of a single cord segment are united in a single structure as they exit from the spinal canal through the intervertebral foramen (Fig. 14.4). Because a spinal nerve is surrounded by this bony structure, it is particularly vulnerable to local compression by tumor, a herniated nucleus pulposus, or arthritic changes in the bone. Flexion of the spinal cord or traction on a peripheral nerve (e.g., with disk herniation or local tumor) can stretch and irritate a spinal nerve and cause pain.

Each spinal nerve is derived from a segment of the spinal cord, and the names of the nerves correspond to the names of the segments. Because there are only seven

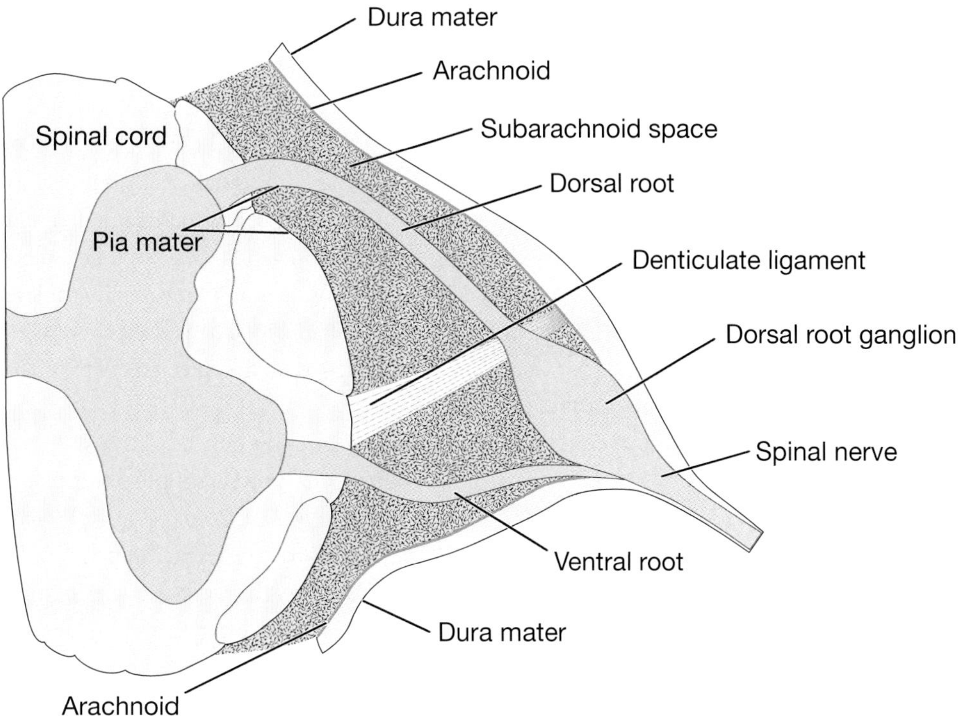

Fig. 14.4. Meningeal relations at the spinal level. The denticulate ligaments attach the spinal cord to the dura mater laterally.

cervical vertebrae, 1) spinal nerves C1 through C7 exit above the pedicle of the vertebra of the same number, 2) spinal nerve C8 emerges between vertebrae C7 and T1, and 3) caudal to T1, a spinal nerve exits below the vertebra of the same number.

Early in development, each spinal cord segment is at the same level as the corresponding vertebra. With growth, the vertebral column elongates more than the spinal cord does and the spinal roots are displaced caudally. The roots of rostral cord segments are displaced less than those of caudal segments. Therefore, the lumbar and sacral nerves have long spinal roots that descend within the dural sac to reach their vertebral level of exit. These long roots are called the cauda equina because they resemble a horse's tail.

Because of the difference in length between the vertebral column and the spinal cord, care must be taken to specify vertebral level or spinal segment level when indicating the location of a lesion. Generally in a neurologic problem, the affected spinal segment is defined first, and then an attempt is made to correlate this with the appropriate vertebral level. However, in cases of vertebral lesions, the level of vertebral involvement is often seen on a neuroimaging study such as plain radiography, computed tomography (CT), or magnetic resonance imaging (MRI), and then the level of a possible spinal cord injury is determined. The general guidelines for locating the level of a spinal cord injury with respect to the vertebrae are as follows:

- The cervical enlargement at the C7 cord segment is centered at the C7 vertebral level.
- Between T1 and T10, add 2 to the number of the vertebral spine to determine the spinal cord segment at the same location.
- The lumbar segments of the spinal cord are approximately at the level of the spinous processes of T11 and T12.
- Sacral and coccygeal segments are at the level of the Ll spinous process.

The dorsal roots transmit sensory input from cutaneous, somatic, muscular, and visceral receptors. The cell bodies of these axons are in the dorsal root ganglia. Each spinal nerve is distributed to a well-defined area of skin called a *dermatome* (Fig. 14.5 and Table 14.1). Dermatomes of adjacent spinal nerves overlap. This overlap accounts for the variation in sensory loss of patients with spinal nerve lesions. The ventral roots contain the myelinated axons of the motor neurons innervating the somatic musculature; these axons are distributed to specific groups of muscles called *myotomes* (Table 14.2).

Meninges

The spinal cord is ensheathed by the pia mater, arachnoid, and dura mater. The arachnoid is a nonvascular membrane separated from the pia mater by the subarachnoid space, which contains cerebrospinal fluid.

The spinal cord is anchored to the inner surface of the dura mater by a series of lateral collagenous bands, called denticulate ligaments, derived from the pia mater (Fig. 14.2). From 18 to 24 of these ligaments firmly attach the pia mater midway between the dorsal and ventral roots to the arachnoid and the dura mater on each side of the spinal cord. The dural sheath terminates at the level of the vertebra S2. A pial extension, the filum terminale, arises from the caudal tip of the conus medullaris and pierces the end of the dural sac. It continues as connective tissue, the coccygeal ligament, and attaches to the periosteum of the coccyx. The spinal dura mater is a continuation of the meningeal layer of the cranial dura mater. The periosteum of the vertebrae corresponds to the outer layer of the cranial dura mater.

Blood Supply

The spinal cord is supplied by one anterior spinal artery and two *posterolateral* (posterior) *spinal arteries* (Fig. 14.6). Spinal cord arteries are branches of the vertebral arteries and six to eight radicular arteries derived from segmental intercostal, lumbar, and sacral arteries.

These vessels pass through the intervertebral foramen and divide into anterior and posterior radicular arteries. Radicular arteries are most frequent on the left side in the thoracic and lumbar segments. One anterior radicular artery in the lumbar region, the artery of Adamkiewicz, is larger than others. It usually originates at the level of vertebral segments T9 to T12 and travels on the left side to supply the lumbar enlargement (see Chapter 12).

The spinal arteries run the length of the spinal cord and are interconnected by anastomoses that form an irregular plexus which circles the surface of the spinal cord and sends short branches into the cord. Sulcal branches from the anterior spinal artery in the anterior median

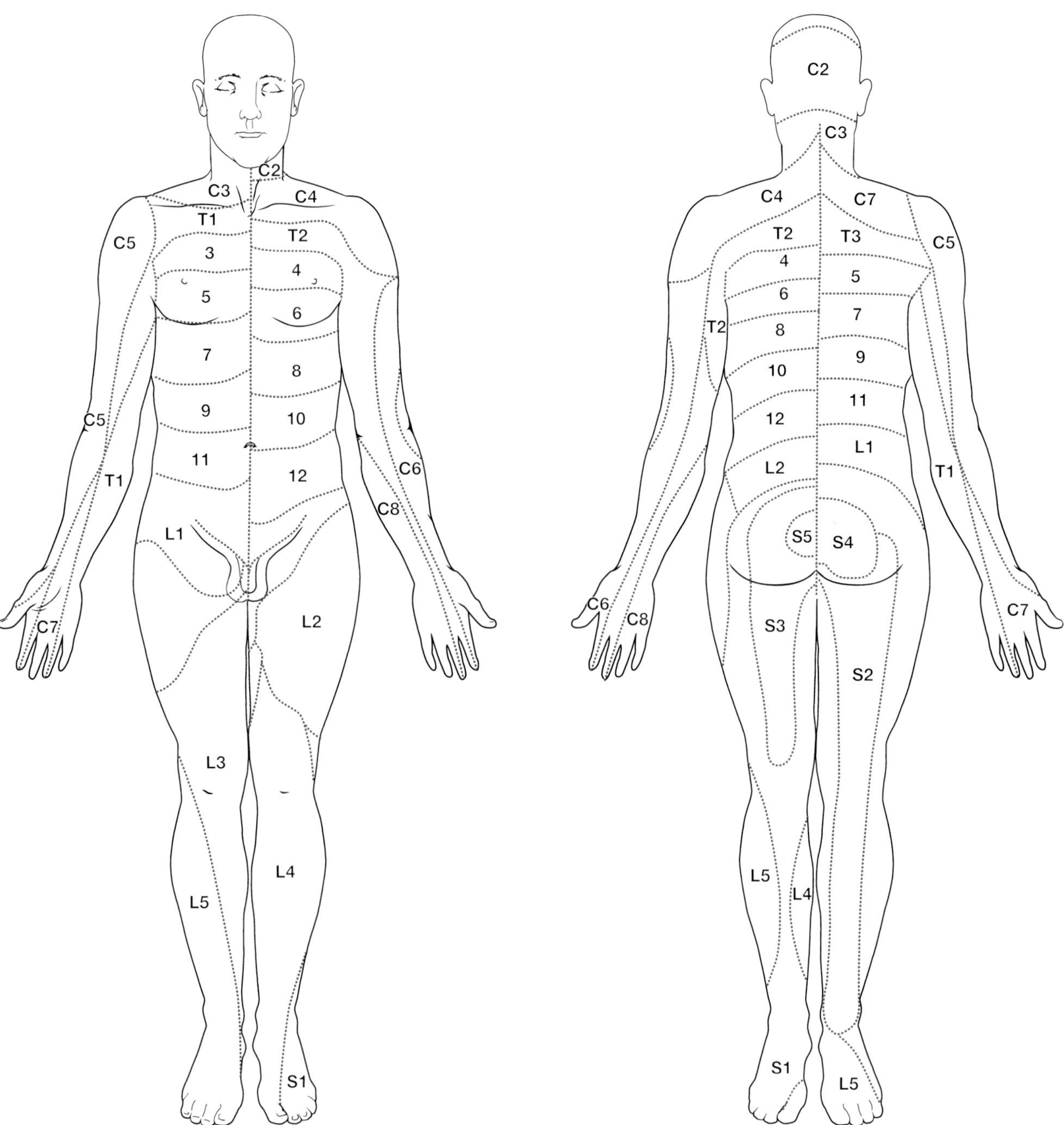

Fig. 14.5. Cutaneous distribution of spinal nerves (dermatomes).

Table 14.1. Dermatomes Useful for Segmental Localization

Spinal nerve root and segment	Area of the skin
C2	Occiput
C3	Neck
C4	Upper shoulder
C5	Lateral shoulder
C6	Thumb
C7	Middle finger
C8	Little finger
T1	Inner arm
T4-T5	Nipple
T10	Umbilicus
L1	Inguinal fold, scrotum
L2	Lateral thigh
L3	Knee
L4	Inner leg and internal malleolus
L5	Outer Leg
	Dorsum of the foot
S1	Lateral foot and heel
S2, S3	Dorsum of the legs and thigh
S4, S5	Perineum

fissure go alternatively right and left. Branches of the anterior spinal artery supply the ventral and intermediate gray matter and the white matter of the ventrolateral (anterolateral) and dorsolateral (posterolateral) quadrants of the spinal cord. The posterior spinal arteries supply the dorsal horn and the posterior (dorsal) columns (Fig. 14.7). At the level of cervical cord, the anterior spinal artery is supplied primarily by branches of the vertebral artery, but below this level, its continuity depends on anastomotic branches it receives from the anterior radicular arteries. The greatest length between radicular arteries occurs at the level of the thoracic segments. Thus, these segments are at highest risk for ischemia with occlusion of one radicular artery. Spinal cord segments T1 to T4 and L1 are the most vulnerable segments. Spinal cord infarction results from the occlusion of one intercostal artery, which can be a consequence of a dissecting aortic aneurysm or aortic surgery.

Table 14.2. Myotomes Listed by Spinal Nerves and Main Muscles

Spinal nerve root	Muscle (nerve)
C1–C6	Neck flexors and extensors, diaphragm
C5	Infraspinatus (suprascapular)
	Deltoid (axillary)
	Supinator (radial)
	Biceps (musculocutaneous)
C6	Biceps (musculocutaneous)
	Pronators (median)
C7	Triceps (radial)
	Wrist and finger extensors (radial)
	Wrist and finger flexors (median)
C8, T1	Thenar (median)
	Hypothenar (ulnar)
	Interossei (ulnar)
T6–L1	Abdominal muscles (intercostal)
L3, L4	Iliopsoas (femoral)
	Quadriceps (femoral)
	Thigh adductors (obturator)
L5	Gluteus medius (superior gluteal)
	Internal hamstring (sciatic)
	Anterior tibial (peroneal)
	Toe dorsiflexors (peroneal)
	Posterior tibial (tibial)
S1	Gluteus maximus (inferior gluteal)
	External hamstring (sciatic)
	Gastrocnemius-soleus (posterior tibial)
	Toe flexors (posterior tibial)
S3, S4	External anal sphincter (pudendal)

- The vascular supply of the spinal cord consists of one anterior and two posterolateral arteries derived from branches of the vertebral arteries and radicular arteries.
- Spinal cord segments T1 to T4 and L1 are the segments most vulnerable to ischemia and infarction.

Veins draining the spinal cord have a general distribution similar to that of spinal arteries and consist of anterior and posterior longitudinal venous

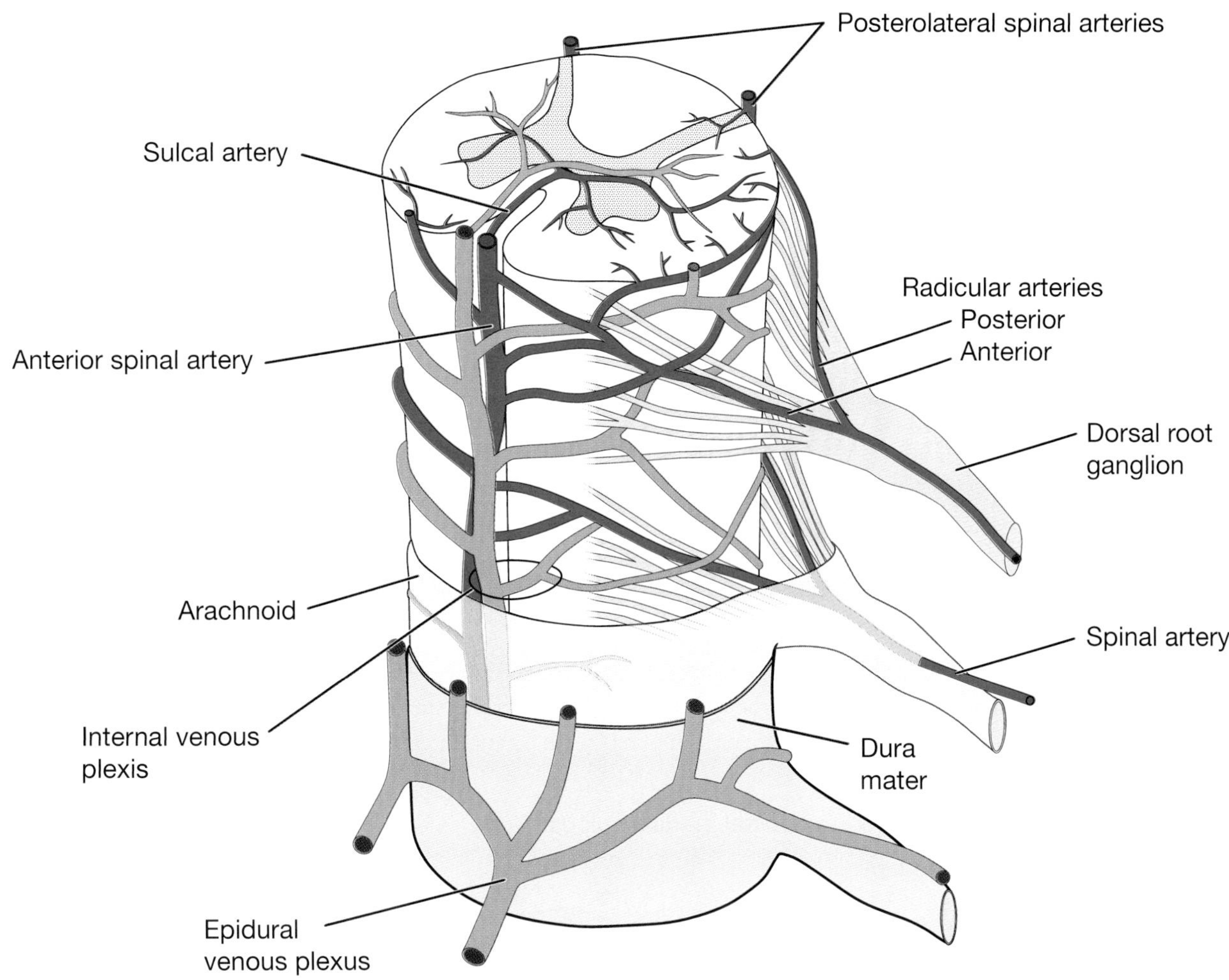

Fig. 14.6. Arterial supply of a spinal cord segment by radicular arteries.

trunks, which are connected to each other by coronal veins that circle the spinal cord, forming an irregular plexus. This spinal venous plexus communicates with the occipital and marginal sinuses and with the basal plexus of veins above the level of the foramen magnum. The *epidural venous plexus* is located between the dura mater and the vertebral periosteum and consists of anterior and posterior venous channels that are interconnected at many levels from the clivus to the sacral region. At each intervertebral space, these channels are connected with thoracic, abdominal, and intercostal veins. Because the spinal venous network does not have any valves, blood flowing into the epidural channels may pass directly into the systemic venous system and vice versa. This venous system provides a route by which metastases arising in abdominal and pelvic organs can reach the nervous system.

Internal Morphology

General Organization of the Spinal Cord

A cross section of the spinal cord shows a central H-shaped gray area surrounded by white matter (Fig. 14.8). The gray matter consists of a longitudinally continuous matrix of neuronal cell bodies, dendrites, myelinated and

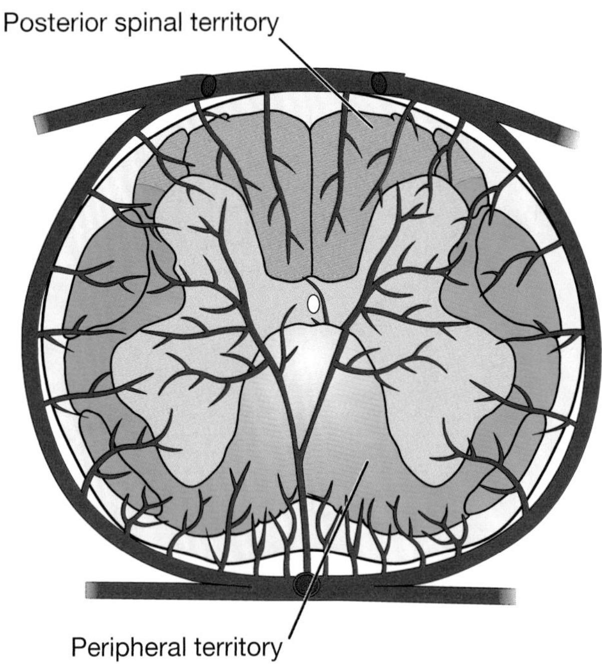

Fig. 14.7. Diagram of a transverse section of the spinal cord illustrating the area of supply of the anterior and posterior (red) spinal arteries and the peripheral zone (green) supplied by the circumferential vessels.

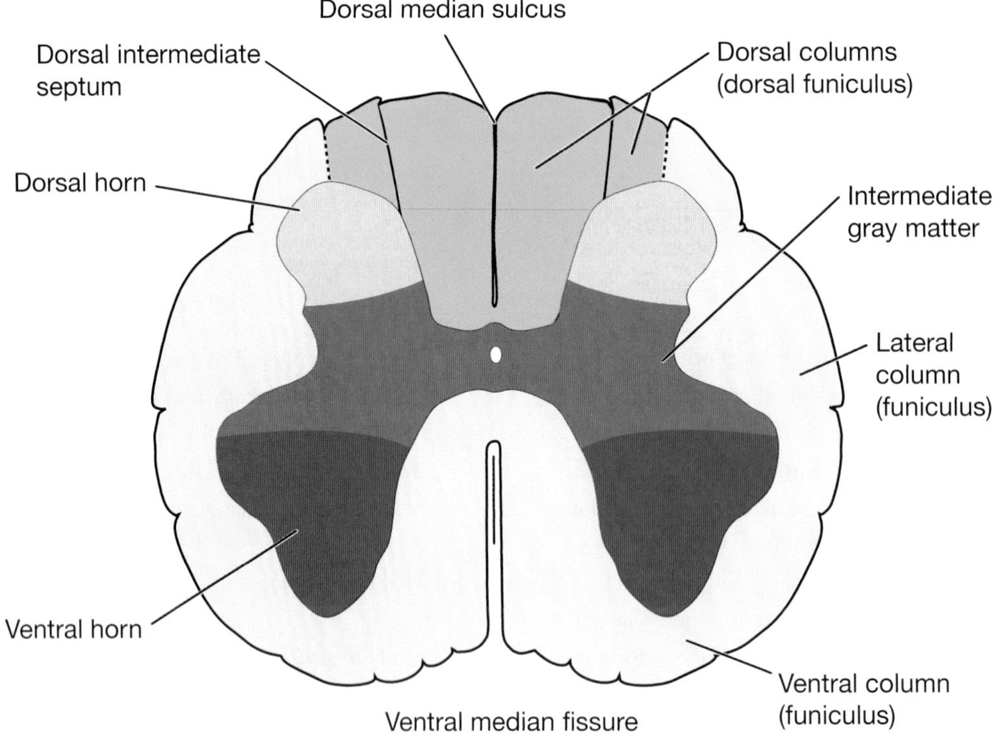

Fig. 14.8. Cross section of the spinal cord showing the major divisions of the gray matter and white matter.

unmyelinated axons, and glial cells. The spinal gray matter is divided into dorsal horns, intermediate gray matter, and ventral horns. The interconnecting gray matter in the midline is separated into a dorsal gray commissure and a ventral gray commissure by the central canal. The dorsal horn contains sensory neurons and interneurons; the ventral horn contains motor neurons and interneurons; and the intermediate gray matter contains primarily interneurons. A lateral projection of the intermediate gray matter, the lateral horn, is present in spinal segments T1 through L2 and contains the preganglionic sympathetic neurons.

The spinal white matter consists of longitudinally arranged myelinated and unmyelinated nerve fibers, with an abundance of myelin that gives it a glistening white appearance. It is subdivided into three columns (or funiculi): the anterior (or ventral), lateral, and posterior (or dorsal) columns (Fig. 14.8). The white matter contains all the ascending and descending pathways that connect the neurons of the gray matter with other levels of the nervous system (Fig. 14.9). Each lateral column includes a dorsolateral and a ventrolateral quadrant. Each anterior column contains descending projections from the brainstem to the motor neurons and interneurons that control the neck and axial musculature bilaterally. The anterolateral quadrant contains the spinothalamic and spinobulbar tracts, which are ascending axons that originate in the contralateral dorsal horn, and descending brainstem motor pathways that control segmental reflexes. The dorsolateral quadrant contains several pathways; the most important is the *lateral corticospinal tract*, which controls voluntary movements of the ipsilateral limbs. Each dorsal column contains predominantly ascending first-order axons from ipsilateral dorsal root ganglion neurons that innervate mechanoreceptors and proprioceptors.

At cervical levels, the dorsal column includes the *gracile fascicle,* which conveys input from the lower limb

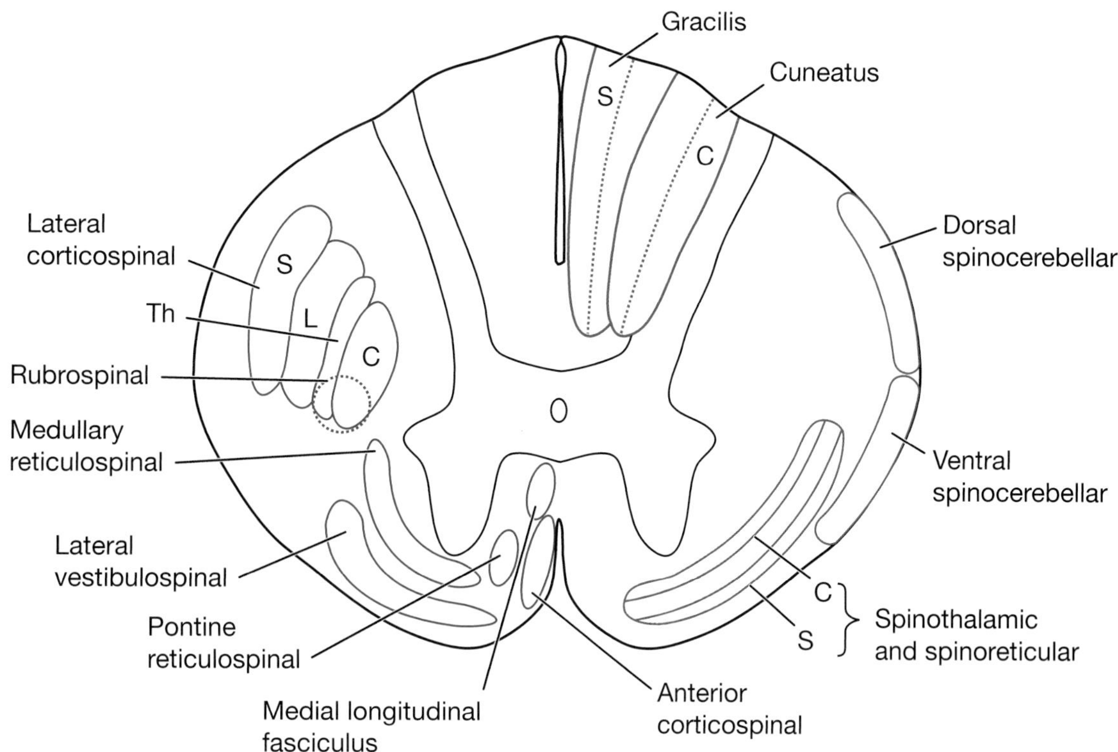

Fig. 14.9. Major ascending (blue) and descending (red) tracts of the spinal cord white matter. C, cervical; L, lumbar; Th, thoracic; S, sacral.

and lower trunk, and the *cuneate fascicle,* which conveys input from the upper limb and upper trunk. Involvement of the major pathways of the ventrolateral quadrant (spinothalamic tract), dorsolateral quadrant (corticospinal tract), and dorsal columns provides the main clues for the transverse localization of lesions at the spinal level. In addition to these three major pathways, the spinal white matter contains many other functionally relevant pathways, including brainstem motor pathways in the anterior and anterolateral quadrants and the dorsal and ventral *spinocerebellar pathways* toward the periphery of the dorsolateral and ventrolateral quadrants. Descending autonomic pathways are located in a narrow band in the lateral columns. The white matter immediately surrounding the gray matter contains fibers that interconnect different segments of the spinal cord. These are the *propriospinal fibers.* The main components of the spinal gray matter and white matter are listed in Table 14.3.

Variations in the Configuration of the Spinal Cord at Different Segments

The variations in the configuration of the gray and white matter of the spinal cord at different segments help in identifying the level of a section of the cord (Fig. 14.10). The spinal cord is oval at cervical segments, nearly circular at thoracic and lumbar segments, and almost quadrangular at sacral segments. These variations result from differences in the relative sizes of the gray and white matter. The variations in internal morphology can be summarized as follows:

1. The proportion of white matter to gray matter progressively decreases from the cervical to the sacral segments.

   This is due to a progressive reduction in the size of the corticospinal tract, with axons leaving the tract and entering the ventral horn as the tract descends

Table 14.3. Main Components of the Spinal Cord

	Gray matter, neurons	White matter, tract
Dorsal horn	Second-order sensory Interneurons	--
Intermediate gray matter	Interneurons Spinocerebellar Preganglionic autonomic	--
Ventral horn	Motor neurons Interneurons	--
Ventrolateral quadrant	--	**Spinothalamic** Spinobulbar Vestibulospinal Reticulospinal Ventral spinocerebellar Autonomic
Dorsolateral quadrant	--	**Corticospinal** Rubrospinal Dorsal spinocerebellar
Dorsal columns	--	**Gracile and cuneate**

Bold type: important for clinical localization of lesions at the transverse spinal level.

from the cervical to the sacral levels. There is also a progressive increase in the size of the spinothalamic and dorsal column pathways, with axons joining these pathways as they ascend from the sacral to the cervical levels.

2. The size of the ventral horn is larger in the segments of the cervical and lumbar enlargements, which supply the muscles of the upper and lower extremities, respectively, than in the thoracic and sacral segments.
3. At the cervical and upper thoracic levels, a dorsal intermediate sulcus separates the gracile fascicle (medial) from the cuneate fascicle (lateral).

Because the cuneate fascicle conveys primary afferents from the upper extremity and upper trunk, it is not present below the upper thoracic level.

4. Thoracic segments have a well-marked lateral horn containing the intermediolateral cell column of preganglionic sympathetic neurons.

Functional Anatomy of the Gray Matter

Types of Spinal Cord Neurons

The two main types of neurons in the spinal gray matter are projection neurons and interneurons. The projection neurons include 1) *second-order sensory neurons* in the

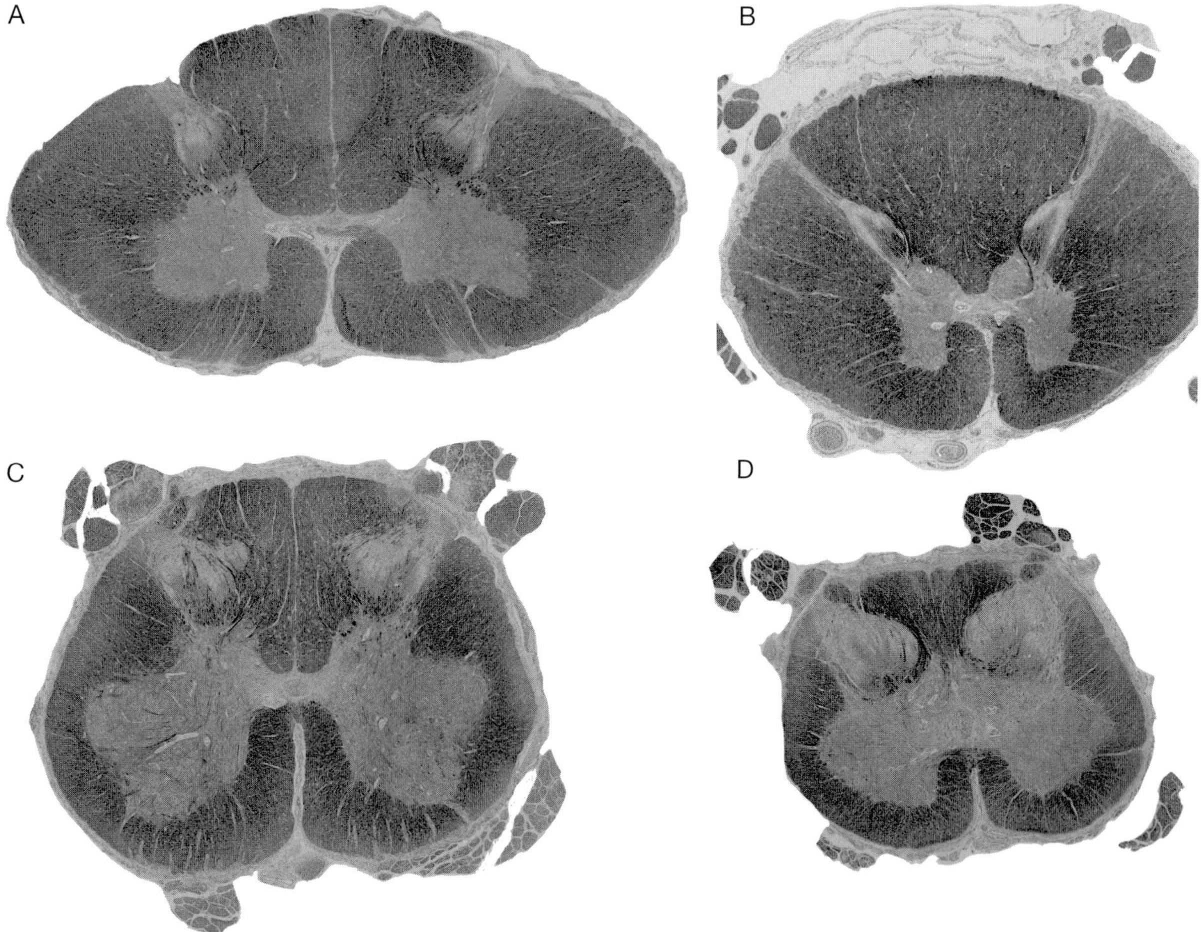

Fig. 14.10. Myelin-stained cross sections of the spinal cord showing the various shapes and relative proportions of white matter (dark areas) and gray matter (light areas) at various levels. *A*, Cervical; *B*, thoracic; *C*, lumbar; *D*, sacral.

dorsal horn and intermediate gray matter that project to the thalamus, brainstem, or cerebellum and have L-glutamate as the neurotransmitter; 2) *motor neurons* in the ventral horn that have acetylcholine as the neurotransmitter and project to skeletal muscles; and 3) *preganglionic neurons* of the intermediate gray matter that have acetylcholine as the neurotransmitter and project to autonomic ganglia. The interneurons include 1) *local interneurons* with axonal projections that remain on the same side and within a segment of the spinal cord; 2) *commissural neurons* whose axons cross the midline to terminate in the contralateral gray matter; and 3) *propriospinal neurons* whose axons project rostrally or caudally in the surrounding white matter for several segments before terminating in the gray matter. All these interneurons are located throughout the spinal cord, particularly in the intermediate gray matter, and constitute the bulk of spinal neurons. By receiving information from primary afferents, dorsal horn neurons, motor neurons, and descending pathways, the interneurons integrate segmental and intersegmental activity that control spinal sensory processing and motor and autonomic outputs. Interneurons may have excitatory or inhibitory effects on other spinal neurons; most inhibitory interneurons have γ-aminobutyric acid (GABA) or glycine (or both) as a neurotransmitter. The neurotransmitter of excitatory interneurons is glutamate.

- The dorsal horn contains second-order sensory neurons that receive input from the dorsal roots and project to supraspinal centers.
- The ventral horn contains somatic motor neurons, and the lateral horn contains preganglionic neurons; both horns receive input from primary afferents and descending pathways and project through the ventral roots.
- Spinal interneurons predominate in the intermediate gray matter and receive and integrate segmental, propriospinal, and suprasegmental information.

The neurons of the spinal cord are organized into functional clusters, or columns, that extend longitudinally for various distances and form specific nuclei. The spinal gray matter is divided into 10 cytoarchitectonic cell layers, or *laminae of Rexed*, on the basis of neuronal size, cell density, staining characteristics, and input and output (Fig. 14.11). The neurons in each lamina have specific patterns of connectivity (Table 14.4).

> Laminae I through V are located in the dorsal horn and subserve sensory functions; laminae VI and VII are located in the intermediate gray matter and are involved with reflex activity; laminae VIII and IX are in the ventral horn and are involved with motor function; and lamina X surrounds the central canal and contributes to sensory and autonomic functions.

Dorsal Horn

Neurons in laminae I, III, IV, and V are projection neurons that send axons across the midline in the anterior spinal commissure to ascend contralaterally in the *spinothalamic* and *spinoreticular* (also called spinobulbar) *tracts* (see Chapter 7). Neurons of lamina I (the marginal zone) convey pain, temperature, and visceral sensation; those in laminae III and IV convey tactile information; and those in lamina V convey both nociceptive and tactile information. Some neurons also project ipsilaterally through the dorsal column or dorsolateral quadrant. Lamina II, also known as the *substantia gelatinosa*, contains local neurons that regulate the activity of neurons in other dorsal horn laminae.

Intermediate Gray Matter

The intermediate gray matter, laminae VI and VII, is functionally heterogeneous. Neurons in lamina VI contribute to the spinothalamic tract. Between spinal cord segments T1 and L1, lamina VI contains the neurons of Clarke column, which conveys proprioceptive and tactile information via the ipsilateral dorsal spinocerebellar tract to the cerebellum. Lamina VII contains different types of interneurons. A lateral extension of lamina VII between spinal segments T1 and L2 forms the lateral horn, which contains the intermediolateral cell column of preganglionic sympathetic neurons. At spinal segments S2 to S4, lamina VII contains the *sacral parasympathetic nucleus*.

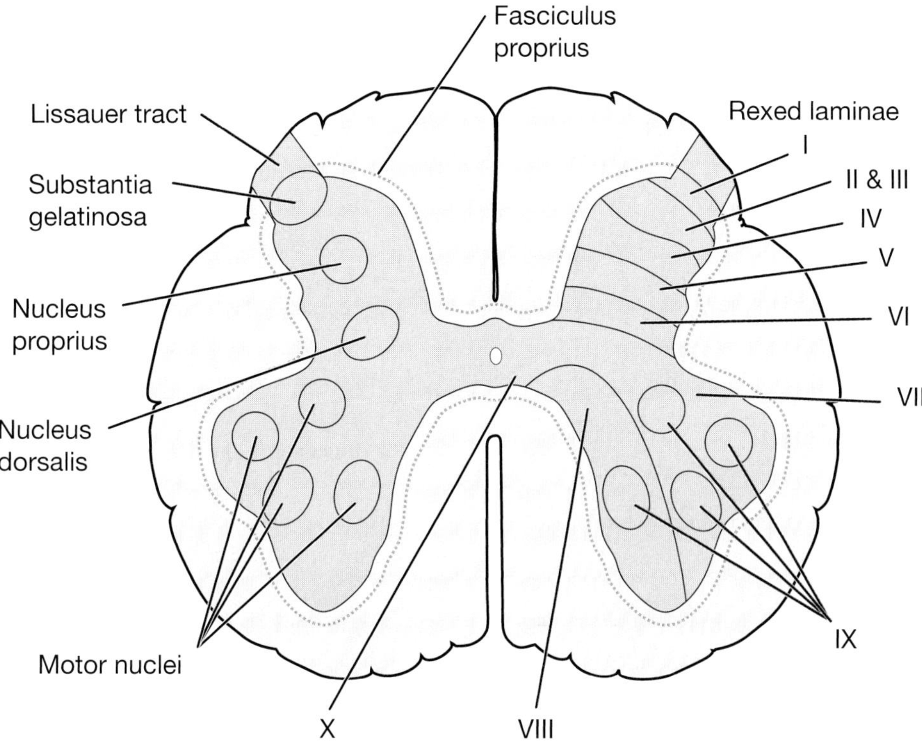

Fig. 14.11. Groups of nuclei (*left*) and the laminae of Rexed (*right*) of the gray matter of the spinal cord.

Ventral Horn

The ventral horn includes laminae VIII and IX. Lamina VIII contains motor interneurons and propriospinal neurons that receive input from primary muscle afferents and descending motor pathways from the brainstem and cerebral cortex. Lamina IX contains the motor neurons that project to the skeletal muscles (see Chapters 8 and 13).

> Spinal motor neurons are somatotopically organized in distinct functional columns within lamina IX. Those innervating the axial musculature are in the extreme ventromedial portion of the lamina, those innervating the distal limb muscles are clustered in the dorsolateral sector, and those innervating the girdle musculature occupy an intermediate position. Extensor motor neurons are ventral to flexor motor neurons.

The spinal innervation of somatic muscles follows a strict myotomal organization, as follows: C1 to C3 motor neurons innervate the cervical muscles; C3 and C4 motor neurons, the diaphragm (*phrenic motor neurons*); C5 to T1 motor neurons, the upper limb; T2 to L1 motor neurons, the intercostal and abdominal muscles; L3 to S2 motor neurons, the lower limb; and S2 to S4 motor neurons (*Onuf nucleus*), the external sphincter and pelvic floor musculature (Table 14.2).

- Laminae I, III, IV, and V of the dorsal horn contain second-order sensory neurons that project through the spinothalamic and spinoreticular (spinobulbar) tracts.
- Lamina II (substantia gelatinosa) contains excitatory and inhibitory interneurons.
- Laminae VI and VII in the thoracic and lumbar cord contains Clarke column and the intermediolateral cell column.
- Lamina VIII contains motor interneurons.
- Lamina IX contains different pools of somatotopically organized motor neurons innervating skeletal muscles.

Table 14.4. Main Components of the Gray Matter Laminae and Their Function

Lamina	Cell type	Function
I	Nociceptive Thermoreceptive Visceroceptive	Relay of modality-specific input to contralateral thalamus (spinothalamic tract) and internal regulation system (spinoreticular tracts)
II	Excitatory and inhibitory interneurons	Local control of nociceptive transmission
III-IV	Low-threshold mechanoreceptive	Relay of tactile and proprioceptive input via spinothalamic tract, dorsal column, and dorsolateral quadrant
V-VI	Wide dynamic range neurons	Relay of multimodal input to contralateral thalamus (spinothalamic tract)
VII	Motor interneurons	Segmental reflexes
	Clarke column (T1–L2)	Relay of proprioceptive input from lower limb to ipsilateral cerebellum (dorsal spinocerebellar tract)
	Intermediolateral cell column (T1–L2)	Preganglionic sympathetic
	Sacral parasympathetic neurons (S2–S4)	Preganglionic parasympathetic to pelvic viscera
VIII	Motor interneurons	Relay and integration of segmental and descending inputs to motor neurons
IX	Motor neurons	Final common pathway for reflex, postural, and voluntary movements
X	Wide dynamic range neurons	Relay of visceral pain and visceral reflexes

Sensory Pathways in the Spinal White Matter

The white matter contains all the ascending or descending pathways that connect the neurons of the gray matter with other levels of the central nervous system (Table 14.5 and Fig. 14.9).

Dorsal Root Entry Zone

The dorsal roots enter the dorsolateral aspect of the spinal cord and break up into small rootlets. As the primary dorsal root afferents approach the *dorsal root entry zone*, the axons become segregated. The large myelinated axons of dorsal root ganglion neurons conveying information from skin mechanoreceptors and muscle proprioceptors form a medial bundle that enters the dorsal column. Collaterals of these axons end in deep laminae of the dorsal horn. The small-diameter myelinated or unmyelinated axons from nociceptive, thermoreceptive, and visceroreceptive dorsal root ganglion neurons form a lateral bundle that terminates directly in laminae I and II.

Propriospinal System

The white matter immediately surrounding the gray matter contains axons from interneurons that interconnect different segments of the spinal cord at variable distances from each other. These are termed *propriospinal fibers*, and they form the *fasciculi proprii*. The tract of Lissauer consists of collaterals of primary small myelinated and unmyelinated dorsal root fibers and a large number of propriospinal pathways that interconnect different levels of the substantia gelatinosa.

Table 14.5. Main Pathways of the Spinal Cord White Matter and Their Function

Anatomy	Pathway	Function
Dorsal (posterior)	Gracile and cutaneous	Tactile discrimination Vibration Joint position sense Feedback for fine motor control of fingers
Dorsolateral	Spinocervical	Contributes to touch and vibration sense
	Dorsal spinocerebellar	Proprioceptive and exteroceptive input from lower limb to ipsilateral cerebellum
	Corticospinal	Motor neuron recruitment Fractionated control of finger movements Inhibits antigravity reflexes
	Rubrospinal	Contributes to control of forearm and hand
	Dorsolateral reticulospinal	Inhibits flexor reflexes
	Monoaminergic	Modulation of nociceptive, autonomic, and motor functions
Ventrolateral	Spinothalamic	Relay of pain, temperature, and visceral sensation to thalamus
	Spinoreticular	Relay of pain, temperature, and visceral sensation to internal regulation and consciousness systems
	Medullary reticulospinal	Mediates cortical inhibition of muscle stretch reflexes
	Lateral vestibulospinal	Facilitates extensor postural reflexes
	Autonomic	Supraspinal control of preganglionic neurons
Ventral	Medial vestibulospinal and tectospinal	Control of neck movements for head-eye coordination
	Pontine reticulospinal	Facilitates antigravity reflexes
Propriospinal	Propriospinal	Multilevel sensory and motor integration

Dorsal Columns

The dorsal columns contain predominantly ascending first-order axons from dorsal root ganglion neurons that innervate low-threshold skin mechanoreceptors and muscle and joint proprioceptors of the same side of the body. These axons form the *direct dorsal column pathway* that terminates in the dorsal column nuclei of lower medulla. The dorsal columns also contain a *postsynaptic dorsal column pathway* that consists of axons of second-order mechanoreceptive neurons in laminae III and IV. At cervical and upper thoracic levels, each dorsal column consists of a medially located gracile fascicle, which conveys input from the lower limb to the gracile nucleus, and the cuneate fascicle, which conveys input from the upper limb to the cuneate nucleus. Below midthoracic levels, each dorsal column consists only of a gracile fascicle. The second-order axons from the gracile and cuneate nuclei decussate in the medulla and ascend in the contralateral medial lemniscus. The dorsal column–medial lemniscus system is critical for tactile discrimination, vibration sense, and proprioception necessary for fine motor control, particularly of the fingers (see Chapter 7).

Dorsolateral Quadrant: Dorsal Spinocerebellar Tract

The dorsolateral quadrant contains several ascending pathways containing second-order axons from dorsal horn neurons that receive input from skin mechanoreceptors and proprioceptors. The most important is the *dorsal spinocerebellar tract*. It originates from neurons in Clarke column at spinal segments T1 to L2 and conveys feedback input from proprioceptors and low-threshold skin mechanoreceptors of the lower limb to the ipsilateral cerebellum. This pathway is critical for maintenance of station and gait.

The dorsolateral quadrant also contains the spinocervical tract. This consists of second-order axons from low-threshold mechanoreceptive neurons in laminae III and IV. It terminates ipsilaterally in the lateral cervical nucleus in the upper cervical cord and contributes axons to the lemniscal system.

Ventrolateral Quadrant: Spinothalamic and Spinoreticular Pathways

The major sensory pathways in the ventrolateral quadrant are the spinothalamic and spinoreticular (or spinobulbar) tracts. The *spinothalamic tract* is the major pathway for transmission of conscious pain, temperature, visceral, and sexual sensation to the brain. This tract consists of axons from neurons in the dorsal horn and intermediate gray matter that receive primary afferent input from the dorsal root ganglion. These second-order spinothalamic axons ascend one to two segments as they decussate in the ventral spinal commissure to ascend in the contralateral ventrolateral quadrant to reach the thalamus. Therefore, lesions that affect these decussating axons produce contralateral deficits of pain and temperature sensation in dermatomes located one or two segments below the lesion. As these axons decussate, they become somatotopically arranged in the spinothalamic tract: the cervical segments are represented medially, followed by the thoracic, lumbar, and sacral segments, which are represented progressively more laterally.

The spinothalamic tract is functionally heterogeneous and arises from different types of neurons in the dorsal horn and the intermediate gray matter. Different types of neurons in lamina I convey pain, temperature, and visceral sensations. Neurons in laminae III and IV convey crude tactile information, and neurons in lamina V convey both pain and tactile information. Neurons in the intermediate gray matter provide tactile information for motor control. The spinothalamic tract is the main, but not the only pathway, for transmission of pain sensation. A pathway in the midline of the dorsal columns conveys pain sensation from midline visceral structures. This explains the failure of anterolateral chordotomy, which is used for management of intractable cancer pain, to relieve midline visceral pain.

The *spinoreticular*, or *spinobulbar*, pathway also originates from the dorsal horn and intermediate gray matter and primarily ascends contralaterally in the ventrolateral quadrant. This pathway, also functionally heterogeneous, terminates in areas of the posterior fossa and supratentorial level that are part of the internal regulation and consciousness systems. They include the nucleus of the solitary tract, parabrachial nucleus, ventrolateral medullary reticular formation, and periaqueductal gray matter of the midbrain. These areas initiate autonomic and pain modulatory responses either directly or by projections to the hypothalamus and amygdala, which also receive direct input from the dorsal horn (see Chapter 9).

- The dorsal columns are important for tactile discrimination, vibration sense, and proprioception (including joint position sense) of the ipsilateral body.
- The dorsal spinocerebellar tract conveys proprioceptive input from the lower extremity to the ipsilateral cerebellum; this input is needed for the control of gait.
- The spinothalamic tract is critical for the sensations of pain and temperature of the contralateral body.
- The spinoreticular (spinobulbar) pathway conveys pain, temperature, and visceral sensations to areas involved in visceral control, emotional and adaptive responses, pain modulation, and behavioral arousal.

Motor and Autonomic Pathways of the Spinal White Matter

Motor Pathways in the Ventral Column and Ventrolateral Quadrant

The ventral column and ventrolateral quadrant of the spinal cord contain descending brainstem motor pathways that control the axial muscles of the neck and trunk and the proximal muscles of the extremities. These pathways are referred to as the *medial motor pathways*. They arise from the vestibular nuclei, superior colliculus, and reticular formation of the pons and medulla and descend bilaterally in the spinal cord. The pathways descending in the ventral columns, including the *medial vestibulospinal tract* and *tectospinal tract*, coordinate neck movements with eye movements. The pathways descending in the ventrolateral quadrant, including the *lateral vestibulospinal tract* and *reticulospinal tracts*, control postural reflexes, muscle tone, and gait. The ventral columns also contain uncrossed corticospinal fibers that contribute to the control of axial and proximal muscles bilaterally.

Motor Pathways in the Dorsolateral Quadrant

The dorsolateral quadrant of the spinal cord contains crossed pathways controlling voluntary movements of the distal portion of the extremities. The most important pathway is the *lateral corticospinal tract* that originates from several motor areas of the contralateral frontal lobe (see Chapter 8). Approximately 80% to 90% of corticospinal axons decussate at the junction of the medulla and spinal cord and descend in the dorsolateral quadrant of the spinal cord. In humans, the corticospinal tract has three main functions: 1) to allow recruitment of motor neuron pools in response to increased effort, 2) to inhibit antigravity reflexes that may interfere with execution of voluntary movements, and 3) to control fractionated movements of the distal part of the limb, particularly the fingers.

The dorsolateral quadrant also contains the *rubrospinal tract*, which originates from magnocellular neurons of the contralateral red nucleus. It terminates in the cervical segments of the spinal cord. This pathway is of uncertain functional significance in humans, but it does cooperate with the corticospinal tract in facilitating flexor movements of the elbow and hand.

- The ventral column and ventrolateral quadrant of the spinal cord contain brainstem motor pathways that control postural reflexes, muscle tone, and gait.
- The lateral corticospinal tract is the main descending spinal motor pathway in humans.

Descending Pathways from the Consciousness and Internal Regulation Systems

Areas of the brainstem that are part of the consciousness and internal regulation systems project to the spinal cord. These include monoaminergic pathways and pathways involved in the control of autonomic function. The monoaminergic pathways arise from norepinephrine neurons in the locus ceruleus and serotonergic neurons in the raphe nuclei, and they descend in the dorsolateral quadrant of the spinal cord. These monoaminergic pathways have multiple functions. They modulate the relay of nociceptive information in the dorsal horn, spinal reflexes, and activity of motor neurons and preganglionic neurons.

Several descending projections originate from structures of the internal regulation system, including the paraventricular nucleus and lateral hypothalamic area, raphe nuclei, and rostral ventrolateral medulla. All these pathways descend in a narrow band in the lateral columns, close to the gray matter. They activate and coordinate the activity of preganglionic sympathetic and sacral parasympathetic neurons that mediate several segmental autonomic reflexes. These pathways also include axons from medullary respiratory neurons that activate phrenic and other respiratory motor neurons and axons from neurons in the pontine micturition center that control the micturition reflex. Descending monoaminergic inputs control pain transmission, motor neuron excitability, and spinal reflexes.

- Pathways from the hypothalamus and brainstem that control sympathetic, respiratory, and micturition neurons descend in the lateral quadrant of the spinal cord.

Spinal Cord Physiology

The major functions of the spinal cord are 1) local regulation of sensory processing and relay of this information to rostral levels; 2) integration and mediation of descending motor commands with local reflexes for voluntary movements, maintenance of posture, and generation of motor patterns for locomotion; and 3) generation of segmental visceral reflexes and integration of descending commands for coordinated control of visceral organs.

Sensory Processing

Primary (first-order) afferents from the dorsal root ganglion enter the spinal cord through the dorsal root entry zone, where they divide into a medial bundle of large myelinated afferents and a lateral bundle of small myelinated and unmyelinated afferents. From this common entry, the dorsal root fibers branch to ascend and descend in the white matter and to arborize in the gray matter. The pathways for the different sensory modalities diverge as they ascend in the spinal cord to higher centers (see Chapter 7).

Inputs From Low-Threshold Skin Mechanoreceptors and Proprioceptors

The large myelinated axons from dorsal root ganglion neurons relay input from low-threshold skin mechanoreceptors and proprioceptors. The low-threshold skin mechanoreceptor afferents (Aα and Aβ fibers) convey information about skin pressure, skin stretch, flutter, and vibration that is necessary for the tactile recognition of objects. Proprioceptive afferents that signal joint position and movement innervate mainly muscle spindles (type Ia and II afferents) and joint receptors.

All these large myelinated afferents bifurcate into ascending and descending branches that have different patterns of connections. They may 1) ascend directly in the ipsilateral dorsal column (direct dorsal column pathway); 2) synapse on dorsal horn neurons in laminae III and IV and then ascend in the dorsal column (postsynaptic dorsal column pathway), dorsolateral funiculus, and spinothalamic tract; 3) synapse on lamina II interneurons for segmental modulation of pain transmission; 4) ascend in the dorsal column to synapse on Clarke column neurons or intermediate gray matter neurons that give rise to spinocerebellar tracts; and 5) synapse on interneurons and motor neurons in the ventral horn to trigger segmental muscle stretch reflexes.

Afferents From Nociceptors, Thermoreceptors, and Visceral Receptors

The small myelinated (Aδ) and unmyelinated (C) afferents from primary nociceptors, thermoreceptors, and visceral receptors and mechanosensitive and chemosensitive muscle (type III-IV) afferents bifurcate into ascending and descending branches that run longitudinally in Lissauer tract; within two or three segments, the axons leave the tract to enter the dorsal horn and intermediate gray matter. At this level, they may 1) synapse on second-order neurons in laminae I, V, and VI that project primarily through the contralateral spinothalamic and spinobulbar tracts; 2) synapse on interneurons in lamina II involved in the segmental modulation of pain; 3) activate polysynaptic flexor reflexes; and 4) activate, through interneurons, preganglionic neurons that mediate segmental visceral reflexes.

Relay of Sensory Information in the Dorsal Horn

Neurons in laminae I and V are the main source of axons in the spinothalamic tract (Fig. 14.12). Lamina I receives monosynaptic input from Aδ and C afferents and contains several classes of neurons, including *nociceptive-specific*, *polymodal nociceptive*, thermoreceptive (*cold-sensitive*), and viscerosensitive neurons and neurons that receive muscle afferents. These different populations of lamina I neurons convey these modality-selective sensations to the thalamus through the spinothalamic tract and to the brainstem, hypothalamus, and amygdala.

Lamina V contains *wide dynamic range neurons* that receive direct input from large-diameter Aβ and small-diameter Aδ fibers and polysynaptic input from C fibers relaying to excitatory neurons of lamina II. Thus, lamina V neurons integrate afferent input from nociceptors, tactile receptors, and proprioceptors and convey this information through the spinothalamic tract.

- Lamina I spinothalamic neurons provide modality-specific nociceptive, thermoreceptive, and viscerosensitive inputs to the thalamus.

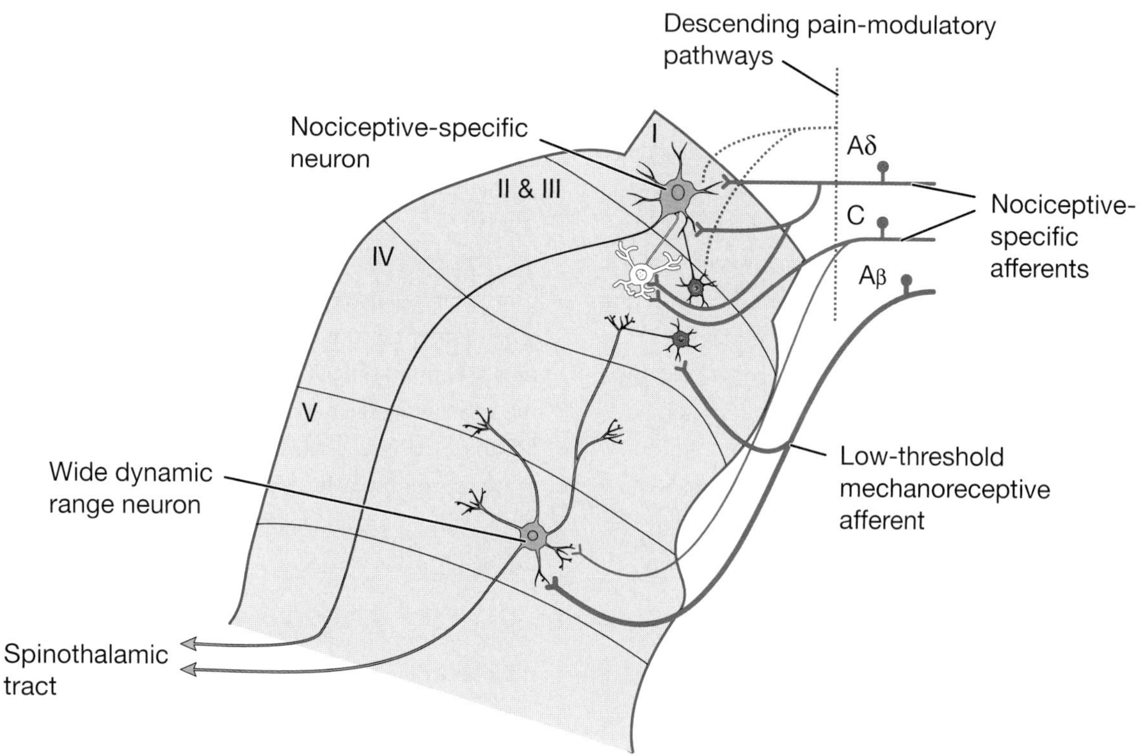

Fig. 14.12. Neurons in laminae I, III-IV, and V are the main sources of the axons in the spinothalamic tract. Lamina I receives monosynaptic input from Aδ and C afferents and contains several classes of neurons, including nociceptive-specific, polymodal nociceptive, thermoreceptive (cold sensitive), and viscerosensitive neurons. Laminae III-IV neurons (not shown) receive nonnociceptive input and project through the spinothalamic tract and postsynaptic dorsal column pathway. Lamina V contains wide dynamic range neurons that receive direct input from large-diameter Aβ and small-diameter Aδ fibers and polysynaptic input from C fibers relaying on excitatory neurons in lamina II. Lamina II, or the substantia gelatinosa, has a major role in modulation of nociceptive transmission. It contains both excitatory and inhibitory local circuit neurons. Lamina II neurons receive input from nociceptive C afferents and low-threshold tactile afferents as well as descending noradrenergic and serotonergic input from the brainstem involved in the central control of pain transmission in the dorsal horn.

- Lamina V spinothalamic neurons respond both to noxious and innocuous stimuli.

Transmission of Afferent Input to the Dorsal Horn: Windup Phenomenon, Central Sensitization, and Mechanisms of Pain

Primary afferents to the dorsal horn are excitatory, with L-glutamate as neurotransmitter. These axons elicit fast, short-lasting excitation. Some nociceptive afferents also release neuropeptides, such as substance P and calcitonin gene-related peptide. In response to repetitive stimulation of primary nociceptive afferents, spinothalamic neurons undergo physiologic changes that result in sensitization to the afferents. This is called the *windup phenomenon*, which results in increased spontaneous activity, decreased threshold, and enlargement of the receptive fields of spinothalamic neurons. This *central sensitization* mechanism underlies neuropathic and central pain disorders. These disorders are characterized by spontaneous (generally, burning) pain, decreased threshold for pain sensation (*hyperalgesia*), and perception of an innocuous stimulus (such as touch) as painful (*allodynia*). These are the manifestations of chronic pain disorders that result from damage to a peripheral nerve or dorsal roots or from a central lesion that affects the spinothalamic system.

Normally, transient stimulation of nociceptors causes the release of L-glutamate. In response to repetitive stimulation, nociceptive C afferents also release substance P, which reduces K^+ conductances and thus depolarizes the spinothalamic neuron. This allows glutamate to activate *N*-methyl-D-aspartate (NMDA) receptors, producing an influx of Ca^{2+} that, in turn, activates protein kinases and triggers the production of nitric oxide and prostaglandins and the expression of immediate early genes.

Substantia Gelatinosa and Regulation of Nociceptive Transmission in the Dorsal Horn

Lamina II, or the substantia gelatinosa, has a major role in the modulation of nociceptive transmission. It contains both excitatory and inhibitory local circuit neurons (Fig. 14.12). Excitatory neurons have L-glutamate as a neurotransmitter, and inhibitory neurons have GABA or glycine. In addition, local lamina II neurons contain different types of neuropeptides, including opioid peptides. Lamina II neurons receive input both from nociceptive C afferents and low-threshold tactile afferents. These neurons also receive input from noradrenergic and serotonergic cells in the brainstem, which mediate central control of pain transmission in the dorsal horn. The substantia gelatinosa is thus the site of integration of segmental and suprasegmental influences that control the transmission of nociceptive input in the dorsal horn. These descending influences may inhibit or facilitate the transmission of pain sensation.

- Repetitive activation of nociceptive input produces central sensitization of spinothalamic neurons, which is the basis of neurogenic pain.
- The substantia gelatinosa integrates segmental and suprasegmental influences that control the transmission of nociceptive input in the dorsal horn.

Motor Functions of the Spinal Cord

The segmental motor apparatus of the spinal cord consists of topographically organized groups of ventral horn motor neurons located in lamina IX and interneurons in laminae VII and VIII. These neurons receive and integrate segmental afferents, primarily from muscle, and descending motor pathways from the cerebral cortex and brainstem (Fig. 14.13).

Motor Neurons, Motor Units, and the Size Principle

The ventral horn motor neurons, also referred to as *motoneurons* or lower motor neurons, are the final common pathway for segmental motor control. They are arranged somatotopically in lamina IX, and the large expansion of the lateral motor neuron pools that innervate the distal limb muscles is reflected in the expansion of the ventral horn at the cervical and lumbar enlargements. An alpha motor neuron, its axon, and all the muscle fibers that it innervates constitute a motor unit (see Chapters 8 and 13). The function of the motor unit, including the biochemical and contractile properties of the muscle, depends on the motor neuron type.

There are two main types of alpha motor neurons

and, thus, two main types of motor units. Small motor neurons have a low threshold of activation, fire at low frequency, and have small myelinated axons. The muscle fibers they innervate generate slow, low-twitch tensions and are resistant to fatigue (type I). These motor units are involved in the tonic contraction of muscle for long periods and are called tonic, or *slow twitch*, motor units. In contrast, large motor neurons have a high threshold of activation, fire at high frequency, and have large axons. The muscle fibers they innervate generate large twitch tensions but fatigue easily (type II). These are the phasic, or *fast twitch*, motor units.

The force of muscle contraction is modulated both by controlling the firing frequency of active units and by activating or deactivating motor units. With increasing force of muscle contraction, individual motor units first increase their firing frequency, and as more force is generated, other motor units are activated. This is referred to as *recruitment*. Normally, a second motor unit is recruited when the firing of the first unit attains approximately 10 to 15 Hz. Recruitment occurs according to the *size principle*: during voluntary or reflex muscle contraction, motor neurons start firing in the order of increasing size, with small motor neurons recruited early and large motor neurons later.

- The motor unit is the final common pathway for all movement.

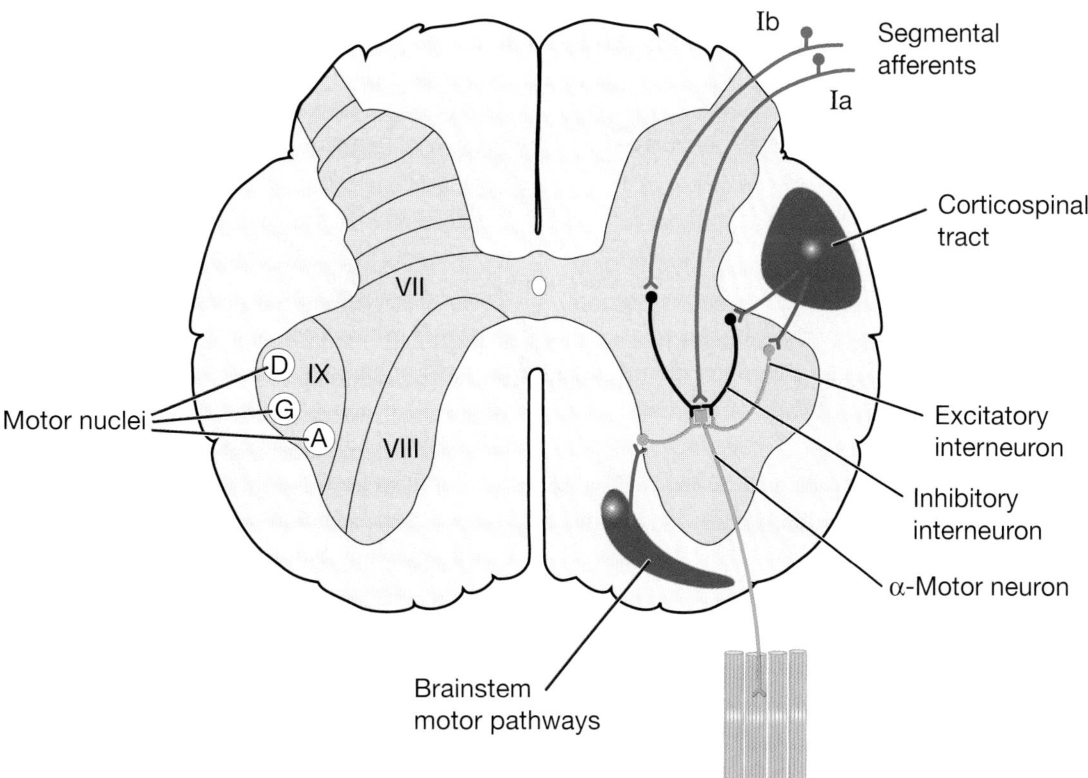

Fig. 14.13. The segmental motor apparatus of the spinal cord consists of topographically organized groups of ventral horn motor neurons, located in lamina IX, and excitatory and inhibitory interneurons in laminae VII and VIII. The motor neurons are organized into functional columns that innervate axial (A), girdle (G), or distal (D) limb muscles. Most of the influence on motor neurons and segmental reflexes is by way of interneurons, which receive and integrate input from segmental afferents and descending motor pathways from the cerebral cortex and brainstem.

- Small motor neurons have a low threshold of activation; fire at low frequency; innervate low twitch, fatigue-resistant type I muscle fibers; and are recruited early.
- Large motor neurons have a high threshold of activation; fire at high frequency; innervate fast twitch, fatigable (type II) muscle fibers; and are recruited late.

Segmental Spinal Reflexes

The segmental motor apparatus of the spinal cord is involved in two types of activity: reflex activity, including phasic and tonic stretch reflexes that control posture and voluntary movement, and complex motor synergies, such as locomotion. The activity of spinal motor neurons is regulated by two main influences, namely, segmental afferents and descending inputs. With few exceptions, these influences control the activity of the motor neurons through excitatory and inhibitory interneurons (see Chapter 8).

Primary afferents from muscle and other peripheral receptors trigger three main types of reflexes: 1) muscle stretch reflexes, 2) Golgi tendon organ reflexes, and 3) polysynaptic flexor reflexes. These reflexes are described in more detail in Chapter 8, and only some important features are emphasized here. The main components of the segmental reflexes that affect motor neurons are summarized in Table 14.6.

Table 14.6. Segmental Influences on Motor Neurons

		Golgi tendon	Multisynaptic	
	Stretch reflex	**reflex**	**Proprioceptive**	**Nociceptive**
Receptor	Muscle spindle	Golgi tendon organ	Muscle spindle, joint receptors	Skin and muscle nociceptors
Stimulus	Change in muscle length	Tension generated by active contraction	Various mechanical inputs	Noxious inputs
Afferents	Ia	Ib	II, III-V FRAs	Nociceptive III-IV muscle FRAs
Interneuron	Ia inhibitory	Ib inhibitory	Multiple excitatory or inhibitory	Multiple excitatory or inhibitory
Effect on agonist motor neurons	Monosynaptic excitation	Disynaptic inhibition	Polysynaptic excitation or inhibition	Polysynaptic excitation of ipsilateral flexors and contralateral extensors
Effect of antagonist	Disynaptic (reciprocal) inhibition	Excitation or inhibition	Excitation or inhibition	Polysynaptic inhibition of ipsilateral extensors and contralateral extensors
Function	Length servomechanism	Tension servomechanism	Locomotion	Withdrawal

FRAs, flexor reflex afferents.

The muscle stretch reflex, or myotatic reflex, is the most relevant reflex physiologically and clinically. It is triggered by muscle stretch or lengthening. This activates receptors in the muscle spindles, including nuclear bag receptors innervated by Ia afferents that respond to rapid change in length and nuclear chain receptors innervated by type II afferents that respond to continuous stretch. Activation of Ia afferents produces monosynaptic excitation of the alpha motor neuron pools that innervate the corresponding muscle, resulting in muscle contraction (Fig. 14.14). Thus, this reflex constitutes a length feedback mechanism. The Ia afferent input is also important for maintaining the optimal excitability of the alpha motor neuron during any motor activity.

The physiologic range of useful spindle signals is maintained by the gamma motor neurons that innervate intrafusal muscle fibers (Fig. 14.15). Fusimotor activity produces an internal change in length and local stiffening of the intrafusal fiber, so that more stretch is transmitted to the portion of the spindle innervated by the Ia and II afferents. Fusimotor control maintains the sensitivity of the muscle spindle receptors and thus provides a servoassistance mechanism during muscle contraction. Most postures and slow movements are made with *coactivation* of alpha and gamma motor neurons.

In addition to exciting alpha motor neurons to produce a monosynaptic stretch reflex, Ia afferents activate alpha motor neurons that innervate the synergistic muscles and disynaptically inhibit the alpha motor neurons that innervate the antagonist muscles. This process, called *reciprocal inhibition*, is mediated by the *Ia inhibitory interneuron*. Reciprocal inhibition is important

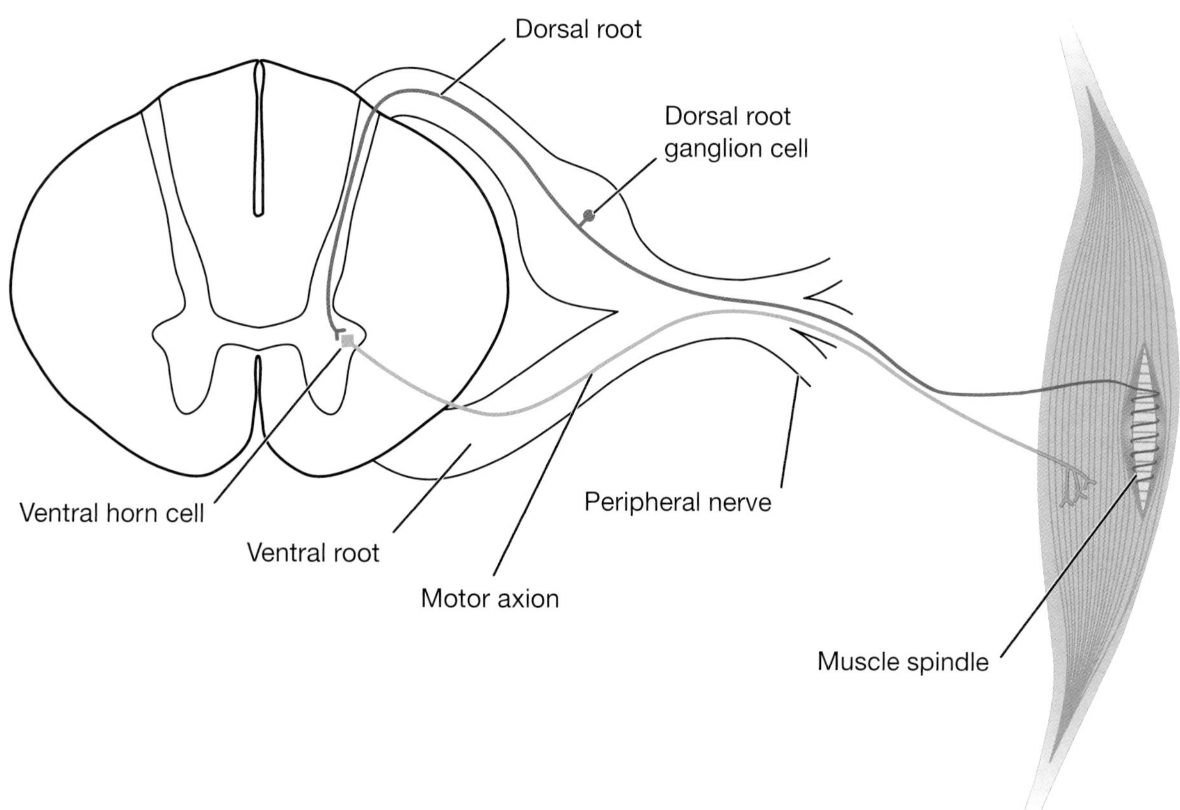

Fig. 14.14. Pathway for the monosynaptic stretch reflex. Group I afferents from muscle spindles, activated by muscle stretch, activate the alpha motor neuron innervating the same muscle.

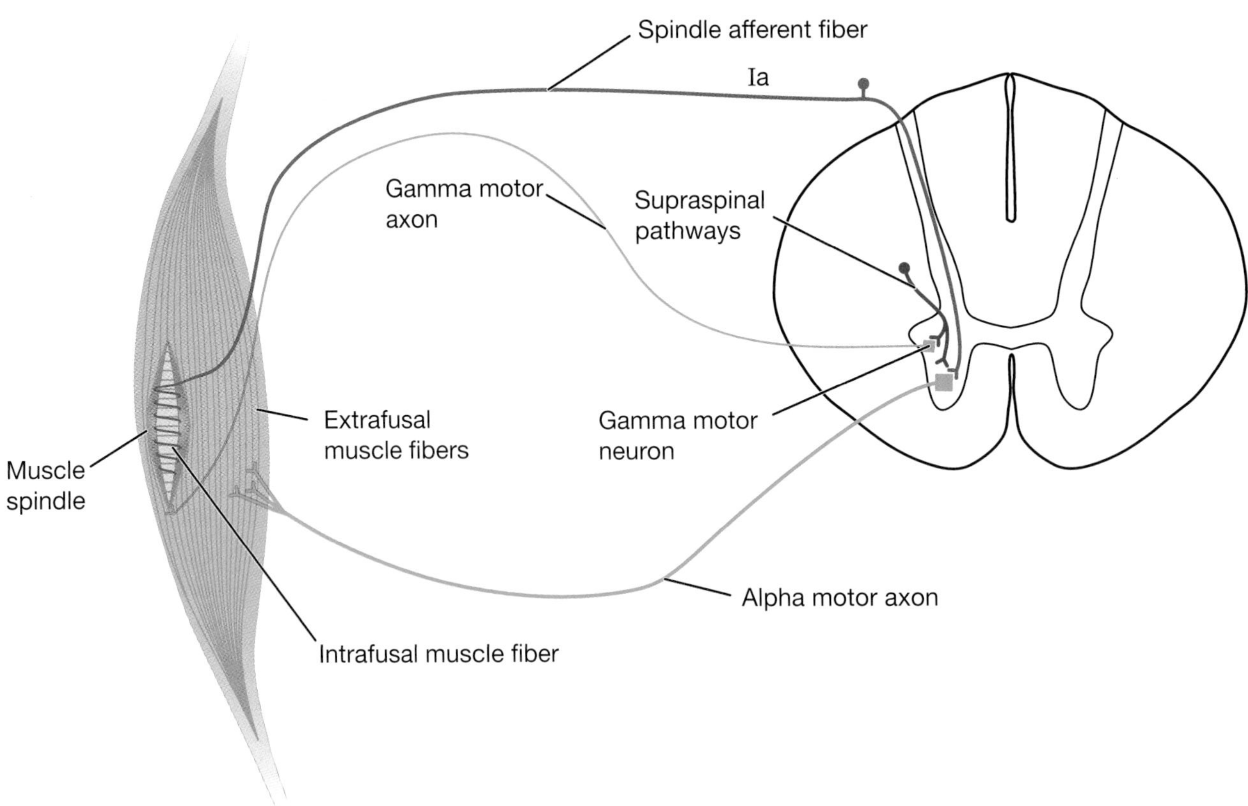

Fig. 14.15. Gamma motor neurons, which are coactivated with alpha motor neurons during most movements, innervate the intrafusal fibers and maintain the excitability of the muscle spindle despite shortening of the muscle. This gamma servoassistance mechanism is important for maintaining maximal activity of the alpha motor neuron.

for balancing the activity of the agonist and antagonist muscles that act on a joint (Fig. 14.16).

The Golgi tendon organ reflex provides a tension servomechanism. These receptors are generally silent in relaxed muscles and in response to passive stretch, but their discharge increases as muscle contraction increases tension at the level of the tendon. Input from Golgi tendon organs is carried by Ib afferents, which disynaptically inhibit the alpha motor neuron that innervates the corresponding muscle. This inhibition is mediated by *Ib inhibitory interneurons* and results in relaxation of the homonymous muscle, providing a tension feedback (Fig. 14.17). However, during locomotion, activation of Ib afferents from extensor muscles facilitates the homonymous extensor motor neuron. This is important in maintaining extension of the lower extremity during the stance phase of locomotion.

Flexor reflex afferents comprise group II muscle spindle afferents, groups III and IV muscle afferents, and skin afferents. These afferents trigger multiple polysynaptic reflexes. Polysynaptic proprioceptive reflexes integrate inputs from muscle, joint, and cutaneous afferents that may be triggered, for example, by contact of the foot on the ground. Flexor type II afferents converge with supraspinal commands on common spinal interneurons. Polysynaptic proprioceptive reflexes control the adjustment in motor neuron activity needed to maintain equilibrium and to generate a pattern of leg muscle activation during locomotion. Activation of nociceptive afferents from the skin elicits the nociceptive flexion reflex, which results in withdrawal of the limb from a noxious stimulus. This polysynaptic reflex activates ipsilateral flexor motor neurons and reciprocally inhibits the ipsilateral extensor motor neurons. Typically, the activation of flexor motor neurons is widespread so that flexor muscles at the ankle, knee, and hip contract to withdraw the entire limb (Fig. 14.18). Contralateral to the side of stimulation, flexor motor neurons are inhibited and extensor motor neurons are excited. This crossed extensor reflex stabilizes the body as the limb ipsilateral to the stimulus is flexed.

- The monosynaptic muscle stretch reflex, triggered by activation of muscle spindle Ia afferents, provides

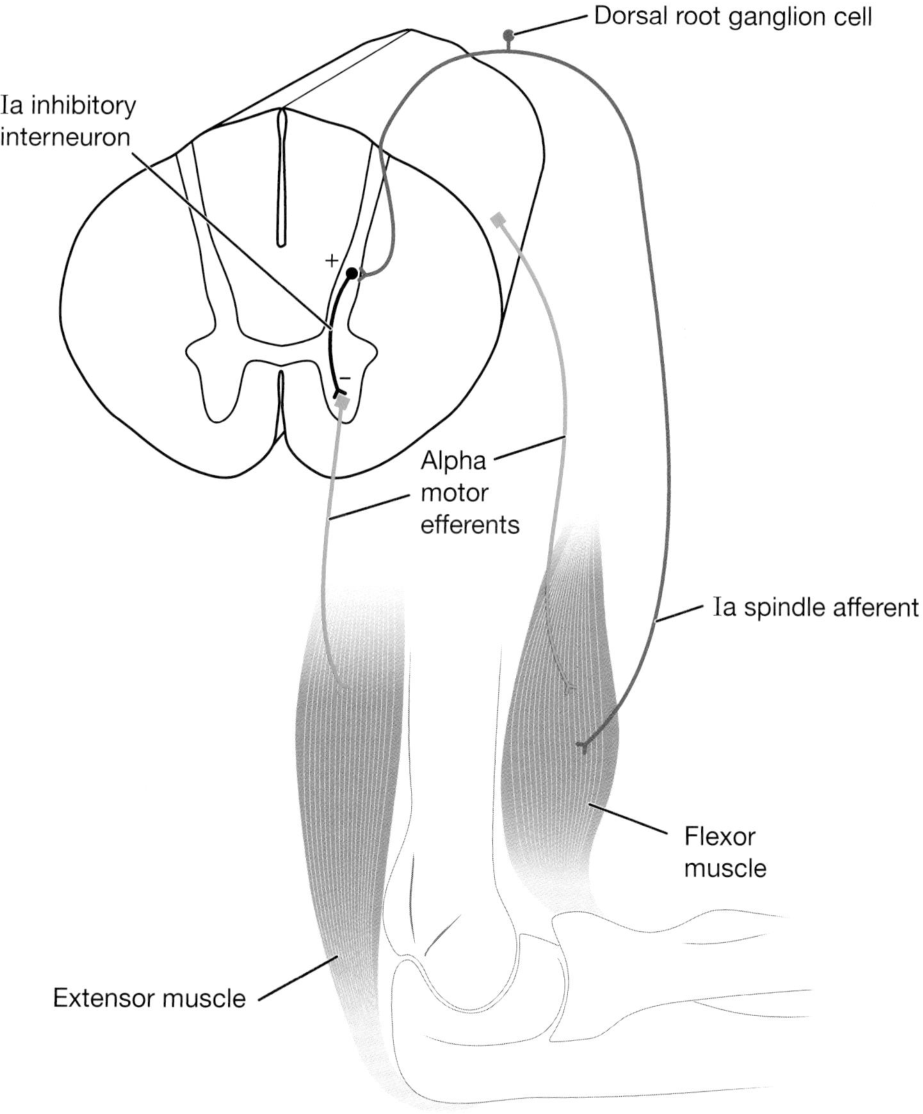

Fig. 14.16. Reciprocal inhibition, mediated by Ia inhibitory interneurons, is critical for controlling the activity of antagonist muscle groups acting on a given joint. In this figure, a Ia afferent from an arm flexor (biceps) elicits, through the Ia inhibitory interneuron, a disynaptic inhibition of the alpha motor neuron innervating the arm extensor (triceps) acting on the same joint.

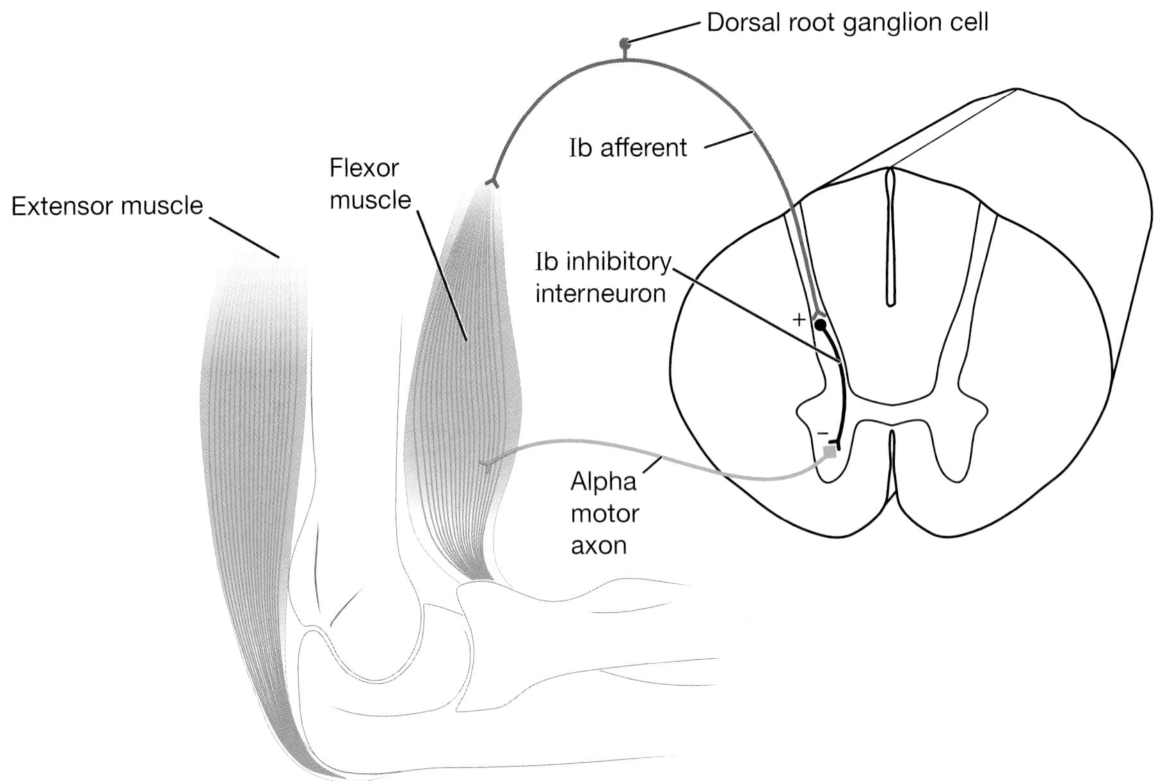

Fig. 14.17. Golgi tendon organ reflex. Group Ib afferents, activated by muscle tension, inhibit through the Ib inhibitory interneuron, the alpha motor neuron innervating the muscle, thus providing a tension servomechanism.

a length servomechanism and maintains the optimal excitability of the alpha motor neuron.

- Gamma motor neurons are coactivated with alpha motor neurons and, by input to intrafusal fibers, maintains the excitability of the muscle spindle during contraction.
- The Golgi tendon organs reflex, mediated by Ib afferents, provides a tension servomechanism.
- Flexor reflex afferents trigger polysynaptic proprioceptive reflexes that are critical for locomotion and nociceptive reflexes that mediate withdrawal from noxious stimuli.

Interneurons as Gain Control Devices

An important role of spinal interneurons is the control of the gain of segmental reflexes. As discussed above, Ia inhibitory interneurons activated by muscle spindle afferents mediate reciprocal inhibition between motor neuron pools that innervate antagonist muscles acting on a joint, and Ib inhibitory interneurons activated by Golgi tendon organ afferents decrease the activity of the motor neuron to control the force of contraction. Two other important types of inhibitory interneurons are *presynaptic inhibitory interneurons* and *Renshaw cells* (Fig. 14.19). Presynaptic Ia inhibitory neurons form GABAergic axoaxonic synapses with primary Ia afferents, which decreases neurotransmitter release and, thus, the gain of the muscle stretch reflex. Renshaw interneurons are activated monosynaptically by collaterals of motor neuron axons. In turn, Renshaw cells project to the same or related motor neurons and inhibit them. This is called *recurrent inhibition.*

Interneurons as Integrative Units

Spinal interneurons have a critical role in integrating the input from multiple primary afferents and descending pathways and in transforming all this input into specific patterns of activation or inhibition of selective pools of motor neurons. Individual spinal reflexes triggered by muscle spindles, Golgi tendon organs, or flexor reflex afferents are integrated, through interneurons, with descending motor commands from supraspinal centers (Fig. 14.20). Individual interneurons receive converging input from multiple types of afferents and descending pathways, and because of its divergent connections, a single interneuron may influence the activity of many motor neurons. This allows synergistic multijoint movement of a limb.

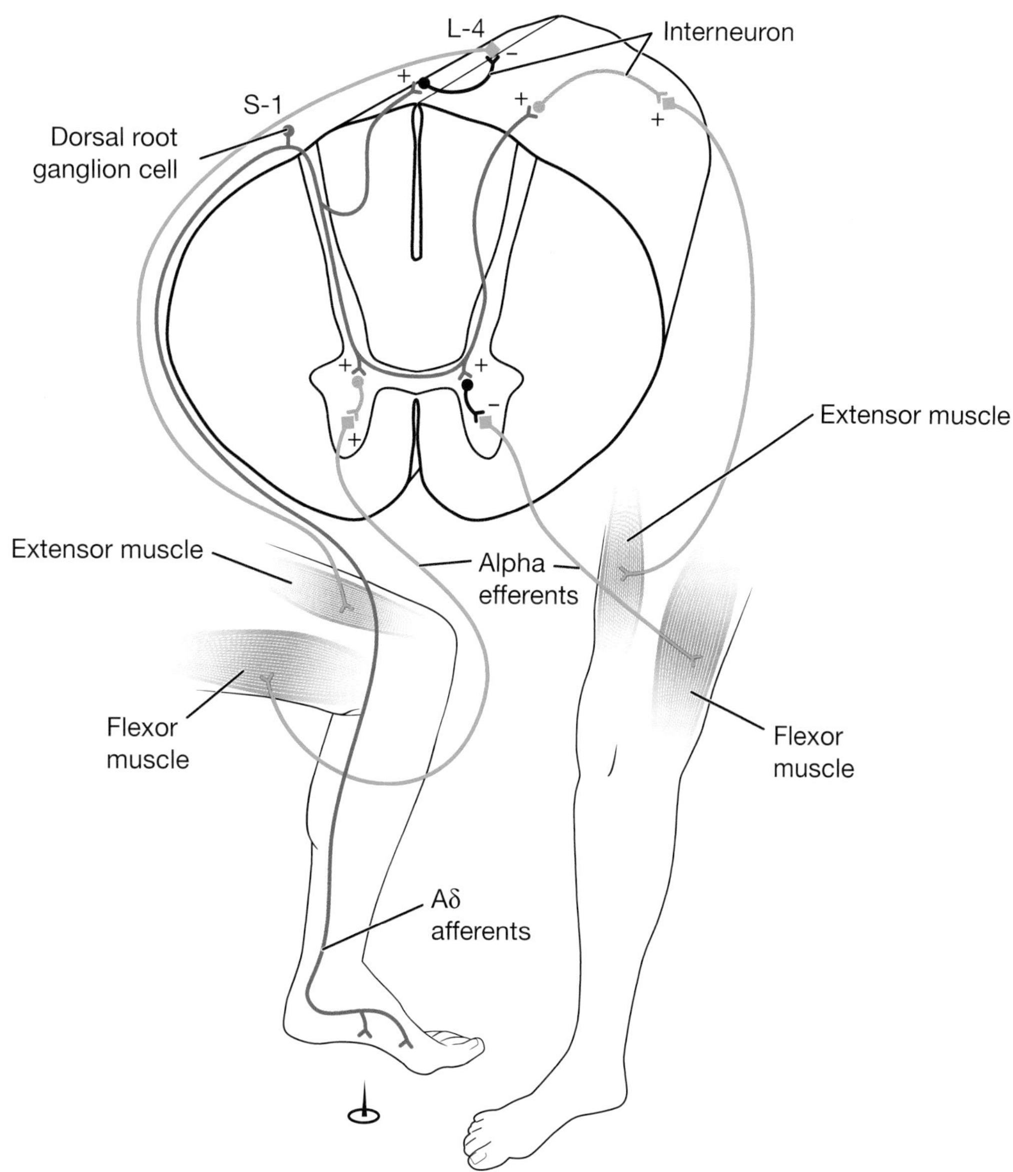

Fig. 14.18. Scheme of the nociceptive flexor reflex pathway. Nociceptive skin afferents from the foot activate, through a polysynaptic excitatory pathway, all motor neuron pools that lead to ipsilateral flexion (withdrawal) of the limb. If the stimulus is sufficiently intense, this reflex is associated with extension of the contralateral limb (crossed extensor reflex). These multisynaptic reflexes are also triggered by proprioceptive input and are important in locomotion.

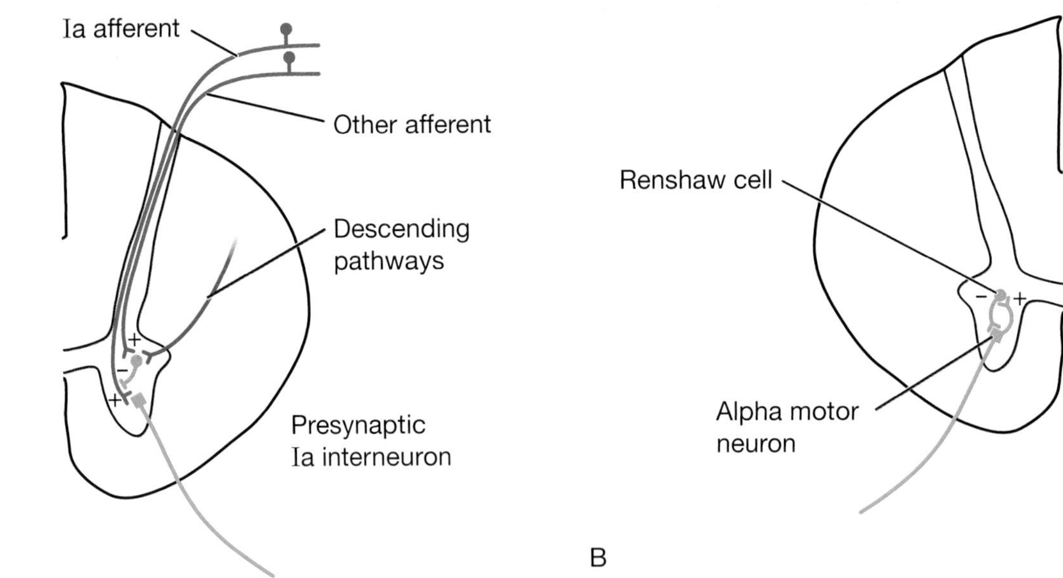

Fig. 14.19. Examples of inhibitory interneurons in the spinal cord. *A*, Presynaptic inhibitory neurons are activated by other afferents or descending inputs and form axoaxonic synapses on Ia (or other) afferents, inhibiting the release of neurotransmitter. *B*, Renshaw cells are activated by a collateral of a motor neuron axon. The Renshaw cell, in turn, synapses on the motor neuron and inhibits it.

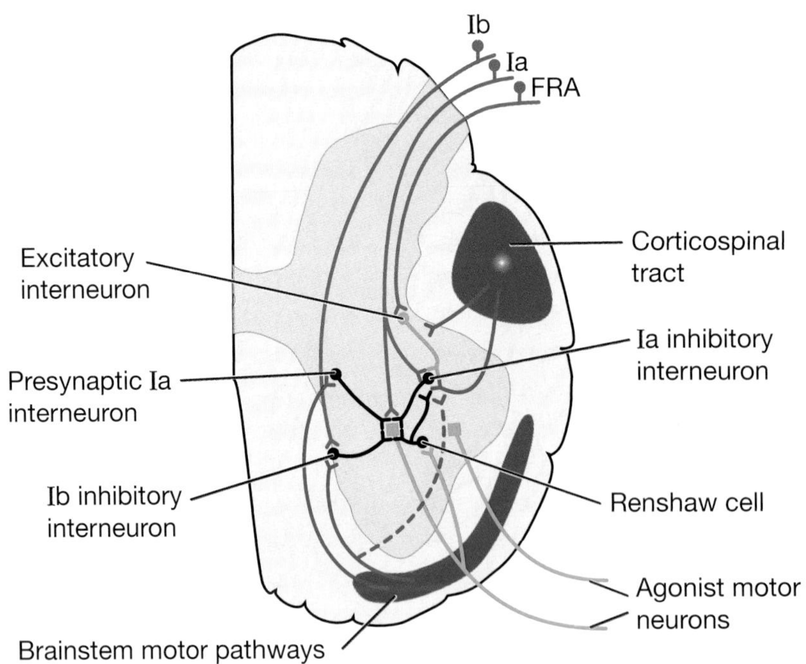

Fig. 14.20. Convergence of segmental and descending afferent input onto spinal interneurons. The individual interneurons integrate the input from several sources and coordinate the activity of many motor neuron pools. FRA, flexor reflex afferent.

Spinal Interneurons as the Central Pattern Generators for Locomotion

Locomotion in mammals depends on a *central pattern generator* located in the spinal cord and involving segmental networks of excitatory and inhibitory interneurons distributed in the intermediate gray matter across all lumbar and lower thoracic segments. These interneurons can generate rhythmic bursts of reciprocal activity in flexor and extensor motor neurons, even without sensory input or descending influences. However, despite this intrinsic ability to generate a rhythmic pattern of locomotion, the normal pattern is regulated by segmental afferent input and, in humans, it is also dependent on supraspinal input.

> After spinal cord injury, there are plastic changes in the number, size, distribution, and efficacy of the remaining synapses on all neuron types in the spinal cord. After complete transection, the isolated lumbosacral cord is capable of producing well-coordinated treadmill locomotion, and this activity improves with training. When patients with a complete or incomplete mid to low thoracic spinal cord injury step on a treadmill while being supported by a harness that can adjust weight bearing, extensor and flexor leg muscles are activated (measured as electromyographic activity). Robotic assistive devices can be used to guide the kinematics of the limbs and thus expose the spinal cord to new patterns of motor activity associated with a particular motor task. Improvement may occur independently of the time since injury and persist beyond the input of the assistive device.

- Spinal inhibitory interneurons regulate the gain of all spinal reflexes.
- Spinal interneurons integrate multiple primary afferents and descending motor pathways and coordinate the activity of multiple motor neuron pools in a flexible manner according to the specific motor task.
- Interneurons in the spinal cord form a pattern generator network that can generate locomotion even without segmental afferents or supraspinal input.

Descending Control of the Spinal Motor Apparatus

Spinal reflex patterns and locomotor central pattern generators are subjected to progressively increasing control from supraspinal levels during the course of development. The supraspinal motor pathways that originate in the cerebral cortex and brainstem control the spinal motor apparatus (motor neurons and interneurons of the reflex pathways) and serve three major functions: 1) to maintain erect body posture, 2) to perform independent, flexion movements of the limbs important in voluntary actions and locomotion, and, in humans, 3) to provide independent control of the fingers. These functions are differentially controlled by various descending pathways (see Chapter 8). The main descending motor pathways are summarized in Table 14.7.

The pathway most important for maintenance of the erect posture against gravity is the *lateral vestibulospinal tract*. It originates in the lateral vestibular nucleus, descends ipsilaterally in the ventrolateral quadrant through the length of the spinal cord, and terminates in laminae VII and VIII, where it activates directly and through interneurons the gamma and alpha motor neurons that innervate the extensor axial and proximal limb muscles and mediate all antigravity reflexes.

The reticular formation of the medial dorsal tegmentum of the lower pons and medulla is the origin of the *reticulospinal tracts*. These tracts reach all spinal cord segments either directly or through the propriospinal system and terminate primarily on interneurons in lamina VIII and adjacent portions of lamina VII. The *pontine reticulospinal tract*, sometimes called the medial reticulospinal tract, descends ipsilaterally in the ventral funiculus and activates the alpha motor neurons that innervate the antigravity muscles responsible for erect posture, including flexors of the upper limb and extensors of the lower limb.

The medullary reticular formation contains different groups of neurons that receive excitatory input from the cerebral cortex and upper brainstem and, through reticulospinal projections to interneurons, inhibit several segmental reflexes that may interfere with the execution of specific motor acts. The *lateral medullary reticulospinal tracts* course bilaterally in the ventrolateral funiculus and inhibit segmental stretch reflexes, particularly those

Table 14.7. Main Descending Motor Pathways and Their Function

Pathway	Origin	Central connections	Function
Corticospinal	Primary motor cortex Premotor cortex Supplementary motor cortex Anterior cingulate motor area	Collateral inputs to red nucleus, reticular formation, pontine nuclei, and dorsal column nuclei	Motor neuron recruitment Inhibits antigravity muscles Fractionated control of finger movement
Rubrospinal	Red nucleus (magnocellular)	Receive input from motor cortex and cerebellar nuclei	Contributes to control of forearm and hand muscles
Lateral vestibulospinal	Lateral vestibular nucleus	Input from otolith organs, neck proprioceptors, and cerebellum	Activates extensor motor neurons for antigravity postural reflexes
Medullary reticulospinal	Medullary reticular formation	Requires excitatory input from premotor and supplementary motor cortices	Inhibits muscle stretch reflexes that may interfere with voluntary movements
Dorsolateral reticulospinal	Medullary reticular formation	Motor cortex, red nucleus, pedunculopontine nucleus	Inhibits interneurons of flexor reflex afferent pathways to make them available for locomotion
Pontine reticulospinal	Pontine reticular formation	Vestibular nuclei Proprioceptors	Facilitates antigravity reflexes
Medial vestibulospinal	Medial vestibular nuclei	Semicircular canals Cerebellum	Controls neck movements for head-eye coordination
Tectospinal	Superior colliculus	Frontal eye fields	

involving extensor motor neurons. The activity of these medullary reticulospinal neurons depends on excitatory input from the premotor cortex and supplementary motor area. This corticoreticulospinal system suppresses stretch reflexes that would otherwise interfere with the smooth and rapid execution of voluntary movements. The *dorsolateral reticulospinal tract* tonically inhibits segmental polysynaptic reflexes triggered by flexor reflex afferents and Ib afferents. This releases interneurons from segmental reflex function and makes them responsive to descending inputs during locomotion.

The most important descending motor pathway in the spinal cord is the lateral corticospinal tract. This pathway arises from several motor areas of the cerebral cortex and has two main functions in humans: to provide general background excitation that allows the recruitment of motor neuron pools in response to increased effort and to control fractionated movements of the distal portion of the limbs, particularly the digits (see Chapter 8). Most corticospinal control of the spinal motor output is exerted through interneurons, which allow the motor cortex to influence complex patterns of muscle contraction by controlling segmental spinal reflexes. Corticospinal axons may activate presynaptic inhibitory neurons that control the input from Golgi tendon organs, type II afferents from muscle spindles, and some cutaneous afferents. The cerebral cortex facilitates the initiation of voluntary action by inhibiting the motor neurons of antigravity muscles (flexors in the upper limb and extensors in the lower limb) and exciting the motor neurons of the antagonists (extensors in the upper limb and flexors in the lower limb). This inhibition is also mediated by cortical input to the medullary reticular formation, including the origin of the lateral reticulospinal pathway. Although most corticospinal axons synapse on interneurons in the intermediate gray matter, many pyramidal cells of the primary motor cortex synapse directly on motor neurons that innervate the distal hand muscles.

The motor cortex controls upper limb motor neurons not only by synapsing directly on spinal motor neurons and on interneurons but also through collateral projections to the red nucleus, the origin of the *rubrospinal tract*, and to cervical propriospinal neurons. The rubrospinal tract may contribute to the activation of flexor motor neurons of elbow and wrist muscles.

- The functions of the supraspinal motor pathways are to maintain erect posture, facilitate flexor movements of the limbs for voluntary action and locomotion, and, in humans, to provide independent control of finger movement.
- The lateral vestibulospinal tract facilitates extensor antigravity reflexes and is essential for maintaining erect posture.
- The medullary reticulospinal tracts are activated by the cerebral cortex and inhibit, through interneurons, segmental muscle reflexes that may interfere with the execution of voluntary motor acts or locomotion.
- The corticospinal tract directly activates motor neurons that control the intrinsic hand muscles and, through interneurons, inhibits the motor neurons of antigravity muscles (flexors in the upper limb and extensors in the lower limb) and excites the motor neurons of the antagonists.

Integration of Segmental and Supraspinal Influences on Muscle Tone, Stretch Reflexes, and Cutaneous Reflexes

Muscle tone is the resistance offered by the muscles to continuous stretch, as elicited by passive flexion or extension of a joint (see Chapter 8). In relaxed normal individuals, fusimotor activity and muscle stretch reflexes do not contribute to muscle tone, and resistance to joint rotation is moderate and uniform at all speeds and is due mainly to the viscoelastic properties of the muscles and joints. However, tone also depends importantly on the level of arousal and increases when stretch reflexes are reinforced through mental concentration or contraction of the involved muscle. This depends on facilitatory support of tonic muscle stretch reflexes by corticospinal pathways activated by muscle spindle afferents through the lemniscal system, *long loop reflexes*.

The muscle stretch reflex, or *tendon jerk*, is one of the most important objective clinical signs of the integrity of the segmental motor apparatus. It is elicited by percussion of a tendon, typically the biceps, brachioradialis, triceps, patellar (quadriceps), or Achilles tendon. This directly stretches the relevant muscle, activates the primary muscle spindle endings, produces a synchronized Ia afferent volley from that muscle, and activates the corresponding motor neuron pools, thus eliciting muscle contraction. Consequently, these reflexes have a major localizing value for lesions in a single spinal cord segment or peripheral nerve. The tonic and phasic stretch reflexes are under strong inhibitory control by the corticomedullary reticulospinal system.

The nociceptive flexion reflex, a phylogenetically primitive protective reflex, is triggered by stimulation of nociceptive afferents in the skin and mediated by polysynaptic pathways. In adults, the circuit of this reflex is incorporated into the more complex volitional movements initiated by motor cortex, including locomotion. Because the flexion reflex is polysynaptic, activation of the flexor motor neurons is typically widespread, and as a result, flexor muscles at the ankle, knee, and hip, for example, contract to withdraw the entire limb. The corticospinal pathway facilitates the interneuronal pathways activated by the flexor reflex afferents, but the dorsolateral medullary reticulospinal pathway inhibits it. A function of the corticospinal tract may be selecting the synaptic actions of the flexion reflex afferents appropriate for a particular task.

- Muscle tone depends on arousal and motor set; in this setting, it involves tonic stretch reflexes assisted by long loop reflexes.

- The tendon jerk, or muscle stretch reflex, is an important, objective sign of the integrity of the segmental motor apparatus, including the afferent and efferent components.

Autonomic Function

Preganglionic Sympathetic Neurons and Segmental Sympathetic Reflexes

Preganglionic sympathetic neurons are organized into different functional units in the intermediolateral cell column of the spinal cord (see Chapter 9). These include muscle vasomotor, skin vasomotor, sudomotor, and visceromotor units. Although these neurons may be activated by segmental afferents, supraspinal influences coordinate the activity of specific subsets of sympathetic neurons according to the task. Several parallel pathways descending from the hypothalamus and brainstem differentially control the functionally defined subpopulations of preganglionic neurons. For example, muscle vasoconstrictor neurons are activated by input from rostral ventrolateral medulla and are necessary for maintaining arterial blood pressure, and skin vasoconstrictor neurons receive input from the medullary raphe neurons and mediate responses to cold. In humans, sympathetic vasomotor activity in skeletal muscles is finely regulated by baroreflex activity; however, the vasomotor and sudomotor activity in the skin is regulated mainly by environmental temperature and emotional state.

Preganglionic neurons are the effectors of segmental somatosympathetic and viscerosympathetic reflexes. These reflexes may be triggered by skin, muscle, or visceral afferents that generally synapse on local interneurons. For example, the activation of skin nociceptors excites sympathetic vasoconstrictor neurons (somatosympathetic reflex). Preganglionic neurons in spinal segments T11 to L2 are activated by low-frequency input from the bladder that signals bladder filling and triggers relaxation of the bladder detrusor muscle and contraction of the bladder neck, allowing storage of urine (continence reflex) (see Chapter 9).

Micturition

The preganglionic parasympathetic neurons that control the function of the bladder, rectum, and sexual organs are located in the sacral parasympathetic nucleus in spinal segments S2 to S4. Normally, the activity of these neurons is reciprocally regulated with that of the sacral motor neurons of Onuf nucleus, which innervate the external sphincter muscles. The micturition reflex normally is triggered by bladder distention above a certain threshold and is coordinated by neurons in the *pontine micturition center*. Descending axons from neurons in this center coordinate the activation of the sacral preganglionic neurons that innervate the bladder detrusor muscle and, through local interneurons, the inhibition of motor neurons in Onuf nucleus that innervate the external sphincter muscle. This coordinated action produces complete emptying of the bladder. Although bladder afferents may also activate a sacral micturition reflex, this is normally overridden by the pontine micturition center.

- Preganglionic sympathetic neurons form functionally different units that generate patterns of sympathetic activation determined by supraspinal inputs.
- Preganglionic neurons receive segmental afferent input that can trigger segmental reflexes.
- The normal micturition reflex is coordinated by the pontine micturition center.

Clinical Correlations

Diseases at the spinal level, like those at other levels, can be classified as focal or diffuse. Focal disease may be segmental, as with lesions of the spinal nerve in the intervertebral foramen, or it may be a combination of segmental and longitudinal symptoms and signs if the pathways in the spinal cord are involved. In focal lesions, localization depends on the unique combination of segmental and intersegmental signs. Diffuse disease may involve only a single system, for example, the motor system in motor neuron disease, or multiple systems, as in some degenerative and inflammatory disorders.

Segmental Manifestations of Focal Lesions at the Spinal Level

Focal lesions at the spinal level are characterized by segmental signs or symptoms specific for a particular level of the spinal canal. These may be due to damage to a spinal nerve, a dorsal or ventral nerve root, a single vertebra, or a single spinal cord segment. Lesions of the spinal nerves are often due to (or related to) disease of the vertebral column. Many of their clinical features are similar to those of peripheral nerve lesions. However, lesions of spinal nerves are recognized by their dermatomal or myotomal pattern of distribution.

Sensory Manifestations

With segmental lesions, there is sensory loss of *all* modalities in a dermatomal distribution. This is usually best recognized in regard to pain, temperature, or touch. There may be *paresthesia* (pins-and-needles sensation) from spontaneous firing of the larger axons, or spontaneous lancinating or burning pain, hyperalgesia, or allodynia, due to abnormal firing of small-diameter nociceptive axons. The pain is often perceived outside the distribution of the spinal nerve because of central sensitization of spinothalamic neurons. Irritable spinal nerves are more sensitive to stretch, and pain is produced when the extremities are put in certain positions, for example, in a *straight leg raising test.*

Lower Motor Neuron Weakness

Involvement of the alpha motor neurons or ventral root of a segment produces findings of lower motor neuron (final common pathway) damage. These include weakness, hypotonia, atrophy, and fasciculations in the corresponding myotome. Atrophy occurs after the lesion has persisted for sufficient time. Fasciculations, which are the clinically detectable manifestation of irritability of the affected axons and thus the entire motor unit, are commonly associated with fibrillation potentials, which are only detectable with electromyography and are the manifestation of denervation of individual muscle fibers. Because the lesion is proximal to the origin of the posterior branch of the spinal nerve innervating the paraspinal muscles, the paraspinal muscles are involved as well as other proximal muscles. Paraspinal involvement does not occur with lesions that involve the peripheral nerve.

Reflex Loss

Muscle stretch reflexes may be lost if either the sensory component (primary large myelinated dorsal root afferents from muscle spindles) or the motor component (motor neurons or their axons in the ventral root) of the reflex arc is damaged. Therefore, these reflexes are an important segmental sign of spinal nerve or spinal cord disease (Table 14.8).

Autonomic Involvement

Autonomic fibers are also involved by segmental lesions, but because of more extensive overlap, autonomic disturbances do not occur with lesions of single spinal nerves. However, there may be segmental loss of sweating in the affected dermatome. Bilateral sacral spinal nerve or cauda equina damage, however, denervates the bladder detrusor muscle, producing a *flaccid bladder*. This is a hypotonic bladder with large capacity and postvoid residual urine. These lesions also affect the innervation of the external sphincters, which is manifested by overflow urinary or fecal incontinence.

Table 14.8. Stretch Reflexes

Reflex	Spinal level and spinal nerve	Plexus	Peirpheral nerve
Biceps jerk	C5, C6	Brachial	Musculocutaneous
Triceps jerk	**C7**, C8	Brachial	Radial
Knee jerk	L3, L4	Lumbar	Femoral
Ankle jerk	**S1**, L5	Lumbar	Femoral

Bold type, spinal nerve that provides major innervation.

Vertebral Pain

Focal symptoms at the spinal level are commonly segmental signs of associated vertebral column involvement. For example, neck, thoracic spine, or low back pain is often associated with restricted motion because of spasms of the paraspinal muscles and tenderness of a vertebra to palpation. When a lesion affects the dorsal root or spinal nerve, the pain also radiates in the distribution of the dermatome innervated by the segment.

- Localization to a specific spinal level may be on the basis of the following:
  - Pain in a dermatomal or myotomal distribution and associated with signs of irritability of the nerve root to mechanical stimuli
  - Variable sensory loss for all modalities in a dermatomal distribution
  - Flaccid weakness, atrophy, and fasciculations in a myotomal distribution
  - Loss of segmental reflexes
  - Segmental autonomic impairment, such as loss of sweating, or a flaccid bladder

Intersegmental Manifestations of Spinal Cord Lesions

The most convincing evidence of a focal lesion at the spinal level is the presence of segmental signs in association with intersegmental signs due to involvement of the long ascending or descending pathways of the spinal cord. There are three major types of intersegmental signs: 1) a long tract sensory level, reflecting involvement of the spinothalamic tract, dorsal column, or both, 2) a long tract motor level, reflecting involvement of the corticospinal and brainstem motor pathways, and 3) autonomic involvement below the level of the lesion.

Dorsal Column Involvement

Lesions that affect the dorsal column impair tactile discrimination and object recognition (*astereognosia*), vibration sense, and joint position sense on the same side of the body below the level of the lesion. Cervical cord lesions (involving the gracile and cuneate fascicles) affect these sensory modalities in both the upper and lower limbs, whereas thoracic and lumbar lesions (involving only the gracile fasciculus) affect only the lower limbs.

Spinothalamic Tract Involvement

Because the spinothalamic tract crosses to the opposite side within two or three segments of its origin, a lesion that affects the ventrolateral quadrant of the spinal cord causes loss of pain and temperature sensations of the contralateral body below the level of the lesion. The dermatomal level of sensory loss is located two segment levels below the level of the lesion. Bilateral lesions produce bilateral loss of pain and temperature sensations below the level of the lesion as well as loss of visceral and sexual sensations.

Thus, there are fundamental differences between lesions of the peripheral nerves or dorsal roots and lesions in the spinal cord. Peripheral or dorsal root lesions commonly affect all sensory modalities, including pain, temperature, vibration, joint position, and touch, on the same side of the body as the lesion. In contrast, with lesions of the spinal cord, these sensory modalities are dissociated. Dorsal column lesions affect tactile discrimination, vibration, and joint position sense on the same side, whereas spinothalamic tract lesions affect pain and temperature sensation on the opposite side. This is called *sensory dissociation*. This and a dermatomal *sensory level* below which sensation is impaired are the hallmarks of a lesion at the spinal level.

Descending Motor Pathway Involvement

Lesions that affect the lateral portion of the spinal cord produce the *upper motor neuron syndrome*. This is the consequence of the interruption of corticospinal and parallel corticoreticulospinal input to spinal interneurons and motor neurons. The upper motor neuron syndrome includes weakness, loss of dexterity, enhanced muscle stretch reflexes, enhanced muscle tone, release of flexor reflexes, and the extensor plantar response (*Babinski sign*). With spinal lesions, these manifestations are ipsilateral below the level of the lesion. The distinctive features of the lower motor neuron syndrome (occurring at the segment of the spinal lesion) and the upper motor neuron syndrome (occurring below the level of the spinal lesion) are summarized in Table 14.9.

A cardinal element of the upper motor neuron syndrome is *spasticity*. This is a velocity-dependent increase in tonic stretch reflexes and muscle tone associated with

Table 14.9. Summary of Findings in Lower and Upper Motor Neuron Disease

Finding	Lower motor neuron[a]	Upper motor neurons[b]
Strength	Decreased	Decreased
Atrophy	Present	Absent
Fasciculations	Present	Absent
Tone	Decreased	Increased
Stretch reflexes	Decreased	Increased
Clonus	Absent	Present
Superficial reflexes	Absent	Absent
Babinski sign	Absent	Present

[a]Segmental finding of involvement of the final common pathway (motor unit).
[b]Suprasegmental finding of involvement of the corticospinal and corticoreticulospinal pathways.

exaggeration of the phasic muscle stretch reflexes and clonus. Spasticity reflects increased excitability of the motor neuron pools involved in the muscle stretch reflex. This increased excitability is due to the loss of activity of spinal inhibitory interneurons from the interruption of the medullary reticulospinal system.

The loss of descending corticospinal and reticulospinal control of the flexor reflex afferent pathways produces other features of the upper motor neuron syndrome. These include the *clasp-knife response*, which refers to the phenomenon in which the increased resistance to passive movement, present with initial stretch, subsides with continuous stretch. The lack of supraspinal control of the polysynaptic nociceptive flexor reflex appears as an exaggeration of the *triple flexion reflex*. In the newborn, this reflex includes the toe extensors, which physiologically are flexors. Normally, after age 2 years, the toe extensors are no longer part of the reflex. Instead, in response to noxious stimulation of the sole, the toes may curl down, because of segmental reflex activation of the small muscles of the foot underlying the stimulated skin. When the function of the corticospinal tract is impaired, noxious stimulation of the sole elicits an extension of the great toe; this extensor plantar response is the *Babinski sign*. Exaggeration of the flexor reflex in spinal lesions may also manifest with *flexor spasms*, which may be triggered by noxious somatic and other stimuli (including bladder distention).

The exaggeration of the intersegmental flexion reflex responses is in sharp contrast to the inhibition of segmental nociceptive reflexes that occurs with the upper motor neuron syndrome. The *abdominal reflexes*, elicited by stimulating the skin of the abdomen, and the *cremasteric reflex*, normally induced by stimulating the skin along the inner side of the thigh, cannot be elicited after a corticospinal tract lesion.

- Dorsal column lesions impair tactile discrimination, vibratory sense, and joint position sense on the same side of the body below the level of the lesion.
- Spinothalamic tract lesions in the ventrolateral quadrant of the spinal cord impair pain and temperature sensations on the opposite side of the body below the level of the lesion.
- Lesions affecting the corticospinal and reticulospinal pathways produce weakness, spasticity, exaggerated muscle stretch reflexes (including clonus), and the Babinski sign, and they abolish abdominal cutaneous reflexes.
- The upper motor neuron syndrome occurs contralateral to a lesion at the supratentorial or posterior fossa level but is ipsilateral to a lesion at the spinal level.

Involvement of Descending Autonomic Pathways

Unilateral involvement of the descending autonomic pathways that synapse on the preganglionic neurons in spinal segment T1 that innervate the superior cervical ganglion and control the pupil produces an ipsilateral *Horner syndrome*. Interruption of the descending input to preganglionic neurons that control sudomotor function impairs thermoregulatory sweating (*anhidrosis*) ipsilaterally below the level of the lesion.

Because of the bilateral innervation of the blood vessels and bladder, only bilateral or midline lesions affecting the descending autonomic pathways impair cardiovascular control or produce a neurogenic bladder. Lesions that affect the descending vasomotor pathways above spinal segment T5 produce *orthostatic hypotension* and abolish skin vasomotor responses below the level of the lesion, thus impairing the response to either a cold or a hot environment. Interruption of these supraspinal pathways also impairs the modulation and coordination of the activity of preganglionic sympathetic neurons and their response to segmental input. In patients with chronic bilateral or midline lesions above spinal segment T5, stimulation of the skin, muscle, or viscera innervated by segments below the lesion may cause massive reflex activation of all sympathetic outputs and produce severe hypertension. This is called *autonomic dysreflexia*.

Bilateral involvement of the spinal cord, usually due to a midline lesion, is typically manifested as neurogenic bladder (Table 14.10). Lesions at the cervical or thoracic level that affect the connections between the pontine micturition center and the reflex apparatus in the sacral cord produce a *spastic bladder*. This is the consequence of uncoordinated activation of sacral preganglionic parasympathetic neurons and somatic motor neurons by segmental input from the bladder, leading to a segmental micturition reflex in which contraction of the bladder detrusor muscle is not accompanied by relaxation of the external sphincter, as normally occurs with input from the pontine micturition center. This *detrusor-sphincter dyssynergia* produces hypertrophy of the bladder wall, decreased bladder volume, and compliance. In contrast, lesions that affect the sacral cord (conus medullaris), such as bilateral sacral spinal nerve or cauda equina damage, denervate the bladder detrusor muscle, resulting in a *flaccid bladder*. Other typical manifestations of spinal lesions producing neurogenic bladder include neurogenic bowel (usually causes constipation) and erectile dysfunction.

Localization of Lesions at the Spinal Level

Combinations of segmental and long tract signs permit the identification of the site of spinal cord disease with some accuracy. Characteristic patterns of abnormality are as follows:

1. Upper cervical: This pattern includes long tract signs in the upper and lower extremities for motor and sensory modalities and spastic (reflex) bladder dysfunction.
2. Middle and lower cervical: Segmental signs of motor and sensory dysfunction appear in the upper extremities along with long tract signs in the lower extremities and spastic bladder dysfunction.
3. Thoracic: Long tract signs in the lower extremities appear with a segmental sensory finding (level of sensation) in the trunk and spastic bladder dysfunction.

Table 14.10. Types of Neurogenic Bladder Occurring With Lesions at the Spinal Level

	Spastic (upper motor neuron)	Flaccid (lower motor neuron)
Clinical symptoms		
Urgency	Present	Absent
Incontinence	Present	Present
Retention	Late in evolution	Initial manifestation
Anal reflex	Present	Absent
Urodynamics		
Bladder capacity	Decreased	Increased
Bladder tone	Increased	Decreased
Uninhibited contractions	Present	Absent
Detrusor-sphincter dyssynergia	Present	Absent
Lesion location	Cervical or thoracic cord	Conus medullaris or cauda equina
Common causes	Trauma, multiple sclerosis	Extruded intervertebral disk, neoplasms

Clinical Problem 14.1.

A 57-year-old woman began to notice problems walking about 1 year ago. She felt that her gait was becoming stiff and slow. The problem has been progressive since that time. More recently, she has also noted weakness in the left hand, especially when she tries to grip something with it. Neurologic examination shows atrophy and weakness in the left hand muscles. The left triceps reflex is absent. Reflexes are increased in the left leg. There is mild weakness in the left leg, especially in hip and knee flexion and about the ankle. Tone is increased in the left leg, and the Babinski sign is elicited on the left. Motor examination findings on the right side are normal.

a. What is the location of the lesion?
b. What is the possible pathologic basis?
c. What sensory finding would you expect in the patient's hands?
d. In which foot would you expect to find impaired joint position and vibration sense?
e. In which foot would you expect the patient to have loss of pain and temperature sensations?
f. Why is bladder function spared with this lesion?

4. Lumbar and upper sacral: This pattern includes segmental motor and sensory signs in the lower extremities with spastic bladder dysfunction.
5. Conus medullaris: Segmental signs appear in the lower extremities with a flaccid (nonreflex) bladder.
6. Cauda equina: There is pain and asymmetrical motor and sensory involvement of multiple roots, generally associated with a flaccid bladder.

Clinical Syndromes

The term *radiculopathy* refers specifically to disease of the nerve root located within the vertebral column and spinal canal. The distribution of dermatomal deficits (sensory loss of all modalities) and myotomal deficits (weakness atrophy, fasciculations, or reflex loss, or a combination of these) allows localization of the root involved. A disorder that affects the spinal cord is referred to as *myelopathy*. Isolated or combined involvement of long pathways in the spinal white matter may produce specific syndromes that have localizing value in determining the transverse extent of the lesion.

Radiculopathy

Localized nerve root disease may produce pain and purely sensory deficits in a dermatomal distribution, purely motor deficits in a myotomal distribution, or both, depending on whether the dorsal root or ventral root or both are affected. Because the nerve roots and spinal nerves have the same segmental derivation, disease of the spinal nerve (in which the dorsal and ventral roots have joined) is also commonly referred to as a radiculopathy.

Polyradiculopathy

Diffuse involvement of spinal nerves is referred to as *polyradiculopathy*. Proximal weakness, which is seen more often in muscle disease, may also occur in polyradiculopathy, but there usually are additional abnormalities such as reflex and sensory loss. Polyradiculopathy may be

Clinical Problem 14.2.

A 30-year-old man had acute onset of severe back and right leg pain after falling while carrying a sack of bagels. His symptoms have worsened over the 4 weeks since onset. Neurologic examination showed a lack of sensation to pinprick and touch on the lateral aspect of his leg, but normal knee and ankle muscle stretch reflexes. There is mild weakness of hip abductors, hamstrings, ankle dorsiflexors, and toe extensors on the right. He experiences severe pain when he coughs or when his leg is elevated.

a. What are the site and type of the lesion?
b. What neural structure is involved?
c. In a patient with footdrop, at what sites could the lesion be located?
d. What produces pain on straight leg raising?

difficult to recognize clinically, but the involvement of paraspinal muscles at multiple levels, as shown with electromyography, is strong evidence of it.

One form of polyradiculopathy is *Guillain-Barré syndrome*, a subacute, inflammatory disorder with segmental demyelination predominantly in nerve roots. Another important example of polyradiculopathy is *cauda equina syndrome*, which usually is caused by a mass lesion, for example, a large midline vertebral disk herniation or neoplasm, that affects the lumbrosacral roots bilaterally. Features of this syndrome include severe pain, the straight leg raising sign, and asymmetrical motor and sensory involvement of multiple lumbar and sacral roots, leading to areflexia and a flaccid bladder.

Clinical Problem 14.3.

A 47-year-old woman developed lower back pain within the last year after planting her garden. Despite rest, the back pain has slowly worsened. Three months ago, after a long "driving" vacation, she began to notice pain in the right groin and anterior thigh. This also worsened and was followed in several weeks by similar pain in the left groin and thigh. Three to four weeks ago, she began to have trouble climbing stairs and her legs felt weak. For the last week, her husband has had to assist her in climbing the stairs and getting out of the car. In the last 2 or 3 days, her legs have felt "dead and swollen." This morning she was brought to the hospital because she was unable to get out of bed.

Neurologic examination showed weakness in both legs, right greater than left. The knee and ankle muscle stretch reflexes were absent bilaterally, and muscle tone was reduced in both legs. The anal reflex was absent. No Babinski sign was elicited. All forms of sensation were reduced in both lower extremities. Flexion at the hip of either lower extremity with the knee extended produced severe pain.

a. What are the segmental signs and symptoms?
b. What structure is most likely involved?
c. What is the pathologic basis?
d. At what vertebral level is the nervous system involved?
e. Eighteen hours after admission, the nurse reports that the patient has not urinated and asks you if there is a neurologic explanation. What would your answer be? Why?

Dorsal Column Syndrome

The dorsal columns may be affected directly at the level of the spinal cord or be involved because of wallerian degeneration that results from a disease affecting the dorsal root ganglia or the dorsal roots. Dorsal column lesions impair tactile discrimination, vibration sense, and joint position sense below the level of the lesion. Lack of proprioception compromises the sensory feedback essential for maintaining posture, gait, and motor coordination. This results in *sensory ataxia*, which is characterized by the Romberg sign, pseudoathetosis, impaired stereognosis, and loss of fine control of finger movements in the absence of visual clues.

The effects of intrinsic spinal cord lesions that involve the dorsal columns are difficult to distinguish from those that affect the large myelinated nerve fibers or dorsal root ganglion neurons conveying discriminative touch, vibration, and joint position sense in the dorsal columns. However, unlike spinal cord lesions, lesions of the dorsal root ganglion or the dorsal root affect all primary large myelinated afferents, not only those that ascend in the dorsal columns but also those that contribute to the dorsolateral quadrant and spinocerebellar pathways and those that mediate segmental muscle stretch reflexes. Thus, lesions of large dorsal root ganglion cells or large myelinated afferents produce a more severe sensory ataxia than lesions of only the dorsal columns. Furthermore, unlike pure dorsal column lesions, lesions of large dorsal root ganglion cells or large myelinated afferents also abolish muscle stretch reflexes.

Commissural and Central Spinal Cord Syndromes

Midline lesions that affect the central gray matter of the spinal cord interrupt the crossing spinothalamic axons bilaterally at the level of the anterior spinal commissure.

Clinical Problem 14.4.

A 52-year-old woman presents to you because of gait unsteadiness. She reports that 3 years ago she began complaining to her doctor of a "pins and needles" sensation in her feet and hands; this gradually spread to her knees and elbows. For the past 18 months, she has had progressive difficulty with gait. On neurologic examination, her gait is unsteady. Although she stands alone quite well, she nearly falls when asked to close her eyes. Position sense is mildly impaired in the fingers and severely impaired in the feet. Vibration sense is absent to the iliac crest. Touch, pain, and temperature sensations are normal, including in the perianal region. Muscle stretch reflexes are normal. An electromyographic nerve conduction study shows normal sensory potentials in the lower extremities.

a. What is the name of the syndrome?
b. What are the possible locations of lesions producing the syndrome?
c. Define the location of the lesion in this patient, whether or not it is a mass lesion, and the possible pathologic substrate.
d. How do the muscle stretch reflexes and electromyographic findings help to localize the lesion in this patient?

The result is bilateral loss of pain and temperature sensations in the dermatomes located approximately two segments below the lesion. Sensory modalities conveyed by the dorsal column (tactile discrimination, vibration sense, and joint position sense) will be spared. This is called the *commissural syndrome*. If the lesion expands to involve the ventral horns, a lower motor neuron syndrome (flaccid weakness, atrophy, and fasciculations) of the corresponding myotomes will develop. Involvement of the descending motor pathways may produce an upper motor neuron syndrome (weakness, spasticity, hyperreflexia, and Babinski sign) below the level of the lesion.

Clinical Problem 14.5.

A 60-year-old woman first noted numbness of all fingers of the right hand 2 1/2 years ago. Clumsiness of the right hand developed shortly thereafter. Defective appreciation of temperature with the right hand had been noted 1 1/2 years ago, and 7 months before admission, a similar numbness of all fingers of the left hand developed. At the same time, she noticed stiffness of both lower extremities and this was associated with unsteadiness on rapid turning. On neurologic examination, mental status and cranial nerve function were intact. Fasciculations and a minor degree of atrophy were present in the muscles of both shoulders. Fasciculations were not present in the lower extremities. Strength was decreased bilaterally as follows: moderate weakness in shoulder abductors and elbow flexors and extensors. There was marked weakness of intrinsic hand muscles. The lower extremities had minimal weakness. Spasticity was noted on passive motion of the lower extremities, and her gait was spastic. The triceps, quadriceps, and Achilles tendon reflexes were increased bilaterally. Plantar responses were extensor bilaterally. Pain and temperature sensations were decreased at the C4 to T1 dermatomes bilaterally, with total loss of these sensations in her right hand and lower arm. However, touch sensation was intact in these dermatomes.

a. What are the level and type of the lesion?
b. Which systems and which subdivisions of each are involved?
c. Which cord segments are involved and at what transverse location?
d. What is the most likely cause?

Hemicord Syndrome (Brown-Séquard Syndrome)

Lesions that involve one-half of the spinal cord affect 1) the dorsal and ventral roots at this level, producing ipsilateral segmental loss of all sensory modalities in the corresponding dermatome and flaccid weakness in the corresponding myotome; 2) the dorsal columns, causing loss of tactile discrimination, joint position sense, and vibration sense on the same side below the level of the lesion; 3) the spinothalamic tract, causing loss of pain and temperature sensation on the contralateral side of the body below the level of the lesion; 4) the descending motor pathways, producing weakness, increased muscle tone, and hyperreflexia below the level of the lesion, together with the Babinski sign; and 5) the autonomic pathways, causing lack of sweating ipsilateral to the lesion. Arterial blood pressure and bladder functions are not affected by unilateral spinal cord lesions.

Clinical Problem 14.6.

A 53-year-old man has had difficulty in the lower extremities since being wounded in the Vietnam War by shrapnel in the back. He complains of weakness in the left leg and sensory changes in both legs. Neurologic examination shows weakness in the left hip flexors, hamstrings, and foot dorsiflexor muscles. Muscle stretch reflexes are increased at the knee and ankle, and the Babinski sign is elicited on the left. The motor examination is normal for both upper extremities and the right lower extremity. Touch, pinprick, and temperature sensations are lost in the left T4 dermatome and pinprick and temperature sensation are lost in the right lower trunk and lower extremity. Also, joint position sense and vibration sense of the toes are lost on the left side.

a. What are the segmental findings?
b. What are the intersegmental findings?
c. What level of the spinal cord is affected?
d. What side of the spinal cord is affected?
e. What is the extent of the lesion?
f. Would you expect to observe Horner syndrome on the side of the lesion?
g. Would you expect impaired bladder function as a consequence of the lesion?

Anterior Spinal Artery Syndrome

The anterior spinal artery supplies essentially all portions of the spinal cord except the dorsal columns and dorsal horns. Below the cervical level, the arterial supply of the cord depends on anastomoses of radicular arteries. Because of this, the anterior two-thirds of the spinal cord, particularly segments T1 to T4 and the upper lumbar segments, is particularly susceptible to ischemic lesions due to intercostal artery occlusion, as occurs during dissection of or surgery on an abdominal aneurysm. An infarction

Clinical Problem 14.7.

A 55-year-old man with a history of hypertension and atherosclerosis suddenly became aware of the inability to get up from a chair and walk. He was unable to move his legs. He had poorly localized mid-low back pain. He was hospitalized and required urinary catheterization.

Neurologic examination showed flaccid paralysis, with hypotonia of the lower abdominal muscles, hip flexors, hip adductors, and knee extensors. There was weakness of other muscles of the lower extermities, but with increased tone (spastic). Reflexes were normal in the arms, absent at the knees, and hyperactive at the ankles. He had Babinski signs bilaterally. Pain and temperature sensations were absent over the lower back, abdomen, below the umbilicus, and in both lower exremities, but not in a small area around the anus. Joint position sense and vibration sense were normal. All findings were symmetrical.

a. What are the segmental signs and symptoms?
b. What are the intersegmental signs and symptoms?
c. What is the location of the lesion?
d. What is the longitudinal extent of the lesion?
e. What is the likely pathologic substrate?
f. Why are joint position sense and vibration sense spared?
g. What is the name of this syndrome?

in the distribution of the anterior spinal artery affects the ventral funiculus and ventrolateral and dorsolateral quadrants bilaterally. Because these areas contain the spinothalamic and descending motor pathways, the result is bilateral loss of pain and temperature sensations and upper motor neuron signs bilaterally below the level of the lesion. There also are bilateral segmental signs of ventral horn and ventral root involvement at the level of the lesion, including flaccid weakness and atrophy in the corresponding myotomes and lack of segmental reflexes. The bladder is affected. In contrast, dorsal column function is spared.

Transverse Myelopathy

Transverse involvement of the spinal cord affects all motor, sensory, and autonomic functions below the level of the lesion. The term used to describe the clinical consequences of acute and severe spinal cord injury as occurs after traumatic spinal cord transection or a severe ischemic or fulminant inflammatory lesion is *spinal shock*. Acute focal spinal cord lesions abruptly interrupt all descending excitatory influences on spinal cord motor neurons and interneurons. This results in paralysis and loss of muscle stretch reflexes below the level of the lesion. After a few days to a few weeks, the spinal neurons gradually regain their excitability.

The first reflexes to reappear are flexion reflexes, especially in response to stimulation of the plantar surface of the foot (Babinski sign). After 3 to 4 weeks, flexion reflexes can be triggered from a broader area and are more generalized. After several months, hyperexcitability develops to the point that plantar stimulation may induce flexion responses on both sides of the body. After recovery from spinal shock, a patient who has had a major spinal cord injury is left with deficits that are a function of the level of the lesion. In general, the patient has severe lower motor neuron weakness at the level of the lesion and upper motor neuron weakness below the level of the lesion. The primary task of the physician, after localizing the lesion and minimizing the damage, is to enable the patient to achieve maximal use of whatever function remains. Some of the effects of spinal cord lesions are listed in Table 14.11.

These motor deficits are associated with the loss of all sensory modalities below the level of the lesion. In these conditions, the preservation of pinprick sensation in the perianal region, called *sacral sparing*, is clinically useful because it indicates that the spinal cord lesion is not complete but rather spares the peripheral rim of white matter that contains the spinothalamic fibers representing the sacral dermatomes.

In addition to motor and sensory deficits, transverse spinal cord lesions affect autonomic functions because

Clinical Problem 14.8.

A 37-year-old man was involved in an automobile accident. Immediately after the accident, he could not move his lower extremities and had loss of sensation up to a level just below the nipples bilaterally. An examination in the emergency department showed flaccid paralysis of both lower extremities and loss of pinprick sensation in both lower extremities and up to a level 2 cm below the nipples. The patient had no perception of passive toe or knee movement when his eyes were closed. Muscle tone was flaccid in the lower extremities, and lower extremity muscle stretch reflexes were absent. Examination of the upper extremity was normal. He required urinary catheterization. One month later, neurologic examination showed hyperreflexia, spasticity of tone, and the Babinski sign in both lower extremities. Sensory and motor strength findings were unchanged.

a. What is the level of the lesion?
b. What segment is affected, and what is the transverse extent of the lesion?
c. How do you explain the occurrence of flaccid paraplegia and arreflexia immediately after the lesion?
d. What type of bladder dysfunction would you expect to find with recovery of spinal cord excitability?
e. What serious manifestations may occur as a consequence of bladder distention, fecal impaction, or other sensory stimulation below the level of the lesion?

Table 14.11. Functional Consequences of Lesions of Spinal Cord Segments

Segment	Deficit	Independence	Aids required
C4, C5	Quadriplegia Impaired respiration Spastic bladder AD, OH	None	Respiratory assistance Wheelchair
C6, C7	Quadriplegia Spastic bladder AD, OH	Minimal May abduct shoulders	Wheelchair Hand splints
C8, T1	Hand weakness Paraplegia Spastic bladder AD, OH	Personal care Drive car	Wheelchair Special braces
T2, T3	Paraplegia Spastic bladder AD, OH	Complete	Wheelchair Leg braces
T12, L1	Paraplegia Spastic bladder	Complete	Wheelchair Leg braces
L4, L5	Paraplegia Spastic bladder	Complete	Foot braces
S2, S3	Flaccid bladder	Complete	Catheter

AD, autonomic dysreflexia; OH, orthostatic hypotension.

the descending regulatory influence on preganglionic neurons and autonomic reflexes is interrupted. In acute stages (spinal shock) thermoregulatory sweating and skin vasomotor responses are lost below the level of the lesion; thus, patients are at high risk for experiencing marked hyperthermia or hypothermia in response to changes in ambient temperature. Also because these patients are not able to maintain resting arterial blood pressure, they have orthostatic hypotension. Acute interruption of input from the pontine micturition center produces a flaccid bladder. However, with recovery of the excitability of the sacral micturition reflex arc, a spastic bladder develops.

With chronic bilateral or midline lesions above spinal segment T5, stimulation of the skin, muscle, or viscera innervated by segments below the lesion may cause a massive reflex activation of all sympathetic output. This dramatic complication is called *autonomic dysreflexia*. Its mechanism is generalized reflex sympathetic activation triggered by various visceral or somatic noxious or innocuous stimuli below the spinal lesion, most commonly distention of the bladder or bowel. The most serious manifestation of autonomic dysreflexia is severe hypertension. Other manifestations include headache, flushing, and excessive sweating below the level of the lesion. This potentially serious complication can be prevented with appropriate nursing care and early recognition of urinary catheter obstruction, fecal impaction, decubitus ulcers, and other potential triggers of autonomic dysreflexia.

Pathologic Bases of Lesions at the Spinal Level

Structures at the spinal level may be affected by focal or diffuse lesions. Focal lesions may be progressive (mass) or nonprogressive (nonmass) and include traumatic, vascular, inflammatory, and neoplastic lesions. Multifocal lesions are commonly inflammatory. Diffuse lesions may be inflammatory, metabolic, or degenerative.

Focal Lesions

Focal lesions at the spinal level may be nonprogressive, as in trauma or infarction, or progressive (mass). Progressive focal lesions may be vascular (hematoma), inflammatory (abscess, granuloma, or demyelinating plaque), or neoplastic or they may be intervertebral due to disk extrusion. Depending on the transverse extent of the lesion, it may produce various combinations of deficits involving the intersegmental dorsal column and spinothalamic and corticospinal tracts and produce the different clinical patterns described above. In these cases, the clinical history indicates focal progressive deficits of acute, subacute, or chronic temporal profile.

It is of particular importance to determine if a lesion is extrinsic (extramedullary) to the spinal cord or roots, producing neurologic deficits by mechanical compression, or if it is intrinsic (intramedullary), directly causing the loss of neurons, axons, or myelin (or a combination of these). Extrinsic spinal cord lesions are more common than intrinsic ones and often can be removed surgically, with recovery of some or all function. Therefore, in any case of a focal disorder at the spinal level, the presence of a compressive lesion should be excluded first. Neuroimaging techniques, including MRI and myelography with CT, provide important information about the location and pathologic nature of the lesion.

Extrinsic lesions arise outside the substance of the spinal cord and compress it. These lesions include epidural or intradural extramedullary lesions. Extrinsic lesions commonly damage the dorsal or ventral roots and, thus, are usually associated with radicular pain. Important examples of epidural lesions are disk extrusion, hematoma, abscess, and neoplasm. Ruptured intervertebral disks compress the nerve roots (Fig. 14.21) and, at the cervical or thoracic level, they may also compress the spinal cord. Extrinsic neoplastic disorders at the spinal level include primary neoplasms arising from the meninges (meningioma) or nerve roots (schwannoma) or, more commonly, metastases, which often involve the epidural space (Fig. 14.22).

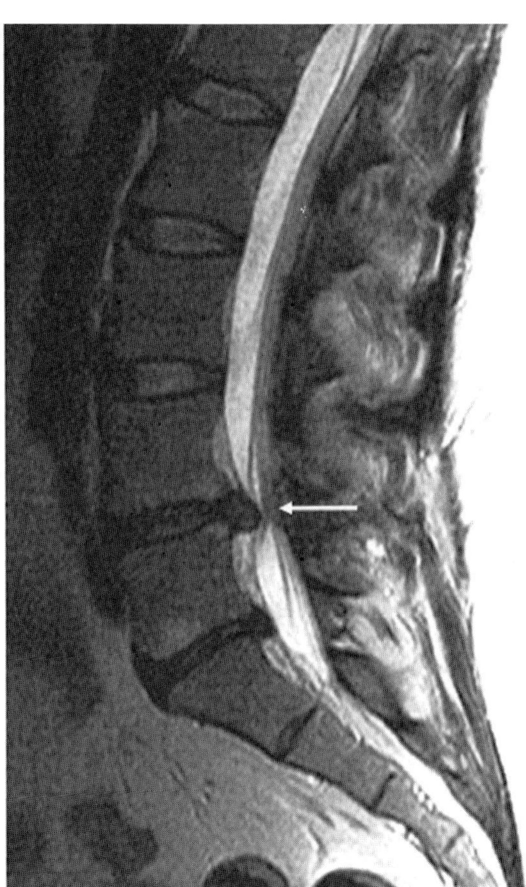

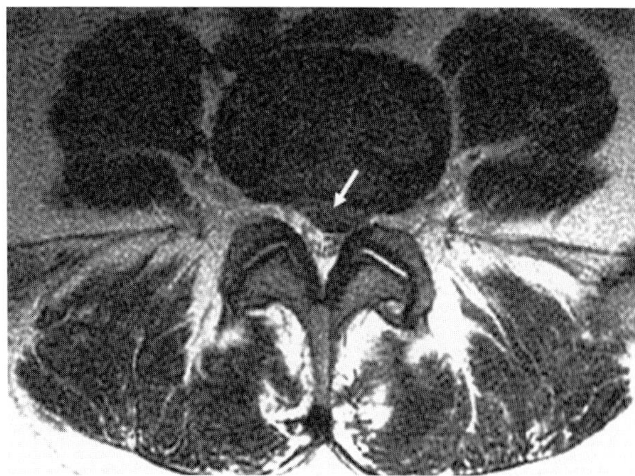

Fig. 14.21. T2-weighted magnetic resonance image of the lumbar spine in the sagittal (*left*) and transverse (*right*) planes showing a large extruded intervertebral disk (*arrow*), with epidural compression and displacement of the cauda equina.

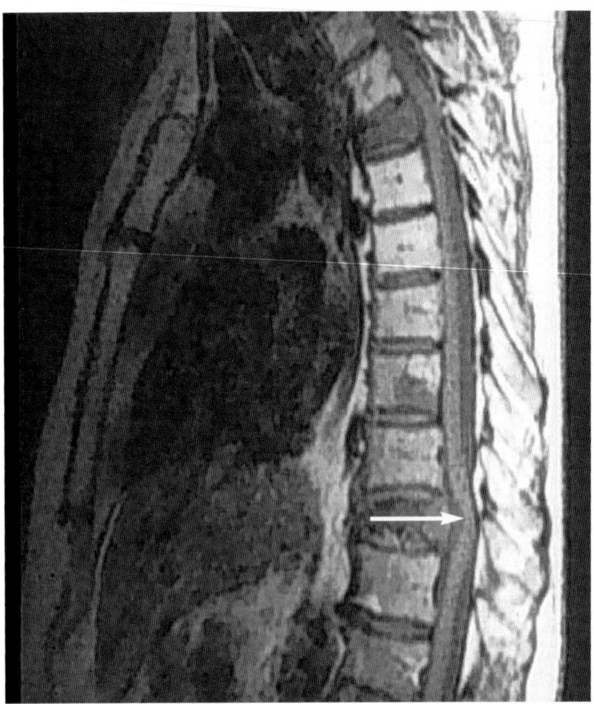

Fig. 14.22. T1-weighted magnetic resonance image of the thoracic cord showing vertebral metastasis with epidural compression (*arrow*) of the spinal cord.

Intrinsic lesions arise within the substance of the spinal cord and often spare the more peripheral tracts in the cord. Although sensory symptoms are prominent, they are often painless. Intrinsic lesions preferentially damage first the more medially located corticospinal and spinothalamic fibers representing the cervical dermatomes, and the more laterally located corticospinal and spinothalamic fibers representing the sacral dermatomes may be spared. Thus, sacral sparing may be found in cases of a syrinx or tumor in the cervical cord gray matter.

Important examples of intrinsic lesions include traumatic lesions such as spinal cord transaction, vascular lesions such as spinal cord infarction, and inflammatory demyelinating lesions. Large demyelinating lesions of the spinal cord may produce a focal subacute deficit that may be progressive, suggesting a mass lesion. However, a focal, progressive, and subacute profile may also indicate an epidural abscess. The most common intrinsic spinal cord neoplasms are astrocytoma and ependymoma (Fig. 14.23).

Multifocal Lesions: Multiple Sclerosis

Multiple sclerosis is an immune disorder characterized by focal areas of demyelination and inflammation in the white matter of the central nervous system. Although the spinal cord is commonly involved, particularly the cervical segments (Fig. 14.24), the lesions may also occur in the optic nerves, brainstem, and cerebral hemispheres. The focal lesions typically develop over a few days, and the symptoms may resolve over a few days to weeks or the lesion may leave a persistent deficit.

Diffuse Lesions

Many inflammatory, degenerative, or metabolic disorders may involve the spinal cord diffusely. A typical example of a diffuse inflammatory lesion at the spinal level is a viral infection of the spinal gray matter (*poliomyelitis*), which generally is associated with meningeal inflammation. Infections such as those caused by poliovirus or West Nile virus cause the loss of spinal motor neurons in multiple segments. This results in asymmetrical weakness, atrophy, and lack of reflexes of trunk and limb muscles in

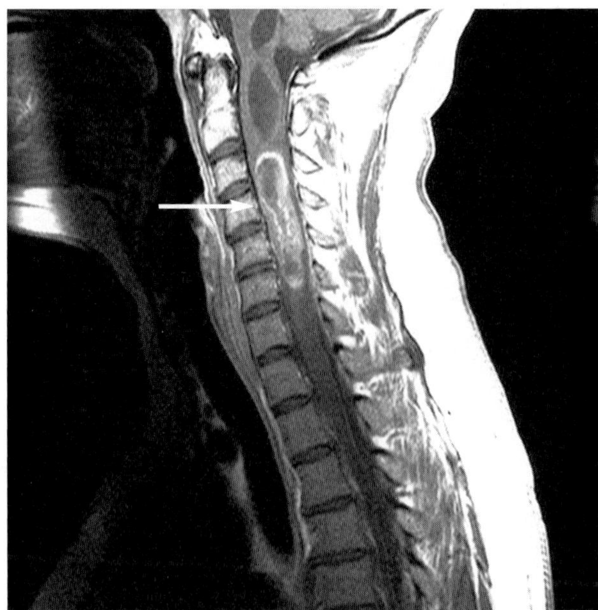

Fig. 14.23. T1-weighted magnetic resonance image of the cervical cord showing a gadolinium-enhancing intramedullary lesion suggestive of an ependymoma (*arrow*).

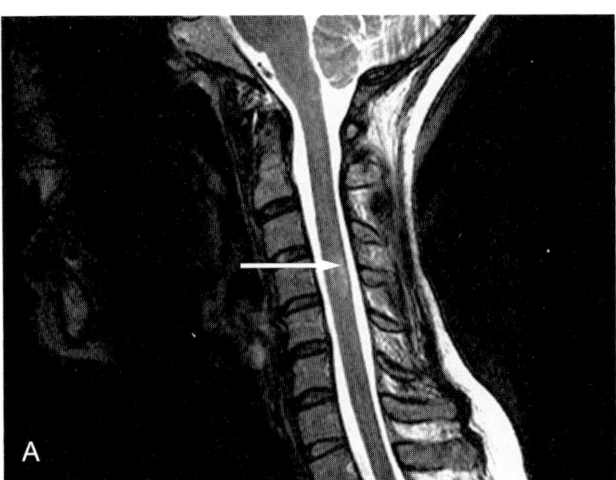

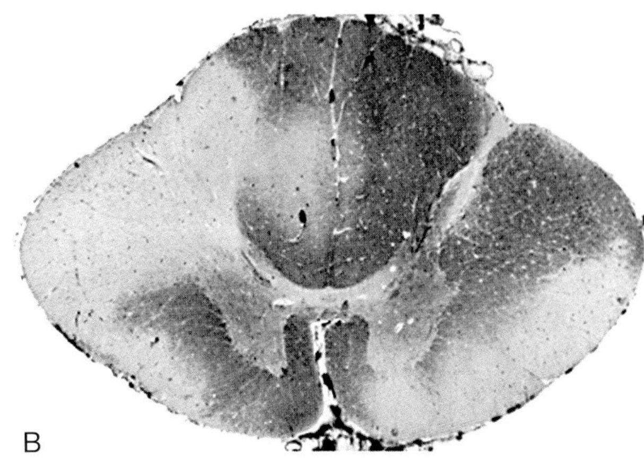

Fig. 14.24. *A*, Sagittal T2-weighted magnetic resonance image of the cervical cord showing a focal area of increased T2 signal (*arrow*) suggestive of a demyelinating disease such as multiple sclerosis. *B*, Coronal section of the upper thoracic cord stained with Luxol fast blue to show myelin. The several focal areas of myelin loss in the posterior, posterolateral, and anterolateral quadrants of the spinal cord are suggestive of multiple sclerosis.

different combinations and with different degrees of severity. The presence of lower motor neuron findings in cervical, thoracic, lumbar, or sacral myotomes reflects the diffuse nature of the disorder.

Motor neuron disease, such as *amyotrophic lateral sclerosis*, is an example of a degenerative single system disorder in the spinal cord. In amyotrophic lateral sclerosis, progressive destruction of the motor neurons in the ventral horn is associated with degeneration of the corticospinal tract. This produces a combination of lower motor neuron findings (weakness, atrophy, and fasciculations), usually in more than one myotome in two or more limbs, and upper motor neuron signs. In some cases, the combination of lower motor neuron weakness affecting the upper limbs and upper motor neuron findings in the lower limbs should prompt the search for a focal lesion at the cervical level.

However, not all diffuse, progressive system diseases of the spinal level (or elsewhere) are degenerative. Vitamin B_{12} deficiency may affect the long axons of the central nervous system, primarily those of the dorsal columns and corticospinal tracts, resulting in myelin loss and, if untreated, axonal degeneration. The manifestations typical of vitamin B_{12} deficiency reflect the combined involvement of the dorsal columns and corticospinal tracts (Fig. 14.25). The large myelinated axons in peripheral nerves and cerebral white matter are also affected. The clinical findings include subacute or chronic progressive sensory ataxia, with upper motor neuron signs (such as the Babinski sign), lower motor neuron signs (depressed ankle reflexes), paresthesia, and occasionally dementia.

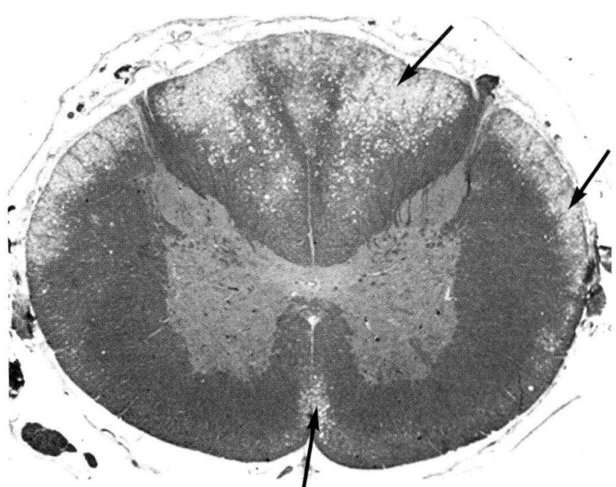

Fig. 14.25. Coronal section of the cervical cord stained with hematoxylin-eosin showing degeneration of the dorsal columns in combination with that of the lateral and anterior corticospinal tracts (*arrows*) from vitamin B_{12} deficiency.

Clinical Problem 14.9.

A 52-year-old woman is hospitalized because of ataxia and mental symptoms. She is unable to give a history, but her husband relates that for the last 3 years she has complained of a pins-and-needles sensation in her feet and hands that gradually spread to her knees and elbows. For the last 18 months, she has had progressive gait ataxia and weakness of the legs. For about the same length of time, she has had mental symptoms. Initially, she was irritable and uncooperative. Currently, she has impaired memory, thinks her husband is trying to poison her, and is confused at night. She is also incontinent of urine and stool.

On examination, she has multiple cognitive deficits consistent with dementia. She has gait ataxia. The Romberg sign is present. Both legs are moderately and symmetrically weak. Muscle stretch reflexes are normal in the arms and absent in the legs. The Babinski sign is present bilaterally. Position sense is impaired in her toes. Vibration sense is absent in her legs. Touch, pain, and temperature sensations are not significantly impaired. She has a urinary catheter in place.

a. What are the location and type of the lesion(s)?
b. What sensory pathways are involved?
c. Why are tendon reflexes absent, but the Babinski sign is present?
d. What laboratory tests are indicated for this patient?

Additional Reading

Craig AD. How do you feel? Interoception: the sense of the physiological condition of the body. Nat Rev Neurosci. 2002;3:655-666.

Davidoff RA. Skeletal muscle tone and the misunderstood stretch reflex. Neurology. 1992;42:951-963.

Gilman S. Joint position sense and vibration sense: anatomical organisation and assessment. J Neurol Neurosurg Psychiatry. 2002;73:473-477.

Willis WD, Westlund KN. Neuroanatomy of the pain system and of the pathways that modulate pain. J Clin Neurophysiol. 1997;14:2-31.

Woolsey RM, Young RR. The clinical diagnosis of disorders of the spinal cord. Neurol Clin. 1991;9:573-583.

Chapter 15
Part A

The Posterior Fossa Level

Brainstem and Cranial Nerve Nuclei

Objectives

1. Identify the major anatomical features of the medulla, pons, and midbrain as described in the text, and state their function.
2. Name and identify the nuclei and peripheral portions of cranial nerves III through XII. Describe their functions and the signs and symptoms that indicate their dysfunction.

Introduction

The posterior fossa level contains all the structures located within the skull below the tentorium cerebelli and above the foramen magnum (Fig. 15A.1). These structures are derivatives of the embryonic mesencephalon, metencephalon, and myelencephalon and include portions of all the systems discussed in previous chapters.

The major structures of this level are the brainstem (medulla, pons, and midbrain), cerebellum, and segments of cranial nerves III through XII, before their emergence from the skull. The brainstem, the central core of the posterior fossa level, is a specialized rostral extension of the embryonic neural tube that preserves, even in the mature state, many of the longitudinal or intersegmental features of the spinal cord and also provides for segmental functions of the head.

This chapter describes the general anatomy of the posterior fossa, the anatomy and functions of cranial nerves III through XII, and the internal anatomy of the medulla, pons, and midbrain. The cerebellum, new systems at the level of the posterior fossa, and clinical examination with clinical correlations are discussed in part B of this chapter.

Overview

The brainstem contains ascending and descending pathways traveling to or from the thalamus, hypothalamus, cerebral cortex, cerebellum, cranial nerve nuclei, and spinal cord. The main sensory pathways include those that originate in the spinal cord (the spinothalamic tracts, dorsal column–lemniscal system, and spinocerebellar pathways) as well as those that arise from cranial nerves or their nuclei (the descending tract of the trigeminal nerve, the trigeminothalamic tract, and the lateral lemniscus). The main motor pathways include the direct activation pathways (the corticospinal and corticobulbar pathways) and the indirect activation pathways (reticulospinal, rubrospinal, and vestibulospinal pathways). Other important intersegmental pathways at this level include the medial longitudinal fasciculus, the ascending and descending fibers of the consciousness and internal regulation systems, and many of the structures of the ocular motor, auditory, and vestibular systems.

The brainstem traditionally is subdivided into three parts: the *medulla* (derived from the myelencephalon), which contains the motor neurons for swallowing, tongue movement, talking, and certain visceral motor functions; the *pons* (derived from the metencephalon), which contains the nuclei associated with motor, sensory, and

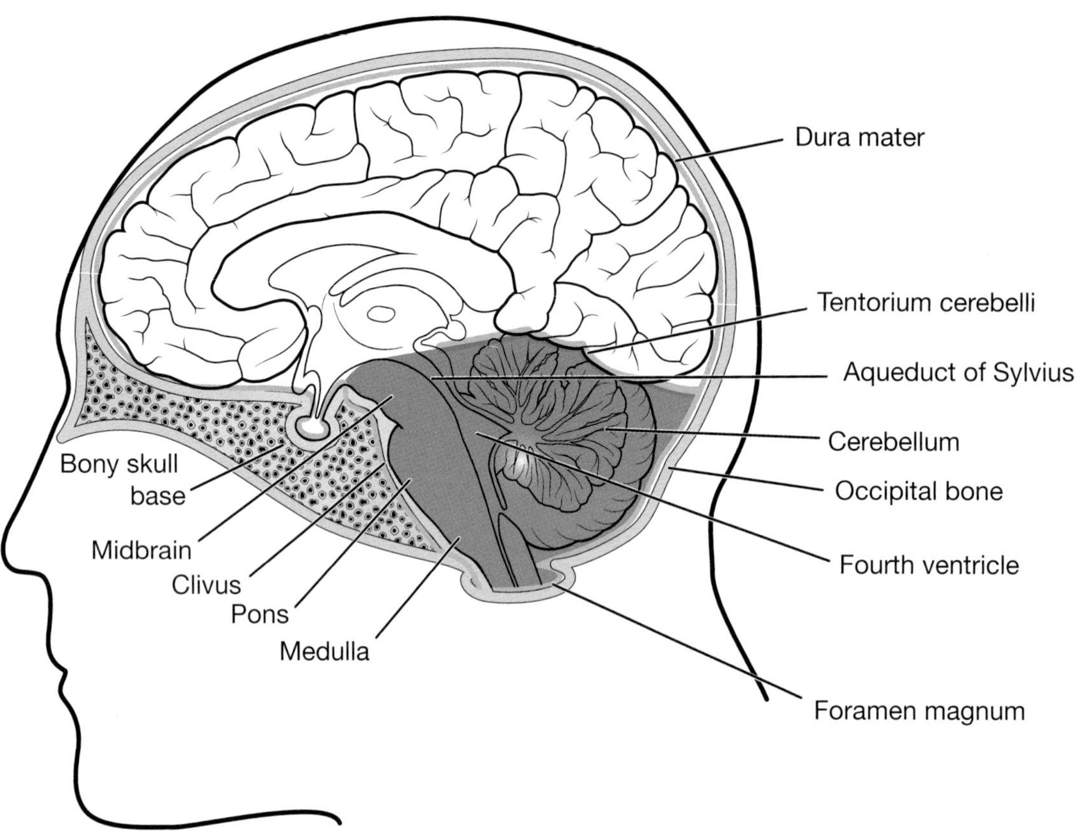

Fig. 15A.1. The posterior fossa (red area) is bordered by the foramen magnum, tentorium cerebelli, clivus, and occipital bones.

parasympathetic innervation of the face and abduction of the eye; and the *midbrain* (derived from mesencephalon), which contains the nuclei of the ascending reticular activating system, the nuclei that govern eye movements (except abduction), and the fibers involved in pupillary constriction and accommodation.

Although the tubular configuration of the central nervous system is greatly altered in the brainstem, the general relationships between systems developing in the inner tube region (primitive, indirect, diffuse) and the outer tube region (newer, direct, discrete) can still be discerned. The anatomical structure that typifies the inner tube region is the reticular formation, a complex group of nuclei and interconnections that extends throughout the core of the brainstem. In each of the three major subdivisions of the brainstem, the reticular formation is divided into medial, intermediate, and lateral zones. The relative importance of these zones and the functions they serve differ at each level. The major functional components of the reticular formation are discussed in the following sections that describe each of the subdivisions of the brainstem.

The cerebrospinal fluid system is represented at the posterior fossa level by the aqueduct of Sylvius, the fourth ventricle, the meninges, the extraventricular subarachnoid cisterns, and the cerebrospinal fluid itself.

The entire blood supply to the posterior fossa level is derived from the vertebrobasilar arterial system, which supplies paramedian arteries and short and long circumferential arteries to the brainstem and cerebellum. The major long circumferential arteries are the posterior inferior cerebellar arteries at the medullary level, the anterior inferior cerebellar arteries at the pontine level, and the superior cerebellar arteries at the midbrain level.

The brainstem has 10 pairs of cranial nerves (Fig. 15A.2), which perform segmental functions comparable to the functions of spinal nerves. The portions of these nerves contained within the cranium are considered part of the posterior fossa level, and the segments distal to the bones of the skull are considered part of the peripheral level. The location and general function of the cranial nerves at the posterior fossa level are summarized in Table 15A.1.

General Anatomy of the Posterior Fossa Level

Posterior Cranial Fossa and Tentorium

The posterior cranial fossa is formed by the occipital bones at the base of the skull and the temporal bones anteriorly and laterally (Fig. 15A.3). The inferior limit of the posterior fossa is the foramen magnum, where the cervical cord merges with the medulla. The rostral limit of the posterior fossa is the *tentorium cerebelli*, which lies between the cerebellum and the occipital lobe. The tentorium is attached posteriorly and posterolaterally to the transverse sinus and anterolaterally to the petrous ridge. The anterior border is not attached to bone but forms the tentorial notch, through which the midbrain passes to merge with the diencephalon.

Systems Contained in the Posterior Fossa Level

The neural structures of the posterior fossa level consist of cranial nerves III through XII, midbrain, pons, medulla, and cerebellum. Each of the longitudinal systems is represented at this level.

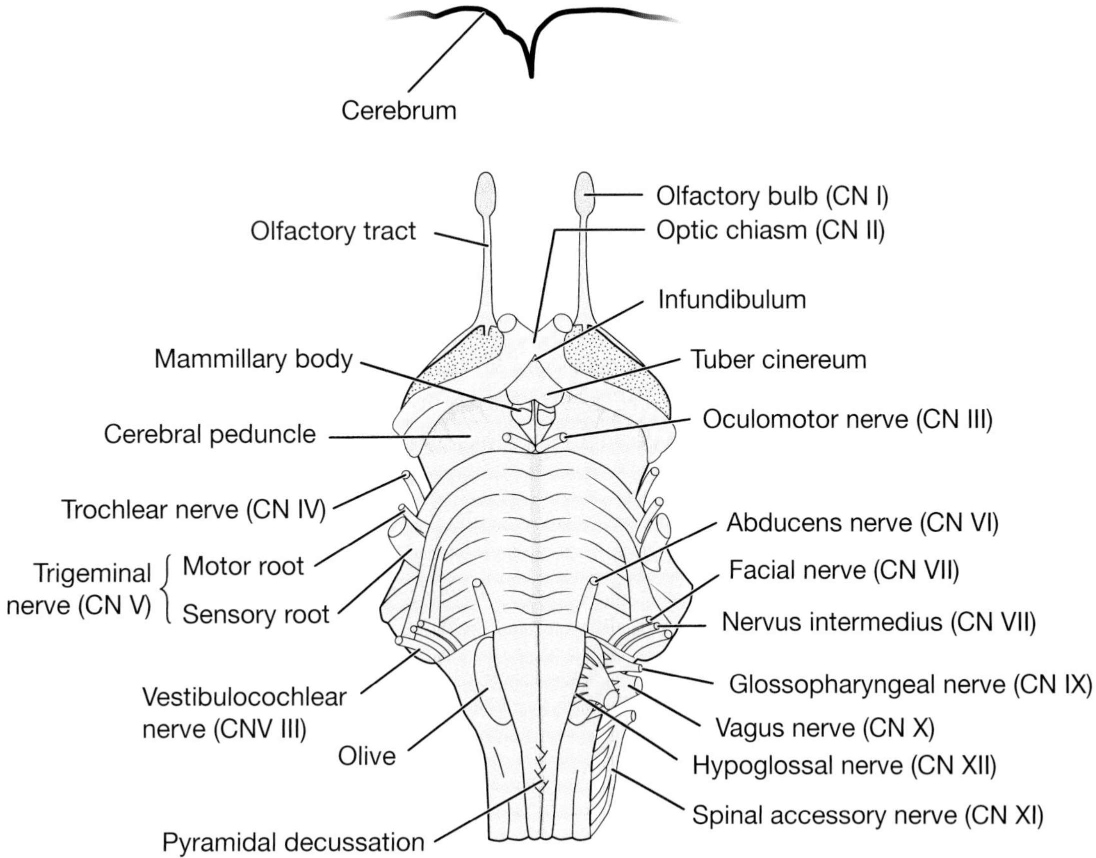

Fig. 15A.2. Ventral (anterior) view of the brainstem showing the cranial nerves. (Only cranial nerves III through XII are at the posterior fossa level.) CN, cranial nerve.

Table 15A.1. Location and General Function of Cranial Nerves at the Posterior Fossa Level

Level	Cranial nerve		General function
Medulla	XII	Hypoglossal	Motor to muscles of tongue
	XI	Spinal accessory	Motor to sternocleidomastoid and trapezius muscles
	X	Vagus	Motor to muscles of soft palate, pharynx, and larynx; parasympathetic fibers to thoracic and abdominal viscera; sensory fibers from pharynx and external auditory meatus; visceral sensory fibers from thoracic and abdominal cavities
	IX	Glossopharyngeal	Motor to stylopharyngeus muscle; sensory from pharynx and tongue; taste from posterior tongue
Pons	VIII	Vestibulocochlear	Hearing and equilibration
	VII	Facial	Motor to muscles of facial expression; parasympathetic to salivary glands; taste from anterior tongue
	VI	Abducens	Motor to lateral rectus muscle of eye
	V	Trigeminal	Sensory from face; motor to muscles of mastication
Midbrain	IV	Trochlear	Motor to superior oblique muscle of eye
	III	Oculomotor	Motor to medial, superior, and inferior recti and inferior oblique muscles of eye, and levator palpebrae of eyelid; parasympathetic to constrictors of pupil

Cerebrospinal Fluid System

Cerebrospinal fluid flows into the posterior fossa through the *aqueduct of Sylvius*, a narrow canal in the midbrain between the third and fourth ventricles. The fourth ventricle is located at the level of the medulla and pons, which form the ventricular floor. The roof of the fourth ventricle is the ventral midline portion of the cerebellum. Cerebrospinal fluid leaves the fourth ventricle through the *foramen of Magendie* (at the caudal end of the ventricle) and through the two *foramina of Luschka* (at each lateral angle of the ventricle) to enter the subarachnoid space, where it circulates through the cisterna magna, cerebellopontine, prepontine, interpeduncular, and ambient cisterns.

Sensory System

The brainstem contains ascending pathways mediating 1) pain and temperature (spinothalamic system), 2) conscious proprioception and discriminative sensation (dorsal column–lemniscal system), 3) unconscious proprioception (ventral and dorsal spinocerebellar systems), and 4) touch (spinothalamic and dorsal column–lemniscal systems). Also, sensory input from the face and head enters at this level.

Consciousness System

The central core of the brainstem contains the reticular formation and its ascending projection pathways. The brainstem, with other areas of the nervous system, serves the important function of mediating consciousness, attention, and the wake-sleep cycle.

Motor System

All subdivisions of the motor system are represented at the posterior fossa level. The lower motor neurons of several cranial nerves contain the final common pathway to muscles of the head and neck. The direct activation pathways are represented by the corticospinal tracts, which descend through the brainstem and decussate in the lower medulla en route to the spinal cord, and the corticobulbar pathways, which provide supranuclear innervation to brainstem motor nuclei. The indirect activation pathways

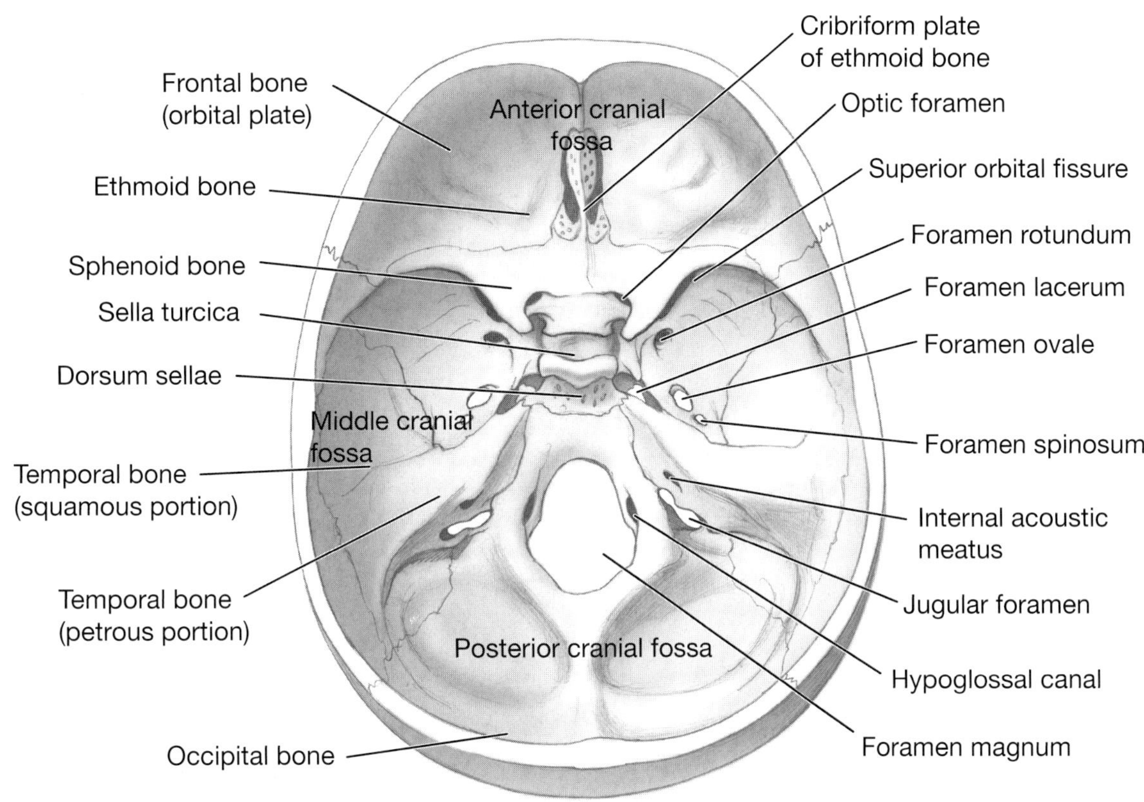

Fig. 15A.3. Base of the skull, showing major bones and foramina.

in the brainstem consist of the reticulospinal, rubrospinal, and vestibulospinal tracts, descending pathways arising in the brainstem. Much of the cerebellar control circuit is located at this level, and portions of the basal ganglia control circuit (substantia nigra and red nucleus) are present in the midbrain.

Internal Regulation System

The posterior fossa contains visceral sensory relay nuclei (particularly the nucleus solitarius), reticular formation, and preganglionic parasympathetic neurons.

The intermediate zone of the medullary reticular formation contains interneurons and neurons that project to preganglionic sympathetic neurons and to spinal motor neurons that control respiration. The lateral zone contains the central pattern generators that integrate complex motor patterns involving multiple cranial nerves to produce such actions as swallowing and vomiting. In addition to the reticular formation and the ascending and descending pathways that regulate visceral function, the posterior fossa level contains the preganglionic parasympathetic fibers contained in cranial nerves III, VII, IX, and X.

Vascular System

The structures in the posterior fossa receive their blood supply from the vertebrobasilar arterial system (Fig. 15A.4). The vertebral arteries enter the cranial cavity through the foramen magnum and then course rostrally along the ventrolateral surface of the medulla, where they give off branches to form the anterior spinal artery, which descends on the ventral aspect of the lower medulla to the cervical spinal cord. At the level of the pons, the two vertebral arteries merge to form the basilar artery,

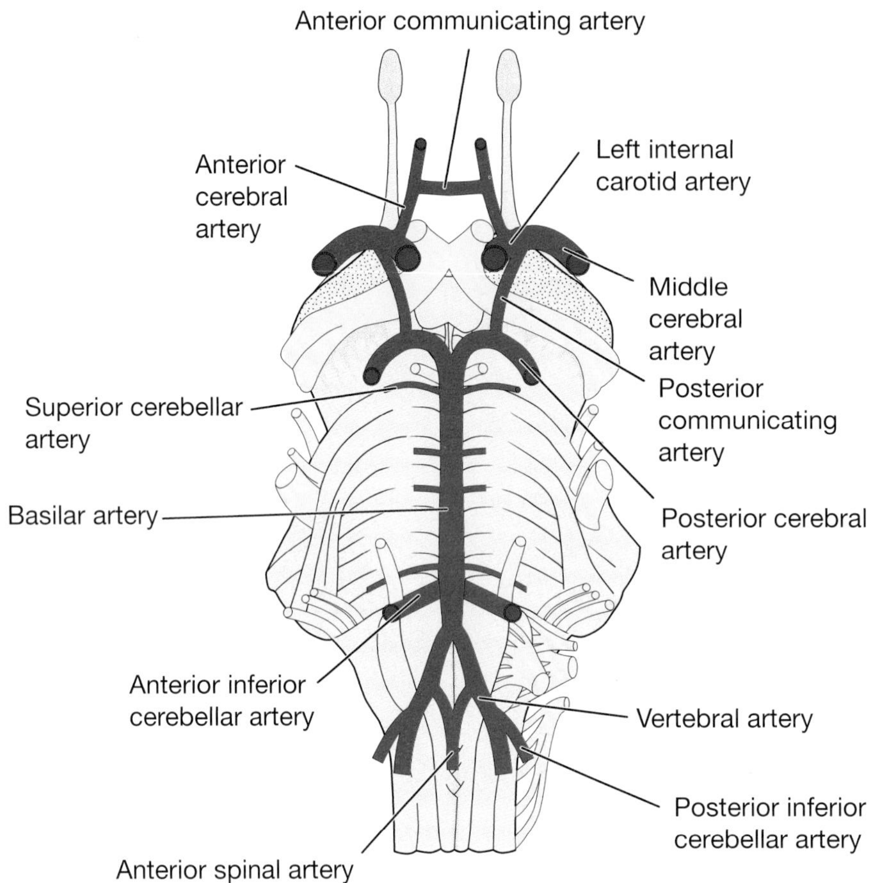

Fig. 15A.4. Blood supply to posterior fossa structures from the vertebral and basilar arteries.

which continues rostrally to the upper midbrain level, where it branches to form the posterior cerebral arteries.

Branches of the vertebral and basilar arteries are subdivided into three groups that supply each level of the brainstem and the cerebellum. The paramedian zone on either side of the midline is supplied by *paramedian branches*, the intermediate zone is supplied by *short circumferential branches*, and the lateral zone is supplied by *long circumferential branches* (Fig. 15A.5). The paramedian and lateral zones are often involved by vascular lesions, which can cause major clinical deficits. The paramedian area of the medulla is supplied by paramedian branches of the anterior spinal artery, and the intermediate zone is supplied by the vertebral arteries. The paramedian areas of the pons and midbrain are supplied by the paramedian branches of the basilar artery. The lateral areas of the brainstem are supplied by three pairs of long circumferential arteries: the *posterior inferior cerebellar artery*, a branch of the vertebral artery that supplies the lateral area of the medulla and the posterior inferior aspect of the cerebellum; the *anterior inferior cerebellar artery*, a branch of the basilar artery that supplies the lateral area of the pons and the anterior inferior aspect of the cerebellum; and the *superior cerebellar artery*, a branch of the basilar artery that supplies the lateral area of the midbrain and the superior surface of the cerebellum.

Other Systems

Three other special systems are found primarily at the posterior fossa level: 1) the ocular motor system, which mediates eye movement; 2) the auditory system, which mediates hearing; and 3) the vestibular system, which

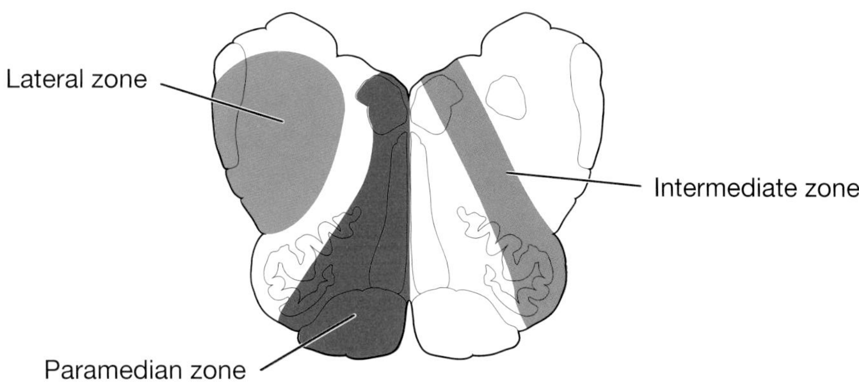

Fig. 15A.5. Blood supply of the medulla. The lateral zone is supplied by the posterior inferior cerebellar artery, the paramedian zone is supplied by the anterior spinal artery, and the intermediate zone is supplied by the vertebral artery.

mediates balance and equilibrium. These systems are discussed in part B of this chapter.

Embryologic Organization of the Brainstem

The primitive neural tube displays an anatomical organization similar to that of the spinal cord, with functional areas for sensation (alar plate) and motor activity (basal plate) separated by the sulcus limitans. Within these sensory and motor areas, the brainstem is divided further into somatic and visceral regions (Fig. 15A.6). This organizational framework is grafted onto the concepts mentioned above that relate older, more diffuse pathways to the inner tube of the brainstem and newer, more direct, and discrete pathways to the outer tube of the brainstem.

These functional divisions exist as rostrocaudal cell columns from which cranial nerve nuclei are derived. Some cranial nerves contain components from more than one of these columns. The appearance of new structures in the brainstem and the enlargement of the embryonic neural canal into the fourth ventricle displace some of these nuclear columns from their embryonic position. The location of the cell columns in the adult brainstem and the cranial nerves arising from each is shown in Figure 15A.7. These functionally oriented cell columns provide an important framework for learning the intrinsic anatomy of each of the major subdivisions of the posterior fossa. The components of each of these cell columns, found in each of the cranial nerves, are listed in Table 15A.2.

- The posterior fossa contains structures below the tentorium cerebelli, including the brainstem (medulla, pons, midbrain), cranial nerves III through XII, and the cerebellum.
- The longitudinal systems extend through the brainstem, including the sensory, motor, consciousness, internal regulation, cerebrospinal fluid, and vascular systems.
- Three new systems occur at the level of the posterior fossa:
    - The ocular motor system appears in the posterior fossa and mediates conjugate eye movement.
    - The auditory system mediates hearing.
    - The vestibular system mediates balance and equilibrium.
- The posterior fossa structures receive their blood supply from the vertebrobasilar arterial system.
- The presence of the fourth ventricle in the brainstem displaces the motor and sensory columns from their embryonic dorsal and ventral positions in the spinal cord to a medial motor column and lateral sensory column.

The Medulla

The medulla oblongata is the portion of the brainstem that extends from the level of the foramen magnum to the caudal border of the base of the pons. Many of the

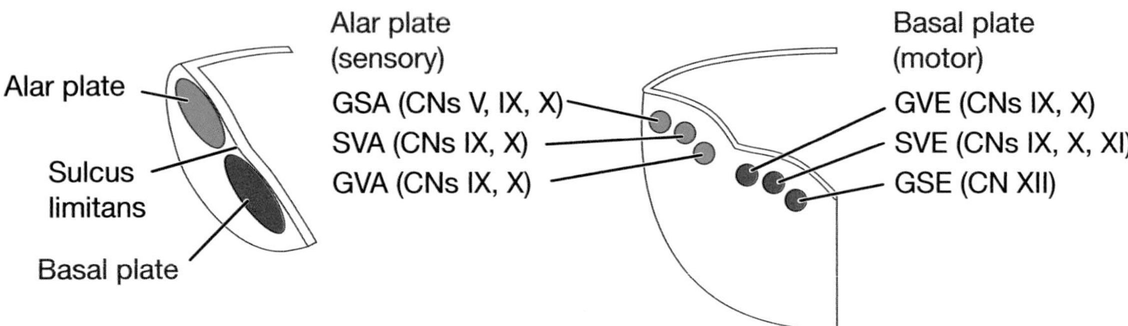

Fig. 15A.6. Alar and basal plates of the brainstem at the level of the medulla in a 5-week (*left*) and 10-week (*right*) embryo (see Table 15A.2). CN, cranial nerve; GSA, general somatic afferent; GSE, general somatic efferent; GVA, general visceral afferent; GVE, general visceral efferent; SVA, special visceral afferent; SVE, special visceral efferent.

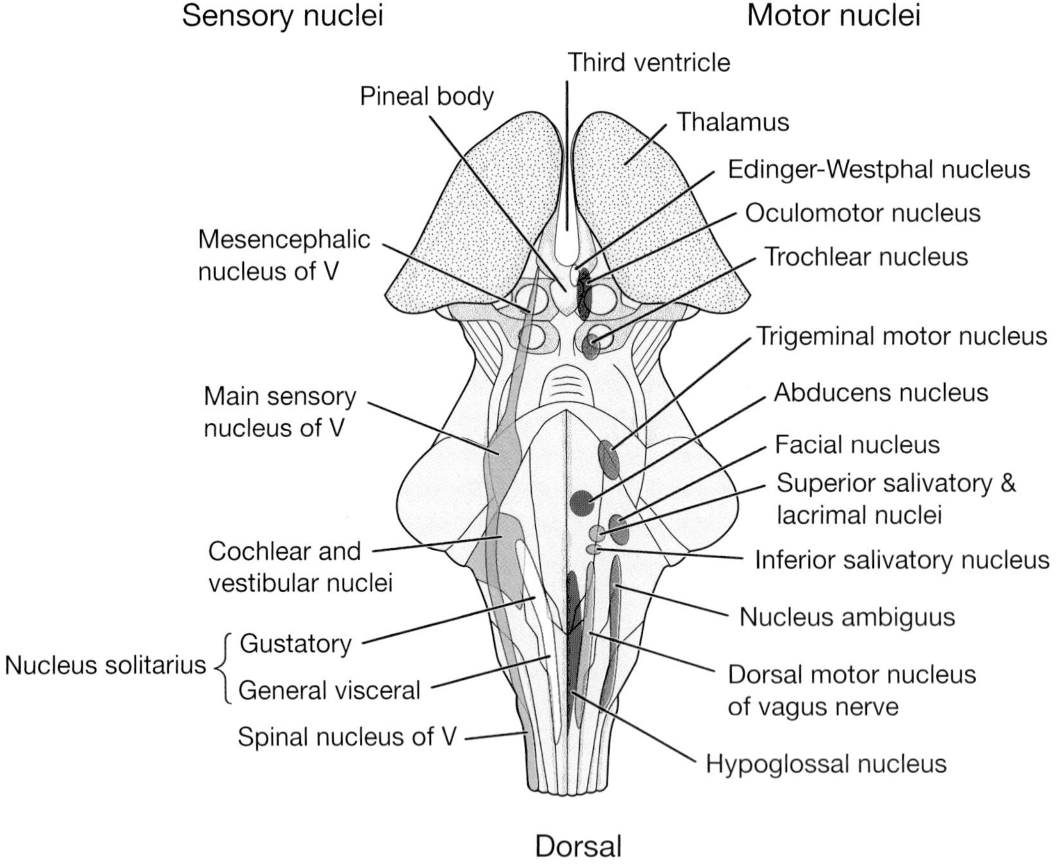

Fig. 15A.7. Location of cell columns in the brainstem. Sensory nuclei are shown on the left and motor nuclei on the right.

Table 15A.2. Components of the Cranial Nerves

Component	Function	Cranial nerve
Efferent	Motor	
General somatic efferent (GSE)	Somatic striated muscles	III, IV, VI, XII
General visceral efferent (GVE)	Parasympathetic glands and smooth muscles	III, VII, IX, X
Special visceral efferent (SVE)	Branchial arch muscles	V, VII, IX, X, XI
Afferent	Sensory	
General somatic afferent (GSA)	Somatesthetic senses	V, IX, X
Special somatic afferent (SSA)	Vision, hearing, and balance	II, VIII
General visceral afferent (GVA)	Pharynx and viscera	IX, X
Special visceral afferent (SVA)	Smell, taste	I, VII, IX, X

features of the medulla are similar to those of the spinal cord (Fig. 15A.8). The major ascending and descending pathways present in the spinal cord are also present in this area; however, several important changes occur in this region, including 1) the location of the corticospinal tracts in the ventromedial portion of the medulla (the medullary pyramids), 2) the termination of the fasciculi gracilis and cuneatus in their respective nuclei and the subsequent course of the axons of the second-order neurons in the medial lemniscus, 3) the replacement of the zone of Lissauer by the descending tract of the trigeminal nerve (spinal tract of V), 4) the replacement of the central gray portion of the spinal cord by the reticular formation, 5) the entrance of the dorsal spinocerebellar tracts into the inferior cerebellar peduncle, and 6) the replacement of the central canal of the spinal cord by the fourth ventricle.

Anatomical Features

Additional important anatomical features of the medulla include the following:

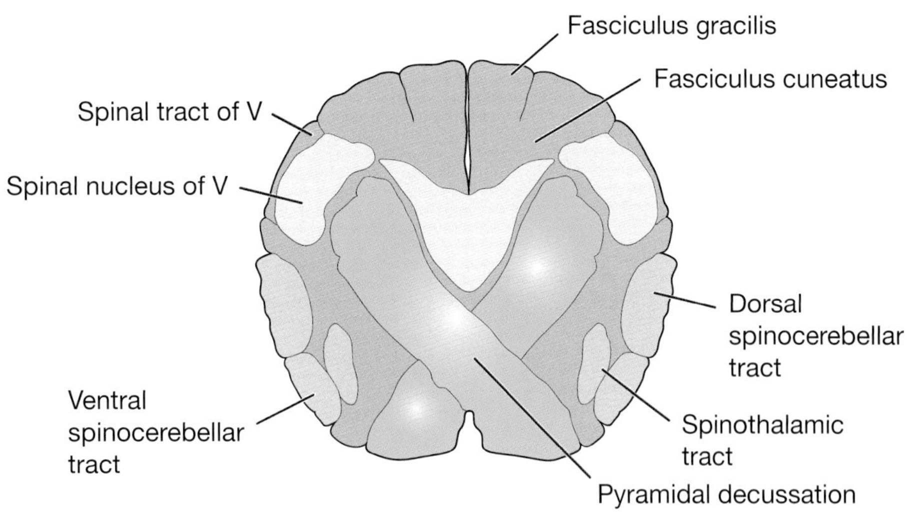

Fig. 15A.8. Cross section of caudal medulla at the decussation of the pyramids.

Decussation of the Pyramids
At the lower end of the medulla, most of the fibers in the descending corticospinal pathways cross to the opposite side of the brainstem before descending in the spinal cord as the lateral corticospinal tracts (Fig. 15A.8).

Decussation of the Medial Lemniscus
In the caudal medulla, rostral to the pyramidal decussation, second-order axons from the *nuclei gracilis* and *cuneatus* sweep ventromedially around the central gray matter as the *internal arcuate fibers*. These fibers cross the midline and continue rostrally as the medial lemniscus (Fig. 15A.9).

Inferior Olivary Nuclei
The convoluted bands of cells in the ventrolateral portion of the medulla are the *inferior olivary nuclei* (Fig. 15A.10), which receive fibers from the dentate nucleus of the cerebellum, red nuclei, basal ganglia, and cerebral cortex. Axons from the inferior olivary nuclei form the olivocerebellar tract, which travels through the inferior cerebellar peduncle to the opposite cerebellar hemisphere. The inferior olive is a major relay station for cerebellar pathways. It provides tonic cerebellar support for reflex movements and triggers phasic motor programs in the cerebellum.

Medial Longitudinal Fasciculus
This fiber tract is located in the paramedian region of the brainstem dorsal to the medial lemniscus. The medial longitudinal fasciculus extends rostrally from the upper midbrain level to the cervical cord and transmits information for the coordination of head and eye movements.

Inferior Cerebellar Peduncle (Restiform Body)
The *inferior cerebellar peduncle* is one of the three major connections between the cerebellum and brainstem. It is located in the dorsolateral portion of the medulla and contains dorsal spinocerebellar, olivocerebellar, vestibulocerebellar, and reticulocerebellar fibers and cerebellovestibular fibers.

Hypoglossal Nerve (Cranial Nerve XII)

Function
The *hypoglossal nerve* is a motor nerve that innervates the intrinsic muscles of the tongue. Its nucleus is part of the general somatic efferent group of cranial nerve nuclei.

Anatomy
The hypoglossal nucleus is located in the paramedian area of the caudal medulla in the floor of the fourth ventricle. The fibers course ventrally and exit from the ventral aspect

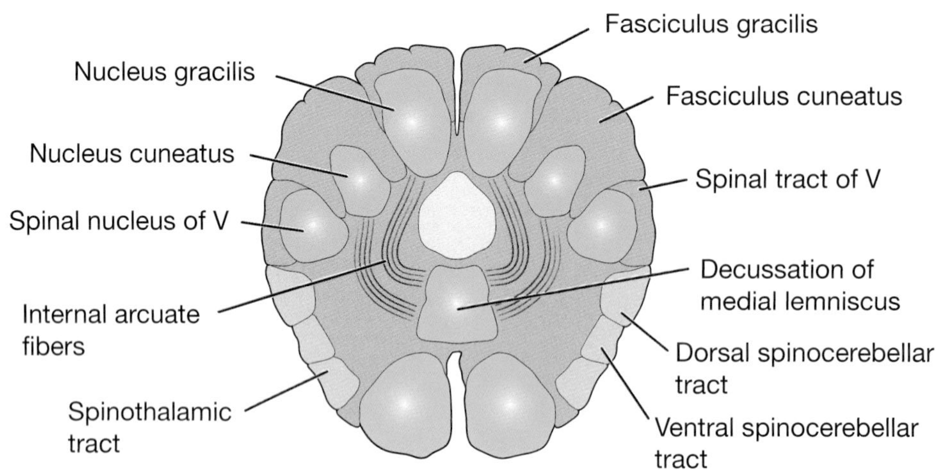

Fig. 15A.9. Cross section of caudal medulla at the decussation of the medial lemnisci.

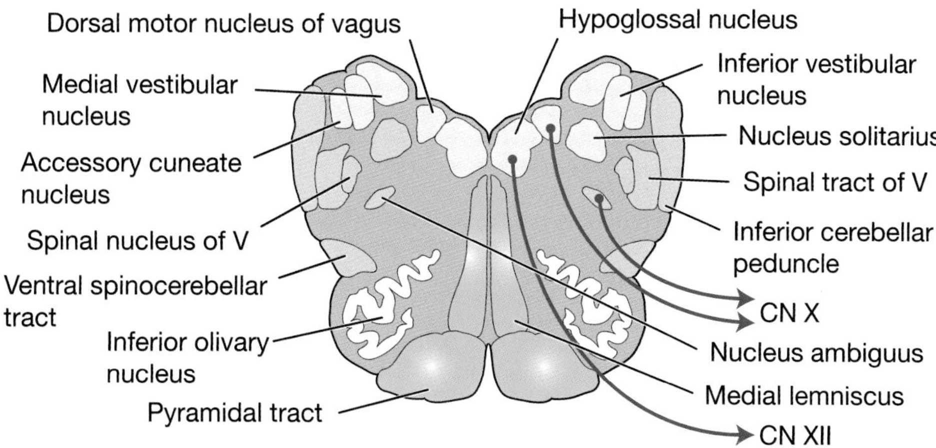

Fig. 15A.10. Cross section of middle medulla at the origin of the hypoglossal and vagus nerves. CN, cranial nerve.

of the medulla, between the medullary pyramids and the olive. After exiting from the brainstem, the fibers pass through the hypoglossal canal in the occipital condyle and innervate the striated muscles of the tongue (Fig. 15A.11).

Pathophysiology

Diseases involving the hypoglossal nucleus or cranial nerve XII are associated with atrophy, paresis, and fasciculations of tongue muscles. Unilateral weakness causes the tongue to deviate toward the side of the weakness when protruded. Involvement of upper motor neuron pathways innervating the hypoglossal nuclei produces slowing of alternating movements of the tongue and weakness, without atrophy. The structure and function of the hypoglossal nerve are summarized in Table 15A.3.

Spinal Accessory Nerve (Cranial Nerve XI)

Function

The spinal accessory nerve is a motor nerve that innervates the sternocleidomastoid and trapezius muscles. It is a special visceral efferent nerve innervating striated muscles derived from branchial arches.

Anatomy

Cranial nerve XI arises mainly from cell bodies in the ventral gray horn of the upper five cervical cord segments (Fig. 15A.12). The nerve ascends in the spinal canal lateral to the spinal cord, enters the skull through the foramen magnum, where it is joined by the minor accessory component that originates in the *nucleus ambiguus*, and leaves the cranial cavity through the jugular foramen to innervate the sternocleidomastoid and trapezius muscles. The accessory component passes to the vagus nerve below the jugular foramen and innervates the muscles of the larynx and pharynx.

Pathophysiology

The spinal accessory nerve may be compressed by lesions in the region of the foramen magnum (where the nerve enters the skull) or in the region of the jugular foramen as it exits from the skull. Signs of dysfunction of cranial nerve XI include weakness of head rotation (sternocleidomastoid muscle) and inability to elevate or shrug the shoulder (trapezius muscle) on the side of the lesion. The sternocleidomastoid muscle rotates the face to the opposite side so that damage to the spinal accessory nerve results in weakness in turning the head toward the side contralateral to the lesion. The structure and function of the spinal accessory nerve are summarized in Table 15A.4.

Vagus Nerve (Cranial Nerve X)

Function

The *vagus nerve* is a mixed nerve with special visceral efferent, general visceral efferent, general somatic afferent,

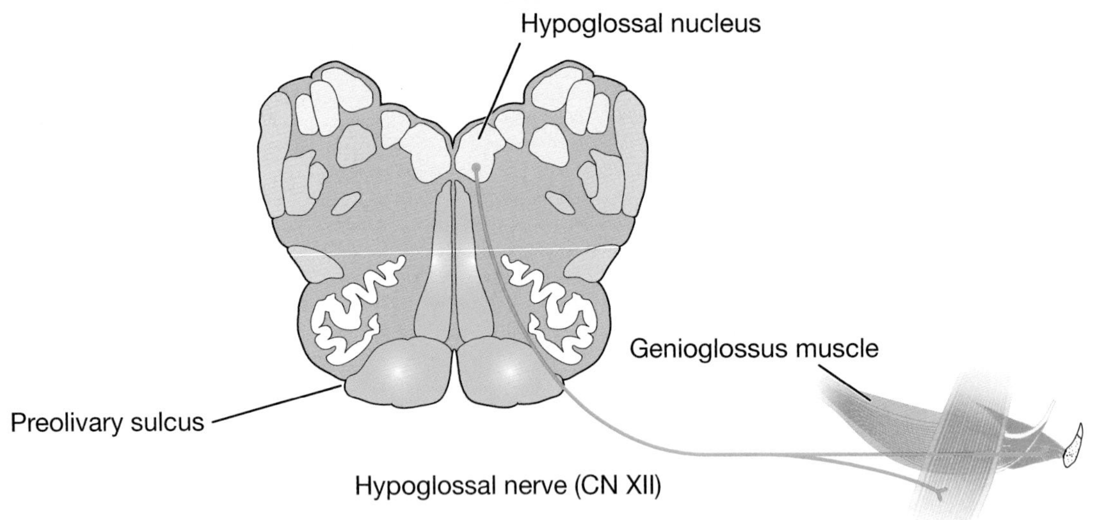

Fig. 15A.11. Origin, course, and distribution of the hypoglossal nerve. CN, cranial nerve.

general visceral afferent, and special visceral afferent functions. The functions of cranial nerve X are innervation of the striated muscles of the soft palate, pharynx, and larynx derived from branchial arches (special visceral efferent); parasympathetic innervation of the thoracic and abdominal viscera (general visceral efferent); sensory innervation of the external auditory meatus (general somatic afferent); sensory innervation of the pharynx, larynx, and thoracic and abdominal viscera (general visceral afferent); and innervation of taste receptors on the posterior pharynx (special visceral afferent).

Anatomy

The special visceral efferent fibers of the vagus nerve that innervate the striated muscles of the soft palate, pharynx, and larynx arise from the nucleus ambiguus located in the lateral medullary region dorsal to the inferior olivary nucleus (Fig. 15A.13). The general visceral efferent component of the vagus nerve contains preganglionic parasympathetic fibers arising in the *dorsal motor nucleus* to supply the thoracic and abdominal viscera. Preganglionic vagal neurons innervating the heart are located in the area of the *nucleus ambiguus*. These preganglionic fibers synapse

Table 15A.3. Structure and Function of the Hypoglossal Nerve

Component	Function	Nucleus of origin or termination	Ganglion	Foramen	Signs of dysfunction
GSE	Motor innervation of tongue	Hypoglossal		Hypoglossal	Tongue weakness, with deviation of tongue to weak side

GSE, general somatic efferent.

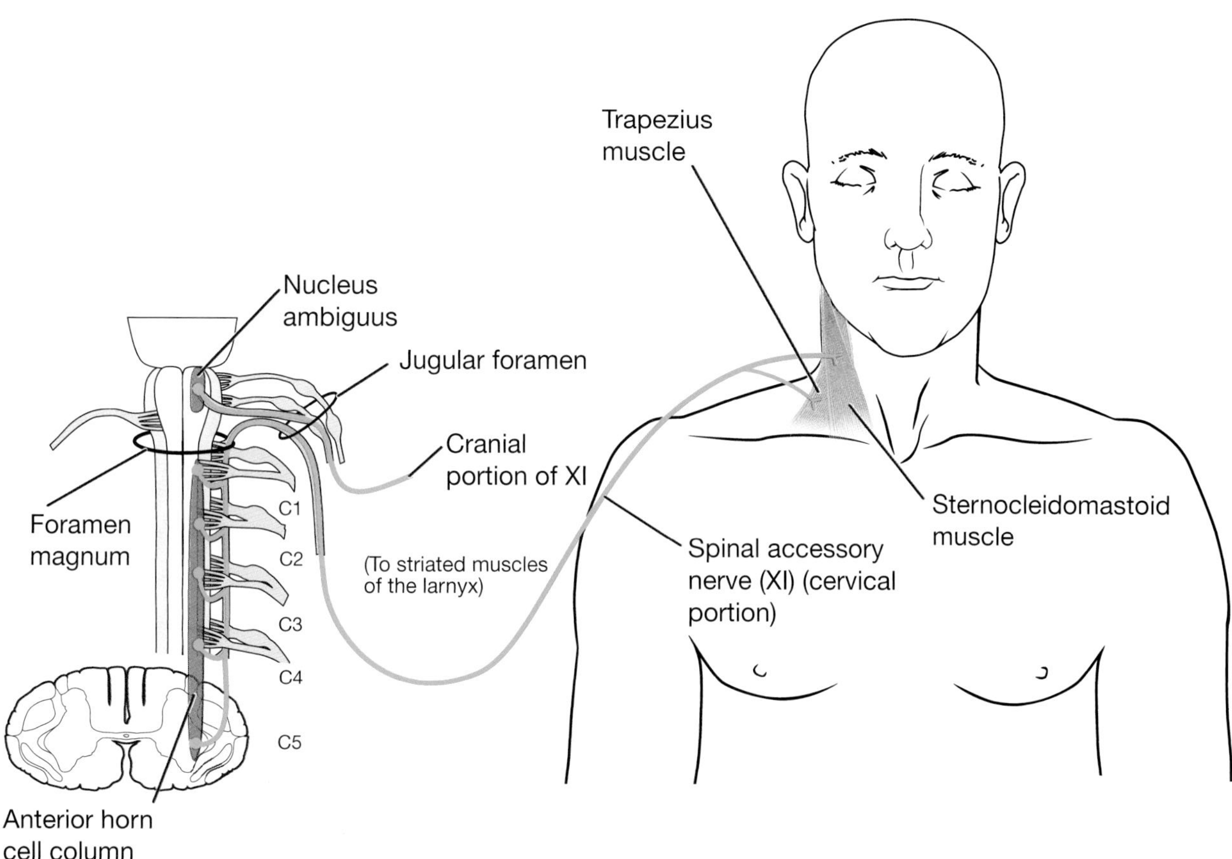

Fig. 15A.12. Spinal accessory nerve (green). Origin of axons in the upper cervical cord and their course to the trapezius and sternocleidomastoid muscles are shown on the left. Nuclei of origin in the medulla are also shown on the left.

Table 15A.4. Structure and Function of the Spinal Accessory Nerve

Component	Function	Nucleus of origin or termination	Ganglion	Foramen	Signs of dysfunction
SVE					
Spinal	Motor to sterno-cleidomastoid and trapezius muscles	Anterior horn of cervical cord		Jugular	Weak shoulder elevation and head rotation toward side of weak sternocleidomastoid
Bulbar	Motor to pharyngeal and laryngeal muscles	Nucleus ambiguus		Jugular	Joins vagus below jugular foramen (see Table 15A.5)

SVE, special visceral efferent.

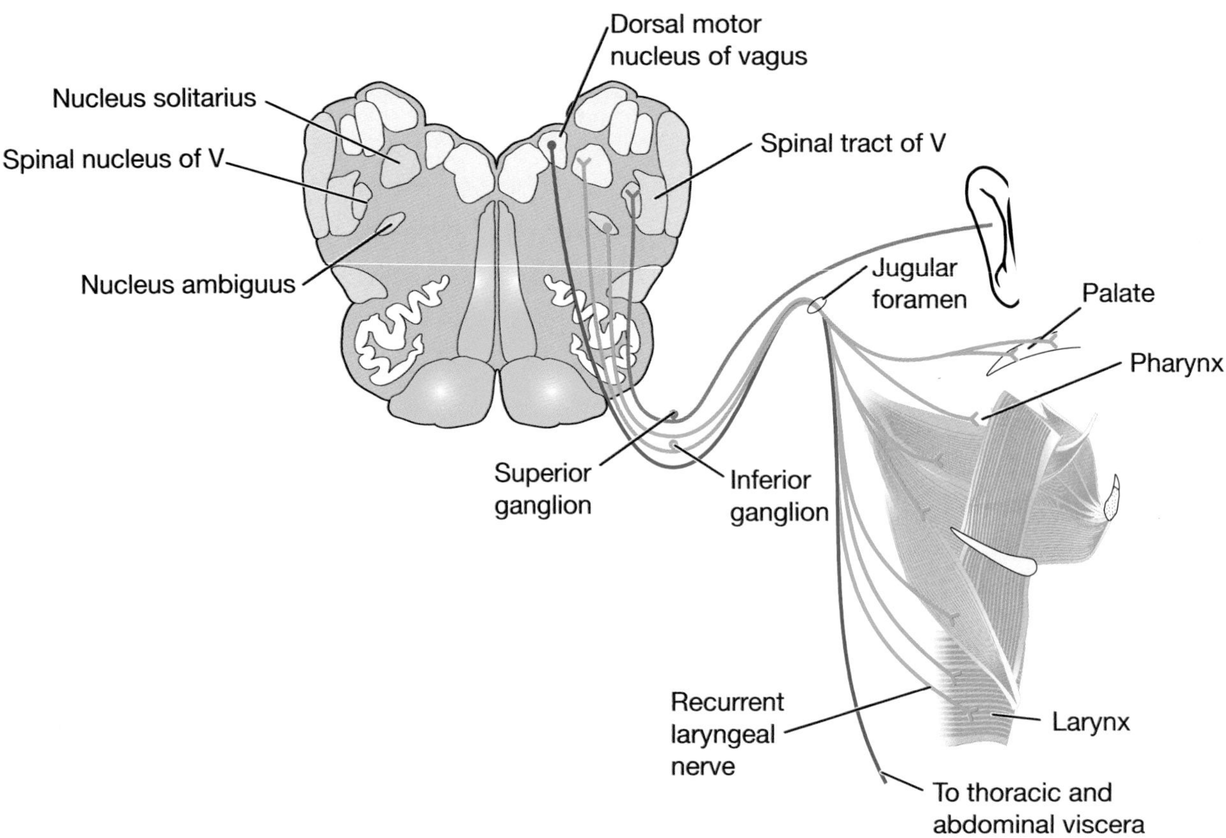

Fig. 15A.13. Motor and sensory nuclei of the vagus nerve and the course and distribution of some of the special visceral and general visceral efferent fibers to thoracic and abdominal viscera.

with postganglionic neurons in the cardiac, pulmonary, esophageal, or celiac plexuses or within the visceral organs themselves.

The afferent fibers in the vagus nerve arise from three different sources: 1) general somatic afferent fibers carrying general sensation from the external auditory meatus have cell bodies in the *superior (jugular) ganglion*, and central processes from this ganglion enter the medulla with the vagus and terminate in the spinal nucleus of the trigeminal nerve; 2) general visceral afferent fibers carrying information from abdominal and thoracic viscera have their cell bodies in the *inferior (nodose) ganglion*, and the central processes terminate in the caudal aspect of the *nucleus solitarius*; and 3) special visceral afferent fibers in the vagus nerve carrying taste from the posterior pharynx also have cell bodies located in the inferior (nodose) ganglion; the central processes terminate in the rostral aspect of the nucleus solitarius.

The vagus nerve emerges from the lateral aspect of the medulla, dorsal to the olive, and leaves the skull through the jugular foramen. The superior and inferior ganglia of the vagus nerve are located in (or just below) the jugular foramen. The nerve then passes down the neck near the carotid artery and jugular vein. At the base of the neck, it passes in front of the subclavian artery. At this point on the right side, the right vagus nerve gives off the *right recurrent laryngeal nerve*, which loops below and behind the subclavian artery and runs upward to the larynx to innervate most of the laryngeal muscles on the right side. On the left side, the vagus nerve descends in front of the arch of the aorta and gives off the *left recurrent laryngeal nerve*, which loops under the arch of the aorta and then runs upward to the larynx to innervate most of the laryngeal muscles on the left side. After giving off the recurrent laryngeal nerves, the vagus nerve descends into the thoracic and abdominal cavities to supply the esophagus, heart, lungs, and abdominal viscera.

Pathophysiology

Because of the dual innervation of many viscera and the ability of viscera to function within certain limits independently of innervation, unilateral disease processes that involve the vagus nerve do not produce visceral symptoms. Instead, the neurologic signs usually consist of weakness of the striated muscles of the larynx and pharynx and difficulty in swallowing and speaking. Injury to the recurrent laryngeal nerves results in vocal cord paresis and a hoarse voice. The structure and function of cranial nerve X are summarized in Table 15A.5.

Glossopharyngeal Nerve (Cranial Nerve IX)

Function

The *glossopharyngeal nerve* is also a mixed nerve, with special visceral efferent, general visceral efferent, general somatic afferent, general visceral afferent, and special visceral afferent components. The functions of cranial nerve IX are innervation of the stylopharyngeus muscle of the pharynx (special visceral efferent); parasympathetic innervation of the parotid gland (general visceral efferent); sensory innervation of the back of the ear (general sensory afferent); sensory innervation of the pharynx, tongue, eustachian tube, carotid body, and carotid sinus (general visceral afferent); and innervation of taste receptors on the posterior one-third of the tongue (special visceral afferent).

Anatomy

The special visceral efferent fibers to the stylopharyngeus muscle originate in the nucleus ambiguus (Fig. 15A.14).

Table 15A.5. Structure and Function of the Vagus Nerve

Component[a]	Function	Nucleus of origin or termination	Ganglion	Foramen	Signs of dysfunction
SVE	Motor to muscles of soft palate, pharynx, and larynx	Nucleus ambiguus		Jugular	Hoarseness, dysphagia, decreased gag reflex
GVE	Parasympathetic to thoracic and abdominal viscera	Dorsal motor nucleus of CN X		Jugular	Visceral disturbance, tachycardia
GSA	Sensation: external auditory meatus	Spinal nucleus of CN V	Superior (jugular)	Jugular	Decreased sensation: external auditory meatus
GVA	Sensation: pharynx, larynx, and thoracic and abdominal viscera	Nucleus solitarius	Inferior (nodose)	Jugular	Decreased sensation: pharynx
SVA	Taste: posterior pharynx	Nucleus solitarius	Inferior (nodose)	Jugular	Not clinically significant

CN, cranial nerve.
[a]See Table 15A.2 for definition of abbreviations.

The general visceral efferent components of the glossopharyngeal nerve carry preganglionic parasympathetic fibers that arise in the *inferior salivatory nucleus* and terminate in the *otic ganglion*. Postganglionic fibers from this ganglion supply the parotid salivary gland; stimulation increases salivary flow.

The afferent fibers carried in the glossopharyngeal nerve arise from three sources: 1) general somatic afferent fibers, carrying general sensation from behind the ear, have cell bodies in the superior ganglion; their central processes terminate in the spinal nucleus of the trigeminal nerve; 2) general visceral afferent fibers carrying sensation from the pharynx and information from the carotid body baroreceptors; and 3) special visceral afferent fibers carrying taste sensation from the posterior tongue. The latter two components arise from cell bodies in the *inferior* (*petrosal*) *ganglion* and have central processes that terminate in the nucleus solitarius. Within the medulla, there are segmental reflex connections between the pharyngeal sensory fibers and the motor neurons supplying the muscles of the pharynx to mediate the gag reflex.

The glossopharyngeal nerve emerges from the medulla, dorsal to the inferior olivary nucleus, and passes through the jugular foramen (which is also the location of its ganglia) to innervate peripheral structures. The

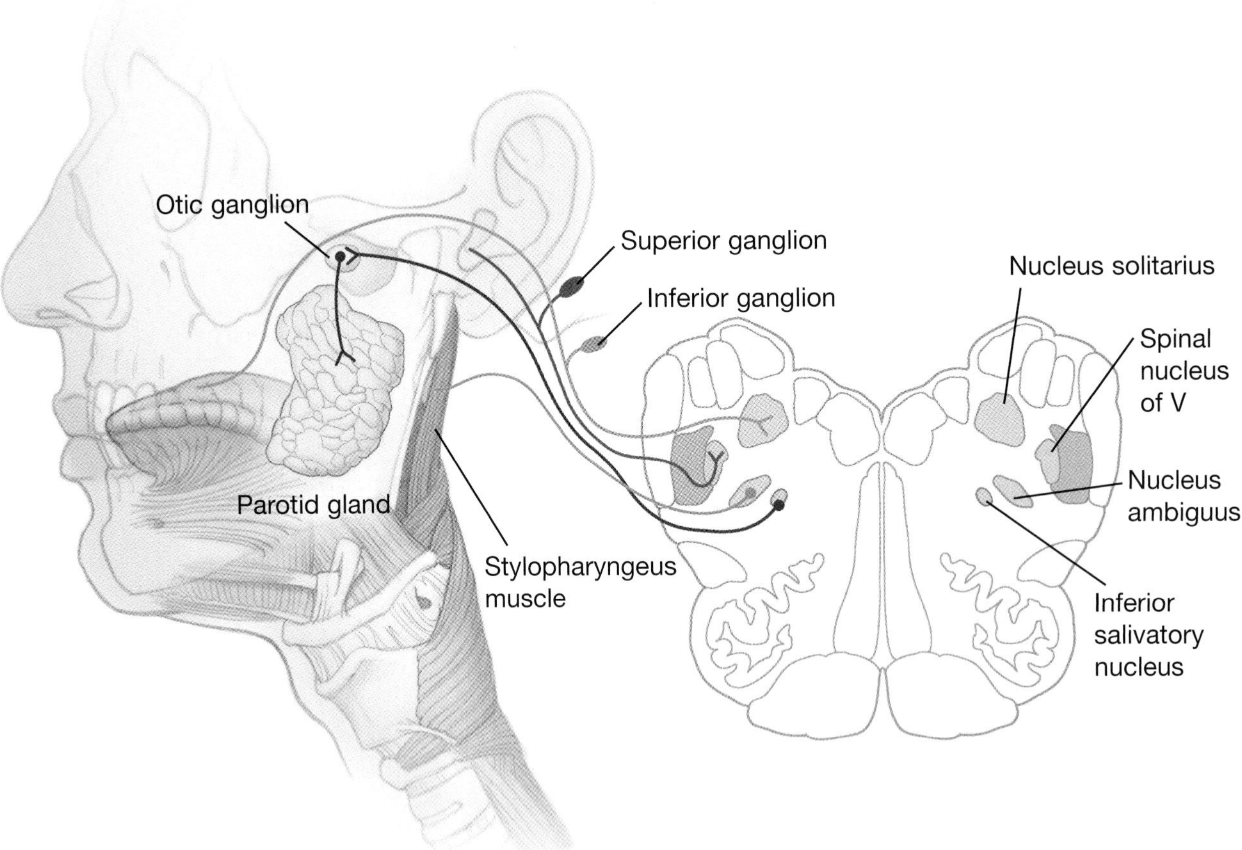

Fig. 15A.14. Motor and sensory nuclei of the glossopharyngeal nerve in the medulla and the course and distribution of the special visceral efferent fibers to the stylopharyngeus muscle and general visceral efferent fibers to the parotid gland.

components and structure of the glossopharyngeal nerve are similar to those of the vagus nerve (Table 15A.6).

Pathophysiology

Isolated lesions of the glossopharyngeal nerve are rare but, with or without damage to the vagus nerve, result in loss of pharyngeal sensation and the gag reflex. Occasionally, lesions produce a paroxysmal pain syndrome of unknown cause called *glossopharyngeal neuralgia*. In this disorder, the patient experiences brief attacks of severe pain that usually begin in the throat and radiate down the side of the neck in front of the ear and to the back of the lower jaw. Occasionally, the pain may begin deep in the ear. Attacks of discomfort may be precipitated by swallowing or protruding the tongue.

Reticular Formation

The reticular formation of the medulla occupies much of the core area, in which it is dispersed among the tracts and nuclei described above. This location reflects its primitive, indirect, diffuse organization as opposed to the phylogenetically newer direct, discrete motor and sensory pathways that occupy the ventral and lateral surfaces of the medulla. In transverse sections, the medullary reticular formation can be divided into three zones: medial, intermediate, and lateral. The medial zone projects to spinal motor neurons, predominantly through the ipsilateral lateral reticulospinal tract (an indirect activation pathway). The intermediate zone projects to preganglionic sympathetic neurons in the spinal cord to influence vasomotor tone. It also projects to spinal motor neurons that innervate respiratory muscles and is one of several brainstem centers involved in the control of respiration. The lateral zone contains the central pattern generators concerned with coordination of complex reflexes involving multiple cranial nerves important in swallowing and vomiting.

Clinical Correlations: Medulla and Lower Cranial Nerves

Bulbar and Pseudobulbar Palsy

Dysfunction of the motor components of the cranial nerves of the lower portion of the brainstem (particularly the medulla, or "bulb") occurs with either upper or

Table 15A.6. Structure and Function of the Glossopharyngeal Nerve

Component[a]	Function	Nucleus of origin or termination	Ganglion	Foramen	Signs of dysfunction
SVE	Motor to stylopharyngeus muscle	Nucleus ambiguus		Jugular	Not clinically significant
GVE	Parasympathetic to parotid gland	Inferior salivatory nucleus	Otic	Jugular	Decreased salivation
GSA	Sensation: back of ear	Spinal nucleus of CN V	Superior	Jugular	Decreased sensation: back of ear
GVA	Sensation: pharynx, tongue, carotid receptors	Nucleus solitarius	Inferior (petrosal)	Jugular	Decreased gag reflex
SVA	Taste: posterior 1/3 of tongue	Nucleus solitarius	Inferior (petrosal)	Jugular	Decreased taste

CN, cranial nerve.
[a]See Table 15A.2 for definition of abbreviations.

lower motor neuron lesions. Lesions affecting lower motor neurons (final common pathway) produce *bulbar palsy*, which is manifested as flaccid weakness of the muscles associated with talking, chewing, swallowing, and movements of the tongue and lips. Supranuclear lesions, involving cortical or subcortical components of the direct or indirect activation pathways, produce upper motor neuron dysfunction of the bulbar musculature, manifested as slow movements and a harsh, strained speech pattern. Because most bulbar motor nuclei receive bilateral cortical input, unilateral supranuclear lesions do not usually produce significant bulbar dysfunction. However, bilateral supranuclear lesions result in severe paresis of bulbar muscles characterized by spastic weakness with dysarthria, dysphagia, and reduced mouth and tongue movements. This involvement of bulbar function by bilateral supranuclear lesions is called *pseudobulbar palsy*.

Jugular Foramen Syndrome

Cranial nerves IX, X, and XI leave the skull with the jugular vein through the jugular foramen (Fig. 15A.15). A lesion (usually a mass lesion) in or adjacent to the jugular foramen may affect all three cranial nerves and cause ipsilateral weakness of the pharyngeal and laryngeal muscles (cranial nerve X), decreased sensation of the ipsilateral pharynx (cranial nerve IX), and weakness of the ipsilateral trapezius and sternocleidomastoid muscles (cranial nerve XI). One cause of this syndrome is chemodectoma arising in chemoreceptors along the jugular vein.

Vomiting

Vomiting is a complex stereotyped motor behavior integrated at the level of the medulla; it involves coordinated activation of neurons controlling gastrointestinal, respiratory, upper airway, and postural muscles. The neuronal network coordinating vomiting is located in the dorsolateral reticular formation of the medulla and has connections with the area postrema, nucleus solitarius, nucleus ambiguus, dorsal motor nucleus of the vagus, and respiratory neurons. These neuronal networks, referred to as *central pattern generators*, can be involved in more than one physiologic function, including breathing, vomiting, coughing, and sneezing. Vomiting is primarily the

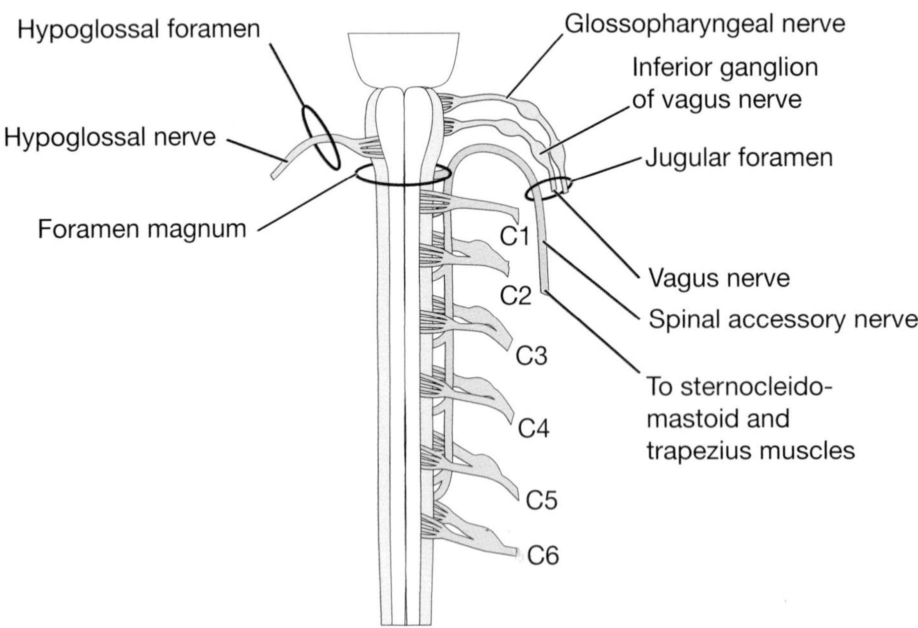

Fig. 15A.15. Ventral view of the medulla and the spinal accessory, vagus, and glossopharyngeal nerves exiting together through the jugular foramen. Spinal roots of C1-C6 are also shown.

result of changes in intra-abdominal and intrathoracic pressures generated by synergistic activation of the diaphragm (inspiratory) and abdominal (expiratory) muscles. Relaxation of the stomach and retrograde contraction of the proximal small intestine serve as a buffer to dilute the acidic contents of the stomach before it passes through the esophagus and mouth. Vomiting can be triggered by input to the vomiting center from the gut, oral cavity, blood, vestibular system, and higher brain centers. Vagal afferents detect emetic stimuli in the gut, including stimuli that activate mechanoreceptors and chemoreceptors in the distal stomach and proximal small intestine. These vagal afferents project primarily to the nucleus of the tractus solitarius and the area postrema. The area postrema, located in the floor of the fourth ventricle, lacks the blood-brain barrier and functions as a chemoreceptor trigger zone. Its neurons detect emetic substances in the blood and cerebrospinal fluid. Antineoplastic drugs and dopamine agonists activate the area postrema, and this is the basis for the vomiting induced by these agents. Patients with posterior fossa lesions, particularly neoplasms involving the dorsal medulla, may present with vomiting, even in the absence of signs of increased intracranial pressure.

Clinical Problem 15A.1.

A 50-year-old man was well until 6 months previously when he noted some difficulty swallowing. Food seemed to stick in the right side of his throat, and liquids occasionally entered the right side of his nose. In the last 3 months, he has noted progressive hoarseness of his voice and difficulty in reaching overhead with his right arm. Neurologic examination showed that the soft palate sagged on the right side. When the left posterior pharynx was stimulated, the soft palate pulled upward and to the left. When the right side was similarly stimulated, nothing happened and the patient said he could barely feel the touch. Indirect laryngoscopy showed that the right vocal cord did not move with phonation. Muscle testing revealed weakness and atrophy of the right trapezius and sternocleidomastoid muscles. Results of the rest of the examination were normal.

a. What are the location and type of lesion?
b. What neural structures are involved?
c. Through what foramen do these structures leave the skull?
d. What other structure also passes through this foramen?
e. Name one lesion that can produce the above syndrome.

- The medulla oblongata is the portion of the brainstem extending from the level of the foramen magnum to the caudal border of the base of the pons.
- Unique to the medulla are the decussation of the pyramids, decussation of the medial lemniscus, inferior olivary nuclei, nucleus ambiguus, nucleus solitarius, inferior cerebellar peduncle, and cranial nerves IX through XII.
- The hypoglossal nerve (cranial nerve XII) is a general somatic efferent nerve that exits from the preolivary sulcus and passes through the hypoglossal canal of the skull to innervate the muscles of the tongue.
- The spinal accessory nerve (cranial nerve XI) has a spinal component (special visceral efferent) that arises from the upper five cervical segments, enters the foramen magnum, and exits through the jugular foramen to innervate the sternocleidomastoid and trapezius muscles. The cranial portion (special visceral efferent) arises from the nucleus ambiguus and, along with cranial nerves IX and X, innervates muscles of the pharynx and larynx.
- The functions of the vagus nerve (cranial nerve X) are innervation of the striated muscles of the soft palate, pharynx, and larynx (special visceral efferent); parasympathetic innervation of the thoracic and abdominal viscera (general visceral efferent); sensory innervation of the external auditory meatus (general somatic afferent); sensory innervation of the pharynx, larynx, and thoracic and abdominal viscera (general visceral afferent); and innervation of

taste receptors on the posterior pharynx (special visceral afferent).

- The functions of the glossopharyngeal nerve (cranial nerve IX) are innervation of the stylopharyngeus muscle of the pharynx (special visceral efferent); parasympathetic innervation of the parotid gland (general visceral efferent); sensory innervation of the back of the ear (general somatic afferent); sensory innervation of the pharynx, tongue, eustachian tube, carotid body, and carotid sinus (general visceral afferent); and innervation of taste receptors on the posterior one-third of the tongue (special visceral afferent).
- The nucleus ambiguus is dorsal to the inferior olivary nucleus and contains cell bodies of axons in cranial nerves IX, X, and XI that carry motor fibers (special visceral efferent) to muscles of the pharynx and larynx.
- The nucleus solitarius lies ventral to the dorsal motor nucleus of the vagus and receives sensory information regarding taste (special visceral afferent) and sensory information from the viscera (general visceral afferent).

The Pons

The pons is the portion of the brainstem bound ventrally by the rostral and caudal borders of the basis pontis (Fig. 15A.2). In cross section, it is divided into two general areas. The ventral area is called the *basis pontis*, formed by transversely oriented crossing (pontocerebellar) fibers of the middle cerebellar peduncle and bundles of rostrocaudally running fibers of the corticospinal, corticobulbar, and corticopontine tracts. Small collections of neurons, the pontine nuclei, are dispersed in the basis pontis and are the origin of the axons that form the pontocerebellar fibers that congregate laterally as the *middle cerebellar peduncle*.

The area of the pons dorsal to the basis pontis and ventral to the fourth ventricle is the *tegmentum*, which contains the spinothalamic tracts, medial lemnisci, and the medial longitudinal fasciculi. The reticular formation and the pathways related to the consciousness and internal regulation systems are concentrated in the core of the pontine tegmentum. The tegmentum also contains structures related to the following cranial nerves: acoustic and vestibular divisions of cranial nerve VIII, facial nerve (cranial nerve VII), abducens nerve (cranial nerve VI), and trigeminal nerve (cranial nerve V). The location of many of these structures is shown in Figure 15A.16.

Auditory Nerve (Cranial Nerve VIII)

Cranial nerve VIII (also called the auditory, vestibulocochlear, or statoacoustic nerve) consists of two divisions: one mediates auditory sense, and the other mediates vestibular sense. Because these two divisions are grossly inseparable in their course from the brainstem to the *internal auditory meatus*, they traditionally are considered a single nerve (Fig. 15A.17). However, they represent the peripheral connections of two functionally distinct sensory systems and have separate peripheral receptors and central connections and pathways. Therefore, the two divisions are discussed separately.

Acoustic Division of Cranial Nerve VIII

Function

The acoustic division of cranial nerve VIII is an afferent nerve that conducts impulses from the inner ear structures related to hearing. Hearing is a special somatic afferent function.

Anatomy

Fibers in this division of cranial nerve VIII arise from cell bodies in the *spiral ganglion* of the cochlea in the inner ear (Fig. 15A.17). The nerve, composed of the central axons of these first-order neurons, enters the dorsolateral medulla at the pontomedullary junction. The axons bifurcate on entering the brainstem and synapse in both the *dorsal* and *ventral cochlear nuclei* located at that level. The subarachnoid space from the internal auditory meatus to the dorsolateral medulla, through which cranial nerve VIII courses, is bordered by the base of the pons and the ventral surface of the cerebellar hemisphere and is called the *cerebellopontine angle cistern*. Pathways arising from the cochlear nuclei relay auditory information through the brainstem to the medial geniculate body of the thalamus bilaterally and from there to the auditory cortex of

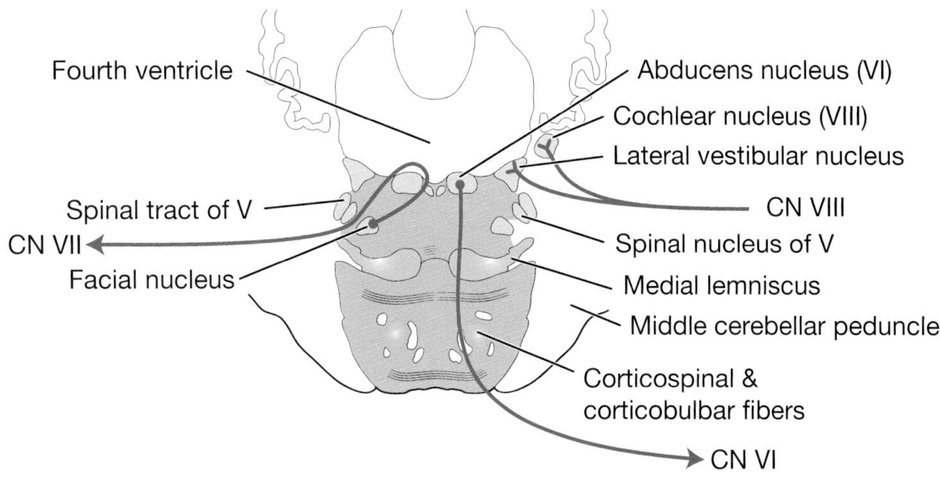

Fig. 15A.16. Cross section of caudal pons at the level of cranial nerves VI and VII. CN, cranial nerve.

the temporal lobes (see The Auditory System in part B of this chapter).

Pathophysiology

Lesions of the acoustic division of cranial nerve VIII produce unilateral loss of hearing. The physiology and pathophysiology of hearing are discussed below (see The Auditory System in part B of this chapter). The structure and function of the auditory division of cranial nerve VIII are summarized in Table 15A.7.

Vestibular Division of Cranial Nerve VIII

Function

The vestibular division of cranial nerve VIII is an afferent nerve that conducts gravitational and rotational

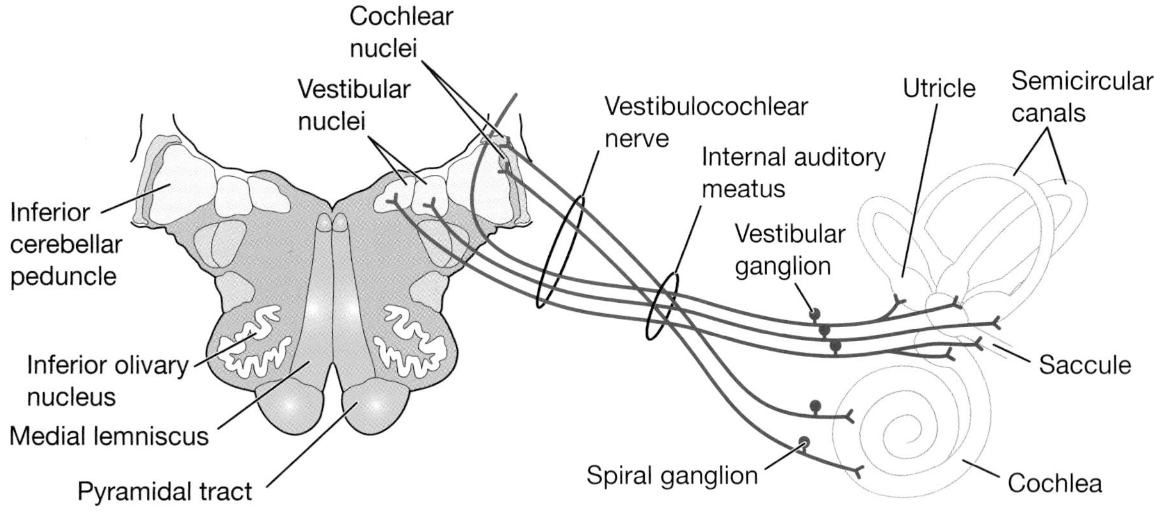

Fig. 15A.17. Vestibulocochlear nerve. The cell bodies are located in ganglia near the cochlea and semicircular canals, with the primary afferents terminating in lateral medulla and pons (pontomedullary junction).

Table 15A.7. Structure and Function of the Acoustic Division of Cranial Nerve VIII

Component	Function	Nucleus of origin or termination	Ganglion	Foramen	Signs of dysfunction
SSA	Hearing	Dorsal and ventral cochlear nuclei	Spiral	Internal auditory meatus	Decreased hearing

SSA, special somatic afferent.

information from the inner ear. This information is necessary for maintaining proper balance and equilibrium, which are special somatic afferent functions.

Anatomy

Fibers in this division of cranial nerve VIII arise from bipolar cells in the *vestibular (Scarpa) ganglion* located in the internal auditory canal. The peripheral axons of these ganglion cells innervate sensory receptors located in the organs of balance (utricle, saccule, and semicircular canals) in the inner ear. The central processes of the axons travel to the brainstem with the auditory division of cranial nerve VIII and synapse in the vestibular nuclei located beneath the floor of the fourth ventricle in the rostral medulla and caudal pons (Fig. 15A.17). Pathways arising from the vestibular nuclei conduct information to the cerebellum, spinal cord, reticular formation, and, through the medial longitudinal fasciculus, to the nuclei of cranial nerves III, IV, and VI (see The Vestibular System in part B of this chapter).

Pathophysiology

Lesions of the vestibular division of cranial nerve VIII cause the sensation of vertigo (hallucination of rotatory movement) or dysequilibrium. The physiology and pathophysiology of equilibrium are discussed below. The structure and function of the vestibular division of cranial nerve VIII are summarized in Table 15A.8.

Facial Nerve (Cranial Nerve VII)

Function

The *facial nerve* innervates the muscles of facial expression, which are derived from branchial arch mesoderm. This is the special visceral efferent component of the nerve. The facial nerve also has a general visceral efferent component consisting of preganglionic parasympathetic fibers that synapse on postganglionic neurons which innervate the lacrimal, submaxillary, and submandibular glands. A special visceral afferent component innervates taste receptors on the anterior two-thirds of the tongue.

Table 15A.8. Structure and Function of the Vestibular Division of Cranial Nerve VIII

Component	Function	Nucleus of origin or termination	Ganglion	Foramen	Signs of dysfunction
SSA	Balance and equilibrium	Vestibular nuclei	Vestibular	Internal auditory meatus	Dysequilibrium, vertigo

SSA, special somatic afferent.

Anatomy

The special visceral efferent fibers that innervate the striated muscles of the face arise in the *facial nucleus* located in the lateral tegmentum of the pons (Fig. 15A.16 and 15A.18). Axons from this nucleus first course medially and then arch dorsally, forming a loop, or genu, around the abducens nucleus before proceeding to the lateral surface of the caudal pons, where they emerge medial to cranial nerve VIII. The looping of the facial nerve fibers around the abducens nucleus causes a slight bulge, the *facial colliculus*, on each side of the midline in the floor of the fourth ventricle.

As the facial nerve leaves the pons, two separate nerve roots are apparent: the larger division carries the special visceral efferent component supplying the facial muscles, and the smaller division, the *nervus intermedius*, carries the general visceral efferent and special visceral afferent components. The parasympathetic fibers of the facial nerve originate in the superior salivatory nucleus and, after joining the fibers from the facial nucleus, emerge from the pons to end on postganglionic neurons that innervate the lacrimal, sublingual, and submandibular glands (Fig. 15A.19).

The special visceral afferent component of the facial nerve mediates taste from the anterior two-thirds of the tongue. The cell bodies of the first-order neurons of this component are located in the *geniculate ganglion*, a name derived from its position at a bend in the facial canal. The central axons from this ganglion enter the pons as part of the nervus intermedius. In the pons, the axons turn caudally to synapse, along with other taste fibers, in the rostral aspect of the nucleus of the tractus solitarius.

Both divisions pass through the cerebellopontine angle cistern and leave the cranial cavity through the internal auditory meatus and enter the facial canal of the temporal bone. The special visceral efferent fibers to the face continue through the horizontal and then vertical parts of the canal, exiting at the *stylomastoid foramen* below the ear (Fig. 15A.19). In addition to innervating the muscles of facial expression, a small branch is given off to the stapedius muscle, a tiny striated muscle in the middle ear. The nervus intermedius does not traverse the entire facial canal. In the

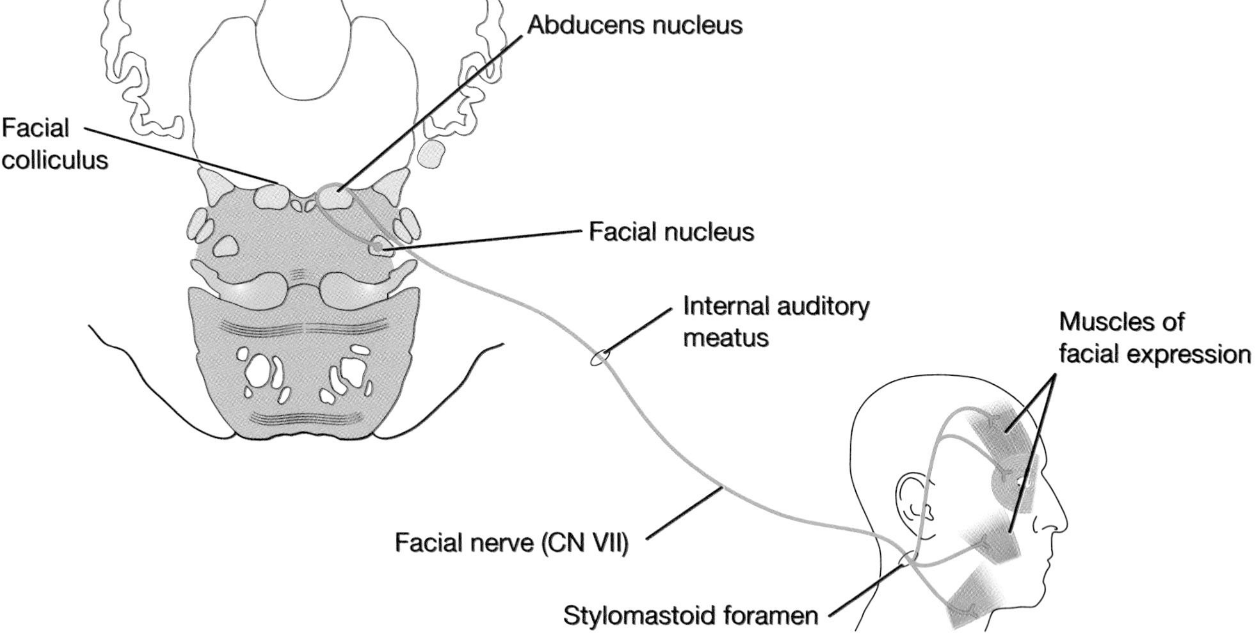

Fig. 15A.18. Facial nerve nucleus in the pons and the course and distribution of motor axons. The loop of the facial nerve over the abducens nucleus forms the facial colliculus in the floor of the fourth ventricle. CN, cranial nerve.

region of the geniculate ganglion, it splits into two branches: the *greater (superficial) petrosal nerve* (general visceral efferent fibers for the lacrimal gland) and the chorda tympani (general visceral efferent fibers for the salivary glands and special visceral afferent fibers for taste).

The preganglionic parasympathetic fibers in the greater petrosal nerve synapse in the *sphenopalatine ganglion*. Postganglionic cholinergic fibers from this ganglion innervate the lacrimal gland. The chorda tympani nerve leaves the facial canal in its vertical segment, enters the middle ear cavity, arches over the tympanic membrane, and emerges from the petrous bone to join the lingual branch of cranial nerve V on its way to the tongue. The preganglionic parasympathetic fibers leave the lingual nerve and synapse in the *submandibular ganglion*. Postganglionic cholinergic fibers supply the sublingual and submandibular salivary glands.

Pathophysiology

The most conspicuous result of disorders of the facial nerve is weakness of the muscles of facial expression. Loss of taste on the anterior two-thirds of the tongue may also occur. Facial weakness, however, may also result from lesions involving the direct activation pathway descending from the cerebral cortex to the facial nucleus. It is clinically important to distinguish between *upper motor neuron* (central) facial weakness involving the lower half of the face and *lower motor neuron* (peripheral) facial weakness involving both the upper and lower halves of the face.

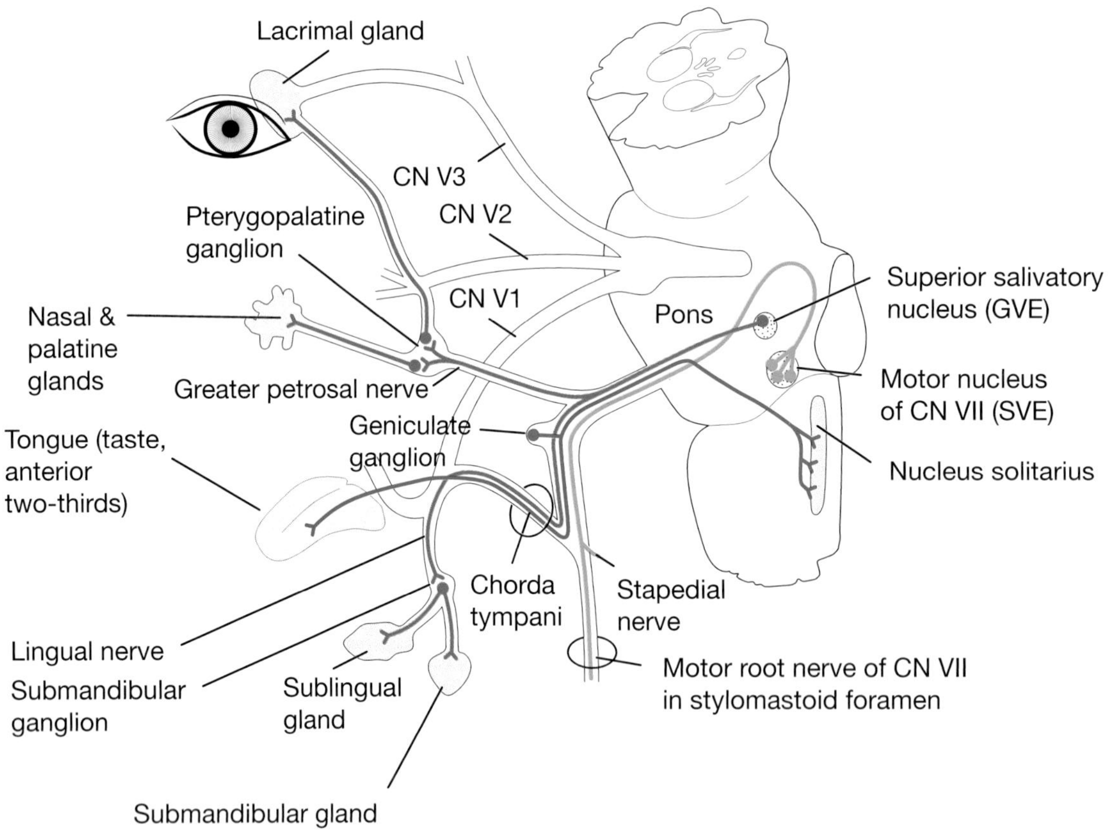

Fig. 15A.19. Course of visceral efferent and afferent divisions of the facial nerve. CN, cranial nerve; GVE, general visceral efferent; SVE, special visceral efferent; V1-V3, ophthalmic, maxillary, and mandibular divisions, respectively, of CN V. (Modified from Parent A. Carpenter's human neuroanatomy. 9th ed. Baltimore: Williams & Wilkins; 1996. Used with permission.)

A relatively common disorder that produces peripheral facial weakness is *Bell palsy*. Although the cause is usually unproved, it is thought to result from inflammation of the facial nerve in the facial canal. Patients with this condition exhibit weakness of both upper and lower facial muscles, including weakness of eye closure, a feature not seen in upper motor neuron facial weakness. Also, depending on the site of involvement of the nerve in the facial canal, patients may have decreased lacrimation and salivation, decreased taste sensation, and hyperacusis (increased sensitivity to noise because of weakness of the stapedius muscle).

The structure and function of the facial nerve are summarized in Table 15A.9.

Abducens Nerve (Cranial Nerve VI)

Function

The abducens nerve is a general somatic efferent nerve that innervates the *lateral rectus muscle* of the eye. Contraction of this muscle produces lateral movement (abduction) of the eyeball.

Anatomy

The abducens nucleus is located in the general somatic efferent cell column at the midpontine level, beneath the floor of the fourth ventricle and near the midline (Fig. 15A.16). The axons take a ventral and slightly caudal course through the tegmentum and basis pontis to emerge on the ventral surface near the pontomedullary junction. The nerve then ascends ventral to the base of the pons, traverses the lateral wall of the cavernous sinus (along with cranial nerves III, IV, and the first division of V), and leaves the cranial cavity through the superior orbital fissure to supply the lateral rectus muscle of the eye (Fig. 15A.20).

Pathophysiology

Lesions affecting the abducens nerve produce weakness of the lateral rectus muscle, with inability to abduct the eye, causing double vision (diplopia) (see the Ocular Motor

Table 15A.9. Structure and Function of the Facial Nerve

Component[a]	Function	Nucleus of origin or termination	Ganglion	Foramen	Signs of dysfunction
SVE	Motor to muscles of facial expression and stapedius	Facial nucleus		Internal auditory meatus, stylomastoid	Facial weakness, hyperacusis
GVE	Parasympathetic				
	Lacrimal gland	Superior salivatory nucleus	Sphenopalatine	Internal auditory meatus	Decreased tearing
	Salivary glands	Superior salivatory nucleus	Submandibular	Internal auditory meatus	Decreased salivation
SVA	Taste: anterior 2/3 of tongue	Nucleus solitarius	Geniculate	Internal auditory meatus	Decreased taste

[a]See Table 15A.2 for definition of abbreviations.

System in part B of this chapter). Because the intracranial course of cranial nerve VI is unusually long, the nerve may be affected by many pathologic processes involving the pons, the base of the skull (clivus), the cavernous sinus, the superior orbital fissure, or the orbit. The structure and function of the abducens nerve are summarized in Table 15A.10.

Trigeminal Nerve (Cranial Nerve V)

Function

The *trigeminal nerve* is the sensory nerve of the face. It is a mixed nerve containing general somatic afferent and special visceral efferent components. In addition to conveying touch, pain, temperature, and proprioceptive information (general somatic afferent) from the face, this nerve provides motor innervation (special visceral efferent) to the muscles of mastication, which are derived from branchial arch mesoderm.

Anatomy

The general somatic afferent fibers that mediate touch, pain, and temperature sense arise from cell bodies in the trigeminal (gasserian or semilunar) ganglion that lies in a dural fold called *Meckel cave* on the medial petrous ridge (Fig. 15A.21). Axons travel centrally from the ganglion to enter the lateral aspect of the pons. Fibers mediating touch synapse directly in the *main (chief) sensory nucleus of V* located in the dorsolateral tegmentum of the pons. Second-order neurons from this nucleus ascend in both crossed and uncrossed pathways, the trigeminothalamic tracts, to synapse in the ventral posteromedial nucleus of the thalamus.

Pain and temperature fibers do not synapse in the main sensory nucleus but turn caudally to descend through the dorsolateral medulla and upper three or four segments of the cervical spinal cord as the *spinal (descending) tract of the trigeminal nerve* (Fig. 15A.21). Axons in this tract synapse on cell bodies of second-order neurons in the underlying *nucleus of the spinal (descending) tract of the trigeminal nerve*. The general somatic afferent fibers in cranial nerves IX and X, from the skin of the external ear, join the spinal tract of V where they enter the medulla. The fibers from the mandibular division are located most dorsally in the spinal tract of the trigeminal nerve and those from the ophthalmic division are

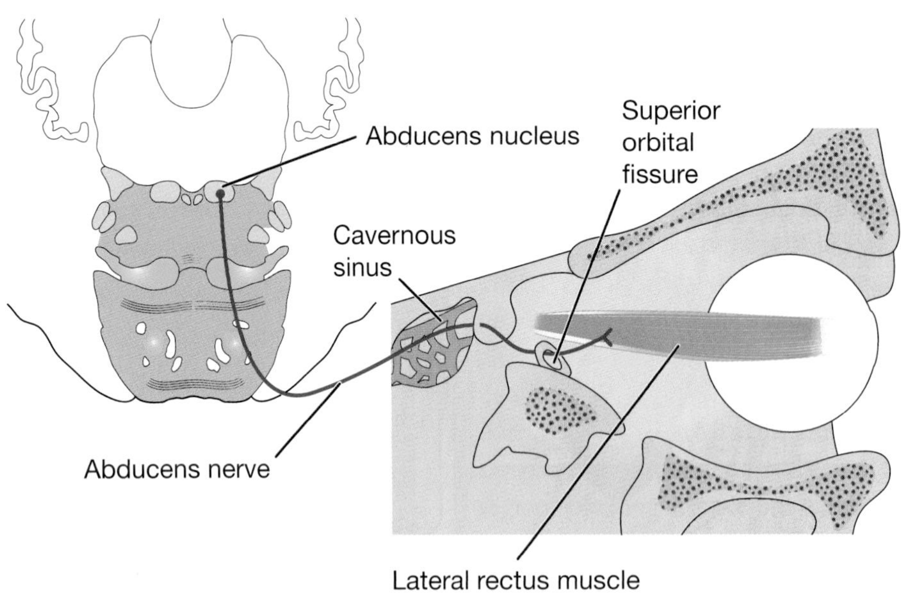

Fig. 15A.20. The abducens nerve arises from the abducens nucleus in the pons and has a long intracranial course to the lateral rectus muscle, passing through the cavernous sinus and superior orbital fissure.

Table 15A.10. Structure and Function of the Abducens Nerve

Component	Function	Nucleus of origin or termination	Ganglion	Foramen	Signs of dysfunction
GSE	Motor to lateral rectus muscle	Abducens		Superior orbital fissure	Diplopia, medial deviation of eye

GSE, general somatic efferent.

most ventral as the tract descends through the caudal pons and medulla. Second-order fibers from the spinal nucleus of V cross to the opposite side of the medulla and ascend to the thalamus as the *ventral trigeminothalamic tract*, which is near the medial lemniscus. These fibers synapse in the ventral posteromedial nucleus of the thalamus, where third-order neurons send axons to the parietal lobe.

Proprioceptive fibers in the trigeminal nerve, unlike all other first-order sensory neurons, arise from cell bodies located in the central nervous system. These cell bodies form the mesencephalic nucleus of the trigeminal nerve and lie along the lateral border of the rostral fourth ventricle and aqueduct of Sylvius. The peripheral axons of these unique first-order neurons innervate receptors in the muscles of mastication (and perhaps other muscles) and travel without synapse through the trigeminal ganglion to enter the lateral pons along with the rest of the nerve. Central axons from the mesencephalic nucleus synapse directly in the motor nucleus of V to mediate the monosynaptic jaw reflex.

The special visceral efferent fibers that innervate the muscles of mastication arise from cell bodies in the *motor nucleus of V*, located medial to the main sensory nucleus (Fig. 15A.22). Axons course ventrolaterally and exit from the lateral surface of the pons as the motor root, medial to the sensory root. These fibers run along the ventral aspect of the trigeminal ganglion and join the mandibular (third) division of the trigeminal nerve to exit the skull through the foramen ovale. They innervate the temporalis, masseter, medial and lateral pterygoid, and tensor tympani muscles. The temporalis, masseter, and medial pterygoid muscles close the jaw, the lateral pterygoid muscles open and facilitate lateral movement of the jaw, and the tensor tympani, a small muscle in the middle ear, dampens vibration of the eardrum.

From the trigeminal ganglion, sensory fibers of cranial nerve V course peripherally in three major divisions: the *ophthalmic division* (V1) passes through the superior orbital fissure to innervate the upper face; the *maxillary division* (V2) exits the skull through the foramen rotundum to innervate the midface; and the mandibular division (V3), joined by the motor root, exits through the foramen ovale to innervate the lower face.

Pathophysiology

Lesions involving cranial nerve V produce loss of facial sensation and, if the motor fibers are involved, weakness of the masticatory muscles, which causes the jaw to deviate to the side of the weakened muscles when the jaw is opened.

Trigeminal neuralgia (tic douloureux) is a disorder characterized by transient, brief, repetitive paroxysms of pain in the distribution of one or more branches of cranial nerve V. The pain is severe and is either spontaneous or triggered by relatively minor sensory stimulation of the face. Although various pathologic changes have been noted in the trigeminal ganglion, nerve, or root entry zone in the pons, the cause of the syndrome is unknown.

Two reflexes tested as part of the neurologic examination involve cranial nerve V: the jaw jerk and corneal reflex. The *jaw jerk* is the only muscle stretch reflex that can be elicited in the head. It is mediated entirely by the mandibular branch of cranial nerve V. Tapping the jaw briefly stretches the muscles of mastication. Proprioceptive

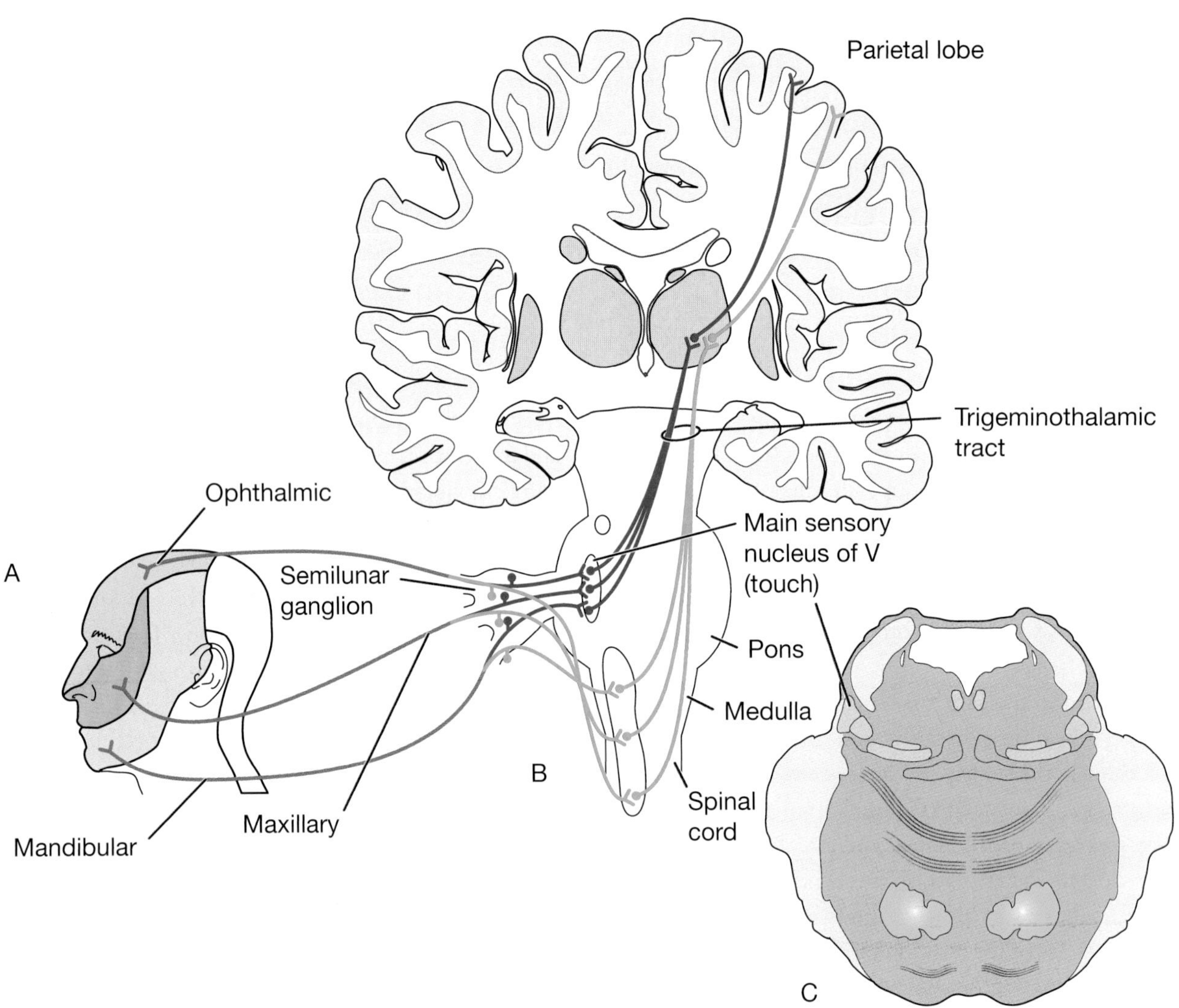

Fig. 15A.21. Trigeminal nerve. *A*, Peripheral distribution of each of the three divisions of cranial nerve V. *B*, Horizontal section with the course and distribution of sensory axons. *C*, Cross section through mid pons.

impulses travel centrally, synapse in the motor nucleus of V, and activate reflex contraction of the jaw muscles. The clinical usefulness of this reflex in detecting lesions affecting the reflex arc is limited by the frequent difficulty in eliciting it in healthy persons. Therefore, it is regarded as abnormal only when it is hyperactive, which occurs with bilateral upper motor neuron lesions affecting the direct and indirect activation pathways to the motor nucleus of V.

The *corneal reflex* is elicited by touching the cornea of one eye with a piece of cotton. The afferent limb of this reflex is the ophthalmic division of cranial nerve V. The observed result of this maneuver is an apparently simultaneous blink of both eyes, both the side stimulated (direct reflex) and the side not stimulated (consensual reflex). This response implies bilateral activation of facial nucleus neurons related to the orbicularis oculi muscles through complex central connections. Lesions involving the ophthalmic division of cranial nerve V, the tegmentum of the pons, or the facial nerve alter this reflex. The structure and function of the trigeminal nerve are summarized in Table 15A.11.

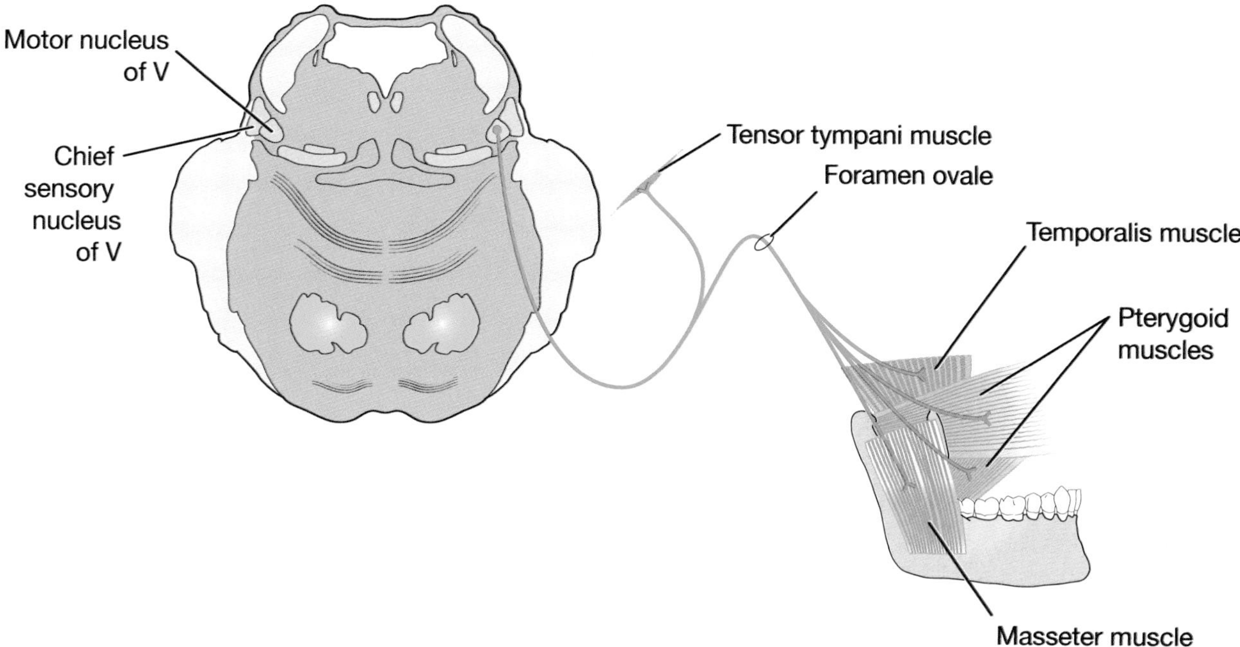

Fig. 15A.22. Motor division of the trigeminal nerve with its nucleus in the pons and the course of the axons to the muscles of mastication.

Reticular Formation

The pontine reticular formation, located in the core of the tegmentum, is continuous with the reticular formation of the medulla caudally and the midbrain rostrally. As in the medullary reticular formation, different functional zones can be distinguished in transverse sections. The medial zone at this level is concerned primarily with the ocular motor system and the reticulospinal system. The role of the paramedian pontine reticular formation in the coordination of eye movements is discussed below. The lateral pontine reticular formation contains neurons of the internal regulation system, including those that modulate the micturition reflex. The pontine reticular formation also contains several neuronal groups of the consciousness system, including the raphe nuclei and locus ceruleus.

- The pons is the portion of the brainstem bound ventrally by the rostral and caudal borders of the basis pontis and is associated with cranial nerves V through VIII.
- Cranial nerve VIII has two divisions: one mediates auditory sense, and the other mediates vestibular sense (equilibrium and balance).
- The facial nerve (cranial nerve VII) innervates the muscles of facial expression (special visceral efferent), provides parasympathetic output (general visceral efferent) to the lacrimal, submaxillary, and submandibular glands, and carries taste (special visceral afferent) from the anterior two-thirds of the tongue.
- Bell palsy, due to inflammation of the facial nerve in the facial canal, produces peripheral facial weakness. Patients may also experience decreased lacrimation and salivation, decreased taste sensation, and hyperacusis.
- The abducens nerve (cranial nerve VI) is a general somatic efferent nerve that exits the pons ventrally, traverses the cavernous sinus and superior orbital fissure, and innervates the lateral rectus muscle of the eye.
- The trigeminal nerve (cranial nerve V) contains general somatic afferent (facial sensation) and special visceral efferent (motor output to muscles of mastication) components.

Table 15A.11. Structure and Function of the Trigeminal Nerve

Division of trigeminal nerve V	Component	Function	Nucleus of origin or termination	Ganglion	Foramen	Signs of dysfunction
Ophthalmic	GSA	Sensation: forehead pain	Spinal nucleus of V	Gasserian (semilunar)	Superior orbital fissure	Decreased forehead pain Decreased corneal reflex
(V1)		Touch: forehead	Main sensory nucleus of V	Gasserian (semilunar)	Superior orbital fissure	Decreased forehead touch Decreased corneal reflex
Maxillary	GSA	Sensation: cheek pain	Spinal nucleus of V	Gasserian (semilunar)	Rotundum	Decreased cheek pain
(V2)		Touch: cheek	Main sensory nucleus of V	Gasserian (semilunar)	Rotundum	Decreased cheek touch
Mandibular	GSA	Sensation: jaw pain	Spinal nucleus of V	Gasserian (semilunar)	Ovale	Decreased jaw pain
(V3)		Touch: jaw	Main sensory nucleus of V	Gasserian (semilunar)	Ovale	Decreased jaw touch
		Proprioception	Mesencephalic nucleus		Ovale	Decreased jaw jerk
	SVE	Motor to muscles of mastication	Motor nucleus of V		Ovale	Weakness of muscles of mastication, decreased jaw jerk

GSA, general somatic afferent; SVE, special visceral efferent.

Clinical Problem 15A.2.

A 25-year-old man awoke one morning and noted that the left side of his face seemed weak. On looking in a mirror, he saw that he could not retract the left corner of his mouth as well as he could retract the right corner. He also noticed that he could no longer close his left eye completely or smile with the left side of his face. Neurologic examination showed no abnormality except for the following: at rest, the left side of his face drooped and the left palpebral fissure was wider than on the right. The left side of his forehead did not wrinkle when he tried raising his eyebrows. He could not close his left eye completely. When he attempted to show his teeth, his mouth pulled to the right. Results of testing for sensations of pain, temperature, and touch of the face were normal. Taste was absent on the left side of his tongue. Strips of filter paper were placed in the conjunctival sacs; the strip on the right side became moist within a few minutes, and the one on the left side remained dry.

a. What are the location and type of lesion?
b. Why was taste involved?
c. Why was lacrimation decreased?
d. What is the name of this clinical entity?

- The three sensory nuclei of the trigeminal nerve are the spinal nucleus (pain and temperature sensation of the face), chief or principal sensory nucleus (touch and vibratory sense of the face), and mesencephalic nucleus (unconscious proprioception).
- Trigeminal neuralgia (tic douloureux) is characterized by transient, brief, repetitive paroxysms of pain in the distribution of one or more branches of the trigeminal nerve.

The Midbrain

The midbrain is the portion of the brainstem located between the pons and diencephalon. The major external anatomical features that mark its boundaries are the cerebral peduncles ventrally and the quadrigeminal plate, featuring the paired inferior and superior colliculi, dorsally. In transverse section, the midbrain is divided dorsoventrally into three main regions: tectum (dorsal), tegmentum, and base (ventral) (Fig. 15A.23). Its derivation from the primitive neural tube is highlighted most clearly by its tubular cavity, the *aqueduct of Sylvius*.

The *tectum*, or roof, of the midbrain lies above the transverse plane of the aqueduct of Sylvius. The tectum is made up of two paired structures, the *inferior* and *superior colliculi*, collectively called the *corpora quadrigemina*. The inferior colliculi act as a relay station for auditory fibers that pass to the thalamus through the brachium of the inferior colliculus. The superior colliculi are associated with ocular motor control. The aqueduct of Sylvius, a remnant of the neural canal, is surrounded by a zone of periaqueductal gray matter.

The *tegmentum* is the area ventral to the aqueduct and dorsal to the substantia nigra. The major longitudinal

Clinical Problem 15A.3.

A 60-year-old woman had a myocardial infarction. Several days later, she complained to the nurse that she had an abrupt onset of seeing double whenever she looked to the left and that she was having difficulty using her right arm. Testing of cranial nerves showed paralysis of the left lateral rectus muscle. Her speech was slightly slurred, and the left nasolabial fold was flattened. She could not close her left eye tightly, and she could not raise her eyebrow on the left as high as on the right. Facial sensation and taste were normal. Testing of the extremities showed weakness of the right arm and leg, with hyperactive reflexes and a Babinski sign on the right. There was loss of joint position and vibration sense in the right arm and leg.

a. What are the location and type of lesion?
b. What anatomical structures are involved?
c. What is the pathologic nature of the lesion?

pathways in the tegmentum of the midbrain are the lateral lemniscus, spinothalamic tract, medial lemniscus, medial longitudinal fasciculus, indirect activation pathways of the motor system, descending pathways of the internal regulation system, and projection pathways of the reticular formation. It also contains the nuclei of cranial nerves III and IV and their axons, the red nuclei, and the decussation of the superior cerebellar peduncles (Fig. 15A.23 *A*).

At the midbrain level—perhaps more clearly than at other brainstem levels—the primitive concentric organization of the neural tube can be recognized. The phylogenetically older multisynaptic pathways concerned with internal regulation, consciousness, and other primitive functions occupy the inner regions close to the aqueduct; the newer, more direct, and functionally discrete pathways concerned with somatic motor and sensory functions lie more peripherally.

The Superior Cerebellar Peduncle (Brachium Conjunctivum) Efferent fibers from the dentate nucleus of the cerebellum pass rostrally, and near the dorsal surface of the midbrain, just caudal to the inferior colliculi, they can be identified grossly as the *superior cerebellar peduncles*. From this

A

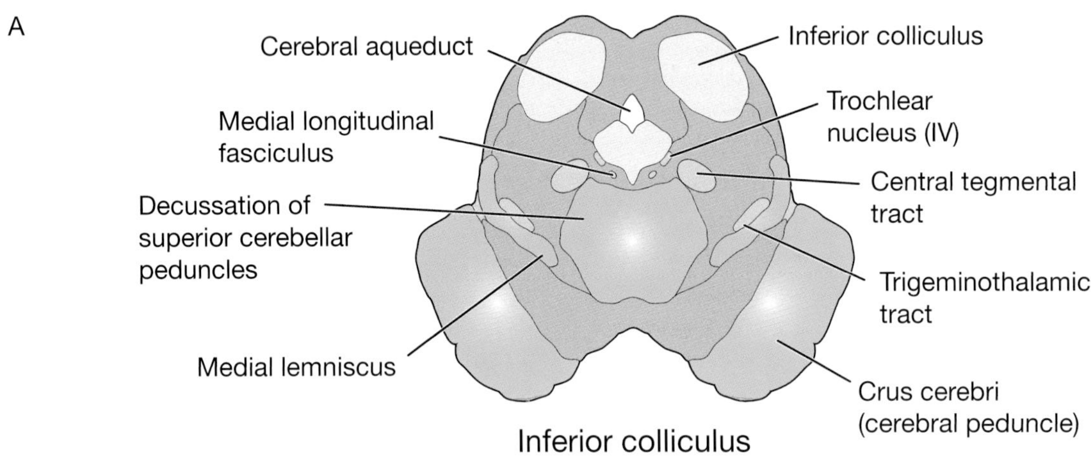

B

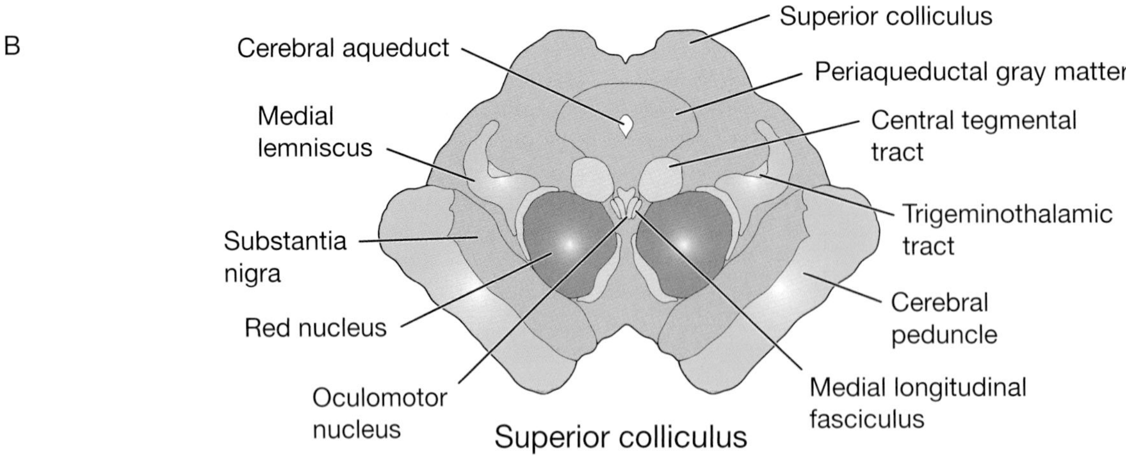

Fig. 15A.23. Cross section of the midbrain. *A*, Caudal midbrain (level of the inferior colliculus). *B*, Rostral midbrain (level of the superior colliculus).

point, they pass ventrally into the tegmentum of the midbrain. In caudal midbrain (level of the inferior colliculus), they cross to the opposite side, forming the *decussation of the brachium conjunctivum* (Fig. 15A.23 *A*). The fibers then proceed to the red nucleus and thalamus.

The Red Nucleus

The red nucleus is a large oval mass of gray matter in the central portion of the tegmentum on each side at the level of the superior colliculus (Fig. 15A.23 *B*). When viewed in a freshly cut brain, the nucleus is slightly red because of the density of its capillaries and high iron content. The red nuclei receive fibers from the cerebellum and the cerebral cortex and give rise to 1) descending fibers that synapse in the ipsilateral inferior olivary nucleus, from which fibers project to the contralateral cerebellar cortex; and 2) the rubrospinal tract, which crosses in the ventral tegmental decussation caudal to the red nucleus and descends to the spinal cord.

The Basis Pedunculi

The base of the midbrain, called the *basis pedunculi*, consists of the cerebral peduncles (containing the corticospinal, corticobulbar, and corticopontine tracts) and the substantia nigra, which is dorsal to each cerebral peduncle (Fig. 15A.23). The substantia nigra is dark because of its melanin-containing neurons. It is related functionally to the basal ganglia as part of the indirect activation pathway of the motor system.

Clinical Problem 15A.4.

A 35-year-old woman presents with sudden numbness of the left arm and leg, right-sided limb incoordination, and difficulty walking. Her examination shows a reduction to pain, temperature, and vibratory sense of the left arm and leg. She has right hemiataxia and gait ataxia. A magnetic resonance imaging scan of the brain is shown in Figure 15A.24.

a. What is the anatomicopathologic nature of this lesion?
b. If the lesion is not in the cerebellum, why does the patient have ataxia?

Trochlear Nerve (Cranial Nerve IV)

Function

The *trochlear nerve* is a general somatic efferent nerve that innervates the superior oblique muscle of the eye. Contraction of this muscle causes downward movement of the eye when the eye is in the adducted position and intorsion in the primary position.

Anatomy

The trochlear nucleus lies at the level of the inferior colliculus, just ventral to the periaqueductal gray matter and dorsal to the medial longitudinal fasciculus. Its axons pass dorsolaterally and caudally around the periaqueductal gray matter. They cross caudal to the tectum and emerge from the dorsal aspect of the midbrain on the side opposite of their origin. This is the only completely crossed cranial nerve and the only cranial nerve to emerge from the dorsal surface of the brainstem (Fig. 15A.25). The nerve passes around the midbrain to enter the lateral wall of the cavernous sinus. It enters the orbit through the superior orbital fissure to innervate the superior oblique muscle.

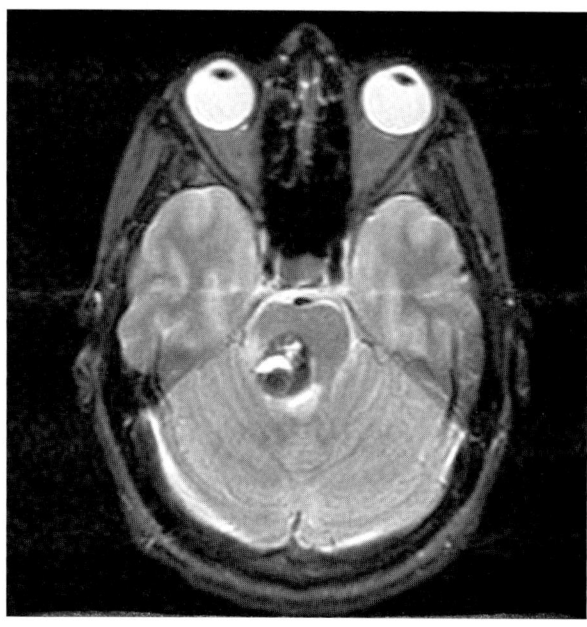

Fig. 15A.24. Magnetic resonance imaging scan of the brain.

Pathophysiology

Lesions of the trochlear nerve cause weakness of the superior oblique muscle, causing diplopia on downward and inward gaze. The patient may compensate for the torsional imbalance caused by the unopposed action of the inferior oblique muscle by tilting the head to the opposite side. Isolated injury to the trochlear nerve may occur where it runs along the edge of the tentorium cerebelli toward the cavernous sinus. This often results from head trauma. Otherwise, the nerve is usually involved along with cranial nerves III, V, and VI by lesions of the cavernous sinus, superior orbital fissure, or orbit. The structure and function of the trochlear nerve are summarized in Table 15A.12.

Oculomotor Nerve (Cranial Nerve III)

Function

The *oculomotor nerve* is a mixed motor nerve that provides general somatic efferent fibers to the following muscles of the eye: superior rectus, inferior rectus, medial rectus, inferior oblique, and levator palpebrae superioris. The oculomotor nerve also supplies general visceral efferent (parasympathetic) fibers to the iris and the ciliary muscle controlling the lens of the eye.

Anatomy

The general somatic efferent fibers of cranial nerve III arise from the oculomotor nucleus, which is ventral to the aqueduct at the level of the superior colliculus (Fig. 15A.26). The nucleus is composed of subnuclei for each of the muscles innervated. All the projections are ipsilateral except for those to the superior rectus muscle (which are crossed) and those to the levator palpebrae superioris muscle (which come from a single midline nucleus). Axons pass ventrally through the tegmentum and base of the midbrain and emerge in the interpeduncular fossa.

The general visceral efferent fibers that provide preganglionic parasympathetic innervation to the iris arise in a small subnucleus, the *Edinger-Westphal* nucleus, at the rostral end of each oculomotor nucleus. These fibers join the general somatic efferent fibers and, after emerging from the interpeduncular fossa, pass through the lateral wall of the cavernous sinus and superior orbital fissure into the orbit (Fig. 15A.26). The general somatic

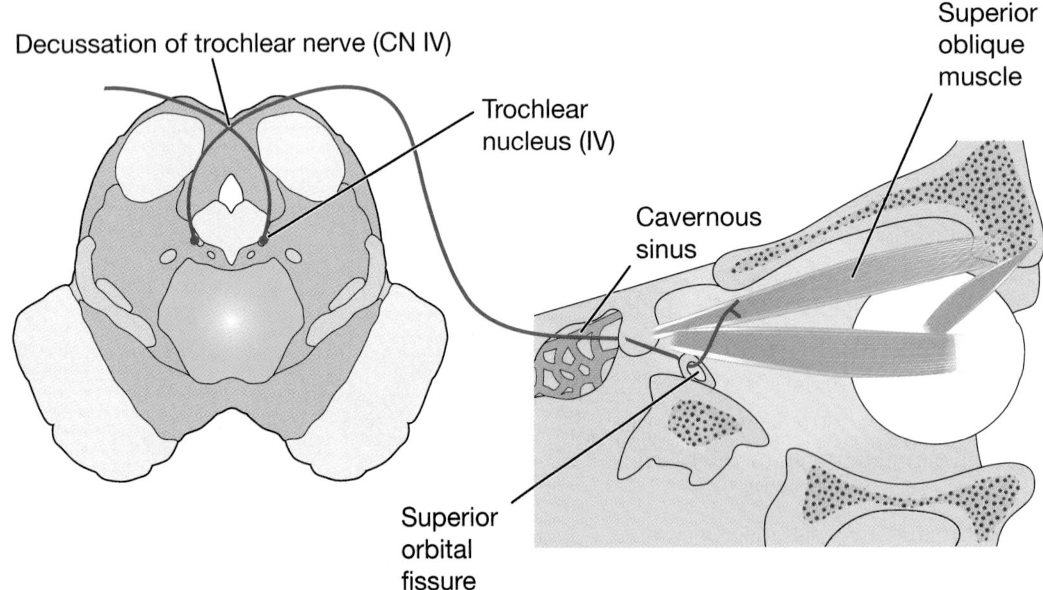

Fig. 15A.25. Trochlear nerve. Cross section of caudal midbrain showing the trochlear nucleus and the course and distribution of its axons to the superior oblique muscle of the opposite eye. CN, cranial nerve.

Table 15A.12. Structure and Function of the Trochlear Nerve

Component	Function	Nucleus of origin or termination	Ganglion	Foramen	Signs of dysfunction
GSE	Motor to superior oblique muscle	Trochlear nucleus on opposite side		Superior orbital fissure	Diplopia

GSE, general somatic efferent.

efferent fibers continue directly to the extraocular muscles and innervate them, and the general visceral efferent fibers synapse in the ciliary ganglion. Postganglionic fibers from this ganglion proceed to the pupilloconstrictor muscle of the iris and the ciliary body.

Pathophysiology

Lesions involving the general somatic efferent component of cranial nerve III produce weakness of all voluntary eye muscles except the lateral rectus and superior oblique and cause diplopia. The eye tends to deviate downward and outward because of the unopposed action of the lateral rectus and superior oblique muscles, and ptosis is often present because of weakness of the levator palpebrae superioris muscle. In rare cases in which the nucleus itself is the site of the lesion, there is weakness of the contralateral superior rectus and bilateral ptosis in addition to ipsilateral third nerve palsy.

Ptosis caused by weakness of the levator palpebrae superioris must be distinguished from ptosis due to lesions

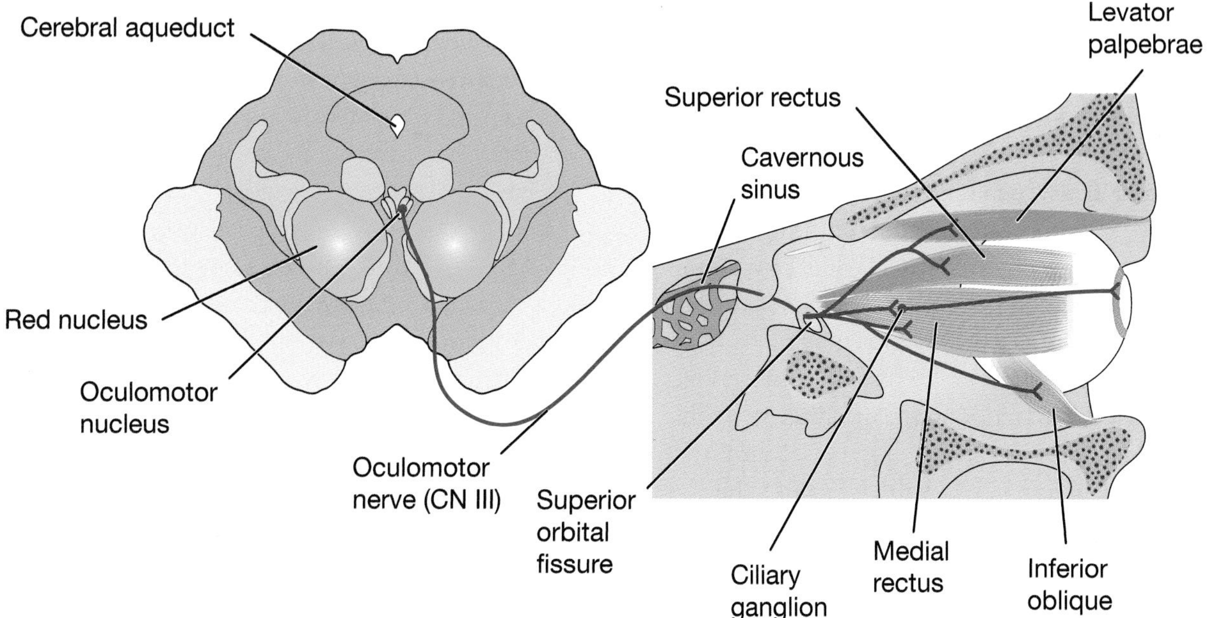

Fig. 15A.26. Oculomotor nerve. Cross section of upper midbrain with the oculomotor nucleus and course and distribution of axons to the extraocular muscles. CN, cranial nerve.

affecting the sympathetic innervation of the eye. The postganglionic sympathetic fibers are from the superior cervical sympathetic ganglion. They ascend into the cranial cavity along the internal carotid artery and join cranial nerve III in the cavernous sinus. Damage to these sympathetic fibers causes mild ptosis because of loss of innervation of the smooth muscle in the upper lid (Müller muscle); the damage also causes *miosis* (pupillary constriction). In contrast, lesions of the general visceral efferent component of cranial nerve III cause loss of the parasympathetic innervation of the eye and produce *mydriasis* (pupillary dilatation).

Observation of pupillary size and testing of the pupillary light reflex are an integral part of the neurologic examination. The size of the pupil is influenced by many factors, primarily the intensity of light falling on the retina. The afferent pathway of the pupillary light reflex is conducted by the optic nerve (cranial nerve II) (Fig. 15A.27). The fibers from each retina partially decussate in the optic chiasm and proceed in the optic tract and brachium of the superior colliculus to the pretectal area, from which fibers pass to the Edinger-Westphal nucleus on both sides. From the Edinger-Westphal nucleus, the efferent limb of the pupillary light reflex continues in the oculomotor nerve (Fig. 15A.27).

The normal pupil constricts briskly when light is shown on the ipsilateral retina. This is the *direct light reflex*. Because of the partial decussation of the optic pathway in the optic chiasm and again in the pretectal area, the contralateral pupil also constricts; this is the *consensual light reflex*. Unilateral lesions of the optic nerve do not produce anisocoria (unequal pupils) but diminish both the direct and the consensual light reflex when the involved eye is tested. However, moving the light source rapidly from the normal eye (with a strong direct and consensual light reflex) to the involved eye (with a diminished reflex) can make it appear as if the pupils actually dilate in response to light. Of course, they are only moving to a less constricted state because of decreased detection of light in the involved eye. Both pupils again constrict briskly when the light source is moved back to the normal eye. This phenomenon can be demonstrated repeatedly by moving the light source back and forth from the involved to the uninvolved eye. This response identifies the *afferent pupillary defect*, which is due to decreased conduction in the afferent limb of the pupillary light reflex.

Lesions that involve the parasympathetic innervation of the eye cause ipsilateral mydriasis and loss of the direct pupillary light reflex with preservation of the consensual reflex on testing the involved eye (and the reverse on testing the uninvolved eye). Anisocoria also occurs with lesions involving the sympathetic innervation of the pupil, resulting in ipsilateral miosis with normal pupillary light reflexes. This pupillary abnormality is usually accompanied by other features of Horner syndrome, including mild ptosis due to denervation of Müller muscle (see above) and decreased sweating on the ipsilateral face from the loss of sympathetic innervation of sweat glands. The structure and function of the oculomotor nerve are summarized in Table 15A.13. The functions of ocular nerves (cranial nerves III, IV, and VI) are summarized in Table 15A.14.

Reticular Formation

Perhaps more clearly than at other levels of the brainstem, the reticular formation in the midbrain is concentrated around the inner tube, which surrounds the neural canal derivative, the aqueduct of Sylvius. Its most conspicuous component is the periaqueductal gray matter, which is concerned predominantly with the central modulation and control of pain and with integrating responses to stress. The rostral interstitial nucleus of the medial longitudinal fasciculus (important in the coordination of vertical eye movements), the raphe nuclei and mesopontine cholinergic nuclei (important in the consciousness system), and other specific nuclei in the midbrain reticular formation are discussed in connection with the systems in which they perform important functions.

- The midbrain is the portion of the brainstem located between the pons and diencephalon. It contains three main cross-sectional regions: the tectum (dorsal), tegmentum, and base (ventral).
- Unique features of the midbrain include the superior cerebellar peduncle, red nucleus, substantia nigra, corpora quadrigemina, basis pedunculi, and cranial nerves III and IV.

Clinical Problem 15A.5.
A 45-year-old woman presented with acute, progressively worsening diplopia (double vision) and drooping of the right eyelid. Neurologic examination showed ptosis of the right eye. The right pupil was 7 mm compared with the approximately 2 mm of the left pupil. The right pupil did not react to light directly or consensually. The patient had difficulty with right medial and upward gaze.

a. What are the location and type of lesion?
b. What neural structure is involved?
c. Name a potential cause of this presentation.

- The trochlear nerve (cranial nerve IV) is a general somatic efferent nerve that innervates the superior oblique muscle of the eye, which functions to intort and depress the eye.
- The oculomotor nerve (cranial nerve III) innervates the superior rectus, inferior rectus, medial rectus, inferior oblique, and levator palpebrae superioris muscles (general somatic efferent) and pupilloconsrictor muscles and the ciliary muscle (general visceral efferent).
- The light reflex involves cranial nerve II as the afferent limb and cranial nerve III (general visceral efferent component) as the efferent limb of the reflex. A direct and consensual response to light is expected.

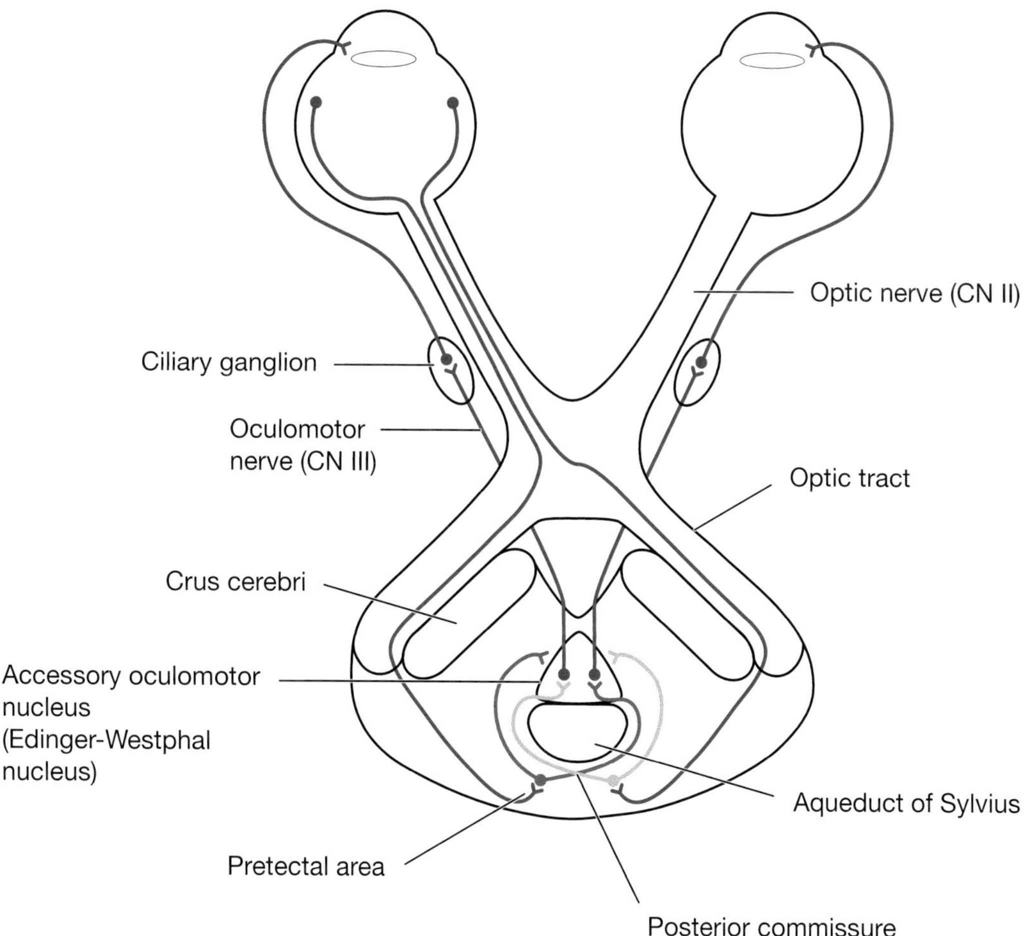

Fig. 15A.27. Pathway of the pupillary light reflex. The afferent arm is the optic nerve, and the efferent arm is the oculomotor nerve. CN, cranial nerve.

Table 15A.13. Structure and Function of the Oculomotor Nerve

Component	Function	Nucleus of origin or termination	Ganglion	Foramen	Signs of dysfunction
GSE	Motor to medial rectus, superior rectus, inferior rectus, inferior oblique, and levator palpebrae	Oculomotor		Superior orbital fissure	Diplopia, ptosis
GVE	Parasympathetic to pupilloconstrictor muscles, ciliary muscle	Edinger-Westphal	Ciliary	Superior orbital fissure	Mydriasis, loss of direct pupillary light reflex, loss of lens accommodation

GSE, general somatic efferent; GVE, general visceral efferent.

Table 15A.14. Functions of the Ocular Nerves

		Normal function		
Nerve	Muscle	Primary position[a]	Secondary position[b]	Dysfunction
III	Medial rectus	Adduction		Eye is deviated down and out with complete paralysis of CN III (usually associated with ptosis and mydriasis)
	Superior rectus	Elevation	Intorsion	
	Inferior rectus	Depression	Extorsion	
	Inferior oblique	Extorsion	Elevation	
IV	Superior oblique	Intorsion	Depression	Limitation of downward gaze when eye is looking medially, extorsion of eye
VI	Lateral rectus	Abduction		Eye is deviated medially

[a]Refers to the action of the muscle when the eye is positioned in the plane of the muscle and then contracted.
[b]Refers to the action of the muscle when the eye is gazing forward in the orbit.

Chapter 15
Part B

The Posterior Fossa Level

Cerebellar, Auditory, and Vestibular Systems

Objectives

1. Identify the major anatomical features of the cerebellum as described in the text, and state its function.
2. Outline the physiologic and anatomical features of the auditory and vestibular systems, and identify the signs and symptoms of their dysfunction.
3. Describe the actions of the ocular muscles, the significance of diplopia, the anatomy of the pupillary light reflex, and the significance of nystagmus, the oculocephalic reflex (doll's eye phenomenon), and ptosis.
4. List the major herniations of the brain, and briefly describe the mechanisms by which they produce symptoms.

Introduction

The brainstem and cranial nerves III through XII are discussed in part A of this chapter. The focus of part B is on the anatomy of the cerebellum and the three systems characteristic of the posterior fossa level: the ocular motor, auditory, and vestibular systems. The clinical examination and clinical correlations at the level of the posterior fossa are also discussed in part B.

Overview

The cerebellum (a derivative of the metencephalon) is dorsal to the pons and medulla and consists of a midline vermis and two lateral hemispheres. The cerebellum is divided functionally and anatomically into three lobes: the flocculonodular lobe, responsible for equilibrium and balance; the anterior lobe, responsible for gait and posture; and the large posterior lobe, responsible for coordinated movements of the extremities.

The major components of three special systems are found at this level. The ocular motor system is represented by cranial nerve nuclei III, IV, and VI; their axons traveling to the extraocular muscles; the medial longitudinal fasciculus; and the fibers for supranuclear control of eye movement descending from the cerebral cortex. The auditory system is represented by the auditory nerves, cochlear nuclei, trapezoid bodies, and multiple bilateral pathways that ascend to the inferior colliculi en route to the thalamus and temporal cortex. The vestibular system is represented by the vestibular nerves, vestibular nuclei, and their multiple connections with the cerebellum, spinal cord, medial longitudinal fasciculus, and structures at the supratentorial level.

Lesions can be localized precisely at the posterior fossa level when there is a combination of intersegmental and segmental involvement. Lesions at the posterior fossa level are unique in that unilateral brainstem lesions may produce neurologic signs and symptoms involving the ipsilateral side of the face and the contralateral side of the body. Other types of neurologic dysfunction that help localize a lesion at the posterior fossa level are disturbances of cerebellar function or involvement of the intracranial portions of cranial nerves III through XII.

The Cerebellum

The *cerebellum* is the largest structure in the posterior fossa. It is dorsal to the pons and medulla and forms the roof of the fourth ventricle. The cerebellum is an embryonic derivative of the metencephalon, and although it is derived from the alar plate (rhombic lip) and is important in the integration of unconscious proprioception, it is closely related functionally to the motor system and is the central structure in the cerebellar control circuit (see Chapter 8).

Gross Anatomy

The cerebellum is composed of two lateral lobes, the *cerebellar hemispheres*, and a midline portion, the *vermis* (Fig. 15B.1). The cerebellum is also divided transversely into three lobes, with each one containing a portion of the vermis and the adjacent hemisphere.

1. The *anterior lobe* consists of the vermis and cerebellar hemispheres anterior to the primary fissure.
2. The *flocculonodular lobe* consists of the most caudal lobule of the vermis, the nodulus (in the roof of the fourth ventricle), and the flocculus.
3. The *posterior lobe* consists of the rest of the cerebellum and includes the cerebellar tonsils, which are apparent on the inferomedial aspect of the cerebellar hemispheres just above the foramen magnum.

Functional Anatomy

Clinically, it is convenient to discuss the cerebellum in the context of its functional anatomy. The vermis of the anterior and posterior lobes forms the midline cerebellar zone, which receives the spinocerebellar afferents and is concerned mainly with the muscle synergies involved in walking. The terms *paleocerebellum*, reflecting its phylogenetic origin, and *spinocerebellum*, reflecting its major functional connections, roughly correspond to this zone. The lateral zone corresponds to most of the cerebellar hemisphere, including the major part of the posterior lobe. It receives the corticopontocerebellar afferents and is also referred to as the *neocerebellum* or *corticocerebellum*. The lateral zone is involved in the coordination of ipsilateral limb movement. Between the midline zone and the lateral zone of each hemisphere, anatomists recognize an intermediate zone, which projects through the globose and emboliform nuclei to the nuclei of the indirect

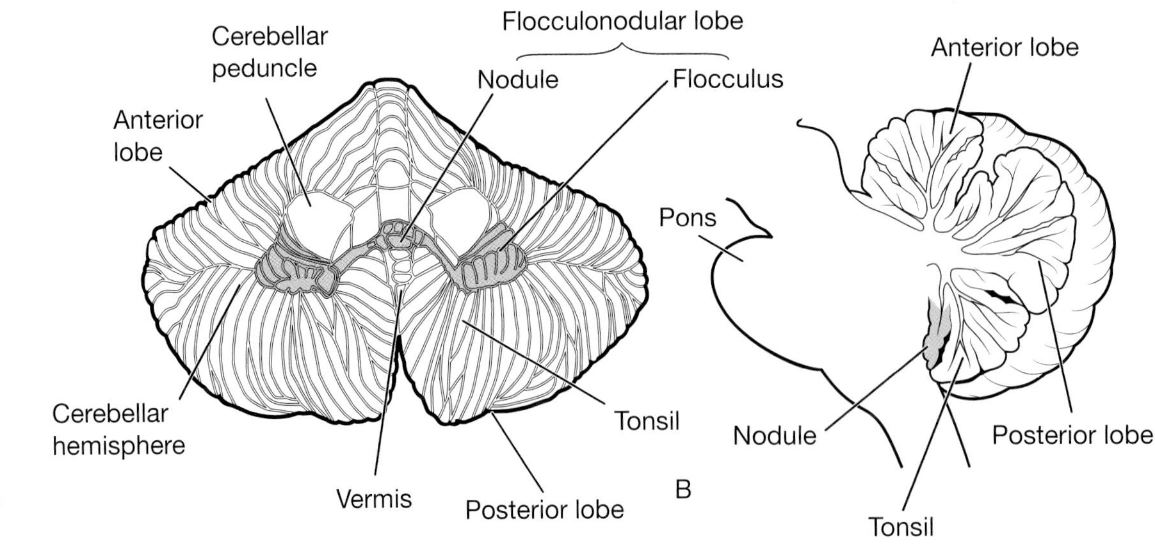

Fig. 15B.1. Lobes of the cerebellum from the inferior surface (*A*) and in a midsaggital section (*B*).

activation pathways; the clinical relevance of this region in humans is unknown. The flocculonodular lobe receives input from the vestibular system and is also referred to as the *archicerebellum* or *vestibulocerebellum*. It is concerned primarily with coordination of head and eye movements and the maintenance of equilibrium.

The Cerebellar Peduncles

The cerebellum is connected to the brainstem by three pairs of peduncles that contain cerebellar afferents and efferents (Fig. 15B.2).

The *inferior cerebellar peduncle* (*restiform body*) contains both afferent and efferent fibers. It carries most of the information the cerebellum receives from the spinal cord and medulla. The important afferent pathways reaching the cerebellum through this peduncle are the dorsal spinocerebellar and cuneocerebellar tracts (carrying proprioceptive input that does not reach consciousness) and the vestibulocerebellar, reticulocerebellar, and olivocerebellar pathways. The main efferent fibers are the cerebellovestibular and cerebelloreticular pathways.

The *middle cerebellar peduncle* (*brachium pontis*) contains only afferent fibers, which originate in the contralateral pontine nuclei. The pontine nuclei receive afferents from the ipsilateral cerebral cortex through the corticopontine tract. The corticopontocerebellar connections establish a pathway whereby each cerebellar hemisphere is influenced by the contralateral cerebral hemisphere.

The *superior cerebellar peduncle* (*brachium conjunctivum*) contains both afferent and efferent fibers and is the main outflow pathway from the cerebellum. The only afferent component in this peduncle is the ventral spinocerebellar tract. Efferent fibers originating in the dentate nucleus constitute the bulk of the superior cerebellar peduncle. In caudal midbrain, these fibers cross, forming the decussation of the brachium conjunctivum, and proceed to the contralateral red nucleus, thalamus, and inferior olivary nucleus. The fibers descending to the inferior olivary nucleus are in the central tegmental tract. As a result of the connections described above, two loops are extablished: the cortico-ponto-cerebello-dentato-thalamo-cortical pathway and

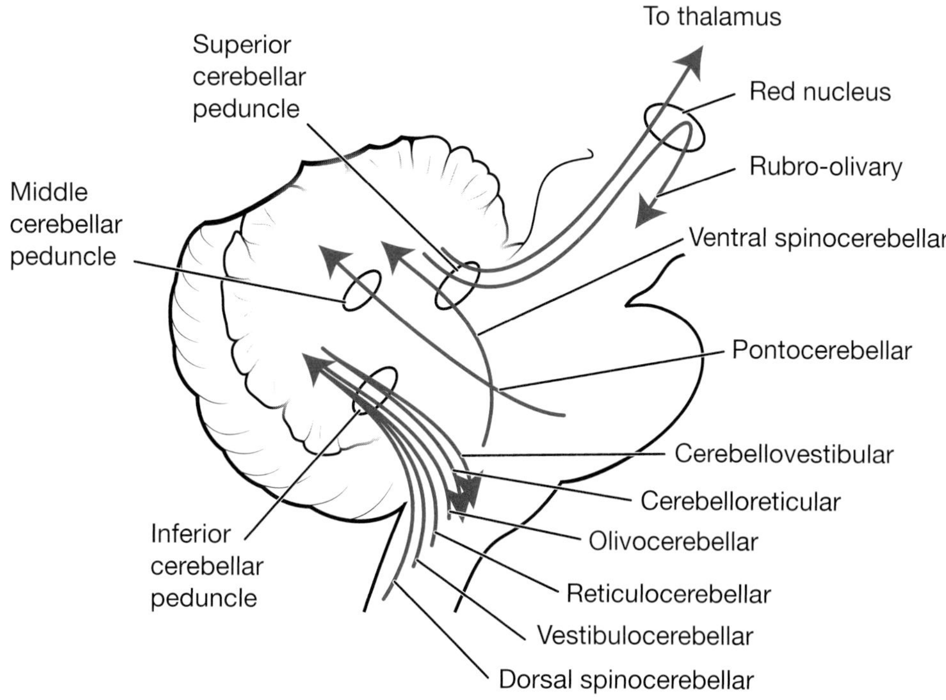

Fig. 15B.2. Afferent and efferent fibers in the cerebellar peduncles.

the cerebello-dentato-rubro-olivo-cerebellar pathway. Their roles in monitoring and modulating the activity of the motor system are not completely understood.

Internal Anatomy

The cerebellar cortex is a highly convoluted structure. The individual convolutions are referred to as *folia* rather than gyri. Deep to the cerebellar cortex is white matter that consists of the fiber tracts entering and leaving the cortex. Four paired nuclei lie within the deep cerebellar white matter: the *dentate*, *emboliform*, *globose*, and *fastigial nuclei*. They are relay stations for efferent fibers from the cerebellar cortex and are the origin of most of the efferent pathways from the cerebellum (Fig. 15B.3).

Histologically, the cerebellar cortex consists of three layers: the *molecular layer*, *Purkinje cell layer*, and *granule cell layer* (Fig. 15B.4). The outermost is the molecular layer; it consists mainly of axons and dendrites, among which are a small number of neurons called *basket cells* and *stellate cells*. The middle layer consists of a single layer of large goblet-shaped *Purkinje cells*. The innermost (granule cell) layer is composed of densely packed small neurons called *granule cells* and scattered larger neurons called *Golgi cells*.

Afferent fibers entering the cerebellar cortex terminate as either *mossy fibers* or *climbing fibers*. The mossy fibers represent the cerebellar afferent fibers from all sources except the inferior olivary nucleus. They synapse on the dendrites of granule cells and Golgi cells. Axons of the granule cells, in turn, enter the molecular layer and synapse on Purkinje cell dendrites. Purkinje cell dendrites arborize in a fanlike fashion perpendicular to the long axis of the folium. Granule cell axons enter the molecular layer and bifurcate to run, as *parallel fibers*, 2 to 3 mm in each direction in the long axis of the folium. Thus, each parallel fiber can synapse with the dendrites of up to 500 Purkinje cells as well as with dendrites of basket cells and stellate cells. The Golgi cell dendrites also ramify in the molecular layer and are excited by the parallel fibers of the granule cells. Golgi cell axons end in the granule cell layer and form inhibitory synapses on granule cells. Activation of a single incoming mossy fiber can produce excitation of a small, rectangular array of Purkinje cells, because the mossy fiber contacts multiple granule cells

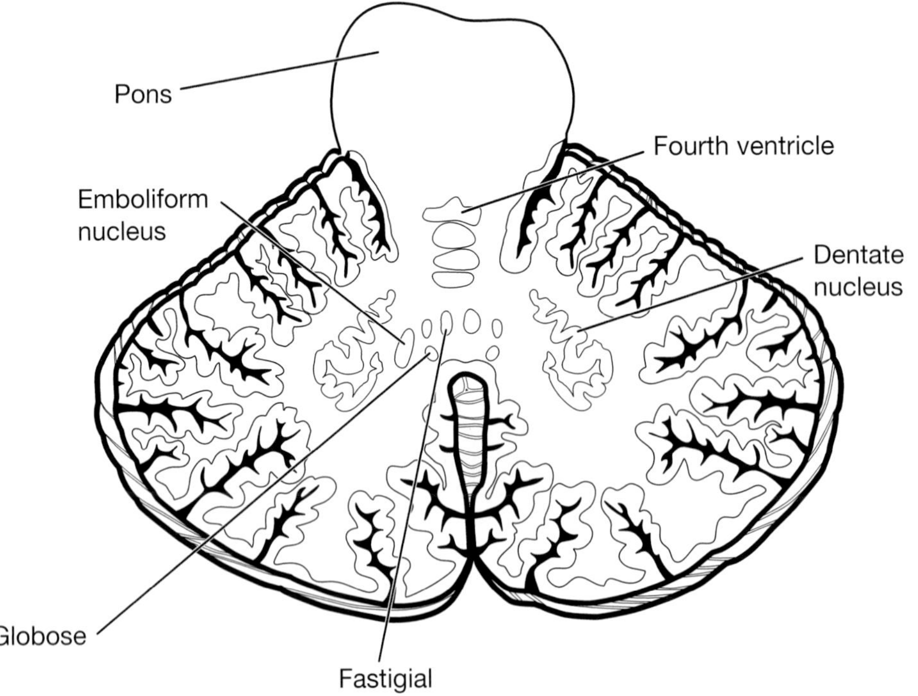

Fig. 15B.3. Cerebellar nuclei in horizontal section.

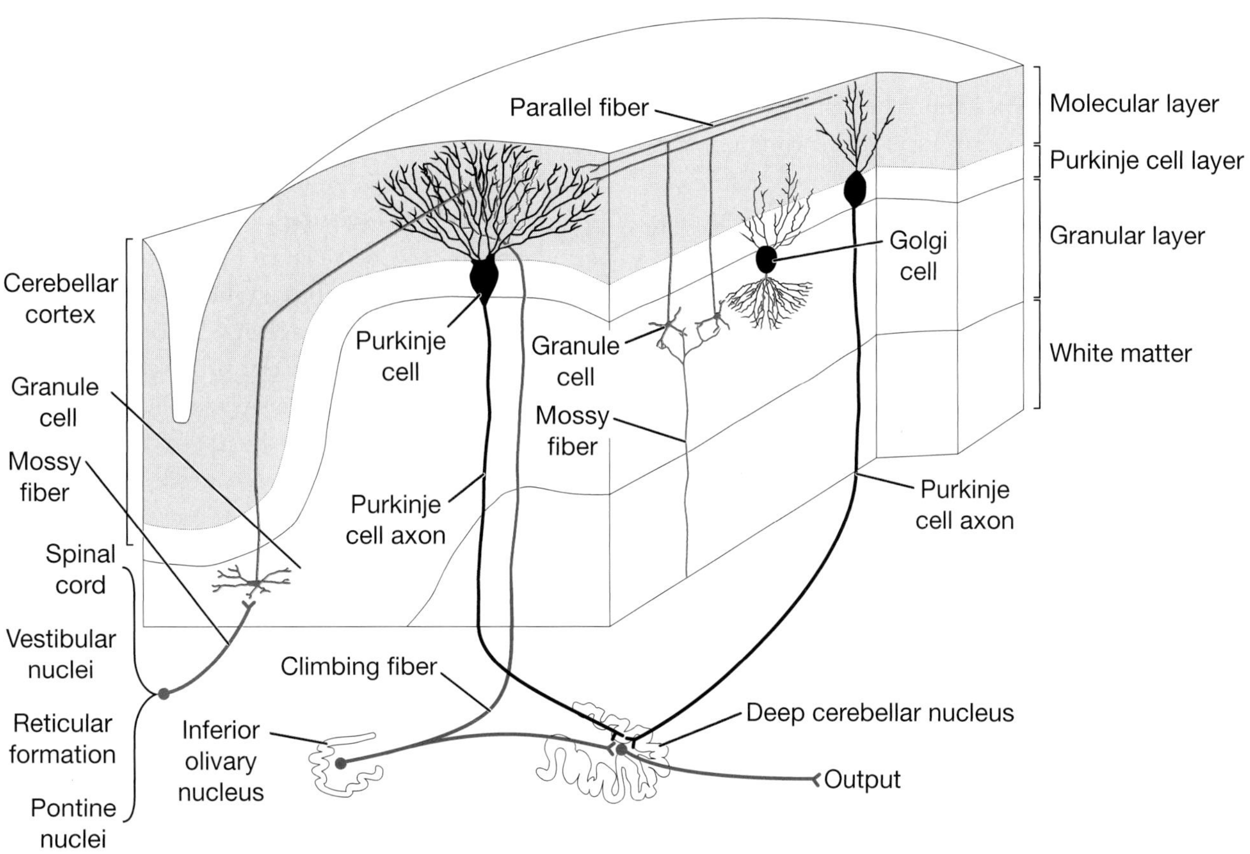

Fig. 15B.4. Cell layers and connections of the cerebellar cortex.

whose parallel fibers contact multiple Purkinje cells. The mossy fiber synapses and parallel fiber synapses are excitatory. All the other neurons activated by parallel fibers (Golgi, basket, and stellate cells) are inhibitory to Purkinje cells. Because of the spatial organization of the cerebellar cortex, these inhibitory neurons create a simultaneous intense inhibition of Purkinje cells surrounding the activated zone. The mossy fiber system constantly modulates cerebellar activity during voluntary movement.

The axons of the olivocerebellar pathway end as climbing fibers. They synapse directly on Purkinje cells by an array of terminal axon branches that wind around and "climb" the Purkinje cell body and dendritic tree. The climbing fiber input to Purkinje cells, like the granule cell input, is excitatory. The climbing fiber system signals errors in motor performance and adapts Purkinje cell firing to the new circumstance. It is important in motor learning.

All output from the cerebellar cortex is by the axons of the Purkinje cells, which project to the deep cerebellar nuclei and form inhibitory synapses. A few Purkinje cell axons go directly to the vestibular nuclei.

Pathophysiology

As described in Chapter 8, disturbances of cerebellar function are manifested as loss of balance and equilibrium or as a disorder in the modulation of the range, force, rate, and direction of movement. The flocculonodular lobe is primarily responsible for balance and equilibrium, and lesions in this region of the cerebellum result in an inability to sit or stand without swaying or falling (*truncal ataxia*). The anterior lobe is primarily responsible for posture and coordination of gait. Lesions involving this region result in an unsteady, staggering gait (*gait ataxia*). The posterior lobe is primarily responsible for coordination of ipsilateral voluntary movements of the extremities. Lesions of this region result in loss of motor coordination of the extremities, dysmetria, and, if the dentate nucleus or its outflow pathway (the brachium conjunctivum) is involved, intention tremor (*limb ataxia*).

- The cerebellum is dorsal to the pons and medulla and forms the roof of the fourth ventricle and is composed of two lateral lobes, the cerebellar hemispheres, and a midline portion, the vermis.
- Three pairs of cerebellar peduncles connect the cerebellum with the brainstem: inferior cerebellar peduncle (restiform body), middle cerebellar peduncle (brachium pontis), and superior cerebellar peduncle (brachium conjunctivum).
- The cerebellum contains four pairs of deep nuclei: dentate, emboliform, globose, and fastigial.
- The cerebellum can be divided on the basis of its functional anatomy: the vestibulocerebellum, spinocerebellum, and corticocerebellum.
- Histologically, the cerebellar cortex consists of three layers: the molecular layer, Purkinje cell layer, and granule cell layer.
- Afferent fibers entering the cerebellar cortex terminate as either mossy fibers or climbing fibers.
- All output from the cerebellar cortex is by the axons of the Purkinje cells, which project to the deep cerebellar nuclei and form inhibitory synapses. A few Purkinje cell axons go directly to the vestibular nuclei.
- Cerebellar dysfunction may be manifested as loss of balance and equilibrium or as a disorder in the modulation of the range, force, rate, and direction of movement.

Systems at the Posterior Fossa Level

In addition to the major longitudinal systems discussed in other chapters, three additional special systems, the ocular motor, auditory, and vestibular, are located in the posterior fossa level.

Clinical Problem 15B.1.

A 10-year-old boy was evaluated because of trouble with coordination of his left side. He had been well until 3 months earlier, when he experienced severe headaches. Two months ago, he began to note that his left hand shook when he reached for an object. One month before admission, he noted increasing clumsiness of his left leg. Because of headaches, nausea and vomiting, and increased clumsiness of his left arm and leg, he was examined. Examination showed that his optic nerve heads were swollen and that he took frequent missteps with his left leg and had an intention tremor on finger-to-nose and heel-to-shin testing. Muscle tone was slightly decreased on the left, but strength and sensation were intact.

a. What are the location and type of lesion?
b. What specific area of the neuraxis seems to be involved?
c. What signs and symptoms suggest the presence of increased intracranial pressure?
d. Name the most common lesion occurring in children that can produce this syndrome.

The Ocular Motor System

The ocular motor system controls eye movements and is part of the motor system. Its major components, particularly the final common pathway (lower motor neurons), are located at the posterior fossa level; however, as with other parts of the motor system, the pathways for supranuclear control originate at the supratentorial level. Vision itself is exclusively a supratentorial function. The anatomy and physiology of the visual system are discussed with that level (see Chapter 16 Part A).

Eye movement is accomplished through the action of the extraocular muscles, which are activated by cranial nerves III, IV, and VI. Most of the input to the nuclei of these cranial nerves is through the paramedian reticular formation of the brainstem, which determines the activity of lower motor neurons for both reflex and voluntary eye movements. Input to the reticular formation for voluntary and pursuit movements comes by way of descending supranuclear pathways from the frontal eye fields and parieto-occipital visual cortex, respectively. Reflex movements are mediated by input from the vestibular nuclei in the medulla to the abducens nucleus (cranial nerve VI) and then through the medial longitudinal fasciculus to the trochlear (cranial nerve IV) and oculomotor (cranial nerve III) nuclei. Input from the retina travels to the superior colliculus and the pretectal region and then to the brainstem reticular formation.

Lesions at the supratentorial, posterior fossa, or peripheral level can produce ocular motor disorders such as paresis of one or more extraocular muscles, resulting in *diplopia*, *gaze paresis*, or *nystagmus*.

Physiology

Different neural mechanisms are used for eye movements that subserve different functions. *Saccadic eye movements* are rapid reflex movements that bring a visual image to the fovea. *Smooth pursuit* movements keep the fovea focused on a moving target. *Vergence movements* maintain the visual image on the fovea when objects move toward the eyes (convergence) or away from them (divergence). *Vestibulo-ocular reflexes* hold images steady on the retina during brief head rotations. *Optokinetic movements* hold stable images on the retina as long as possible when object-filled space is moving past the eyes and then quickly refixates on the next available target.

Each of these eye movements is mediated by the nuclei of cranial nerves III, IV, and VI and coordinated through neurons in the brainstem *paramedian reticular formation*. The different pathways acting on the reticular formation to produce these movements have not been fully clarified, but some of the anatomical features of the various control systems are well defined.

Anatomy

The five major areas of ocular motor control are 1) the nuclei of cranial nerves III, IV, and VI, 2) the brainstem paramedian reticular formation, 3) the superior colliculus and pretectal region, 4) the vestibular connections through the abducens nucleus and medial longitudinal fasciculus, and 5) the cortical eye fields.

The anatomy of the oculomotor, trochlear, and abducens nuclei and nerves forming the final common pathway of the ocular motor system is described in part A of this chapter. The medial and lateral recti muscles turn the eye inward and outward, respectively. The superior and inferior recti muscles move the eye up and down when it is turned outward, and the inferior and superior oblique muscles move the eye up and down when it is turned inward (Table 15B.1). The muscles that turn the two eyeballs are yoked in pairs so that the eyes move conjugately in exactly the same direction with exactly the same velocity and force. This principle of equal innervation of yoked pairs of extraocular muscles is known as *Hering's law*. For example, the left medial rectus and right lateral rectus muscles are the yoked pair for right lateral gaze, and when looking to the right, the right superior rectus and left inferior oblique are the yoked pair for upward gaze. When the eye is turned outward, the oblique muscles produce more torsion than up and down movement. Similarly, when the eye is turned inward, the action of the superior and inferior recti becomes primarily torsional (Fig. 15B.5 *A*). Ocular movements are tested by asking the patient to look in the six cardinal directions of gaze, as shown in Figure 15B.5 *B*.

The brainstem paramedian reticular formation is located along the midline and paramedian core of the brainstem from the midbrain to the medulla and receives input from all prenuclear areas concerned with eye movements, including the vestibular nuclei, superior colliculi, pretectal region, cerebellum, and cortical eye fields. This region consists of small scattered nuclei that have different firing patterns with different types of eye movement. On the basis of their effect on the firing pattern of the neurons of cranial nerve nuclei III, IV, and VI, the neurons in these cell groups are classified as *pause cells*, *burst cells*, and *tonic cells* (Table 15B.2).

The control of conjugate horizontal eye movements is integrated primarily at the level of the pons and the control of vertical eye movements, at the level of the midbrain (Table 15B.2). The abducens nucleus of the pons not only contains the motor neurons that innervate the ipsilateral lateral rectus muscle but also commissural neurons. Axons of the commissural neurons cross the midline at the level of the pons and ascend in the *contralateral*

Table 15B.1. Functions of the Ocular Nerves

Cranial nerve	Muscle	Normal function: Primary position[a]	Normal function: Secondary position[b]	Dysfunction
III	Medial rectus	Adduction		Eye is deviated down and out, with complete paralysis of cranial nerve III usually associated with ptosis and mydriasis
	Superior rectus	Elevation	Intorsion	
	Inferior rectus	Depression	Extorsion	
	Inferior oblique	Extorsion	Elevation	
IV	Superior oblique	Intorsion	Depression	Limitation of downward gaze when eye is looking medially, extorsion of eye
VI	Lateral rectus	Abduction		Eye deviated medially

[a]Primary position refers to the action of the muscle when the eye is positioned in the plane of the muscle and then contracted.
[b]Secondary position refers to the action of the muscle when the eye is gazing foward in the orbit.

medial longitudinal fasciculus to innervate the motor neurons in the midbrain oculomotor nucleus that innervate the medial rectus muscle. Thus, excitation of the abducens nucleus produces ipsilateral deviation of gaze by direct activation of ipsilateral lateral rectus motor neurons and indirect activation of contralateral medial rectus motor neurons through the medial longitudinal fasciculus. Conjugate vertical gaze is integrated by connections between different neurons in the oculomotor nucleus in rostral midbrain (innervating the superior and inferior recti and inferior oblique muscles) and the trochlear nucleus in caudal midbrain (innervating the superior oblique muscle). Upward gaze depends on activation of the superior rectus and inferior oblique muscles, and downward gaze depends on activation of the inferior rectus and superior oblique muscles. Some of the interconnections between the corresponding motor neurons cross the midline in the *posterior commissure.*

These basic circuits for conjugate horizontal and vertical gaze are activated by different gaze control systems, including the *vestibulo-ocular reflex*, *saccadic system*, *smooth pursuit-optokinetic system*, and *convergence system* (Table 15B.3). Maintenance of the eyes in a particular position in the orbit depends on tonic input from neurons located in the vestibulocerebellum and other components of a central network referred to as the *neural integrator.* The neural integrator includes neurons in the vestibulocerebellum and medial vestibular nucleus, in the *nucleus prepositus hypoglossi* in rostral medulla (containing tonic neurons for horizontal eye movements), and in the *interstitial nucleus of Cajal* in the midbrain (containing tonic neurons for vertical eye movements). These groups of tonic neurons are located in the dorsal midline reticular formation (Table 15B.2).

The *vestibulo-ocular reflex* maintains the image on the fovea during rapid head movement. This involves conjugate movement of the eyes in the direction opposite to that of head movement. Also, the velocity of eye movement is equal to that of head movement. The receptors for this reflex are in the vestibular organs (see below). For example, in the horizontal vestibulo-ocular reflex, rotation of the head to the right produces slow conjugate rotation of the eyes to the left. This reflex involves vestibular input from the right ear that relays in the ipsilateral vestibular nucleus and crossed excitatory connections of the vestibular nucleus with the contralateral abducens nucleus (Fig. 15B.6 *A*).

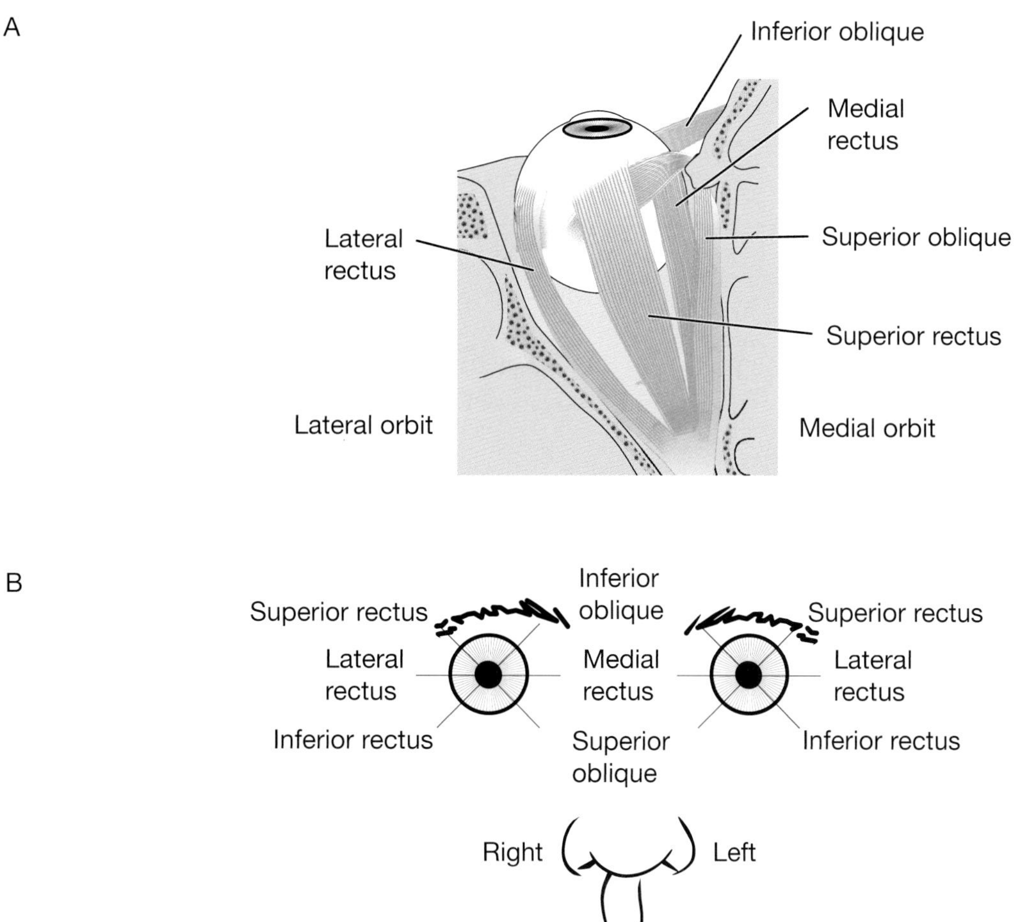

Fig. 15B.5. *A*, Attachment of eye muscles as seen from above (left eye). *B*, Eye movement produced by each muscle.

Table 15B.2. Location of Control Cells for Horizontal and Vertical Conjugate Eye Movements

Movement	Level of integration (cranial nerve nucleus)	Saccadic burst cells	Tonic cells	Pause cells
Horizontal	Pons (abducens)	Pontine paramedian reticular formation	Flocculonodular lobe Medial vestibular nucleus Nucleus prepositus hypoglossi (rostral medulla)	Raphe nuclei
Vertical	Midbrain (oculomotor, trochlear)	Rostral interstitial nucleus of the medial longitudinal fasciculus	Flocculonodular lobe Medial vestibular nucleus Interstitial nucleus of Cajal	Raphe nuclei

Table 15B.3. Systems Controlling Conjugate Gaze

Type of eye movement	Main function	Control mechanism	Effect
Vestibular (vestibulo-ocular reflex)	Holds images steady on the fovea during brief head rotations	Semicircular canals and vestibular nuclei	Conjugate deviation of eyes opposite to direction of head rotation
Smooth pursuit	Holds image of a moving target on the fovea	Visual pathway and parieto-occipital cortex Vestibulocerebellum	Conjugated deviation toward direction of movement of object (ipsilateral to parieto-occipital cortex)
Optokinetic	Holds images of the target steady on the retina during sustained head rotation	Visual pathway and parieto-occipital cortex, vestibulocerebellum, vestibular nuclei	Maintains deviation of eyes initiated by the vestibulo-ocular reflex
Saccade	Brings the image of an object of interest onto the fovea	Frontal eye fields Superior colliculus Pontine paramedian reticular formation	Rapid conjugate deviation toward opposite side
Nystagmus quick phase	Directs the fovea toward the oncoming visual scene during self-rotation; resets the eyes during prolonged rotation	Cortical	Quick deviation toward stimulated labyrinth (vestibular) Quick deviation toward inhibited cerebellum (cerebellar)
Vergence	Moves the eyes in opposite directions (disconjugate) so that images of a single object are placed on both fovae	Unknown direct input to oculomotor neurons, likely via interneurons	Accommodation to near targets

The vestibular and optokinetic systems control compensatory eye movements to head rotation and movement of the visual environment. When the semicircular canals are stimulated by head movement, signals are sent to the appropriate combination of cranial nerves III, IV, and VI for compensatory eye movement in the opposite direction. If one looks at a target and shakes the head from side to side, the eyes can be maintained on the target through this mechanism. It does not require any cortical input and, in fact, can be seen in comatose patients. The pathway from the vestibular nuclei to cranial nerves III, IV, and VI is largely through the medial longitudinal fasciculus (Fig. 15B.6 *A*).

The *smooth pursuit system* keeps the fovea focused on a moving target. In this case, visual input from the retina is integrated, through the thalamus, in both the primary visual cortex and parieto-occipital cortex (Fig. 15B.7) (see Chapter 16). Axons from these cortical regions descend ipsilaterally to activate neurons in pontine nuclei that project to the contralateral flocculonodular lobe, which in turn projects to the medial vestibular nucleus. The final effect is slow conjugate eye movement toward

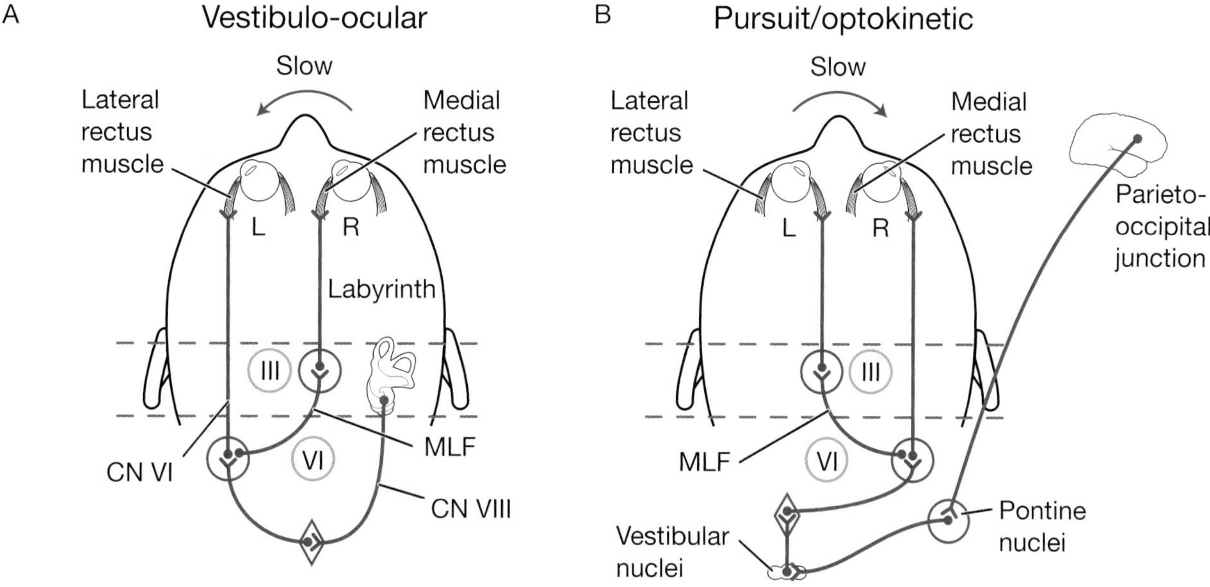

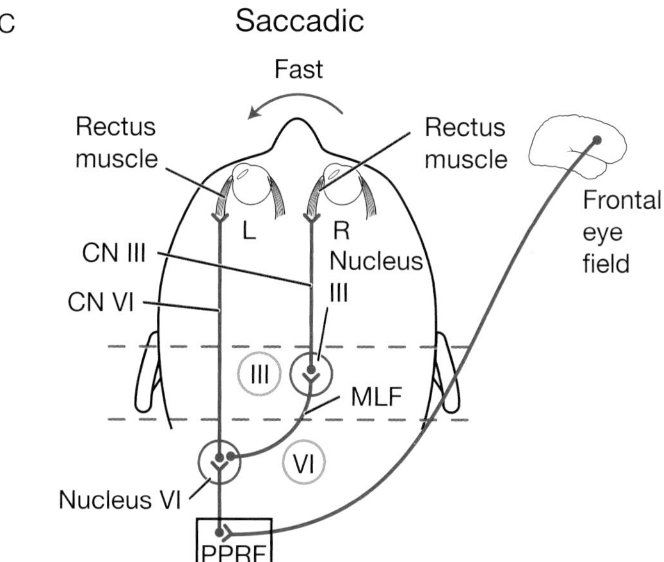

Fig. 15B.6. Three systems for lateral gaze. *A*, Vestibulo-ocular reflex. *B*, Pursuit/optokinetic system. *C*, Saccadic system. (CN, cranial nerve; MLF, medial longitudinal fasciculus; PPRF, pontine paramedian reticular formation.)

the side of the cortex stimulated (Fig. 15B.6 *B*).

The parieto-occipital eye field is located at the parieto-occipital junction of each hemisphere (Brodmann area 19) (Fig. 15B.7). This eye field is responsible for involuntary smooth pursuit movements in which the eyes are fixated on an object and maintain visual fixation as the object moves (Fig. 15B.6 *B*). Fibers from area 19 project to nuclei in the pretectal region and to the superior colliculus and from there to the reticular formation. Voluntary fixation on a visual target is broken when the target reaches the limit of the visual field. The eyes then make a quick movement in the opposite direction to fixate on a new target. This movement is called *optokinetic nystagmus* and depends on an intact parieto-occipital eye field.

The *saccadic system* rapidly brings visual images to the fovea. Saccades can be voluntary in response to a command, a remembered target, or a reflex in response to visual, auditory, or somatosensory stimuli. Control of voluntary saccades depends on the *frontal eye fields* (Fig. 15B.7) (see Chapter 16), whereas reflex saccades involve the *superior colliculus*. The frontal eye fields and superior colliculus project to the brainstem.

When the eyes are still, pause cells located in the raphe nuclei fire tonically and inhibit the burst cells. When the eyes make a rapid movement, or saccade, the pause cells are inhibited. Burst cells then fire briefly, driving the eyes to their new position. Tonic cells also begin to fire, and their discharge frequency is just enough to hold the eye at the new desired position. The pulse created by the firing of the burst neuron and the step created by the firing of tonic neurons drive the eye to the new position and hold it there. The burst neurons for horizontal saccades are located in the *pontine paramedian reticular formation* near the abducens nucleus, and the burst neurons for vertical eye movements are located in the *rostral interstitial nucleus of the medial longitudinal fasciculus*.

The frontal eye field is in the posterior portion of the middle frontal gyrus (Fig. 15B.7). It is responsible for the voluntary control of conjugate saccades (Fig. 15B.6 *C*). Fibers from this region project to the pontine reticular formation and the superior colliculus. Stimulation of the frontal eye field produces conjugate deviation of the eyes to the opposite side, and acute destruction of this cortical area results in conjugate deviation of the eyes toward the side of the lesion.

The superior colliculus and the pretectal region receive input from the retina, cortical eye fields, and inferior colliculus, which is a relay station in the auditory pathway. Fibers from these regions connect with the reticular formation and mediate eye movements in response to targets picked up in the peripheral vision and in response to sound. The superior colliculi map the visual and auditory environment, which helps in the localization of objects and sounds in space.

Eye movements usually have to be conjugate to maintain a visual image on the fovea of both eyes; however, if the object moves closer to the observer, the eyes converge to maintain the image on the fovea. When the object moves away, the eyes diverge. The anatomy and physiology of convergence movements are not well understood. They are slow and seem to be mediated by pontine and medullary structures but not by the medial longitudinal fasciculus.

Two other reflexes normally accompany convergence: accommodation and miosis. Both are mediated by the Edinger-Westphal nucleus, the origin of the parasympathetic fibers of the oculomotor nerve. These fibers travel with cranial nerve III to the ciliary ganglion, where they synapse on postganglionic cells that innervate the ciliary muscle. This muscle relaxes the tension on the lens,

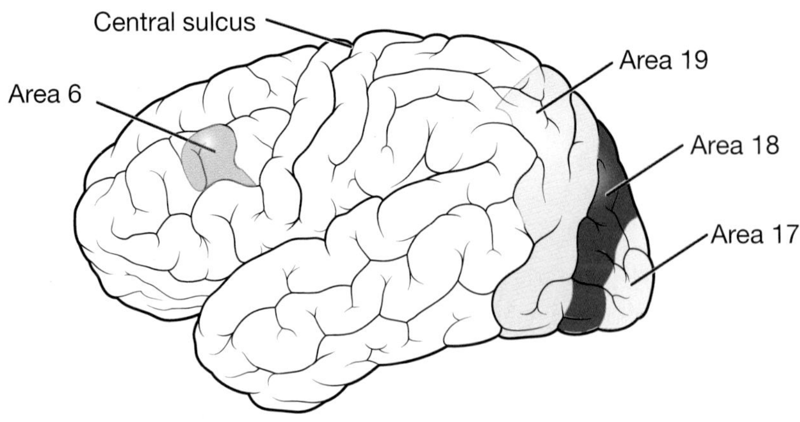

Fig. 15B.7. Cortical eye fields. The frontal eye fields are located in area 6. Area 17 is primary visual cortex. Areas 18 and 19 are visual association cortices.

allowing it to round up and shorten its focal distance. Parasympathetic activity also causes contraction of the circular muscle of the iris, causing constriction of the pupil.

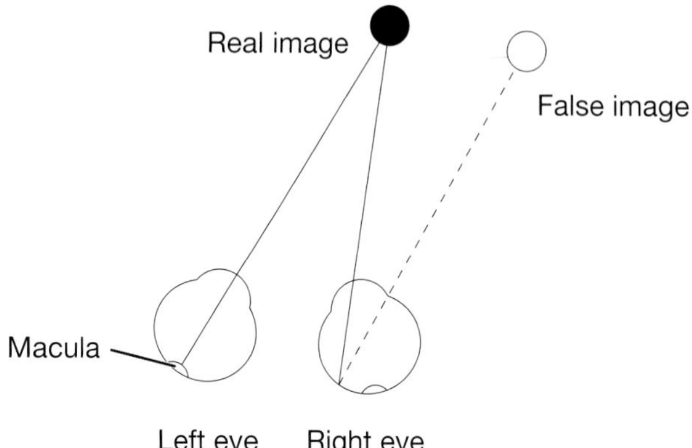

Fig. 15B.8. Diplopia occurs when the images of one object fall on different parts of the two retinas. The brain interprets this as seeing two images. In this example, the right lateral rectus muscle is paretic, and the patient cannot rotate the right eye to the right. The image of the object falls on the nasal aspect of the retina of the right eye, and the brain interprets this as a second image (false image) to the right of the real image.

Pathophysiology

Disturbances of ocular movements are important localizing signs in neurologic diagnosis. Lesions of the final common pathway occur at either the posterior fossa level (nucleus or nerve) or the peripheral level (nerve, neuromuscular junction, or muscle) and produce diplopia. Supranuclear or prenuclear control over the final common pathway is affected by lesions of the brainstem, vestibular system, cerebellum, or cortical eye fields.

Diplopia, or double vision, occurs when an image no longer falls on exactly corresponding areas of the two retinas. The brain interprets this as seeing two images instead of one (Fig. 15B.8). Diplopia usually occurs from a lesion that affects one or more of the ocular nerves or extraocular muscles. The affected eye shows restricted movement in the field of the weak muscle, and the patient reports maximal separation of the images in the direction of gaze of the weak muscle.

Prenuclear brainstem lesions can produce various gaze disorders. Lesions of the paramedian pontine reticular formation interrupt horizontal conjugate eye movements toward the side of the lesion. This occurs because the pontine paramedian reticular formation sends fibers to the ipsilateral abducens nucleus and from there, through the medial longitudinal fasciculus, to the contralateral oculomotor nucleus, specifically to the neurons innervating the medial rectus muscle. Lesions in the rostral interstitial nucleus of the medial longitudinal fasciculus affect both upward and downward vertical gaze. The fibers from this nucleus that mediate upward gaze pass dorsally through the posterior commissure to the oculomotor nucleus, so that a lesion here may affect only upward gaze.

In addition to lower motor neurons, the abducens nucleus contains internuclear neurons that send axons through the contralateral medial longitudinal fasciculus to the oculomotor nucleus. Therefore, a lesion in the medial longitudinal fasciculus prevents adduction of the eye on the side of the lesion when the patient attempts to gaze toward the opposite side. This clinical syndrome is called *internuclear ophthalmoplegia* (Fig. 15B.9). A lesion in the abducens nucleus itself, however, produces an ipsilateral conjugate gaze palsy similar to that caused by a lesion of the pontine paramedian reticular formation. However, in this case, the paralysis of the ipsilateral lateral rectus muscle is disproportionately severe.

The interactions between the vestibular and ocular motor systems are most evident clinically in a phenomenon called *nystagmus* (Table 15B.4). Nystagmus is a combination of slow eye movements in one direction, followed by quick saccades in the opposite direction. It occurs normally with stimulation of the vestibular system, for example, when a person is rotated rapidly in a circle and then stopped. A normal response to a moving visual environment is *optokinetic nystagmus*, for example, when a person watches a passing train. The eyes make a following movement along the path of the train and then a quick saccade back to the primary position. Nystagmus can also be a sign of disease in the vestibular end organ or in the vestibulocerebellar pathways in the brainstem.

The most important clinical feature of cortical ocular motor control is the tonic influence of the frontal eye field on the contralateral pontine paramedian reticular

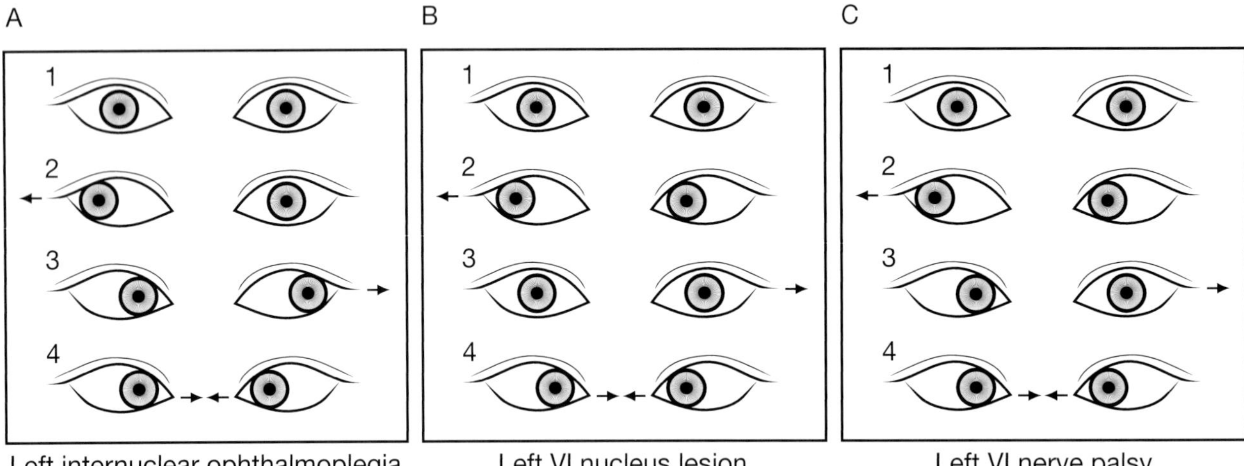

Fig. 15B.9. Pathologic eye movements. *A*, Left internuclear ophthalmoplegia. When viewing in the direction of the arrow in *2*, to the right, the left eye cannot adduct. However, the patient is able to abduct the left eye (*3*) and to converge the eyes (*4*). *B*, Left cranial nerve VI nucleus lesion. A lesion of this nucleus involves the axons innervating the ipsilateral lateral rectus muscle but also axons that cross the midline and project through the medial longitudinal fasciculus to the neurons in the oculomotor nucleus that innervate the medial rectus muscle. The result is the inability to abduct the left eye and adduct the right eye (*3*). *C*, Left cranial nerve VI palsy. In contrast to a nuclear lesion, a left cranial nerve VI palsy results in inability to abduct the left eye (*3*); however, the right eye could adduct because the medial longitudinal fasciculus is still intact.

formation, causing the eyes to tend to deviate toward the opposite side (Fig. 15B.6 *C*). Normally, the influence from the two sides is balanced. Supratentorial lesions involving the frontal eye fields produce loss of voluntary conjugate gaze to the opposite side. When the lesion is acute, the eyes may be forcefully, conjugately deviated toward the side of the lesion. An irritative lesion (i.e., a focal seizure) can cause tonic deviation of the eyes to the opposite side. When lesions affect the parieto-occipital eye field, the optokinetic response toward the side of the lesion is abolished. This is demonstrated by moving a striped tape or rotating a striped drum in front of the patient's eyes. When the stripes move toward the normal side, the eyes follow and then jerk back to pick up the next stripe. When the stripes move toward the abnormal side, the eyes do not move.

- The ocular motor system controls eye movements.
- The control of conjugate horizontal eye movements is integrated by the abducens nucleus, which has two types of neurons, one that innervates the ipsilateral lateral rectus muscle and a second whose axon crosses midline and ascends in the medial longitudinal fasciculus to the contralateral oculomotor (cranial nerve III) nucleus.
- Conjugate vertical gaze is integrated by connections between neurons in the oculomotor nucleus and the trochlear nucleus.
- Eye movement and maintenance of gaze requires pause cells, burst cells, and tonic cells.
- Saccadic eye movements are voluntary or reflexive rapid movements that bring a visual image to the fovea and are controlled by the frontal eye fields, which drive eyes to the opposite side.
- Smooth pursuit movements keep the fovea focused on a moving target.
- Vestibulo-ocular eye movements involve conjugate movement of the eyes in the direction opposite to that of head movement to keep the image steady on the fovea during movement. This reflex involves vestibular input to the contralateral abducens nucleus.

Table 15B.4. Examples of Nystagmus

Type of nystagmus	Lesion	Slow eye deviation	Direction of nystagmus (quick phase)
Pendular	Visual system	None	Oscillation to both sides
Optokinetic	None (physiologic)	Toward a moving target	Toward primary position
Vestibular	Vestibular organs or vestibular nerve	Toward the side of the inactive labyrinth, because of predominance of the contralateral vestibular drive to ocular motor neurons	Toward side of more active labyrinth
Cerebellar (gaze-evoked)	Flocculonodular lobe May also occur with muscle fatigue or effects of drugs	Toward the neutral position despite attempt to maintain eccentric gaze, because of inability of ipsilateral cerebellum to provide tonic gaze-holding command ("leaky integrator")	Toward side of cerebellum with lesion Toward direction of gaze
Downbeat	Craniocervical junction	Upward because of lack of tonic stimulation from posterior semicircular canals	Downward
Dysconjugate (internuclear ophthalmoplegia)	Medial longitudinal fasciculus	Inability to adduct ipsilateral eye during attempted lateral gaze	Saccade of abducting eye

- Diplopia (double vision) occurs from a lesion that affects one or more of the ocular nerves or extraocular muscles.
- Internuclear ophthalmoplegia results from a lesion of the medial longitudinal fasciculus.

The Auditory System

The auditory system is represented at the posterior fossa and supratentorial levels. The auditory structures transform mechanical energy (sound) into action potentials and relay them to the brainstem and cerebral cortex. Auditory information is used for communication.

Sound waves are transformed into electrical signals by the structures in the inner ear. Afferent impulses pass centrally in the acoustic division of cranial nerve VIII and, after synapse in the cochlear nuclei, ascend bilaterally through a multisynaptic brainstem pathway to *primary auditory cortex* in the anterior *transverse gyrus of Heschl* in the temporal lobe. Relay nuclei in the brainstem include the *superior olivary nuclei*, *nucleus of the lateral lemniscus*, *inferior colliculus*, and *medial geniculate body*. Although lesions central to the cochlear nuclei result in some alteration of auditory function, unilateral loss of hearing occurs only with lesions of cranial nerve VIII or the peripheral receptors.

The Ear

The receptors for the auditory system are in the ear, which is subdivided into three major regions (Fig. 15B.10): 1) the *external ear* consists of the pinna, which collects and directs sounds through the external auditory canal; 2) the *middle ear*, or tympanic cavity, contains the tympanic membrane (eardrum) and auditory ossicles, which convert sound waves into waves in a fluid-filled chamber; and 3) the *inner ear*, or labyrinth, which is a series of fluid-filled membranous channels in the petrous portion of the temporal bone. The membranous labyrinth duplicates the shape of the bony labyrinth and is divided into two

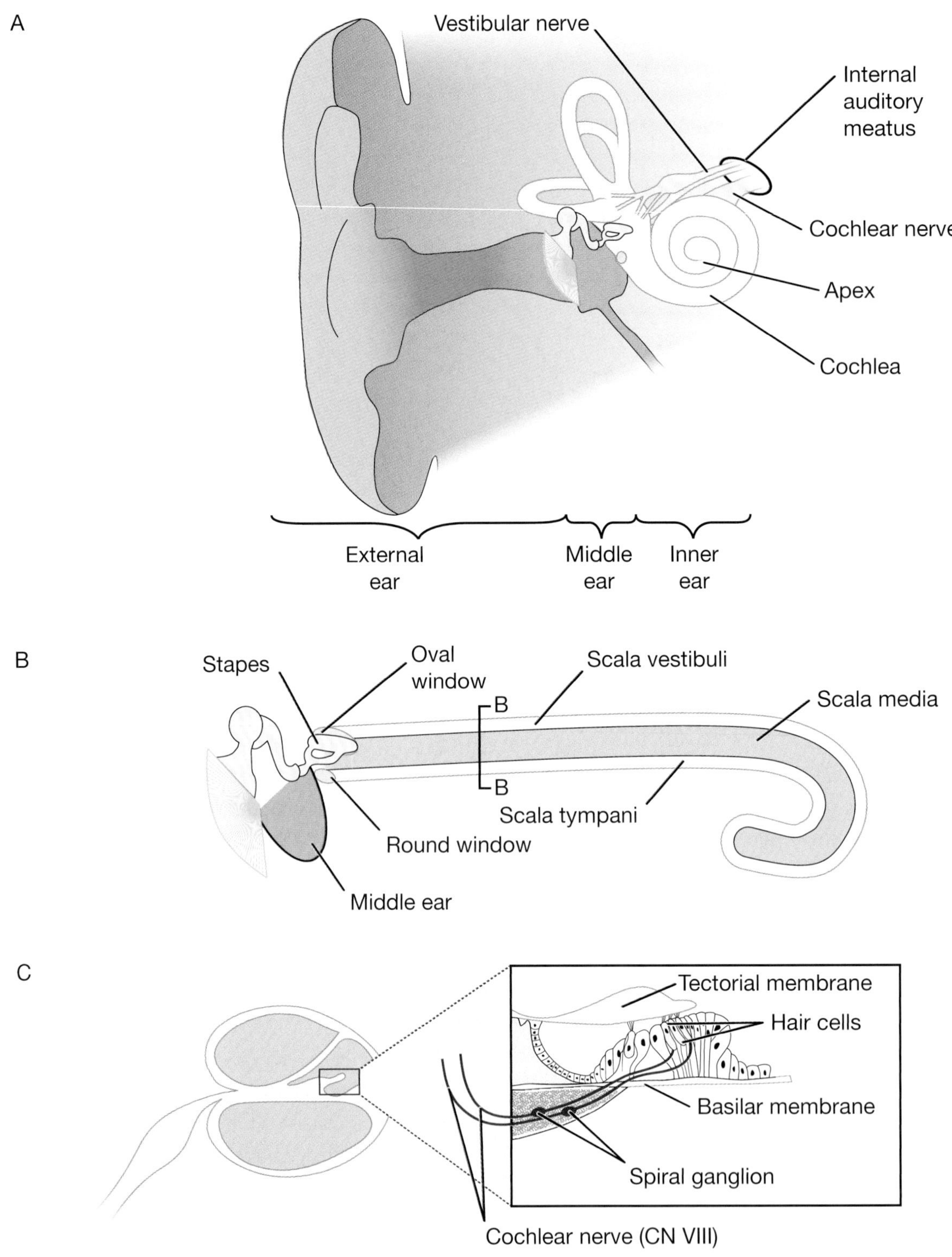

Fig. 15B.10. *A*, Structures of the external, middle, and inner ear. *B*, Cochlea uncoiled, showing the three chambers. *C*, Cross section of the cochlea (B-B in *B*) showing the three chambers and the basilar membrane. *Inset*, Close-up view of the organ of Corti. CN, cranial nerve.

channels, one containing endolymph and the other containing perilymph. The ionic composition of these two fluids is different. Perilymph is similar to cerebrospinal fluid, whereas endolymph has a high potassium and low sodium content. The labyrinth is further divided into the cochlea and vestibule, which consists of the utricle, the saccule, and the three semicircular canals. The cochlea contains the receptors for sound, and the vestibule contains the receptors of the vestibular apparatus.

Anatomy

The cochlea contains three parallel chambers and is shaped like a snail, coiled 2¾ turns from the base to the apex (Fig. 15B.10). The two outer chambers, the *scala vestibuli* and *scala tympani*, contain perilymph and are in continuity at the apex of the coil. The middle chamber, the *scala media* (also called the cochlear duct), contains endolymph.

The scala vestibuli and scala media are separated by the vestibular (Reissner) membrane, and the scala tympani and scala media are separated by the basilar membrane. At the base of the cochlea, the scala vestibuli ends at the oval window and the scala tympani ends at the round window. The *organ of Corti* lies on the surface of the basilar membrane and contains mechanically sensitive hair cells, the auditory receptors. These cells have processes called *stereocilia* and generate electrotonic potentials in response to movement of the basilar membrane produced by sound waves. The base of the hair cell is enmeshed in a network of nerve endings of the cochlear nerve. The cochlear nerve fibers emerge from the coils of the cochlea in the central axis of the coil and join together to form the acoustic division of cranial nerve VIII. The cell bodies of these first-order neurons for hearing are located in the *spiral ganglion* in the axis of the helix. Fibers pass centrally, enter the brainstem, and synapse in the dorsal and ventral cochlear nuclei (Fig. 15B.11).

From the cochlear nuclei, axons of second-order neurons travel by several pathways to the thalamus. Some fibers enter the reticular formation and participate in the alerting functions of the consciousness system. Some fibers ascend directly in the ipsilateral lateral lemniscus, and others synapse in the *nuclei of the trapezoid body* or the *superior olivary nuclei* in the ventral tegmentum of the pons (Fig. 15B.11). Many, but not all, of these fibers cross to the opposite side in the trapezoid body before passing rostrally. Thus, each lateral lemniscus contains auditory fibers that conduct information from both ears. Some of the fibers synapse in the nucleus of the lateral lemniscus en route to the inferior colliculus. At the inferior colliculus, some fibers again synapse, and a few may pass to the opposite side. Fibers traveling in the brachium of the inferior colliculus end in the medial geniculate body of the thalamus, which gives rise to axons that pass through the sublenticular portion of the internal capsule to go to the auditory cortex of the anterior transverse gyrus (Heschl gyrus) in the temporal lobe (Fig. 15B.11). Because of the partial decussation of auditory fibers, sound entering each ear is transmitted to both cerebral hemispheres.

Physiology

The ear converts sound waves in the external environment into action potentials in the auditory nerves. Sound waves entering the external auditory canal move the tympanic membrane (Fig. 15B.12). This movement is transmitted to the ossicles (malleus, incus, and stapes) of the middle ear, which amplify and transform the movements of the eardrum into smaller and more forceful movements of the footplate of the stapes, which rests against the oval window of the inner ear. The movement of the stapes against the oval window produces traveling pressure waves in the perilymph of the scala vestibuli. At the apex of the cochlea, these waves pass into the scala tympani and are dissipated by movement of the round window. As the sound waves enter the perilymph of the scala vestibuli, they are transmitted through the vestibular membrane to the endolymph of the scala media. This causes displacement of the basilar membrane, which in turn stimulates the hair cells in the organ of Corti. The movement of the stereocilia in the hair cells generates electrotonic potentials that are converted into action potentials in the auditory nerve fibers.

From the base to the apex, the basilar membrane gradually decreases in width and increases in tension. Because of this, different portions of the basilar membrane respond to different frequencies. The base responds to high frequencies and the apex to low frequencies. Thus, the cochlea mechanically separates the activation of different hair cells by different frequencies.

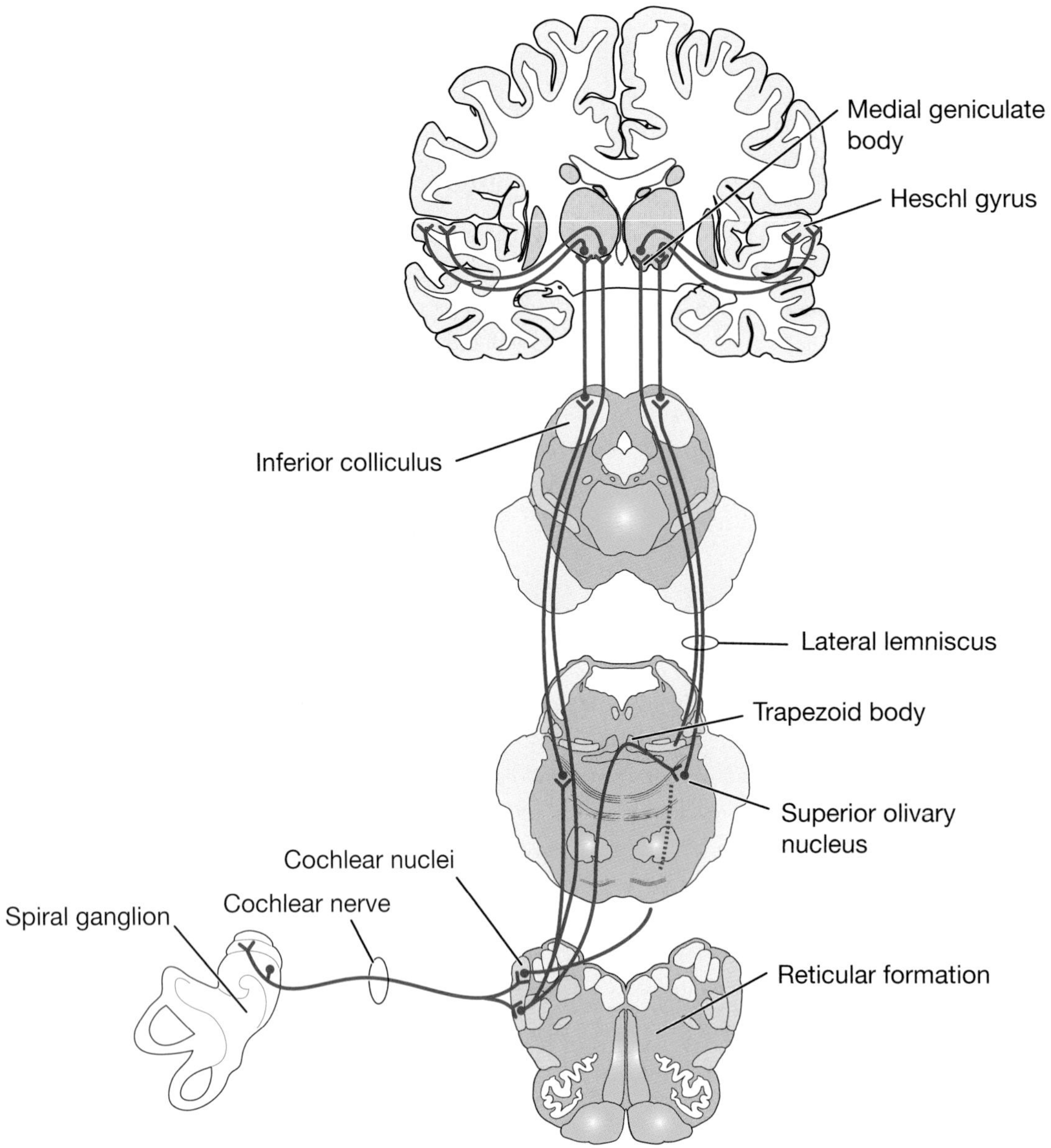

Fig. 15B.11. Auditory pathways. Auditory impulses can ascend directly in the ipsilateral lateral lemniscus or synapse in the trapezoid body or superior olivary nucleus. They also may cross to the opposite side and ascend in the contralateral lateral lemniscus. Fibers thus ascend bilaterally to the inferior colliculus, medial genticulate body, and auditory cortex.

Pathophysiology

Patients with disease of the auditory division of cranial nerve VIII or its receptors complain of *tinnitus* (buzzing or ringing sensation in the ear) or loss of hearing. These can be important symptoms and signs in localizing a pathologic process to the posterior fossa level. Lesions within the central nervous system seldom produce a notable alteration in hearing. Therefore, unilateral hearing loss commonly indicates disease in the ipsilateral ear or in cranial nerve VIII. It is important to distinguish

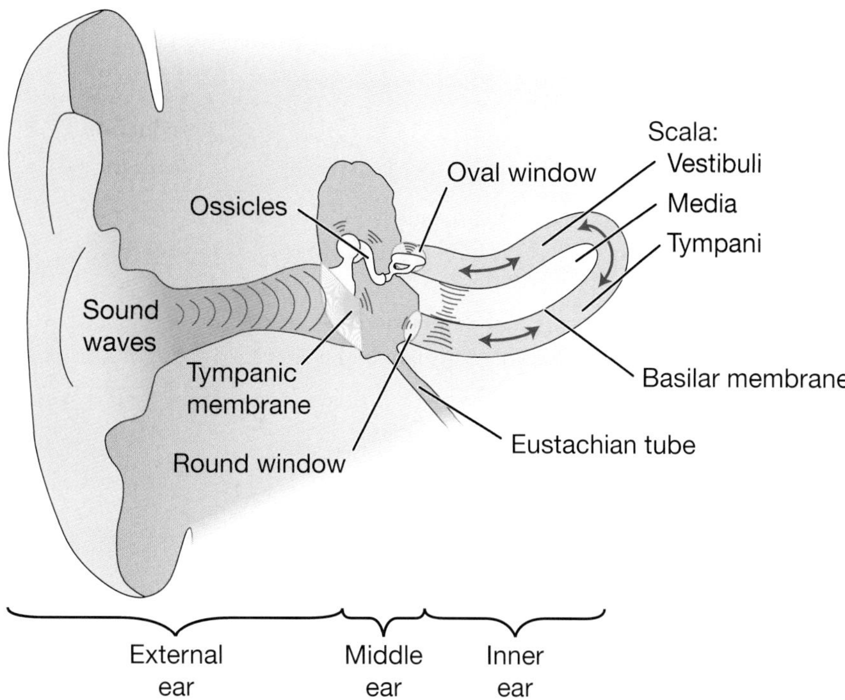

Fig. 15B.12. The sound waves move the tympanic membrane, and this mechanical force is transmitted by the ossicles to the footplate of the stapes. The movement of the stapes against the oval window is eventually transmitted to the endolymph, producing movement of the basilar membrane.

between the types of hearing deficit found in ear disease and in neural disease. *Conduction deafness* is due to disease of the external or middle ear that prevents sound waves being transmitted to the cochlea. *Sensorineural deafness* is due to disease of the cochlea or the auditory nerve or its nuclei. The distinction can often be made with a tuning fork, by performing the Weber and Rinne tests, as outlined in Table 15B.5. Audiometric testing identifies the frequencies most impaired. Middle ear disease is associated with low-frequency loss, and nerve damage is associated with high-frequency loss.

Patients with lesions central to the cochlear nuclei do not complain of hearing loss. Although bilateral lesions of the inferior colliculi, medial geniculate bodies, or anterior transverse gyri produce hearing loss, examples of these are so rare as to be of no practical clinical importance. Unilateral lesions in the region of the auditory receptive areas of the cerebral cortex do not cause hearing loss, but they produce a deficit in sound localization or discrimination. Focal seizures involving the cortical auditory receptive area in the temporal lobe produce hallucinations of sound. Electrical potentials evoked by click stimulation, called *brainstem auditory evoked potentials*, can be recorded on the scalp from the structures along the auditory pathway (Fig. 15B.13). Abnormalities in these potentials can identify and localize lesions in the auditory system.

- The auditory structures transform mechanical energy (sound) into action potentials and relay them to the brainstem and cerebral cortex.
- Important components of the auditory system include the following:
  - Ear (external, middle, and inner ear)
  - Acoustic division of cranial nerve VIII
  - Central processing: cochlear nuclei, superior olivary nuclei, trapezoid body, nucleus of the lateral lemniscus, inferior colliculus

Table 15B.5. The Weber and Rinne Tests for Unilateral Deafness

Test	Method	Normal response	Conduction deafness	Sensorineural deafness
Weber	Base of vibrating tuning fork placed on vertex of skull	Heard equally in both ears (or center of the head)	Sound is louder in abnormal ear	Sound is louder in normal ear
Rinne	Each ear is tested separately—base of vibrating tuning fork is placed on the mastoid region until subject no longer hears sound (bone conduction), then held in air next to the ear (air conduction)	Air conduction is better than bone conduction	Bone conduction is better than air conduction in involved ear	Air conduction is better than bone conduction in involved ear

- Thalamic relay nucleus: medial geniculate body
- Cerebral cortex: primary auditory cortex in the anterior transverse gyrus of Heschl in the temporal lobe

- Unilateral loss of hearing is found only with lesions of cranial nerve VIII or the peripheral receptors.
- Unilateral lesions in the region of the auditory receptive areas of the cerebral cortex do not cause hearing loss, but they produce a deficit in sound localization or discrimination.

The Vestibular System

The vestibular structures provide the nervous system with information about gravity, rotation, and acceleration that is necessary for maintenance of balance and equilibrium. These structures are located primarily in the posterior fossa.

Receptors that detect gravitational pull, rotational movements, and acceleration are located in the utricle, saccule, and semicircular canals of the inner ear. They transmit information to the central nervous system through the vestibular division of cranial nerve VIII. Numerous connections exist between the vestibular nuclei and the cerebellum, spinal cord, reticular formation, medial longitudinal fasciculus, and cerebral cortex to allow integration of vestibular impulses with other sensory information for normal balance and equilibrium. Lesions affecting the vestibular structures cause a sense of imbalance (dysequilibrium). *Vertigo* is a highly specific symptom of vestibular system dysfunction. *Nystagmus* also occurs with lesions of the vestibular system.

Anatomy and Physiology

The receptors for the vestibular system are enclosed in the vestibular portion of the labyrinth in the utricle, the saccule, and the three semicircular canals (Table 15B.6 and Fig. 15B.14). The receptors are *hair cells* that respond to mechanical movement and initiate impulses that are transmitted in the vestibular division of cranial nerve VIII to the vestibular nuclei in the medulla and pons. The cell bodies of the first-order neurons are in the vestibular ganglion located in the internal auditory meatus. Movement of the hair cell stereocilia in one direction produces local potentials that increase the frequency of the action potentials in the nerve; movement in the opposite direction inhibits nerve discharge. The hair cells in the utricle and saccule respond to positional and gravitational change, and those in the semicircular canals respond to rotational or angular acceleration.

The utricle and saccule contain endolymph and specialized areas of epithelium called *maculae* in their

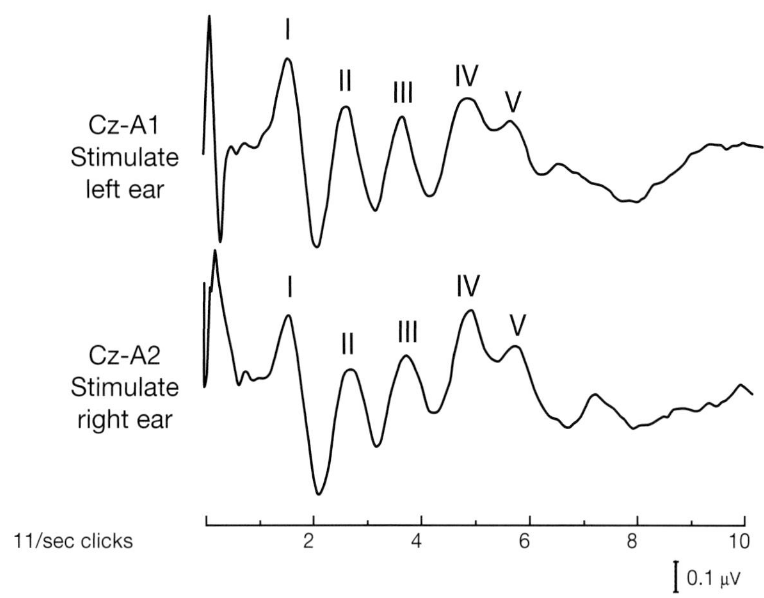

Fig. 15B.13. Normal brainstem auditory evoked potentials (I-V) in a 26-year-old man. *Top*, The response of the left ear. *Bottom*, The response of the right ear. (The responses represent an average of 2,048 samples with summation of two superimposed responses.) Cz, central vertex area; A1, left ear; A2, right ear.

walls (Fig. 15B.14). Each macula is a tuft of ciliated columnar epithelial cells embedded in a gelatinous matrix that contains small calcified particles (otoliths).

When the head is tilted from the vertical position, gravitational pull on the otoliths distorts the hair cells and initiates an action potential in the vestibular nerve. The three semicircular canals monitor acceleration in any plane. At one end of each canal is an enlargement called the *ampulla* (Fig. 15B.14). The ampulla contains a specialized region of epithelium, the crista, similar to the maculae in

Table 15B.6. Comparison of Function and Connections of Vestibular Organs

Organ	Semicircular canals (lateral, superior, posterior)	Otolith organ (utricle and saccule)
Receptor	Hair cells in crista ampullaris	Hair cells in macula
Stimulus	Rotatory (angular) acceleration	Linear acceleration Gravity
Afferent	Vestibular nerve	Vestibular nerve
Vestibular nuclei	Superior, medial	Lateral, medial, inferior
Main function	Vestibulo-ocular reflex	Increased tone of antigravity muscles via vestibulospinal tracts
Effects of lesion	Rotational vertigo	Illusion of linear acceleration, loss of postural tone, head and ocular tilt

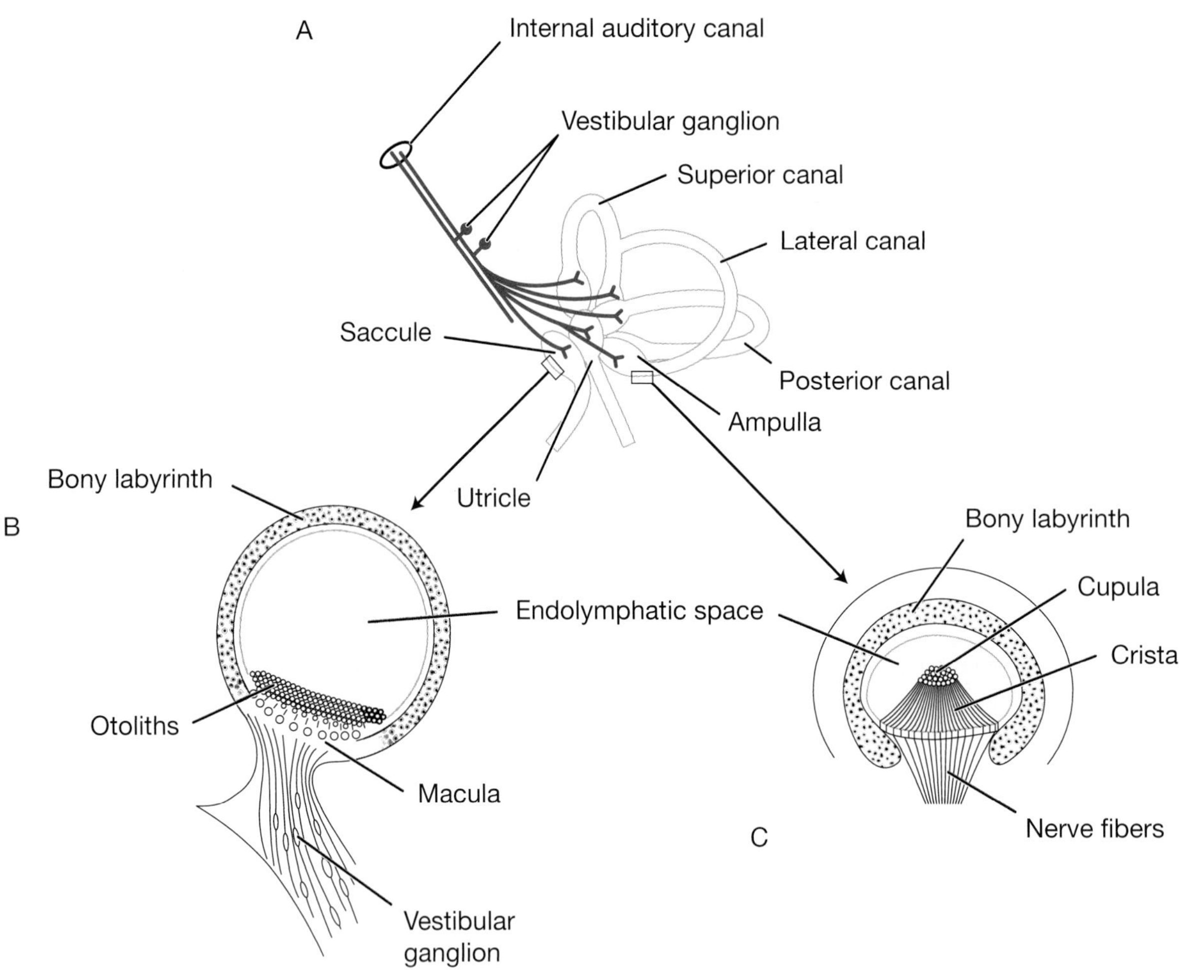

Fig. 15B.14. Vestibular receptors. *A*, Nerve supply to vestibular receptors (utricle, saccule, and semicircular canals). *B*, Macula of utricle and saccule. *C*, Ampulla of semicircular canals.

the saccule and utricle. The *crista* is on a transverse ridge that projects into the lumen of the semicircular canal. During rotational movement, the endolymph in the semicircular canal moves and distorts the crista, thus stimulating the hair cells and initiating action potentials. Each semicircular canal lies in a different plane so that each one is sensitive to rotation about a different axis.

Fibers of the vestibular division of cranial nerve VIII synapse in the *superior*, *medial*, *lateral*, and *inferior vestibular nuclei* located in the floor of the fourth ventricle. These nuclei have connections with several areas of the central nervous system. Some fibers of the vestibular nerve pass directly to the cerebellum through the inferior cerebellar peduncle. Others synapse in the inferior and medial vestibular nuclei before entering the cerebellum and terminating in the flocculonodular lobe. The flocculonodular lobe, in turn, sends fibers to the lateral vestibular nucleus, the origin of the lateral vestibulospinal tract and a portion of the medial vestibulospinal tract, to regulate muscle tone in response to changing position. All the vestibular nuclei send fibers to the reticular formation, which can modify activity in the internal regulation and consciousness systems. The medial longitudinal fasciculus receives fibers from the vestibular nuclei for coordination of head and eye movements (Fig. 15B.6). Pathways ascending to the cerebral cortex are not clearly defined. However, vestibular function is represented in the temporal lobes.

Pathophysiology

Input from the vestibular apparatus on each side is continuous and balanced. When receptor activity is altered by motion, the pattern of afferent impulses changes and a subjective sensation of motion is produced. When sensations of motion are consistent with other sensory input, they are perceived as a correct response to a changing environment. When a lesion renders a portion of the vestibular system either hypoactive or hyperactive, the centrally integrated afferent impulses are not in accord with other sensory stimuli, and dysequilibrium is experienced. Dizziness, light-headedness, giddiness, and wooziness are common but nonspecific examples of dysequilibrium and frequently are not associated with disease of the vestibular system. However, vertigo, that is, the hallucination of rotatory movement, is a highly specific form of dysequilibrium and is suggestive of disease of the vestibular system. Rarely, vertigo is a manifestation of focal seizures involving the temporal lobe. More often, it is a manifestation of disease of the peripheral receptors, vestibular nerve, or brainstem. Thus, vertigo is an important neurologic symptom of disease at the level of the posterior fossa or the ear. Vertigo caused by disorders of the vestibular system is often accompanied by nausea, vomiting, ataxia, and nystagmus because of the resulting dysfunction of the reticular, cerebellar, and ocular motor connections of the vestibular system described above.

Vestibular system function is evaluated by caloric stimulation and by testing oculocephalic reflexes. In *caloric testing*, the external canal of each ear is irrigated with either warm or cold water. The temperature gradient of the water causes convection currents and movement of the endolymph in the semicircular canals. If the labyrinth, vestibular nerves, medial longitudinal fasciculus, and oculomotor system in the brainstem are intact, nystagmus occurs. Quantitative electrical measurement of the direction and amplitude of the eye movements produced in caloric testing is used in electronystagmography to help define the location and severity of vestibular lesions. The *oculocephalic* (*doll's eye*) *reflexes* are tested by rapidly turning the head from side to side or up and down. This movement stimulates the semicircular canals and causes the eyes to move conjugately in the opposite direction. Clinical caloric testing and doll's eye movements are commonly used to test the integrity of brainstem pathways in patients with altered states of consciousness. Abnormal results are helpful in localizing the responsible lesion to the posterior fossa level.

- The vestibular structures provide the nervous system with information about gravity, rotation, and acceleration that is necessary for maintaining balance, posture, and equilibrium and for maintaining steady vision with change in position.
- Important components of the vestibular system include the following:
  - Receptors: hair cells within the semicircular canals (angular acceleration) and otoliths (linear acceleration)
  - Cranial nerve: vestibular division of cranial nerve VIII
  - Central nuclei: superior, medial, lateral, and inferior vestibular nuclei
  - Vestibulo-ocular connections: the vestibulocerebellum (flocculonodular lobe) and vestibular input to nuclei of cranial nerves III, IV, and VI.
  - Vestibulospinal connections: lateral and medial vestibulospinal tracts
  - Vestibulo-cortical connections: cerebral cortex (temporal lobes)
- The oculocephalic (doll's eye) reflex involves rapidly turning the head from side to side or up and down. This movement stimulates the semicircular canals and causes the eyes to move conjugately in the opposite direction.
- Vertigo may result from dysfunction of the vestibular system.

Clinical Correlations

Lesions that involve the posterior fossa level are associated with abnormalities in cranial nerve, cerebellar, or brainstem function. Because components of each of the major longitudinal systems are found at this level, dysfunction in any of these systems may be present. Lesions in all etiologic categories are found at this level, and the pathologic nature of these lesions can be determined, as at other levels, by applying the general principles of neurologic diagnosis outlined in Chapter 4.

Before the specific manifestations of lesions involving a particular level of the brainstem are described, it is helpful to consider symptom complexes that are common to involvement of multiple levels or of posterior fossa structures as a whole, specifically dysarthria and coma.

Dysarthria

Dysarthria, or motor speech impairment, must be distinguished clearly from aphasia, a disorder of symbolic language function discussed in Chapter 16. Clear speech involves closely coordinated and modulated activity of muscles supplied by cranial nerves V, VII, IX, X, and XII as well as the respiratory muscles, especially the diaphragm, innervated by the phrenic nerve (spinal level C4) (Table 15B.7). The activation, modulation, and coordination of this output are controlled by the direct activation pathway through the corticobulbar tracts, by the indirect activation pathways, and by cerebellar control circuits. Thus, dysarthria can take many forms depending on the structures or combination of structures involved.

The most common types are outlined in Table 15B.8. Lesions of the final common pathways of cranial nerves V, VII, IX, X, or XII cause *flaccid dysarthria*. Although the manifestations vary depending on the specific nerve or combination of nerves involved, typical features include breathy voice, hypernasality, and articulatory imprecision.

Table 15B.7. Components of Speech Production

Component	Nerve	Muscle
Respiration	Phrenic	Diaphragm, intercostal
Phonation	CN X (inferior laryngeal)	Laryngeal
Resonation	CNs IX, X	Palate
Articulation	CN V	Masseter, pterygoid
	CN VII	Orbicularis oris, buccinator
	CN XII	Tongue

CN, cranial nerve.

Spastic dysarthria is the result of bilateral corticobulbar tract lesions and is characterized by a strained hoarseness, hypernasality, and a slow articulatory rate. These two speech patterns are typically seen in patients with bulbar and pseudobulbar palsy (Table 15B.9). Lesions of the cerebellum produce *ataxic dysarthria*, that is, irregular articulatory breakdowns and, less frequently, voice tremor and loss of loudness of the voice. Lesions of the basal ganglia circuits cause *hypokinetic* and *hyperkinetic dysarthrias*. Hypokinetic dysarthria is characteristic of Parkinson disease and related syndromes and features low-volume,

Table 15B.8. Types of Dysarthrias

Type	Lesion	Clinical features
Flaccid	CNs V, VII, IX, X, XII	Breathy voice, hypernasality, articulatory imprecisions
Spastic	Corticobulbar pathway	Strained voice, hypernasality, slow articulatory rate
Ataxic	Cerebellar control circuit	Irregular articulatory breakdowns (scanning), slow rate
Hypokinetic	Substantia nigra Basal ganglia (parkinsonism)	Reduced voice volume, monopitch, rapid, indistinct articulation
Hyperkinetic	Basal ganglia (dystonia, chorea)	Unpredictable interruptions and distortion of phonation, resonation, and articulation

CN, cranial nerve.

Table 15B.9. Differences Between Bulbar and Pseudobulbar Palsies

	Bulbar	Pseudobulbar
Location of lesion	Lower motor neuron (CNs V, VII, IX, X, XII)	Upper motor neuron (corticobulbar tract, bilateral)
Type of dysarthria	Flaccid	Spastic
Tongue atrophy/fasciculations	Yes	No
Masseter reflex	Normal or ↓	Exaggerated
Gag reflex	Absent	Exaggerated
Emotional lability	No	Yes

CN, cranial nerve.

monotonous, rapid speech with indistinct articulation. Hyperkinetic dysarthria occurs in dystonias and choreas in which there are uncontrolled and unpredictable movements of the laryngeal, pharyngeal, lingual, and facial muscles that interrupt and distort phonation, resonation, and articulation.

Coma

The pathophysiology of coma is discussed in Chapter 10. However, because coma is a common result of lesions in the posterior fossa, it is useful to comment on certain specific features of coma of brainstem origin. Coma due to lesions of the brainstem can be identified and localized more precisely by the presence of associated disturbances in brainstem function outside the consciousness system. These include dysfunction of the descending motor pathways resulting in disturbances in posture and tone, dysfunction of the ocular motor system, and disturbances in control of respiratory and cardiovascular functions. The effects on these systems when different levels of the brainstem are involved are outlined in Table 15B.10.

Decorticate and decerebrate posturing involve abnormally increased muscle tone in the extremities mediated by the rubrospinal and vestibulospinal pathways. In *decorticate posturing* due to damage of the rostral brainstem (rostral to the red nucleus), flexor tone is increased more than extensor tone in the upper extremities, resulting in flexion of the arms. *Decerebrate posturing* occurs with lesions at or caudal to the red nucleus but rostral to the vestibular nuclei. Extensor tone is increased in all four limbs because of the uninhibited influence of the vestibulospinal pathway. Lesions at or caudal to the vestibular nuclei abolish the excitatory influence of all these pathways.

The effects of various lesions on the size and reactivity of the pupil can be deduced from recognizing that the sympathetic influence on pupillary dilatation originates with neurons in the hypothalamus whose axons descend the length of the brainstem. In contrast, the parasympathetic fibers that mediate pupillary constriction originate in the midbrain and leave the brainstem at that level with cranial nerve III. Any lesion that isolates one or the other results in either abnormally dilated or constricted pupils, whereas a lesion that affects both sets of fibers results in a mid-position, unreactive pupil.

The *oculovestibular reflex* refers to the effects on eye movements by caloric stimulation of the labyrinth. In normal subjects, caloric stimulation produces nystagmus. In coma due to cerebral damage rostral to the midbrain, the refixation, or fast, phase of nystagmus is absent, and the expected response to caloric stimulation, if the brainstem between the vestibular nuclei and the oculomotor nuclei is intact, is conjugate ocular deviation. If the ear is irrigated with cold water, the eyes will deviate slowly toward the stimulated ear. This occurs because cold water inhibits vestibular discharge from the stimulated ear, which results in the relative predominance of the contralateral labyrinth.

Table 15B.10. Levels of Brainstem Involvement in Patients With Coma

Level	Posture	Pupils	Oculovestibular response	Respiration, blood pressure
Between cortex and midrain	Decorticate	Miotic, reactive	Slow phase present, fast phase absent	Cheyne-Stokes, normal or elevated
Midbrain (rostral to red nucleus)	Decorticate	Midposition, nonreactive	Slow phase present, fast phase absent	Cheyne-Stokes
Midbrain (caudal to red nucleus) and pons (rostral to vestibular nuclei)	Decerebrate	Pinpoint, reactive	Slow phase present, fast phase present	Central neurogenic hyperventilation, hypertension, tachycardia, sweating
Caudal pons and rostral medulla (caudal to vestibular nuclei)	Flaccid	Midsize	Absent	Apneustic respiration
Medulla	Flaccid	Midsize, nonreactive	Absent	Irregular, bradycardia, hypotension

This drives the eyes toward the side of cold irrigation. With brainstem lesions at or caudal to the level of the ocular motor nuclei, the response will be distorted or absent.

Brainstem centers that participate in the regulation of respiration and cardiovascular reflexes are discussed in Chapter 9. Normal rhythmic respiration appropriately responsive to changes in blood chemistry (especially carbon dioxide level and pH) requires the integrated function of all levels of the nervous system. Loss of cerebral influence because of lesions rostral to the red nucleus results in a periodic breathing pattern characterized by waxing-and-waning hyperpnea alternating with short periods of apnea. This is called *Cheyne-Stokes respiration*. Midbrain and rostral pontine lesions are suggested by sustained hyperpnea called *central neurogenic hyperventilation*. Lesions in the lower brainstem cause slow, arrhythmic, or periodic breathing patterns, including *apneustic breathing* (long inspiratory pauses), respiration alternans, and *ataxic* (*Biot*) *breathing*.

Ischemic Lesions of the Brainstem

The blood supply of the brainstem is derived from the vertebrobasilar arterial system. The pattern of supply to each level is relatively constant, with the midline region being supplied by small penetrating paramedian branches of the vertebral and basilar arteries and the lateral area being supplied by larger circumferential branches: the posterior inferior cerebellar artery at the level of the medulla, the anterior inferior cerebellar artery at the level of the pons, and the superior cerebellar artery at the level of the midbrain. Ischemic lesions involving the brainstem usually occur either in the paramedian region or in the lateral region. Infarction of the paramedian region involves the descending motor pathways, medial lemniscus, and the nuclei of cranial nerves III, IV, VI, or XII. Infarction of the lateral region involves the cerebellum, cerebellar pathways, descending sympathetic pathways, the lateral spinothalamic tract, and the nuclei of cranial nerves V, VII, VIII, IX, or X.

Vascular Lesions of the Medulla

The paramedian region of the medulla is supplied by vessels from the anterior spinal and vertebral arteries. Infarction in the paramedian medulla involves the medullary pyramids, medial lemniscus, and cranial nerve XII, resulting in contralateral hemiparesis, impaired conscious proprioceptive sensation, and ipsilateral tongue weakness (Fig. 15B.15).

The lateral regions of the medulla and portions of the cerebellum are supplied by the posterior inferior cerebellar artery. Occlusion or thrombosis of this artery (or its parent vertebral artery) produces infarction of the lateral medulla and results in a constellation of signs and symptoms referred to as *Wallenberg syndrome* (Fig. 15B.15). This syndrome includes dysarthria and dysphagia due to involvement of the nucleus ambiguus, ipsilateral impairment of pain and temperature in the face due to involvement of the descending nucleus and tract of cranial nerve V, contralateral loss of pain and temperature in the trunk and extremities due to involvement of the spinothalamic tract, ipsilateral Horner syndrome due to involvement of the descending sympathetic fibers in the lateral part of the brainstem, ipsilateral limb ataxia due to involvement of the inferior cerebellar peduncle, and vertigo due to involvement of the vestibular nuclei or vestibulocerebellar fibers in the tegmentum of the medulla.

Vascular Lesions of the Pons

An infarct of the paramedian area of the pons results in ipsilateral sixth nerve palsy due to involvement of axons arising in the abducens nucleus, ipsilateral facial weakness due to involvement of the facial nerve as it passes around the abducens nucleus, contralateral hemiparesis due to involvement of the corticospinal tracts in the

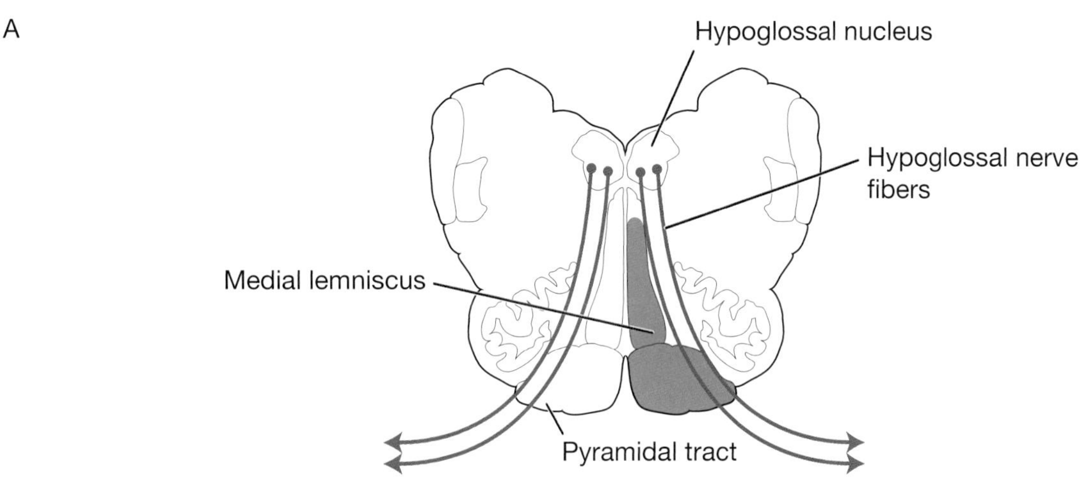

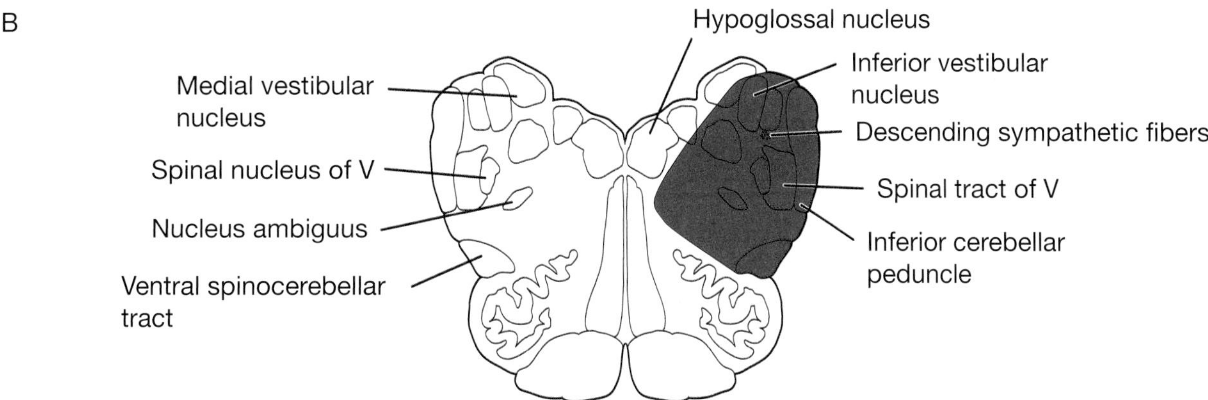

Fig. 15B.15. *A*, Paramedian infarct of medulla (green area). *B*, Lateral medullary infarct of medulla (red area) (Wallenberg syndrome).

basis pontis, and contralateral impairment of conscious proprioception due to involvement of the medial lemniscus (Fig. 15B.16).

An infarct of the lateral portion of the pons causes ipsilateral facial paralysis due to involvement of the facial nucleus; impairment of touch, pain, and temperature on the same side of the face due to involvement of the main sensory nucleus and descending nucleus and tract of cranial nerve V; loss of pain and temperature sensation on the contralateral side of the body due to involvement of the spinothalamic tract; ipsilateral deafness due to involvement of the nuclei of cranial nerve VIII; ipsilateral Homer syndrome due to involvement of the descending sympathetic fibers; and ipsilateral cerebellar signs due to involvement of the middle cerebellar peduncle.

Vascular Lesions of the Midbrain

Infarction of the lateral midbrain is uncommon; however, ischemic lesions involving the paramedian region (Fig. 15B.17) are seen occasionally and produce diplopia, ptosis, and mydriasis due to involvement of cranial nerve III and contralateral hemiparesis due to involvement of the cerebral peduncle. This constellation of symptoms is called *Weber syndrome.*

Clinical Problem 15B.2.

A 70-year-old woman had sudden onset of weakness of her right arm and leg and difficulty in moving her tongue. When evaluated in the emergency department a few hours later, she had weakness of her right arm and leg and decreased ability to perceive proprioceptive and tactile stimuli on the right. When her tongue was protruded, it deviated to the left.

a. What are the location and type of lesion?
b. What structures are involved?
c. What is the pathologic nature of the lesion?

Neoplasms of the Posterior Fossa

Certain tumors of the posterior fossa are encountered more commonly in children and adolescents than in older adults. Ependymomas and medulloblastomas frequently arise in the region of the fourth ventricle and are associated with ataxia, nausea, and vomiting. As these lesions increase in size, they obstruct the outflow of cerebrospinal fluid from the ventricular system and cause noncommunicating hydrocephalus and signs of increased intracranial

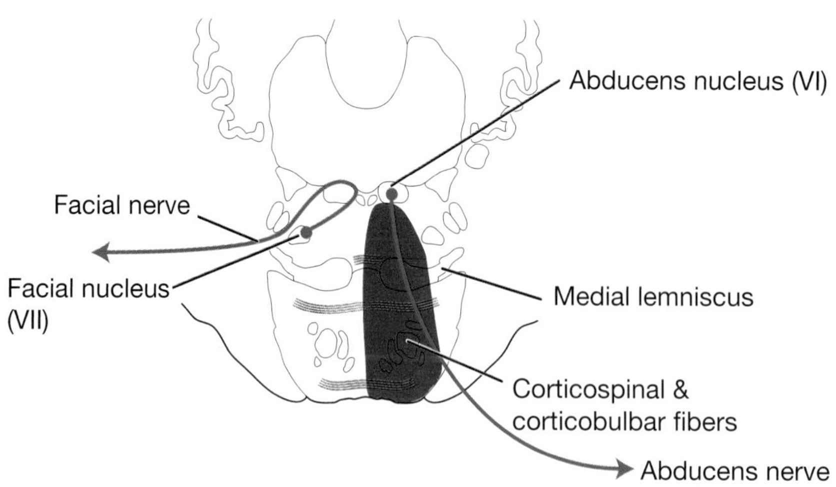

Fig. 15B.16. Paramedian infarct of pons (red area) with involvement of cranial nerves VI (abducens nerve) and VII (facial nerve), medial lemniscus, and corticospinal tract.

Clinical Problem 15B.3.

A 68-year-old woman, previously in good health, suddenly became extremely nauseated and dizzy, as if the room were spinning around her. She remained conscious and could describe her symptoms to a companion, who noted that her voice was hoarse. Examination in the emergency department several hours later showed the following abnormalities: the patient could not sit or stand because of vertigo. She was anxious and perspiring, except on the left side of her face. Her left pupil was small, and her left eyelid drooped slightly. Horizontal and rotatory nystagmus was noted. The left palate drooped, and the left gag reflex was absent. There was loss of pain and temperature sensation on the left side of her face, but touch sensation was preserved. Muscle strength and stretch reflexes were normal in the extremities. There was moderate incoordination of her left arm and leg. Sensory examination showed loss of pain and temperature sensation in her right arm, trunk, and leg.

a. To what anatomical portion of the posterior fossa does this process localize: medulla, pons, midbrain, or cerebellum?
b. What is the specific site of the lesion?
c. What artery supplies the involved area?
d. What anatomical structures are responsible for the loss of pain and temperature sensation on the left side of the face and on the right side of the trunk?
e. What is the cause of the ptosis, miosis, and anhidrosis on the left?

Clinical Problem 15B.4.

A 73-year-old woman with diabetes mellitus entered the hospital because of abrupt onset of double vision and left-sided weakness. Examination several hours later showed that the pupil was 4 mm on the right and 3 mm on the left. The direct and consensual light responses of the right pupil were less brisk than those of the left. There was slight ptosis of the eyelid on the right. On following a light with her eyes, she reported seeing two images when the light was moved directly to her left and to her right and upward. A red glass was placed over her right eye. When the light was moved to the left, the red image was seen to the left of the white image. When the light was moved to her right and upward, the red image was above the white image. In each instance, the separation increased as the light was moved further to the periphery of her vision. The only other abnormalities on neurologic examination were slight drooping of the left corner of her mouth and slight weakness of her left arm and leg, with hyperactive deep tendon reflexes, reduced abdominal reflexes, and the Babinski sign on the left.

a. What are the location and type of lesion?
b. What anatomical structures are involved?
c. Diplopia testing indicated weakness of which muscles?
d. Why was the pupillary light reflex altered?
e. What is the pathologic nature of the lesion?

pressure. Astrocytomas of the cerebellum also are common in childhood; they arise in the cerebellar hemisphere (resulting in ipsilateral limb ataxia). These tumors, which frequently have a cystic structure, display a unique biologic behavior. The early diagnosis and surgical removal of cerebellar astrocytomas, in contrast to astrocytomas of other locations, are associated with a good prognosis.

Astrocytomas also arise from glial cells located within the substance of the brainstem and result in a brainstem or pontine glioma (Fig. 15B.18). These tumors involve either the base or the tegmentum and are usually associated with progressive (often bilateral) symptoms of cranial nerve, motor, and sensory dysfunction. If the reticular formation is affected, consciousness is altered.

Certain tumors arise outside the parenchyma of the brainstem (extra-axial tumors), often from the meninges

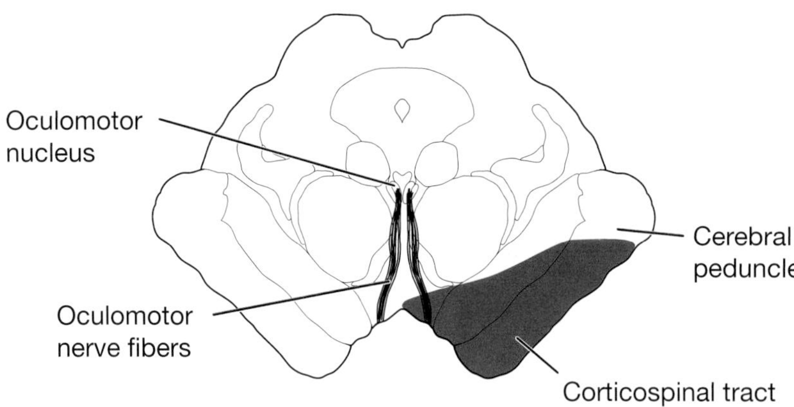

Fig. 15B.17. Paramedian infarct (red area) of midbrain (Weber syndrome), with involvement of cranial nerve III (oculomotor nerve) and cerebral peduncle.

(meningiomas) or the supporting cells in the cranial nerves. Extra-axial tumors initially alter cranial nerve function and secondarily affect brainstem function by compression or direct invasion. The most common tumor in this group is the vestibular schwannoma. Although it is commonly referred to as acoustic neuroma, the tumor arises from Schwann cells in the vestibular division of cranial nerve VIII in virtually all cases (Fig. 15B.19). The tumors frequently are bilateral in central, or type II, neurofibromatosis. Early signs of a vestibular schwannoma are unilateral tinnitus, decreased hearing, and disequilibrium. As the tumor enlarges, ipsilateral facial paresis, loss of the corneal reflex, and ipsilateral limb ataxia occur. With further increase in size, additional signs of brainstem compression and increased intracranial pressure may develop. These tumors are usually visualized with computed tomographic scanning and, even when very small, magnetic resonance imaging scanning.

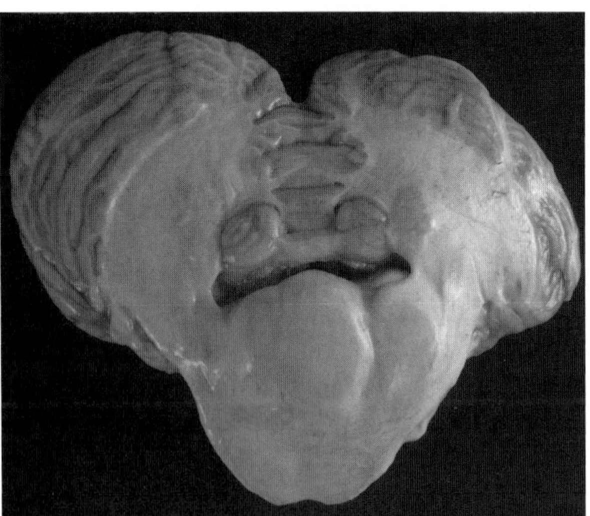

Fig. 15B.18. Gross specimen of brainstem glioma. Transverse section showing diffuse asymmetric enlargement.

Herniations of the Brain

Expanding supratentorial mass lesions may secondarily affect the structures located in the posterior fossa. The cranial cavity is a closed space and cannot accommodate to changes in intracranial volume. In the presence of a supratentorial or posterior fossa mass, intracranial pressure increases and, with further expansion, the brain adjusts to the increased volume by an alteration in shape and a slight shift in position. With further compression and shift, the function in areas of the nervous system remote from the expanding mass is also compromised and the clinical condition deteriorates further. The changes in shape and position that occur from intracranial mass lesions are called *herniation of the brain.*

Uncal Herniation

Uncal herniation characteristically occurs when unilateral, expanding supratentorial lesions, especially in the middle fossa, shift the mediobasal edge of the uncus of the hippocampal gyrus toward the midline and over the free edge of the tentorium, compressing the adjacent midbrain (Table 15B.11 and Fig. 15B.20 *A*). Cranial nerve III and occasionally the posterior cerebral artery on the side of the herniating temporal lobe are compressed by the overhanging swollen uncus. The clinical sign resulting from compression of cranial nerve III is an ipsilateral third nerve paresis, usually beginning with dilatation of the pupil. Compression of the contralateral cerebral peduncle against the free edge of the tentorium can cause hemiparesis ipsilateral to the expanding lesion. Midbrain compression also affects the ascending reticular activating system, and there is progressive loss of consciousness. If the posterior cerebral artery is compressed, infarction of the occipital lobe occurs, producing homonymous hemianopia.

Central or Transtentorial Herniation

This type of herniation is a further progression of uncal herniation and is associated with parasagittal or bilateral supratentorial masses. It consists of the caudal displacement of the diencephalon, midbrain, and pons (Table 15B.11 and Fig. 15B.20 *B*). Caudal displacement of the basilar artery (which is attached to the circle of Willis by the posterior cerebral arteries) does not occur to the same degree, resulting in stretching and shearing of paramedian perforating vessels, with secondary infarction and hemorrhage in the brainstem. This type of herniation blocks the flow of cerebrospinal fluid through the aqueduct of Sylvius, thus further increasing the volume of the supratentorial contents. The clinical signs of central herniation are oculomotor paresis, progressive alteration of consciousness, and decerebrate rigidity. Because mass lesions rarely are directly in the midline, some degree of lateral shift and uncal herniation nearly always accompanies transtentorial herniation.

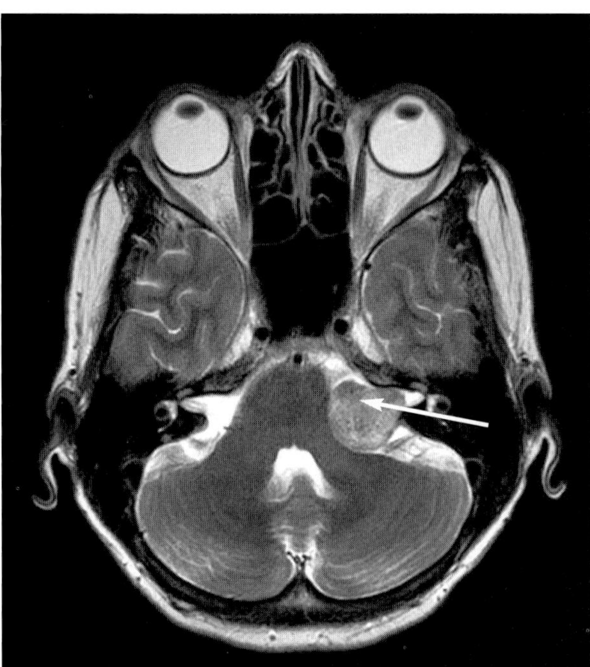

Fig. 15B.19. Vestibular schwannoma. Computed tomographic scan of the posterior fossa at the level of the pons showing a tumor (*arrow*) in the cerebellopontine angle compressing the pons.

Tonsillar or Foramen Magnum Herniation

As a result of an expanding mass in the posterior fossa or further progression of uncal or transtentorial herniation, the cerebellar tonsils herniate through the foramen magnum, with compression of the medulla (Fig. 15B.20 *C*). Signs of tonsillar herniation include neck pain and stiffness, the result of stretching and irritation of the lower cranial nerves supplying the neck muscles; progressive loss of consciousness from involvement of the ascending reticular activating system; generalized flaccidity; alteration of vital signs, with slowing of the pulse and vasomotor instability; and periodic or irregular respiration, the result of involvement of visceral centers in the medulla.

The three types of herniation of the brain are summarized in Table 15B.11 and Figure 15B.20.

- Dysarthria is a motor speech impairment that may result from impairment of any portion of the motor system.
- Coma may result from a posterior fossa lesion that involves the ascending reticular activating system.
- Decorticate posturing is due to damage of the rostral brainstem (rostral to the red nucleus) and results in increased flexor tone in the upper extremities and increased extensor tone in the lower extremities.
- Decerebrate posturing occurs with lesions at or caudal

Clinical Problem 15B.5.

A 13-year-old girl awoke one morning complaining of a left earache and dull generalized headache. Her temperature was 102°F (38.9°C) orally. Her condition did not improve with aspirin and bed rest. That evening, she was taken to her family physician, who diagnosed acute otitis media and gave her an injection of penicillin. For the next several days, she continued to have some ear drainage and mild left-sided ear pain and headache. During the next week, she had increasingly severe headaches, with nausea and vomiting. One day before admission, she experienced progressive weakness of the right face, arm, and leg and difficulty with speaking. She also seemed to have difficulty in thinking of what word she wanted to say, and she had difficulty in understanding what people were saying to her.

a. At this point, what are the suspected location and type of lesion?

When evaluated at the local hospital, she was stuporous but could be aroused by strong stimuli. Her left pupil was dilated and reacted poorly to light. The right pupillary reflex was intact. The left eye was deviated down and out, and she had ptosis of the left eyelid. During the examination, her right hemiparesis became much worse.

b. What is the reason for the change in level of consciousness?
c. How do you explain the eye findings?
d. Why was there worsening of the hemiparesis?
e. What is the term used to describe the above process?

It was decided to send the patient to the nearest neurosurgical facility, which was several hours away. On arrival at the second hospital, she was comatose. Respirations were deep and rapid. Her temperature was 105°F (40.6°C). Her pupils were slightly dilated and did not react to light. Her jaw was slightly clenched. Her spine was extended and arched posteriorly. Her arms were stiffly extended and the fists clenched. Her legs were also stiffly extended.

f. The findings present at this point suggest involvement at what level of the neuraxis?
g. What term describes her body position and tone?
h. What term describes the process producing this clinical picture?

to the red nucleus but above the vestibular nuclei and results in increased extensor tone in all four limbs.

- Acute onset and focal neurologic deficits are likely to represent a vascular cause of dysfunction. Vascular lesions of the posterior fossa present with specifically recognizable syndromes.

Neurologic Examination of the Posterior Fossa Level

The integrity of the posterior fossa is examined by testing the function of each of the major longitudinal systems found at this level (see Chapters 6-11) and the functions associated with the ocular motor, auditory, and vestibular systems and cranial nerves III through XII.

The Ocular Motor System and Cranial Nerves III, IV, and VI

Neurologic examination of the eyes begins with observing the size and bilateral symmetry of the palpebral fissures, especially looking for ptosis. The size, shape, and symmetry of the pupils are noted. The pupillary light reflex is tested by shining a light into each eye while observing the direct and consensual pupillary responses. The near reflex is tested by bringing a target toward the patient's nose and by observing pupillary constriction and eye convergence.

The position, alignment, and stability of the eyes when the patient attempts to gaze straight ahead (primary position) are observed. Abnormalities include inability

Table 15B.11. Herniations of the Brain

Type	Location	Cause	Anatomical structures involved	Clinical effects
Uncal	Tentorial notch, midbrain	Mass lesion in temporal lobe or middle fossa	Parahippocampal gyrus and uncus	
			Oculomotor nerve	Paresis of cranial nerve III
			Cerebral peduncle	Hemiparesis
			Midbrain ascending reticular activating system	Coma
			Posterior cerebral artery	Homonymous hemianopia
Central (transtentorial)	Tentorial notch, midbrain	Mass lesion in frontal, parietal, or occipital lobe	Midbrain and pons	Decerebrate rigidity
		Progression of uncal herniation	Ascending reticular activating system	Coma
Tonsillar (foramen magnum)	Foramen magnum, medulla	Mass lesion in posterior fossa	Cerebellar tonsils	Neck pain and stiffness
		Progression of uncal or transtentorial herniation	Indirect activation pathways	Flaccidity
			Ascending reticular activating system	Coma
			Vasomotor centers	Alteration of pulse, respiration, blood pressure

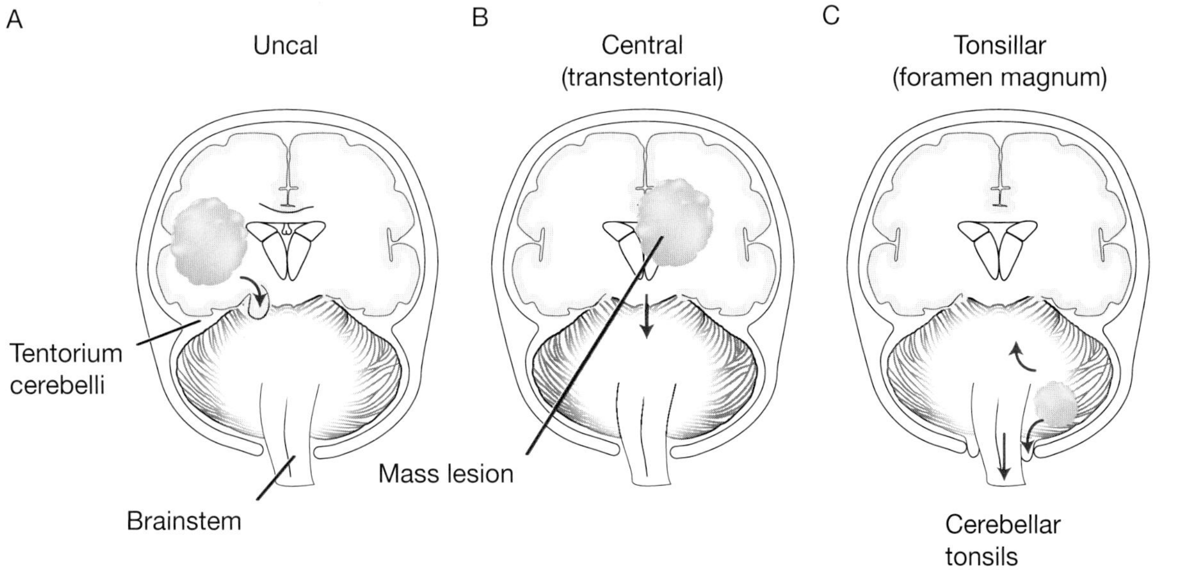

Fig. 15B.20. Herniations of the brain. *A*, Uncal herniation. *B*, Central herniation. *C*, Tonsillar (foramen magnum) herniation.

to maintain the primary position because of conjugate deviation, misalignment of the eyes because of monocular deviation, and spontaneous nystagmus. Eye movement is tested in the six cardinal directions, first with both eyes fixing on the target and then testing each eye with the other covered. Subtle muscle weakness can be demonstrated by placing a red glass in front of one eye while the patient follows a white light. This inhibits the reflex tendency of the brain to fuse identical images if possible and allows clearer identification of the field of gaze in which the image separation (diplopia) is greatest, thus identifying the weak muscle. Nystagmus is also examined for in each direction of gaze.

Sensory function is examined by testing the patient's ability to perceive pinprick and light touch applied to the skin supplied by the three divisions of the trigeminal nerve. The corneal reflex (which also involves cranial nerve VII) is tested by asking the patient to look to one side while the cornea is gently touched with a wisp of cotton, brought toward the cornea from the opposite direction. The normal response is prompt, bilateral blinking.

Motor function is tested by having the patient open the jaw. In the presence of unilateral pterygoid weakness, the jaw deviates to the weak side. The patient is also asked to bite firmly while the examiner palpates the masseter and temporalis muscles on each side. The jaw jerk is tested by placing the examiner's forefinger on the relaxed jaw and by striking the finger with a reflex hammer.

Cranial Nerve VII

Examination of the facial nerve begins with observing the patient's facial expressions. As the patient talks and smiles, facial asymmetry or reduced contraction becomes apparent. Specific muscle groups are then examined. The frontalis muscles are tested by asking the patient to wrinkle the forehead; strength can be assessed by attempting to smooth the wrinkles on each side. The orbicularis oculi can be tested by asking the patient to close the eyes tightly and then to try opening them. The lower facial muscles are tested by asking the patient to smile or show the teeth. Taste is not examined unless a peripheral facial nerve lesion is suspected. It is tested by having the patient protrude the tongue and then asking him or her to identify sugar, salt, or other substances applied to the side of the tongue.

The Auditory and Vestibular Systems and Cranial Nerve VIII

Audiometry provides the best means of examining hearing, but a rough estimate of the functioning of the acoustic system can be made by determining if the patient can hear the sound of a watch or the sound produced by rubbing the forefinger and thumb together in front of the ear. Auditory acuity of one side is compared with that of the other. The Weber and Rinne tests should be performed (Table 15B.5).

Vestibular function ordinarily is not examined unless disease of cranial nerve VIII, sensory ataxia, or brainstem disease is suspected. Caloric testing (irrigating the outer ear canal with cold water and observing for nystagmus, conjugate deviation of the eyes, or subjective vertigo) is a convenient means of testing vestibular function but usually is reserved for comatose patients.

Cranial Nerves IX and X

The glossopharyngeal and vagus nerves are often tested together by listening to the patient talk and inquiring about difficulty in speaking or swallowing. A soft, breathy voice associated with the nasal escape of air is suggestive of weakness in the oropharynx, whereas a hoarse or husky voice suggests a lesion of the nerve supply to the larynx. The patient is also asked to open the mouth and say "ah." Normally, the palate rises in the midline; unilateral palatal weakness causes the uvula to deviate toward the intact side. The gag reflex is examined by touching the back of the throat with a tongue blade and noting the contraction of the pharyngeal muscles.

Cranial Nerve XI

The sternocleidomastoid muscle is tested by asking the patient to turn the head to the side, against resistance applied by the examiner to the patient's jaw. The contracting muscle (on the side opposite the turn of the head) can be observed and palpated. The trapezius muscle is examined by having the patient elevate the shoulders against resistance applied by the examiner.

Cranial Nerve XII

The patient is asked to protrude the tongue in the midline and then to wiggle it from side to side. With upper motor neuron lesions, there is slowing of the alternate motion rate of the tongue. With unilateral lower motor neuron weakness, ipsilateral atrophy and fasciculations develop and the protruded tongue deviates toward the side of the lesion.

Clinical Problem 15B.6.

A 55-year-old man had noted progressive difficulty in swallowing and talking during the past year; liquids had tended to go down his trachea or out his nose, and he had felt that his trouble with speech was due to his tongue "not working right." Neurologic examination showed fasciculations and atrophy of the tongue bilaterally. He had trouble protruding his tongue and moving it from side to side. When he was asked to say "ah," his palate showed only minimal elevation. When asked to say "ka-ka-ka," he had nasal emission of speech. When asked to show his teeth, he was noted to have bilateral facial weakness, left greater than right, and he could not whistle. Also, slight distal extremity weakness and fasciculations were seen. Deep tendon reflexes were reduced, but the Babinski sign was present bilaterally. Results of the rest of the examination were normal.

a. What are the location and site of the lesion?
b. What system(s) is (are) involved?
c. What component(s) of the system(s) is (are) involved?
d. Name one disorder that can produce this syndrome.

Speech

Verbal communication includes both cognitive and motor skills. The cognitive aspects of verbal communication are considered language and are described in Chapter 16. Some motor speech disorders may result from disease of the brainstem and cranial nerves (flaccid dysarthria) or cerebellum (ataxic dysarthria). Spastic, hypokinetic, and hyperkinetic dysarthrias result from disease at the supratentorial level.

Tests for disorders of speech, the dysarthrias, are commonly administered at the same time as the testing of cranial nerve function. Speech can be evaluated by listening to spontaneous speech or by having the patient repeat the syllables pa-pa-pa (facial muscle and nerve function), ta-ta-ta (tongue and hypoglossal nerve function), and ka-ka-ka (pharyngeal muscle and cranial nerve IX and X function). The syllables pa-ta-ka-pa-ta-ka test cranial muscle coordination (cerebellar function).

Additional Reading

Baloh RW, Honrubia V. Clinical neurophysiology of the vestibular system. 2nd ed. Philadelphia: FA Davis; 1990.

Hudspeth AJ. The cellular basis of hearing: the biophysics of hair cells. Science. 1985;230:745-752.

Ito M. The cerebellum and neural control. New York: Raven Press; 1984.

Leigh RJ, Zee DS. The neurology of eye movements. 2nd ed. Philadelphia: FA Davis; 1991.

Rhoton AL Jr. Cerebellum and fourth ventricle. Neurosurgery. 2000;47(Suppl 3):S7-S27.

Chapter 16
Part A

The Supratentorial Level

Thalamus, Hypothalamus, and Visual System

Objectives

1. Name the divisions of the diencephalon, list the components of each division, and localize the structures on a diagram, a brain model, or a magnetic resonance imaging scan.
2. Name the functions of the thalamus.
3. List the functional groups of thalamic nuclei and their connections.
4. List the clinical manifestations of thalamic lesions.
5. Describe the general organization and functions of the hypothalamic nuclei.
6. Describe the clinical significance of the pituitary gland, and list the hormones secreted by the anterior and posterior lobes and their functions.
7. Describe how a mass lesion in the region of the hypothalamus may affect vision, ocular motility, and endocrine function.
8. Describe the function of the pineal gland.
9. Locate the following on a diagram: cornea, sclera, iris, ciliary body, lens, vitreous humor, retina, and choroid.
10. Describe the mechanism of phototransduction, the functions of rods and cones, and the basic intrinsic circuit of the retina.
11. Describe the anatomy of the visual pathways.
12. Describe the differences between the parvicellular and magnicellular components of the visual pathway.
13. Describe the visual field defect resulting from a lesion of each of the following: optic nerve, optic chiasm, optic tract, optic radiations, and occipital cortex.
14. Define hemianopia, quadrantanopia, homonymous, macular sparing, scotoma, and visual hallucination.
15. Given a visual field defect, localize the lesion.
16. Define and describe the significance of papilledema.

Introduction

The supratentorial level includes all structures located within the skull and above the tentorium cerebelli. These structures develop from the embryonic prosencephalon and, therefore, include derivatives of the diencephalon and telencephalon (Fig. 16A.1). The telencephalon includes the cerebral cortex and basal ganglia and the white matter of the cerebral hemispheres that connect these structures with each other and with other areas of the central nervous system. Telencephalic structures are discussed in Part B of this chapter. The diencephalon consists of the thalamus, hypothalamus, optic nerves, pituitary gland, and pineal gland. The thalamus is critical for the relay, gating, and integration of information that reaches the cerebral cortex. Through connections with the cerebral cortex, brainstem, pituitary, and pineal gland, the hypothalamus is important in the control of circadian rhythms, the sleep-wake cycle, homeostasis, and reproduction. The visual system, a derivative of the diencephalon, provides input to the cerebral cortex for the identification of objects and motor control under visual guidance.

This chapter discusses the anatomy, physiology, and clinical correlates of the diencephalic components of systems at the supratentorial level.

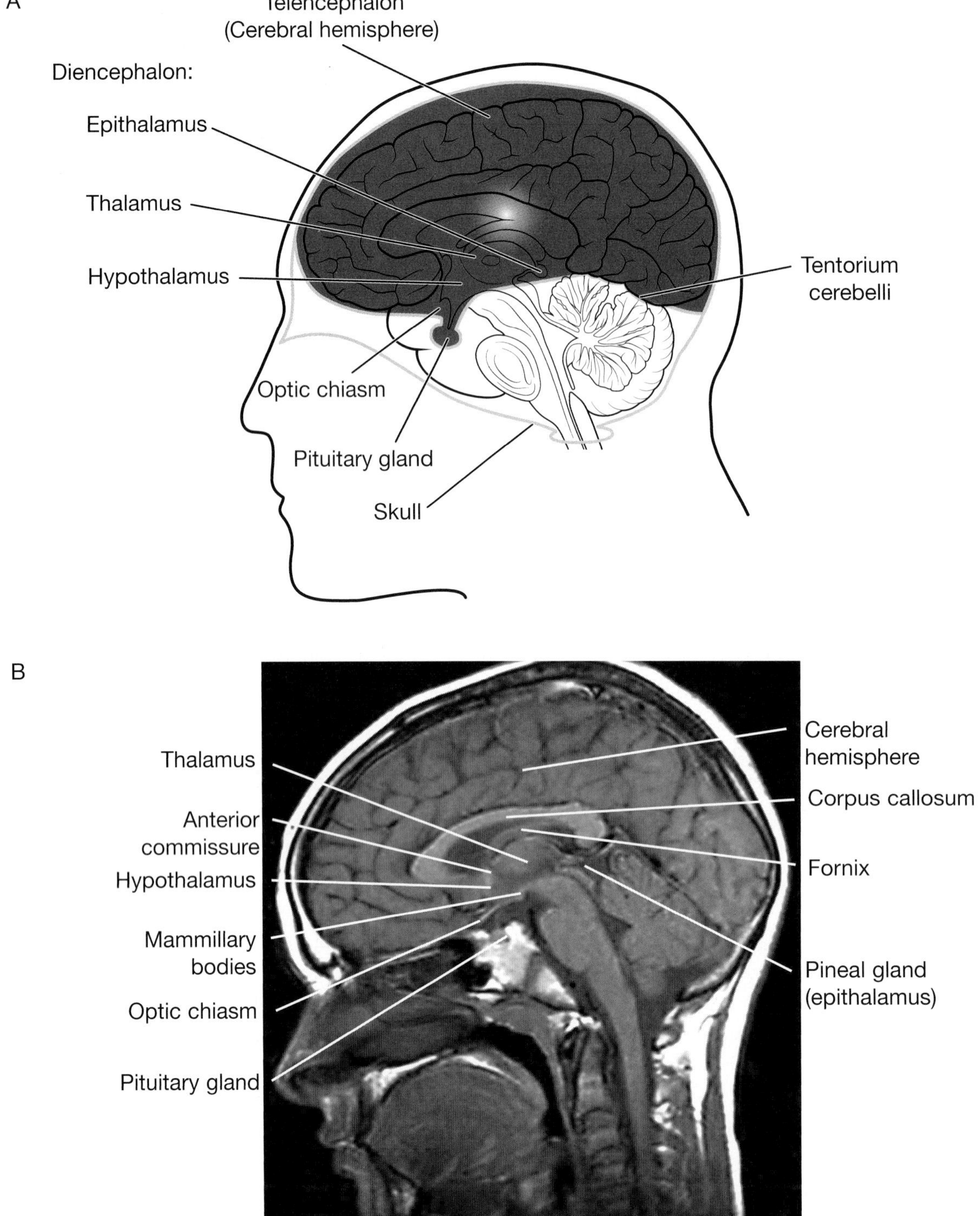

Fig. 16A.1. *A*, The supratentorial level (red area) includes the diencephalon and telencephalon. *B*, Sagittal T1-weighted magnetic resonance image showing components of the supratentorial level. The diencephalon includes the thalamus, hypothalamus (including the mammillary bodies), epithalamus (corresponding to the pineal gland), and optic chiasm. The structures of the telencephalon shown here include the medial aspect of the cerebral hemisphere, corpus callosum, and fornix.

Overview

The diencephalon consists of the structures located between the midbrain and cerebral hemispheres and surrounding the third ventricle (Fig. 16A.2). The diencephalon is bound superiorly by the floor of the lateral ventricles, corpus callosum, and fornix and laterally by the internal capsule. Anteriorly, it extends to the region of the foramen of Monro, and caudally, it merges with the tegmentum of the midbrain. The diencephalon includes the *thalamus* (also referred to as dorsal thalamus or thalamus proper), *ventral thalamus* (also referred to as perithalamus), *hypothalamus*, and *epithalamus*. The thalamus is the largest structure in the diencephalon and surrounds the upper and posterior portions of the third ventricle. The thalamus consists of nuclei that act as relay and integrating stations for sensory input to the cerebral cortex. Through reciprocal connections with the cerebral cortex, the thalamus is part of the circuits involved in motor control and higher cognitive functions. The ventral thalamus includes the *reticular nucleus of the thalamus*, which is a component of the consciousness system and is involved in mechanisms of arousal and sleep (see Chapter 10). Just ventral to the thalamus is the *subthalamic nucleus*, a component of the basal ganglia circuits.

The hypothalamus is inferior and anterior to the thalamus and is separated from it by the hypothalamic sulcus, a groove in the wall of the third ventricle that extends from the foramen of Monro to the aqueduct of Sylvius. The hypothalamus contains several nuclei that regulate visceral and endocrine functions, body temperature, blood osmolality, food intake, and sleep. Therefore, it is a critical component of both the internal regulation system (Chapter 9) and the consciousness system (Chapter 10). The inferior aspect of the hypothalamus, visible on the ventral surface of the brain, consists of the *tuber cinereum* and mammillary bodies. The *pituitary gland* is attached to the tuber cinereum by the pituitary stalk. The hypothalamus controls endocrine function by its projections to the pituitary gland. The *epithalamus* forms part of the roof of the diencephalon and lies superior and posterior to the thalamus. It includes the habenular nuclei, which are limbic

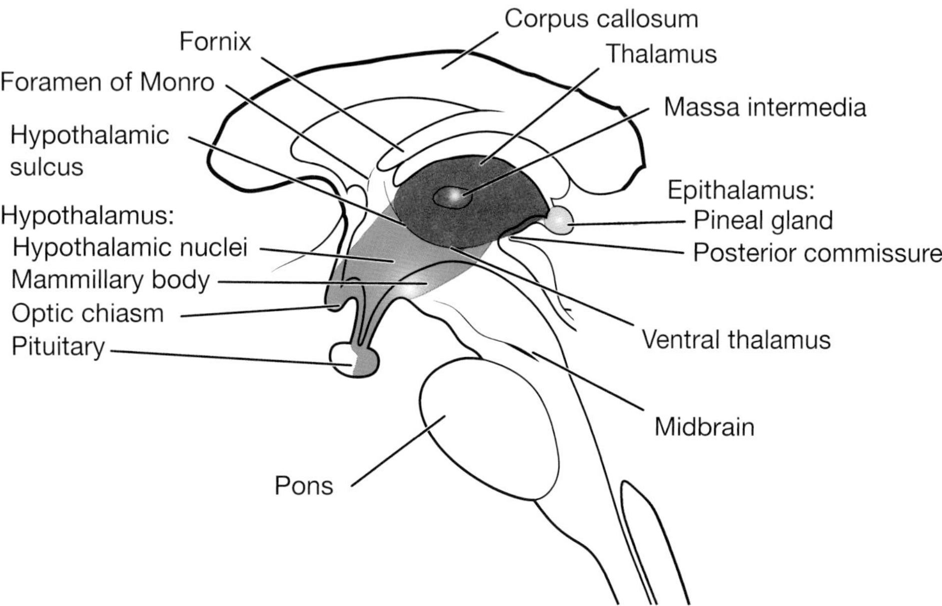

Fig. 16A.2. Diencephalon and its four subdivisions: thalamus (thalamus proper) (red), ventral thalamus, hypothalamus (green), and epithalamus (yellow). The anterior pituitary (white) is not part of the hypothalamus.

components of the basal ganglia circuits. Another part of the epithalamus is the *pineal gland*, which secretes melatonin.

The neural components of the *visual system*, including the retina and optic nerves, are derived from the diencephalon. The optic nerves project to the thalamus, which relays the information to the cerebral cortex for visual perception. At the cortical level, visual information is further analyzed for form, color, position, and movement of the object. Thus, the visual system consists of diencephalic and telencephalic components. The optic nerves also project to the hypothalamus, to control circadian rhythms, and the midbrain, to trigger the pupillary light reflex and reflex eye movements.

Disorders affecting the diencephalon and visual pathways have different clinical manifestations. For example, unilateral lesions of the thalamus impair contralateral sensory or motor functions and produce a contralateral visual field loss, whereas midline lesions affect consciousness. Hypothalamic lesions affect endocrine function and the sleep-wake cycle and disrupt homeostasis. Disorders of the pituitary cause different endocrine syndromes. Focal lesions of the visual pathway have important localizing value.

- The diencephalon includes the dorsal thalamus, ventral thalamus, hypothalamus, epithalamus, and portions of the visual system.

Thalamus

The thalamus consists of multiple nuclear groups and has four fundamental functions: 1) it relays input from each sensory pathway (except olfaction), the basal ganglia, and the cerebellum to specific areas of the cerebral cortex; 2) it associates multiple sensory modalities and relays this integrated information to areas of the cerebral cortex involved in attention and executive functions; 3) it filters ("gates") and modulates the access of sensory information to the cerebral cortex according to the sleep-wake cycle; and 4) it coordinates the activity of widespread areas of the cerebral cortex for cortical arousal and cognitive functions.

Anatomy

The thalamus is ovoid and forms the superior and posterior walls of the third ventricle. The anterior end of the thalamus is narrow, and the posterior end is broad. The Y-shaped *internal medullary lamina* divides the thalamus into anterior, medial, and lateral regions. These regions together with the enlarged posterior region form the main anatomical subdivisions of the thalamus (Fig. 16A.3). The left and right thalami are occasionally connected in the midline by the interthalamic adhesion, or *massa intermedia*.

The thalamus (thalamus proper, dorsal thalamus), contains the relay nuclei for sensory, motor, and association pathways and has reciprocal connections with the cerebral cortex. The ventral and lateral portions of the thalamus are surrounded by the ventral thalamus (sometimes referred to as the perithalamus), which consists of the *reticular thalamic nucleus*. The nucleus projects to the thalamus but not to the cerebral cortex; however, it receives input from the cortex and collaterals from the thalamic nuclei.

The nuclei of the thalamus are subdivided into three groups, according to their connections and functions: thalamic relay nuclei, associative nuclei, and nonspecific nuclei (Table 16A.1).

Specific Relay Nuclei

The specific thalamic relay nuclei are located in the anterior, lateral, and ventral portions of the thalamus. Each one receives input from a specific pathway and projects to a specific area of the cerebral cortex, with which the nucleus is reciprocally connected (Fig. 16A.4).

The *anterior* nuclear group of the thalamus (and its superior extension, called the lateral dorsal nucleus) is a component of the memory circuit of the hippocampal formation. It receives input from the hippocampal formation through the fornix, either directly or by a relay in the mammillary bodies of the hypothalamus, and projects primarily to the cingulate cortex (Fig. 16A.4).

The nuclei of the lateral region of the thalamus relay input from the substantia nigra pars reticulata, globus pallidus, cerebellar nuclei, and medial lemniscus and project to prefrontal, premotor, motor, and somatosensory areas of the cerebral cortex. The most anterior of these nuclei, the *ventral anterior nucleus*, receives input from the substantia nigra pars reticulata and projects to the

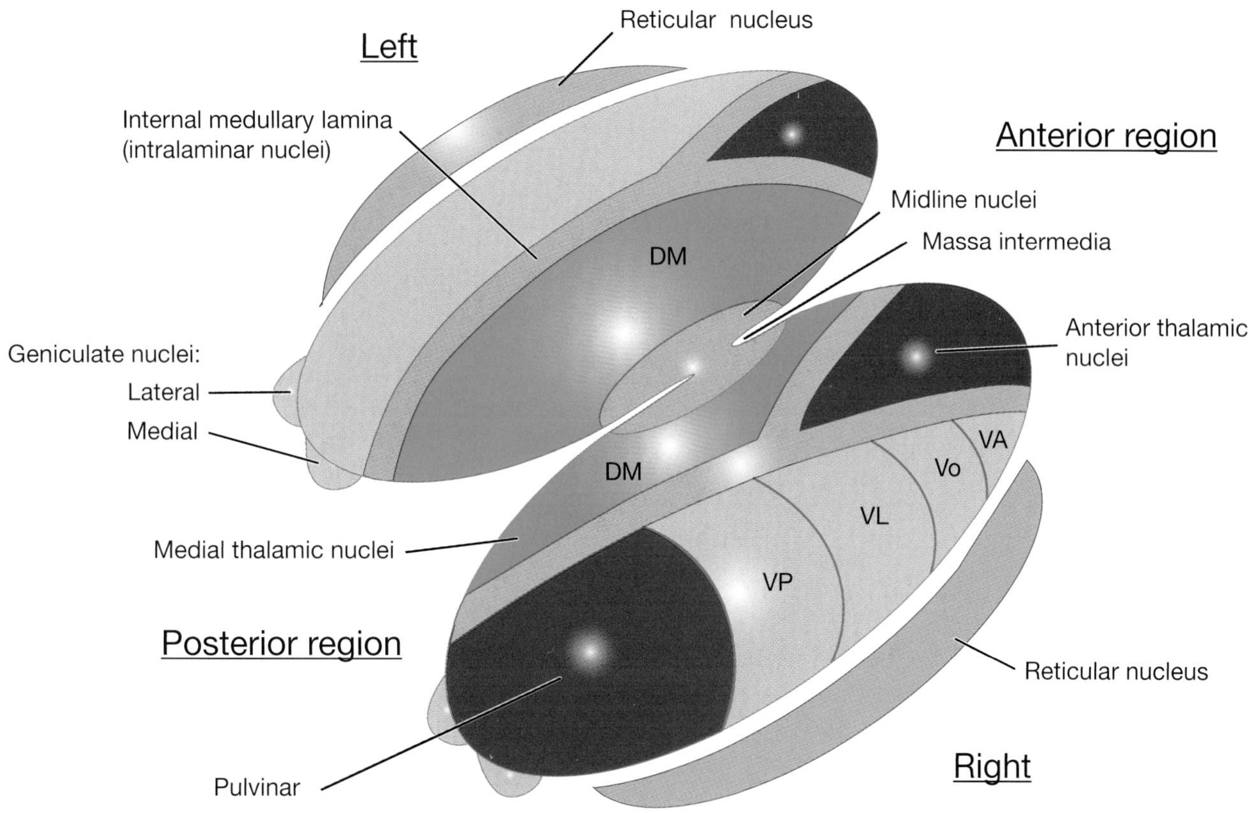

Fig. 16A.3. The major regions of the thalamus and their nuclei, as defined by their input and output: anterior; medial (dorsomedial nucleus [DM]); lateral, including the ventral posterior (VP), ventral lateral (VL, also called ventral intermedius); ventral oral (Vo), and ventral anterior (VA) nuclei; and posterior, corresponding to the pulvinar. The medial and lateral geniculate nuclei are located in this posterior region, just below the pulvinar. The intralaminar and midline nuclei are a functionally distinct group. The reticular nucleus corresponds to the ventral thalamus.

prefrontal cortex and frontal eye fields. The *ventral oral nucleus* receives input from the internal segment of the globus pallidus and projects to the supplementary motor area. The *ventral lateral*, or *ventral intermedius*, *nucleus* receives input from cerebellar nuclei and projects to the premotor and motor cortices. The *ventral posterior complex* includes several subnuclei that receive somatosensory input from the medial lemniscus and the spinothalamic and trigeminothalamic tracts and project to the primary somatosensory area in the postcentral gyrus. The rostral portion of the ventral posterior complex receives proprioceptive information, and the caudal portion receives tactile information. This nuclear complex includes the *ventral posterolateral nucleus*, which is the site of termination of somatosensory pathways representing the trunk and limbs, and the *ventral posteromedial nucleus*, which is the site of termination of trigeminothalamic pathways representing the head.

Immediately medial to the ventral posteromedial nucleus in the basal portion of the thalamus is the *ventral-posteromedial thalamic region*, which receives taste, visceral, pain, and temperature information from the spinothalamic tract and parabrachial nucleus and relays this information to the insular cortex. The *medial geniculate nucleus* receives auditory input from the inferior colliculus, through the brachium of the inferior colliculus, and

Table 16A.1. Summary of Thalamic Nuclei

Thalamic nucleus	Input	Target
Relay nuclei		
Anterior	Hippocampus Mammillary bodies	Cingulate cortex
Ventral anterior	Substantia nigra pars reticulata	Prefrontal cortex Frontal eye fields
Ventral oral	Globus pallidus (internal segment)	Supplementary motor area
Ventral lateral (ventral intermedius)	Cerebellar nuclei	Premotor and motor cortices
Ventral posterior	Medial lemniscus and spinothalamic and trigeminothalamic tracts	Primary sensory cortex
Ventral medial	Spinothalamic tract Parabrachial nucleus	Insular cortex
Medial geniculate	Inferior colliculus	Auditory cortex
Lateral geniculate	Optic tract	Primary visual cortex
Association nuclei		
Pulvinar	Superior colliculus Primary visual, auditory, and somatosensory cortices	Posterior parietal and lateral temporal association cortices
Dorsomedial (mediodorsal)	Prefrontal cortex Amygdala Substantia nigra Spinothalamic tract	Prefrontal cortex
Nonspecific nuclei		
Intralaminar	Globus pallidus Spinothalamic tract Reticular formation	Striatum Cerebral cortex
Midline	Hypothalamus Amygdala Reticular formation	Anterior cingulate cortex Hippocampus
Ventral thalamus		
Reticular nucleus	Cerebral cortex Reticular formation Thalamic nuclei	Thalamic nuclei

projects to the primary auditory cortex in the superior temporal gyri of Heschl. The *lateral geniculate nucleus* relays visual information from the optic tract and projects to the calcarine (primary visual) cortex of the occipital lobe.

All these relay nuclei are reciprocally connected with the specific areas of the cerebral cortex to which they project. The myelinated axons that interconnect the thalamus and cerebral cortex form part of the *internal capsule*. Connections with the prefrontal, premotor, and cingulate cortices occupy the *anterior limb* of the internal capsule and connections with the somatosensory cortex occupy the *posterior limb*, just posterior to the descending corticospinal fibers. Projections from the medial geniculate nucleus form the *auditory radiations* in the sublenticular portion of the posterior limb of the internal capsule. The lateral geniculate nuclei give rise to the *optic*

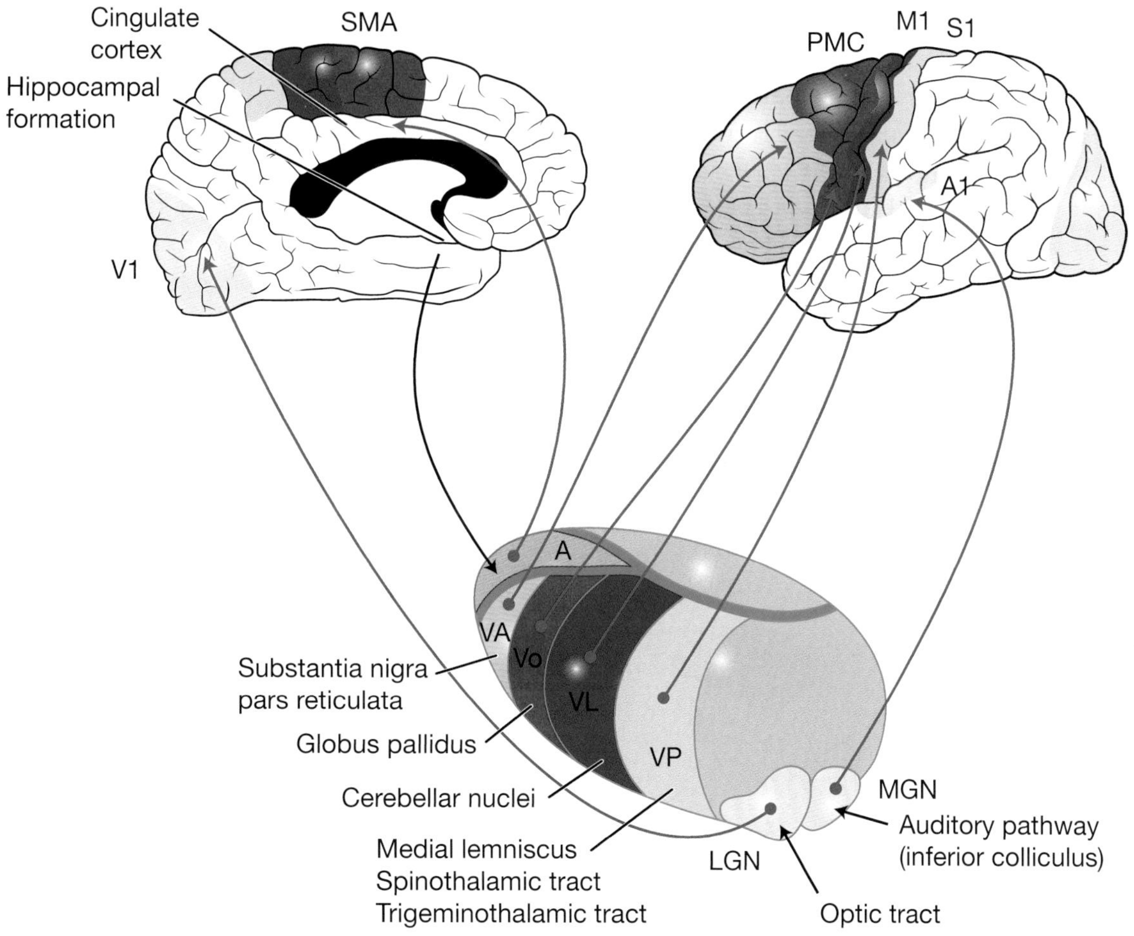

Fig. 16A.4. Main connections of the specific thalamic relay nuclei. The anterior (A) nuclear group receives input from the hippocampal formation via the fornix (both directly and from the mammillary bodies) and projects to the cingulate gyrus. The ventral anterior (VA) nucleus relays input from the substantia nigra pars reticulata to the prefrontal cortex and frontal eye fields; the ventral oral (Vo) relays input from the internal segment of the globus pallidus to the supplementary motor area (SMA). The ventral lateral (VL), or ventral intermedius, relays cerebellar input to the premotor (PMC) and primary motor (M1) cortices. The ventral posterior (VP) relays input from the medial lemniscus, spinothalamic tract, and trigeminal system to the primary sensory cortex (S1). The lateral geniculate nucleus (LGN) relays retinal input to the primary visual cortex (V1), and the medial geniculate nucleus (MGN) receives auditory input from the inferior colliculus and projects to the primary auditory cortex (A1).

radiations, which are in the *retrolenticular* portion of the posterior limb of the internal capsule.

Association Nuclei

The *association nuclei* of the thalamus are the largest nuclei of the thalamus and are reciprocally connected with association areas of the cerebral cortex (Fig. 16A.5). An important association nucleus is the *pulvinar*, located at the posterior pole of the thalamus. The pulvinar (and the lateral posterior nucleus) receives visual, somatosensory, and auditory inputs from the corresponding cortical sensory areas and from the superior colliculus and distributes this integrated information to association areas in the posterior parietal and lateral temporal cortices. Through these projections, the pulvinar is critical for mechanisms of spatial attention. The *mediodorsal* (or *dorsomedial*) *nucleus* corresponds to the medial thalamic region and is reciprocally connected with the frontal cortex. It receives input from the amygdala, substantia nigra pars reticulata, and superior colliculus and projects to the prefrontal cortex, frontal eye fields, and cingulate cortex. This nucleus is an essential link in prefrontal lobe circuits involved in attention, decision making, and behavioral planning.

Nonspecific Thalamic Nuclei

The third group of thalamic nuclei is the so-called nonspecific thalamic nuclei. These nuclei differ from the other thalamic nuclei in their morphology and patterns of connections. For example, these nuclei have important reciprocal connections with the basal ganglia and project to various regions of the cerebral cortex. The nonspecific thalamic nuclei include the *intralaminar nuclei*, which are located within the Y-shaped internal medullary lamina. They receive input from the globus pallidus and spinothalamic tract and project to the striatum and widespread areas of the cerebral cortex. The *midline nuclei* are located medially in thalamus and abut the third

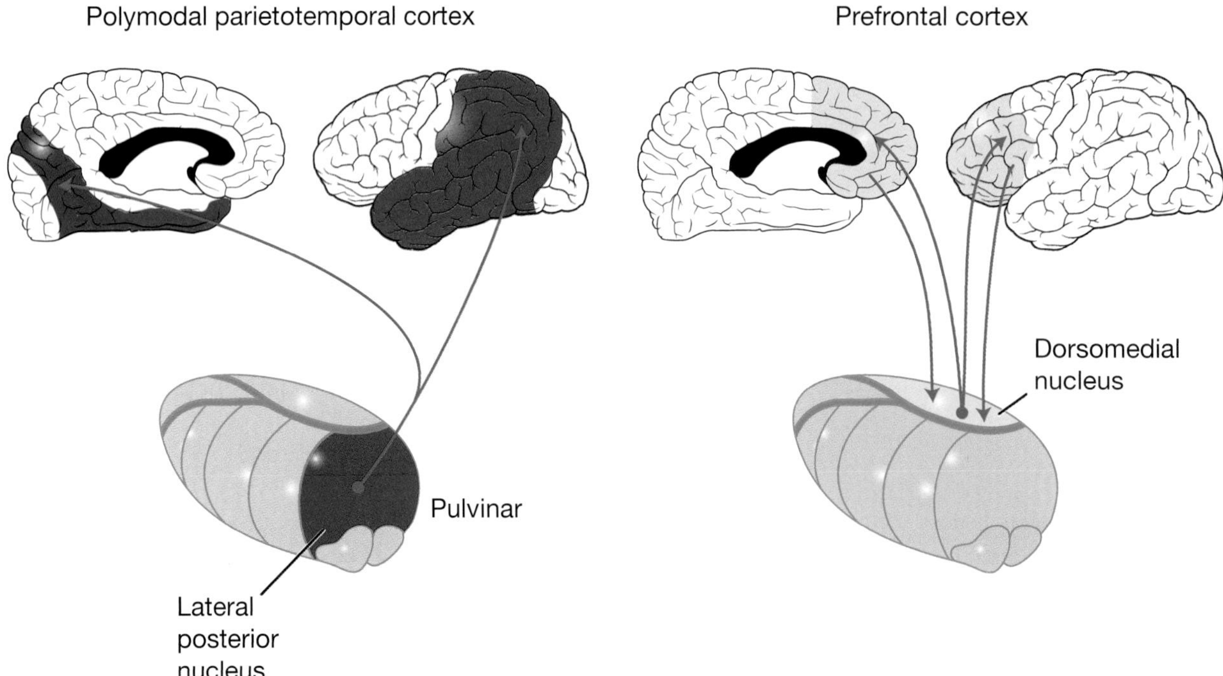

Fig. 16A.5. Association thalamic nuclei. The pulvinar (and the lateral posterior nucleus) receives input from the visual, somatosensory, and auditory cortices and projects to polymodal association areas of the posterior parietal and lateral temporal lobes. The dorsomedial (mediodorsal) nucleus has reciprocal connections with prefrontal cortex.

ventricle. These nuclei are part of circuits that interconnect the limbic portions of the basal ganglia, hypothalamus, anterior cingulate gyrus, and insula.

All the thalamic nuclei consist of excitatory projection neurons that have L-glutamate as the neurotransmitter. These neurons project to the cerebral cortex and receive input from the cortical areas to which they project.

Reticular Nucleus of Thalamus

The reticular nucleus of thalamus is derived embryologically from the ventral thalamus. Unlike the nuclei of dorsal thalamus, the reticular nucleus does not project to the cerebral cortex but instead to the thalamic nuclei. The reticular nucleus consists of highly interconnected GABAergic neurons that receive collaterals from all thalamocortical and corticothalamic fibers that traverse it. The relations of the thalamic relay nuclei, reticular nucleus, and cerebral cortex are summarized in Figure 16A.6.

Physiology

The thalamus serves as a relay station, gates information going to the cerebral cortex, and coordinates the activity of the cortex. Reciprocal excitatory thalamocorticothalamic loops between the different thalamic nuclei and the cerebral cortex regulate the relay of information and coordinate the activity initiated in different parts of the cerebral cortex involved in a specific task.

The reticular nucleus of thalamus receives excitatory collateral input from the cerebral cortex and the thalamic relay nuclei. The highly interconnected GABAergic neurons of the reticular nucleus inhibit the thalamocortical relay neurons in thalamus, regulating their firing pattern and thus their ability to relay information to the cerebral cortex. This coordinated inhibitory activity, maintained through cortical input to the reticular nucleus, is critical for synchronization of thalamocortical activity during non–rapid eye movement (NREM) sleep. The activity of these corticothalamocortical loops during wakefulness and the different sleep stages is regulated by cholinergic and monoaminergic input from the basal forebrain, hypothalamus, and brainstem, which reaches the reticular and relay thalamic nuclei as well as the cerebral cortex directly, as described in Chapter 10 (the Consciousness System).

As mentioned in Chapter 10, thalamic neurons exhibit two types of activity: 1) tonic firing that allows precise transmission of information from subcortical sources to the cerebral cortex, typical of active states of the thalamocortical circuits (wakefulness and rapid eye movement [REM] sleep), and 2) rhythmic burst firing that prevents transmission of sensory information to the cerebral cortex and is typical of inactive states, such as NREM sleep. The transition from one firing pattern to the other depends on the presence or absence of excitatory input from cholinergic and monoaminergic nuclei in the reticular formation.

- The thalamus acts as a relay area and gateway for information transfer to the cerebral cortex.
- Corticothalamocortical loops allow synchronized activity in the cerebral cortex.

Clinical Correlations

Vascular Disorders

The blood supply to the posterior thalamus is from branches of the posterior cerebral and posterior communicating arteries. Discrete lesions that destroy the ventral posterior nucleus of the thalamus produce contralateral hemianesthesia, with loss of all sensory modalities in the trunk, limbs, and face. This is often the result of an infarction due to hypertensive vascular disease or thrombosis of one of the thalamogeniculate branches of the posterior cerebral artery. The initial stage of contralateral hemianesthesia after a thalamic infarct may, in turn, be followed by partial return of sensation associated with a very unpleasant burning sensation; this is referred to as the *thalamic syndrome*.

The nuclei located medially in the thalamus can be affected bilaterally by infarction in the territory of paramedian perforating branches of the posterior cerebral artery. This produces an impaired state of consciousness with excessive somnolence; it is associated with deficits in memory and vertical gaze.

- A unilateral lesion in the ventral posterior portion of thalamus produces a sensory loss of all modalities on the contralateral face and body.

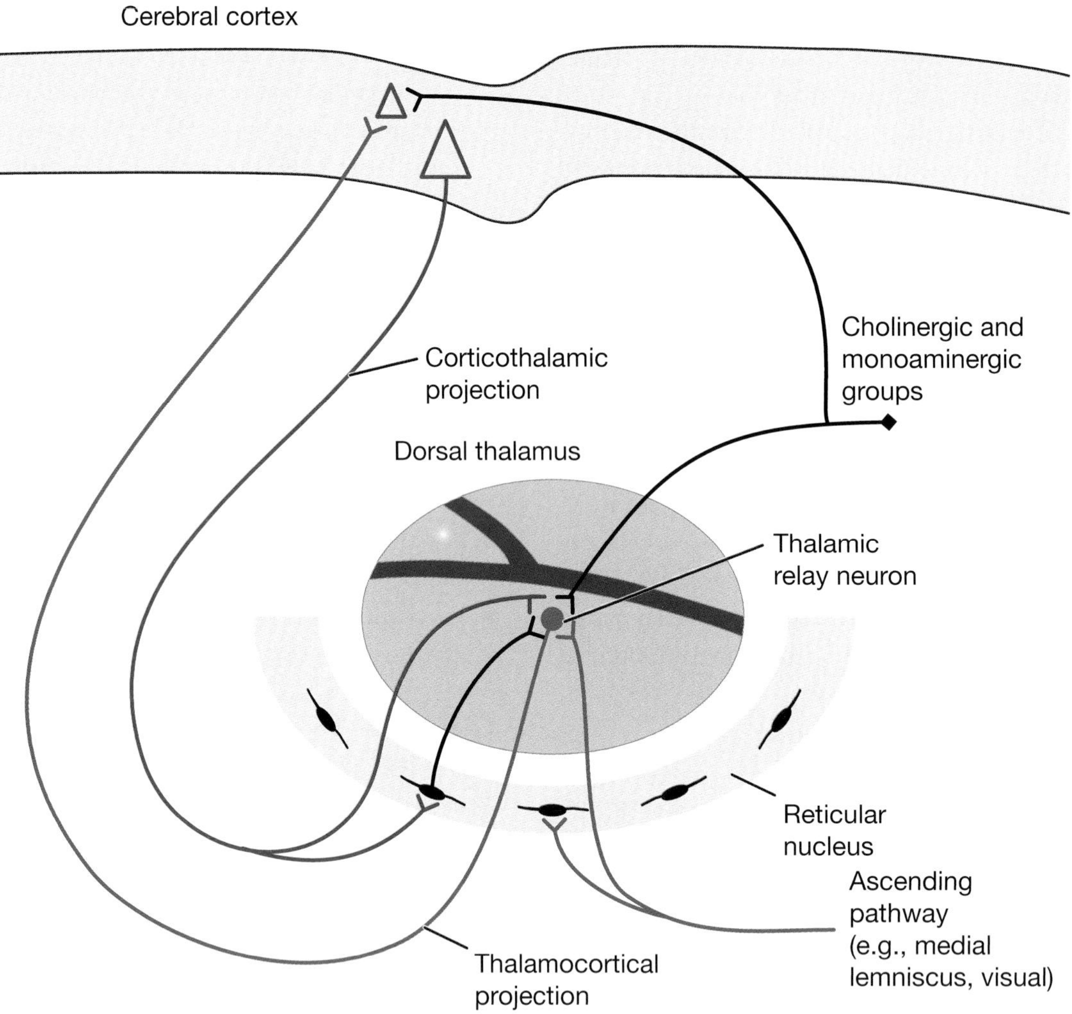

Fig. 16A.6. Reciprocal thalamocortical interactions. The projection neurons of the thalamic relay nuclei receive excitatory input and send an excitatory projection to a restricted area of the cerebral cortex. Pyramidal neurons in this cortical area send a reciprocal projection to the thalamic relay nucleus and a collateral projection to the thalamic reticular nucleus. The thalamic reticular nucleus also receives an excitatory collateral projection from the thalamocortical neuron (not shown) and sends an inhibitory GABAergic projection to the thalamic relay neuron. These reciprocal thalamocorticothalamic interactions gate the relay of information at the level of the thalamus and control thalamocortical synchronization. These functions change during the sleep-wake cycle under the modulatory influence of cholinergic and monoaminergic neurons of the brainstem, which project to the thalamic relay and reticular nuclei as well as to the cerebral cortex.

- A midline thalamic lesion can cause somnolence and can impair memory.

Other Disorders

Motor function can be altered by lesions of the thalamic motor relay nuclei. Discrete neurosurgical lesions placed in the ventral lateral thalamic nucleus disrupt connections between the cerebellum and the cerebral cortex and thereby decrease the tremor of some patients who have cerebellar disease, Parkinson disease, or essential tremor.

A prion disease, *fatal insomnia*, is associated with selective lesions of the anterior and dorsomedial thalamic

Clinical Problem 16A.1.

A 70-year-old man with hypertension had sudden onset of numbness of the entire left side of his body and face. When evaluated in the emergency department several hours later, he was unable to perceive pinprick, temperature, touch, proprioception, and vibration sensation over the left side of the face and body. Speech and motor function were intact.

a. Where is the lesion?
b. What is the lesion?
c. What vessels supply the affected area?
d. One month later, the patient developed a disagreeable burning sensation whenever he was touched on the left side of the body. What is this syndrome called?

nuclei. The clinical manifestations include progressive intractable insomnia, sympathetic hyperactivity, and disruption of circadian rhythms.

Hypothalamus and Pituitary Gland

The hypothalamus is a component of the internal regulation and consciousness systems. It integrates cortical, visceral, humoral, and sensory inputs and initiates coordinated responses that regulate the sleep-wake cycle, homeostasis, adaptation to environmental stimuli, and reproduction.

Anatomy

Hypothalamus

The hypothalamus is anterior and inferior to the thalamus and separated from it by the hypothalamic sulcus. The hypothalamus extends from the region of the optic chiasm to the caudal border of the mammillary body. The region in front of the optic chiasm is called the *preoptic area*, which has a telencephalic origin but forms a functional unit with the hypothalamus. The anterior edge of the third ventricle corresponds to the *lamina terminalis*, which extends from the anterior commissure dorsally to the optic chiasm ventrally. From anterior to posterior, the hypothalamus is subdivided into the preoptic-anterior, tuberal, and mammillary or posterior regions (Fig. 16A.7). The highly vascularized ventral portion of the tuberal region, which corresponds to the tuber cinereum, and the mammillary bodies form the floor of the third ventricle and are visible on the ventral surface of the brain.

Pituitary Gland

The pituitary gland, or *hypophysis*, is anatomically and functionally related to the hypothalamus and attached to it at the tuber cinereum by the *infundibulum*, or *pituitary stalk*. The hypophysis lies within a bony-walled cavity, the sella turcica ("Turkish saddle"), in the sphenoid bone at the base of the brain (Fig. 16A.7). The pituitary stalk is between the optic chiasm and the mammillary bodies. Its relation to the optic chiasm is clinically important because enlargement of the pituitary gland may compress the fibers in the optic chiasm. The pituitary gland consists of the anterior lobe, or *adenohypophysis*, and the posterior lobe, or *neurohypophysis*. Although both lobes are part of a single gland, each has a different embryologic origin. The anterior lobe arises from a neuroectodermal ridge in the oral region, *Rathke pouch*, and the posterior lobe, together with the pituitary stalk, are from a downward evagination of the embryonic diencephalon. The anterior lobe fuses with the posterior lobe, and it is controlled by the hypothalamus through a system of portal vessels.

Anatomical Relations of the Hypothalamus and Pituitary Gland

An important anatomical relation of the hypothalamo-pituitary region is with the *cavernous sinus*. This venous structure is lateral to the pituitary gland and contains the internal carotid arteries and cranial nerves III, IV, VI and the ophthalmic and maxillary divisions of cranial nerve V (Fig.16A.8). This relation is important because with lateral enlargement, the pituitary may compress the carotid artery and these cranial nerves. Another important relation is with the *optic chiasm*, which is immediately anterior to the pituitary stalk.

The hypothalamus is connected with all areas of the

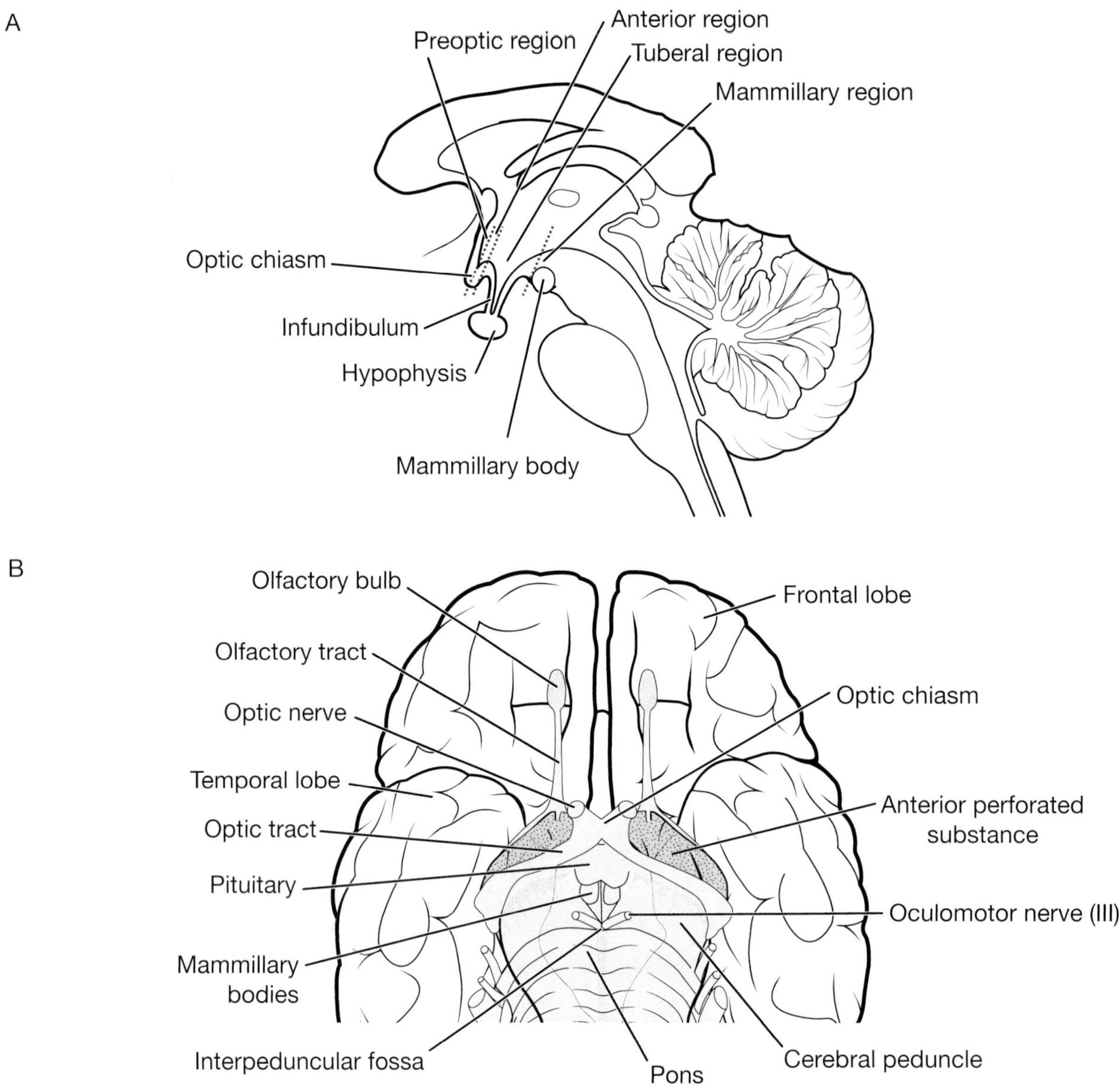

Fig. 16A.7. Gross anatomy of the hypothalamus and pituitary region. *A*, Midline section showing the different regions of the hypothalamus, the pituitary gland in the sella turcica, and the mammillary bodies. *B*, Base of the brain showing the optic chiasm, pituitary, and mammillary bodies.

brainstem and cerebral hemispheres, including the amygdala and hippocampus. The most prominent fiber tract is the *fornix*. It originates in the hippocampal formation and ends in the mammillary body, which projects through the *mammillothalamic tract* to the anterior nuclear group of the thalamus. These pathways are important in learning and memory.

Physiology

The hypothalamus is the effector structure of the diencephalon and has a critical role in homeostasis, including thermoregulation, osmoregulation, regulation of immune responses, and the control of food intake, reproduction, biologic rhythms (including the sleep-wake cycle), and integrated responses to stress. All these functions,

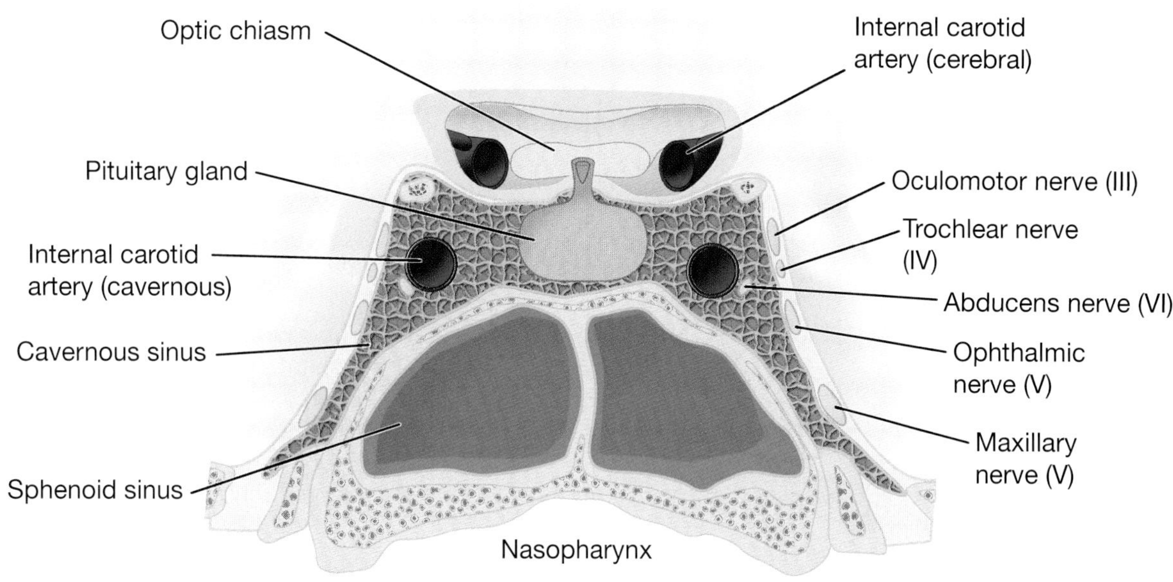

Fig. 16A.8. Coronal section through the base of the brain. The structures adjacent to the pituitary gland in the cavernous sinus include cranial nerves III, IV, V (ophthalmic and maxillary divisions), and VI and the carotid arteries. The optic chiasm and tract are adjacent to the pituitary stalk.

essential for survival, depend on the ability of different hypothalamic nuclei to initiate the appropriate autonomic, endocrine, and behavioral responses to challenges from the internal and external environments.

From the functional standpoint, the hypothalamus is subdivided into three longitudinally arranged zones: the periventricular, medial, and lateral zones (Fig. 16A.9). The periventricular zone, adjacent to the wall of the third ventricle, contains nuclei involved in neuroendocrine control through connections with the pituitary or median eminence. The medial zone, medial to the fornix, contains several nuclei involved in thermoregulation, osmoregulation, control of food intake, and reproduction. The lateral zone, lateral to the fornix, contains hypothalamic nuclei that through connections with the cerebral cortex and brainstem are involved in the control of the sleep-wake cycle and food intake. The lateral zone contains the *medial forebrain bundle*, which interconnects the hypothalamus with brainstem cholinergic and monoaminergic nuclei and limbic structures of the telencephalon. Although each of these longitudinal zones contains several nuclei with different connections and functions, they are closely interconnected and interact to generate the integrated autonomic, endocrine, and behavioral responses dependent on the hypothalamus. All these zones contain nuclei that project to autonomic nuclei in the brainstem and spinal cord. The function and dysfunction of hypothalamic nuclei are summarized in Table 16A.2.

- The hypothalamus includes periventricular, medial, and lateral zones that are interconnected and control endocrine, autonomic, and behavioral functions.

Neuroendocrine Control

The neuroendocrine functions of the hypothalamus are mediated by two neurosecretory systems, the magnicellular and the parvicellular neurosecretory systems (Fig. 16A.10). Neurosecretion is the release of a chemical transmitter from an axon terminal into a blood vessel. The *magnicellular system* consists of neurons in the *supraoptic* and *paraventricular* nuclei that synthesize either *vasopressin* (also called antidiuretic hormone) or *oxytocin*. These peptides are transported down the axons, through

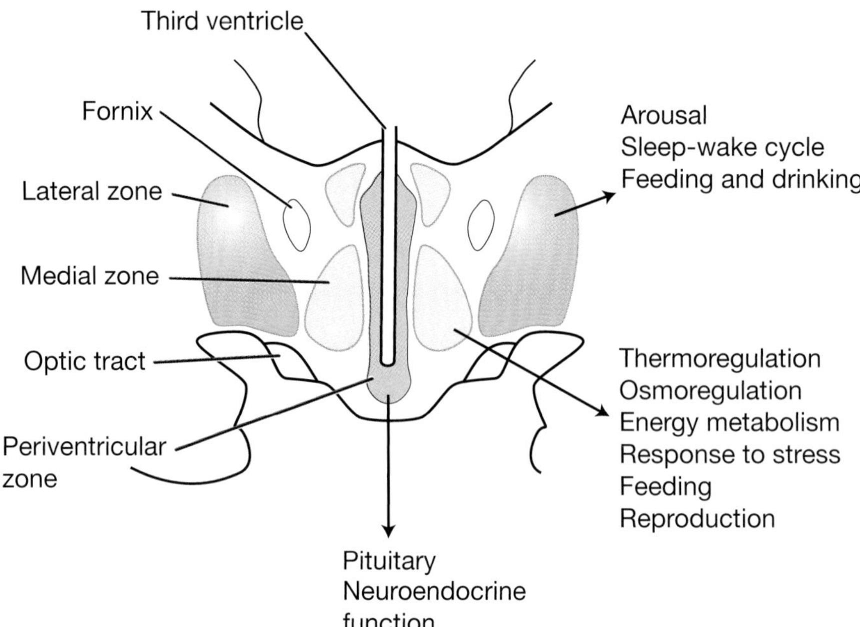

Fig. 16A.9. Functional subdivisions of the hypothalamus shown in the transverse plane.

Table 16A.2. Function and Dysfunction of Hypothalamic Nuclei

Nucleus	Function	Dysfunction
Suprachiasmatic	Circadian rhythms	Disruption of circadian rhythms
Magnicellular supraoptic and paraventricular	Secretion of arginine vasopressin (antidiuretic hormone) and oxytocin	Diabetes insipidus Inappropriate secretion of antidiuretic hormone
Medial preoptic and anterior	Thermoregulation Osmoregulation	Hyperthermia or hypothermia Hypernatremia, salt-wasting syndrome, thirst disorders
Parvicellular paraventricular, medial preoptic, and arcuate (infundibular)	Control of anterior pituitary secretion	Hypopituitarism Cushing syndrome Acromegaly Amenorrhea/galactorrhea Infertility, impotence Sexual precocity
Arcuate (infundibular)	Inhibition of food intake	Obesity
Lateral	Stimulation of food intake	Anorexia
Ventrolateral preoptic	Sleep induction	Insomnia
Posterior lateral hypothalamic area	Arousal	Somnolence Narcolepsy

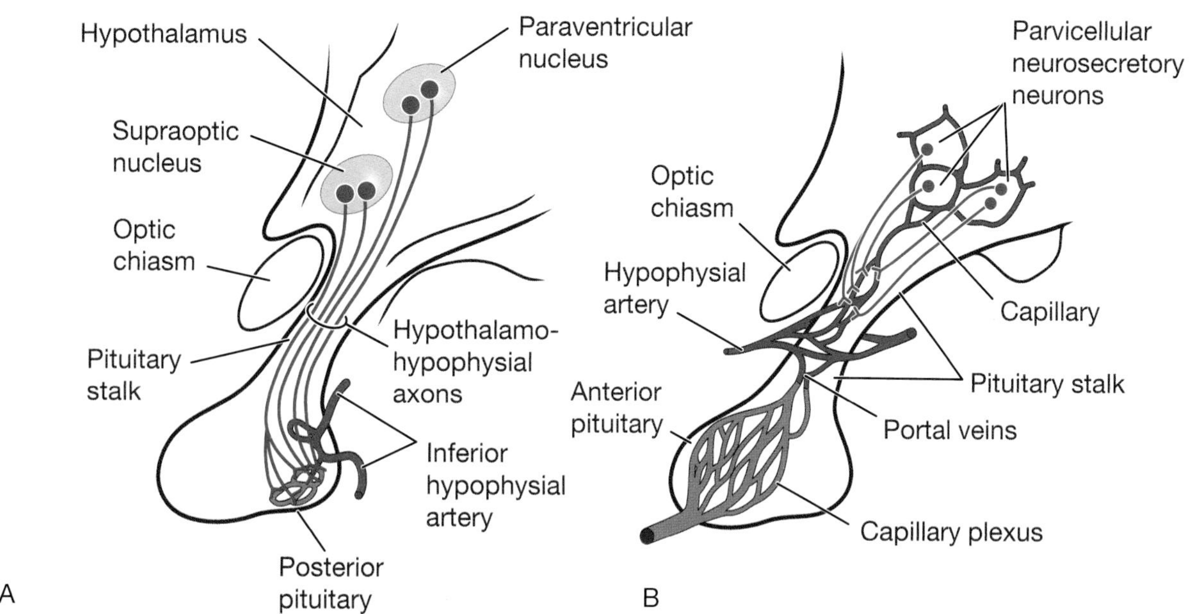

Fig. 16A.10. Neuroendocrine systems of the hypothalamus. *A*, Magnicellular system. Neurons of the supraoptic and paraventricular nuclei synthesize arginine-vasopressin or oxytocin and send axons through the pituitary stalk to secrete these hormones into capillaries in the posterior pituitary. *B*, Parvicellular system. Neurons of the periventricular preoptic, paraventricular, and arcuate nuclei synthesize releasing or inhibitory factors and their axons deliver these factors to the portal circulation at the level of the median eminence. The portal circulation delivers these factors to the anterior pituitary to control hormonal secretion by the pituitary endocrine cells.

the pituitary stalk, to nerve terminals in the posterior lobe for storage or release. Vasopressin regulates water metabolism and blood osmolality by increasing water reabsorption in the kidney. Oxytocin enhances the contractility of 1) uterine musculature during and after delivery and 2) the myoepithelial cells of the breast ducts in lactating women, thus facilitating milk ejection.

The *parvicellular system* includes neurons in the *medial preoptic*, *paraventricular*, and *infundibular* (or *arcuate*) nuclei in the periventricular zone of the hypothalamus. These neurons synthesize different regulatory hormones that may facilitate or inhibit the secretion and release of hormones by endocrine cells in the anterior pituitary gland. This hypothalamic control is exerted on the anterior pituitary gland through a *vascular mechanism* that involves a portal circulation which connects the hypothalamus and the anterior lobe. This portal circulation consists of hypophysial arteries in the *median eminence* giving rise to capillaries that drain into a series of parallel veins coursing down the pituitary stalk. On reaching the anterior lobe, these veins form a capillary plexus that supplies blood to the anterior lobe. The parvicellular hypothalamic neurons release regulatory hormones from their nerve endings in the median eminence. The regulatory substances enter the capillaries of the portal circulation, travel down the pituitary stalk through the portal veins, and finally reach the capillary plexus of the anterior pituitary gland, where they stimulate or inhibit specific groups of anterior pituitary endocrine cells. Important features of anterior pituitary cells, including their hormones, functions, and their regulation by the hypothalamus are outlined in Table 16A.3.

Autonomic Control

The most important autonomic output of the hypothalamus arises from the paraventricular nucleus, with important contributions from the lateral hypothalamic area and nuclei of the medial zone. All these nuclei contain a mixed population of neurons that form part of the internal regulation system and control the activity of preganglionic parasympathetic or sympathetic neurons of the brainstem and spinal cord. The hypothalamic control of sympathetic output is important in coordinating the activity of effectors such as blood vessels, sweat glands, and peripheral endocrine organs with the circumstances (see Chapter 9).

For example, in response to heat, the hypothalamus activates sympathetic sudomotor neurons and inhibits skin vasoconstrictor neurons, whereas in response to hypoglycemia, it activates sudomotor and skin vasoconstrictor neurons and the secretion of epinephrine from the adrenal medulla.

Thermoregulation

The medial preoptic and anterior hypothalamic regions contain thermosensitive neurons, including warm-sensitive neurons that initiate a heat-loss response (skin vasodilatation and sweating) and inhibit cold-sensitive neurons that initiate heat-gain responses (skin vasoconstriction, shivering, lipolysis, increased muscle metabolism, and release of thyroid hormones). These responses likely involve polysynaptic pathways that relay in the posterior hypothalamus and brainstem.

The febrile response is an integrated response coordinated by the hypothalamus. It consists of an increase in body temperature, shivering, malaise, sleepiness, and anorexia and is associated with increased secretion of vasopressin and corticosteroids. All these responses are attributed to effects of circulating cytokines, which can gain access to the hypothalamus, including the medial preoptic and paraventricular nuclei, by activating vagal afferents relaying in the medulla or through the vascular organ of the lamina terminalis, a circumventricular organ that lacks the blood-brain barrier.

Table 16A.3. Anterior Pituitary Hormones

Cell type	Hormone (standard abbreviation)	Main hypothalamic regulatory hormone(s)	Function
Somatotroph	Growth hormone (GH)	Growth hormone-releasing hormone Somatostatin (inhibits release)	Linear growth Intermediate metabolism
Lactotroph	Prolactin (PRL)	Dopamine (inhibits release)	Breast growth and development Lactogenesis
Corticotroph	Corticotropin (ACTH)	Corticotropin-releasing hormone (CRH)	Functional integrity and steroidogenesis of adrenal cortex (glucocorticoids, mineralocorticoids, and sexual steroids)
Thyrotroph	Thyrotropin (TSH)	Thyrotropin-releasing hormone (TRH) Somatostatin (inhibits release)	Integrity and function of thyroid gland; secretion of thyroxin and triiodothyronine
Gonadotroph	Luteinizing hormone (LH) Follicle-stimulating hormone (FSH)	Gonadotrophin-releasing hormone	Gonadal function, sexual maturation, gametogenesis, sex steroid production

Water Metabolism (Osmoregulation)

The hypothalamus is critical for coordinating the mechanisms of water and sodium homeostasis. Behavioral mechanisms include thirst and salt appetite, and reflex mechanisms involve the secretion of vasopressin from the magnicellular supraoptic and paraventricular neurons and the control of autonomic output to maintain osmolarity and blood pressure and to modify renal losses of sodium and water. For example, the physiologic responses to hyperosmolarity include thirst, decreased salt appetite, and increased water retention by the antidiuretic action of vasopressin.

The hypothalamus contains osmoreceptor neurons, which are specialized neurons that transduce osmotic changes into electrical signals. Osmoreceptors are located in the area of the lamina terminalis in the anteroventral wall of the third ventricle and include structures such as the subfornical organ, which lacks a blood-brain barrier and responds to circulating signals such as angiotensin II. Angiotensin II stimulates thirst, salt appetite, and vasopressin release in response to hypovolemia. The osmotic control of magnicellular vasopressin neurons results from their intrinsic properties, synaptic inputs, and paracrine actions of the surrounding glia.

Food Intake

The hypothalamus is important in the control of feeding and energy metabolism. It contains neurons whose activity changes according to the levels of blood glucose and other circulating signals, for example leptin (a circulating anorexigenic signal from adipose tissue) and insulin. These neurons also respond to input from the gastrointestinal tract that reaches them indirectly from vagus nerve afferents that relay in the brainstem. The hypothalamic neurons that control food intake include neurons in the *arcuate nucleus* that are stimulated by leptin and inhibit feeding. Neurons in the posterior lateral hypothalamus synthesize *hypocretin* (also called *orexin*), are inhibited by leptin, and stimulate feeding. Both the arcuate and the lateral hypothalamic neurons project to the paraventricular nucleus, which also contains neurons that stimulate food intake.

These glucose- and leptin-sensitive neurons of the arcuate nucleus, lateral hypothalamus, and paraventricular nucleus regulate food intake and energy metabolism in part through output to autonomic centers of the brainstem and spinal cord that control the endocrine secretion of the adrenal gland and the islets of the pancreas.

Reproductive Function

The hypothalamus affects sexual function and reproduction by controlling the secretion of *gonadotropin-releasing hormones* and *prolactin* and specific sexual behaviors. Important regions include the medial preoptic area, which contains a sexually dimorphic nucleus, and the ventromedial nucleus. The neurons in these areas have an abundance of receptors for sex steroids (estrogens and androgens).

Response to Stress

The paraventricular nucleus of the hypothalamus is the critical effector for the stress response. It receives input from limbic structures involved in emotion and from brainstem monoaminergic nuclei that respond to both internal and external stressors, including pain, hypoglycemia, hypotension, and circulating cytokines released during inflammation. The paraventricular nucleus has three types of effector neurons: magnicellular neurons that release vasopressin, neurons that activate sympathetic activity, and neurons that synthesize *corticotropin-releasing hormone* and release it into the capillaries of the median eminence. This hormone activates anterior pituitary cells that produce *adrenocorticotropic hormone* (ACTH, also called *corticotropin*), which stimulates the secretion of glucocorticoids from the adrenal cortex.

Sleep-Wake Cycle

The lateral hypothalamus can be considered the diencephalic component of the reticular formation. Nuclei of the lateral hypothalamus are involved in the control of arousal and motivated behavior (see Chapter 10). The *ventrolateral preoptic nucleus* is a sleep-promoting area that sends inhibitory GABAergic projections to the ascending cholinergic and monoaminergic arousal systems and particularly to the histamine-producing neurons of the *tuberomammillary nucleus* in the posterior lateral hypothalamus, which are essential for arousal. The posterior lateral hypothalamus also contains neurons that synthesize hypocretin (orexin) and project to and activate monoaminergic brainstem neurons, preventing abrupt transitions between wakefulness and sleep. These neurons also stimulate food intake.

Circadian Rhythms

The circadian pacemaker is the *suprachiasmatic nucleus* of the hypothalamus. Its neurons have an intrinsic circadian rhythm, and they control endocrine, autonomic, and behavioral functions, including the sleep-wake cycle and diurnal variations in body temperature through projections to other hypothalamic nuclei. The circadian activity of the suprachiasmatic nucleus is entrained to the light-dark cycle of day and night by a direct projection from the retina. An important example of circadian rhythm is the secretion of *melatonin* by the pineal gland. The *pineal gland*, derived from a dorsal evagination of the roof of the diencephalon, is in the dorsal wall of the posterior part of the third ventricle. It is the main structure of the epithalamus.

> The suprachiasmatic nucleus controls the release of melatonin from the pineal gland through a polysynaptic pathway that involves the paraventricular nucleus, intermediolateral cell column, and superior cervical ganglion. This sympathetic ganglion innervates the pineal gland and stimulates melatonin production. Light activates the suprachiasmatic nucleus, which in turn inhibits the paraventricular nucleus and, thus, melatonin secretion. As a consequence, melatonin secretion peaks during the night and is minimal during daytime.

- The hypothalamus is critical for thermoregulation, osmoregulation, regulation of immune responses, and the control of food intake, reproduction, biological rhythms (including the sleep-wake cycle), and the integrated response to stress.
- The endocrine output of the hypothalamus involves vascular connections with the pituitary gland.

Clinical Correlations

Disorders of the Hypothalamus

Lesions that affect the hypothalamus and surrounding structures can be encountered in all areas of medical practice because these lesions can affect endocrine, reproductive, visual, or homeostatic function (or a combination of these). Disorders of the hypothalamus are manifested by disturbances of thermoregulation, osmotic balance, endocrine function, feeding behavior, and state of alertness. For example, lesions of the preoptic area may produce hypothermia, hyperthermia, or poikilothermia (fluctuations in body temperature). Hypothalamic thermoregulatory disorders may be subclinical, chronic, or paroxysmal, associated or not with excessive sweating. Hypothalamic disorders may also affect osmoregulation. Failure of secretion of antidiuretic hormone produces *diabetes insipidus*, in which excessive quantities of dilute urine are excreted. Inappropriate secretion of antidiuretic hormone causes retention of water and can produce hyponatremia. Hypothalamic disease can also affect thirst or produce excessive loss of sodium in the urine. Hypothalamic lesions may affect feeding behavior. Lesions in the ventromedial portion of the hypothalamus may be associated with excessive feeding and obesity, whereas those in the lateral part of hypothalamus result in anorexia. Lesions in posterior lateral hypothalamus that include the hypocretin-synthesizing neurons produce narcolepsy, characterized by inappropriate episodes of daytime sleepiness.

If the hypothalamic control of pituitary function is impaired, then endocrine function is abnormal. Lesions of the pituitary stalk that interrupt hypothalamopituitary connections may decrease the secretion of all pituitary hormones except prolactin, which is increased. The explanation for this is that the hypothalamus secretes releasing factors for all pituitary hormones but also releases dopamine, which tonically inhibits the release of prolactin. Because the hypothalamus forms the lower third of the wall of the third ventricle, mass lesions of the hypothalamus may cause obstructive hydrocephalus. Hypothalamic lesions that impinge on the optic chiasm produce homonymous hemianopia, as described below.

Clinical Problem 16A.2.

A 10-year-old boy had become fat and listless during the last year. He also drank water and urinated excessively. For the last several months, he complained of headaches and experienced nausea and vomiting on arising in the morning. Neurologic examination showed an obese boy with papilledema and bitemporal hemianopia.

a. Where is the primary lesion?
b. What is the lesion?
c. What areas and functions of the hypothalamus are affected by this lesion?
d. What hormones are affected by this lesion?
e. How do you explain the papilledema and bitemporal hemianopia?

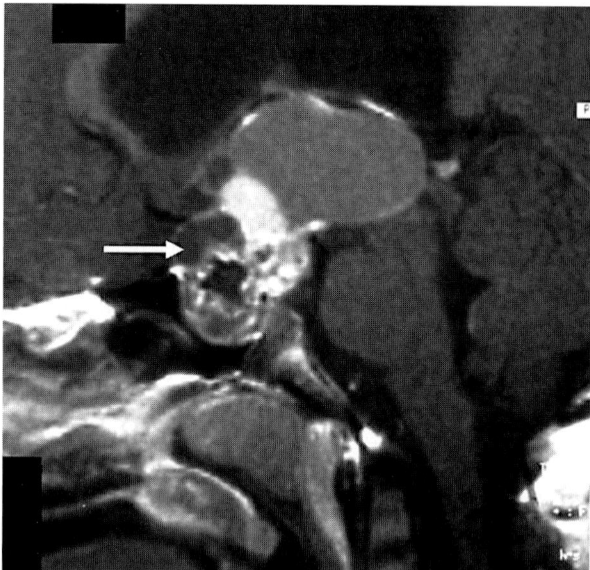

Fig. 16A.11. Sagittal magnetic resonance image (T1 sequence with gadolinium) showing a large tumor (*arrow*) in the pituitary region.

Endocrine Manifestations of Pituitary Lesions

Lesions of the pituitary gland cause endocrine disorders characterized by the increased or decreased secretion of pituitary hormones. Increased secretion is a manifestation of benign tumors affecting the anterior pituitary cells; these are called *pituitary adenomas*. Decreased secretion results from compression (by the adenoma), vascular or immune lesions, and impaired hypothalamic function (Fig. 16A.11).

A pituitary adenoma arises from anterior pituitary cells. These biologically active tumors are classified on the basis of specific secretory granules shown by electron microscopy and hormone content shown by immunostaining (immunoperoxidase or immunofluorescence). Tumors that are acidophilic on routine staining usually are associated with either the secretion of somatotropin or prolactin. Basophilic tumors produce corticotropin, thyrotrophin, or gonadotrophin. Although all the tumors mentioned contain densely granulated cells, similar hormonal activity may occur in less densely granulated tumors, called *chromophobe adenomas*. Many other chromophobe adenomas contain identifiable hormone granules, but there is no clinical evidence of trophic hormone excess. These tumors may grow to be enormous and produce clinical effects by compressing the normal pituitary gland and adjacent structures.

Examples of endocrine disorders include the following:

1. Prolactin. Unlike other pituitary hormones, prolactin is under tonic inhibitory control by dopaminergic neurons in the hypothalamus. Excessive prolactin secretion may result either from pituitary adenomas or lesions that interrupt the hypothalamopituitary connections. Prolactin activates milk secretion and inhibits sexual hormones; therefore, hyperprolactinemia causes *amenorrhea-galactorrhea* syndrome in women and hypogonadism and impotence in men. If a woman is prolactin deficient post partum, she will not be able to lactate.
2. Growth hormone. Increased secretion causes *gigantism* in children and *acromegaly* (enlargement of the face, hands, and feet) in adults. Decreased secretion during childhood causes dwarfism.
3. Corticotropin. Increased corticotropin secretion produces *Cushing syndrome*, which is due to excessive secretion of steroid hormones from the adrenal

cortex. Its features include obesity, hirsutism, vascular striae, hypertension, diabetes mellitus, and bone and muscle loss. Decreased secretion of ACTH results in hypoadrenalism, with generalized weakness, hypotension, and decreased tolerance to stress.

4. Thyroid-stimulating hormone. Decreased secretion results in *hypothyroidism*, with loss of hair, dry skin, slow pulse, loss of energy, mental apathy, decreased cold tolerance, and slow relaxation of deep tendon reflexes. Increased secretion of thyroid-stimulating hormone can cause enlargement of the thyroid gland (goiter) and *hyperthyroidism*.
5. Gonadotropic hormone. Decreased secretion produces amenorrhea and decreased libido, amenorrhea, or impotence. This is usually the result of the inhibitory effects of excessive prolactin secretion rather than being a primary deficit of gonadotrophin secretion.

Manifestations of the Involvement of Neighboring Structures

The three most common mass lesions of the hypothalamopituitary region are *pituitary adenoma*, *craniopharyngioma*, and *aneurysm* of the internal carotid artery. Craniopharyngioma arises from an embryonic remnant of Rathke pouch and is usually located in the region of the pituitary stalk or sella, near the hypothalamus and pituitary gland.

In addition to the clinical manifestations described above, mass lesions may produce symptoms or signs due to compression of neighboring structures, particularly the optic chiasm, cavernous sinus, third ventricle (in the case of the hypothalamus), and sella turcica (in the case of the pituitary). Involvement of the optic chiasm serves as an important localizing sign of lesions in this area. This causes a characteristic visual field defect, bitemporal hemianopia, that is due to the interruption of crossing fibers from the nasal portions of the retina (conveying input from the temporal portions of the visual field). Lateral expansion of a pituitary lesion or a lesion involving the internal carotid artery in the cavernous sinus can compress cranial nerves III, IV, and VI, and the opthalmic and maxillary divisions of cranial nerve V. The results are diplopia and loss of sensation over the forehead and cheek. Whereas a mass lesion in the hypothalamus may cause obstructive hydrocephalus, one in or near the sella can cause enlargement of the sella turcica or can erode its bony margins, which can be seen on radiographs of the skull.

- Lesions in the hypothalamopituitary region may compress the optic chiasm (producing bitemporal hemianopia) and the cavernous sinus.
- Hypothalamic lesions may cause obstructive hydrocephalus.
- Pituitary lesions can cause the sella turcica to enlarge.

The Visual System

The visual system transforms visual representations of the external world into a pattern of neural activity that the person can use. Its peripheral receptive structures are in the eye, and the central pathways are in the diencephalon and telencephalon. The eye is a peripheral receptor organ specialized to respond to visual stimuli. It has nonneural

Clinical Problem 16A.3.

A 30-year-old woman noted the onset of amenorrhea 1 year ago. In the last 6 months, she has tired easily, has not been able to tolerate stress or cold weather, and has lost weight. Physical examination showed a dull, apathetic, thin woman with low blood pressure, slow pulse, bitemporal hemianopia, and deep tendon reflexes with a slow relaxation phase.

a. Where is the primary lesion?
b. What structures are affected by the lesion?
c. Which lobe of the pituitary gland is involved?
d. What hormones are secreted by this lobe? What regulates these hormones?
e. Which hormones are affected in this patient?
f. What structures are near the pituitary gland?
g. How do you explain the visual symptoms?
h. What is the lesion?

components whose function is the transmission of light stimuli to the retina, which contains the receptors and neurons that respond to light stimuli.

Nonneural Structures of the Eye

Most of the nonneural structures of the eye are derivatives of embryonic ectoderm, but the muscles that control the eye are mesodermal in origin. The nonneural structures include the cornea, sclera, anterior chamber, iris, lens, and vitreous humor (Fig. 16A.12). The *cornea* is a transparent membrane that covers the anterior part of the eye and joins the opaque white sclera at the limbus. The *sclera* is a supporting tissue that covers the rest of the eyeball. The extraocular muscles attach to the sclera. The *iris* is a circular diaphragm with a central aperture, the *pupil*, through which light enters to reach the retina. The *ciliary body* supports the *lens*, a biconvex, transparent, elastic structure that accommodates for vision at varying distances. The *vitreous humor* is a transparent gelatinous material that separates the lens and retina and serves to hold both in place. The *choroid* lies between the sclera and the retina and functions to decrease the scatter of light inside the eye.

These nonneural structures transmit light rays and focus them on the retina. The iris opens or closes in response to varying intensities of light, thus controlling the illumination of the retina. The lens inverts the image. The configuration of the lens also changes to focus light rays from near or distant objects on the retina. The response to a near object is complex and includes convergence of the eyes, increased convexity of the lens (*accommodation*), and pupillary constriction. Accommodation is necessary for focusing the image on the retina.

- The nonneural peripheral structures of the eye consist of the cornea, sclera, iris, pupil, lens, and vitreous humor.
- The nonneural structures transmit light rays and focus them on the retina.

The Retina

The retina is an extension of the brain and performs the first stages of visual processing. It is derived from the embryonic optic vesicle, an evagination of the embryonic diencephalon (see Chapter 2). As the optic vesicle grows, it forms a two-layered cup, with the outer layer becoming the retinal pigment epithelium and the inner layer becoming the retina.

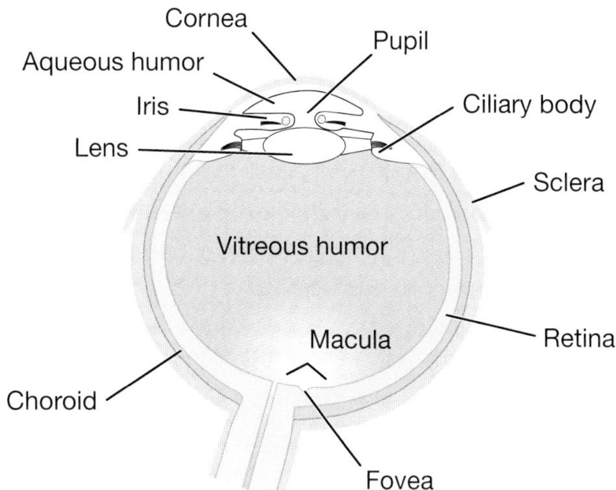

Fig. 16A.12. The nonneural structures of the eye form the anterior portion and outer coats. The retina and optic nerve are the neural components.

Histology

The main cell groups in the retina are the photoreceptor cells, bipolar cells, ganglion cells, horizontal cells, and amacrine cells. These cells are stratified in well-demarcated layers (Fig. 16A.13). From the outer to inner layer, they are the photoreceptor cell layer, outer nuclear layer, outer plexiform layer, inner nuclear layer, inner plexiform layer, and ganglion cell layer. Nuclear layers contain cell bodies, and plexiform layers contain dendrites and synapses. The photoreceptor cell layer is bound by the retinal pigment epithelium and Bruch membrane. The ganglion cell layer is the innermost layer and lies adjacent to the vitreous humor. The nerve fiber layer lies just inside the ganglion cell layer and is bound by the internal limiting membrane.

Light has to travel across the inner layers before reaching the photoreceptor cells in the outer layer. The photoreceptor cells include the *rods* and *cones*, which convert light into an electrical response. Photoreceptors consist of an outer segment containing a photosensitive pigment, an inner segment, a cell body located in the outer nuclear layer, and a synaptic terminal in the outer plexiform layer, where these cells synapse with bipolar cells and horizontal cells. The cell bodies of *bipolar cells* are in the inner nuclear layer. These cells convey information from the photoreceptors to the *ganglion cells* (ganglion cell layer). The synapses between the bipolar and ganglion cells are in the inner plexiform layer. Ganglion cell axons form the optic nerve, the output cells of the retina. The flow of information from photoreceptors to bipolar cells is regulated by *horizontal cells* at the level of the outer plexiform layer. The flow of information from bipolar cells to ganglion cells is regulated by *amacrine cells* at the level of the inner plexiform layer.

The thickness of the retina and its cell density vary from the central visual axis to the peripheral regions. The maximal density of cones is in the *macula lutea*, a specialized region at the posterior pole of the eye. The center of the macula, the *fovea centralis*, is responsible for sharpest visual acuity. At this level, unlike in peripheral retina, the overlying structures (bipolar cells, ganglion cells, and blood vessels) are swept to the side and light has an uninterrupted path to the cones. In addition, the receptor cells are packed together tightly and have nearly a one-to-one ratio with ganglion cells.

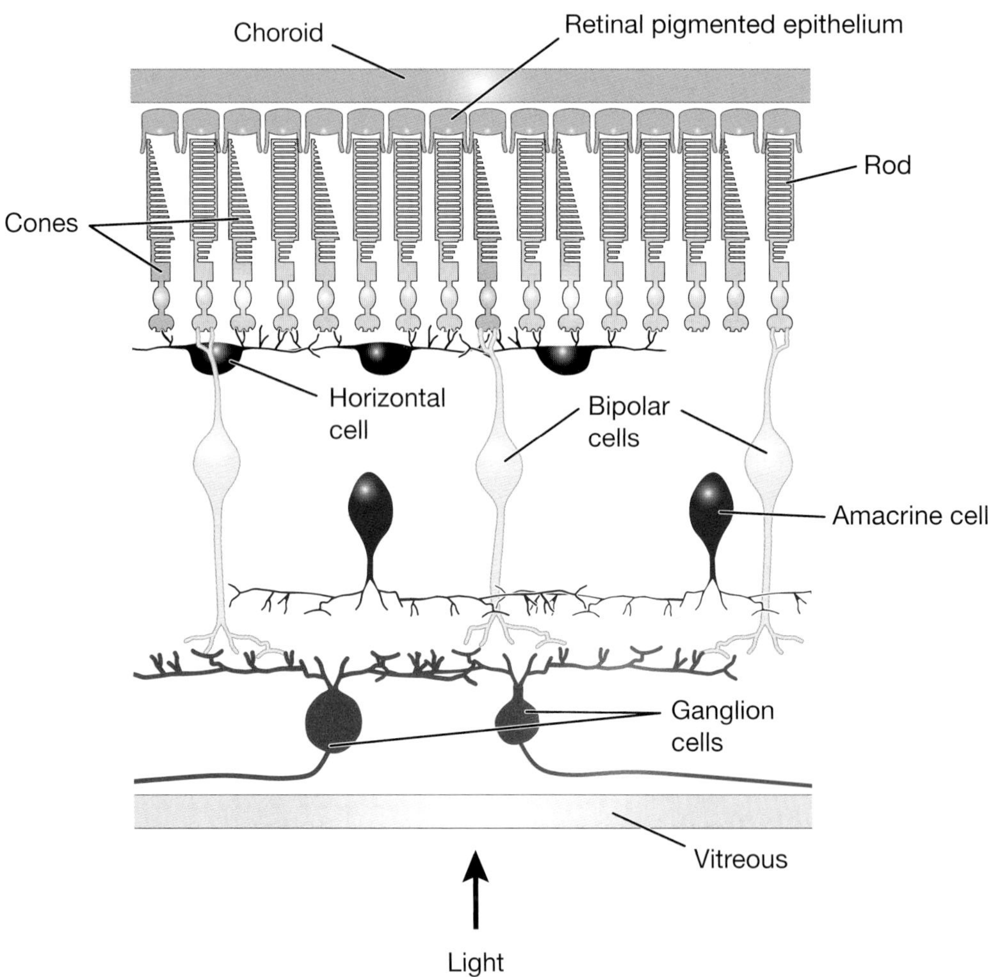

Fig. 16A.13. The main cell groups in the retina are the photoreceotor cells, bipolar cells, ganglion cells, horizontal cells, and amacrine cells. These cells are stratified in well-demarcated layers. The photoreceptor cell layer, the outermost layer, is bound by retinal pigmented epithelium. The ganglion cell layer, the innermost layer, is adjacent to the vitreous humor. Light has to travel across the inner layers to reach the photoreceptor cells in the outer layer.

Physiology

The outer segments of the rods and cones consist of membranous disks that contain *photopigment*, which is a protein, called *opsin*, bound to 1-*cis* retinal, a derivative of vitamin A. Rods contain the photopigment *rhodopsin*. They occur predominantly in the peripheral retina, are exquisitely sensitive to light, and are active in dim light, *scotopic vision*. Cones, in contrast, are concentrated in the fovea and are involved in vision at high levels of light, *photopic vision*, including color vision. Cones contain one of three different types of visual pigments (opsins) that absorb maximally at the red, green, or blue band of the spectrum.

> The red and green opsins are products of two genes located in tandem on chromosome X. Mutations that affect these genes produce X-linked color blindness.

The transduction of the light signal depends on interactions between the photons and the photopigment and leads to the closure of a cation channel in the photoreceptor cells. In darkness, photoreceptor cells are depolarized by a persistent influx of sodium and calcium. This phenomenon, called *dark current*, allows the tonic release of glutamate at the synapses between photoreceptors and bipolar cells. The dark current is turned off by light, decreasing the release of glutamate at the photoreceptor–bipolar cell synapse.

The decrease in intracellular calcium initiated by light triggers various mechanisms that block activation of rhodopsin, interrupting the light signal. This is referred to as *photoreceptor adaptation*. Because bright light blocks regeneration of rhodopsin, vision is reduced for 10 to 15 minutes after a person enters a dark room. As rhodopsin is regenerated in the rods, the eye becomes adapted to light.

> The dark current depends on opening of a cyclic guanosine monophosphate (cGMP)-gated cation channel that is open in darkness. The tonically released glutamate from the photoreceptors exerts two opposite effects on two types of bipolar cells: it inhibits the so-called on-bipolar cells and activates the off-bipolar cells. Light produces isomerization of the retinal; this results in activation of rhodopsin to metarhodopsin. Activated metarhodopsin is a G protein-coupled receptor coupled to the G protein called transducin. Transducin activates a cGMP phosphodiesterase, which decreases the level of cGMP and closes the cGMP-gated cation channel in photoreceptors. Light-induced hyperpolarization of photoreceptors transiently interrupts the tonic release of glutamate from these cells.

The signal from the cones and rods is conveyed by bipolar cells to the ganglion cells. The receptive field of a ganglion cell is a circular area on the retina. According to the response to light, ganglion cells are subdivided into *on-center cells*, which respond best to a small spot of light shined on a field surrounded by darkness, and *off-center cells*, which respond to reduced brightness of a small region relative to its surround. Thus, the visual system is designed to respond to contrast rather than to absolute light intensity. Visual acuity depends on a mechanism of lateral inhibition in which the light stimulus activates only a small group of photoreceptors and, thus, bipolar and ganglion cells, while the surrounding cells are inhibited. This mechanism of lateral inhibition is mediated by *horizontal cells*.

The two types of bipolar cells are *on-bipolar cells* and *off-bipolar cells*. On-bipolar cells are activated by light and, in turn, activate on-center ganglion cells. Off-bipolar cells are active during darkness and excite off-center ganglion cells. During daylight, cones directly activate the on-bipolar–ganglion cell pathway. As light intensity decreases, the rods become active. During dim light, the rods activate the on-bipolar cells through *AII amacrine cells*.

According to the response to visual stimuli, ganglion cells are subdivided into different types. P-type ganglion cells receive input from a few cones, have high spatial resolution, and can respond to colors. In contrast, M-type cells collect input from several rods and have poor spatial resolution but high sensitivity to dim light and movement. The ganglion cell axons form the optic nerve (cranial nerve II).

- **The retina consists of photoreceptors, bipolar cells, and ganglion cells whose activity is controlled by horizontal cells and amacrine cells.**

- Rods contain rhodopsin and are used for vision under dim light (scotopic vision); cones are active at high levels of light (photopic vision) and are involved in color vision.
- Visual acuity is greatest in the central fovea, where the density of cones is greatest, and decreases in the peripheral regions.
- Visual information is transmitted by the photoreceptor–bipolar cell–ganglion cell pathway in the retina.
- The axons of the retinal ganglion cells form the optic nerve.

Visual Pathways

The visual structures within the cranial cavity at the supratentorial level include the optic nerve and optic chiasm, the optic tracts, and the lateral geniculate nuclei in the diencephalon and the optic radiations and occipital cortex in the telencephalon (Fig. 16A.14).

Diencephalic Structures

The axons of ganglion cells in the retina converge at the optic disc, become myelinated, and then leave the back of the eye through the lamina cribrosa, forming the optic nerve. The optic nerve leaves the orbit through the *optic canal* and enters the cranial cavity. Although the optic nerve is considered a cranial nerve (cranial nerve II), it is actually a nerve tract, similar to other tracts in the central nervous system, and consists of axons with myelin sheaths formed by oligodendroglia cells rather than by Schwann cells. Thus, diseases such as multiple sclerosis that affect the myelin of the central nervous system produce similar lesions in the optic nerve.

After the optic nerves pass through the optic canals, they unite to form the *optic chiasm*, beyond which the axons continue as the *optic tracts*. Within the chiasm, the optic fibers partially decussate: the fibers from the nasal half of each retina cross to the opposite side and those from the temporal half of each retina remain uncrossed. As the fibers from the inferior nasal retina cross, they loop forward a short distance into the opposite optic nerve. In binocular vision, each visual field, right and left, is projected upon one-half of both right and left retinas. Thus, the images of objects in the right field of vision are projected on the right nasal and left temporal halves of the two retinas. In the chiasm, the fibers from these two retinal segments are combined to form the left optic tract, which then represents the complete right field of vision. By this arrangement, the whole right visual field is projected upon the left hemisphere, and the left visual field is projected upon the right hemisphere (Fig. 16A.14).

- The optic nerve axons from the nasal half of each retina (conveying input from the temporal visual field) decussate in the optic chiasm.

After the partial decussation in the optic chiasm, the optic fibers, now called the *optic tracts*, continue laterally and posteriorly to terminate in the *lateral geniculate body* (or nucleus) in the thalamus. Axons from the lateral geniculate nucleus form the *geniculocalcarine tract*, which terminates in the primary visual cortex. The different layers of the lateral geniculate body project to different layers in the visual cortex.

From the initial stages in the retina, the visual pathway is segregated into various subsystems involved in the analysis of different aspects of an image. P-type retinal ganglion cells respond primarily to shapes and color and project to the dorsal, or *parvicellular* (*P*), laminae of the lateral geniculate body. M-type ganglion cells respond primarily to the movement of the object and project to the ventral, or *magnicellular* (*M*), laminae of the lateral geniculate body. These different laminae project to different portions of the primary visual cortex.

A small group of ganglion cells that receive input from the blue cones project to the koniocellular laminae intercalated between the parvicellular and magnicellular laminae.

- Each optic tract transmits information from the contralateral visual field to the corresponding lateral geniculate body.
- Information about either object color and form or object position and movement is conveyed over parallel pathways that originate from different types of ganglion cells and terminate in different layers of the lateral geniculate body.

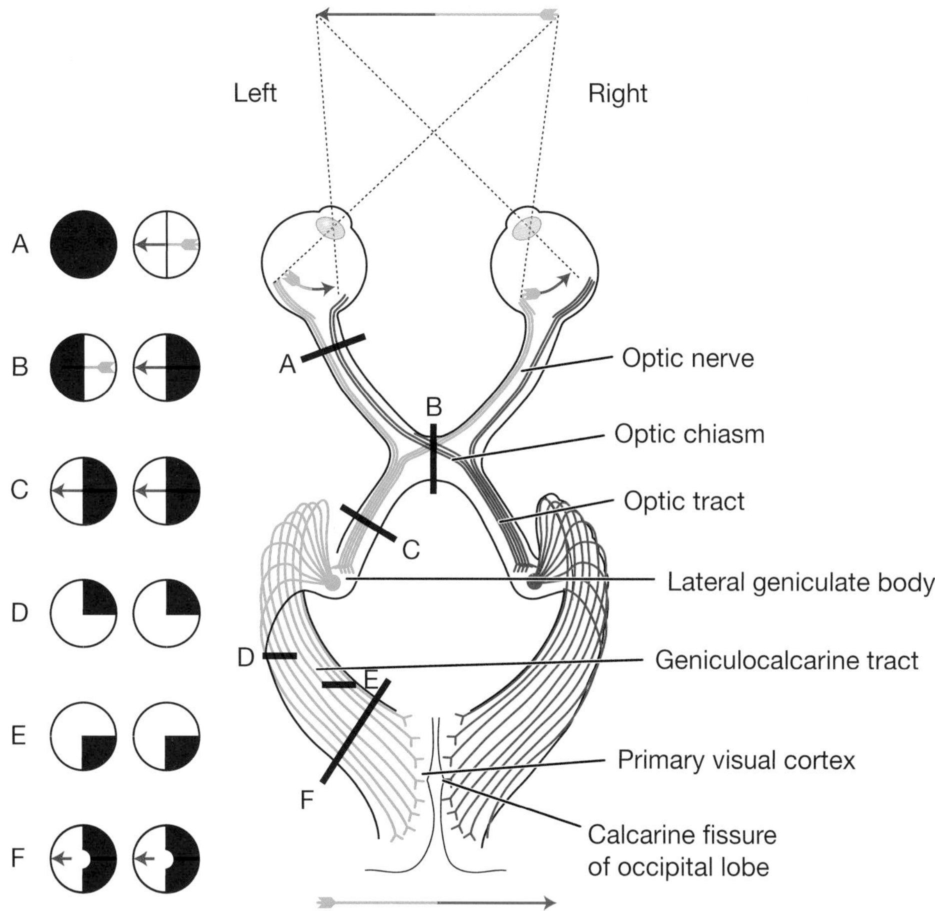

Fig. 16A.14. Visual pathway as seen from the base of the brain. The visual impulses from the right half of the visual field project to the left half of each retina and to the left occipital lobe. On the left are the visual field defects (black areas) produced by lesions affecting the optic nerve (A), optic chiasm (B), optic tract (C), optic radiation in the temporal lobe (D), optic radiation in the parietal lobe (E), and occipital cortex (F).

The majority of the optic tract axons synapse in the lateral geniculate body, which relays visual information to the visual cortex; however, a few fibers leave the optic tract before it reaches the thalamus. Some of these axons terminate in the *superior colliculus*, which is involved in reflex saccadic eye movements and limb movement during orientation responses to external stimuli. The superior colliculus also projects to the *pulvinar* of the thalamus, which is connected with areas of the posterior parietal cortex involved in visual attention. Other optic tract axons synapse in the pretectal nuclei (located just rostral to the superior colliculi). These nuclei, through the Edinger-Westphal parasympathetic nuclei and oculomotor nerves (cranial nerve III), mediate the pupillary *light reflex* (pupillary constriction). Ganglion cell axons also project to the suprachiasmatic nucleus by way of the *retinohypothalamic tract*. This pathway is essential for the entrainment of circadian rhythms by the light–dark cycle.

A small group of special ganglion cells is activated directly by light, independently of the photoreceptor–bipolar cell pathway. These photoreceptive ganglion cells contain a pigment called *melanopsin* and project directly to the suprachiasmatic nucleus.

- The retina projects to the superior colliculus for orienting responses and visual attention, to the pretectal nucleus for the light reflex, and to the suprachiasmatic nucleus for entrainment of circadian rhythms.

Telencephalic Structures

The geniculocalcarine tract arises from the lateral geniculate body, passes through the retrolenticular portion of the internal capsule, and forms the *optic radiation*. These axons terminate in the *calcarine cortex* of the occipital lobe, which is the primary visual area. This area is also referred to as striate cortex because of its morphology. The upper, or dorsal, fibers of the optic radiations convey information from the lower half of the contralateral visual field, course posteriorly in the parietal lobe, and terminate in the superior calcarine cortex. The lower, or ventral, fibers convey information from the upper half of the contralateral visual field, loop anteriorly and laterally around the temporal horn in the temporal lobe (Meyer loop), and then turn posteriorly to end in the inferior calcarine cortex (Fig. 16A.15).

- The optic radiation arises from the lateral geniculate nucleus and travels through the parietal and temporal lobes to the primary visual cortex in the occipital lobe.
- The visual images impinging on the retina are inverted so that the superior part of the visual field projects to the inferior half of the retina and the inferior visual field projects to the superior half of the retina.
- Fibers from the upper half of the retina form the superior part of the optic radiations, which run in the parietal lobe and terminate in the superior calcarine cortex.
- Fibers from the lower half of the retina form the inferior part of the optic radiations, which run in the temporal lobe and terminate in the inferior calcarine cortex.

The calcarine cortex is topographically organized, with the superior half of the visual field represented in the inferior calcarine cortex and the inferior visual field represented in the superior calcarine cortex (Fig. 16A.16). In addition, most of the posterior portion of the occipital pole is concerned primarily with macular (central) vision, with the more anterior part of visual cortex devoted to peripheral vision.

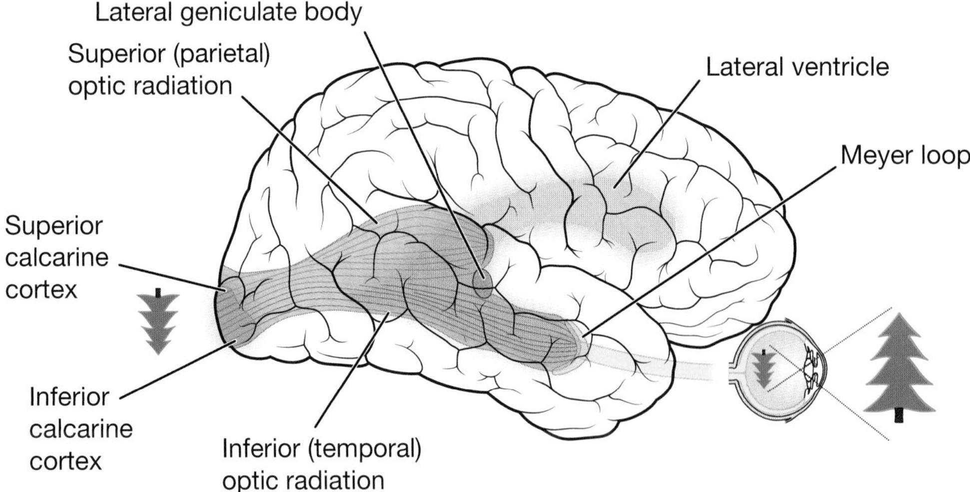

Fig. 16A.15. The course of the superior and inferior optic radiations. Fibers from the upper part of the retina (which receives input from the inferior visual field) form the superior optic radiation (located in the parietal lobe) and terminate in the superior calcarine cortex. Fibers from the inferior part of the retina (which receives input from the superior visual field) form the inferior optic radiation (located in the temporal lobe) and terminate in the inferior calcarine cortex.

- The visual images impinging on the retina are inverted so that the superior visual field projects to the inferior part of the retina and the inferior visual field projects to the superior part of the retina.
- The superior part of the visual field projects to the inferior calcarine cortex, and the inferior visual field projects to the superior calcarine cortex.
- The posterior part of the occipital pole is concerned with central vision.
- The anterior part of the visual cortex is concerned with peripheral vision.

The visual submodalities are segregated in calcarine cortex. The different layers of the lateral geniculate nucleus project to different layers of the calcarine cortex. Neurons of the different layers project to different *visual association areas* (extrastriate cortex). Cortical visual processing is discussed in Part B of this chapter. Briefly, however, neurons of primary visual (calcarine) cortex that receive input primarily from the magnicellular (M) layers of the lateral geniculate nucleus and respond to the position and motion of the object project to the visual association areas in the posterior parietal cortex. This constitutes the *dorsal visual stream*, which is involved in processing the position and motion of the object in space ("where") to generate appropriate eye and limb movements toward the object. In contrast, neurons in the primary visual cortex that receive input from the parvicellular (P) layers of the lateral geniculate nucleus and respond to the color and shape of the object project to visual association areas in the inferior temporal cortex. This constitutes the *ventral visual stream*, which is involved in processing of the form and color ("what") of the object required for recognizing and naming the object. Information conveyed by the dorsal and visual streams is eventually integrated at a higher level of processing to obtain an integrated perception of the visual scene.

- The primary visual cortex projects to visual association areas of the posterior parietal cortex for analysis of the location and motion of the object required to guide movements.
- The primary visual cortex projects to visual association areas of the inferior temporal cortex for analysis of the color and form of the object required for recognizing and naming the object.

Clinical Correlations

Testing of the Visual System

Visual system testing requires attention to four aspects of visual function: the appearance of the nonneural components of the eye, visual acuity, visual field, and

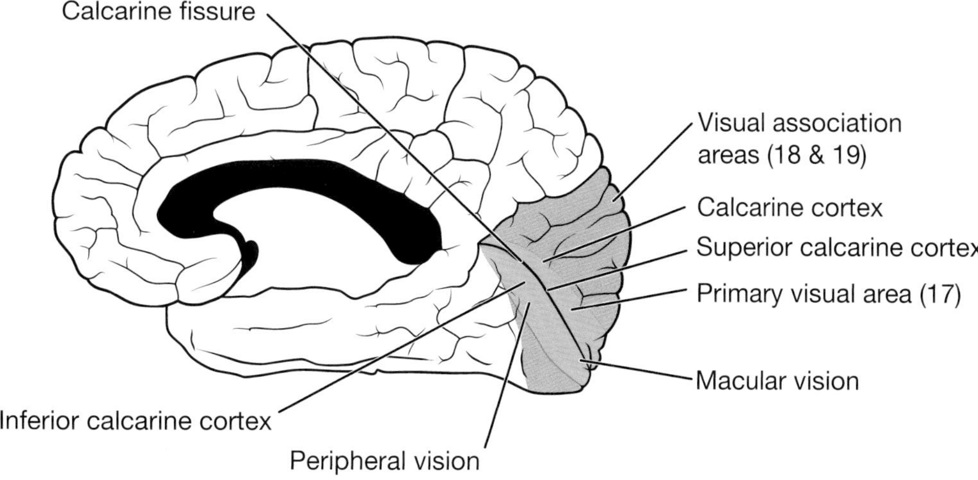

Fig. 16A.16. Medial aspect of the occipital lobe showing the superior and inferior calcarine cortices separated by the calcarine fissure, located in the primary visual area (V1, area 17, or striate cortex), and the visual association areas (areas 18 and 19, or peristriate cortex).

ophthalmoscopic examination of the optic fundus. The nonneural structures are examined by direct inspection of the external appearance and by visualization of internal features, such as the lens, with the ophthalmoscope. Tests of the extraocular muscles are described in Chapter 15.

The resolving power of vision depends on the ability of the retina to distinguish a separation between two images, and it is measured as *visual acuity*. Visual acuity is tested separately in each eye for near and distant vision. A patient who wears glasses should be tested with and without the glasses. Eye charts (the Snellen chart) are available that are read at fixed distances. The smallest print size the patient can read is compared with what a person with normal vision can read at the same distance, and acuity is reported as a comparison of these numbers. For example, visual acuity of 20/200 means that the patient can read at 20 feet what a person with normal vision can read at 200 feet. With major visual loss, acuity can be tested with large objects such as fingers or hands.

The examination of the *visual fields* allows the site of visual loss to be localized in the visual pathways (Fig. 16A.14). Visual fields are tested by confrontation in which the examiner faces the patient and compares his or her visual field with the patient's. Each eye is tested separately by having the patient look straight ahead at the examiner's nose while a target (usually a finger) is moved in the field of vision. Two methods of testing can be used. In one, a finger is wiggled and gradually brought in from the periphery in all four quadrants of the visual field to determine where it is first seen. In the second, one to four fingers are briefly extended in each of the four quadrants, and the patient is asked to identify the number of fingers shown. With uncooperative patients or those who cannot respond directly, the field can be tested grossly by swiftly moving the hand toward the eye from one direction and looking for defensive blinking. Very precise plots of the visual field can be obtained with a perimeter or tangent screen.

An integral part of the evaluation of the visual system is the assessment of the *pupillary light reflex*. As mentioned in Chapters 9 and 15, the afferent arm of this reflex is the optic nerve. The fibers from each retina partially decussate in the optic chiasm and enter the optic tracts, but instead of going to the lateral geniculate nucleus, they proceed through the brachium of the superior colliculus to the pretectal area. This area contains neurons that project bilaterally to the Edinger-Westphal nucleus. The Edinger-Westphal nuclei contain the cell bodies of the preganglionic parasympathetic fibers that travel in cranial nerve III and synapse postganglionic neurons in the ciliary ganglion to elicit pupillary constriction. The normal pupil reacts briskly when light is shone on the ipsilateral retina (direct reflex) and, because of the partial decussation of the optic pathways at the levels of the optic chiasm and pretectal area, the contralateral pupil also constricts (consensual reflex). Unilateral lesions of the optic nerve do not produce anisocoria (unequal pupils) but impair both the direct and consensual light response when the affected eye is tested. In this situation, moving the light source rapidly from the normal eye (with a strong direct and consensual light reflex) to the affected eye (with diminished reflex) can make it appear that the pupil actually dilates in response to light. Instead, the pupil moves to a less constricted state because of decreased detection of light in the eye with optic nerve disease. Both pupils again constrict briskly when the light source is moved back to the eye with a normal optic nerve. This phenomenon can be demonstrated repeatedly by moving the light source back and forth from the affected to the unaffected eye. This response identifies an *afferent pupillary defect* that indicates a lesion in the ipsilateral optic nerve.

Both *optic fundi* should be examined routinely with an ophthalmoscope as part of a neurologic examination. The optic disc, blood vessels, and retina should be examined. The optic disc should be examined for any variation in its usual yellow color and flat appearance with distinct margins. In papilledema, the margins are blurred and elevated; in optic atrophy, the disc is pale. The arteriolar caliber and appearance and the venous pulsation should be examined. Areas of exudates, hemorrhage, and abnormal pigmentation may be seen in the retina.

A low-amplitude, surface-positive electrical potential can be recorded over the occipital areas in response to a visual stimulus. This is the *visual evoked potential*. The best stimulus for eliciting a consistent visual evoked response is a black and white checkerboard pattern with rapid reversal of the black and white checks. With amplification and computer averaging of a hundred or more successive responses, the evoked response is clearly distinguished from random background electroencephalographic activity (Fig. 16A.17). The major surface-positive potential occurs approximately 100 milliseconds after the stimulus. A latency of the response prolonged beyond the upper limit of normal suggests delayed conduction in the visual pathway of that eye.

Disorders of the visual system produce specific, readily identifiable visual defects that depend on the part of the visual system damaged. Knowledge of these defects permits precise localization of many lesions involving the visual system. Damage may occur at any site along the visual pathways.

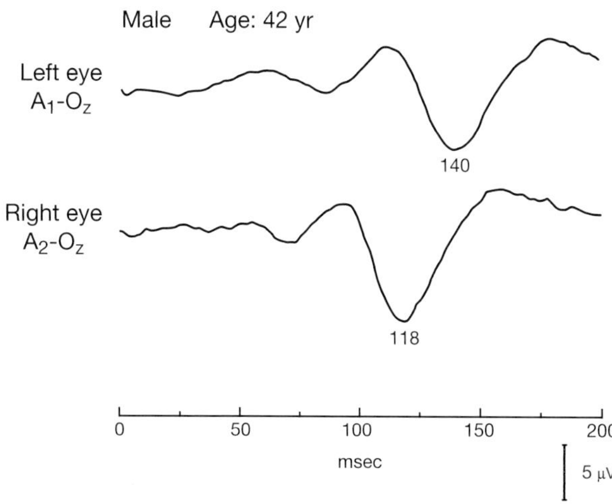

Fig. 16A.17. Visual evoked response to checker board pattern reversal stimuli in a 42-year-old man with multiple sclerosis. Stimulation of the left eye (*top tracing*) shows an abnormal peak-positive response with a latency of 140 milliseconds due to demyelination of the optic nerve. Stimulation of the right eye (*bottom tracing*) shows a normal response with a latency of 118 milliseconds. Responses represent an average of 128 responses. (Recording electrodes: A1, left ear; A2, right ear; Oz, midline occipital).

Eye Disease

Most visual system disorders are due to abnormalities in the nonneural structures of the eye and are abnormalities in visual acuity from the inability to focus visual images properly. Common examples are nearsightedness (*myopia*) and farsightedness (*hypermetropia*), distortion of light rays by diseases of the cornea or lens (*cataract*), and increased pressure within the eye (*glaucoma*). Each of these causes monocular visual loss (unless both eyes are involved) and can be identified by tests of visual acuity and direct inspection of the eye.

Retinal Disease

Disorders of the retina also cause monocular visual loss, often with reduced visual acuity. Both *retinal detachment* and *retinal degeneration* are associated with progressive loss of vision. A focal lesion of the retina causes a *scotoma*, or blind spot. Vascular diseases involving the retina are also reflected in visible changes in the retinal arteries with arteriosclerosis, small emboli, or hemorrhages. A transient loss of vision in one eye due to decreased blood supply is called *amaurosis fugax* (see Chapter 12). In elderly persons, it usually is the result of atherosclerotic disease in the ipsilateral internal carotid artery. Vitamin A deficiency causes a deficiency of retinene (a precursor of retinal) and thus rhodopsin, which results in *night blindness*, the inability to see in the dark. Similar symptoms occur with selective degeneration of the rods, as in paraneoplastic retinal degeneration.

- Amaurosis fugax is the transient loss of vision in one eye due to decreased blood supply.

Optic Nerve Disease

Focal lesions may involve a single optic nerve to produce a *negative scotoma*, in which part of the visual world is missing. Some disorders of the optic nerve head may be seen with the ophthalmoscope. *Optic neuritis* is an inflammation of the optic nerve and may be associated with blurring of the optic disc margin and decreased visual acuity. Patients with optic neuritis have impaired color vision (especially for red) and an impaired light reflex, both direct and consensual, when light is shone on the affected eye. In some cases, optic nerve involvement is detected only by the presence of an afferent pupillary defect. An important cause of optic neuritis is demyelinating disease, for example, multiple sclerosis. The optic nerve also can be affected by ischemic lesions that produce *ischemic optic neuropathy*, as in arteritis or atherosclerosis. *Papilledema*, a sign of increased intracranial pressure, is seen as swelling and elevation of the optic disc, with blurring of the disc margin. *Optic atrophy* is seen as a pale optic disc and occurs with chronic compressive, inflammatory, or degenerative disease of the retina or nerve (see Chapter 7).

- Lesions that involve the optic nerve include optic neuritis, ischemic optic neuropathy, papilledema, and optic atrophy.
- Optic neuritis is an inflammation of the optic nerve and frequently occurs in demyelinating disease.
- Ischemic optic neuropathy occurs with vasculitis or atherosclerosis.
- Papilledema is a sign of increased intracranial pressure.
- Optic atrophy occurs with degenerative diseases or as a consequence of chronic compression or inflammation.

Clinical Problem 16A.4.

A 23-year-old secretary developed visual blurring one morning while working on a computer. She noticed that the colors looked "washed-out." The next day her vision was worse, and she started complaining of pain behind the right eye. Visual testing showed that her visual acuity was 20/20 in the left eye and 20/400 in the right eye. Her pupils were symmetrical and both reacted to light, although the right pupil did not react as briskly. When the doctor swung the light between the two eyes, the right eye appeared to transiently dilate. On ophthalmoscopic examination, the optic fundus was normal.

a. What is the likely location of the lesion?
b. How do you explain the pupillary findings?
c. Magnetic resonance imaging of the patient's head showed multiple white matter lesions in the corpus callosum, periventricular region, and middle cerebellar peduncle. For the patient described here, what is the significance of these findings?
d. What abnormality would you expect in the visual evoked responses?

Optic Chiasm

Lesions of the optic chiasm cause several kinds of defects. Most commonly, the crossing fibers from the nasal portions of the retina are involved, with consequent loss of the two temporal fields of vision (*bitemporal hemianopia*). Rarely, both lateral angles of the chiasm are compressed; in these cases, the nondecussating fibers from the temporal retinas are affected, and the result is loss of the nasal visual fields (*binasal hemianopia*) (Fig. 16A.14).

Optic Tract and Optic Radiations

Lesions that affect the optic tract, lateral geniculate body, or optic radiations on one side produce *homonymous* defects in the opposite visual field. For example, a lesion of the optic tract or optic radiation on the right side produces a homonymous field defect in the left visual field of both eyes. Complete destruction of the optic tract or optic radiation on one side produces a complete *homonymous hemianopia*, that is, complete loss of vision in the opposite half of the visual field of each eye. A lesion in the temporal lobe on one side destroys the fibers running in the lower portion of the optic radiation, causing a *superior quadrantic field defect*, that is, loss of vision in the superior quadrant of the visual fields of the opposite side ("a pie in the sky"). A lesion in the parietal lobe destroys the superior optic radiations and produces an *inferior quadrantic field defect*, that is, loss of vision in the inferior visual fields of the opposite side.

- Lesions involving the optic tract, the lateral geniculate body, or the optic radiation on one side produce a homonymous defect in the opposite visual field.
- Lesions affecting the optic tract, the lateral geniculate body, or the optic radiation produce homonymous defects in the opposite visual field.
- A lesion of the optic radiation in the temporal lobe on one side can produce a superior quadrantic field defect.
- A lesion of the optic radiation in the parietal lobe on one side can produce an inferior quadrantic field defect.

Axons mediating the pupillary light reflex and other visual reflexes leave the optic tract at or before the lateral

Clinical Problem 16A.5.

What type of visual field defect might be expected in each of the following clinical situations?

a. A 47-year-old woman with a large tumor in the pituitary region
b. An 81-year-old man with hypertension who had an occlusion in a perforating branch of the right posterior cerebral artery
c. A 44-year-old woman with a right parietal lobe tumor
d. A 14-year-old boy with an abscess of the left temporal lobe after a chronic infection of the left middle ear

geniculate nucleus to terminate in the pretectal area. Therefore, unlike optic tract lesions, optic radiation lesions spare the pupillary light reflex.

Occipital Lobe

Lesions that affect the visual cortex in the occipital lobe on one side also cause homonymous loss of vision in the contralateral visual field. Because the visual fibers are topographically ordered in the occipital lobe, lesions here cause *congruent* visual field defects, that is, exactly the same loss in the fields of the two eyes. Bilateral destruction of the occipital lobes produces *cortical blindness*. In some cases, visual loss is denied by these patients but some perception of movement remains (*blindsight*).

- Lesions that affect the visual cortex and occipital lobe on one side cause a homonymous loss of vision in the contralateral visual field.
- Bilateral destruction of the occipital lobe produces a form of blindness in which visual loss may be denied but some perception of movement is preserved.

Disorders of occipital cortex can also be associated with subjective transient anomalies of vision such as scintillating scotomata, visual hallucinations, and illusions. These are described in Chapter 16B.

Additional Reading

Benarroch EE. Paraventricular nucleus, stress response, and cardiovascular disease. Clin Auton Res. 2005;15:254-263.

Boulant JA. Role of the preoptic-anterior hypothalamus in thermoregulation and fever. Clin Infect Dis. 2000;31 Suppl 5:S157-S161.

McCormick DA. Neurotransmitter actions in the thalamus and cerebral cortex and their role in neuromodulation of thalamocortical activity. Prog Neurobiol. 1992;39:337-388.

Saper CB. Hypothalamus. In: Paxinos G, editor. The human nervous system. Philadelphia: Elsevier; 2003. pp. 389-414.

Chapter 16
Part B

The Supratentorial Level
Telencephalon

Objectives

1. List the components of the cerebral hemispheres.
2. Localize the limbic, paralimbic, and neocortical areas of the cerebral cortex.
3. Describe the basic connectivity among primary, association, paralimbic, and limbic areas of the cerebral cortex.
4. Describe columnar organization, parallel processing of information, and plasticity of the cerebral cortex.
5. Define projection fibers, commissural fibers, and association fibers.
6. Locate the internal capsule on a gross specimen, and describe what occurs with a lesion of the internal capsule.
7. Identify the components of the basal ganglia on a brain specimen, a diagram, and a magnetic resonance image of the brain and describe their main connections.
8. Localize the amygdala, anterior cingulate cortex, and orbitofrontal cortex, and describe their basic connections and function.
9. Localize the hippocampus, entorhinal cortex, and parahippocampal region, and describe their basic connectivity.
10. Describe the role of the hippocampus and parahippocampal region in memory. Define anterograde and retrograde amnesia.
11. List the structures involved with olfaction, and provide examples of lesions affecting these structures.
12. Localize on a diagram or brain specimen and describe the functions of the lateral prefrontal, orbitofrontal, lateral premotor, and supplementary motor cortices; the frontal eye fields; Broca area; primary somatosensory cortex; primary visual cortex; primary auditory cortex; Wernicke area; posterior parietal cortex; and inferior occipitotemporal cortex.
13. Describe cortical sensory loss. Define agnosia, and describe its various types and the cortical lesions producing the different types of somatosensory, visual, and auditory agnosia.
14. Define apraxia. Localize the lesions producing ideomotor apraxia, dressing apraxia, constructional apraxia, and oculomotor apraxia.
15. Define aphasia and its types, and localize the lesion that produces each type. Define motor speech apraxia.
16. Define dementia, confusional state, and mental retardation.
17. Differentiate partial seizures from generalized seizures.
18. Describe absence seizures and generalized tonic-clonic seizures.
19. Given the clinical manifestations of a partial seizure, localize the site of origin of the seizure.
20. List the deficits produced by lesions affecting each of the following: the frontal, parietal, occipital, and temporal lobes.

Introduction

The supratentorial level consists of two main anatomical regions: the diencephalon and the telencephalon. The diencephalon consists of the thalamus, hypothalamus, optic nerves, pituitary gland, and pineal gland. The visual system includes components of the diencephalon and telencephalon. The anatomy, physiology, and clinical correlations of lesions affecting the diencephalon and visual pathways are described in Chapter 16A.

The telencephalon forms the cerebral hemispheres, which consist of the cerebral cortex, basal ganglia, and subcortical white matter tracts that interconnect areas of the cerebral cortex with one another and with the basal ganglia, thalamus, brainstem, and spinal cord (Fig. 16B.1).

The cerebral cortex contains projection neurons and local interneurons. The phylogenetically older portions of the cerebral cortex occupy the medial portion of the cerebral hemispheres and are components of the so-called limbic system. They include the amygdala and hippocampal formation, which have a critical role in emotion and memory. The olfactory system is intimately related to these limbic structures. The phylogenetically newer components of the cerebral cortex constitute the neocortex, which occupies the lateral aspect of the cerebral hemispheres. The neocortex includes most of the frontal, parietal, temporal, occipital, and insular lobes and is involved in the processing of sensory information, object recognition, motor programing and control, language, attention, decision making, and control of behavior. Connecting the limbic areas with the neocortex are paralimbic areas, located on the medial part of the hemispheres. Normal function of the cerebral cortex depends on interactions of different cortical areas with each other and the basal ganglia through the thalamus. This chapter

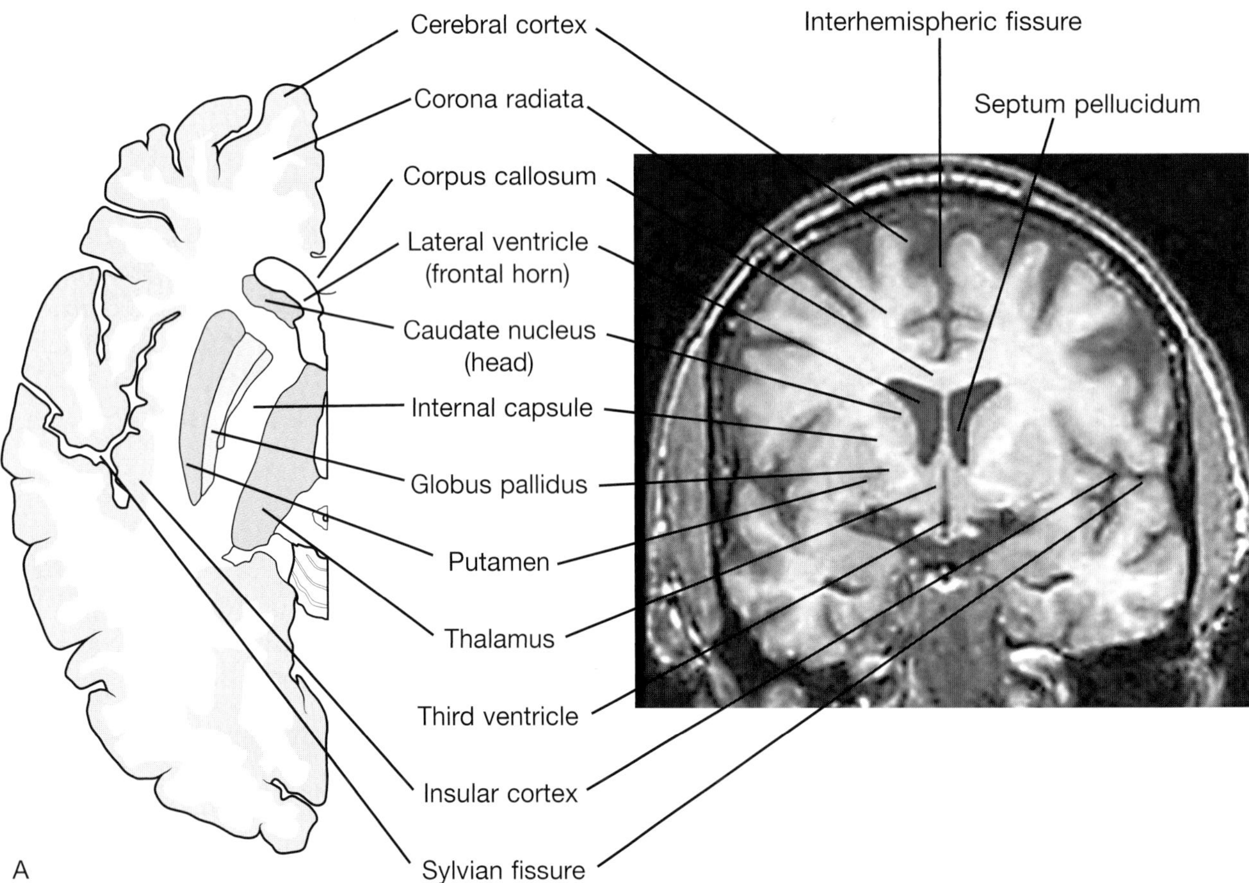

Fig. 16B.1. Main structures of the telencephalon. *A*, Diagram of an axial section (*left*) and a coronal T1-weighted magnetic resonance image (*right*). *B*, Diagram (*left*) and T2-weighted magnetic resonance image (*right*) of an axial section.

discusses the anatomy, physiology, and clinical correlates of these telencephalic areas.

Overview

The telencephalon arises from lateral evaginations of the most rostral portion of the embryonic neural tube (prosencephalon) and gives rise to the cerebral hemispheres. The two cerebral hemispheres fill most of the cranial cavity above the tentorium cerebelli and are separated by the falx cerebri. Each cerebral hemisphere consists of cerebral cortex, subcortical white matter, and basal ganglia, as well as the thalamus (a diencephalic structure) (Fig. 16B.1). The outermost layer of the cerebral hemispheres is the *cerebral cortex*, which contains neurons that have migrated to this location during embryonic development. These neurons form a thin mantle of gray matter that covers the outer surface of the cerebral hemispheres, forming the gyri of the brain. The *subcortical white matter* is a dense collection of axons that connect areas within the cerebral hemispheres with each other and with other areas of the central nervous system. Immediately adjacent to the ventricles, near the thalamus, are the *basal ganglia* (or more properly, basal nuclei). The ventral portion of the telencephalon constitutes the *basal forebrain*, which provides widespread input to the cerebral cortex and is intimately connected with the limbic system.

Two main sulci, the *central sulcus* and *sylvian fissure*, divide each cerebral hemisphere into frontal, parietal, occipital, and temporal lobes (Fig. 16B.2). The frontal lobe is anterior to the central sulcus, and the parietal and occipital lobes are posterior to it. The sylvian fissure separates the temporal lobe from the frontal and parietal lobes. The insular lobe is buried in the sylvian fissure, being covered by the frontal and parietal opercula and the temporal lobe (Fig. 16B.1). The *frontal lobe* has executive and

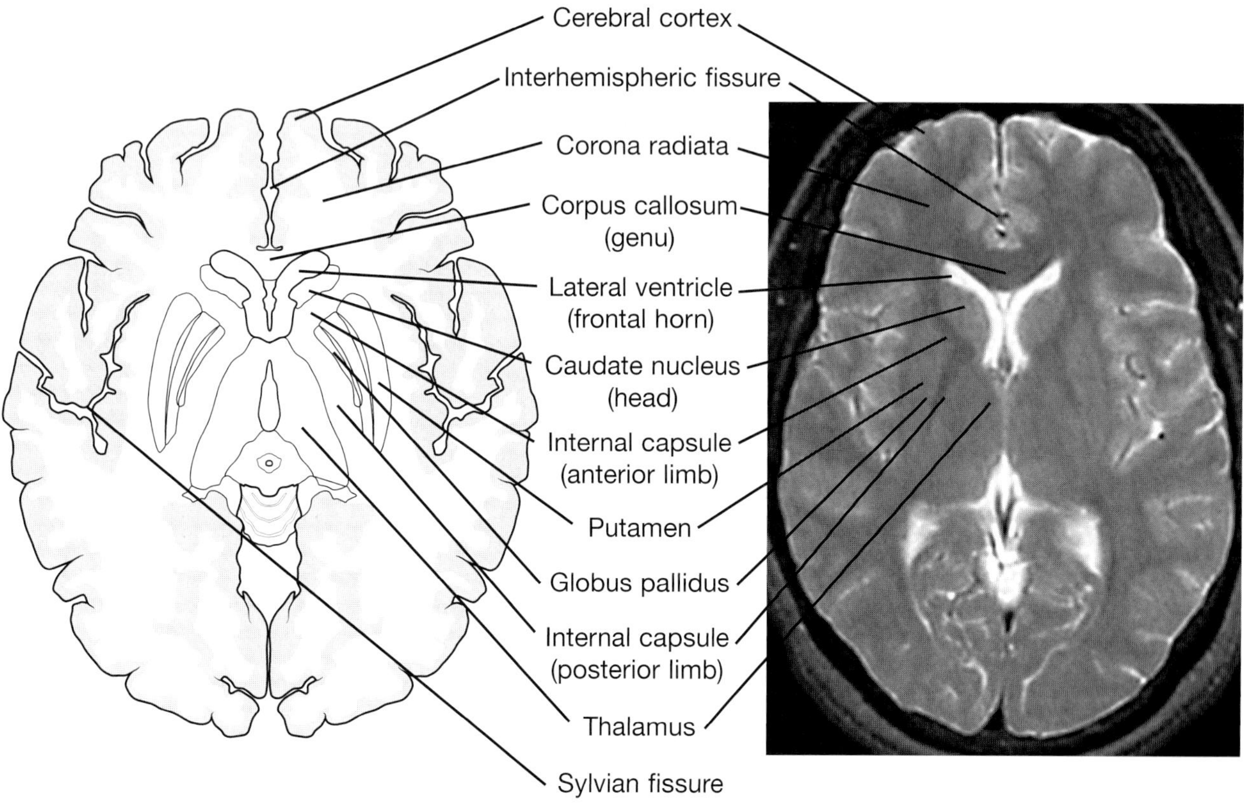

B

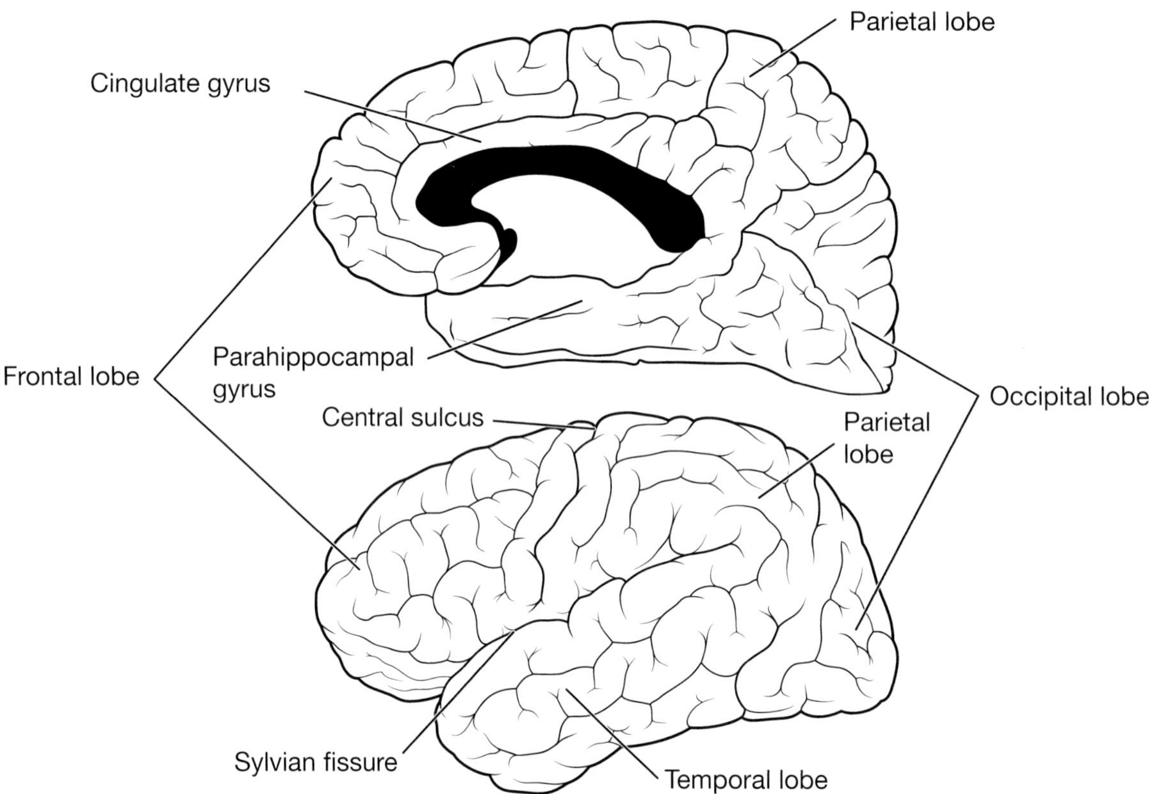

Fig. 16B.2. Diagram of the cortical lobes. Medial (*top*) and lateral (*bottom*) views of the cerebral hemisphere. The parahippocampal and cingulate gyri are part of the limbic system.

motor functions. It includes the *prefrontal cortex*, which is involved in attention, decision making, and control of affective behavior, and the premotor and motor areas, which are involved with the programming and execution of limb movements, control of gaze, and speech production. The *parietal lobe* includes the somatosensory area in the postcentral gyrus and the *posterior parietal cortex*, which integrates somatosensory, visual, and auditory information for visuospatial attention and control of motor function. The *temporal lobe* is functionally complex. Its superior aspect, the *transverse gyri*, is the primary auditory cortex; its lateral aspect includes auditory and association areas required for object recognition and naming. Its inferior aspect is critical for visual recognition of objects and faces. The *insular lobe* is involved in pain, visceral, and taste sensation. The *occipital lobe* contains the visual areas in the *calcarine cortex* and surrounding cortex. The right and left hemispheres have specialized functions. The dominant (usually, left) hemisphere is involved with language and calculation, and the right hemisphere is involved with visuospatial functions.

The phylogenetically older portions of the cerebral cortex are located on the medial wall of the cerebral hemispheres and are components of the limbic system (Fig. 16B.2). The medial aspect of the temporal lobe includes the *hippocampus* and the surrounding parahippocampal gyrus, both of which are essential for learning and memory, and the *amygdala*, which is critical for emotion. Both the hippocampal formation and the amygdala have important connections with the *cingulate gyrus*, which is adjacent to the corpus callosum and is involved in behavioral drive, motivation, and visuospatial memory. Together, the parahippocampal and cingulate gyri form the *limbic lobe* of the medial wall of the cerebral hemisphere.

Two special sensory systems are associated with the supratentorial level: the *olfactory system*, which has direct access to the limbic structures, and the *visual system*, which includes diencephalic and telencephalic components.

Disorders of the cerebral hemispheres may impair function or produce excessive electrical activity manifested as seizures or do both. These abnormalities may be diffuse or focal. Mental retardation, dementia, and confusional state reflect widespread impairment of cortical function. Diffuse cortical hyperexcitability produces generalized seizures. Focal lesions in primary motor or sensory areas of the cerebral cortex produce contralateral deficits, including hemiparesis, cortical somatosensory loss, or visual field defects. Lesions in sensory association areas produce different types of *agnosia* (inability to recognize an object), but lesions in the parietal cortex and premotor cortex produce *apraxia* (inability to perform complex learned motor acts). In addition, focal lesions of association areas may produce side-specific deficits. In general, lesions in the left hemisphere may produce *aphasia* (language deficit), whereas lesions in the right hemisphere produce visual attention deficits. Lesions of the prefrontal cortex are manifested as impaired attention and decision making or changes in personality and behavior or both. Lesions of the medial temporal lobe cause memory loss (*amnesia*). Focal lesions can produce abnormal synchronized activity in cortical areas, giving rise to focal (or partial) seizures.

Cerebral Cortex

Functional Anatomy

Cytoarchitectonics

From the phylogenetic, cytoarchitectonic, and functional standpoint, the cerebral cortex is subdivided into limbic cortex, paralimbic cortex, and neocortex (Fig. 16B.3). The basis for this cytoarchitectonic subdivision is the degree of differentiation of the cell layers of the cerebral cortex. This differentiation was also the basis for the subdivision of each lobe into histologically distinct areas by the German anatomist Brodmann.

The *limbic cortex* is the most primitive cortical area and includes the amygdala and hippocampal formation, both of which are located in the medial temporal lobe. The *paralimbic cortex* has a degree of differentiation intermediate between the limbic cortex and neocortex. It includes the *parahippocampal cortex* and *cingulate cortex* of

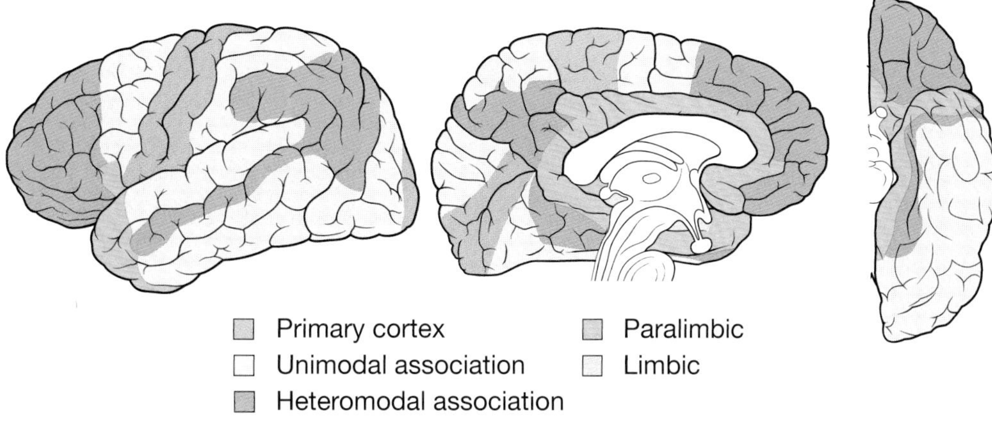

Fig. 16B.3. Cytoarchitectonic subdivisions of the lateral, medial, and inferior aspects of the cerebral cortex on the basis of phylogenetic origin, differentiation of cortical layers, and connectivity patterns. Primary cortex, unimodal association cortex, and heteromodal association cortex constitute neocortex. (Modified from Grabowski TJ, Jr., Anderson SW, Cooper GE. Disorders of cognitive function. Continuum. 2002;8(2). Used with permission.)

the medial wall of the hemisphere and portions of the frontal and temporal lobes and the insula. The *neocortex* is the most differentiated cortex and occupies the lateral surface of the cerebral hemisphere, forming most of the frontal, parietal, temporal, and occipital lobes. The neocortex includes the primary sensory and motor areas and two types of association areas. Modality-specific association areas, called *unimodal association cortex*, surround each primary area and are related to each sensory modality. Surrounding these unimodal areas is *heteromodal* (or multimodal) *association cortex* that receives and integrates input from several sensory modalities.

Each lobe is divided into different gyri and contains areas with different cytoarchitectural features and functions.

The frontal lobe contains primary, association, paralimbic, and limbic areas (Fig. 16B.4). It includes the primary motor cortex (M1) located in the precentral gyrus (area 4) and the lateral premotor and supplementary motor areas (lateral and medial area 6, respectively). Most of the frontal lobe is occupied by the prefrontal cortex, which is subdivided into the *dorsolateral prefrontal cortex* (heteromodal cortex that includes the superior, middle and inferior frontal gyri and frontal pole), and the *orbitomedial prefrontal cortex*, which is paralimbic cortex. In the left hemisphere, the inferior frontal gyrus contains Broca area (area 44).

The parietal lobe contains the primary somatosensory cortex (S1) in the postcentral gyrus (areas 3a, 3b, 1, and 2), which is surrounded by unimodal somatosensory

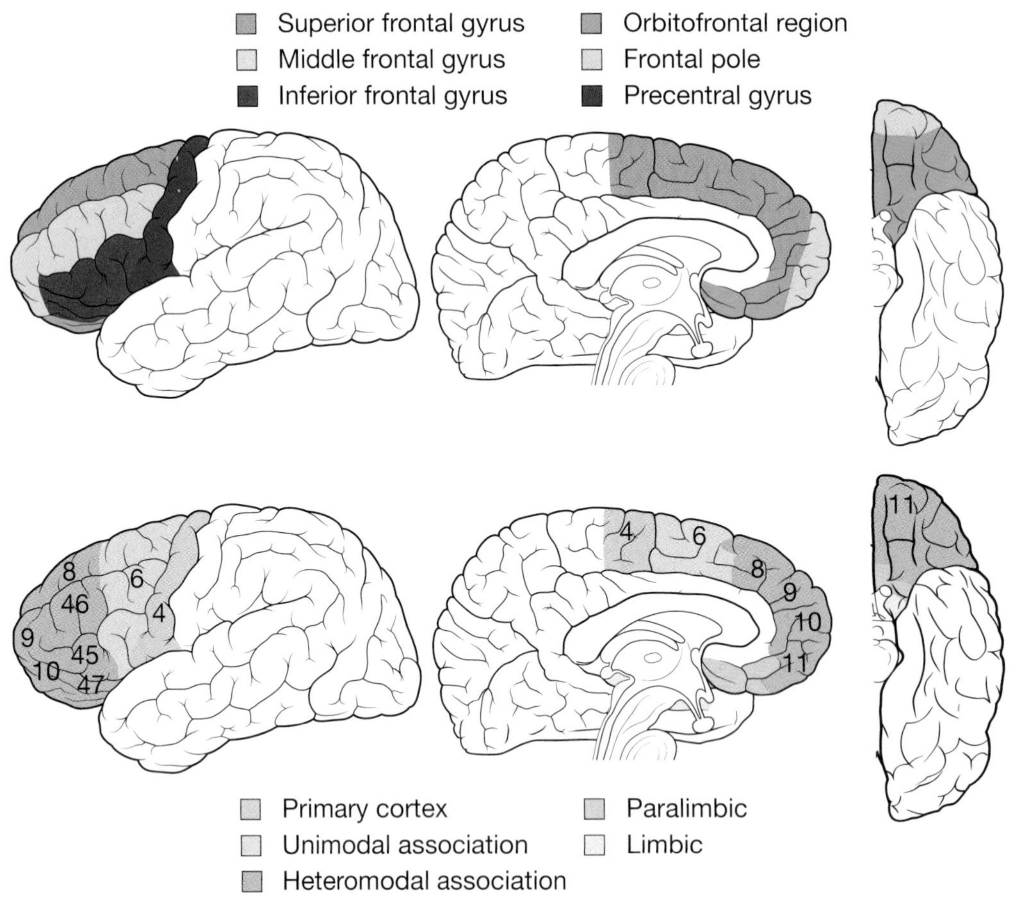

Fig. 16B.4. Anatomical (*upper*) and functional (*lower*) subdivisions of the frontal lobe. (Modified from Grabowski TJ, Jr., Anderson SW, Cooper GE. Disorders of cognitive function. Continuum. 2002;8(2). Used with permission.)

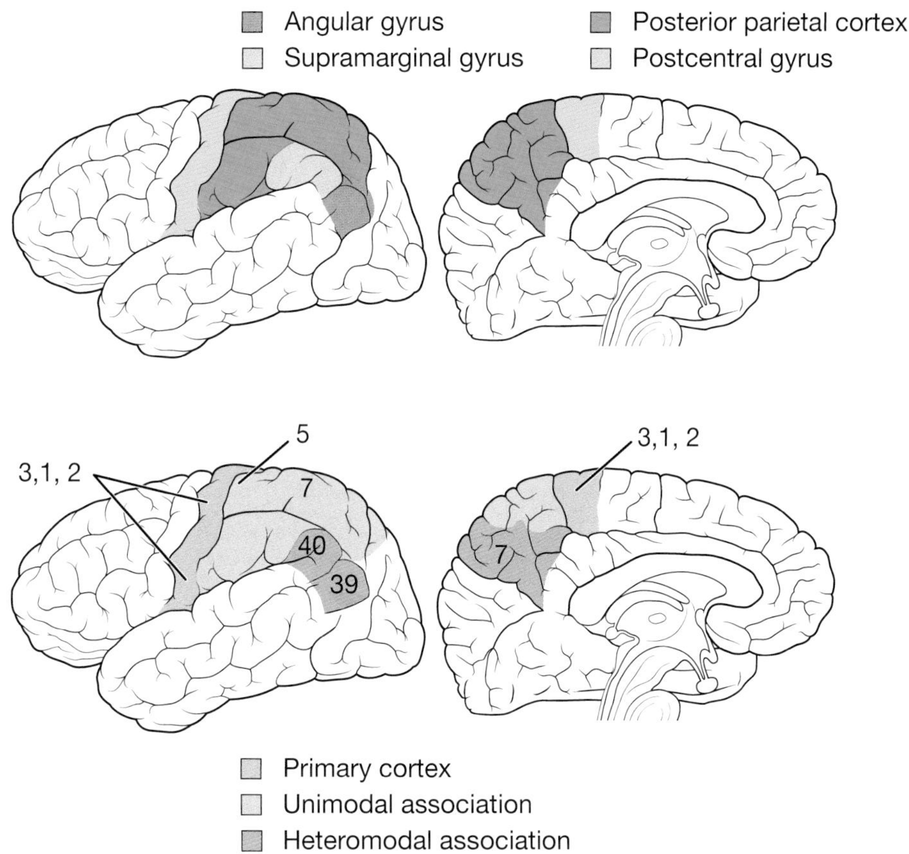

Fig. 16B.5. Anatomical (*upper*) and functional (*lower*) subdivisions of the parietal lobe. (Modified from Grabowski TJ, Jr., Anderson SW, Cooper GE. Disorders of cognitive function. Continuum. 2002;8(2). Used with permission.)

association areas. Most of the parietal lobe consists of the *posterior parietal cortex*, which is a heteromodal sensory association area (Fig. 16B.5). It includes the superior parietal lobule and the inferior parietal lobule separated by the *intraparietal sulcus*. The inferior parietal lobule includes the *supramarginal gyrus* and *angular gyrus*.

The temporal lobe is cytoarchitectonically and functionally heterogeneous (Fig. 16B.6). The superior aspect contains the *transverse gyri of Heschl*, which correspond to the primary auditory cortex (area 41), surrounded by the unimodal auditory association area (area 42). The lateral aspect of the temporal lobe contains the superior and medial temporal gyri, which are heteromodal sensory association areas. The posterior portion of the superior temporal gyrus and adjacent supramarginal gyrus in the left hemisphere correspond to *Wernicke area*. The inferior aspect of the temporal lobe and adjacent parts of the occipital cortex (inferior occipitotemporal cortex) are a unimodal visual association area and include the *lingual gyrus* and *fusiform gyrus*. The medial portion of the temporal lobe contains the amygdala and hippocampus. Immediately adjacent to the hippocampus is the *entorhinal cortex*, which is part of the parahippocampal gyrus.

The occipital lobe contains the primary visual cortex (V1, calcarine or striate cortex, area 17) and the unimodal visual association areas (extrastriate areas 18 and 19) (Fig. 16B.7).

The medial portion of the cerebral hemisphere contains the cingulate gyrus (including and anterior and posterior cingulate cortical areas) and the parahippocampal gyrus, including the entorhinal cortex. Although they

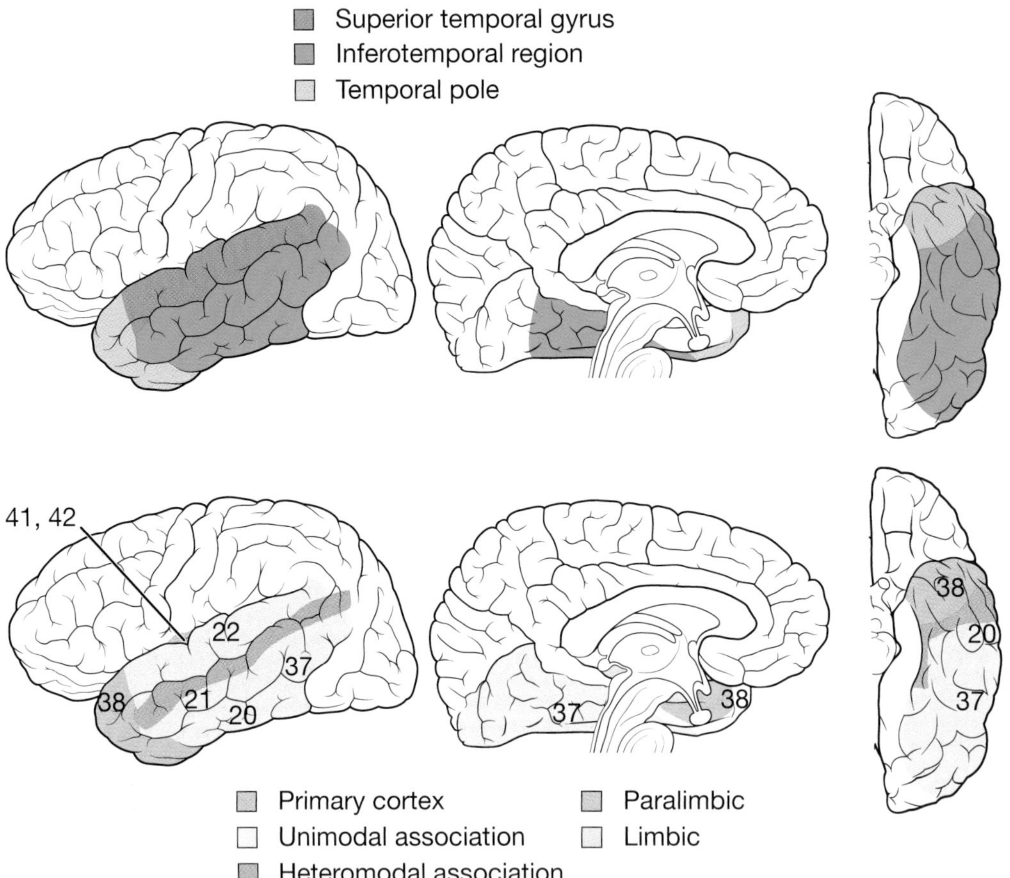

Fig. 16B.6. Anatomical (*upper*) and functional (*lower*) subdivisions of the temporal lobe. (Modified from Grabowski TJ, Jr., Anderson SW, Cooper GE. Disorders of cognitive function. Continuum. 2002;8(2). Used with permission.)

are paralimbic areas, they are classically referred to as the limbic lobe (Fig. 16B.8).

- The cerebral cortex is subdivided into limbic, paralimbic, and neocortical regions.
- The limbic regions include the amygdala and hippocampus.
- The neocortex includes primary, unimodal, and heteromodal association areas.
- The paralimbic cortex connects association areas of the neocortex with the limbic cortex.

Histology

The two main types of cortical neurons are *pyramidal cells* and several varieties of local *interneurons* (Fig. 16B.9). Pyramidal cells are excitatory projection neurons; their axons project to other areas of the cerebral cortex or to subcortical structures. Local interneurons are inhibitory and control the excitability of the pyramidal cells in the different layers of the cerebral cortex.

Cortical pyramidal cells originate from the ventricular zone and migrate radially to reach different layers of the cerebral cortex. These neurons have an apical dendrite that extends to the pial surface and basal dendrites; all these dendrites contain dendritic spines. Pyramidal neurons are excitatory and contain L-glutamate. Local interneurons arise from the ganglionic eminence and reach the cerebral cortex through tangential migration. They have γ-aminobutyric acid (GABA) as a neurotransmitter. In general, these neurons are multipolar and lack

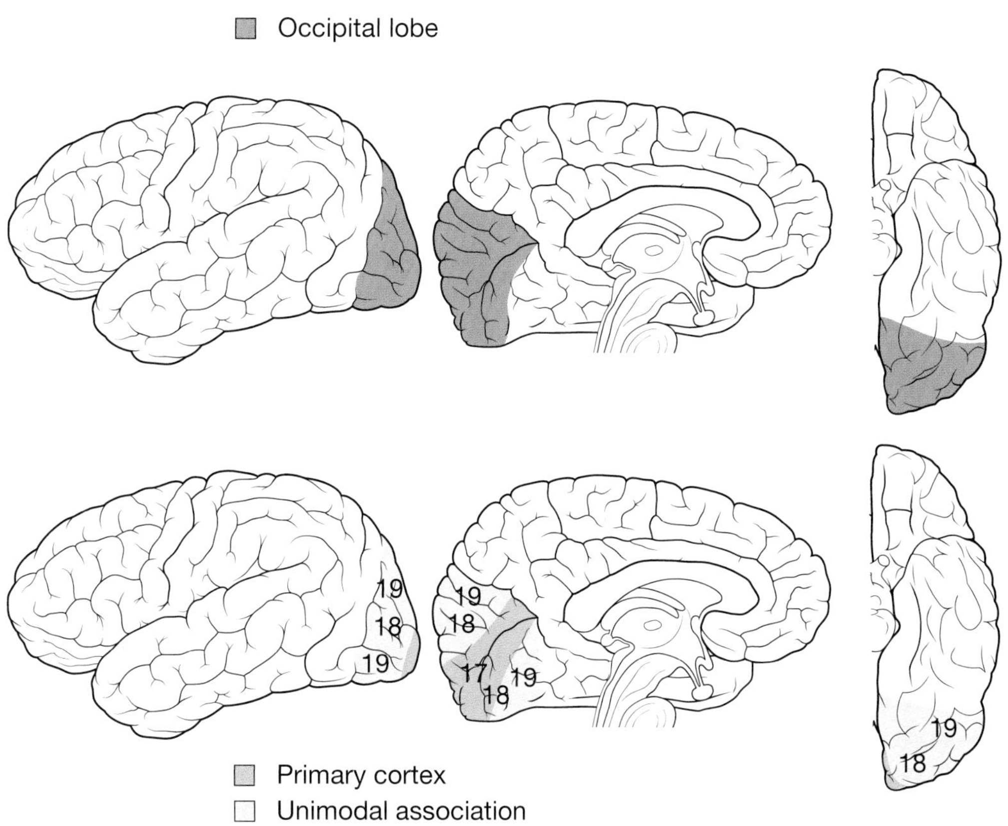

Fig. 16B.7. Anatomical (*upper*) and functional (*lower*) subdivisions of the occipital lobe. (Modified from Grabowski TJ, Jr., Anderson SW, Cooper GE. Disorders of cognitive function. Continuum. 2002;8(2). Used with permission.)

dendritic spines. Their axons may extend vertically or horizontally. Local interneurons are interconnected with each other, forming extensive networks in the cerebral cortex. In primary cortical sensory areas, special neurons called spiny stellate neurons (glutamatergic cells) receive input from the thalamus and activate pyramidal neurons.

- The two main types of cortical neurons are pyramidal cells and local interneurons.
- Pyramidal cells are excitatory projection neurons that have L-glutamate as a neurotransmitter.
- Local interneurons are inhibitory and have γ-aminobutyric acid (GABA) as a neurotransmitter.

Cortical cells are organized into horizontal laminae or layers that vary in number from three in the hippocampus to six in the neocortex (Fig. 16B.10).

Layer I, the superficial layer, contains the apical dendrites of pyramidal cells as well as local interneurons and receives projections from thalamic and brainstem neurons.

Layer II, the external (outer) granular layer, contains local interneurons and pyramidal cells that project to contralateral cerebral cortex (commissural fibers).

Layer III, external (outer) pyramidal layer, contains pyramidal cells that give rise to commissural or association fibers.

Layer IV, the internal (inner) granular layer, has closely packed spiny stellate cells that receive input from thalamocortical fibers and project to pyramidal neurons. This layer is highly developed in primary sensory cortical areas; the cortex in these regions is called granular cortex.

Layer V, the internal (inner) pyramidal layer, contains the large pyramidal cells that project to the basal ganglia, brainstem, and spinal cord. This layer is prominent in motor areas at the expense of layer IV; motor areas are referred to as agranular cortex. The most prominent example is primary motor cortex (area 4), which contains the giant pyramidal cells of Betz that project to the spinal cord.

Layer VI, or multiform layer, contains pyramidal neurons that project to the thalamus.

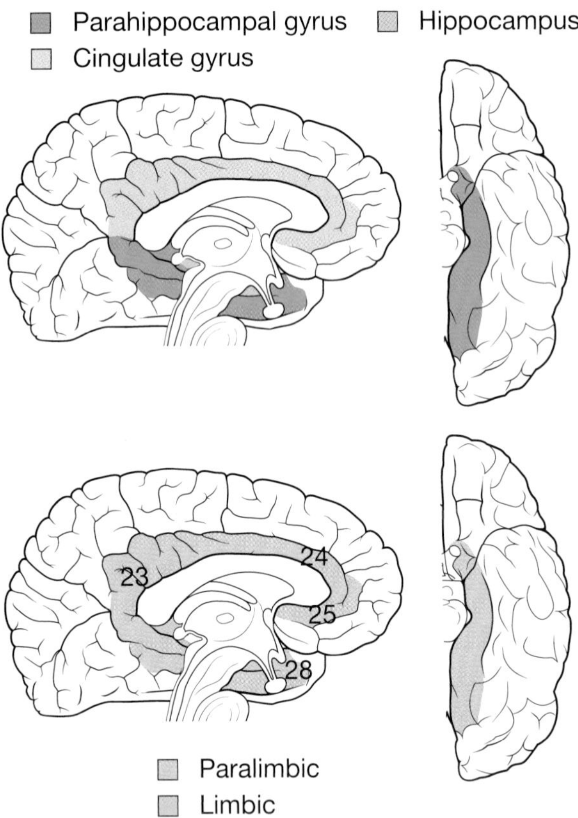

Fig. 16B.8. Anatomical (*upper*) and functional (*lower*) subdivisions of the limbic lobe. (Modified from Grabowski TJ, Jr., Anderson SW, Cooper GE. Disorders of cognitive function. Continuum. 2002;8(2). Used with permission.)

Extrinsic Connectivity

The cerebral cortex has a basic pattern of connectivity. Input from thalamocortical relay nuclei terminate primarily in layer IV. In primary sensory cortices, these axons synapse on the spiny stellate excitatory neurons, whose axons synapse on and excite pyramidal neurons in layers II and III. Layer II and III pyramidal neurons also receive input from and project to other cortical areas. Pyramidal neurons in layer V project to the basal ganglia, brainstem, or spinal cord, and those in layer VI project to the thalamus. Input from intralaminar thalamic or brainstem nuclei of the consciousness system terminate in layer I, synapsing on the apical dendrites of pyramidal neurons of all layers.

Columnar Organization of the Cerebral Cortex

An important feature of the neocortex is its organization into functional modules, or columns. A *column* is a vertical cylinder of cortical tissue that includes all six layers and represents the functional unit of cortex. Cortical neurons in each column receive input from other columns, thalamic relay nuclei, and brainstem areas of the consciousness system. In primary sensory cortices, all neurons in a given column have a similar peripheral receptive field and response characteristics. They receive input from a particular set of thalamic neurons and are interconnected by the local excitatory spiny stellate neurons in layer IV. Within a column, there are recurrent excitatory interactions between pyramidal cells of deep layers V and VI and superficial layers II and III.

Columns that have similar properties are interconnected with each other over widespread areas of the cerebral cortex. Generally, the activation of a column is associated with inhibition of the surrounding columns. This is mediated by interneurons that project horizontally for various distances across several columns. This lateral inhibitory mechanism is important for sensory discrimination and fine motor control.

- Columns are the functional units of the cerebral cortex.
- Cells within a column receive similar input and have similar properties.
- Columns that have a similar function are linked by corticocortical connections.

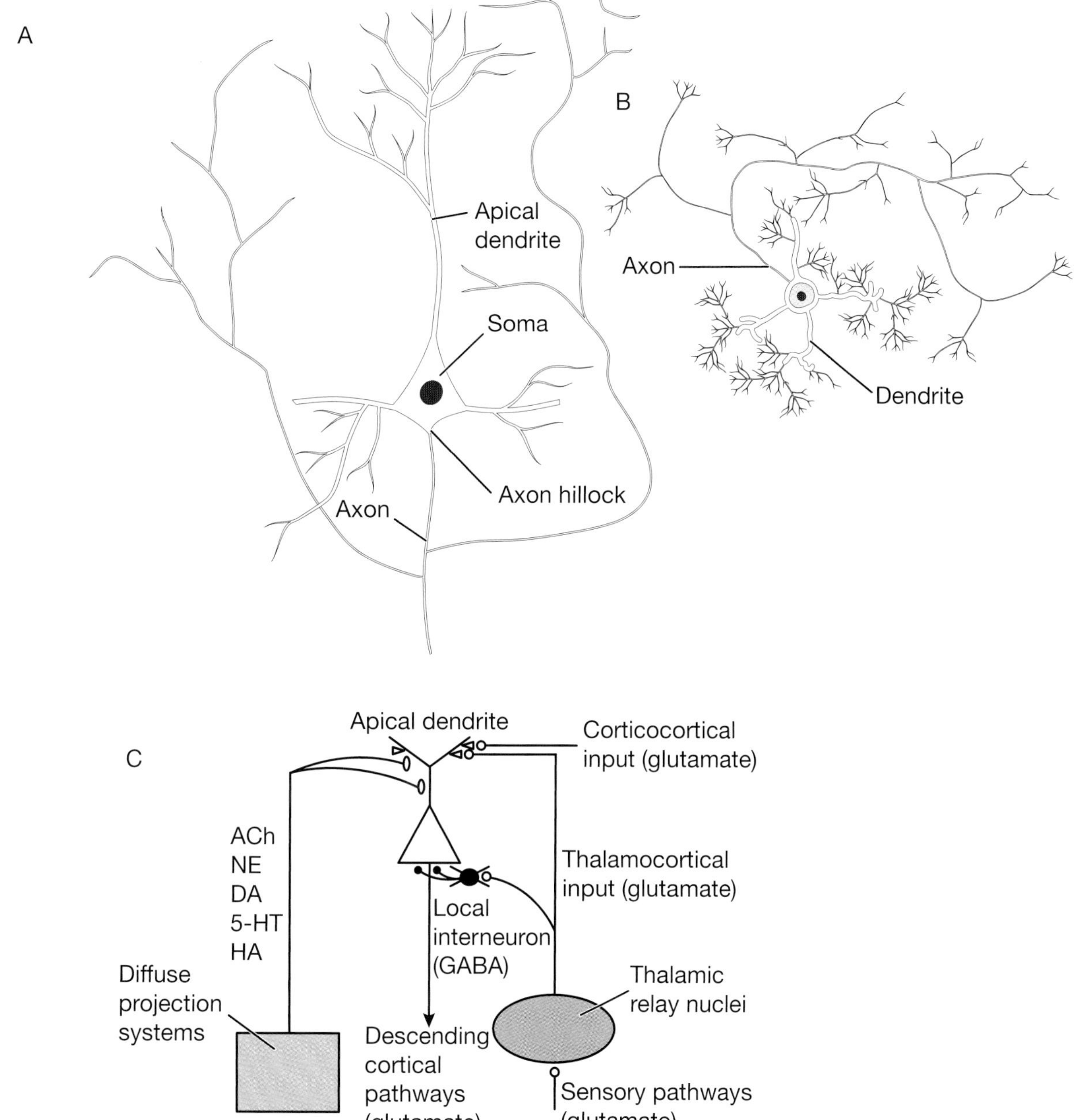

Fig. 16B.9. The two types of neurons in the cerebral cortex. *A*, Pyramidal cells constitute the majority of neurons in the cerebral cortex. They are excitatory projection neurons that have L-glutamate as the neurotransmitter. Typically, they have an apical dendrite and basal dendrites, all with dentritic spines. *B*, Local interneurons lack dendritic spines and have γ-aminobutyric acid (GABA) as the neurotransmitter. Several types of interneurons synapse on different parts of pyramidal cells. *C*, Pyramidal cells receive excitatory glutamatergic input from other pyramidal cells (corticocortical projections) and the thalamus (thalamocortical projections). Excitatory inputs terminate on dendritic spines. Pyramidal cells receive inhibitory GABAergic input from different types of local interneurons, which do not synapse on spines. Ascending projections from structures of the consciousness system, including neurons producing acetylcholine (ACh), norepinephrine (NE), dopamine (DA), serotonin (5-HT), and histamine (HA), modulate the response of pyramidal cells to excitatory and inhibitory inputs.

- Lateral inhibitory interactions are critical for sensory discrimination and fine motor control.

Hierarchical Processing of Information in the Cerebral Cortex

The processing of information in the cerebral cortex is hierarchical (Fig. 16B.11). Sensory information reaching the primary sensory areas is processed first in the unimodal sensory association areas. Whereas neurons in the primary cortical areas respond to specific features of a sensory stimulus, such as a point or shape, neurons in unimodal areas respond to combinations of features, allowing representation of the whole object. For example, neurons of the primary visual cortex respond to points or bars of light, whereas neurons in progressively more hierarchical areas of unimodal visual association cortex respond selectively to specific combinations of features that characterize an object or a face.

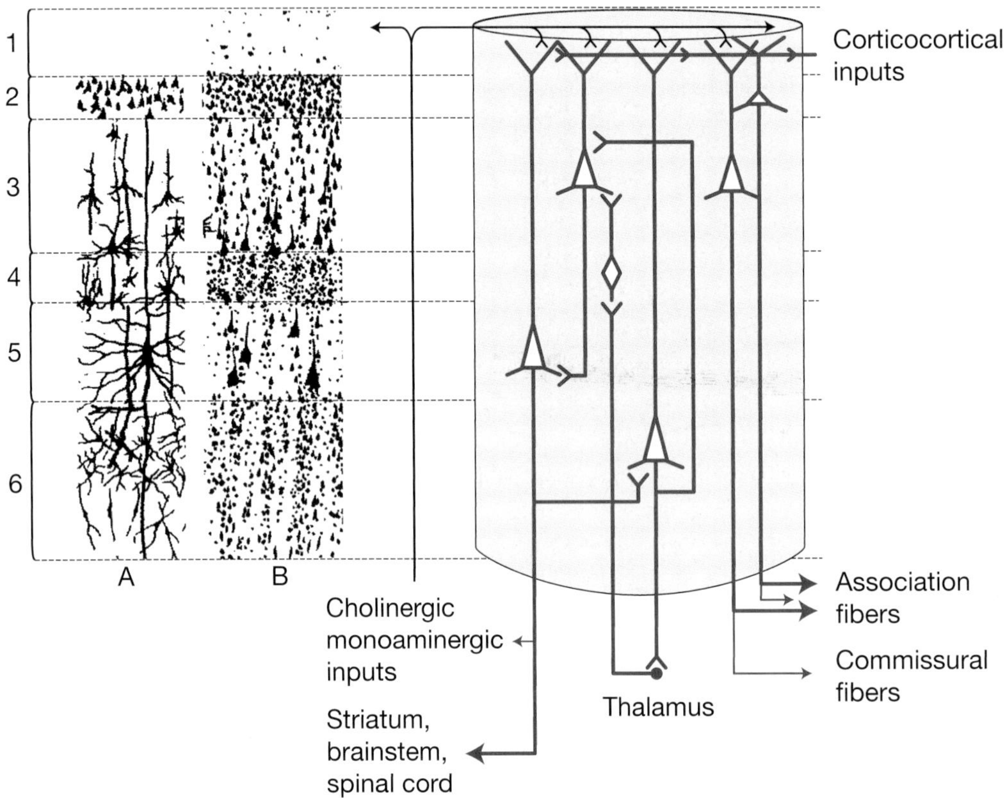

Fig. 16B.10. *Left*, Laminar structure of the neocortex as shown with Golgi (*A*) and Nissl staining (*B*). This is prototypical six-layered cortex, as in areas of association cortex. *Right*, Basic excitatory connectivity pattern within a functional column of neocortex. Input from a thalamic relay nucleus terminates primarily in layer 4, which contains spiny stellate excitatory neurons that project to pyramidal neurons in layers 2 and 3. These neurons project to pyramidal neurons in layer 5, which in turn activate pyramidal neurons in layer 6. These neurons send recurrent excitatory projections to layers 2 and 3. The excitatory interactions within a column are controlled by different types of local interneurons (not shown), which also mediate lateral inhibition of surrounding columns. The apical dendrites of pyramidal cells reach layer 1, where they receive input from other cortical areas, thalamic intralaminar nuclei, and cholinergic and monoaminergic systems of the brainstem, hypothalamus, and basal forebrain. Cortical pyramidal cells give rise to extrinsic connections: layer 2 cells to intrahemispheric corticocortical association fibers, layer 3 cells to interhemispheric commissural fibers, layer 5 cells to corticostriate, corticorubral, corticopontine, corticobulbar, and corticospinal fibers, and layer 6 cells to corticothalamic fibers.

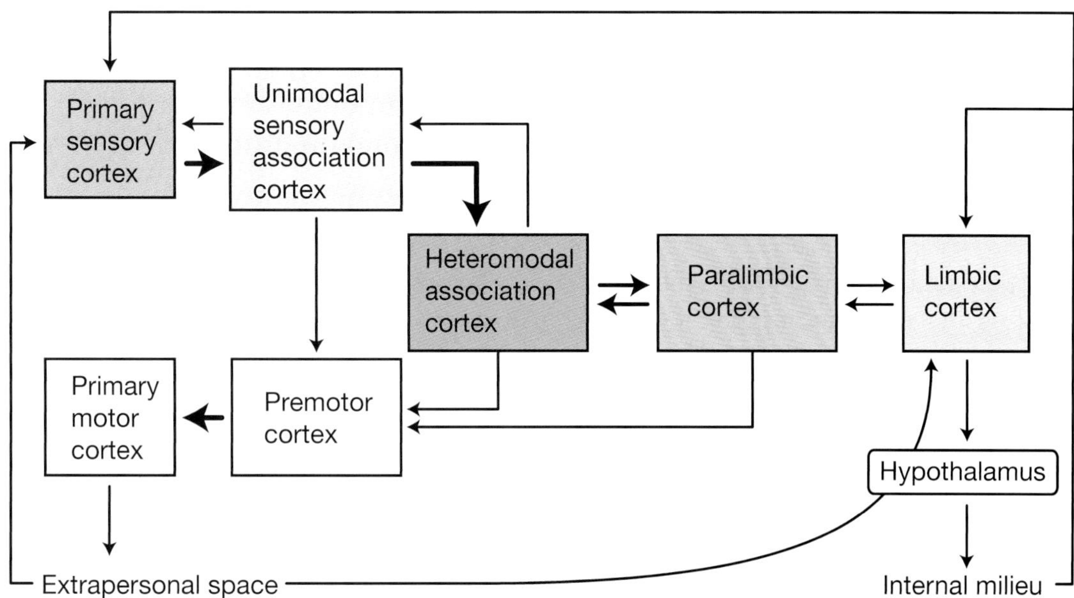

Fig. 16B.11. Hierarchical processing of information in the cerebral cortex. Sensory information is processed serially from primary sensory, to unimodal sensory, to heteromodal sensory association areas in the posterior parietal and lateral temporal cortices. These areas project to both heteromodal association areas of the frontal lobe (prefrontal cortex) and paralimbic areas, which provide input to the hippocampus and amygdala. The prefrontal cortex projects to premotor areas (unimodal motor association areas), which activate primary motor cortex. Note the feedback connections between the paralimbic, heteromodal, and unimodal areas.

Different unimodal sensory areas project to heteromodal sensory association areas in the posterior parietal cortex and lateral temporal cortex. These heteromodal areas contain neurons that respond to specific combinations of visual, somatosensory, and auditory stimuli. Neurons in posterior parietal cortex are involved in visuospatial orientation and those in lateral temporal cortex are important in object recognition and identification required for naming.

Heteromodal sensory areas are reciprocally connected with the heteromodal areas of the prefrontal cortex and with the paralimbic areas. Neurons in prefrontal cortex are involved in executive function and control of behavior and project to the premotor and supplementary motor areas that, in turn, control the activity of primary motor cortex. The paralimbic areas, including the orbitofrontal, cingulate, and parahippocampal cortices, are reciprocally connected with both heteromodal association neocortex and limbic cortex, including the hippocampus (involved in memory) and amygdala (involved in emotion).

- Sensory information is processed hierarchically in the cerebral cortex.
- Unimodal sensory association areas receive input from several columns of the corresponding primary areas, allowing feature extraction and object recognition.
- Processing of unimodal sensory information in heteromodal, paralimbic, and limbic areas is critical for object identification and naming, emotional response to the object, memory, and motor control.

Parallel Processing of Information

Processing of sensory information from each modality occurs in two parallel streams involving the parietal and temporal lobes. This has been characterized best for the visual system. Input from primary visual cortex is processed in a *dorsal stream* involving neurons in the unimodal visual association cortex of the posterior parietal lobe that respond to object location and motion (i.e., "where" is the object) and a *ventral stream* involving neurons in the unimodal visual association cortex of the inferior occipitotemporal region that respond to object shape and color and allow object identification (i.e., "what" is the object). Information from the ventral stream is processed in the premotor cortex for visual guidance of eye and limb movement, and information from the ventral stream is used for object recognition, naming, emotional response, and memory (Fig. 16B.12).

- Sensory processing occurs in a dorsal (parietal) stream involved with object location and a ventral (temporal) stream involved with object identification.

Reciprocal Interactions in the Cerebral Cortex

There is a reciprocal flow of information between primary and association sensory and motor areas of the neocortex and between neocortical association areas and the limbic system. Feedback projections from the prefrontal and posterior parietal cortices to the unimodal and primary sensory areas are critical for mechanisms of *selective attention* to a specific sensory stimulus at the expense of distracting stimuli. Reciprocal input from the limbic system to the paralimbic and then heteromodal cortex provides emotional bias to sensory processing and contributes to recognition of the object.

- Feedback projections from the prefrontal and posterior parietal cortices to the unimodal sensory areas are critical for attention.

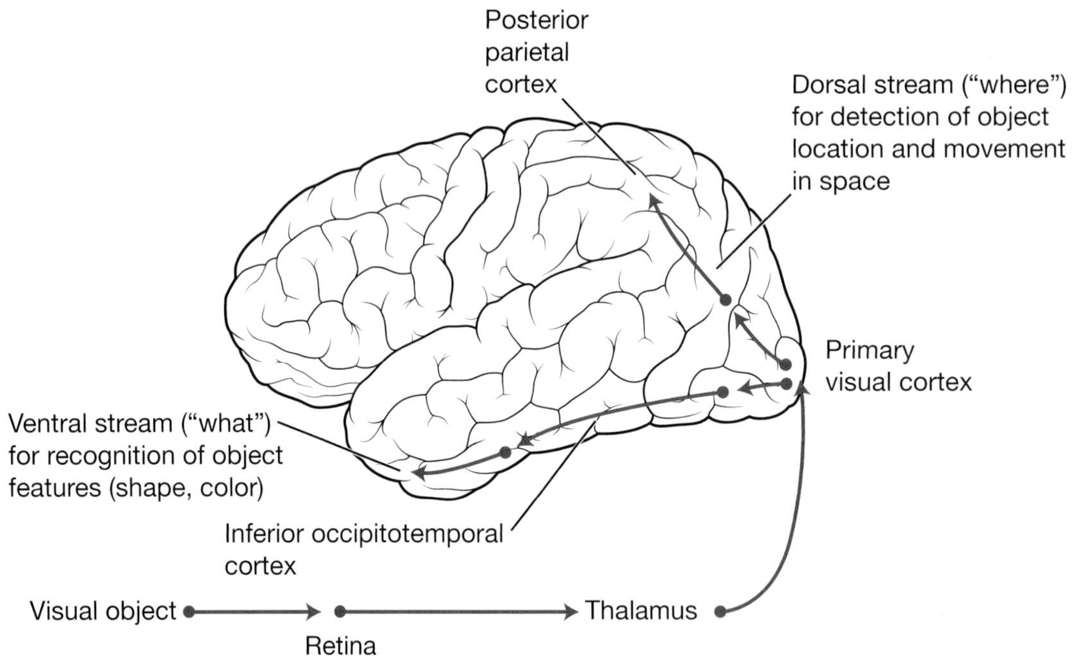

Fig. 16B.12. Parallel processing of visual information. Visual information reaching primary visual cortex is processed further in dorsal and ventral streams. The dorsal (occipitoparietal) stream reaches the posterior parietal cortex and is involved in analysis of the position and movement of the object. This information is used to guide movements of the limbs or the eyes toward the object. The ventral (occipitotemporal) stream involves progressive processing steps in the inferior occipitotemporal cortex (fusiform and lingual gyri) and is involved in the analysis of color and shape of the object. This information is used for recognizing the object, including faces, which is required for naming, emotion, and memory of the object. Similar parallel processing occurs in the somatosensory and auditory systems.

Distributed Networks of the Cerebral Cortex

Every cortical function depends on the parallel and simultaneous processing of information by anatomically separate networks that involve widespread areas of neocortex, paralimbic cortex, and limbic cortex that interact through their specific cortical and subcortical connections. For example, language involves structures in the left posterior superior temporal and inferior frontal cortices, caudate nucleus, and thalamus. Therefore, even though a lesion in a specific area of the hemisphere produces a specific deficit, this does not mean that this area is necessarily the seat of the function affected. Instead, the area may be a nodal component of a complex network involved in that function.

> There is evidence that widespread separated neuronal networks are simultaneously engaged in a particular task. The mechanism by which this occurs forms the binding problem. Functional binding may occur through synchronized, high-frequency rhythmic activity (gamma activity) in widespread neuronal populations and depend on interactions between highly interconnected cortical GABAergic interneurons and reciprocal corticothalamocortical loops.

- Cortical activity involves the simultaneous interaction of widespread, distributed, but temporally linked cortical networks.

Cortical Plasticity

The ability of the cerebral cortex to undergo anatomical and functional change in response to environmental circumstances is called *cortical plasticity*. This phenomenon is essential for establishing connections during development of the nervous system, but it also occurs in the cerebral cortex throughout life. Thus, the cortical representations of sensory and motor maps may change in size and distribution in response to peripheral injury or to training. Cortical plasticity may explain recovery of function after a large hemispheric lesion.

Connections Through the Subcortical White Matter

A large proportion of the cerebral hemispheres consists of myelinated axons that interconnect one area of cerebral cortex with numerous other areas of cortex and with subcortical areas. These axons include *projection fibers* that connect the cerebral cortex and subcortical structures, *commissural fibers* that connect homologous areas in the two cerebral hemispheres, and *association fibers* that connect cortical areas within the same hemisphere.

Projection Fibers

The projection fibers that connect subcortical and cortical areas form a compact group of axons called the *internal capsule*. The internal capsule is a broad band flanked medially by the thalamus and caudate nucleus and laterally by the globus pallidus and putamen (Fig. 16B.13). In horizontal sections, it is a V-shaped structure consisting of an anterior limb, posterior limb, and a junction called the genu. The projection fibers in the internal capsule relay afferent input from the thalamus to the cerebral cortex and efferent output from the cerebral cortex to all subcortical structures.

The afferent projection fibers arise largely from the thalamus and are called *thalamic radiations*. Axons traveling to the frontal lobe are in the anterior limb of the internal capsule, fibers projecting to the motor and premotor areas are in the genu and posterior limb, and fibers carrying sensory information to the parietal cortex are also in the posterior limb. The optic radiations are in the *retrolenticular portion* of the internal capsule, and the auditory radiations are in the *sublenticular portion*. As the axons spread out from the internal capsule to reach all areas of the cortex, they form the *corona radiata*.

The efferent projection fibers from the cerebral cortex pass through the corona radiata into the internal capsule en route to the thalamus, basal ganglia, hypothalamus, red nucleus, and brainstem reticular formation. The largest group constitutes the motor pathway projecting from the precentral gyrus. These axons go through the posterior limb of the internal to the motor nuclei in the brainstem and spinal cord. The genu of the internal capsule contains the descending axons to the motor cranial nerve nuclei (*corticobulbar pathway*). The *corticospinal fibers* are located in the posterior limb adjacent to the genu. A second large efferent projection is to the pontine nuclei, the *corticopontine fibers*, which relay information to the cerebellum via the pontine nuclei. The descending motor

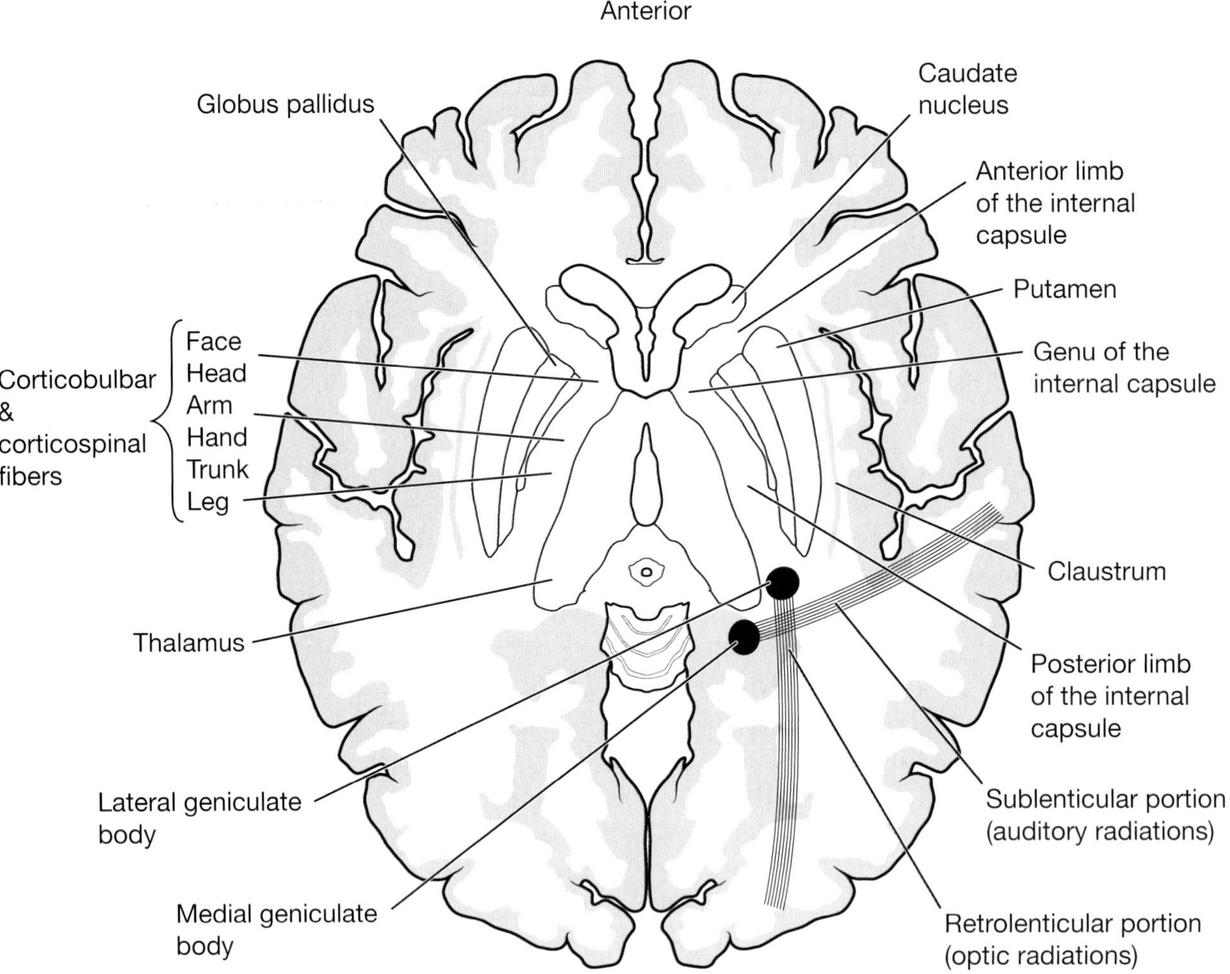

Fig. 16B.13. Internal capsule. The anterior limb contains fibers going to and from the prefrontal cortex; the genu, corticobulbar pathways; and the posterior limb, corticospinal and somatosensory thalamic projections. The retrolenticular portion of the internal capsule contains the optic radiation, and the sublenticular portion, the auditory radiation.

pathways in the posterior limb of the internal capsule form the cerebral peduncles at the level of the midbrain.

- The internal capsule contains the projection pathways between cortical and subcortical structures.
- The afferent projections from the thalamus to the primary sensory cortical areas are called the thalamic radiations and occupy different portions of the posterior limb of the internal capsule.
- Motor projections from the cerebral cortex occupy the genu and posterior limb of the internal capsule, just anterior to the somatosensory thalamic radiations.

Commissural Fibers

Commissural fibers connect homologous areas in the two hemispheres, integrating the activity of the two sides (Fig. 16B.14). Most of these axons pass through the *corpus callosum*, which is the large bundle of fibers that forms the roof of the lateral ventricles. The corpus callosum consists of an anterior portion, or *genu*, a *body*, and a posterior portion, or *splenium*. Two smaller commissures connect areas in the temporal lobes: the *anterior commissure*, anterior to the third ventricle, interconnects anterior temporal areas, and the *hippocampal commissure* interconnects the hippocampal formation of the two sides.

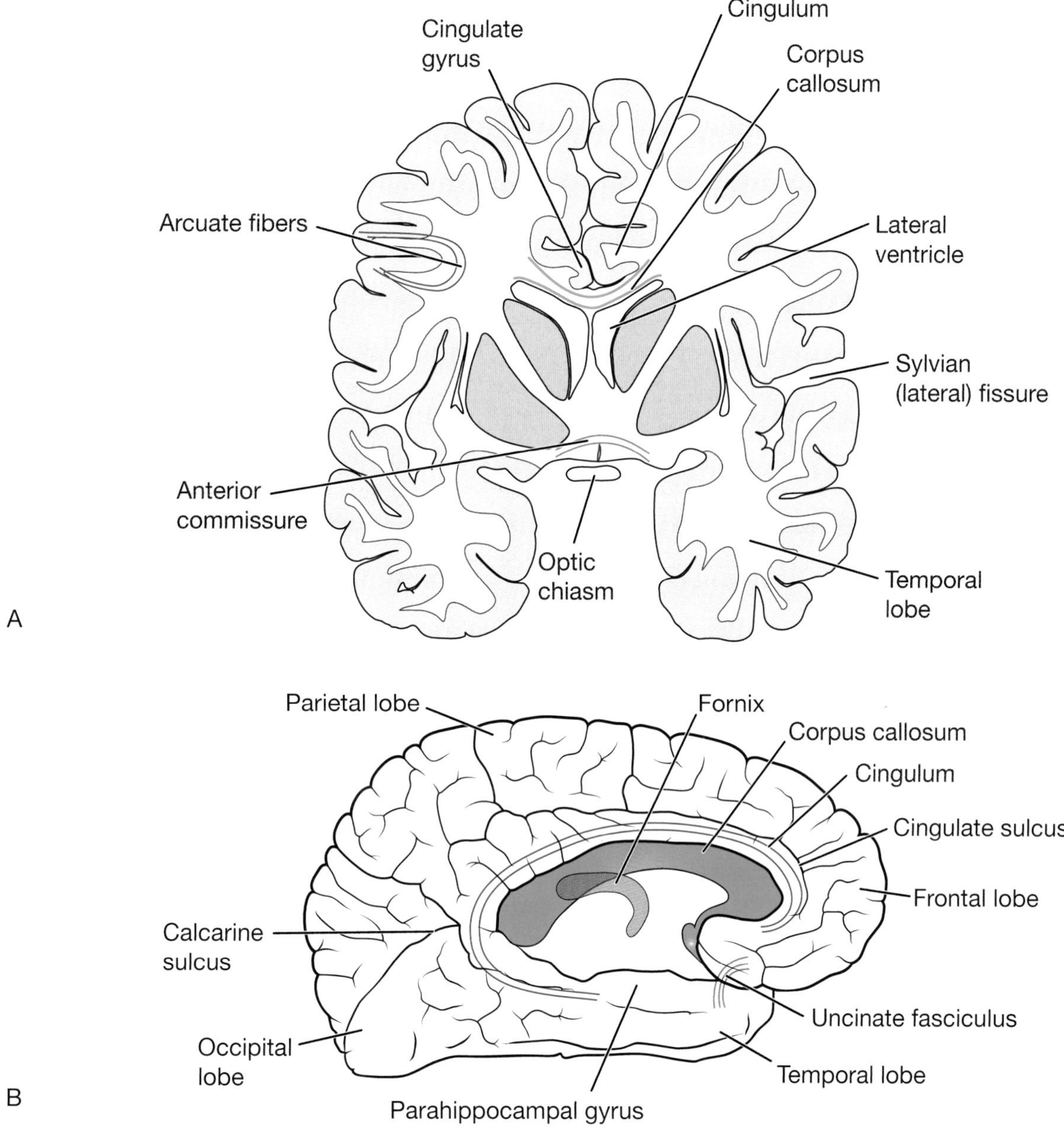

Fig. 16B.14. *A*, Coronal section through the cerebral hemispheres. Commissural fibers (corpus callosum and anterior commissure) connect both cerebral hemispheres. The arcuate fibers, or U fibers, are short association fibers that connect gyri. *B*, Medial view of the cerebral hemisphere. Examples of long association fibers are the cingulum and uncinate fasciculus.

- The corpus callosum connects homologous areas of the two hemispheres.
- The anterior commissure and hippocampal commissure connect areas of the temporal lobes.

Association Fibers

Fiber tracts known as association pathways run longitudinally within a hemisphere, correlating the activity of different lobes. These include the *superior longitudinal fasciculus* and the *inferior longitudinal fasciculus*, which connect the posterior parietotemporo-occipital regions with the frontal lobe, the *uncinate fasciculus*, which interconnects the temporal and frontal lobes, and the *cingulum*, which interconnects the medial surface of the frontal, parietal, and temporal lobes. Short association fibers that connect adjacent gyri are called *arcuate*, or *U, fibers* (Fig. 16B.14).

Cortical Interactions With the Basal Ganglia

The function of the cerebral cortex depends not only on intracortical connections but also on cortical-subcortical circuits that involve the thalamus and basal ganglia.

Anatomy and Basic Connectivity of the Basal Ganglia

The anatomy, basic connections, and function of the basal ganglia (basal nuclei) are discussed in Chapter 8. Briefly, the basal ganglia include the *striatum* and *globus pallidus* (Fig.16B.15). The striatum includes the *caudate nucleus*, *putamen*, and *nucleus accumbens*. The caudate and the putamen are separated by the internal capsule. The caudate consists of a head, body, and tail and is intimately related to the walls of the lateral ventricle. The nucleus accumbens, or limbic striatum, is located in the ventral portion of the striatum and forms part of the basal forebrain. The *globus pallidus* ("pale") is separated from both the thalamus and the substantia nigra by the internal capsule. The globus pallidus consists of external and internal segments. The globus pallidus and putamen together are referred to as the *lenticular nucleus* because of the shape. However, the two nuclei have different connections and functions. The basal ganglia circuits include two functionally related structures: the *subthalamic nucleus* and *substantia nigra*.

The basal ganglia circuits have a basic pattern of connectivity. The cerebral cortex, particularly the frontal lobe, sends excitatory input to the striatum. The striatum contains GABAergic inhibitory neurons that project to both the external and internal segments of the globus pallidus. The internal segment sends a GABAergic inhibitory projection to the thalamic nuclei that project to different portions of the frontal lobe. The subthalamic nucleus contains excitatory neurons that also project to both segments of the globus pallidus. The subthalamic nucleus receives a direct excitatory projection from the cerebral cortex and a reciprocal inhibitory projection from the external segment of the globus pallidus (Fig. 16B.15) (see Chapter 8).

Parallel Cortical-Basal Ganglia-Thalamocortical Circuits

The cerebral cortex and the basal ganglia are involved in different parallel reentrant *cortical-basal ganglia-thalamocortical circuits*. These circuits involve different portions of the frontal lobe, striatum, globus pallidus, subthalamic nucleus, and thalamus. The *motor circuit* involves the motor and supplementary motor cortices, putamen, specific portions of the globus pallidus and subthalamic nucleus, and the ventral oralis nucleus of the thalamus, which projects back to the supplementary motor area. This circuit controls the initiation of selected motor programs while simultaneously inhibiting the execution of competing motor programs (see Chapter 8). The *ocular motor circuit* involves the frontal eye fields, caudate nucleus, and substantia nigra pars reticulata (which is functionally homologous to the internal segment of the globus pallidus) and, through the superior colliculus, controls saccadic eye movements (see Chapter 16A). The *cognitive*, or *association*, *circuit* involves the prefrontal cortex, head of the caudate nucleus, substantia nigra pars reticulata, and dorsomedial nucleus of the thalamus. This circuit is involved in executive functions, including planning and monitoring behavior. The *limbic circuit* involves the orbitofrontal and anterior cingulate cortices, nucleus accumbens, and ventral pallidum. This circuit is important in controlling emotional and motivated behavior.

The cerebral cortex also participates in functional loop interactions with the cerebellum.

Cerebrocerebellar interactions involve the relay of cortical information by the pontine nuclei to the contralateral cerebellum and output from the cerebellar nuclei to the contralateral thalamus, which relays information back to the cerebral cortex. Similar to the reciprocal connections with the basal ganglia, several reentrant cortical-pontocerebellar-thalamocortical circuits involve the cerebellar hemispheres. For example, a "motor" circuit involves motor and premotor cortices and the dorsal part of the dentate nucleus; an "association circuit" involves association areas of the cerebral cortex and the ventral part of the dentate nucleus.

- The cerebral cortex participates in parallel cortical-striatopallidal-thalamocortical loops that regulate motor, ocular motor, cognitive, and emotional behavior.

Physiology

Electrophysiology of Cortical Neurons

The activity of pyramidal cells, which constitute the output of the cerebral cortex, depends on 1) their intrinsic membrane properties, 2) the pattern of excitatory input, 3) the level of local GABAergic inhibition, and 4) state-dependent modulation by cholinergic and monoaminergic pathways. Pyramidal cells receive excitatory input from other pyramidal cells in the same column, from other columns (intracortical connections), and from the thalamus. These excitatory axons have L-glutamate as a neurotransmitter and synapse mainly on dendritic spines. Dendritic spines are functional compartments of dendrites that contain voltage- and glutamate-gated calcium channels. They are the site of use-dependent synaptic plasticity, including long-term potentiation and long-term depression (Chapter 6). The activity of pyramidal cells is controlled locally by GABAergic inhibitory neurons. Cholinergic and monoaminergic input from the basal forebrain, hypothalamus, and brainstem modulate the excitability of cortical neurons according to the level of attention, emotion, and sleep-wake cycle.

Basal Ganglia Circuits

Through the basal ganglia, the cerebral cortex exerts dual control on motor behavior. The physiology of the basal ganglia circuits and their role in motor control are

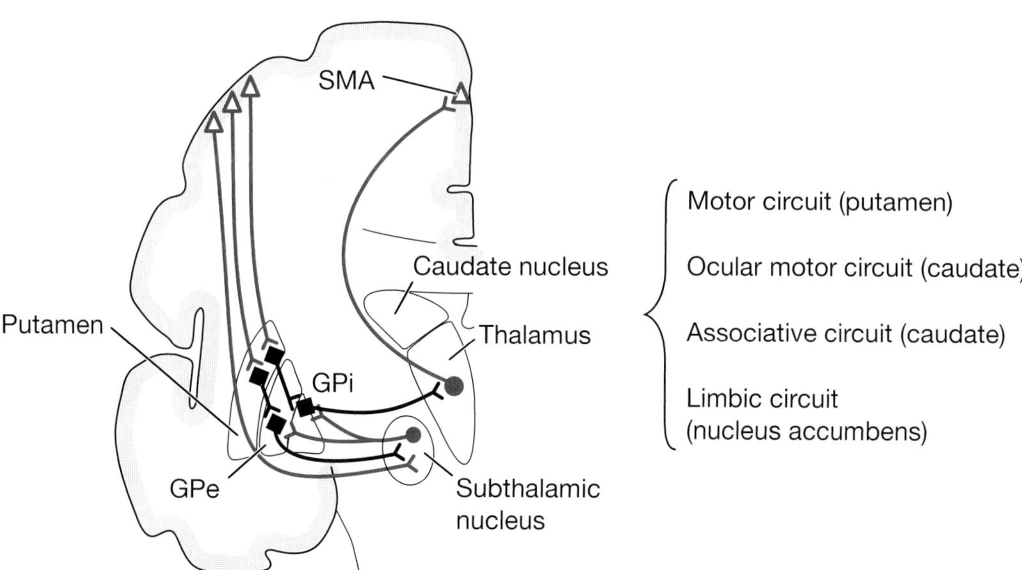

Fig. 16B.15. Diagram of a coronal section of the cerebral hemisphere showing the components of the basal ganglia circuits and their main connections. The basal ganglia include the striatum (caudate nucleus, putamen, and nucleus accumbens [not shown]) and globus pallidus (including an external segment [GPe] and internal segment [GPi]). The cerebral cortex, particularly the frontal lobe, sends excitatory projections to the striatum, which contains GABAergic inhibitory neurons that project to both GPe and GPi. GPi sends a GABAergic inhibitory projection to thalamic nuclei that project to different areas of the frontal lobe. Excitatory neurons in the subthalamic nucleus project to GPi and GPe. The subthalamic nucleus receives direct excitatory projections from the cerebral cortex and reciprocal inhibitory projections from GPe. SMA, supplementary motor area.

discussed in Chapter 8. The main function of cortical-basal ganglia circuits is to facilitate the initiation of a behaviorally relevant motor program while inhibiting that of all other competing motor programs. The initiation of a specific motor program involves an excitatory projection from the cerebral cortex to a subgroup of neurons of the striatum that inhibit the internal segment of the globus pallidus, transiently interrupting the tonic inhibition that this structure exerts on the thalamic and brainstem targets involved in the initiation of motor programs. Suppression of unwanted motor programs or interruption of ongoing motor acts depends on excitatory cortical input to the subthalamic nucleus and a subgroup of neurons in the striatum that inhibit the external segment of the globus pallidus, thus disinhibiting the subthalamic nucleus. The subthalamic nucleus further activates the internal segment of the globus pallidus, leading to increased inhibition of thalamocortical and brainstem motor circuits.

Modulatory Influences on the Cerebral Cortex and Basal Ganglia

The activity of neurons in the cerebral cortex and basal ganglia is regulated by cholinergic and monoaminergic pathways of the consciousness system. Two important examples are the effects of cholinergic and dopaminergic pathways. Cholinergic input from the basal forebrain, including the *nucleus basalis of Meynert*, facilitate synaptic plasticity in cortical neurons and is important in mechanisms of selective attention to sensory stimuli, learning, and memory. Dopaminergic input from the midbrain provides a "reward" signal to the cerebral cortex and basal ganglia to control behavior. Dopaminergic input from the *substantia nigra pars compacta* to the striatum and other components of the basal ganglia circuit facilitates the initiation of behaviorally relevant motor programs, and the dopaminergic input from the *ventral tegmental area* to the prefrontal cortex has an important role in controlling executive functions such as attention, decision making, and motivation.

Other neurotransmitters, including norepinephrine (arising from neurons of the locus ceruleus), serotonin (from neurons of the raphe nuclei), and histamine (from neurons of the tuberomammillary nucleus), modulate the activity of thalamocortical circuits. These monoamines facilitate the relay of thalamic information to the cerebral cortex and increase the signal-to-noise ratio of cortical neurons. Together with the cholinergic system, these monoaminergic systems are critical for cortical arousal (Chapter 10).

Pathophysiology

Seizures

The cellular properties of pyramidal neurons and their pattern of connectivity make the cerebral cortex particularly susceptible to the development of excessive paroxysmal synchronized activity that is manifested as seizures. A *seizure* is a transient disturbance that occurs as a result of an abnormal, excessive, and synchronized discharge of a population of cortical neurons. It is a specific pathophysiologic expression of abnormality at the supratentorial level. The two primary factors that produce seizures are increased excitability of cortical neurons and synchronization of neuronal populations through excitatory connections. Mechanisms that may cause these processes include alteration of intrinsic membrane properties of pyramidal neurons, impairment of local GABAergic inhibitory mechanisms, local changes in neuronal environment, and recurrent synchronized excitation of neuronal populations through reciprocal thalamocortical interactions.

Seizures may be *partial* (*focal*) or *generalized* in distribution. Partial seizures occur with focal lesions such as a vascular disorder, neoplasm, abscess, or trauma and are manifested in different ways with involvement of different cortical areas. Partial seizures may become generalized as a result of synchronizing mechanisms between the two hemispheres, recruitment of synchronizing thalamocortical circuits, or involvement of subcortical structures. Generalized seizures may have a genetic basis or be a consequence of a metabolic, toxic, degenerative, traumatic disorder; they also may develop from focal seizures.

- A seizure is a transient disturbance that is the result of abnormal excessive discharge of cortical neurons; it can be generalized or focal.

Movement Disorders

Because of the reciprocal connections with different parts of the frontal lobe, disorders of the basal ganglia affect not only motor function but also ocular motor, cognitive, and affective functions. The motor effects include the *hypokinetic-rigid syndrome* called *parkinsonism* and *hyperkinetic syndromes*, including chorea, ballismus, and dystonia (Chapter 8). Hypokinetic disorders commonly are the result of impaired dopaminergic input to the striatum, which leads to relative hyperactivity of the "indirect" striatopallidal circuit and subthalamic nucleus and thus inhibition of the thalamus and brainstem targets by the internal segment of the globus pallidus. Hyperkinetic disorders may be due to excessive dopaminergic transmission, loss of selective neuronal populations in the striatum, or lesions of the subthalamic nucleus. In both hypokinetic and hyperkinetic disorders, the synchronization of activity in the basal ganglia circuits is abnormal, leading to impaired information processing in the motor cortex. This explains why the interruption of this oscillatory activity by either subthalamic stimulation or lesions of the subthalamic nucleus or globus pallidus may be beneficial in both Parkinson disease and hyperkinetic disorders.

- Disorders affecting the cortical-basal ganglia-thalamocortical circuits produce motor, ocular motor, cognitive, and behavioral abnormalities.

Limbic System Networks

The limbic system can be subdivided into two main circuits: 1) the anterior limbic circuit involves the amygdala and its connections and is important in the control of emotion and affective behavior and 2) the posterior limbic circuit involves the hippocampal formation and is essential for learning and declarative memory (Fig. 16B.16).

Amygdala and Emotion

Anatomy of the Amygdala

The *amygdala* (from the Greek word for almond) is located just anterior to the hippocampus, deep to the uncus of the temporal lobe. The amygdala consists of several nuclei that are divided into a *basolateral nuclear group*, *centromedial group*, and *olfactory group*. The basolateral group interconnects the amygdala with the cerebral cortex, thalamus, and basal forebrain. This nuclear group also projects to the central nucleus of the centromedial group, which in turn projects to the hypothalamus and brainstem (Fig. 16B.17). The amygdala is connected with the cerebral cortex through the external capsule and with the thalamus, hypothalamus, basal forebrain, and brainstem through the *ventral amygdalofugal pathway* and the *stria terminalis*.

Cortical and thalamic inputs provide sensory information to the basolateral nuclear group of the amygdala. Thalamic input conveys the elemental features of a sensory stimulus, whereas cortical input, from sensory association areas, provides processed sensory information. These two types of sensory information are integrated by neurons in the basolateral complex, which provides the sensory stimulus with emotional significance. These neurons have reciprocal connections with the cerebral cortex, particularly the orbitomedial prefrontal, anterior cingulate, and insular cortices, and hippocampus. These interactions include direct projections or projections through the mediodorsal nucleus of the thalamus or basal forebrain. The basolateral complex projects to the central nucleus of the amygdala, which projects either directly or through the bed nucleus of the stria terminalis to the hypothalamus and brainstem autonomic and motor nuclei. Through these projections, the central nucleus of the amygdala initiates endocrine, autonomic, and motor responses to emotional stimuli (Fig. 16B.17).

Physiology

A fundamental role of the amygdala is to provide a sensory stimulus with emotional significance. Thus, the amygdala is critical for emotional or associative memory, including *conditioned responses*, particularly fear.

The emotional experience stored in the basolateral amygdala generates an integrated emotional response through the connection of the basolateral complex with the central nucleus of the amygdala, which projects to

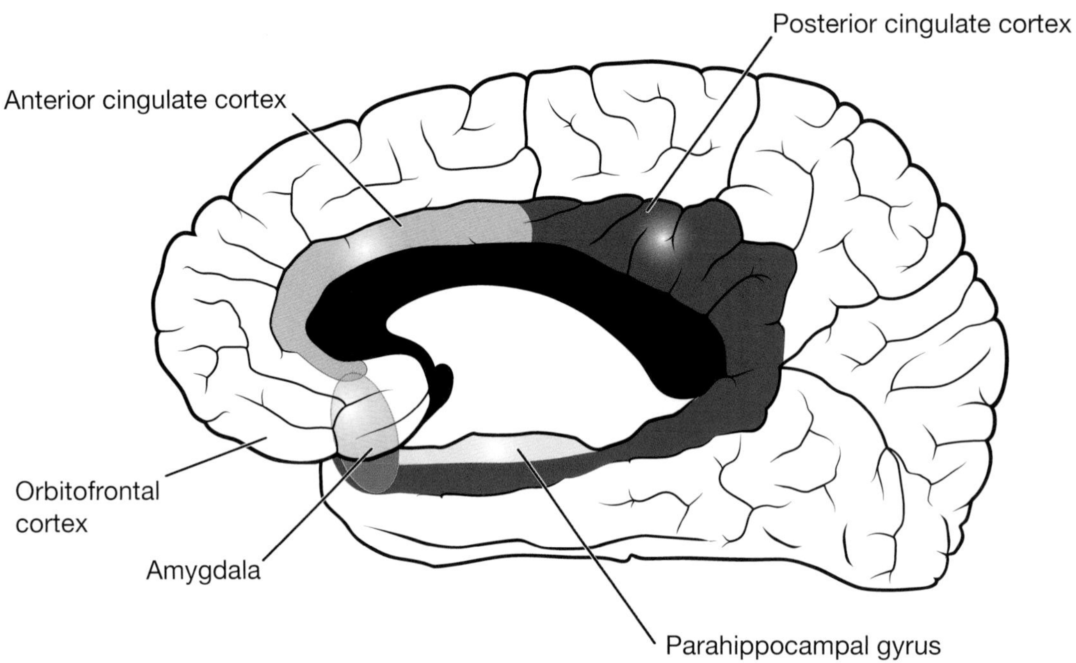

Fig. 16B.16. Telencephalic components of the anterior (salmon) and posterior (red and yellow) limbic circuits. The anterior limbic circuit is centered on the amygdala and includes the orbitofrontal and anterior cingulate cortices. These structures are interconnected with each other and the limbic striatum either directly or through the mediodorsal and midline thalamic nuclei. The anterior limbic circuit is involved in emotion. The posterior limbic circuit is centered on the hippocampus and includes the entorhinal cortex, parahippocampal gyrus, and the posterior cingulate cortex. These structures are interconnected with each other either directly or through the fornix, with a relay in the mammillary bodies and anterior thalamic nucleus. The posterior limbic circuit is involved in declarative (explicit) memory, including autobiographic memory (episodic memory), learning of facts (semantic memory), and spatial memory. (Modified from Benarroch EE. Basic neurosciences with clinical applications. Philadelphia: Elsevier; 2006. Used with permission of Mayo Foundation for Medical Education and Research.)

the hypothalamus and autonomic and motor nuclei of the brainstem. These responses include sympathoexcitation (tachycardia, sweating, mydriasis), secretion of cortisol and epinephrine, and startle. Reciprocal interactions between the amygdala and the cerebral cortex are important for interactions between emotion and cognition. Emotionally driven information from the amygdala can bias attentional processes and sensory perceptions. Projections to the hippocampus may explain why emotionally charged events are more likely to be remembered than emotionally neutral ones, and reciprocal connections with the hippocampus provide context information stored in memory. Input to the anterior cingulate cortex may be important for driving motor responses. The projection from orbitomedial prefrontal cortex to the amygdala is important in inhibiting emotional responses when inappropriate for the social or behavioral context.

Clinical Correlations

Bilateral lesions of the amygdala in humans typically affect the ability to recognize the affective meaning of facial expressions, particularly the expression of fear. More severe lesions may produce the *Klüver-Bucy syndrome*, characterized by the inability to recognize the significance of visual objects, emotional blunting, inappropriate eating behavior, and hypersexuality. Medial temporal lobe seizures that involve the amygdala may produce affective phenomena, particularly fear, perceptual phenomena with an experiential quality, a feeling of reminiscence

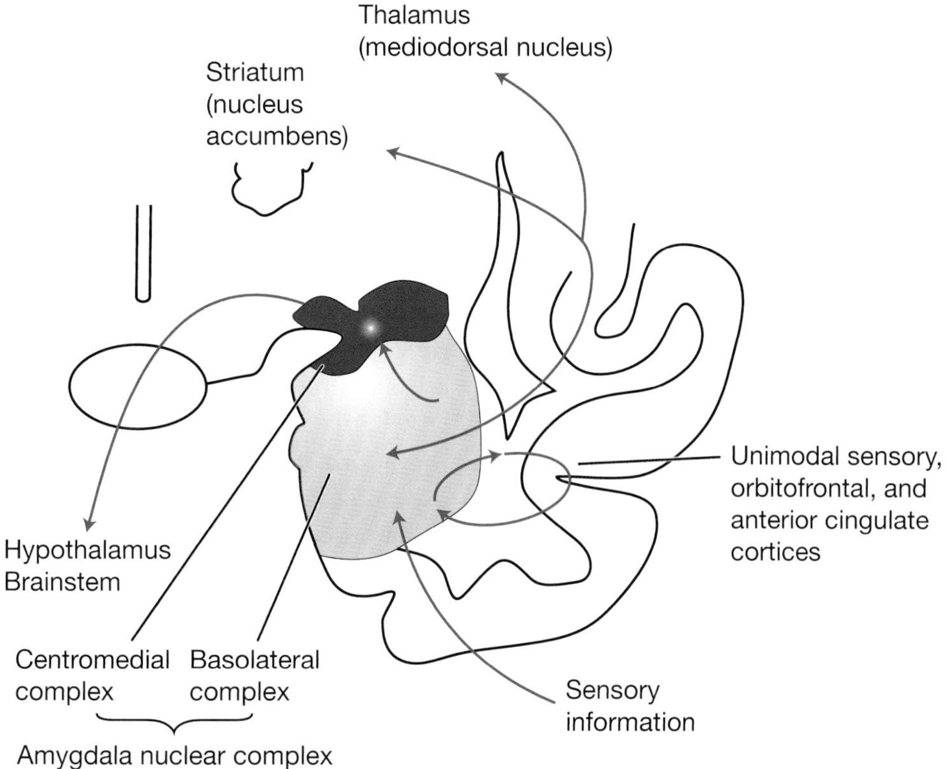

Fig. 16B.17. Main connections of the amygdala. The amygdala consists of several nuclei that are grouped into a basolateral complex, centromedial complex, and olfactory complex (not shown). Nuclei of the basolateral complex receive input from the cerebral cortex and thalamus and are reciprocally connected with these structures as well as with the basal forebrain and limbic striatum, both directly and by relay in the thalamic mediodorsal nucleus. Sensory information is processed in the basolateral complex and tagged with emotional significance. The basolateral complex projects to the central nucleus, which projects to hypothalamic and brainstem nuclei that mediate endocrine, autonomic, and motor responses to emotion, particularly conditioned fear. (Modified from Benarroch EE. Basic neurosciences with clinical applications. Philadelphia: Elsevier; 2006. Used with permission of Mayo Foundation for Medical Education and Research.)

or familiarity with an affective component, autonomic manifestations, and rhythmic oroalimentary automatisms. The amygdala has been implicated in various models of *anxiety disorder*; for example, functional neuroimaging studies have shown abnormal activation of the amygdala in posttraumatic stress disorder.

Bilateral lesions of the orbitomedial prefrontal cortex result in socially inappropriate behavior, impulsivity, and emotional disinhibition, likely by interrupting inhibitory control the prefrontal cortex exerts on the amygdala. The amygdala is important in emotional responses.

- The amygdala is important in emotional responses.
- Lesions of the amygdala result in the inability to recognize emotional facial expressions.
- Lesions of the orbitomedial prefrontal cortex lead to disinhibition of emotional responses.

Hippocampal Formation: Learning and Declarative Memory

Anatomy

The hippocampal formation and parahippocampal cortex, located on the medial aspect of the temporal lobe, are involved in the process of declarative memory. The hippocampal formation consists of the *dentate gyrus*, *cornu Ammonis* (CA1-CA4 areas), and *subiculum* (Fig. 16B.18). Input to the hippocampal formation arises from the *entorhinal cortex*, which conveys information from the neocortex after relay in the parahippocampal gyrus. The function of the hippocampus involves serial, parallel, and reciprocal excitatory connections between all these structures (Fig. 16B.18).

> Neocortical association areas send excitatory projections to the parahippocampal gyrus (parahippocampal and perirhinal cortices), which in turn projects to the entorhinal cortex. The entorhinal cortex conveys this excitatory input to the dentate gyrus or to area CA3 of the hippocampus. Area CA3, which also receives input from the dentate gyrus (mossy fibers), projects to area CA1 (via Schaffer collaterals), and CA1 sends excitatory projections to the subiculum. The subiculum sends excitatory projections to the entorhinal cortex, thus closing a serial multisynaptic excitatory loop.

The highly processed information from the hippocampal formation is transmitted back to the cerebral cortex by both cortical and subcortical routes. The cortical route involves projections from the subiculum to the entorhinal cortex, from the entorhinal to the parahippocampal cortex, and from the parahippocampal cortex to the neocortical association areas. The subcortical route involves axons from area CA1 and subiculum that project through the *fornix* (Fig. 16B.19). The CA1 axons in the

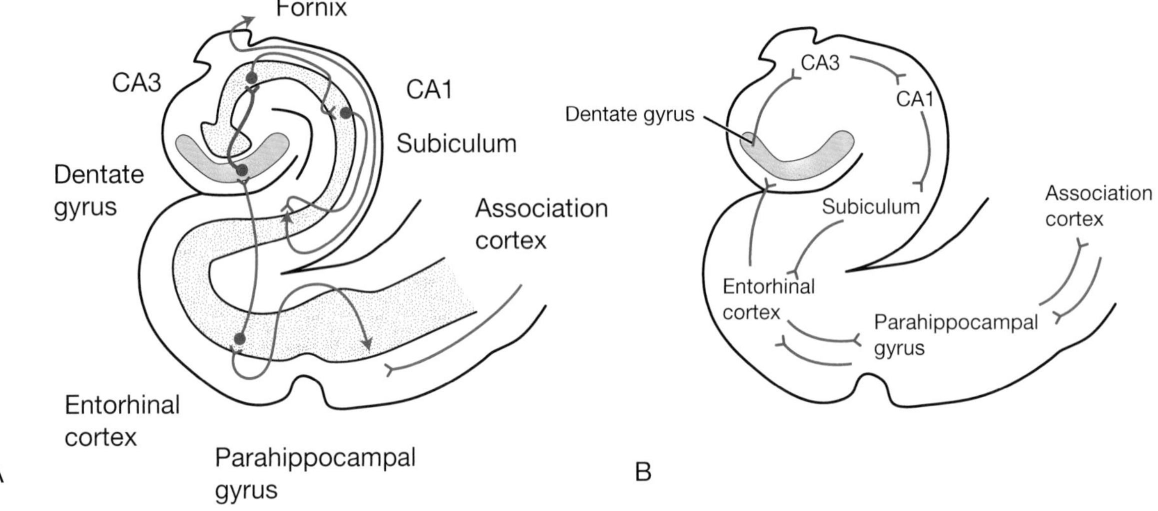

Fig. 16B.18. The medial temporal memory system includes the hippocampal formation, entorhinal cortex, and parahippocampal region. *A*, Association areas of neocortex project to the parahippocampal cortex, which projects to entorhinal cortex. The entorhinal cortex is the gateway for entry of highly elaborated information into the hippocampus. The hippocampal formation comprises the dentate gyrus, hippocampus proper (CA1-CA3 regions), and subiculum. The intrinsic circuit of the hippocampal formation involves feed-forward excitatory connections. Granule cells of the dentate gyrus send excitatory axons (called mossy fibers) to CA3 pyramidal neurons. CA3 pyramidal cells project via Schaffer collaterals to CA1 pyramidal neurons, which project to the subiculum. *B*, There are reciprocal feed-forward and feedback connections among the neocortex, parahippocampal gyrus, and hippocampal formation. Association areas of the neocortex project to the perirhinal and parahippocampal cortices. These, in turn, project to the entorhinal cortex. Neurons of CA1 and subiculum project back to the entorhinal cortex, which relays this input to the parahippocampal cortex, which projects to neocortex.

fornix project to the *septal region*, which contains cholinergic neurons that project back to the hippocampus. The subicular axons in the fornix project to the *mammillary bodies* of the hypothalamus. These nuclei project to the *anterior nucleus* of the thalamus (mammillothalamic tract), which in turn projects to the *cingulate cortex*. The cingulate cortex projects to the parahippocampal formation. This circuit constitutes the classic *Circuit of Papez*.

Physiology: Declarative Memory

The term *memory* encompasses several different processes, each of which has a different anatomical substrate. The hippocampal formation, parahippocampal gyrus, and entorhinal cortex constitute the medial temporal memory system, which is essential for *declarative memory*. Declarative (also called explicit) memory includes the ability to learn, store, and retrieve information about autobiographical events (*episodic memory*), facts and names (*semantic memory*), and places (*spatial memory*).

The hippocampus is critical for the acquisition and maintenance of autobiographical memory and the initial acquisition (*learning*) of general knowledge (semantic memory). Semantic information is stored temporarily in the hippocampus but is eventually translated into a more permanent store in the neocortex, where it may become stabilized. Although hippocampal activation is necessary for the retrieval of episodic memories, the frontal lobes contribute to planning, monitoring, and organizing the retrieval process.

The normal function of the medial temporal memory system depends on connections with the diencephalon and basal forebrain. The entorhinal cortex

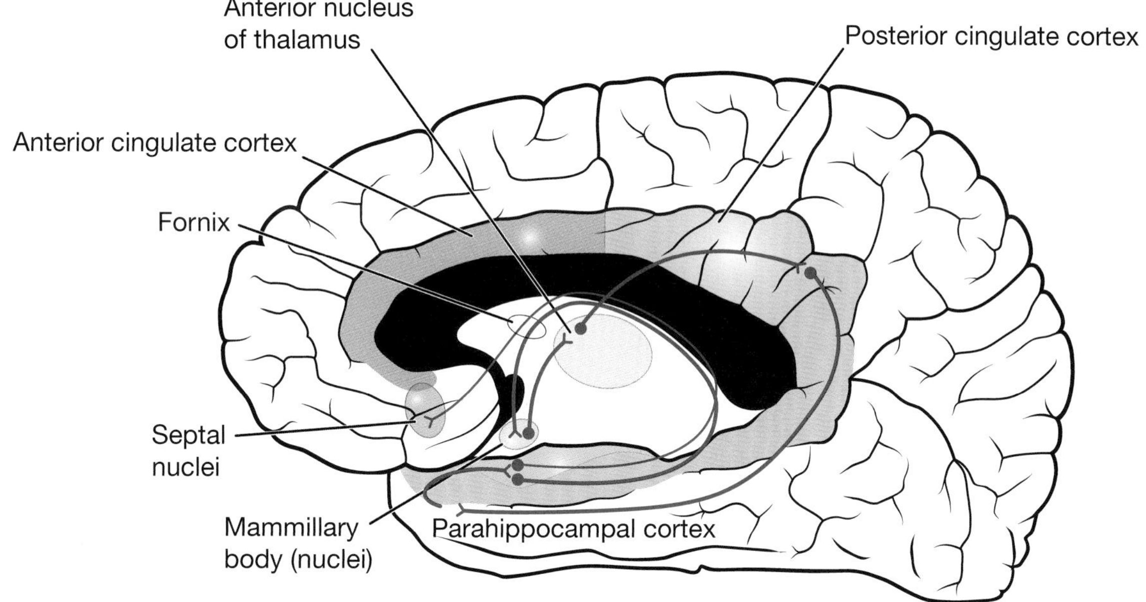

Fig. 16B.19. The hippocampal formation projects to subcortical structures through the fornix, whose axons are from pyramidal neurons of CA1 and particularly the subiculum. The fornix loops over the thalamus and, at the anterior commissure, divides into the precommissural fornix, containing axons from CA1 and terminating in the lateral septal nucleus, and the larger postcommissural fornix, containing axons from the subiculum and terminating in the mammillary body (nuclei). The mammillary body projects to the anterior nucleus of the thalamus, which conveys this information to the cingulate cortex. Cingulate cortex projects back to the parahippocampal gyrus and entorhinal cortex. These regions project to the hippocampal formation. This group of cortical-diencephalic-cortical connections forms the Papez circuit. (Modified from Benarroch EE. Basic neurosciences with clinical applications. Philadelphia: Elsevier; 2006. Used with permission of Mayo Foundation for Medical Education and Research.)

receives input from the midline thalamic nuclei, whereas the major thalamic input to the posterior cingulate cortex and subicular cortex, areas that receive input from the hippocampal formation, is from the anterior nucleus. The mediodorsal nucleus is a central link in the circuits interconnecting the hippocampus, amygdala, and prefrontal cortex. The basal forebrain cholinergic system is also important in memory function.

Clinical Correlations: Amnesia

Loss of declarative memory is called *amnesia*. This usually is due to bilateral damage of the medial temporal cortex, which impairs the ability to learn and store new information. Amnesia is typical of *Alzheimer disease*, the most common degenerative dementia. The memory impairment in this disorder reflects involvement of the entorhinal and perirhinal cortices, followed by that of the hippocampus and the loss of the cholinergic neurons in the basal forebrain. In early stages of the disease, well-established and old memories (remote memory), such as the birth date of a family member or the name of an old friend, are relatively preserved, in part because they often are of a personal nature and quite meaningful to the person and they are stored in association areas of the lateral temporal neocortex. Eventually, as the lateral temporal association neocortex is affected by the disease, the person is unable to recall remote events.

Learning and declarative memory also are selectively impaired by acute or subacute lesions that affect the medial temporal lobe or its connections. Important examples are head injury, herpes simplex encephalitis, and paraneoplastic limbic encephalitis. Impaired learning and declarative memory may also result from midline lesions that affect diencephalic structures (*diencephalic amnesia*). The typical example is *Korsakoff syndrome*, which is caused by thiamine deficiency, as in malnourished patients and those with a history of alcohol abuse. The lesions primarily involve the anterior and dorsomedial thalamic nuclei and the mammillary bodies.

Memory disturbances can be classified on a temporal dimension if they are caused by an abrupt event. The inability to form new memories or to learn new information beginning at the time of the injury is called *anterograde amnesia*. For example, a person who has a head injury may have difficulty remembering events that occur after the injury (this may last for up to several days). In contrast, the inability to recall events that occurred before an injury is called *retrograde amnesia*. Typically, retrograde amnesia has a temporal gradient, with information learned immediately before the injury being more susceptible to disruption because it is less well established. The reversible (within 24 hours) inability to learn new information characterizes *transient global amnesia*. For example, the patient may ask the same question several times. This benign disorder has been associated with migraine. Patients with impaired function of the medial temporal or diencephalic memory system also have

Clinical Problem 16B.1.

An 18-year-old student sustained a closed head injury during a football game and had transient loss of consciousness. Upon recovery, he complained of a headache. The results of computed tomography of the head were normal. On examination 3 days later, he was alert but unable to recall the football game or any event in the 48 hours preceding it. He recalled waking up in the hospital but did not remember the day. On neurologic examination, he was unable to tell what he had for breakfast that morning. When prompted, he said that he had toast and coffee, when in fact he had scrambled eggs and orange juice. He could recall the name of his favorite football team and his birth date. The rest of the neurologic examination was normal.

a. What type of function is affected in this patient?
b. What area of the brain most likely is involved?
c. What are the names for the inability to recall events before or after an injury?
d. Why did he remember the name of the football team and his birth date?
e. What is the term for "filling-up" memory gaps with erroneous information?

confabulations. Confabulations (false memories) consist of intrusion errors or distortions made in response to a challenge to memory.

- Bilateral damage of the medial temporal cortex, including the hippocampus and parahippocampal cortex, or the diencephalic areas connected with them results in the inability to learn new information, leading to the loss of episodic memory.
- Lesions of the lateral temporal lobe interfere with the ability to recall remote events or previously learned facts.

Olfactory System

The olfactory system, unlike other sensory systems, has direct access to the cerebral cortex, without a relay in the thalamus. The rapid access to the amygdala and hippocampal circuit may explain the tendency of some odors to rapidly evoke emotions and memories.

Olfactory Receptors and Nerve

The olfactory receptors lie in the superior nasal mucosa and respond to the chemical structures of many agents that are perceived as smells. The *olfactory nerve* (cranial nerve I) is composed of numerous unmyelinated axons from the receptor cells. The axons penetrate the skull through the cribriform plate and terminate in the olfactory bulb (Fig. 16B.20).

Central Olfactory Pathway

The *olfactory bulb* is a small ovoid structure that lies in the anterior end of the olfactory sulcus on the orbital surface of the frontal lobe. Fibers from the olfactory bulb form the *olfactory tract*, which passes posteriorly and divides into medial and lateral *olfactory striae*. Most olfactory fibers synapse in the *pyriform cortex*, located in the anterior portion of the *uncus*, the chief cortical olfactory area. Others terminate in the orbital cortex and the olfactory (cortical) nucleus of the amygdala.

Clinical Correlations

An important manifestation of focal lesions involving the medial temporal lobe is *complex partial seizures*. By definition, these seizures are associated with transient loss of awareness: the patient is alert but stares into space and is unresponsive to the environment. In many cases, these seizures are preceded by focal symptoms that the patient can describe while still aware and communicative. One of these symptoms is olfactory hallucinations (generally unpleasant, such as the smell of burning rubber), which reflect involvement of olfactory cortex at the level of the uncus or the underlying amygdala (*uncinate seizures*). Other manifestations are oromandibular automatism (such as chewing or licking movements) or more complex motor behaviors, fear or other affective symptoms associated or not with autonomic effects (indicating involvement of the amygdala), and phenomena such as déjà-vu or jamais vu that reflect disturbances of episodic memory (indicating involvement of the hippocampus and parahippocampal cortex).

Several disorders have a relatively selective predisposition for the limbic system. Typical examples are *herpes simplex encephalitis*, rabies, and autoimmune (including paraneoplastic) *limbic encephalitis*. These

Clinical Problem 16B.2.

A 33-year-old right-handed man is evaluated for spells that started 2 weeks ago. Each spell lasts approximately 1 to 2 minutes. During the spell, he experiences an unpleasant odor (as smelling burning rubber). Following this, he felt as if he were in a dream state in which he saw and heard things that he had experienced before. Although some experiences were pleasant, others elicited some fear and he would become pale, sweaty, and tachycardic as if he was experiencing a "panic reaction." He is not able to remember events that were going on around him during these episodes. According to witnesses, he is alert during the episodes but is unresponsive to his environment.

a. What do these spells represent?
b. What is the most likely location of the lesion?
c. What is the anatomical substrate for the olfactory, emotional, autonomic, and cognitive manifestations of the spell?

disorders may manifest as subacute onset of changes in emotional behavior, impaired memory, and complex partial seizures.

As the olfactory nerve fibers go through the cribriform plate, they are particularly susceptible to injury, for example, in head trauma. The olfactory bulb is involved early in some neurodegenerative diseases, including Parkinson disease. The olfactory tract may be affected by a mass lesion on the orbital surface of the brain, for example, an olfactory groove meningioma.

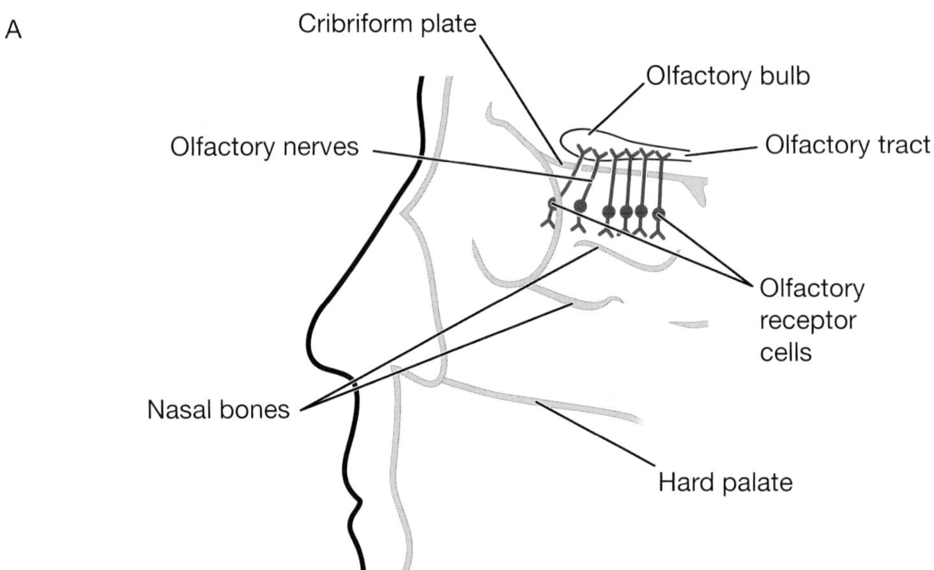

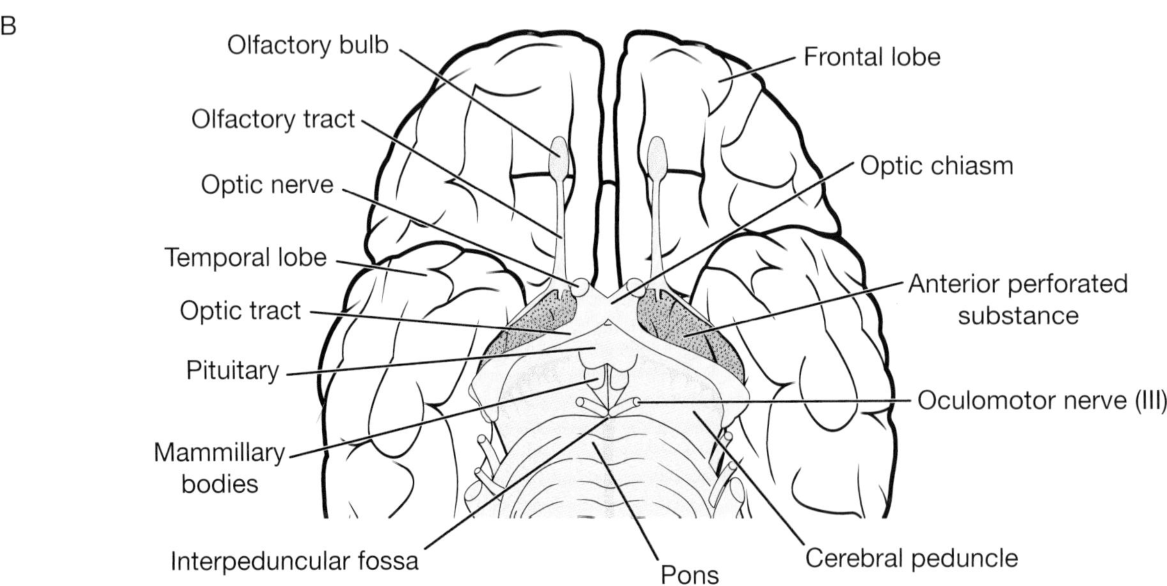

Fig. 16B.20. Olfactory structures. *A*, Lateral view of olfactory nerves penetrating the skull through the cribiform plate to synapse in the ofactory bulb. *B*, Basal view of the brain showing the course of the axons of olfactory bulb neurons in the olfactory tract, which subdivides into a lateral olfactory stria that terminates in the piriform (primary olfactory) cortex and amygdala, at the level of the uncus, and a medial olfactory stria that terminates in the orbitofrontal cortex and septal area.

Neocortical Networks

Several neocortical networks involve interactions among different primary, unimodal, and heteromodal association areas. These networks are important in the following functions: 1) sensory processing and object recognition, 2) directed attention, 3) motor programming and execution, 4) language, and 5) control of behavior. These higher cortical functions depend on the synchronized activity of widespread neurons in each network as well as connections with the thalamus, basal ganglia, and limbic system.

Sensory Processing and Object Recognition

Somatosensory, visual, and auditory information reach the cortex through specific relay nuclei that receive input from the specific sensory pathways described elsewhere in this book. The thalamic projections usually terminate in layer IV of the corresponding primary sensory area. From this primary area, information is sequentially processed in unimodal association and heteromodal association cortical areas. These processing pathways form two partially separated and functionally distinct streams of processing: a dorsal (parietal) stream for object localization and a ventral stream for object recognition.

Somatosensory System

The different areas of the primary somatosensory cortex (areas 3a, 3b, 1, and 2) contain separate somatotopic representations of the contralateral body. The primary area for proprioception is area 3a, and the area for tactile representation is area 3b. Areas 1 and 2 integrate input from both modalities. In combination with proprioceptive information, tactile information from the fingers during *active touch* (tactile discrimination requiring manipulation of the object) is important for recognizing the shape of an object; this is called *stereognosis*. Information from areas 1 and 2 is processed in a dorsal stream that involves areas 5 and 7 of the posterior parietal cortex. The posterior parietal cortex integrates this information with visual information to guide reaching and grasping movements. A ventral stream, through the second somatosensory cortex and insular cortex, connects the somatosensory areas and heteromodal areas required for the tactile recognition of objects.

- The primary somatosensory cortex has separate somatotopic maps for proprioceptive and tactile information and is the first processing stage for tactile recognition of objects and the somatosensory guidance of reaching and grasping movements.

Visual System

Most of the visual cortex is devoted to the analysis of central vision. As discussed in Chapter 16A, the primary visual cortex (area 17, calcarine or striate cortex) is located on the banks the calcarine fissure on the medial aspect and pole of the occipital lobe. Each calcarine cortex has a retinotopic organization, with a complete representation of the contralateral visual field. The macula has a large representation posteriorly in the calcarine cortex, and the peripheral retina is represented more anteriorly. The inferior portion of the calcarine fissure receives the temporal component of the optic radiation and has a representation of the upper half of the contralateral visual field, whereas the superior portion of the calcarine cortex, receiving the parietal component of the optic radiation, has a representation of the lower half. The primary visual cortex is organized into *dominance columns*, which receive preferential input from each eye. Within these columns are cells that respond selectively to a certain orientation or movement of a linear light stimulus. Information about form and color required for object recognition and information about object position and movement in space needed for visually guided motor control are transmitted in parallel channels throughout the visual pathway.

The subchannels within the visual pathway arise from different types of ganglion cells in the retina and terminate in different layers of the lateral geniculate nucleus, which, in turn, project to different sublayers of layer IV of primary visual cortex. The parvicellular (P) pathway arises from retinal ganglion cells that receive input from cones, are highly sensitive to color (red or green), and are specialized for high visual acuity. This pathway terminates in four superficial layers of the lateral geniculate nucleus that project to the deep sublayers of cortical layer IV. The magnicellular (M) pathway

> arises from retinal ganglion cells that receive input primarily from rods and are sensitive to movement of the object. This pathway terminates primarily in two ventral layers of the lateral geniculate that project to the superficial sublayers of cortical layer IV. A koniocellular (K) pathway arises from a group of retinal ganglion cells that receive input from blue cones and project to the intercalated layers of the lateral geniculate nucleus, which, in turn, project to particular compartments called blobs in cortical layers II and III.

Further processing of visual information involves unimodal visual association areas, namely, areas 18 and 19 (extrastriate cortex) in the occipital lobe and areas in the posterior parietal and inferior temporal lobes. The dorsal stream of visual processing involves areas in the middle temporal and middle superior temporal lobe and terminates in the posterior parietal cortex. All these areas contain neurons specialized for analyzing the location and movement of an object. In the ventral stream, the color and form of an object are analyzed in a sequentially hierarchical fashion by neurons located in the occipitotemporal cortex (the fusiform and lingual gyri). At the highest hierarchical level of the ventral stream, neurons respond only to a specific combination of features, such as a specific face or objects (Fig. 16B.21).

- The visual cortex is devoted to the analysis of central vision.
- The visual association area in the occipitotemporal cortex analyzes the form and color of objects.
- The visual association areas in the occipitoparietal and posterior parietal cortices analyze the movement of objects.

Auditory System

In humans, the auditory cortex is located in the transverse temporal gyri of Heschl, which lie on the dorsal surface of the superior temporal gyrus. The middle part of the anterior transverse gyrus (area 41) is the primary auditory receptive area; the remaining part of the transverse gyrus and adjacent parts of the superior temporal area (area 42) are auditory association areas. The auditory cortex is divided into a *core*, a *belt*, and a *parabelt* that participate in the sequential processing of auditory information.

> The core corresponds to the primary auditory area and contains neurons that respond to pure tones of specific frequencies and respond primarily to stimulation of both ears. The neurons are sensitive to the location of the source of the sound. The belt contains neurons that respond to complex sounds. The belt projects to the parabelt, which is located along the lateral surface of the superior temporal gyrus and contains neurons that respond to white noise but not to pure tone.

Although the auditory system consists of bilateral projections beginning with the cochlear nuclei, the left side has a greater capacity for language-related processing, probably from birth. The left superior temporal gyrus is critical for the acoustic processing and extraction of the meaning of spoken language.

Object Recognition and Semantic Knowledge

The recognition of objects, including faces, is necessary for knowledge about the world. This knowledge, called *semantic memory*, depends on the storage of information about the features and attributes (shape, sound, and use) that define an object. Object recognition is the first necessary step for naming, using, and reacting emotionally to an object. Functional neuroimaging studies indicate that information about different object features is represented in a distributed network and stored in widespread areas of the cerebral cortex, particularly in the left hemisphere. The ability of modality-specific visual, somatosensory, or auditory information to activate the relevant multimodal associations that lead to face or object recognition depends on a heteromodal network located in the *anterior middle temporal gyrus* and *temporal pole*.

Clinical Correlations: Agnosias

The inability to identify an object despite being able to perceive it is called *agnosia*. The patient is alert, attentive, not aphasic, and has intact sensation but is unable to

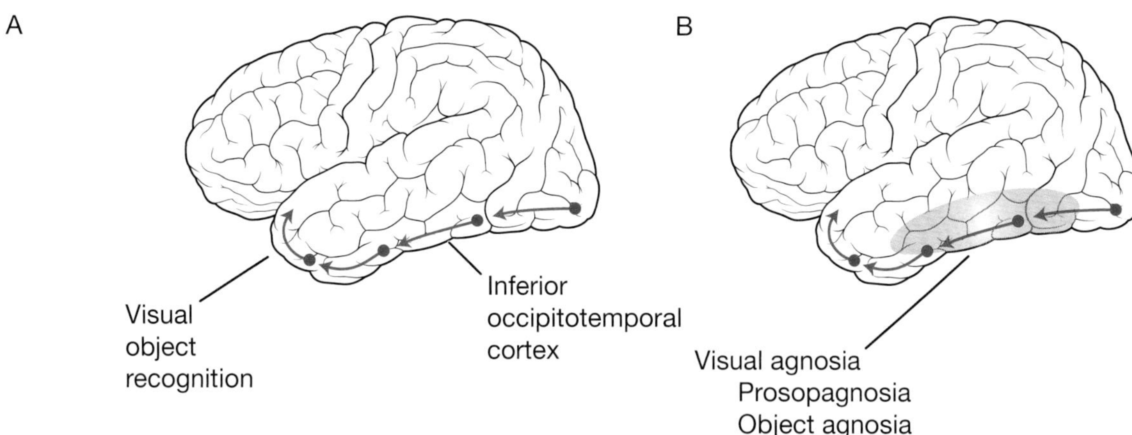

Fig. 16B.21. *A*, Ventral stream of processing of visual information involves several synaptic relays in the inferior occipitotemporal cortex (including the fusiform and lingual gyri), where information about color and shape is processed sequentially, leading to visual recognition of faces and objects. *B*, A unilateral lesion affecting this pathway produces contralateral hemiachromatopsia. Bilateral (or rarely right-sided) lesions interrupting this pathway lead to visual agnosia, including prosopagnosia and object agnosia. The patient cannot recognize faces or objects presented visually but can do so auditorily or tactilely.

tell what the object is. Agnosia occurs with lesions in the unimodal sensory association areas and can involve any of the sensory modalities.

Lesions of the postcentral gyrus that interrupt the connections between the primary and unimodal somatosensory association areas in the parietal lobe cause tactile agnosia, or *astereognosia*. The patient is unable to identify an object by palpating it. This usually is associated with cortical sensory loss, including loss of two-point discrimination, inability to recognize letters or numbers written on the palm of the hand (*agraphesthesia*), inability to localize touch (*atopognosia*), and loss of ability to discriminate weights (*abarognosia*) on the contralateral side.

Lesions of primary visual cortex produce homonymous hemianopsia, but lesions of unimodal visual association cortex have different manifestations depending on whether the dorsal or ventral stream is involved. Lesions of the dorsal visual stream produce *akinetopsia*, in which the patient cannot perceive motion despite relative preservation of other visual modalities. Lesions of the ventral stream that affect the posterior part of the inferior occipitotemporal cortex cause the loss of color perception in the contralateral hemifield, or *hemiachromatopsia*, and different types of

Clinical Problem 16B.3.

A 45-year-old right-handed journalist is evaluated for progressive numbness in his right hand over the past 2 months. He has noticed difficulty holding a pen unless he looks at it. He is unable to retrieve coins or keys from his pockets. Neurologic examination showed impaired joint position and two-point discrimination of the fingers of the right hand. He is unable to identify numbers written on his right palm. With his eyes closed, he cannot identify a key or a coin placed in his right hand, but can do so when the object is placed in his left hand. Touch, vibration, pain, and temperature sensations; motor strength; and reflexes are symmetrically normal.

a. What is the most likely location of the lesion?
b. What is the name given to the inability to recognize objects by touch?
c. How can you differentiate this lesion from one affecting the dorsal columns?

visual agnosia (Fig. 16B.21). The inability to identify familiar faces is called *prosopagnosia*. It is caused most commonly by bilateral lesions of the mid to anterior part of the lingual and fusiform gyri of the inferior occipitotemporal cortex. These patients can recognize a face as a face and sometimes tell if two faces have an identical shape or not, but they cannot recognize familiar faces by visual inspection. The inability to recognize or name an object or to describe its use is *visual object agnosia*. For example, if shown a toothbrush, such a patient is able to describe its length, texture, and color but is not able to name it or to describe its use. However, the patient is able to recognize the object by palpation in the absence of visual clues.

Unilateral lesions of primary auditory cortex do not lead to contralateral deafness because of the bilateral representation of auditory pathways. Lesions in unimodal auditory association cortex or its connections may produce *cortical deafness* (the inability to recognize meaningful verbal and nonverbal auditory patterns), *auditory agnosia* (the inability to describe a sound that can be heard), or *pure word deafness* (the inability to understand or repeat spoken language despite good recognition of environmental sounds and no other language deficit).

Lesions in the anterior middle temporal or temporopolar cortex, particularly on the left side, deprive the person of the ability to associate multimodal information needed to recognize objects. These patients become progressively unfamiliar with objects, leading to progressive loss of knowledge of the world. This is called *semantic dementia*. In this condition, the patient is unable to name the object, not because of a language deficit but because of the inability to recognize the object.

Clinical Problem 16B.4.

A 56-year-old right-handed man is brought for consultation by his wife because of unusual behavior. This morning, he could not recognize her face or that of their children and could identify them only when he heard their voices. On neurologic examination, he is unable to recognize the faces in pictures of the President of the United States or his favorite baseball player. He realizes that they are faces and different from each other.

a. What is the name of this condition?
b. What is the location of the lesion?
c. What cortical network is interrupted?
d. What artery supplies the involved area?

- Agnosia is the inability to recognize an object.
- Patients with agnosia are unable to recognize and, thus, name the object with the use of one sensory modality but can with the use of another sensory modality.
- Prosopagnosia is the inability to recognize individual faces and is the result of lesions (usually bilateral) that affect the inferior occipitotemporal cortex.
- Lesions of the temporopolar or anterior middle temporal cortex, particularly of the left hemisphere, lead to loss of semantic knowledge of the world.

Spatial Attention

Anatomy

The network for directed attention to extrapersonal space includes the posterior parietal lobe, frontal eye fields, and cingulate gyrus and their connections with the pulvinar and caudate nucleus (Fig. 16B.22). Neurons in the posterior parietal lobe, particularly in the *intraparietal sulcus*, receive visual, somatosensory, and auditory information from the respective unimodal sensory association areas through the dorsal stream of sensory processing. These heteromodal posterior parietal neurons also receive input from the *pulvinar*, which transmits information both from unimodal cortical sensory areas and the superior colliculus. Different groups of neurons in the intraparietal sulcus project to the prefrontal eye fields and lateral prefrontal cortex.

Physiology

Neurons of the intraparietal sulcus integrate visual, somatosensory, and auditory information to encode a representation of space. This is forwarded to the premotor cortex and frontal eye fields to initiate reaching and grasping for objects and directing gaze toward contralateral space. The pulvinar of the thalamus, which also receives visual, somatosensory, and auditory information from both the cerebral cortex and superior colliculus, projects to the posterior parietal cortex and is an integral component of the attention network. There are two separate networks for attention. A bilateral network that includes the intraparietal sulcus and the frontal eye fields is involved in orientation toward contralateral space. This network appears to be necessary for binding the different features of an object or scene into a single percept. A ventral frontoparietal network, located in the right hemisphere and including the temporoparietal junction, is involved primarily in directing attention to behaviorally relevant and unexpected sensory stimuli.

Clinical Correlations

Damage to the parietotemporal region, typically in the right hemisphere, produces contralateral *spatial neglect* (Fig. 16B.22). These patients fail to orientate toward or to detect items on their left side, including people or large objects. For example, when asked to draw or copy a figure such as a clock, they may put the numbers only on the right side. This is referred to as *constructional apraxia*. Patients with right parietal lesions may also neglect their own contralateral body parts, failing to use or show any interest in them, for example, dressing only the right side of the body (*dressing apraxia*). These patients may be unaware that they have any problem (*anosognosia*). Less

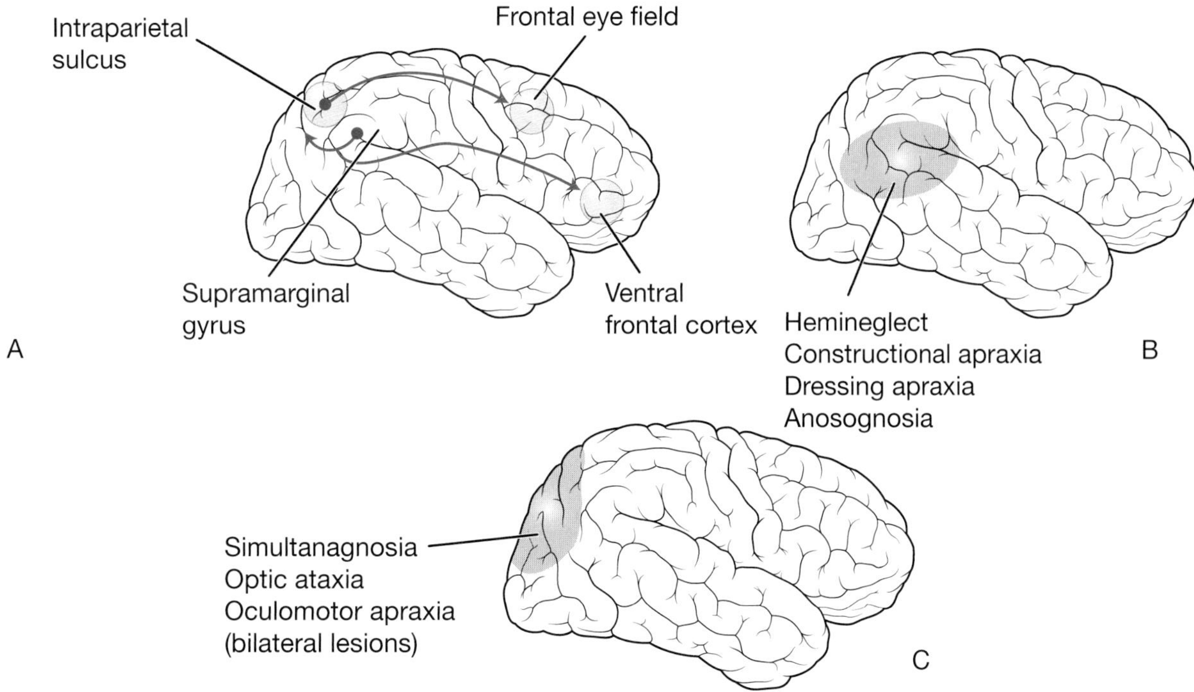

Fig. 16B.22. *A*, Cortical areas involved in spatial attention. They include the intraparietal sulcus that integrates multiple information about position and movement of the object in space and projects to the frontal eye fields, which direct gaze toward the object of interest. These areas are interconnected and form a bilateral network that includes the pulvinar of the thalamus and cingulate cortex and is critical for attention and guidance of movement toward contralateral space. A second group of areas in the right hemisphere, including the inferior parietal lobule (supramarginal gyrus) and ventral frontal cortex, are activated in response to novel, unexpected stimuli. *B*, Lesions of the right inferior parietal lobule (and adjacent superior temporal cortex) produce sensory neglect of the contralateral body, constructional apraxia, dressing apraxia, and anosognosia. *C*, Bilateral lesions of superior parietal cortex and adjacent occipital cortex produce Balint syndrome, characterized by simultanagnosia, oculomotor apraxia, and optic ataxia.

severe degrees of right posterior parietal dysfunction can be detected by the phenomenon of extinction, which is elicited by double simultaneous stimulation of a sensory modality, for example, visual, auditory, or somatosensory.

Patients with bilateral lesions of the superior parietal lobule of the posterior parietal cortex (the *angular gyrus*) may develop a deficit of spatial attention called *Balint syndrome* (Fig. 16B.22). Detecting a target on the neglected side is a problem for these patients when it requires the conjunction of two features, such as color and shape. The three main manifestations of Balint syndrome are *simultanagnosia* (the inability to see more than one object at a time), *oculomotor apraxia* (the fixation of gaze with severe difficulty in voluntarily moving fixation), and *optic ataxia* (the inability to reach toward the correct location of perceived objects).

Clinical Problem 16B.5.

A 65-year-old man is brought in by his wife for evaluation because of his unusual behavior. She became concerned when her husband drove into oncoming traffic and did not realize it. The same day she noticed that he did not eat from the left side of the plate. The patient reports that nothing is wrong, and he is only there at the request of his wife. He did not respond to the medical resident who approached him from the left side, but readily responded when the physician approached him from the right. During a neurologic examination, he put his head through the sleeve of the examining gown. The mental status examination was normal, except when he was asked to draw a clock and he put all the numbers on the right side of the circle. When asked to draw a house, he drew one with a window only on the right side. Strength was normal and symmetrical, and sensation to pinprick and vibratory sense were normal.

a. What are the names of each of these abnormalities?
b. What is the most likely location of the lesion?
c. What artery supplies the affected area?

- The posterior parietal cortex is critical for spatial attention, and the right hemisphere is dominant for selected attention to interpersonal or extrapersonal space.
- Lesions of the right parietal lobe produce contralateral spatial neglect, constructional apraxia, dressing apraxia, anosognosia, or, in less severe cases, extinction with double simultaneous stimulation of both visual fields or both sides of the body.
- Bilateral parieto-occipital lesions produce simultanagnosia, oculomotor apraxia, and optic ataxia (Balint syndrome).

Clinical Problem 16B.6.

A 62-year-old taxi driver was evaluated initially by an ophthalmologist because of visual symptoms. However, he was found to have normal visual acuity and visual fields. He is now referred for neurologic evaluation because of his complaint of not being able to read a road map. Although he is aware of traffic lights, oncoming traffic, and people crossing at an intersection, he cannot perceive all of these things at the same time and has had to stop driving because of this. Although he can see the utensils on the table, he becomes frustrated because he cannot reach or grasp them under visual guidance. When shown a picture of a tennis player hitting a ball, he can detect and name separately parts of the picture, such as the shoes of the player, the racquet, the ball, or the net, but he cannot perceive the picture as a whole. Although he has full eye movements, he cannot follow the examiner's finger with his gaze.

a. What are the names of these clinical manifestations?
b. What component of the visual system is affected?
c. What is the most likely location of the lesion?
d. Is color vision likely to be affected in this patient? Why?

Motor Programming and Execution

Anatomy

Regions of the frontal and parietal lobes are involved in motor control (Chapter 8). The motor regions of the frontal lobe include the primary motor area in the precentral gyrus (area 4), the lateral premotor area (lateral area 6), the supplementary motor area on the medial aspect of the hemisphere (medial area 6), and regions of the anterior cingulate gyrus. These areas contain a somatotopic representation of the contralateral body and project through the corticospinal tract (to control trunk and limb movements) and corticobulbar tract (to control movements of cranial musculature). A second group of motor areas is involved specifically in oculomotor control (Fig. 16B.23). These areas include the *frontal eye fields* (just anterior to the lateral premotor area from the limbs), the *supplementary eye fields* (just anterior to the supplementary motor area), and the parietal eye fields in the intraparietal sulcus. These areas project to the superior colliculus and brainstem generators for conjugate eye movements. The cortical input to all these motor areas arise from the parietal lobe, which provides information for motor control under external clues, and the prefrontal cortex, which provides input for the voluntary initiation of movement in the absence of external clues.

Physiology

Motor programs are a set of commands from the cerebral cortex that are structured before the beginning of the motor act. Through its connections with the frontal lobe, the parietal lobe is an essential component of the central network for motor programming and execution. Neurons of the intraparietal sulcus of the posterior parietal cortex respond to different combinations of visual, somatosensory, auditory, and vestibular input to produce a representation of space. This information is forwarded to different premotor cortical areas that control limb and eye movements.

Motor programs for limb movements initiated in response to visual stimuli are generated by neurons in the intraparietal sulcus. Some of these neurons respond to and integrate visual information about the position, movement, or shape of the object with somatosensory information from the upper limb and then transmit this information to the lateral premotor cortex to initiate the motor programs for reaching to or grasping the object.

The supplementary motor area (medial area 6) and the presupplementary motor area participate in motor learning, selection and preparation of movement, and generation of motor sequences for motivated or goal-directed behavior in the absence of external cues. The primary motor cortex is the main effector area for controlling, through the corticospinal tract, the activity of motor

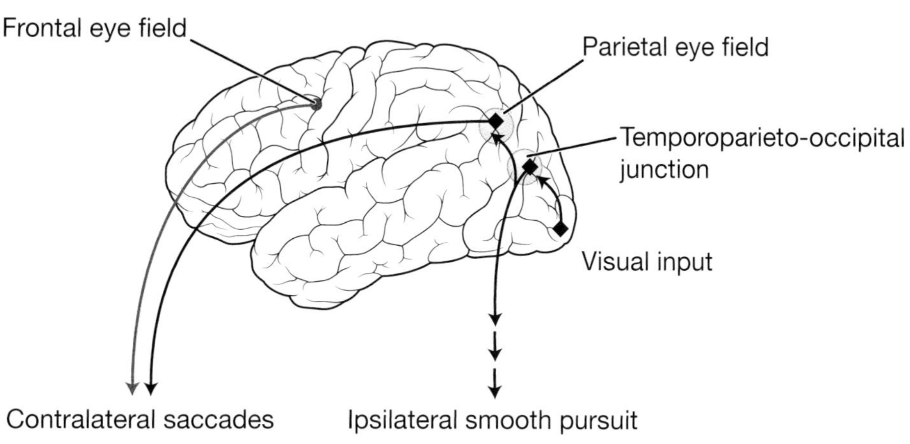

Fig. 16B.23. Cortical structures controlling eye movements.

neurons that innervate the axial and limb muscles. Primary motor cortex is involved in the control of learned, programmed skilled tasks that depend on fractionated hand and finger movements and is the only source of direct corticospinal input to alpha motor neurons.

The two cortical systems that control the brainstem oculomotor networks for conjugate eye movements are the saccadic system and the smooth pursuit system. The rapid conjugate eye movements necessary to bring images of interest onto the macula are called *saccades*. Reflexive saccades are triggered by the presence of an object in extrapersonal space, and voluntary saccades are generated in response to endogenous triggers such as goal-directed behavior. The *smooth pursuit* (tracking) *system* controls eye movements to maintain visual fixation on the object as it moves through the visual field.

The cortical network that controls saccadic eye movements includes the posterior parietal cortex, frontal eye fields, supplementary eye fields, and dorsolateral prefrontal cortex. Neurons in the lateral intraparietal sulcus, referred to as the *parietal eye field*, integrate information about the position and movement of an object in space and the position of the eyes in the orbit and send commands to the frontal eye fields to generate conjugate saccadic or pursuit movements. The frontal eye field is involved in all types of intentional saccades, whereas the parietal eye field is involved primarily in reflexive, visually guided saccades. Stimulation of either the frontal or parietal eye field triggers saccades toward contralateral extrapersonal space. Acute hemispheric lesions of the frontal eye fields produce conjugate deviation of the eyes toward the side of the lesion. The eyes eventually return to the midline because of a compensatory effect of the superior colliculus. However, the patients have residual defects in voluntary saccadic and smooth pursuit movements.

The smooth pursuit system is a complex pathway that involves neurons of the middle temporal and middle superior temporal areas and the temporoparieto-occipital junction (dorsal visual stream). These neurons receive input from primary visual cortex, respond to movement of an object, and initiate slow visual pursuit movements toward *ipsilateral* visual space. The complicated pathway for this includes the pontine nuclei, cerebellar flocculus, and medial vestibular nucleus. Through the action of this system, the eyes of a person casually looking out the window of a moving car automatically fix on some point in the environment and follow the object involuntarily until it approaches the limits of the person's visual fields. When visual fixation is broken, the eyes make a quick conjugate movement (saccade) in the opposite direction to fix on a new point of interest. This involuntary visual pursuit of a moving target is the basis of *optokinetic nystagmus*.

The highest level of motor control involves behavioral drive, the decision to move or not to move, and the selection of motor plans. These functions depend on interactions of the anterior cingulate cortex, involved in emotionally driven behavior, and the prefrontal cortex, which has the executive function for voluntary control of motor behavior according to the goals of the person and the environmental context. These areas project to the premotor areas containing the motor programs that are forwarded to the primary motor cortex and frontal eye fields to initiate voluntary limb and eye movements, respectively.

- The posterior parietal cortex integrates multimodal sensory information, produces a representation of space, and projects to frontal premotor areas to initiate motor programs for limb and eye movements under visual guidance.
- The supplementary motor area is involved in motor learning, selection and preparation of movement, and generation of motor sequences.
- The frontal eye fields are responsible for voluntary and reflex control of conjugate gaze toward contralateral visual space.
- The temporoparieto-occipital cortex initiates smooth pursuit movements toward ipsilateral visual space.
- The prefrontal cortex and anterior cingulate gyrus are involved in selecting motor plans for motivated and goal-directed motor behavior.

Clinical Correlations: Apraxias

Lesions of primary cortical motor areas cause distal motor weakness and lack of dexterity. Lesions of premotor regions produce *apraxia*, which is the inability to perform learned, skilled, purposeful movements in the absence of an attentional disorder, weakness, sensory abnormality, or incoordination. Patients with *ideomotor apraxia* know what to do but not *how* to do it; for example, they have difficulty pantomiming the use of a tool such as a hammer or a toothbrush. Patients with *ideational apraxia* do not know what to do. They cannot perform multiple-step tasks (e.g., hang a picture on a wall), and they use the incorrect tool to perform a task (e.g., use a screwdriver as a toothbrush). Apraxia usually results from lesions in the left hemisphere, mainly the posterior parietal cortex and, less commonly, the premotor or supplementary motor area. Testing for apraxia may involve asking the patient to pretend he or she has a hammer in the hand and to pound a nail. A patient with limb apraxia is unable to perform this act, yet is able to understand the instruction and has normal strength, sensation, and coordination.

- Apraxia is the inability to perform learned skilled movements in the absence of weakness or sensory abnormality.
- Apraxia commonly results from lesions in the posterior parietal or prefrontal cortex in the dominant (usually left) hemisphere.

Clinical Problem 16B.7.

A 66-year-old right-handed carpenter is evaluated for a 3-year history of progressive clumsiness of the right upper limb. The problem started with difficulty writing smoothly, then he began to have difficulty with shaving and using tools. His wife noticed that he tries to reach a cup with his hand rolled into a fist. Now, he is essentially unable to control the use of his right hand. Neurologic examination showed normal motor strength in all four limbs. However, he cannot demonstrate the use of a brush. He demonstrates the use of a screwdriver by rotating his shoulder rather than the elbow and extends the finger to represent the blade of a screwdriver instead of positioning the hand around the screwdriver. The patient was unable to imitate or understand the gestures of the examiner.

a. What is the name of the disorder?
b. What is the most likely location of the lesion?

Language

Anatomy

Language depends on the activity of a distributed neocortical network located around the sylvian fissure (Fig. 16B.24). The left cerebral hemisphere is dominant for language in almost all right-handed persons and in more than two-thirds of left-handed persons. The perisylvian language network has two epicenters. The posterior epicenter is *Wernicke area*, located in the posterior part of the superior temporal gyrus (area 22), superior temporal sulcus, and the adjacent areas of the supramarginal (area 40) and angular (area 39) gyri. Wernicke area receives input from heteromodal association areas of the left temporal lobe devoted to object recognition (semantic knowledge). The anterior epicenter includes *Broca area*, located in the inferior frontal gyrus and including areas 44, 45, and surrounding areas 46 and 47. These two epicenters are interconnected by the *arcuate fasciculus* in the inferior parietal lobe. Broca area receives input from the prefrontal and anterior cingulate cortices.

Physiology

Wernicke area is anatomically and functionally heterogeneous. It functions in the recognition, comprehension, and retrieval of words and renders words in a precise form for the production of spoken or written language. Broca area contains separate regions in the left inferior frontal gyrus involved in different aspects of expressive language, including semantic processing, syntax, and processing of phonemes. The anterior insula is the area critical for speech production (articulation). The lateral prefrontal cortex participates in high-level control of sentence production. The anterior cingulate cortex provides the behavioral drive for the initiation of speech. The right hemisphere has an important role in language comprehension in normal subjects; it participates in processes such as prosody, figurative language, metaphor, and connotative meaning.

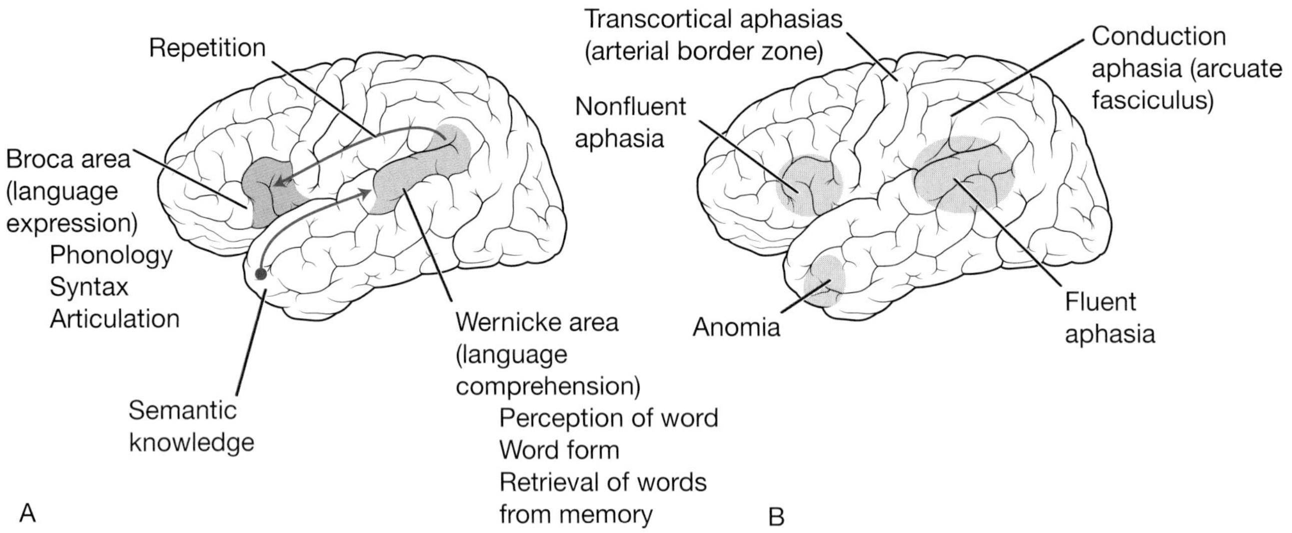

Fig. 16B.24. *A*, The perisylvian language network, located in the left hemisphere of all right-handed and most left-handed persons. *B*, Typical location of lesions producing classic aphasic syndromes. However, in most cases, left hemisphere lesions produce aphasia with mixed features.

Clinical Correlations

Disturbances of language and speech are divided into three types: disorders of central language processing produce *aphasia*, disorders of motor programming of language symbols produce *apraxia of speech*, and disorders of the mechanism of speech produce *dysarthrias*. Aphasia and apraxia of speech are disorders of the supratentorial level. In contrast, dysarthria may occur with disorders of the corticobulbar pathway, basal ganglia, cerebellar control system, or lower motor neurons in the brainstem or disorders at the level of the peripheral nerve, neuromuscular junction, or muscle (Chapter 15).

Aphasia is a disorder of the language network or its connections (usually) in the left hemisphere that impair comprehension, repetition, production, or expression of words or other symbols for communication (including sign language) (Fig. 16B.24). Different types of aphasia have been characterized on the basis of fluency, content, comprehension, and repetition of words (Table 16B.1). Lesions involving Wernicke area produce *fluent aphasia*. These patients produce excessive volume of well-articulated words, but speech conveys little meaning. Lesions in Wernicke area impair the comprehension of spoken or written language. The speech may be unintelligible because of errors in phoneme and word choice, causing *paraphasia* and jargon speech.

Lesions of Broca area or its subcortical connections produce nonfluent aphasia, *Broca aphasia*. This is characterized by loss of speech fluency, agrammatism (inability to organize words into sentences), and telegraphic speech (the nonfluent use of content words without connecting words). Although the patients have normal reception of language, they cannot convert thoughts into meaningful language. These patients may also have hemiparesis of the contralateral face and upper extremity.

Lesions in subcortical white matter of the inferior parietal lobe, including the arcuate fasciculus, that interrupt the connections between Wernicke and Broca areas, produce *conduction aphasia*. This disconnection syndrome is characterized by a major deficit in repetition. However, patients with this type of aphasia can produce intelligible speech and comprehend sentences. Features of Wernicke aphasia and Broca aphasia are combined in *global aphasia*, which is associated commonly with a dense contralateral hemiplegia. The perisylvian aphasias are commonly due to infarctions in the

Table 16B.1. Features of the Main Types of Aphasia

Type	Fluency	Expression	Comprehension	Repetition	Naming	Lesion
Broca	Nonfluent	Impaired	Relatively preserved	Impaired	Impaired	Left frontal operculum
Wernicke	Fluent	Unintelligible (paraphasia)	Impaired	Impaired	Impaired	Left superior temporal and inferior parietal cortices
Conduction	Fluent	Some paraphasia	Preserved	Impaired	May be impaired	Left arcuate fasciculus
Global	Nonfluent	Impaired	Impaired	Impaired	Impaired	Whole perisylvian region
Transcortical						
Motor	Nonfluent	Impaired	Relatively preserved	Normal	Impaired	Arterial border zone
Sensory	Fluent	Unintelligible (paraphasia)	Impaired	Normal	Impaired	Arterial border zone
Anomic	Fluent	Poor content	Preserved	Preserved	Impaired	Left lateral and anterior temporal cortex

territory of the left middle cerebral artery, but they may also be an early manifestation of a neoplastic, inflammatory, or degenerative disorder. In contrast, infarctions in the arterial border zones produce *transcortical aphasias*. These lesions interrupt the connections between the perisylvian language areas and either the prefrontal cortex or lateral temporal cortex. With transcortical aphasias, unlike perisylvian aphasias, repetition is spared (Table 16B.1). Despite this didactic separation among different types of aphasia, most patients have various degrees of involvement of expressive or receptive aspects of language, emphasizing the network concept of cortical function.

All aphasias are associated with word-finding difficulties and difficulty naming objects, a deficit called *anomia*. However, pure anomia may also occur with lesions in areas of the left lateral temporal lobe, including the anterior pole, which are involved in the integration of sensory information for knowledge of the world (semantic knowledge). These patients have progressive impoverishment of language because they have lost knowledge of the meaning of an object and, thus, cannot name it. Substitutions of incorrect words, or *semantic paraphasias*, are particularly common after a left temporal or large left frontal lesion.

Aphasia should be distinguished from other disorders of speech production, including speech apraxia, mutism, and dysarthria. Motor speech apraxia, also called *apraxia of speech*, is a manifestation of lesions restricted to the left insular region in Broca area. This consists of the partial or complete inability to form the articulatory movements of the lips, tongue, and lower jaw for producing individual sounds that make up words. The patient knows what he or she wants to say but is unable to execute the motor aspects of speech. The lack of speech production due to impaired behavioral drive to initiate speech is called *mutism*. It results from bilateral lesions of the prefrontal cortex and anterior cingulate gyrus.

Two syndromes are characterized by the inability to read words, called *alexia*: *alexia with agraphia* and *pure*

Clinical Problem 16B.8.

A 55-year-old right-handed woman is brought to the emergency department by the police because of unusual behavior. When she was at the grocery store, she started talking unintelligibly. She asked for the "luoi" (presumably referring to "oil") and the "froogles" (presumably "noodles") and became very irritated when the grocery assistant did not understand her. On neurologic examination, she was alert and her speech was fluent and nondysarthric. However, she could not follow spoken commands, but she could imitate gestures. She was unable to repeat words, read, or write. The rest of the neurologic examination was normal.

a. What does this disorder represent?
b. What is the most likely location of the lesion?
c. What is the arterial supply of this area?

Clinical Problem 16B.9.

A 65-year-old right-handed lawyer suddenly became mute and agitated. On neurologic examination, he was alert, producing rare guttural sounds but not recognizable words. He could follow occasional simple commands but could not repeat a three-word sentence. He appeared frustrated by his inability to do so. He had mild weakness of the right lower face, weakness of the right upper extremity, and decreased rate of alternate motion in the fingers of the right hand.

a. What does this problem represent?
b. What is the most likely location of the lesion?
c. What artery supplies the affected region?

Three months later, his speech was still nonfluent and poorly articulated. He was unable to control movement of the lips, tongue, and lower jaw for producing words such as "catastrophe."

d. What is the term used to describe the inability to perform articulatory movements to produce speech sounds?

alexia or *alexia without agraphia*. Alexia with agraphia is a deficit in both reading and writing (agraphia) and is associated with damage of the left angular gyrus, which connects the visual cortex with Wernicke area. In pure alexia, or alexia without agraphia, patients have a relatively preserved ability to write but are unable to read what they have written. The classic lesion involves the left calcarine cortex or optic radiation (producing a right hemianopia) and the splenium of the corpus callosum, interrupting the connections from the right to the left occipital association cortex, which provides access to Wernicke area.

Lesions of the left inferior parietal lobule produce agraphia in association with *acalculia* (inability to perform calculations), *finger agnosia* (inability to recognize the fingers), and *left-right disorientation*. This is referred to as *Gerstmann syndrome* (Fig. 16B.25).

- The language network is located in the perisylvian region of the dominant (generally left) hemisphere and includes Wernicke area (involved in word comprehension), Broca area (involved in word production), and their connections.
- Disorders of central language processing produce aphasia.
- Lesions in Wernicke area produce fluent aphasia and impair the comprehension of language.
- Lesions in Broca area produce nonfluent aphasia and impair the expression of language.
- Conduction aphasia selectively impairs repetition of words.
- Most patients with aphasia have mixed features because of the interruption of the language network.
- Anomia occurs in all types of aphasia and, in its pure form, is associated with lesions in the left lateral temporal lobe and temporal pole.
- Disorders of motor programming of language symbols produce apraxia of speech.
- Disorders of the mechanism of speech produce dysarthrias.

Clinical Problem 16B.10.

A 44-year-old school teacher is evaluated for progressive cognitive difficulties over the past 6 months. She could not tell how old her daughter was (but knows her birth date) or calculate how many quarters she needed to operate the laundromat machine. When she tried to read what she had written, her sentences did not make any sense. On neurologic examination, visual acuity and the sensory and motor examinations were normal. Her speech was fluent, but she could not name a dog, car, or van. When asked to write the sentence, "the day is sunny," she wrote "the date is stony." She could not subtract 7 from 93, add 15 to 20, divide 24 by 6, or multiply 5 times 11. She could not name her fingers and could not follow the command "touch your left ear with your right thumb" because of right-left confusion.

a. What types of deficits does this patient have?
b. What is the most likely location of the lesion?
c. What types of lesions can produce this temporal profile of deficit?

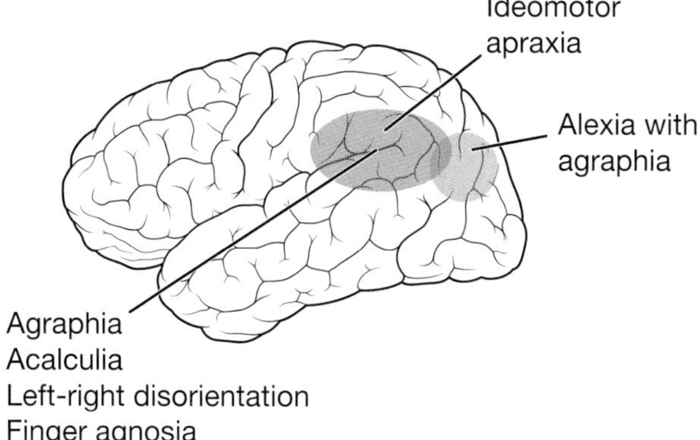

Fig. 16B.25. Manifestations of lesions affecting the left inferior parietal lobule (supramarginal and angular gyri).

- Alexia is the inability to read; alexia with agraphia (inability to write) results from lesions in the left angular gyrus, whereas pure alexia is commonly the result of combined lesions of the left occipital lobe and the splenium of the corpus callosum.
- Lesions of the left inferior parietal lobule produce agraphia, acalculia, left-right disorientation, and finger agnosia (Gerstmann syndrome).

Control of Behavior and Executive Functions

Anatomy

The prefrontal cortex, anterior to the premotor and motor areas, is the largest region of the frontal lobe. It is the site of the confluence of two functional networks. One network is centered in the *dorsolateral prefrontal cortex* and is involved in attention and executive function. The other network is centered in the *orbitomedial prefrontal cortex* and is involved in decision making and the control of affective behavior (Fig. 16B.26). The prefrontal cortex is interconnected with all other heteromodal and paralimbic cortical areas, including the posterior parietal, lateral temporal, and medial temporal cortices. The subcortical input to prefrontal cortex is primarily from the mediodorsal (dorsomedial) nucleus of the thalamus, but this cortical area is also an important target of modulatory dopaminergic input from the ventral tegmental area of the midbrain. The prefrontal cortex projects to the caudate nucleus and amygdala.

- Prefrontal cortex includes lateral and orbitomedial areas.
- Prefrontal cortex has connections with association and paralimbic areas, amygdala, caudate nucleus, dorsomedial nucleus of the thalamus, and midbrain dopaminergic neurons.

Physiology

The lateral prefrontal cortex is involved in goal-directed attention and *working memory*, which is the temporary, online holding of information and its mental manipulation to guide behavior. Working memory involves retaining information for a short time, for example, looking up a telephone number and remembering it briefly

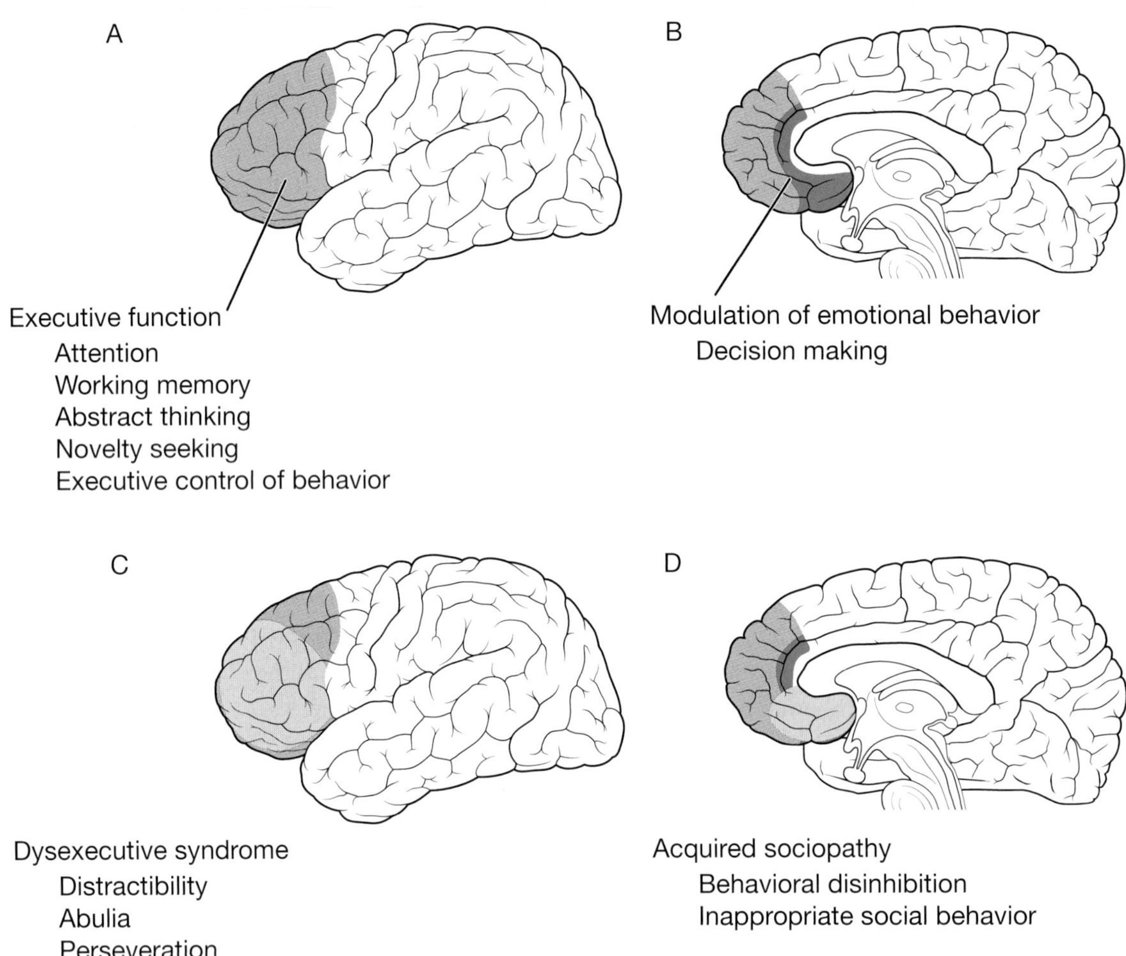

Fig. 16B.26. Functions of the heteromodal dorsolateral prefrontal cortex (salmon area) (*A*) and paralimbic orbitomedial prefrontal cortex (blue area) (*B*). Lesions (gray area) of dorsolateral prefrontal cortex produce a dysexecutive syndrome (*C*), and those of the orbitomedial prefrontal cortex impair decision making and social behavior (*D*).

while dialing it. The lateral prefrontal cortex has a central role in *attention*, which includes the ability to prevent interference from distracting stimuli. It also is necessary for abstraction, retrieval of stored information to guide behavior, novelty seeking, response choice, and behavioral flexibility. All these are referred to as *executive functions*. They are required for stimulus selection and for planning, initiating, maintaining, monitoring, and modifying behavior according to the goal and environmental context.

The orbitomedial prefrontal cortex, through its connections with the amygdala and hypothalamus, has an essential role in the modulation of emotional responses to behaviorally significant events. It links emotional responses related to previous experience or outcomes with selected decisions and behaviors. The anterior cingulate cortex, interconnected with the orbitofrontal cortex, is involved in behavioral drive and the evaluation of the outcomes of the behavior. One of the important functions of the anterior cingulate cortex is to allow the person to infer what another person might think or feel in response to specific events or actions, the *theory of mind*. This ability is critical for social interaction.

Clinical Correlations

Lesions of the prefrontal cortex change cognition and behavior. Because these changes, or abnormalities, occur in the absence of impaired memory, language, motor, or sensory function, they are frequently misinterpreted as a psychiatric illness and may be misdiagnosed until an imaging study is performed. Thus, any marked change in personality or behavior should always raise the suspicion of a prefrontal lobe lesion.

Lateral prefrontal lesions produce a *dysexecutive syndrome* characterized by a deficit of attention, working memory, planning, and response selection. The patients may lack initiative and spontaneity, a condition called *abulia*. They are easily distracted, cannot maintain a train of thought or complete a given task, have little concern for either the past or the future, and have the tendency to spontaneously repeat verbal or motor behaviors despite instructions not to do so, which is called *perseveration*. Patients may develop an external stimulus–bound state in which thinking becomes concrete and behavior is guided by events in the environment. For example, a patient may imitate the gestures of the examiner (*imitation behavior*) or pick up and use objects placed in front of him or her without being asked to do so (*utilization behavior*). This severe lateral prefrontal syndrome most commonly occurs after bilateral damage, for example, from an infiltrating tumor, multiple infarcts, or certain degenerative disorders.

Lesions of the orbitomedial prefrontal cortex affect decision making, personality, and social behavior. The patients are unable to organize future activities and to hold employment; they have an unrealistic favorable view of themselves, diminished capacity to respond to punishment, and a tendency for inappropriate social conduct. They may have either a jocular or humorless attitude, sexually disinhibited humor, inappropriate self-indulgence, perseverative impulse to seek immediate gratification, emotional lability, poor tolerance of frustration, and lack of empathy or concern for others. This is referred to as *acquired sociopathy*. This orbitofrontal syndrome is often the consequence of a traumatic head injury, a tumor in the olfactory groove, or a focal degenerative disorder, but it may also occur with a vascular or inflammatory condition.

- Lesions of the lateral prefrontal cortex impair attention and the planning, initiation, maintenance, monitoring, completion, and context-dependent modification of goal-directed behavior. Conditions associated with lesions of this cortical region include abulia, distractibility, perseveration, imitation behavior, and utilization behavior.
- Lesions of the orbitomedial prefrontal cortex impair decision making and produce socially inappropriate behavior.

Clinical Problem 16B.11.

A 55-year-old right-handed engineer is evaluated for a progressive change in his personality and behavior over the past 6 months. He no longer was interested in reading newspapers or magazines and showed a general lack of initiative and spontaneity. He was asked to leave work because he was unable to complete even simple tasks. He spent his work day wandering around and looking distracted, "as if he had nothing to do." A coworker had complained about the patient making inappropriate comments to her. He has become increasingly irritable and shows no evidence of caring about the feelings of others. He now spends up to 16 hours daily watching TV at home. On neurologic examination, he was inattentive and easily distractible and was not able to provide a coherent history. He sometimes became irritable when asked to perform tasks during the mental status examination. He was unable to repeat 3 digits forward and in 60 seconds could give only two words beginning with the letter B. He has no difficulty with language, calculation, construction, or declarative memory. No motor, sensory, or visual deficits were noted on examination.

a. Where is the most likely location of the lesion?
b. What components of this area are involved?
c. What are the main connections of this area?
d. What are possible causes of this patient's symptoms?

From the description of the different functions of supratentorial networks and effects of lesions, it can be deduced that memory is a complex function with many different components and anatomical substrates (Table 16B.2). Working memory is the ability to hold for relatively short periods information to be used for actions planned in the near future. This is the basis of attention, and it depends on the lateral prefrontal cortex. Declarative memory is the ability to learn and store information about autobiographical events (episodic memory), facts (semantic memory), names, and places; it depends on structures in the medial temporal lobe. Long-term storage occurs in heteromodal neocortical areas, particularly in the lateral and anterior temporal and posterior parietal lobes. The retrieval of stored information to guide behavior is an executive function of lateral prefrontal cortex. Procedural memory (also called implicit memory) is the learning of habits (such as riding a bicycle) and involves motor circuits of the caudate nucleus and dentate nucleus of the cerebellum. Associative (or emotional) memory consists of conditioned responses to emotionally relevant stimuli and involves the amygdala.

Clinical Syndromes of the Cerebral Cortex

Disorders of the cerebral hemispheres may be *diffuse* or *focal* and may be expressed as either *loss of function* (deficit) or *excessive activity* (seizures). Diffuse disorders may consist of altered cognition and behavior, bilateral motor abnormalities, or generalized seizures.

Diffuse Disorders

Important causes of diffuse disorders at the supratentorial level include inflammatory and infectious conditions (e.g., encephalitis), degenerative disorders, toxic or metabolic disorders, and developmental disorders. Their manifestations depend on the location of the lesion (cerebral cortex, basal ganglia, or both) and the underlying lesion. They include generalized seizures, confusion, dementia, mental retardation, and movement disorders.

Table 16B.2. Comparison of Memory Systems

Type of memory	Function	Anatomy
Working memory	Maintains "on-line" information for a short period after transient exposure to stimulus to guide behavior	Prefrontal cortex
Declarative memory		
Episodic	Learning and retrieval of personal events and facts	Medial temporal lobe Medial thalamus, mammillary bodies, basal forebrain cholinergic system
Semantic	General fund of knowledge	Heteromodal association cortex (particularly left lateral and anterior temporal areas)
Priming	Experience of a stimulus influences later processing of the same or related stimulus	Occipital, temporal, parietal, and frontal cortices
Emotional memory	Associative learning of a link between a perceptual stimulus and its emotional significance	Amygdala
Procedural (implicit) memory	Motor skill learning	Striatum, cerebellum

Generalized Seizures

Diffuse hyperexcitability of the cerebral cortex and paroxysmal synchronization through corticothalamocortical loops produce widespread discharges in generalized seizures. These seizures are associated with an alteration of consciousness, which may be brief in absence seizures or prolonged in tonic-clonic seizures. Generalized seizures may result from genetic predisposition (e.g., genetic mutations affecting ion channels) or acquired disorder (developmental, inflammatory, or toxic-metabolic).

In a *generalized tonic-clonic seizure* (classically referred to as grand mal seizures), the patient abruptly loses consciousness and falls as the body stiffens in a tonic contraction. This is followed by symmetrical, clonic jerking of the extremities and head, urinary incontinence, tongue biting, and apnea. After the seizure, the patient is flaccid and unresponsive, with slow return of consciousness through periods of confusion, drowsiness, and headache. The seizure usually lasts 1 to 2 minutes, and the period of altered consciousness afterward may last for 10 to 30 minutes. During the seizure, an electroencephalogram shows generalized, repetitive spike discharges in the tonic phase, spike-and-wave discharges during the clonic phase, and depression of activity followed by slow waves after the seizure (Fig. 16B.27).

A brief generalized seizure that lasts 5 to 30 seconds with impaired consciousness but minimal movement is called an *absence* (petit mal) *seizure*. Usually, the patient abruptly ceases activity, is unresponsive, and stares and sometimes has mild clonic movements of the face or extremities. Absence seizures generally occur in children and can be induced by hyperventilation. They are associated with a characteristic bilateral, synchronous, generalized 3-Hz spike-and-wave pattern on the electroencephalogram (Fig. 16B.28).

Repeated seizures are called *status epilepticus*. This is defined by the presence of repeat seizures without recovery of consciousness in between episodes. Status epilepticus may be convulsive or nonconvulsive. It constitutes a neurologic emergency. Prolonged seizure activity leads to neuronal death from excitotoxicity (Chapter 6).

- Status epilepticus refers to repeated seizures and is a neurologic emergency.

Clinical Problem 16B.12.

A 5-year-old girl is evaluated for spells. During the spells, she stops what she is doing, stares into space, and does not respond to her parents. Each episode lasts 5 to 10 seconds, after which she recovers rapidly and resumes her ongoing activity. The findings on neurologic examination are normal.

a. What do these episodes represent?
b. What does the electroencephalogram show during the episodes?
c. What is the mechanism of these episodes?

Confusional State

Confusional state, or *delirium*, is a state of decreased awareness of the environment that typically reflects deficits in attention. It may be associated with perceptual disturbances (*illusions* or *hallucinations*), increased or decreased psychomotor activity, incoherent speech, and disturbances of the sleep-wake cycle. This clinical syndrome commonly develops over a period of hours to days, tends to fluctuate during the day, and may be reversed if caused by a treatable condition. Causes of confusional state include metabolic encephalopathy, drug intoxication or withdrawal state, infectious process, head injury, diffuse vascular disease, and nonconvulsive status epilepticus. Generalized motor phenomena such as tremor, myoclonus, or seizures may also be present. Patients with dementia may develop an acute confusional state in relation to a systemic triggering factor, such as infection or medication.

- Confusional state is a potentially reversible state of impaired attention and awareness that may result from a metabolic, toxic, vascular, or inflammatory process diffusely affecting the cerebral hemispheres.

Dementia

Dementia is an acquired condition involving a change in cognitive function in an alert person, from a previous level of performance to the point that social and occupational functions are impaired. Most dementias are progressive

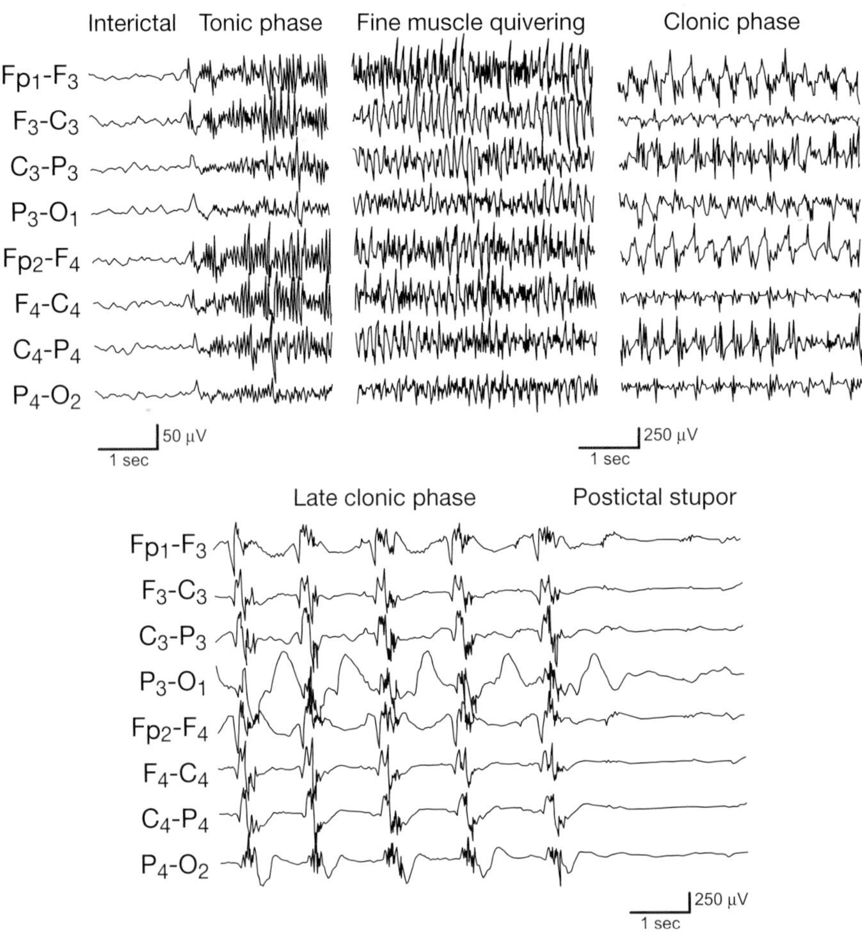

Fig. 16B.27. Electroencephalographic accompaniment of a generalized tonic-clonic seizure. Segments of the recording during different phases of the seizure are shown. Interictal is before the seizure; tonic phase (body stiff) shows repetitive spikes; clonic phase (body jerking) shows spike-and-wave discharges; and postictal phase (after the seizure) shows suppression of activity.

and caused by degenerative disorders of the cerebral cortex. Although degenerative dementias reflect diffuse or bilateral involvement of the cerebral cortex, the initial clinical features may reflect specific involvement of specific cortical areas.

The most common degenerative dementia is Alzheimer disease. Typically, this disorder initially affects medial temporal lobe structures such as the entorhinal cortex and hippocampus (Fig. 16B.29). At this stage, the primary effect is impairment of declarative memory, particularly the learning of new information about recent events and facts. Working memory and procedural memory usually are spared at this early stage. As the disease progresses, neocortical association areas are involved, thus impairing language (particularly naming), calculation, and visuospatial skills. Agnosia and apraxia develop. Behavioral changes, including depression, are frequent. The patient tends to get lost easily, cannot perform household tasks or financial activities, and can no longer drive an automobile. In later stages of the illness, the patient no longer recognizes family members and may become mute. Death is usually due to a complicating illness such as pneumonia or another infection.

Other common types of degenerative dementia are *dementia with Lewy bodies* and *frontotemporal dementia*. Dementia with Lewy bodies is characterized by profound

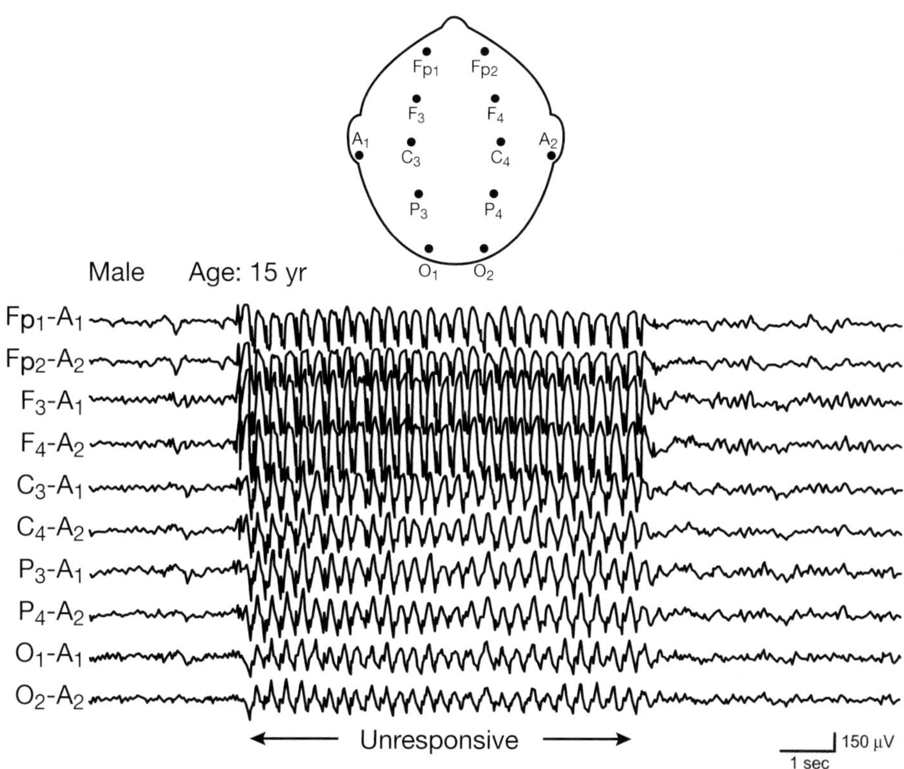

Fig. 16B.28. Electroencephalographic accompaniment during a typical absence seizure consisting of a 3-Hz spike-and-wave pattern, during which the patient was unresponsive.

impairment of visuospatial function early in the disease, fluctuations in cognitive function, and visual hallucinations. Frontotemporal dementia is the second most common dementia after Alzheimer disease in patients younger than 65 years (Fig. 16B.30). Its clinical features vary according to the primary location of the degenerative process. Patients with mainly involvement of the prefrontal cortex present with dysexecutive syndrome, changes in personality and behavior, particularly loss of personal and social awareness, blunting of affect, and loss of insight. They may become markedly apathetic and socially withdrawn, whereas others become more disinhibited. Memory is relatively spared, in contrast to Alzheimer disease. Patients with primary involvement of the left frontotemporal perisylvian region present with *primary progressive aphasia*. Those with lesions in the lateral and anterior temporal cortex, particularly on the left side, have *semantic dementia*. This is characterized by progressive loss of world knowledge, including knowledge about faces, people, objects, and words. Speech becomes progressively more devoid of content and is characterized by frequent vague references to people, objects, and places ("I am going to that place there"). Some forms of dementia affect predominantly the posterior cortical regions. These posterior cortical atrophy syndromes are characterized by profound impairment of visuospatial attention. For example, patients cannot grasp all the elements of a visual scene, such as a picture, but instead describe partial components at a time (simultanagnosia) or shift their gaze to focus on an object in the environment.

These forms of dementia emphasize an important exception to the general rule of pathologic substrate for focal disorders. Whereas chronic, focal, progressive disorders are most frequently the result of a mass lesion (neoplasm), they may also be a manifestation of a focal degenerative disorder. However, this degenerative process eventually affects other areas of the cerebral cortex.

Clinical Problem 16B.13.

A 50-year-old woman had gradual onset of memory loss 3 years ago. This loss has become progressively worse, and now she cannot remember from one minute to the next what she has been doing. She also has had difficulty with various household activities such as sewing, cooking, and washing dishes, even though she says she is not weak or has no trouble with coordination. Neurologic examination showed that she could not recall what numbers had just been presented to her, what she had had for breakfast, or even where she was born. She was unable to perform such activities as pretending to light a cigarette or showing how to use a key.

a. Where is the lesion?
b. What is the disease process?
c. What types of memory function are affected in this patient?
d. What is the difference between dementia and mental retardation?
e. What is the name given to the inability to perform learned complex motor acts in the absence of weakness?

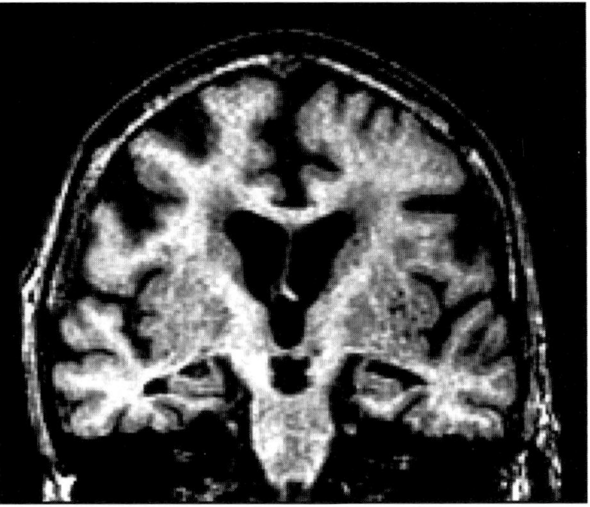

Fig. 16B.29. Coronal T1-weighted magnetic resonance image of the brain of a patient with Alzheimer disease. Note the severe generalized atrophy, involving predominantly the medial temporal and parietotemporal regions.

Some dementias are potentially treatable, most commonly ones due to inflammatory (immune or infectious) or toxic-metabolic disorders. Important examples are the dementias associated with human immunodeficiency virus 1, chronic meningitis, paraneoplastic or other autoimmune disorders, and vitamin B_{12} deficiency).

- Dementia is an acquired condition involving an alteration in cognitive function.
- The most common cause of dementia is Alzheimer disease, characterized by progressive memory loss and difficulty learning new information.
- Dementia with Lewy bodies is characterized by fluctuations in cognitive function and visual hallucinations.
- Frontotemporal dementia may be manifested by a

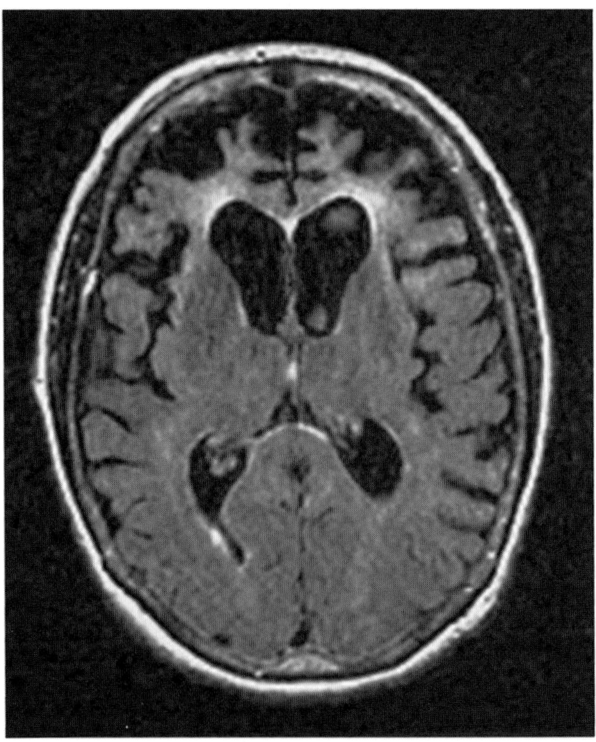

Fig. 16B.30. Axial T1-weighted magnetic resonance image of the brain of a patient with frontotemporal dementia. Note the severe atrophy of the frontal lobes, with relative preservation of other cortical areas.

change in personality and behavior, progressive aphasia, or loss of world knowledge.
- Some dementias have potentially treatable causes.

Mental Retardation

Mental retardation is the failure to develop normal intelligence. It is not a single disease but a group of disorders in which the development of normal intellectual functioning is arrested. Mental retardation may result from a congenital nonprogressive process, an acquired nonprogressive process, or a progressive disease with onset in infancy or childhood. Important examples of mental retardation due to chromosomal abnormalities are *Down syndrome* and *fragile X syndrome.* An important pathologic feature is the presence of cortical neurons with immature dendrites, reduced dendritic arborization, and fewer dendritic spines than normal. Typical examples of genetic biochemical defects are *Tay-Sachs disease* and *phenylketonuria.*

Down syndrome is a chromosomal defect with triplication of a gene on chromosome 21 encoding for the amyloid precursor protein. Children with this syndrome may survive into adulthood and develop Alzheimer disease. Fragile X syndrome is the second most common genetically determined form of mental retardation. The phenotype includes mental retardation, autistic-like behavior, developmental delay, facial abnormalities, and macro-orchidism. This disorder is due to a trinucleotide repeat expansion in a gene on chromosome X encoding for a ribonucleoprotein. Tay-Sachs disease is an inherited autosomal recessive disorder characterized by an excessive accumulation of the lipid ganglioside in neurons of the central nervous system. Also, retinal involvement produces blindness. Infants with this disorder have normal development during the first few months of life but then begin to lose previously acquired abilities. Death is usually caused by infection. Phenylketonuria is an inherited autosomal recessive disorder in which phenylalanine cannot be converted to tyrosine because of an enzymatic defect. The increased levels of phenylalanine cause demyelination in the white matter and ultimately neuronal loss, resulting in retardation and seizures.

Mental retardation has many exogenous causes, such as trauma, anoxia, drugs, toxins, and infections. Important examples are maternal exposure to alcohol during pregnancy or congenital infections with cytomegalovirus or human immunodeficiency virus.

- Mental retardation is a failure to develop normal intelligence and can result from congenital or acquired disorders.

Focal Disorders

Etiology

The cerebral hemispheres are the most common target of focal traumatic, vascular inflammatory, and neoplastic lesions. Focal lesions may be nonprogressive (nonmass), such as an infarct, or progressive (mass lesions), such as a hematoma, abscess, or neoplasm. The most common focal lesions are vascular and neoplastic lesions. Infarctions in the distribution of any major cerebral artery produces specific neurologic effects (see Chapter 12). Mass lesions in the cerebral hemispheres enlarge within the confined space of the cranial cavity and increase intracranial pressure by mass effect and surrounding cerebral edema. Neurologic impairment results from local compression of tissue or neuronal death. Mass lesions may be vascular (hematoma), inflammatory (abscess), or neoplastic. An important example of a focal, progressive, inflammatory lesion is *herpes simplex encephalitis*, which preferentially affects the temporal lobes (Fig. 16B.31). This potentially fatal but treatable condition should be suspected in all patients who have fever, change in mental status, and focal symptoms, including disturbances of language, memory, or behavior. The suspicion is reinforced by the presence of a typical pattern on the electroencephalogram and is confirmed by detection of herpes simplex virus DNA in the cerebrospinal fluid.

Although any cell type in the nervous system may undergo neoplastic change, three major groups of neoplasms account for most brain tumors: gliomas, meningiomas, and metastasis. Astrocytomas and oligodendrogliomas are classified as low-grade or high-grade lesions on the basis of the histologic appearance, namely nuclear atypia, mitotic activity, vascular proliferation, necrosis, and hemorrhage. These features produce characteristic changes visible on neuroimaging studies (Fig. 16B.32). Meningiomas are generally slow growing and produce clinical effects by compressing the brain and neighboring structures (Fig. 16B.33). Although meningiomas have many different histologic appearances, they typically have whorls of cells that may degenerate and calcify to form psammoma bodies. Metastases arise primarily from lung and breast carcinoma and frequently occur in melanoma (Fig. 16B.34). Central nervous system lymphoma is a typical neoplasm in patients with chronic immunosuppression, for example, organ transplant recipients or those with acquired immunodeficiency syndrome.

- The most common neoplasms are astrocytomas, meningiomas, and metastases.

Although focal, chronic progressive neurologic impairment suggests a mass lesion (neoplasm), the main exception at the supratentorial level is focal degenerative disorders, which are progressive but have no mass effect but instead cause focal cerebral atrophy (Fig. 16B.30).

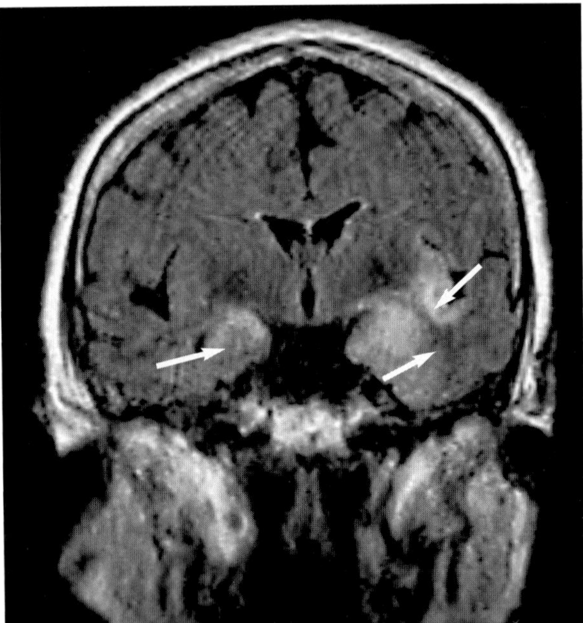

Fig. 16B.31. Coronal T1-weighted magnetic resonance image showing areas of acute hemorrhage (*arrows*) in both temporal lobes and left insular cortex. This is typical of herpes simplex encephalitis.

Focal lesions produce focal disorders that differ in their clinical effects depending on the location of the lesion. These effects include excessive cortical activity (focal or partial seizures), visual field defects, and deficits in motor, sensory, cognitive, or behavioral functions.

Partial Seizures

Seizures that arise from a localized area of the cerebral cortex are called *partial seizures* and are classified as *complex partial seizures* when associated with an alteration of consciousness (awareness) and *simple partial seizures* when awareness is preserved. The symptoms of partial seizures depend on the site of the discharge (Table 16B.3).

- Seizures arising from a localized area of the cortex are called partial seizures.
- Complex partial seizures are associated with an alteration of awareness.
- The symptoms of partial seizures depend on the site of discharge.
- Seizures arising from the temporal lobes are the most common partial seizures and may impair awareness, constituting complex partial seizures.

Observation of symptoms can localize the pathologic process. Seizures in the precentral gyrus of the frontal lobe are associated with clonic movements of the contralateral side of the face or contralateral arm or leg. Seizures in the postcentral gyrus are accompanied by paresthesias or dysesthesias of the contralateral side of the face or the contralateral extremities. Occipital lobe seizures produce unformed visual images or impaired vision. Seizures arising from the temporal and limbic lobes are the most common partial seizures. Symptoms vary and may include strange odors or tastes, formed auditory or visual hallucinations, language and speech disturbances, fear, unusual sensations, mouthing movements, posturing, or automatic behavior. Because there is often an alteration of consciousness, these are complex partial seizures.

A partial seizure may remain localized in a single area or may spread to other areas. It may spread sequentially along a gyrus by way of subcortical fibers and, in the case of the precentral gyrus, involve the face, arm, or leg

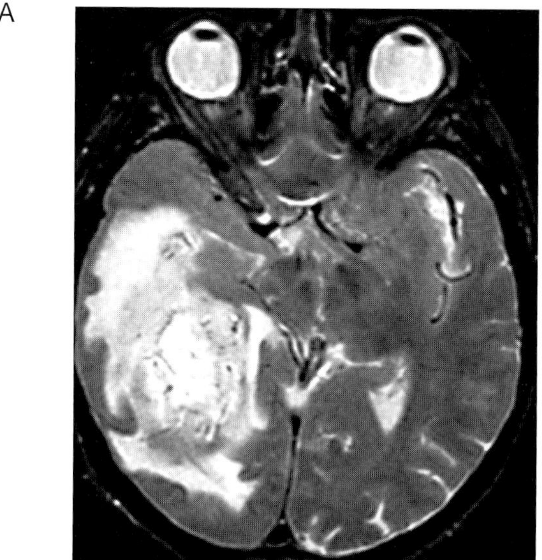

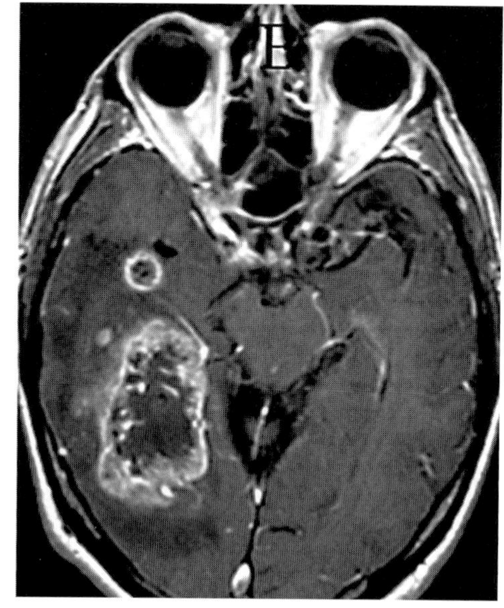

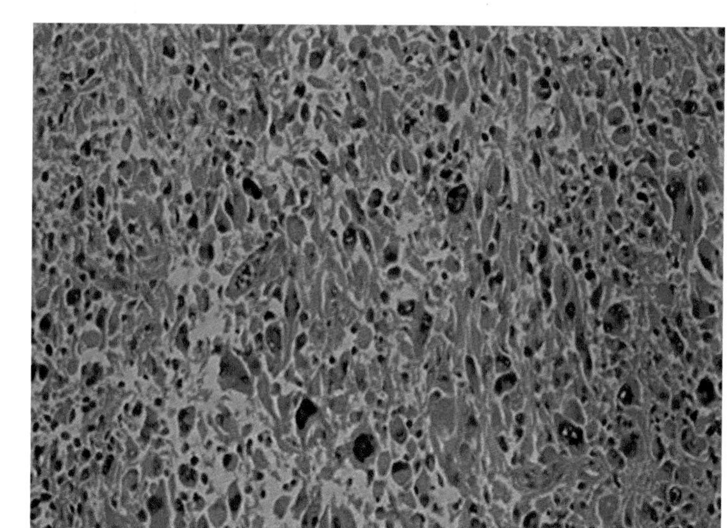

Fig. 16B.32. Axial T2-weighted (*A*) and gadolinium-enhanced T1-weighted (*B*) magnetic resonance images of the brain of a patient with biopsy-proven (*C*) glioblastoma multiforme in the right temporal lobe. Note cerebral edema (in part, reflecting areas of infiltrating tumor cells), contrast enhancement (indicative of increased permeability of blood-brain barrier of abnormally proliferating vessels), and areas of necrosis in the center of the tumor. The biopsy specimen shows nuclear atypia, vascular proliferation, and necrosis.

sequentially in a *jacksonian march*. It may spread from one lobe to another or from one hemisphere to another by way of association or commissural fibers. If focal symptoms precede a generalized seizure, the focal symptoms are called an *aura* and provide evidence of the site of seizure origin.

Visual Field Defects

Visual field defects have localizing value at the supratentorial level. As mentioned in Chapter 16A, the thalamic relay nucleus of the visual pathway is the lateral geniculate nucleus, which projects through the optic radiation to the primary visual (calcarine) cortex of the occipital lobe. The upper, or dorsal, fibers of the optic radiation, conveying information from the lower half of the contralateral visual field, are posterior in the parietal lobe and terminate in the superior lip of the calcarine cortex. The lower, or ventral, fibers, conveying information from the upper half of the contralateral visual field, loop anteriorly and laterally around the temporal horn in the temporal lobe (*Meyer loop*) before turning posteriorly to end in the inferior lip of the calcarine cortex. This has important value for localizing lesions in the cerebral

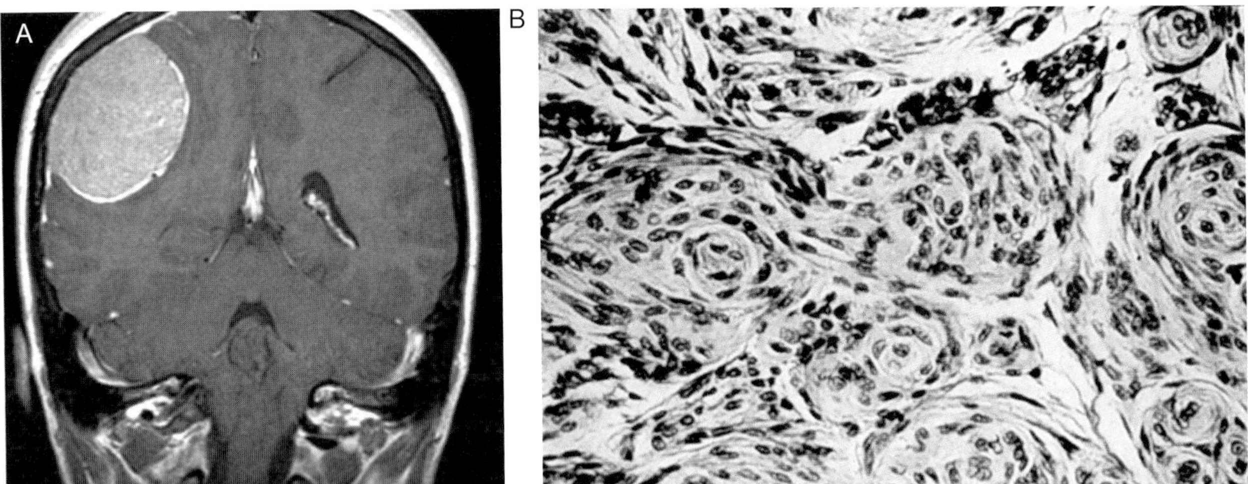

Fig. 16B.33. *A*, Coronal gadolinium-enhanced T1-weighted magnetic resonance image of the brain showing findings typical of a right parietal meningioma. *B*, Biopsy specimen showing the typical whorl formation and elongated cells.

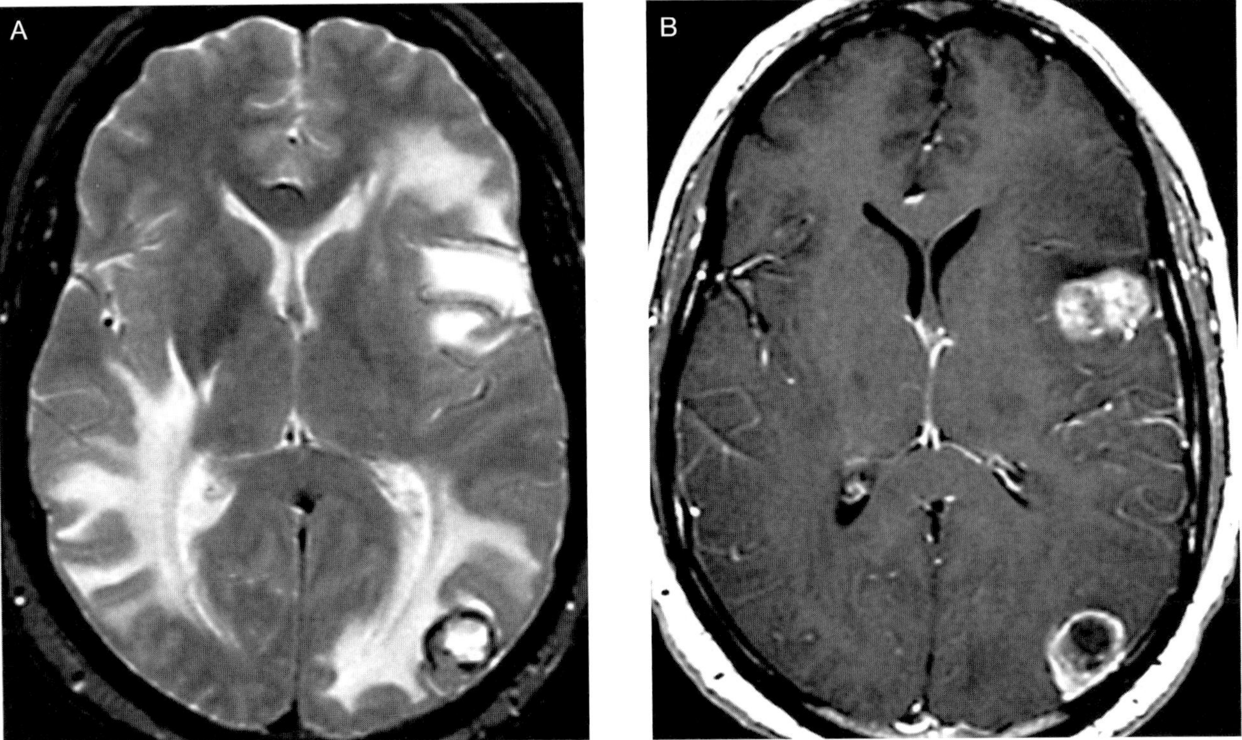

Fig. 16B.34. T2-weighted (*A*) and gadolinium-enhanced T1-weighted (*B*) axial magnetic resonance images of the typical appearance of a brain metastasis. Note the area of hemorrhage in the lesion in the left posterior temporal lobe. Common sources of brain metastases are neoplasms of the lung, breast, colon, kidney, melanoma, and choriocarcinoma.

Table 16B.3. Features of Partial (Focal) Seizures

Site of discharge	Clinical correlate
Frontal lobe	
Precentral gyrus (primary motor cortex)	Focal tonic or clonic movements Postictal paresis (Todd paralysis)
Supplementary motor cortex	Posturing: elevation of arm and deviation of head and eyes toward arm
Frontal eye fields	Deviation of eyes toward contralateral side
Broca area	Speech arrest and postictal aphasia
Cingulate gyrus	Bizarre behavior, automatism, autonomic manifestations
Parietal lobe	
Postcentral gyrus (primary sensory cortex)	Paresthesias and dysesthesias
Posterior parietal cortex	Ipsilateral or contralateral deviation of the eyes
Temporal lobe	
Uncus	Olfactory hallucinations
Medial portion	Impaired awareness, posturing, automatisms, affective and mnemonic phenomena, autonomic phenomena
Lateral surface	Formed visual and auditory hallucinations
Wernicke area	Speech arrest and postictal aphasia
Occipital lobe	Unformed visual hallucinations

hemispheres. Lesions of the optic tract, the lateral geniculate body, or optic radiation on one side produce *homonymous* defects in the opposite visual field. Complete destruction of the optic tract or optic radiation on one side produces a complete *homonymous hemianopia*, that is, loss of vision in the opposite half of the visual field of each eye. Because of the divergent course of axons in the optic radiation, the visual field defect may not be identical in both eyes. This is referred to as an *incongruous* homonymous field defect. A lesion in the parietal lobe destroys the superior optic radiations and produces an *inferior quadrantic field defect*. A lesion in the temporal lobe on one side destroys the fibers in the lower portion of the optic radiation and produces a *superior quadrantic field defect* ("a pie in the sky"). Lesions at the level of the calcarine fissure produce a homonymous hemianopia in the contralateral visual field. Two features may help distinguish homonymous hemianopia due to occipital lesions. One, the defect tends to be similar in both halves of the affected visual field (congruent). Two, because of the dual vascular supply of the pole of the occipital lobe (by branches of the posterior and medial cerebral arteries), the representation of the macula may be spared. This is called *macular sparing*.

Focal disorders may produce disturbances unique to the supratentorial level. Some of these effects reflect focal involvement of a specific area of the cerebral cortex of the contralateral cerebral hemisphere; others indicate involvement of a specific side; and still others are manifestations of bilateral involvement. The following lobar syndromes are due to impairment of the specific functional networks described in the previous section (Table 16B.4).

Frontal Lobe Syndromes

The frontal lobe includes the primary motor cortex, premotor area, supplementary motor area, medial motor area, frontal eye fields, Broca area, lateral prefrontal cortex, and orbitofrontal cortex. Lesions restricted to primary motor cortex impair the ability to perform contralateral fine finger movements or produce paralysis or, in the case of lesions in the paracentral lobule, leg weakness. Acute lesions in primary motor cortex produce flaccid hyporeflexia. Seizures in this region consist of focal tonic or clonic movements (or both) of the contralateral face, arm, or leg. Lesions involving the lateral premotor cortex and supplementary motor area produce hyperreflexia and disinhibition of primitive reflexes, including *forced grasping*. Combined lesions of the motor and premotor cortex area produce spastic hemiparesis. Seizures arising in the supplementary motor area cause a characteristic posturing, with elevation of the arm and deviation of the head and eyes toward the elevated arm.

Acute, bilateral lesions of the anterior cingulate gyrus and supplementary motor area produce *akinetic mutism*.

Lesions of the frontal eye fields impair voluntary and visually guided contralateral saccades. With acute lesions, there is transient conjugate deviation of the eyes toward the affected hemisphere and inability to move the eyes past the midline. Partial seizures in this region cause the eyes to deviate to the opposite side. Lesions of the motor speech (Broca) area may produce nonfluent aphasia or

Table 16B.4. Focal Lobar Syndromes

Lobe	Functional area	Manifestations
Frontal	Motor cortex	Contralateral hemiparesis, focal motor seizures
	Frontal eye fields	Impaired contralateral voluntary saccades
	Left frontal operculum	Nonfluent aphasia, apraxia of speech
	Dorsolateral prefrontal cortex (bilateral)	Dysexecutive syndrome, abulia
	Orbitofrontal cortex (bilateral)	Behavioral disinhibition, sociopathy
Parietal	Somatosensory cortex	Contralateral astereognosia, agraphesthesia, somatosensory seizures
	Optic radiation	Contralateral inferior quadrantanopia
	Left inferior parietal lobule	Agraphia, acalculia, left-right disorientation, finger agnosia (Gerstmann syndrome)
		Conduction aphasia
	Left superior parietal lobule	Apraxia
	Left angular gyrus	Alexia with agraphia
	Right inferior parietal lobule	Contralateral hemineglect, dressing apraxia, constructional apraxia, anosognosia
	Bilateral superior parietal lobule and intraparietal sulcus	Simultanagnosia, optic ataxia, oculomotor apraxia (Balint syndrome)
Temporal	Optic radiation	Contralateral inferior quadrantanopia
	Left superior temporal cortex	Fluent aphasia, auditory agnosia
	Left middle temporal cortex/temporal pole	Semantic dementia, anomia
	Inferior temporo-occipital cortex	Contralateral hemiachromatopsia
		Prosopagnosia, object agnosia
	Medial temporal lobe	Impaired declarative memory (amnesia)
		Complex partial seizures
Occipital		Contralateral homonymous hemianopia
		Cortical blindness (bilateral lesions)
		Unformed visual hallucinations
		Visual illusions

apraxia of speech. Seizures arising in this region result in transient *speech arrest*.

Lesions in the lateral prefrontal cortex produce a dysexecutive syndrome, with impaired attention, distractibility, abulia, perseveration, and impaired motor planning. Features of orbitofrontal lesions are behavioral disinhibition and impaired judgment. When the lesion affects the neighboring olfactory structures, the sense of smell is lost (*anosmia*). Seizures arising in the prefrontal cortical structures are complex partial seizures characterized by bizarre behavior, motor automatisms, and autonomic instability. They may resemble psychogenic seizures.

Clinical Problem 16B.14.

A 54-year-old surgeon is evaluated for progressive change in personality and behavior. He stopped working 2 years ago and was given early retirement because of his inappropriate behavior. He had become irritable and verbally abusive. On one occasion, he started making sexually explicit jokes while operating on a patient and continued the operation despite the anesthesiologist telling him to stop because of the patient's severe hypotension. After retirement, he spent most of his time watching TV. He started craving sweets and has gained approximately 20 lb over the past 5 months. His wife is concerned because he has spent large sums of money buying trivial things he never uses. Last summer, he lost a large sum of money in a casino, despite his wife's attempt to make him stop gambling. On neurologic examination, his memory, calculation, and construction abilities were normal. He became increasingly irritable with the physician during the history and physical examination and decided to leave the office. On his way out, he made an offensive remark to one of the nurses in the corridor.

a. What is the most likely location of the lesion?
b. What are possible causes?
c. How will testing for olfaction help localize the lesion?

Parietal Lobe Syndromes

The parietal lobe includes the primary somatosensory cortex in the postcentral gyrus, the unimodal somatosensory association area, and the multimodal cortex of the posterior parietal lobe. Lesions of primary somatosensory cortex produce contralateral cortical sensory loss characterized by impaired tactile discrimination, touch localization (topognosis), two-point discrimination, weight discrimination (barognosis), recognition of a number written on the hand (graphesthesia), and joint position sense. This cortical sensory loss compromises the use of the hand for manipulating objects and identifying them tactically (astereognosia). Patients with seizures in primary somatosensory cortex present with transient symptoms of numbness or tingling sensation of the contralateral face or body. Lesions of the dorsal (superior) portion of the optic radiation at the level of the parietal lobe produces a contralateral inferior quadrantanopia.

Lateralized syndromes occur with lesions of the heteromodal association area in the posterior parietal cortex. Right-sided lesions of the inferior parietal lobule cause severe sensory neglect of the left hemibody or extrapersonal space, with dressing apraxia and constructional apraxia. Lesions of the left inferior parietal lobule may produce a combination of deficits that includes agraphia, acalculia, finger agnosia, and right-left disorientation (Gerstmann syndrome) as well as ideomotor apraxia. Wernicke aphasia or conduction aphasia may occur with lesions of the left inferior parietal lobule. Bilateral lesions of the superior parietal lobule produce severe deficits in visual attention, including simultanagnosia, optic ataxia, and oculomotor apraxia (Balint syndrome). Lesions of the parietal lobe of either side may be manifested by contralateral agraphesthesia, astereognosia, and inferior quadrantanopia.

Temporal Lobe Syndromes

The temporal lobe includes primary auditory cortex (Heschl gyrus), unimodal auditory and visual association cortices, paralimbic cortex, and limbic cortex. Sound

Clinical Problem 16B.15.

A 65-year-old man had sudden onset of numbness of the right side of his face and right hand. Neurologic examination performed 2 hours later showed that he could not identify objects or written numbers in his right hand, localize sensory stimuli on the right side, or distinguish right from left. Additional testing disclosed that he had difficulty with arithmetic calculations and writing his name.

a. Where is the lesion?
b. What is the lesion?
c. What sensory processing deficits does this patient have?
d. What deficit in motor function may this patient have?
e. What visual field defect would you expect this patient to have?
f. What would be the effects of a similar lesion in the contralateral hemisphere?

stimuli coming into either ear are transmitted to the auditory cortex bilaterally; consequently, a unilateral lesion of auditory cortex does not cause a notable hearing deficit, but the localization of sound in contralateral space is impaired. The superior temporal gyrus (area 22) contains the auditory unimodal association area. Bilateral lesions of this area produce pure word deafness; patients react to environmental noise (i.e., they are not deaf) and recognize written language but cannot understand or repeat spoken language. Damage of Wernicke area in the posterior part of the superior temporal gyrus in the dominant hemisphere produces fluent aphasia characterized by a comprehension deficit for all modalities.

Lesions of temporal visual association cortex in the inferior temporo-occipital cortex may produce achromatopsia, visual agnosia, prosopagnosia, visual anomia, and pure alexia. Focal lesions of the temporal lobe are frequently associated with contralateral superior quadrantanopia, from the interruption of the ventral (inferior) component of the optic radiation.

Bilateral lesions of the medial part of the temporal lobe impair declarative memory. An important effect of focal lesions involving the medial temporal lobe are complex partial seizures, which may be preceded by an aura consisting of olfactory hallucinations, fear or other affective symptoms, and phenomena such as déjà vu or jamais vu that reflect disturbances of episodic memory. If the seizure involves the inferior and lateral apsects of the temporal lobe, the patient may experience complex visual or auditory hallucinations. With these seizures, patients may also have posturing of the contralateral limb and motor automatisms. Postictally, the patient is amnestic of the event and has aphasia, which represent transient dysfunction of the episodic memory and language networks, respectively. Complex partial seizures arising in the medial temporal lobe are the most common form of partial seizures. The most common cause is *mesial temporal sclerosis* (Fig. 16B.35).

Occipital Lobe Syndromes

The occipital lobe includes the primary visual area in the banks of the calcarine fissure on the medial surface of the occipital lobe (area 17) and visual association areas 18 and 19 (peristriate cortex). A lesion of visual cortex of one occipital lobe produces homonymous loss of vision in the contralateral visual field. Bilateral lesions of the occipital lobes produces *cortical blindness*. In some cases, this visual loss is denied by the patient. Patients may retain some perception of movement despite the inability to perceive the object. This phenomenon, called *blindsight*, is mediated by the visual pathway from the superior colliculus to the pulvinar to the posterior parietal cortex.

Disorders of occipital cortex can also be associated with subjective transient anomalies of vision such as scintillating scotomata, visual hallucinations, and illusions. Sensations of flashing lights in the field of vision are *scintillating scotomata*. This condition commonly accompanies migraine headache. Distorted perceptions of external visual stimuli are *visual illusions*. They include macropsia (objects appear larger than normal), micropsia (objects appear smaller than normal), and erythropsia (objects appear to have a red tinge). Compared with visual illusions, *visual hallucinations* are perceptions of

Clinical Problem 16B.16.

Three years ago, a 28-year-old man had onset of transient spells lasting 1 to 2 minutes during which he experienced the sensation of smelling an unpleasant odor. This sensation was immedately followed by the feeling as if he were in a dream state in which he saw and heard things that he had experienced before. He was also aware that he was unable to understand what other people were saying to him during these episodes. In the last year, the spells have changed somewhat, in that he now hears the sound of a bell and at the same time experiences a mental picture of a country scene from his childhood. In the last 3 months, he has been bothered by increasingly severe headaches, nausea, and vomiting. He has difficulty understanding what people are saying to him even when he is not having his spells. Neurologic examination showed bilateral blurring of the optic disc margins, a visual field defect, aphasia, and the Babinski sign on the right.

a. What do the transient spells represent?
b. What was the initial site of origin of the spells?
c. Where is the lesion?
d. What visual field defect would you expect this patient to have?
e. What type of language problem did the patient have?
f. What clues are present that indicate progression of the underlying process?
g. What test would be most helpful for this patient?
h. What might this test show?

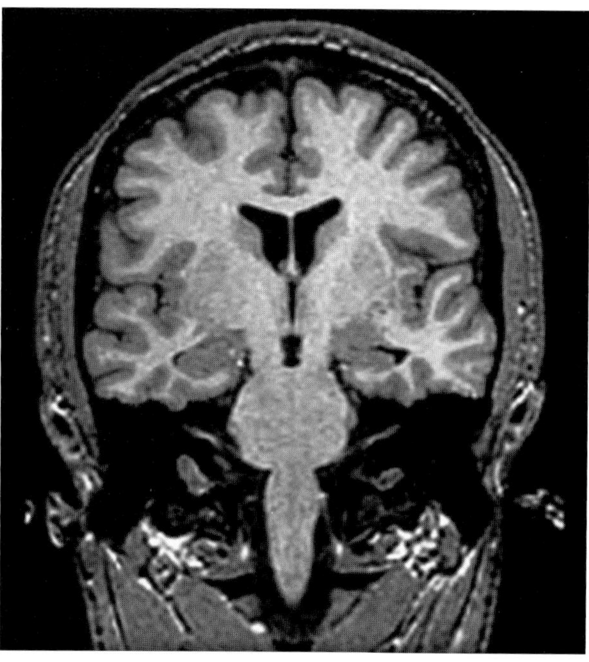

Fig. 16B.35. Coronal T1-weighted magnetic resonance image of the brain of a patient with intractable left temporal lobe seizures. The left hippocampus has atrophied, indicating mesial temporal sclerosis.

visual images for which there is no external stimulus. Simple visual hallucinations, such as flashing or twinkling lights, lines, or angles, can be manifestations of occipital lobe seizures. Formed visual hallucinations in which an actual scene or picture is visualized may be part of a seizure involving the posterior temporal lobes or be an effect of confusional state. Visual hallucinations are also typical with occipital lobe involvement in dementia with Lewy bodies. Although complex visual hallucinations may occur in schizophrenia, complex auditory hallucinations are more common in this and other psychotic states.

Involvement of the visual association (peristriate) cortex affects visuospatial processing, discrimination of movement, and color discrimination. These effects include those described with parietal lesions affecting the "where" pathway (simultagnosia, optic ataxia, oculomotor apraxia) and the inferior temporal cortex lesions affecting the "what" pathway (e.g., contralateral achromatopsia).

Subcortical Lesions

The subcortical white matter and the basal ganglia may be affected by focal or diffuse lesions of the cerebral hemispheres. These lesions interrupt one or several of the cortical-basal ganglia-thalamocortical circuits.

Subcortical White Matter

The subcortical white matter is commonly affected in vascular, demyelinating, and some toxic-metabolic conditions. Important examples include *small-vessel disease* due to hypertension or amyloid angiopathy (Fig. 16B.36), demyelinating disease such as multiple sclerosis, *progressive multifocal leukoencephalopathy* (a viral disease caused by the JC virus in immunosuppressed patients) and *HIV-related dementia*, radiation-induced leukoencephalopathy, and hereditary metabolic disorders (*leukodystrophies*). Important manifestations of these disorders include disturbances of gait and bladder function, spasticity, dementia, and visual impairment.

Lesions of the subcortical white matter of the frontal lobe, for example, hydrocephalus or small lacunar infarcts, may severely impair the automatic control of axial muscles, gait initiation, and automatic gait. Patients have difficulty getting up from a chair and maintaining an erect posture, and difficulty initiating stepping movements. Also, they have a wide-based, short-stepped gait. This *frontal gait disorder* is referred to as *gait apraxia*. Interruption of the inhibitory cortical input to the pontine micturition center produces an uninhibited bladder, characterized by urinary urgency and incontinence.

Basal Ganglia

In many vascular, inflammatory, degenerative, or toxic-metabolic disorders, the basal ganglia circuits may be affected either in isolation or together with the cerebral cortex. The clinical manifestations include motor, oculomotor, cognitive, and behavioral changes in various combinations, depending on the main location of the lesion. As mentioned above, the main motor dysfunctions associated with basal ganglia circuit disorders are parkinsonism and several hyperkinetic syndromes, including chorea, hemiballismus, and dystonia. The typical example of parkinsonism is *Parkinson disease*, which results from the loss of dopaminergic neurons in the substantia nigra pars compacta that synapse in the striatum. Parksinson disease is characterized by hypokinesia, bradykinesia, tremor at rest, and postural instability. Hyperkinetic disorders reflect impaired ability to suppress movements. An important example is *Huntington disease*, which is characterized by chorea resulting from atrophy of the caudate nucleus and, to a lesser extent, the putamen. Oculomotor abnormalities (e.g., inability to initiate saccadic eye movements), cognitive dysfunction (dementia), and psychiatric manifestations (e.g., depression and hallucinations) are also part of both Parkinson disease and Huntington

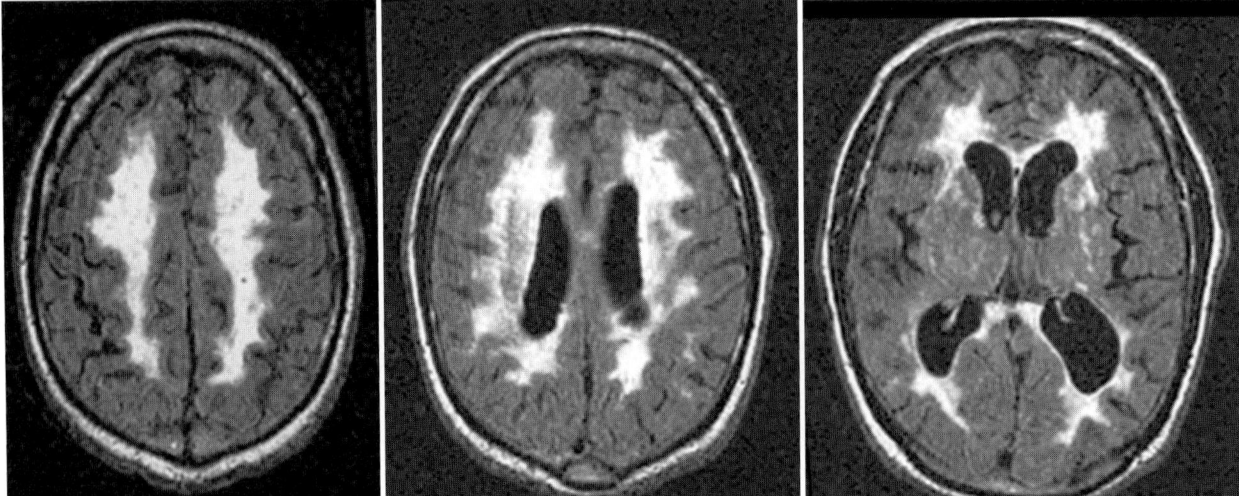

Fig. 16B.36. Axial fluid-attenuated inversion recovery (FLAIR) images of the brain showing severe subcortical white matter involvement by small-vessel disease.

disease. In some disorders, parkinsonism and dystonia in combination with abnormalities of cognition and behavior may reflect a metabolic disorder, as in the case of *Wilson disease.*

An important cause of rapidly progressive dementia associated with both cortical and basal ganglia dysfunction (as well as ataxia) is *Creutzfeldt-Jakob disease.* Typical features of this disorder include rapidly progressive visuospatial abnormalities, followed by cortical blindness, parkinsonism, dystonia, and apraxia. Many patients eventually develop *cortical myoclonus.* Myoclonus is the rapid, jerky movement of the face and limbs that may occur spontaneously or in response to sensory stimuli. Myoclonus has no localizing value because it can occur with lesions of the cerebral cortex, basal ganglia, brainstem, or spinal cord.

> Creutzfeldt-Jakob disease is a typical example of a prion disorder. Prions (from *pro*teinaceous *in*fectious particles) are abnormal forms of proteins normally present in many tissues, including the brain. Interaction between abnormal and normal prion proteins lead to protein precipitation and neuronal cell death. Prion disorders are characterized by abnormalities in the cerebral cortex, basal ganglia, or thalamus detectable on magnetic resonance imaging, periodic discharges on the electroencephalogram, or the presence of the 14-3-3 protein (chaperone protein) in the cerebrospinal fluid.

In some cases, disorders of the basal ganglia mimic disorders of the frontal lobe. Conditions such as depression, obsessive-compulsive disorder, attention-deficit/hyperactivity disorder, tic disorder, and schizophrenia reflect functional impairment of frontal cortex-basal ganglia circuits.

Neurologic Examination

The assessment of functions specific to the supratentorial level includes tests of cranial nerves I and II; evaluation of intellectual function, particularly memory and language; and tests of cortical motor and sensory functions. In addition, the distribution of findings with involvement of longitudinal systems can help localize supratentorial damage. For example, weakness in the face, arm, and leg on one side is evidence of a unilateral cerebral lesion.

Cortical Functions

The specific functions of the cerebral cortex are tested as a group in the mental status examination. The mental status examination is an essential component of the neurologic examination and includes an assessment of the level of consciousness, cognitive functions, cortical motor and sensory functions, and language. Important questions to be asked during history-taking include level of education and whether the patient is right- or left-handed.

Before cognitive function is assessed, the patient's level of alertness (arousal) must be established. Attention and language need to be assessed early in the examination because if they are impaired it will be difficult to interpret the rest of the mental status examination.

Level of Consciousness

The level of consciousness is evaluated by testing the patient's arousal and awareness of (or response to) the external environment. Arousal is tested by assessing the intensity of and responses to verbal, visual, tactile, and painful stimuli (Chapter 11).

Orientation

The patient is asked to give his or her full name, address, current location (building, city, state), and date (day of the week, month, and year).

Attention

The overall ability of the patient to attend to environmental stimuli can be tested by assessing attention span. This can be tested by forward and backward digit spans. The examiner reads to the patient a list of random digits at 1-second intervals, usually starting with a span of 4 digits and going upward. The patient is asked to reproduce exactly the span forward and backward. Normally, patients are able to repeat up to 7 digits forward and 5 digits backward. Other measures of attention include resistance to perseverance (e.g., recitation of the months of the year or days of the week forward and backward); the patient is asked to give common nouns that start with the letter "A," "F," or "S," or to name, in a span of 60 seconds, all animals, vegetables, or fruits he or she can think of. Directed attention is tested, for example, by double simultaneous stimulation of tactile, visual, or auditory sensation.

Language

The four modalities of central language processing are listening, speaking, reading, and writing. Examination of language should assess fluency, comprehension, naming, and repetition. Fluency is the rate of production and accuracy of words. The patient is asked to look at a picture, describe it orally, and write a few sentences about it.

This will disclose word-finding difficulties, production of an incorrect word instead of a target word (*paraphasia*), prosody, and articulation. Fluent aphasias occur with lesions in the left posterior perisylvian region (superior temporal and inferior parietal cortices), whereas nonfluent aphasias occur with anterior lesions (inferior frontal cortex). Auditory comprehension is assessed by asking a patient to perform a series of maneuvers of increased complexity, for example, "open your mouth" or "first look at the ceiling and then point to the floor." Naming is assessed by asking the patient to identify common pictures. Repetition is assessed by asking the patient to repeat sentences such as "No ifs, ands, or buts."

Reading should be evaluated by having the patient either read a paragraph silently and explain the content of the paragraph or, if speech is significantly impaired, point to words and sentences on the printed page spoken by the examiner. Writing can be tested by having the patient write something from dictation or copy a written message. Reading and writing are impaired in aphasia at essentially the same level as auditory comprehension and production of speech. However, impairment of reading (alexia) or writing (agraphia), or both, may occur without aphasia.

- Language is tested by assessing the four modalities of listening, speaking, reading, and writing.

Memory

Several aspects of declarative memory should be assessed separately, including *acquisition* (learning), *retention* (recall after a delayed interval), and *retrieval*. It is usually desirable to assess both verbal (words) and nonverbal (figure) learning. For example, to assess verbal memory, the patient is instructed to learn, retain, and recall four unrelated words such as "apple," "Mr. Johnson," "charity," and "tunnel." After the patient is given the four words, he or she is asked to repeat them immediately afterward (to assess learning) and to recall them after approximately 5 minutes (to assess retention). If the patient cannot recall the words, the examiner may provide cues or prompts, and if this fails, the patient is asked to select a word from a list (recognition test). Similar tests are used for nonverbal material (e.g., pictures). These memory tests assess the function of medial temporal lobe structures (hippocampus and parahippocampal gyrus) as well as related structures (basal forebrain, mammillary bodies, and anterior and dorsomedial thalamic nuclei).

Calculation

Calculation can be assessed by asking the patient to multiply 5 × 13, subtract 7 from 65, divide 58 by 2, and add 11 to 29. More complex arithmetic problems can be used. Calculation assesses primarily left parietal lobe function.

Construction

Constructional tasks depend on perceptual abilities and skilled motor functions. The patient is asked to draw the face of a clock showing 11:15 and to copy a three-dimensional cube. This task relies primarily on the function of the nondominant (generally, right) parietal lobe.

Abstract Reasoning and Conceptual Functions

These tasks depend on complex higher cortical functions integrated at the level of the prefrontal cortex. The patient is required to draw upon acquired knowledge and to apply it to a task in an unfamiliar fashion. This function can be assessed by interpreting similarities in word pairs, such as orange/banana, horse/dog, and table/ bookcase.

Other tasks involve the interpretation of proverbs, such as "People who live in glass houses should not throw stones."

Information

General knowledge of the world, including the name and use of objects and facts, constitutes semantic memory. The long-term storage of learned information involves a widespread cortical network centered in the lateral and anterior portions of the temporal lobes, particularly on the left side. The general fund of information should be tested in the context of the patient's intellectual level, cultural background, and geographic origin. To assess this function, the patient can be asked to name the current president of the United States, the first president of the United States, to state the number of weeks in a year, and to define an island.

Cortical Sensory Processing

Disorders of high-level sensory processing include the inability to recognize an object, that is, agnosia. As a consequence, the patient cannot name the object or describe its use. Agnosia occurs in any of the specific sensory modalities. Tests of somatosensory processing include asking the patient to recognize objects placed on the hand and to recognize a part of the body. In astereognosia, patients are not able to identify objects tactically because of impaired cortical sensory function. In tactile agnosia, the patients are unable to recognize an object despite being able to describe its shape. This occurs with lesions in the left parietal lobe, and it may be associated with left-right confusion or finger agnosia. Finger agnosia can be assessed by asking the patient to "show me your thumb" or "touch your left ear with your right thumb." To test visual processing, the patient can be asked to identify and name pictures or objects. If the patient cannot name the object (because of anomia), object recognition can be tested by asking the patient to demonstrate the use of the object. Auditory processing is assessed by asking the patient to identify a particular sound. Visuospatial localization depends on the nondominant parietal lobe and may be assessed at the bedside by asking the patient to name the states that border his or her own state of residence.

Cortical Motor Function

The ability to perform learned skilled motor acts is called *praxis*, and it can be assessed by asking the patient to perform various tasks on command. This includes demonstrating a gesture (such as a kiss; salute; use of a toothbrush, hammer and nail; or combing the hair). If the patient is unable to perform these tasks, the examiner demonstrates the task and asks the patient to imitate the motion. If the patient is still unable to do so, then an actual object such as a comb or key may be given to him or her. The patient may be asked to perform a sequential task, such as hanging a picture on a wall or finding a number in the telephone book and making a telephone call. These functions generally require the integrity of the left hemisphere, including the posterior parietal, premotor, and supplementary motor areas. Functions performed with the nondominant hand require that the commissural connections, through the corpus callosum, with these areas in the right hemisphere be intact.

Laboratory Assessment of Cortical Function

Additional tests of cortical function include neuropsychologic testing, electroencephalography, and functional imaging studies. Neuropsychologic assessment involves psychometric testing of cortical function with procedures that have a standardized administration and normative references. Neuropsychologic testing generally is used to detect impaired cognitive ability, including learning, memory, attention, language, visuospatial skills, and executive or reasoning functions. Neurocognitive testing is also used in the evaluation of such central nervous system disorders as diffuse encephalopathy, dementia, vascular disorders, stroke, epilepsy, and head injury.

Electroencephalography records the electrical activity of the cerebral cortex and can be used to detect abnormalities of cerebral function and to indicate whether the disturbance is focal or generalized. It is particularly helpful in evaluating patients with seizures, altered states of consciousness, and focal cortical lesions (Chapter 11).

Activity in specific brain regions of humans performing a specific sensory, motor, or verbal task can be studied with functional neuroimaging techniques. These include positron emission tomography (Fig. 16B.37), single photon emission computed tomography, and functional magnetic resonance imaging (Fig. 16B.38). The underlying principle of these techniques is that increased neuronal activity in a particular brain region is coupled to a local increase in cerebral blood flow, oxygen consumption, and glucose metabolism. Thus, changes in blood flow or metabolism detected with any of these functional neuroimaging techniques reflect activation of cortical regions during specific tasks or in pathologic conditions.

- Additional tests of cortical function include neuropsychologic testing, electroencephalography, and functional imaging studies.

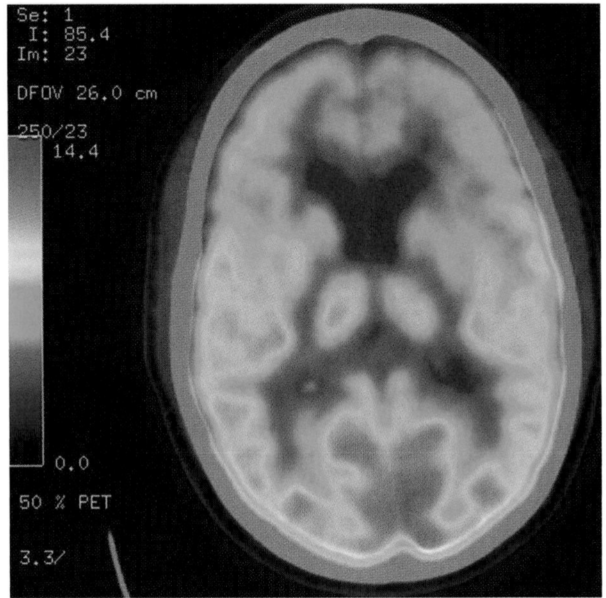

Fig. 16B.37. Fluorodeoxyglucose positron emission tomographic scan of the brain of a patient with frontotemporal dementia. Note the severe bilateral and symmetrical decrease in glucose metabolism in the frontal lobes.

Cranial Nerve I (Olfactory)

Olfaction is tested by having the patient sniff a substance that has an identifiable odor (camphor, coffee, wintergreen) with each nostril separately, while the other nostril is held closed. Because it is not possible to quantify this sensation, the appreciation of the odor is sufficient to exclude anosmia. Intranasal disease is a common cause of impaired olfactory sensation and must be excluded before the diagnosis of neurogenic anosmia is made.

- Cranial nerve I (olfactory) is evaluated by testing the sense of smell.

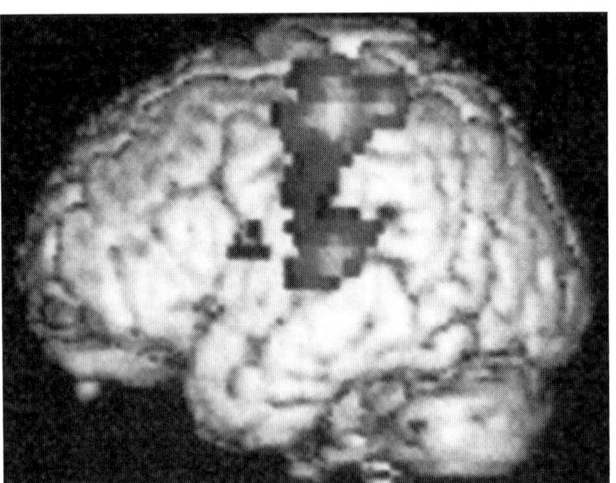

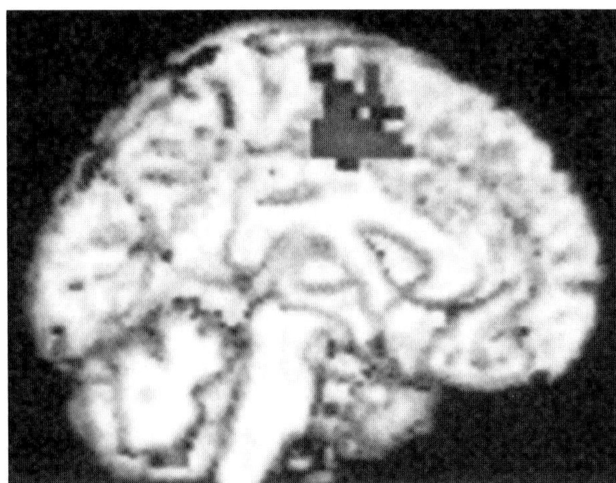

Fig. 16B.38. Normal functional magnetic resonance imaging of the brain of a patient performing alternate finger movements with the right hand. The blood oxygenation level-dependent (BOLD) signal is increased in the left primary motor, premotor, and supplementary motor areas.

Additional Reading

Damasio AR. Aphasia. N Engl J Med. 1992;326:531-539.

Engel J Jr. Seizures and epilepsy. Philadelphia: F. A. Davis Co.; 1989.

Fuster JM. The prefrontal cortex—an update: time is of the essence. Neuron. 2001;30:319-333.

Grabowski TJ Jr., Anderson SW, Cooper GE. Disorders of cognitive function. Continuum. 2002;8(2).

Kanwisher N, Wojciulik E. Visual attention: insights from brain imaging. Nat Rev Neurosci. 2000;1:91-100.

Kopelman MD. Disorders of memory. Brain. 2002; 125:2152-2190.

LeDoux JE. Emotion circuits in the brain. Annu Rev Neurosci. 2000;23:155-84.

Mesulam MM. From sensation to cognition. Brain. 1998;121:1013-1052.

Petersen RC. Aging, mild cognitive impairment, and Alzheimer's disease. Neurol Clin. 2000;18:789-806.

Price CJ. The anatomy of language: contributions from functional neuroimaging. J Anat. 2000;197:335-359.

Squire LR, Zola SM. Structure and function of declarative and nondeclarative memory systems. Proc Natl Acad Sci U S A. 1996;93:13515-13522.

Answers to Clinical Problems

Chapter 1
Integrated Neuroscience for the Clinician

Clinical Problem 1.1

Unresponsive and with no movement

a. Did his heart stop because of an arrhythmia? I need to check his pulse and breathing.
b. His girlfriend dumped him. Did he try to commit suicide? I need to look for signs.
c. Did he fall and injure his brain? I need to check carefully for signs of injury.
d. He has a history of epilepsy. Did he have a seizure?
e. He likes alcohol. Is he "dead drunk"? What does his breath smell like?

Clinical Problem 1.2

Trouble localized to one leg and developing over an hour

a. Did I occlude an artery, with loss of the blood supply to the nerves and muscles in the leg?
b. Did I put pressure on a nerve, damaging the nerves that control sensation and movement?

Chapter 2
Development of the Nervous System (Neuroembryology)

Clinical Problem 2.1

a. Dorsal induction (neurulation)
b. Neural tube and neural crest at 3-4 weeks of gestation
c. Motor (lower limbs and external rectal and urethral sphincters), sensory (lower limbs), and visceral (bladder and rectum)
d. Myelomeningocele
e. Spina bifida, meningocele, cranium bifidum oculta, meningoencephalocele, craniorachischisis, anencephaly; they differ in severity and level of failure of fusion
f. Folic acid

Clinical Problem 2.2

a. Holoprosencephaly
b. Ventral induction of the prosencephalon and cranial and facial structures
c. Sonic hedgehog

Clinical Problem 2.3

a. Microcephaly
b. Neuronal and glial proliferation
c. Ventricular and subventricular zones, external granular layer

Clinical Problem 2.4

a. Tuberous sclerosis
b. The brain, eyes, and skin are all derivatives of the ectoderm.
c. Mutations in tumor suppressor genes

Clinical Problem 2.5

a. Heterotopia
b. Radial migration
c. 12-20 weeks of gestation
d. Lissencephaly (smooth brain) is the lack of development of cortical sulci that reflects impaired neuronal migration.

Clinical Problem 2.6

a. Down syndrome
b. Dendritic development and synaptogenesis
c. Fragile X syndrome, other X-linked forms of mental retardation

Clinical Problem 2.7

a. Myelination
b. Leukodystrophy
c. Oligodendrocytes in the central nervous system and Schwann cells in the peripheral nervous system

Clinical Problem 2.8

a. Dorsal root ganglion and sympathetic ganglion neurons
b. Neural crest
c. Parasympathetic ganglion neurons, enteric neurons, Schwann cells, adrenal medulla, melanocytes, mesoderm of facial structures

Chapter 3
Diagnosis of Neurologic Disorders: Anatomical Localization

Clinical Problem 3.1
Supratentorial, focal, left

Clinical Problem 3.2
Spinal, focal, midline

Clinical Problem 3.3
Posterior fossa, focal, right

Clinical Problem 3.4
Peripheral, focal, right

Clinical Problem 3.5
Posterior fossa, focal, left

Clinical Problem 3.6
Multiple levels, diffuse

Chapter 4
Diagnosis of Neurologic Disorders: Neurocytology and the Pathologic Reactions of the Nervous System

Clinical Problem 4.1
Supratentorial, right, nonmass, vascular (cerebral infarction)

Clinical Problem 4.2
Supratentorial, right, mass, vascular (parenchymal hematoma)

Clinical Problem 4.3
Multiple levels, diffuse, nonmass, vascular (subarachnoid hemorrhage)

Clinical Problem 4.4
Multiple levels, diffuse, nonmass, inflammatory (meningoencephalitis)

Clinical Problem 4.5
Posterior fossa, left, mass, inflammatory (cerebellar abscess)

Clinical Problem 4.6
Multiple levels, diffuse, nonmass, inflammatory (multiple sclerosis)

Clinical Problem 4.7
Supratentorial, left, mass, neoplasm (astrocytoma)

Clinical Problem 4.8
Supratentorial, diffuse, nonmass, degenerative (Alzheimer disease)

Clinical Problem 4.9
Multiple levels, diffuse, nonmass, metabolic (hypoglycemia)

Clinical Problem 4.10
Spinal, right, nonmass, trauma

Clinical Problem 4.11
Posterior fossa, left, nonmass, vascular (lateral medullary infarction)

Clinical Problem 4.12
Posterior fossa, left, mass, neoplasm (acoustic schwannoma)

Clinical Problem 4.13
Multiple levels, diffuse, nonmass, degenerative (amyotrophic lateral sclerosis)

Clinical Problem 4.14
Peripheral, right, mass, neoplasm (sciatic neurofibroma)

Chapter 5
Diagnosis of Neurologic Disorders: Transient Disorders and Neurophysiology

Clinical Problem 5.1

a. Equilibrium
b. Steady state
c. Active transport

Clinical Problem 5.2

a. Ischemia or anoxia impairs ATP production and, thus, the function of the Na^+-K^+ pump. As a result, K^+ accumulates in the extracellular fluid, leading to a decrease in both its concentration gradient and equilibrium potential, thereby reducing the resting membrane potential (which is determined primarily by the equilibirum potential of K^+). The persistent membrane depolarization inactivates voltage-gated Na^+ channels responsible for the generation of action potentials.
b. Recovery occurs from restoration of cerebral blood flow, which leads to the recovery of aerobic metabolism, ATP production, and Na^+-K^+ pump function.

Clinical Problem 5.3
An increase in extracellular K^+ concentration leads to a decrease in the K^+ concentration gradient and, thus, its equilibrium potential, thereby reducing the resting membrane potential (which is determined primarily by the equilibrium potential of K^+). The persistent membrane depolarization inactivates voltage-gated Na^+ channels responsible for the generation of action potentials in skeletal and cardiac muscle.

Clinical Problem 5.4

a. Decreased (by preventing initiation of an action potential)
b. Decreased (by preventing conduction at the nodes of Ranvier)
c. Indirectly decreased (by preventing axon terminal depolarization and opening of voltage-gated Ca^{2+} channels involved in exocytosis)
d. Local anesthesia, treatment of pain, seizures, cardiac arrhythmias

Clinical Problem 5.5
Blockade of voltage-gated Na^+ channels impairs the generation and conduction of action potentials and decreases the probability of neurotransmitter release.

Clinical Problem 5.6
This patient has Lambert-Eaton myasthenic syndrome, a disorder due to autoantibodies that block the presynaptic P/Q-type calcium channels at the level of the neuromuscular junction (causing muscle weakness and impaired muscle stretch reflexes) and autonomic system. This is commonly a paraneoplastic disorder in patients with small cell lung carcinoma.

Clinical Problem 5.7

1. a. No. This mechanism would reduce neuronal excitability.
   b. Yes, this would increase the probability of action potentials being triggered.
2. a. No
   b. Yes. This is the mechanism of action of drugs such as phenytoin and carbamazepine.
   c. Yes. Drugs that potentiate the effects of GABA-activating Cl^- channels, such as benzodiazepines

and barbiturates, are used in the treatment of seizures.

d. No

Clinical Problem 5.8

Loss of myelin results in reduced conduction velocity or conduction block by two mechanisms: 1) increased membrane "leak" of current and 2) impaired clustering of Na^+ channels at the nodes of Ranvier.

Clinical Problem 5.9

1. Peripheral
2. a. No
   b. Yes

Chapter 6 Synaptic Transmission and Neurochemical Systems

Clinical Problem 6.1

a. Multiple levels, diffuse
b. Glutamate
c. Excitotoxicity
d. Blockade of NMDA receptors or Ca^{2+} channels

Clinical Problem 6.2

a. Supratentorial, diffuse
b. GABA
c. Abrupt impairment of inhibitory transmission due to withdrawal of a drug that potentiates GABAergic transmission
d. A benzodiazepine

Clinical Problem 6.3

a. Hippocampal formation
b. Degenerative
c. Acetylcholine
d. Cholinesterase inhibitor

Clinical Problem 6.4

a. Supratentorial
b. Dopamine
c. Parkinson disease
d. Loss of dopaminergic neurons in the substantia nigra pars compacta

Chapter 7 The Sensory System

Clinical Problem 7.1

a. Diffuse, nonmass, inflammatory
b. Dorsal columns
c. Toxic-metabolic: vitamin B_{12} deficiency

Clinical Problem 7.2

a. Peripheral, focal—right, nonmass, traumatic or vascular
b. Lateral femoral cutaneous nerve (see Fig. 7.7)
c. Refer to Figure 7.7

Clinical Problem 7.3

a. Spinal, focal—midline and bilateral, mass, neoplastic
b. Dorsal roots or spinal nerves of C2 segment
c. Structures listed in b and dorsal columns bilaterally
d. The segmental loss at C2 suggests that this is the level of the lesion.
e. The segmental sensory loss would be at the level of the nipples, and the dorsal column deficit would spare the upper extremities and affect the lower extremities.

Clinical Problem 7.4

a. Spinal, focal—midline, mass, neoplastic
b. The second-order axons transmitting pain and temperature impulses (bound for the spinothalamic tracts bilaterally) as they decussate in the ventral white commissure at the involved levels
c. Syringomyelia. However, the same clinical pattern could be produced by an intramedullary neoplasm at that level.

Clinical Problem 7.5

a. Spinal, focal—left, nonmass, traumatic
b. T10 (see Fig. 7.6)
c. Brown-Séquard syndrome

d. The lesion involves only the left side of the spinal cord, affecting the spinothalamic and dorsal column tracts on that side. The sensation of touch ascends in both tracts and, thus, is maintained by the intact tracts on the right side of the spinal cord.
e. Wallerian degeneration occurs in the distal axons when they are severed from their cell bodies. Above the level of the lesion, the left spinothalamic tract would show degeneration up to the level of the thalamus. The left fasciculus gracilis would show degeneration only to the level of its second-order neuron, the nucleus gracilis. The left corticospinal tract would show degeneration below the lesion.

Clinical Problem 7.6

a. Supratentorial, focal—right, nonmass, vascular
b. Thalamus (ventral posterolateral nucleus)
c. In the right thalamocortical radiations

Clinical Problem 7.7

a. Supratentorial, focal—right, mass, neoplastic
b. Focal sensory seizures
c. The lesion is in the primary sensory cortex (postcentral gyrus), producing a cortical sensory loss. Crude perceptions of touch, pain, temperature, and vibration are also integrated in other cortical areas, but discriminative sensations require processing in the parietal sensory cortex.

Chapter 8
The Motor System

Clinical Problem 8.1

a. Spinal, diffuse, nonmass, inflammatory
b. Lower motor neuron (final common pathway)
c. Weakness, atrophy, fasciculations, decreased muscle tone, loss of muscle stretch reflexes
d. Poliovirus, West Nile virus
e. Alpha motor neuron, motor axon, motor nerve terminals, neuromuscular junction, muscle

Clinical Problem 8.2

a. Supratentorial, left, nonmass, vascular
b. Upper motor neuron (motor cortex)
c. Stimulation of the sole of the foot elicits dorsiflexion of the big toe (Babinski sign); abdominal reflexes are abolished.
d. Lack of dexterity of the fingers, difficulty increasing force of contraction
e. Aphasia
f. Bilateral cortical projections to the subdivision of the facial nucleus innervating the forehead

Clinical Problem 8.3

a. Paraparesis involving predominantly extensors of the lower limbs, increased muscle tone, hyperreflexia, clonus, Babinski sign
b. Interruption of descending inputs to spinal Ia presynaptic and Ia inhibitory interneurons
c. Spasticity is a velocity-dependent increase in muscle tone due to exaggerated muscle stretch reflexes caused by an upper motor neuron lesion; it may be associated with a clasp-knife phenomenon. Rigidity is continuous resistance to passive motion (lead pipe resistance) that is associated with parkinsonism but not associated with exaggerated reflexes.
d. Interruption of the input from the micturition center of the pons that activates the sacral parasympathetic neurons innervating the bladder detrusor and inhibits the somatic motor neurons innervating the external sphincter, resulting in an uninhibited bladder (see Chapter 9)
e. Interruption of inputs from low-threshold mechanoreceptors because of a lesion in the gracile fasciculus of the dorsal columns
f. A mass lesion in the thoracic spinal cord

Clinical Problem 8.4

a. Decerebrate posture
b. Bilateral brainstem lesion between the red nucleus and vestibular nuclei
c. Interruption of ascending fibers from the pontine reticular formation to thalamus
d. Structural lesions (e.g., trauma, vascular, inflammatory, neoplasm) or toxic-metabolic lesions (e.g., hypoxia, hypoglycemia, carbon monoxide intoxication). A structural lesion typically has a mass effect

that extends across the midline and affects the components of the consciousness system at the supratentorial level (thalamus, hypothalamus) or posterior fossa level (upper pons and midbrain reticular formation). Toxic and metabolic disorders typically affect the cerebral cortex diffusely, with or without associated diffuse involvement of the brainstem.

Clinical Problem 8.5

a. Supratentorial, right, mass, neoplasm
b. Lesion at the level of the motor cortex and subcortical white matter interrupting the corticospinal tract
c. Astereognosis. It indicates a cortical-type sensory loss due to involvement of the parietal lobe.

Clinical Problem 8.6

a. Weakness in left leg, particularly involving hip and knee flexors and foot dorsiflexors; increase in tone and reflexes in the left leg, left Babinski sign
b. Interruption of descending corticospinal and medullary reticulospinal inputs to spinal Ia presynaptic and Ia inhibitory interneurons
c. Spasticity is a velocity-dependent increase in muscle tone caused by exaggerated muscle sretch reflexes resulting from an upper motor neuron lesion; it may be associated with a clasp-knife phenomenon. Rigidity is continuous resistance to passive motion (lead-pipe resistance) associated with parkinsonism.
d. Weakness and atrophy of left hand muscles, absence of triceps reflex
e. They indicate a segmental spinal lesion at C7 level.
f. Magnetic resonance imaging of the cervical spine

Clinical Problem 8.7

a. Atrophy and fasciculations of the tongue, arms and legs, reduced reflexes of arms and legs
b. Slow-strained speech (spastic dysarthria, Babinski sign)
c. Motor neuron disease
d. Amyotrophic lateral sclerosis

Clinical Problem 8.8

a. Posterior fossa, right, mass, neoplasm
b. Cerebellar control circuit
c. Control of timing of contraction of agonists and antagonists and, thus, the initiation, speed, amplitude, and termination of movement (coordination)
d. Ipsilateral cerebellar hemisphere
e. Flocculonodular lobe
f. Vermis
g. Magnetic resonance imaging of the brain

Clinical Problem 8.9

a. Parkinsonism (hyperkinetic-rigid syndrome), characterized by hypokinesia or akinesia, bradykinesia, rigidity, postural instability, and tremor at rest
b. Parkinson disease, a degenerative disorder characterized by neuronal loss and accumulation of synuclein-containing Lewy bodies in neurons of the substantia nigra pars compacta and other brain regions
c. Drugs that block dopaminergic receptors, toxins such as manganese, other degenerative conditions
d. Basal ganglia control circuit
e. Loss of dopaminergic input to the striatum, which impairs the function of the direct inhibitory pathway and exaggerates the function of the indirect excitatory pathway, with increased activity of the subthalamic nucleus and its target (internal segment of the globus pallidus) resulting in the inability to initiate motor programs
f. Levodopa (in combination with carbidopa), dopaminergic agonists
g. Subthalamic nucleus, internal segment of globus pallidus (ventrolateral part)

Clinical Problem 8.10

a. Supratentorial, diffuse, nonmass, degenerative
b. Chorea
c. Prefrontal cortex and caudate nucleus
d. Huntington disease
e. Bilateral atrophy of the caudate nucleus

Clinical Problem 8.11

a. Supratentorial, right, nonmass, vascular
b. Hemiballismus

c. Subthalamic nucleus
d. The subthalamic nucleus receives excitatory input from the cerebral cortex and inhibitory input from the external segment of the globus pallidus. The subthalamic nucleus elicits tonic excitation of the output neurons of the internal segment of the globus pallidus, which provide a tonic inhibitory output to the thalamus and brainstem to prevent initiation of competing motor programs while executing a selected motor program.
e. The subthalamic nucleus is the preferred target for deep brain stimulation for treatment of Parkinson disease and hyperkinetic movement disorders.

Clinical Problem 8.12
a. Basal ganglia and cerebellar control circuits
b. Degenerative and toxic-metabolic disorders

Chapter 9
The Internal Regulation System

Clinical Problem 9.1
a. Generalized autonomic failure
b. Degenerative diseases, peripheral neuropathies, drugs
c. Sympathetic: orthostatic hypotension, lack of sweating; parasympathetic: urinary retention, constipation, erectile impotence
d. Thermoregulatory and axon reflex sweat tests, heart rate responses to deep breathing, Valsalva maneuver, head-up tilt test
e. Denervation supersensitivity
f. Indicates a peripheral (postganglionic) lesion

Clinical Problem 9.2
a. Excessive activation of muscarinic receptors
b. Peripheral, toxic
c. Intoxication with an anticholinesterase agent
d. Muscarinic antagonists, such as atropine

Clinical Problem 9.3
a. Intoxication with an anticholinergic (muscarinic antagonist) drug
b. Anxiety produces sympathetic activation, which produces tachycardia and mydriasis, but no urinary retention, and may be associated with excessive sweating, unlike in this patient.
c. Blockade of muscarinic cholinergic receptors in the thalamus and cerebral cortex

Clinical Problem 9.4
a. Spinal cord, left
b. Mass, neoplasm
c. Cervical spinal cord motor neurons at C8-T1, descending sympathetic pathway, corticospinal tract
d. Sympathetic fibers
e. Hypothalamus, dorsolateral brainstem, sympathetic chain, superior cervical ganglion, cavernous sinus, orbit
f. Normal response
g. A postganglionic lesion
h. Exaggerated pupillary dilatation

Clinical Problem 9.5
a. Spinal, midline (cauda equina)
b. Mass, neoplasm
c. Flaccid
d. Erectile impotence

Chapter 10
The Consciousness System

Clinical Problem 10.1
a. Narcolepsy with cataplexy
b. Sleep paralysis, hypnagogic hallucinations
c. Intrusion of REM sleep phenomena during wakefulness
d. Loss of hypocretin (orexin) neurons in the posterior lateral hypothalamus

Clinical Problem 10.2
a. Supratentorial, focal right mass, vascular
b. Intracerebral hemorrhage
c. Although unilateral lesions do not ordinarily cause loss of consciousness, a mass lesion (as in this case)

may compress diencephalic structures bilaterally or produce herniation of supratentorial structures (or do both), secondarily involving diencephalic and brainstem structures bilaterally.

d. In addition to focal slow-wave abnormality present over the right hemisphere, more diffuse slowing may be seen.

Clinical Problem 10.3

a. Multiple levels (supratentorial and posterior fossa), nonfocal and diffuse, nonmass, metabolic
b. Widespread areas of the cerebral cortex and portions of the ascending reticular activating system in the cerebral hemispheres, thalamus, and brainstem
c. Hypoglycemia
d. Diffuse, slow-wave abnormality

Clinical Problem 10.4

a. Supratentorial, diffuse, indeterminate. The only abnormality present was transient symptoms. As noted in Chapter 5, transient symptoms alone may be associated with various disorders and do not allow a pathologic diagnosis to be established.
b. Generalized epileptiform abnormalities occurring in repetitive and rhythmic fashion
c. Inflammatory (encephalitis), vascular, neoplastic, degenerative, toxic-metabolic, traumatic
d. The presence of focal seizures would increase the likelihood of an underlying structural lesion involving one cerebral hemisphere. In a patient of this age, a neoplasm should be suspected.

Chapter 11
Cerebrospinal Fluid: Ventricular System

Clinical Problem 11.1

a. By comparison with standardized tables of normal head circumference, 50 cm at 10 months is more than 2 standard deviations above the norm.
b. An increase in the volume of any of the constituents of the skull. At this age, subdural hematomas and hydrocephalus due to several causes are common.
c. Computed tomography and magnetic resonance imaging are safe, noninvasive procedures. This patient has aqueductal stenosis.
d. Noncommunicating hydrocephalus
e. i. Enlargement of the lateral and third ventricles with obstruction at the aqueduct. The fourth ventricle would not be visualized.
   ii. Uniform dilatation of the ventricular system proximal to the blockage (of the lateral and third ventricles, aqueduct, and fourth ventricle)
   iii. Uniform dilatation of the entire ventricular system
   iv. Usually no changes (but the CSF probably would be bloody)

Clinical Problem 11.2

In an infant, intracranial volume can be increased by modest expansion of the sutures, which increases the head size and results in a less significant increase in intracranial pressure. In an adult, such compensation is impossible, and intracranial pressure increases.

Clinical Problem 11.3

a. Multiple levels, diffuse, nonmass, an unidentified inflammation
b. An inflammatory process and a traumatic tap
c. Possibly bacteria; growth of the offending organism
d. In the presence of bacterial meningitis, the CSF glucose level is often significantly decreased because of impaired transport.

Clinical Problem 11.4

a. Spinal, focal-midline, mass, neoplastic
b. Magnetic resonance imaging of the spine, myelography

Chapter 12
The Vascular System

Clinical Problem 12.1

a. Posterior fossa, focal, left (lateral medulla)
b. The following tracts or nuclei (or both) are responsible for this patient's symptoms:

Symptom or sign	Tract or nucleus
Dysarthria, dysphagia (difficulty swallowing), palatal weakness	Nucleus ambiguus
Horner syndrome	Descending hypothalamic fibers that control sympathetic output
Reduced facial pain sensation	Spinal nucleus and tract of V
Reduced arm and leg pain sensation	Spinothalamic tract
Ataxia, vertigo	Inferior cerebellar peduncle

c. The posterior inferior cerebellar artery supplies the dorsolateral medulla.

Clinical Problem 12.2

a. The upper motor neuron weakness of the right arm and face is due to a lesion of the corticospinal tract. With the arm and face predominantly involved, the lesion likely is at the level of the cerebral cortex on the left side. Language expression would be related to the area of Broca of the cerebral cortex of the dominant hemisphere.
b. The left lateral hemisphere of the brain is supplied by the middle cerebral artery.
c. This patient had a transient ischemic attack 1 week before his acute stroke. This attack was a warning sign of the impending stroke. The retina and choroid of the eye are supplied by the ophthalmic artery, a branch of the internal carotid artery. The middle cerebral artery is also a branch of the internal carotid artery. The two clinical events were likely a result of internal carotid artery disease.

Clinical Problem 12.3

Hyperventilation is sometimes used to reduce increased intracranial pressure acutely. This type of therapy potentially could be harmful if used for a prolonged period because hyperventilation decreases carbon dioxide in the blood, producing respiratory alkalosis. Decreased carbon dioxide and alkalosis result in constriction of cerebral blood vessels. Initially, this constriction reduces total cerebral blood volume, thus decreasing intracranial pressure slightly. Over time, however, the prolonged constriction of the blood vessels may cause ischemia.

Clinical Problem 12.4

a. Multiple levels, diffuse, nonmass, vascular. There are no focal abnormalities. The loss of consciousness suggests diffuse involvement of the supratentorial and posterior fossa levels. Full recovery suggests no pathologic change in the central nervous system.
b. Diffuse ischemia (syncope), secondary to decreased cardiac ouput
c. It is the ability of an organ to maintain a constant blood supply in spite of variations in blood pressure. This regulation applies to all but the widest extremes in blood pressure.
d. Only inhalation of carbon dioxide
e. Transient ischemic attacks are episodes of focal neurologic dysfunction; syncope is diffuse ischemia.

Clinical Problem 12.5

a. Multiple levels (supratentorial, posterior fossa, and spinal), diffuse, nonmass, vascular. The diffuse involvement, meningeal signs, and computed tomogram suggest subarachnoid hemorrhage.
b. At this age, the most common cause of nontraumatic subarachnoid hemorrhage is aneurysmal rupture.
c. Computed tomography of the brain is likely to indicate this diagnosis with 92% sensitivity when performed within 24 hours. However, if the imaging findings are negative but the level of suspicion of a subarachnoid hemorrhage is high, an examination of the cerebrospinal fluid to evaluate for red blood cells and xanthochromia is recommended.

Clinical Problem 12.6

a. Supratentorial, focal (right), nonmass, vascular
b. Computed tomography or magnetic resonance imaging

of the brain could show whether it is hemorrhagic or ischemic. Clinical symptoms or signs are unreliable for making this distinction.

c. The lesion is in the distribution of the right posterior cerebral artery.
d. Ischemic stroke or transient ischemic attack may be due to large-vessel disease, small-vessel disease, cardiac abnormalities, or blood coagulation disorders. This patient likely has emboli from the heart because of endocarditis.
e. It is a stroke if the clinical symptoms persist for 24 hours or longer. It is a transient ischemic attack if the symptoms last less than 24 hours.

Chapter 13 The Peripheral Level

Clinical Problem 13.1

a. Weakness, sensory loss, reflex loss, and pain—nerve
b. Foot dorsiflexion and leg abduction weakness, L5 spinal nerve; lateral calf sensory loss, L5 spinal nerve; reduced Achilles reflex, S1 spinal nerve
c. Acute—traumatic or vascular
d. L5 spinal nerve damage (radiculopathy) probably due to herniated disk and the residuals of old S1 spinal nerve damage (radiculopathy)
e. Ongoing denervation of L5 muscles, active spinal nerve damage (radiculopathy)
f. Loss of some fast-conducting peroneal/L5 axons
g. Neurogenic atrophy with fiber-type grouping from reinnervation by collateral sprouting after previous S1 spinal nerve damage (radiculopathy)

Clinical Problem 13.2

a. Absent reflexes, sensory loss, generalized weakness, no fatigability—peripheral neuropathy
b. Diffuse
c. Subacute, progressive—inflammatory/immunologic
d. System
    i. Sensory—numbness, loss of vibration and position sense
    ii. Motor—ascending weakness and shortness of breath
e. Inflammatory demyelinating neuropathy (Guillain-Barré syndrome)
f. Inflammation, myelin swelling, and segmental loss
g. Suppress inflammation, remove offending antibody to clear conduction block, and repair demyelination. Days to weeks

Clinical Problem 13.3

a. Absent reflexes, sensory loss, mild weakness and no fatigability—peripheral nerve
b. Distal
c. Chronic progressive; likely metabolic, toxic, or degenerative
d. System
    i. Sensory—distal numbness, pain, sensory loss, and reflex loss
    ii. Motor—mild distal weakness and reflex loss
    iii. Autonomic—orthostatic hypotension, dry skin
e. Peripheral neuropathy, likely due to diabetes mellitus; need to exclude other metabolic and toxic causes
f. Loss of motor axons, incomplete collateral sprouting, and ongoing denervation
g. Normal study. Small fibers cannot be tested with electromyography and nerve conduction studies.

Clinical Problem 13.4

a. Fatigable cranial and proximal weakness with reduced reflexes—neuromuscular junction
b. Prejunctional
c. Chronic, progressive—degenerative, metabolic, immune-mediated paraneoplastic
d. Lambert-Eaton myasthenic syndrome secondary to small cell carcinoma of the lung
e. Remove offending antibodies and/or enhance quantal release from the nerve terminals
f. Number of quanta of acetylcholine released from the prejunctional nerve terminal and postjunctional membrane response to the acetylcholine
g. Quantal release
h. 10

Clinical Problem 13.5

Weakness with normal findings on electromyography and nerve conduction study because of block of the activation of actin-myosin contraction without calcium

Clinical Problem 13.6

Collateral sprouting of denervated muscle fibers by remaining, undamaged motor neurons and axons

Clinical Problem 13.7

a. Proximal weakness, normal sensation and reflexes—myopathy
b. Subacute, inflammatory
c. Myositis, possibly immune mediated
d. Loss of muscle fibers from many motor units
e. Increase the number of motor units active, and increase the rate of firing in each of them
f. Muscle fiber destruction by inflammation
g. Endomysial and vascular inflammation with muscle fiber destruction and possibly regeneration

Chapter 14
The Spinal Level

Clinical Problem 14.1

a. Spinal (C7-C8 level), left
b. Mass, neoplasm
c. Loss of all sensory modalities (touch, pain, temperature, vibration, and joint position sense)
d. Left (reflecting involvement of the ipsilateral dorsal column [gracile fasciculus])
e. Right (involvement of crossed spinothalamic tract fibers)
f. The lesion is unilateral (the bladder receives bilateral innervation).

Clinical Problem 14.2

a. Spinal, right
b. Right L5 root
c. Contralateral paracentral lobule or corticospinal tract at the supratentorial and posterior fossa levels; ipsilateral lateral column, L5 root, peroneal nerve
d. Traction on the dura mater of the nerve root

Clinical Problem 14.3

a. Radicular pain, sensory loss of all modalities, weakness, lack of reflexes and muscle tone in the limbs, loss of anal reflex
b. Cauda equina
c. Mass lesion (midline intervertebral disk or neoplasm)
d. Below L1
e. Flaccid bladder because of the lack of afferent and efferent input due to cauda equina lesion

Clinical Problem 14.4

a. Sensory ataxia
b. Large myelinated fibers, large dorsal root ganglion cells, large-diameter dorsal root afferents, dorsal columns
c. Spinal lesion, mass, neoplasia
d. Preservation of muscle stretch reflexes make it unlikely that the lesion affects the dorsal root ganglion cells, large myelinated nerve fibers, or dorsal roots. If the reflexes were impaired, a normal sensory potential in nerve conduction studies would indicate a lesion in the dorsal root, as opposed to the dorsal root ganglion or peripheral nerve (see Chapter 13).

Clinical Problem 14.5

a. Spinal (cervical), midline mass, neoplasm
b. Sensory (decussation of the spinothalamic tract), motor (lower motor neuron involvement of the upper limbs, upper motor neuron involvement of the lower limbs)
c. C5–T3 segments bilaterally
d. Syringomyelia (or a low-grade neoplasm such as an astrocytoma or ependymoma)

Clinical Problem 14.6

a. Loss of all sensory modalities in one dermatome
b. Loss of pain and temperature sensation in the right trunk and lower limb (from involvement of the left spinothalamic tract); loss of vibration and joint position sense in the toes of the left foot (from involvement of the left gracicle fascicle); weakness, increased reflexes, and Babinski sign in the left lower limb (from involvement of corticospinal and reticulospinal pathways)
c. T4
d. Left

e. Complete left hemicord
f. No, because the lesion is below T1, where the preganglionic innervation of the pupil arises
g. No, because the lesion is unilateral

Clinical Problem 14.7

a. Weakness and loss of tone in lower abdominal muscles, hip flexors and adductors, and knee extensor muscles; absence of muscle stretch reflexes at the knees
b. Loss of pain and temperature sensation over the back, below the umbilicus, and in both lower limbs; increased tone of leg and foot muscles; increased ankle jerk; Babinski signs
c. Spinal midline
d. T10–L4
e. Infarction in territory of anterior spinal artery
f. The dorsal columns are supplied by paired posterior spinal arteries.
g. Anterior spinal artery syndrome

Clinical Problem 14.8

a. Spinal (thoracic)
b. Entire spinal cord at T6
c. Spinal shock
d. Spastic bladder
e. Autonomic dysreflexia

Clinical Problem 14.9

a. Multiple levels (supratentorial, spinal, peripheral), diffuse, nonmass, degenerative or metabolic
b. Proprioceptive pathway (large fiber—dorsal root ganglion—dorsal column–lemniscal pathway)
c. Loss of muscle stretch reflexes indicates a loss of afferent input from involvement of large myelinated nerves, dorsal root ganglion, or dorsal root. A Babinski sign may still be present because it is triggered by activation of small-diameter flexor reflex afferents mediating the triple flexion reflex, which is disinhibited in this patient by the upper motor neuron lesion.
d. Vitamin B_{12} and homocysteine levels. These findings are highly suggestive of dementia and combined degeneration of the spinal cord due to vitamin B_{12} deficiency.

Chapter 15
The Posterior Fossa Level
Part A: Brainstem and Cranial Nerve Nuclei

Clinical Problem 15A.1

a. Posterior fossa, right, mass, neoplastic
b. Cranial nerves IX, X, and XI on the right
c. Jugular foramen
d. Jugular vein

Clinical Problem 15A.2

a. Posterior fossa, left, nonmass, vascular
b. Special visceral afferent fibers of the facial nerve transmit taste sensation from the anterior two-thirds of the tongue.
c. General visceral efferent fibers of the facial nerve supply the lacrimal gland.
d. Bell palsy

Clinical Problem 15A.3

a. Posterior fossa, left, nonmass, vascular
b. Cranial nerve VI (lateral rectus), cranial nerve VII (facial weakness), medial lemniscus (loss of joint position and vibratory sense), descending motor pathways (hemiparesis)
c. Infarction, left paramedian region of the pons

Clinical Problem 15A.4

a. Posterior fossa, right, nonmass, vascular
b. The superior cerebellar peduncle contains cerebellar fibers traveling mainly from the cerebellum. The superior cerebellar peduncle crosses at the level of the caudal midbrain. Therefore, a lesion at this level may result in typical cerebellar signs such as ataxia. This MRI scan of the brain shows a hemorrhagic lesion, a cavernous malformation, in the caudal midbrain.

Clinical Problem 15A.5

a. Posterior fossa, right, mass, vascular
b. Right cranial nerve III (both general visceral efferent and general somatic efferent components)
c. An enlarging cerebral aneurysm may cause an acute, pupil-involved, third nerve palsy.

Chapter 15
The Posterior Fossa Level
Part B: Cerebellar, Auditory, and Vestibular Systems

Clinical Problem 15B.1

a. Posterior fossa, left, mass, inflammatory (abscess)
b. Cerebellum
c. Headache, nausea, vomiting, papilledema
d. Cerebellar astrocytoma

Clinical Problem 15B.2

a. Posterior fossa, left, nonmass, vascular
b. Left medullary pyramid (weakness), left medial lemniscus (decreased proprioception), left hypoglossal nerve (tongue weakness)
c. Infarction of the left medial medulla in the paramedian zone

Clinical Problem 15B.3

a. Posterior fossa, left, nonmass, vascular
b. Left lateral medulla
c. Left posterior inferior cerebellar artery, a branch of the left vertebral artery (often the site of occlusion in this syndrome)
d. The left descending tract of cranial nerve V, the left spinothalamic tract
e. Involvement of the descending sympathetic pathways en route to the spinal cord (producing Horner syndrome)

Clinical Problem 15B.4

a. Posterior fossa, right, nonmass, vascular
b. Cranial nerve III on the right (diplopia, ptosis, mydriasis), right cerebral peduncle (left hemiparesis)
c. Right medial and superior rectus muscles
d. The efferent limb of the pupillary light reflex travels with the general visceral efferent fibers contained in cranial nerve III.
e. Infarction, right paramedian region of the mesencephalon

Clinical Problem 15B.5

a. Supratentorial, left, mass, inflammatory (abscess)
b. Secondary involvement of the consciousness system by expanding mass lesion causing herniation
c. Compression of cranial nerve III on the left by expanding temporal lobe mass
d. With increasing herniation, there is also secondary compression of the cerebral peduncle.
e. Uncal herniation
f. Mesencephalon, at or caudal to the red nucleus
g. Decerebrate posturing
h. Transtentorial or central herniation

Clinical Problem 15B.6

a. Multiple levels, diffuse, nonmass, degenerative
b. Motor system only, at the posterior fossa and spinal levels
c. Final common pathway (weakness, fasciculations), direct activation pathways (bilateral Babinski sign)
d. Motor neuron disease (amyotrophic lateral sclerosis)

Chapter 16
The Supratentorial Level
Part A: Thalamus, Hypothalamus, and Visual System

Clinical Problem 16A.1

a. Supratentorial right: ventral posterior nucleus of the thalamus
b. Lacunar infarction
c. Posterior cerebral artery
d. Thalamic syndrome

Clinical Problem 16A.2

a. Hypothalamus
b. Mass lesion (craniopharyngioma)
c. Preoptic region (osmoregulation), magnicellular paraventricular and supraoptic nuclei (diabetes insipidus), ventromedial hypothalamus (obesity)
d. Arginine vasopressin (antidiuretic hormone). In this patient, prolactin levels may be increased because of interruption of inhibitory dopaminergic input from the hypothalamus to the anterior pituitary.
e. Papilledema is due to increased intracranial pressure. Bitemporal hemianopia is due to compression of the optic chiasm.

Clinical Problem 16A.3

a. Pituitary gland
b. Optic chiasm
c. Anterior lobe
d. Prolactin, growth hormone, follicle-stimulating hormone, luteinizing hormone, corticotropin hormone, and thyrotropin. These hormones are regulated by substances secreted from parvicellular neurons in the periventricular region of the hypothalamus: dopamine (which tonically inhibits prolactin secretion); gonadotropin-releasing hormone; growth hormone-releasing hormone and somatostatin (which facilitate and inhibit growth hormone secretion, respectively); gonadotropin-releasing hormone (which stimulates follicle-stimulating hormone and luteinizing hormone); corticotropin-releasing hormone (which activates corticotropin secretion), and thyrotropin-releasing hormone (which stimulates thyrotropin secretion)
e. Prolactin, luteinizing hormone, follicle-stimulating hormone, thyrotropin, corticotropin
f. Optic chiasm superiorly, cavernous sinus (containing the internal carotid artery, postganglionic oculosympathetic fibers, and cranial nerves III, IV, V [ophthalmic and maxillary divisions], VI) laterally, and splenoid sinus inferiorly
g. Compression of the optic chiasm
h. Pituitary adenoma

Clinical Problem 16A.4

a. Right optic nerve
b. Impaired visual afferent input to pretectal nucleus (relative pupillary afferent defect) involved in the pupillary light reflex
c. Indicates that the optic nerve lesion is likely due to demyelinating disease (multiple sclerosis) and is optic neuritis
d. Increased latency of the response on the affected side

Clinical Problem 16A.5

a. Bitemporal hemianopia
b. Left homonymous hemianopia
c. Left inferior quadrantanopia
d. Right superior quadrantanopia

Chapter 16
The Supratentorial Level
Part B: Telencephalon

Clincal Problem 16B.1

a. Declarative memory
b. Hippocampal formation
c. Anterograde and retrograde amnesia, respectively
d. Long-term autobiographical and factual memories are stored in association areas (particularly the lateral temporal cortex).
e. Confabulation

Clinical Problem 16B.2

a. Complex partial seizures
b. Medial temporal lobe, including the uncus
c. Olfactory: uncus (including pyriform cortex and subjacent olfactory amygdala); emotional and autonomic: amygdala; cognitive (memory): hippocampus and parahippocampal gyrus

Clinical Problem 16B.3

a. Supratentorial, left primary somatosensory cortex
b. Astereognosia
c. Relative preservation of vibration sense, unlike dorsal column lesions

Clinical Problem 16B.4

a. Prosopagnosia
b. Inferior occipitotemporal cortex (generally bilateral but may be only on the right)
c. Visual recognition network (ventral stream)
d. Posterior cerebral

Clinical Problem 16B.5

a. Spatial neglect, anosognosia, dressing apraxia, constructional apraxia
b. Right parietal lobe
c. Middle cerebral

Clinical Problem 16B.6

a. Simultanagnosia (inability to perceive all components of a visual scene at the same time while perceiving them individually), optic ataxia (inability to perform accurate limb movements under visual guidance), and oculomotor apraxia (inability to direct conjugate gaze toward a visual target)

b. Dorsal visual stream involved in spatial attention
c. Superior parietal lobule and intraparietal sulcus (bilaterally)
d. No. Color and form are processed in the ventral (occipitotemporal) stream.

Clinical Problem 16B.7

a. Ideomotor apraxia
b. Left posterior parietal or frontal premotor cortex

Clinical Problem 16B.8

a. Fluent aphasia
b. Wernicke area (left posterior superior temporal cortex and adjacent inferior parietal cortex)
c. Middle cerebral artery

Clinical Problem 16B.9

a. Apraxia of speech
b. Left frontal operculum and adjacent insula
c. Middle cerebral
d. Dysarthria

Clinical Problem 16B.10

a. Anomia (inability to name), acalculia, agraphia, left-right disorientation (Gerstmann syndrome)
b. Left parietal cortex
c. Neoplastic, vascular (subdural hematoma), focal degenerative

Clinical Problem 16B.11

a. Prefrontal cortex (probably bilaterally)
b. Dorsolateral prefrontal cortex (impaired attention, abulia, executive dysfunction) and orbitofrontal cortex (inappropriate social behavior)
c. Parietal and temporal association areas, paralimbic areas
d. Degenerative (frontal lobe dementia), neoplastic (e.g., malignant astrocytoma, meningioma), trauma

Clinical Problem 16B.12

a. Typical absence seizures (generalized seizures)
b. Diffuse 3-Hz spike-and-wave discharges
c. Increased synchronization in thalamocortical circuits

Clinical Problem 16B.13

a. Supratentorial, diffuse
b. Degenerative disorders, likely Alzheimer disease
c. Declarative memory (including episodic and semantic memory)
d. Dementia is an acquired progressive degenerative disorder; mental retardation is a congenital, static disorder.
e. Apraxia

Clinical Problem 16B.14

a. Orbitofrontal cortex
b. Neoplasm, focal degenerative (frontal lobe dementia)
c. Impaired olfaction indicates interruption of the olfactory pathway at the level of the olfactory bulb or nerve, as occurs with an olfactory groove meningioma.

Clinical Problem 16B.15

a. Left parietal (primary somatosensory cortex and inferior parietal lobule)
b. Vascular (infarction in middle cerebral artery territory)
c. Astereognosia, agraphesthesia, atopognosia, left-right disorientation, agraphia, acalculia
d. Apraxia
e. Right inferior quadrantanopia
f. Impaired cortical sensation in the left hand or left hemisensory neglect, dressing apraxia, constructional apraxia, left inferior quadrantic field defect (may be difficult to assess because of spatial neglect)

Clinical Problem 16B.16

a. Complex partial seizures
b. Uncus
c. Left temporal cortex
d. Right superior quadrantanopia
e. Wernicke aphasia
f. Increased frequency of seizures, development of progressive aphasia, symptoms of increased intracranial pressure
g. Magnetic resonance imaging or computed tomography of the head
h. Neoplasm

Index

('b' indicates a box; 'f' indicates a figure; 't' indicates a table)

A

B

E

F

G

H

I

J

K

L

M

N

O

Q

R

S

U

V

W

X

Z